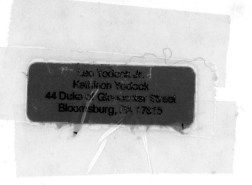
Adult Nurse Practitioner

CERTIFICATION REVIEW

JOHNS HOPKINS UNIVERSITY
SCHOOL OF NURSING

Visit our website at **www.mosby.com**

Adult Nurse Practitioner
CERTIFICATION REVIEW

JOHNS HOPKINS UNIVERSITY
SCHOOL OF NURSING

Volume Editor

ADA ROMAINE DAVIS, PhD, RN, APRN-BC, ELS
Professor Emeritus
Johns Hopkins University School of Nursing
Baltimore, Maryland;
Senior Editor
American Nurses Credentialing Center
Washington, D.C.

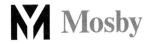

A Harcourt Health Sciences Company

St. Louis   London   Philadelphia   Sydney   Toronto

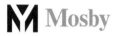

Mosby

A Harcourt Health Sciences Company

Vice President and Publishing Director, Nursing: Sally Schrefer
Executive Editor: Barbara Nelson Cullen
Senior Developmental Editor: Cindi Anderson
Project Manager: Pat Joiner
Production Editor: Rachel E. Dowell
Book Design Manager: Gail Morey Hudson
Cover Designer: Mark A. Oberkrom

Mosby, Inc.
A Harcourt Health Sciences Company
11830 Westline Industrial Drive
St. Louis, Missouri 63146

Printed in the United States of America

Library of Congress Cataloging-in-Publication Data

Adult nurse practitioner certification review / volume editor, Ada Romaine Davis.
     p. ; cm.
  Includes bibliographical references and index.
  ISBN 1-55664-429-9 (alk. paper)
    1. Nursing—Examinations, questions, etc. 2. Nurse practitioners—Examinations, questions, etc. I. Romaine-Davis, Ada, 1929-
    [DNLM: 1. Nursing—Examination Questions. 2. Nurse Practitioners—Examination Questions. WY 18.2 A2438 2001]
RT82.8 .A36 2001
610.73'076—dc21
2001032641

01 02 03 04 05 TG/RDW 9 8 7 6 5 4 3 2 1

Dedication

This *Adult Nurse Practitioner Certification Review* book is dedicated to all those clinicians who have been involved in its conception and development—the administrators of the Johns Hopkins University School of Nursing, the adult nurse practitioner faculty, and of course the students. In particular, of inestimable value to the development and continuation of the Adult Nurse Practitioner Program are the physicians and specialists who volunteer to teach classes in their areas of expertise, year after year. Many are among those who precept our students in the clinical settings. Preceptors are particularly important to students' clinical experiences and attitudes, as well as developing abilities to recognize, diagnose, and treat illnesses. We owe the preceptors more than can ever be repaid.

Our faculty is the most essential part of students' learning. They spend hours teaching, demonstrating procedures, observing students perform physical examinations, developing paper and pencil tests, and grading students' lengthy records of patient histories and physical examinations that are an integral part of nurse practitioner education and expertise. Most are contributors to this book. One person's name is missing from that list—that of Karen Huss, DNSc, RN, CANP, FAAN—a most valuable part of the program, who is a model on whom students can best pattern their professional manner. A special note of gratitude is due her for her special presence in the program and for her exemplary research program.

The following is a list of many of the physicians who worked with us to begin the Adult Nurse Practitioner Program. Without these specialist physicians and nurses, we could not reach our primary goal, which is to prepare nurse practitioners who are able to meet every clinical challenge and to care for patients and their families with warmth and compassion. The administrators and faculty are deeply grateful for your time and expert talents.

Peter B. Terry, *MD, Pulmonary Diseases*
Bevan Yueh, *MD, Otolaryngology (ENT)*
William S. Aronstein, *MD, Ambulatory Medicine*
Norman Beauchamp, *MD, Radiology*
Terrence O'Brien, *MD, Ophthalmology*
Thomas B. Connor, *MD, Ophthalmology*
Peter Rabins, *MD, Gerontology*
John A. Flynn, *MD, Rheumatology*
Charles Angell, *MD, Cardiology*
Amy Gordon, *MD, Gastroenterology*
David C. Foster, *MD, Obstetrics/Gynecology*
Alison R. Molitero, *MD, Hematology*
Ray E. Stutzman, *MD, Urology*
Christine Schneyer, *MD, Endocrinology*
Many Anne Wylie, *MSN, Gerontology*
Carroll Celentano, *RN, NMW, Obstetrics/Gynecology*

Contributors

SUSAN E. APPLING, RN, MS, CRNP
Assistant Professor, Professional Education Programs and Practice, Johns Hopkins University School of Nursing; Nurse Practitioner—Johns Hopkins Breast Center, Baltimore, Maryland

need to do =

2. *Health Care Policy and Professional Issues*
3. *Legal and Ethical Issues*
13. *Gynecologic Disorders*

KATHLEEN LENT BECKER, MS, CRNP
Assistant Professor, The Adult Nurse Practitioner Program, Johns Hopkins University School of Nursing,
Baltimore, Maryland

2. *Health Care Policy and Professional Issues*

ALICE M. BRAZIER, MS, CRNP
Geriatric Nurse Practitioner, Evercare of Maryland,
Baltimore, Maryland

23. *Care of the Aging Adult*

ADA ROMAINE DAVIS, PhD, RN, APRN-BC, ELS
Professor Emeritus, Johns Hopkins University School of Nursing,
Baltimore, Maryland;
Senior Editor, American Nurses Credentialing Center,
Washington, D.C.

1. *Health Promotion and Disease Prevention*
5. *Cardiovascular Disorders*
6. *Neurologic Disorders*
8. *Kidney and Urologic Disorders*
9. *Hepatic and Biliary Disorders*
11. *Acid-Base, Fluid, and Electrolyte Disorders*
12. *Hematologic Disorders*
14. *Reproductive Disorders*
15. *Immunologic Disorders*
16. *Oncologic Disorders*
17. *Musculoskeletal Disorders*
18. *Dermatologic Disorders*
19. *Eye Disorders*
21. *Infectious Diseases*
22. *Psychosocial Disorders*
23. *Care of the Aging Adult*
24. *Genetics*
25. *Study Skills and Test-Taking Strategies*

JULE HALLERDIN, MN, MPH, CNM
Associate Professor, University of the Virgin Islands, Nursing Division,
St. Thomas, U.S. Virgin Islands
13. Gynecologic Disorders

MARY KATHLEEN LEARS, MPH, MSN, RN, CIC
Graduate Student, Public Health (Student Division), School of Hygiene
and Public Health, Instructor, Master's Instruction, Johns Hopkins University
School of Nursing,
Baltimore, Maryland
21. Infectious Diseases

CANDIS MORRISON, PhD, CRNP
Associate Professor, Johns Hopkins University School of Nursing,
Baltimore, Maryland
7. Gastrointestinal Disorders

PHYLLIS LUERS NAUMANN, MSN, MEd, CRNP, BC
Assistant Professor and Coordinator, Johns Hopkins University School of Nursing,
Baltimore, Maryland
10. Endocrine Disorders

PATRICIA O'DONNELL
Ellicott City, Maryland
6. Neurologic Disorders

SHIRLEY E. VAN ZANDT, MSN, RN, MPH, CRNP
Instructor, Johns Hopkins University School of Nursing,
Baltimore, Maryland
20. Ear, Nose, and Throat Disorders

THERESA PLUTH YEO, MSN, MPH, CRNP
Assistant Professor, Johns Hopkins University School of Nursing,
Baltimore, Maryland
4. Respiratory Disorders
5. Cardiovascular Disorders

Reviewers

Harvey H. Baker, RN, CS, ARNP, MPH
Family Nurse Practitioner
Altamont Community Health Center
Altamont, Kansas

Maria Elena Botte, MSN, RN, CDE, CS
Family Nurse Practitioner
Certified Diabetes Educator, In collaboration
    with Hayward K. Zwerling MD, FACP
Endocrinology and Internal Medicine
Lowell, Massachusetts

Patty Campbell, RN, MSN, CCRN, ANPCS
Adult Nurse Practitioner
Emergency Center, Good Samaritan Hospital
Phoenix, Arizona

Sharon G. Childs, MS, CRNP-CS, ONC
Nurse Practitioner, Orthopaedic Nurse Certified
Concentra Medical Centers
Baltimore, Maryland

Carole A. Davis, MS, APRN
Adult Nurse Practitioner
Saint Francis Hospital
Hartford, Connecticut

Sheila A. Dunn, RN, MSN, C-ANP
Adult Nurse Practitioner
Belleville Veterans Clinic
Belleville, Illinois

Michelle Elise Freshman, MSN, MPH, RN, CS
Family Nurse Practitioner, Goddard Center
Boston, Massachusetts

Carol Green-Hernandez, PhD, ANP/FNP-C
Associate Professor
Primary Care Nurse Practitioner Program
The University of Vermont School of Nursing
    and Allied Health
Burlington, Vermont

June L. Helberg, EdD, RN
Associate Professor of Nursing
School of Nursing, University of Rochester
Rochester, New York

Anne M. "Nina" Hyde, APRN
Family Nurse Practitioner
Main Street Pediatrics
Bridgeport, Connecticut

Sharon S. Jamison, CFNP
Family Nurse Practitioner
Ephraim-McDowell Health—Liberty Family
    Medical Center
Liberty, Kentucky

Laima M. Karosas, APRN, MSN, FNP
Family Nurse Practitioner
The Connecticut Hospice
Branford, Connecticut

Judy Kaye, RN, PhD, ACNP, GNP, ANP, CS
Assistant Professor, Administrative & Clinical
    Nursing
University of South Carolina College of Nursing
Columbia, South Carolina

Patricia A. Lamb, RN, MN, CNS
President/Owner
Ophthalmic Nursing Care of Arizona, Inc.
Phoenix, Arizona

Susan B. Leight, EdD, RNCS, C-ANP
Faculty
University of Pennsylvania School of Nursing
Philadelphia, Pennsylvania

Nancy S. Mahan, MS
Director of Residential Services
Bay Cove Human Services
Boston, Massachusetts

Margaret McAllister, PhD, RN, CS, FNP
Faculty and Lecturer
University of Massachusetts
    Boston College of Nursing PhD Program
Boston, Massachusetts

Leona A. Mourad, MS, RN, ONC
Consultant, Mourad Consultant Associates
Adult Nurse Practitioner
Associate Professor Emeritus
Ohio State University
Columbus, Ohio

Jacqueline Rhoads, PhD, RN, ACNP-BC, ANP, CCRN
Professor of Nursing
Louisiana State University
    Health Sciences Center, School of Nursing
New Orleans, Louisiana

Catherine Rhuda, RN. MSN, CS
Adjunct Clinical Instructor
University of Massachusetts, Lowell
Lowell, Massachusetts

Kristyna M. Robinson, PhD, FNPc, RN
Associate Professor, Idaho State University
Pocatello, Idaho

Michele Reneé Susie, RN, BSN, MSN, FNP-C
Family Nurse Practitioner
Community Hospital of Anaconda
Andaconda, Montana

Viva J. Tapper, PhD, ARNP
ANCC Certified Adult Psychiatric Nurse
    Practitioner, University of Washington
Port Townsend, Washington

Susan M. Tucker, MSN, RN, CNAA
Consultant
Roseville, California

Pamela Becker Weilitz, MSN(R), RN, CS, ANP
Adult Nurse Practitioner, Primary Care Practice
Washington University School of Medicine
University Care
St. Louis, Missouri

Carol A. Whelan, APRN, MS, CS, ANP
Assistant Professor, Yale University
New Haven, Connecticut

Jane Williams, MSN, RN, CS, FNP
Manager, Clinical Cancer Prevention
University of Texas MD
Anderson Cancer Center
Houston, Texas

Christy Yates, MSN, CCRN, FNP, WHNP
Family Nurse Practitioner
Fern Creek Medical Center
Louisville, Kentucky

Nancy M. Youngblood, PhD, CRNP
Assistant Professor, Coordinator Family and
    Adult Nurse Practitioner Programs
LaSalle University School of Nursing
Philadelphia, Pennsylvania

Foreword *to the Reader*

The purpose of the *Adult Nurse Practitioner Certification Review* is to provide the most current, accessible, and succinct information available about diseases and conditions that occur in adults. The format therefore is primarily outline, accompanied by boxes, tables, and illustrations to emphasize key concepts. Studying for a certification examination requires hours of preparation. At hand should also be a pathophysiology textbook, to clarify questions that you may have about specific diseases. Understanding the pathophysiologic basis of disease helps you to use "upper-level cognitive processes" (reasoning) to arrive at the correct answers to examination questions. Knowing the pathophysiologic changes that result in particular diseases helps you recall why and how a disease develops. For example, knowing the physiologic effects of hypertension on the circulatory system and the heart enables you to more readily correlate the effects and the developing disease, as well as the signs and symptoms that occur as a result of the effects. The questions attached to each chapter and in the accompanying CD-ROM are not the exact questions that you will have on the certification examination; however, they are similar in content and format and should prepare you to be successful in test-taking. All of the adult nurse practitioners on the faculty of Johns Hopkins University School of Nursing wish you success in passing the examination, personal satisfaction that you will experience in practicing as an adult nurse practitioner, and the rewards that you will derive from seeing your patients' health improve.

Preface

The rapid changes that occur in medical diagnosis, therapy, and technology make it extremely difficult for the average health professional to keep pace with the advances being made continually while at the same time practicing, teaching families and patients, and dealing with crises that come up almost daily regarding families and patients and in the workplace. New advances in treating coronary artery disease are making obsolete those techniques that were used only last month. The completion of the Human Genome Project (HGP) is making possible changes in prevention and diagnosis of diseases that were undreamed of last year. Patients are being cared for in ways that are totally different from those that were standard 2 years ago. A major change is that people are being empowered to take greater responsibility for their own health, through managing weight, implementing more healthful eating patterns, being more active, working to eliminate alcohol and smoking addiction, and learning what to do for themselves when illness or infection occurs. We now know that antibiotics do not cure every infection, but, with patient and reasonable care, the body will cure the infection, using its own defenses. All health professionals, including nurse practitioners, need to be aware of the constant changes occurring and to be prepared to incorporate at least some of the changes in their own practices. To do this, a strong foundation of knowledge and experience is necessary, which takes time and perseverance to develop. Along with clinical expertise, the nurse practitioner needs to know ethical principles, legal ramifications of treating patients, and how health policy develops. No one can be an expert in all of these areas, but knowing the need for these, and how to apply them appropriately in one's own practice, is essential.

Ada Romaine Davis

Contents

Adult Nurse Practitioner

CERTIFICATION REVIEW

JOHNS HOPKINS UNIVERSITY
SCHOOL OF NURSING

Health Promotion and Disease Prevention

GOALS

- Assess protective and predictive factors that influence health.
- Assess genetic factors and risks that influence health.
- Foster strategies for health promotion, risk reduction, and disease prevention across the life span.
- Recognize the need for and implement risk reduction strategies to address social and public health issues, including societal and domestic violence, family abuse, sexual abuse, and substance abuse.
- Use information technologies to communicate health promotion and disease prevention.
- Develop an awareness of complementary modalities and their usefulness in promoting health (e.g., relaxation techniques, stress management).
- Assist patients to access and interpret health information to identify healthy lifestyle behaviors.
- Evaluate the efficacy of health promotion and education methods to use in a variety of settings, with diverse populations.
- Demonstrate sensitivity to personal and cultural definitions of health.

HEALTH PROMOTION AND DISEASE PREVENTION IN PRIMARY CARE

Most health promotion and disease prevention care occurs in the primary care setting. Primary care is a form of care delivery that has the following components:

- It is personalized care.

- It is care that is provided to patients who are entering the health care system for the first time.
- It is comprehensive care, based on knowledge from related disciplines (biology, chemistry, anatomy and physiology, pathophysiology, pharmacology, psychology, and others).
- It provides continuity of care, in that patients are cared for over long periods, whether sick or healthy (i.e., chronic and episodic illness care).
- It is coordinated care, with referrals made to other health care professionals (e.g., medical or surgical specialists, psychologists or psychiatrists, pharmacists, social workers).
- The primary goal in care coordination is to see that the patient receives the right care at the right time, for the least cost in terms of money, time, and effort.
- It is care that incorporates the patient, the family, and the community in terms of water supply, housing, safety, environmental hazards, traffic hazards, and communication.

DEFINITION

Health promotion incorporates the following:
- Identification of health risks
- Reduction of health risks
- Preventive measures
- Screening tests
- Human development across the life span
- Methods to prevent disease: immunization, screening when risk factors are present
- Early diagnosis and treatment

Health promotion applies to all members of a family, with regard to the following:
- Lifestyle behaviors
- Diet and exercise
- Sleep
- Weight
- Genetic makeup
- Family history
- Race
- Substance use: tobacco, alcohol, street drugs
- Obesity
- Other

TYPES OF PREVENTION (Table 1-1)

- Primary: No symptom or disease is evident, but risk factors are present.
- Secondary: Disease is present and can be diagnosed, but no symptoms are present (early disease).
- Tertiary: Disease is diagnosed, and symptoms are present. Treatment is aimed at preventing advance of the disease and avoiding disability resulting from effects of the disease (e.g., rheumatoid arthritis, tuberculosis, diabetes, chronic obstructive pulmonary disease [COPD]).

RISK FACTORS

- Age
- Gender

OBSTACLES TO PROVIDING COMPREHENSIVE PREVENTIVE HEALTH CARE

- Lack of family and community resources
- Patients who do not know about the benefits of preventive health care
- Time limits (e.g., work schedules of both provider and patient)
- Lack of transportation (e.g., unavailability, cost, hours of operation)
- Previously, lack of third-party reimbursement for preventive care
- Under managed care, the health care system administrators now recognize that prevention and treatment of disease at early stages are much less costly than treating advanced disease.

TABLE 1-1
Recommendations for Preventive Care for Asymptomatic, Low-Risk Adults

Preventive Care	U.S. Task Force			American College of Physicians		
	Gender	Age (yr)	Frequency	Gender	Age (yr)	Frequency
PHYSICAL EXAMINATION						
Blood pressure	MF	18+	q 2 yr	MF	18+	q 2 yrs
Clinical breast examination	F	50-69	q 1-2 yr	F	40+	q yr
LABORATORY TESTS						
Papanicolaou test	F	18-65	q 3 yr	F	20-65	q 3 yr
Stool: occult blood	MF	50+	q yr	MF	50-80	q yr
Sigmoidoscopy	MF	50+	q ? yr	MF	50-70	q 10 yr
Mammography	F	50-69	q 1-2 yr	F	50-75	q 2 yr
Cholesterol	M	35-65	q 5+ yr	M	35-65	Once
	F	45-65		F	45-65	
IMMUNIZATIONS						
Tetanus-diphtheria	MF	18+	q 15-30 yr	MF	18+	q 10 yr or once at age 50
Influenza vaccine	MF	65+	q yr	MF	65+	q yr
Pneumococcal vaccine	MF	65+	Once*	MF	65+	Once*
COUNSELING	MF	18+	Routine visits	MF	18+	Routine visits

From Tierney LM, McPhee SJ, Papadakis MA: Recommendations for preventive care for asymptomatic, low-risk adult. In *Current medical diagnosis and treatment,* ed 39, New York, 2000, Lange Medical Books, p 4.
*Reimmunize at age 65 years those high-risk persons whose first immunization was 6 or more years ago.

DECISION ABOUT SCREENING

- Benefits of screening for particular diseases in terms of impact on patient, family, and community
- Identification of those individuals or groups most likely to develop the disease, based on risk factors and screening tests (Table 1-2)
- Available screening tests that are accurate, have no adverse effects, and are acceptable to patients
- Availability of treatment modalities that will significantly alter the course of the disease and improve patients' quality of life

TABLE 1-2
Selected Causes of Death in the United States, 1950 and 1998 (Deaths per 100,000 resident population)

	1950	1998
ALL PERSONS		
All causes	841.5	471.7
NATURAL CAUSES	766.6	422.6
Diseases of the heart	307.2	126.6
Ischemic heart disease	—	79.6
Cerebrovascular diseases	88.8	25.1
Malignant neoplasms	125.4	123.6
Trachea, bronchus, lung	11.1	37.0
Colorectal	—	11.8
Prostate	13.4	13.2
Breast (female only)	22.2	18.8
COPD	4.4	21.3
Pneumonia and influenza	26.2	13.2
Chronic liver disease, cirrhosis	8.5	7.2
Diabetes mellitus	14.3	1995:15.6 3.6
HIV infection	—	4.6*
EXTERNAL CAUSES		
Unintentional injuries	57.5	30.1
Motor vehicle-related injuries	23.3	15.6
Suicide	11.0	10.4
Homicide and legal intervention	5.4	7.3

From National Center for Health Statistics: *Age-adjusted death rates for selected causes of death, according to sex, detailed race, and Hispanic origin: United States, selected years 1950-1998,* DHHS Pub No 00-1232, Washington, DC, U.S. Department of Health and Human Services.
*Declines in death rates are due primarily to earlier diagnosis, improved treatment, and improved drug therapies (i.e., protease inhibitors for HIV infection).

- Treatments that have proven effectiveness, low risk, few side effects, low costs, and patient acceptance

PRINCIPLES OF PREVENTION USE IN SPECIFIC DISEASES

- Assess the impact and degree of support and participation by family members.
- Involve at least one family member (e.g., spouse) in all preventive strategies.
- Be flexible in all aspects of prevention.

Coronary Heart Disease

Incidence
- Annual incidence: estimated 1.5 million persons
- Rate: 67% men; 43% women

Presenting Event
- Myocardial infarction (MI)
- Sudden death

Prevalence
- About 13.5 million persons in the United States have a history of MI or symptomatic coronary heart disease (CHD).
- Between 1 and 2 million men over age 45 have asymptomatic but significant CHD.
- An estimated 7.2% of the U.S. population over age 20 have CHD.
- Postmortem reports show that by age 20 to 24, raised lesions in the coronary arteries are present in the following groups:
  —44% of white men
  —34% of black men
  —11% of white women
  —43% of black women

Cost to Society
- Cost of treatment and lost productivity for all cardiovascular disease in the United States is $151.1 billion, with about $66.4 billion attributed to cost of heart disease alone.

Morbidity and Mortality
- One in every 4.6 deaths in the United States is caused by CHD, accounting for 489,970 deaths each year (30% of all patients with MI).

- Among survivors, 65% do not recover fully.
- About 88% of persons under age 65 are able to return to work.
- Six-year follow-up shows the following:
  —13% of men and 6% of women who have had MI die suddenly.
  —23% of men and 31% of women have a second MI.

Screening and Monitoring
- Assess total cholesterol and high-density lipoprotein (HDL) cholesterol between ages 20 and 30, then every 5 years.
- Those at high risk, based on screening values, should have a complete fasting lipid panel to determine risk status.
- Record blood pressure at each office visit in both arms, with patient sitting and lying.
- Monitor weight for obesity (>20% to 30% above ideal weight).
- Provide written low-fat, low-calorie diet for steady weight loss.
- Recommend 30 to 40 minutes of aerobic exercises three or four times per week.
- Assess stress levels every 6 months.
- Determine fasting blood glucose annually to detect diabetes mellitus.

Preventive Strategies
- Encourage healthy lifestyles for all patients of all ages.
- Identify and reduce risk factors to decrease the incidence of CHD.
  —Serum cholesterol
  —Hypertension
  —Cigarette smoking
  —Sedentary lifestyle
- Consider dietary changes.
  —Low fat
  —Low cholesterol
- High serum cholesterol is strongly correlated with CHD.
- Nonpharmaceutical treatment can result in regression of coronary artery lesions and thus the risk of MI.
  —Very-low-fat diet
  —Exercise program
  —Meditation
  —Relaxation
- Cholesterol-lowering drugs have proven efficacy in reducing the incidence and mortal-

TABLE 1-3

Levels of Low-Density Lipoprotein (LDL): Dietary and Drug Treatment (mg/dl)

Patient Status	Diet	Drug	Ideal LDL
No CHD, fewer than two risk factors	≥160	≥190	<160
No CHD, more than two risk factors	≥130	≥160	<130
CHD present	≥100	≥130	≤100

From Expert Panel on Detection, Evaluation, and Treatment of High Blood Cholesterol in Adults, *JAMA* 269:3015-3023, 1993. *CHD,* Coronary heart disease.

ity of MI in both symptomatic and non-symptomatic patients.

Risk Factors (Table 1-3)
Positive
- Age
  —Men: over 45
  —Women: over 55 or in early menopause without hormone replacement therapy (HRT)
- Family history of CHD (men <55; women <65)
- Cigarette smoking (active and passive)
- Hypertension
- Low high-density lipoprotein (HDL) cholesterol (<35 mg/dl)
- Diabetes mellitus
- Lack of information about early symptoms (e.g., chest pain, fatigue)

Negative
- High HDL cholesterol (60 mg/dl or higher)

Other
- Elevated triglyceride levels
- High-stress personality profile
- Inactive lifestyle
- Oral contraceptive use, especially smokers age 35 and older
- Severe obesity (>30% over ideal weight)
- History of any occlusive vascular disease, peripheral or cerebrovascular

Goals of Treatment
- Control cholesterol (Table 1-4).
- Control hypertension.

TABLE 1-4
Dietary Changes to Reduce Cholesterol and Fat

Foods to Decrease or Eliminate	Recommended Substitutions
Eggs*	Egg whites (2 = 1 egg) Egg substitutes (e.g., Egg Beaters)
Cheese	Whey cheeses Low-fat cottage cheese Low-fat (part skim milk) cheese Nondairy, nonfat cheese
Whole milk	Low-fat or skim milk
Butter, hard margarine	Soft margarine Powdered butter flavoring
Ice cream, sherbets	Ice milks Sorbets or ices
Fatty meats, hot dogs, luncheon meats, bacon, poultry skin, internal organ meats	Lean varieties of red meats Skinned chicken and turkey Fish No frying Meatless meals
Shellfish	Lower-cholesterol seafood: crab, clams, scallops
Chocolate	Cocoa
Highly refined prepared foods	Whole-grain foods, fresh fruits and vegetables
High-fat prepared foods (bakery products; food prepared with coconut, palm kernel, or hydrogenated vegetable oils or animal fat or animal fat or lard)	Homemade or prepared low-fat varieties using unsaturated vegetable oils (soybean, olive, corn, safflower, sesame, sunflower)

From Barker LR, Burton LR, Zieve PD, eds: *Principles of ambulatory medicine*, ed 5, Baltimore, 1999, Williams and Wilkins, p 1140.
*Eggs are not eliminated from the diet to the extent that they were in the early 1990s.

- Cease smoking.
- Improve lifestyle behaviors.

Cerebrovascular Disease
Incidence
- About 500,000 persons have a cerebrovascular accident (CVA, stroke) every year in the United States.
- Incidence increases with age.
  —Persons age 45 to 54: 100 per 100,000 population (1:20 chance of stroke before age 70)
  —Persons age 85: 1800 per 100,000 population

- Significant decreases have occurred in the last 15 to 20 years because of emphasis on risk factor management and lifestyle changes.

Prevalence
About 3.8 million persons have survived stroke and are living in the United States. Millions of other people with significant atherosclerotic cerebrovascular disease are at high risk of stroke.

Cost to Society
- Annual cost of CVA is estimated at $26.2 billion for medical treatment and lost productivity.

Morbidity and Mortality
- One in 15 deaths is caused by stroke, or 149,000 deaths per year.
- Stroke is the third leading cause of death in the United States, after CHD and cancer.
- About 31% of stroke victims die within 1 year of the CVA.
- Stroke is the leading cause of long-term disability.
  —About 40% of stroke survivors require special services (e.g., rehabilitation).
  —About 10% require total care.

Factors Relevant to Prevention
- The major risk factor for stroke is hypertension.
- CHD or atrial fibrillation indicates a high risk for emboli to the brain.
- Diabetes mellitus significantly increases the risk for stroke.
- Transient ischemic attacks (TIAs) are a major risk factor for stroke.
- One in five stroke victims had at least one out of the following four symptoms of TIA within the previous year:
  —Temporary loss of vision (one eye only)
  —Unilateral numbness, tingling
  —Aphasia
  —Focal weakness
- Patients who have carotid artery bruit have a 1% to 3% incidence of stroke each year.
- Aspirin, anticoagulants, and surgery are used to treat carotid bruits, but data are not sufficient to show that these treatments are effective in preventing stroke.

- Additional risk factors include family history, cigarette smoking, oral contraceptive use, hyperlipidemia, and elevated hematocrit.

Screening Recommendations
- Elevated blood pressure (systolic and diastolic) is the most significant risk factor for stroke.
- Cigarette smoking is the second most significant risk factor for stroke.
- For carotid bruit, those over age 40 should be assessed annually.

Preventive Strategies
- Provide treatment for mild but sustained hypertension.
- Tell those who smoke to stop; provide programs and suggestions for cessation.
- Prescribe aspirin prophylaxis for those who have had symptoms of TIA.
- Assess impact of stroke on families.
  —Disability may be both physical and cognitive.
  —Family members may become caregivers.
  —Rehabilitation and care of stroke victims can be costly.
  —Patient's condition may require decision regarding placement in nursing home.

Substance Abuse: Alcohol and Drugs

Definition
Chemical dependency is the continued habitual use of a substance despite serious adverse effects on the user's life.

Incidence
Incidence rates are difficult to assess because of the uncertain or variable level of dependency, development of tolerance, and other factors.

Prevalence
- An estimated 18 million Americans, or 7.5% of the total population, are substance abusers.
- Men make up 17% to 24% of alcohol abusers.
- In a primary care setting, 10% to 20% of patients come for conditions related to alcohol abuse and 2% for other drug dependency.
- Rates of tobacco, alcohol, and drug use among America's young population are increasing alarmingly after a decade of decline.

Cost to Society
- Estimated annual cost of alcohol abuse in the United States is $85.8 billion, including $72.3 billion from lost and decreased productivity and $13.6 billion for cost of care.
- Social costs of problem drinking and drug use are not quantifiable but may equal or exceed medical costs.
- Problems may involve co-workers, family, friends, or police.
- Substance abusers have higher rates of divorce, domestic violence, unemployment, and poverty.
- Effects on children are often permanent.

Morbidity and Mortality
- Patients who are dependent on alcohol have 2½ times the normal overall risk of death.
- Mortality is 30% to 36% higher among men and has more than doubled in women who drink six or more drinks per day.
- More than 100,000 deaths each year are attributable to alcohol abuse; 50% are related to accidental deaths.
- Morbidity for chemical dependency (alcohol or drugs) is substantial, with problems that range from the strong relationship between crime and cirrhosis to the effects of psychosis, depression, cardiomyopathy, peptic ulcer disease, overdose, cancer of directly exposed organs (i.e., lips, mouth, larynx, pharynx, esophagus, stomach, liver), pancreatitis, suicide, various infections (e.g., hepatitis, AIDS, endocarditis, pneumonia), fetal alcohol syndrome in offspring, and accidents.

Factors Relevant to Prevention
- Most adverse consequences result from inappropriate use of alcohol or drugs, not necessarily from actual dependence.
- Legal means to increase the enforcement of drinking and driving laws, increase the price of alcoholic beverages, and increase the legal drinking age have been successful in reducing consumption and the legal consequences of drinking.

- Children of alcoholics have a three times greater risk of alcoholism, regardless of whether they were raised by their biological parents.
- Spontaneous recovery from alcoholism is reported in up to 30% of patients, and treatment recovery rates are as high as 61%, although different groups use different definitions of "alcoholism" and "recovery."

Screening Recommendations

- All patients over age 12 should be screened regularly for alcohol and substance abuse.
- Annual screening sends a strong message to young patients.
- Family history focuses on first-degree relatives.
- The best screening tool is the CAGE Screening Test for Alcoholism or the Michigan Alcoholism Screening Test (MAST), both of which also can be used for drug abusers (Fig. 1-1).
- With CAGE, any two positive responses are suggestive:
  —Cutting down?
  —Annoyed by criticism of your drinking?

Question	Yes	No
• Do you enjoy having a drink now and then?	0	—
• Do you feel you are a normal drinker? (By normal, we mean less than or as much as most people, and you have not gotten into any recurring trouble while drinking.)	—	2
• Have you ever awakened the morning after some drinking the night before, and found that you could not remember part of the evening?	2	—
• Does either of your parents, any near relative, or your spouse, girlfriend, or boyfriend ever worry or complain about your drinking?	1	—
• Can you stop drinking without a struggle after one or two drinks?	—	2
• Do you feel guilty about your drinking?	1	—
• Do friends or relatives think you are a normal drinker?	—	2
• Are you able to stop drinking when you want to?	—	2
• Have you ever attended a meeting of Alcoholics Anonymous (AA)?	5	—
• Have you gotten into physical fights when you have been drinking?	1	—
• Has your drinking ever created problems between you and either your parents or another relative, your spouse, or any girlfriend or boyfriend?	2	—
• Has any family member of yours ever gone to anyone for help about your drinking?	2	—
• Have you ever gotten into trouble at work or school because of your drinking?	2	—
• Have you ever lost a job because of drinking?	2	—
• Have you ever neglected your obligations, your schoolwork, your family, or your job for 2 or more days in a row because you were drinking?	2	—
• Do you drink before noon fairly often?	1	—
• Have you ever been told you had liver trouble or cirrhosis?	2	—
• After heavy drinking, have you ever had severe shaking, heard voices, or seen things that really weren't there?	2 (5 DTs)	—
• Have you ever gone to anyone for help about your drinking?	5	—
• Have you ever been in a hospital because of your drinking?	5	—
• Have you ever been a patient in a psychiatric hospital or a psychiatric ward of a general hospital where drinking was part of the problem that caused the hospitalization?	2	—
• Have you ever been seen at a psychiatric or mental health clinic or gone to any doctor, social worker, or clergy for help with any emotional problem, where drinking was part of the problem?	2	—
• Have you ever been arrested for drunk driving, driving while intoxicated, or driving under the influence of alcoholic beverages or any other drug? If yes, how many times? _____	2	—
• Have you ever been arrested, or taken into custody for few hours, because of drunk behavior, whether due to alcohol or any other drug? If yes, how many times? _____	2	—

Each response scores the number of points listed. A score of 0 to 3 points-probable normal drinker; 4 = borderline; 5 to 9 = 80% likelihood of dependence; 10 or more = 100% likelihood.

Fig. 1-1   MAST questionnaire. (From Seizer ML: The Michigan Alcohol Screening Test: the quest for a new diagnostic instrument, *Am J Psychiatry* 127:1653, 1971.)

—Guilty about your drinking?
—Eye opener event?

Cancer

Incidence (Table 1-5)
Cost to Society
- Estimated total cost of care for cancer is more than $104 billion per year, with $55 billion for medical care and $69 billion in other costs.
- Screening programs account for only $3 to $4 billion of the total cost of medical services for cancer.

Morbidity and Mortality (Table 1-6)
- Cancer is the second leading cause of death, after cardiovascular disease.
- Cancer causes 25% of all deaths.
- Leading causes of deaths from cancer involve the lungs, colon or rectum, breasts, prostate, pancreas, urinary system, lymphoma, and leukemia.
- Between 1930 and 1992 the annual mortality rate for cancer increased from 130 to 172 per 100,000 population, primarily because of lung cancer.

TABLE 1-5
Cancer Cases by Site and Gender

Site	Male	Site	Female
Prostate	317,300	Breast	184,300
Lung	98,900	Lung	78,100
Colon, rectum	76,600	Colon, rectum	65,900
Bladder	38,300	Uterus	34,000
Lymphoma	33,900	Ovary	26,700
Melanoma (skin)	21,800	Lymphoma	16,500
Oral	20,100	Melanoma (skin)	16,500
Kidney	18,500	Cervix uteri	15,700
Leukemia	15,300	Bladder	14,600
Stomach	14,000	Pancreas	13,900
Pancreas	12,400	Leukemia	12,300
Liver	10,800	Kidney	12,100
All sites	**764,300**	**All sites**	**594,850**

US Department of Health and Human Services, Centers for Disease Control and Prevention, National Center for Health Statistics: *Health, United States, 2000 with adolescent health chartbook,* Hyattsville, Md, 2000, National Center for Health Statistics.

TABLE 1-6
Cancer Deaths by Site and Gender

Site	Male	Site	Female
Lung	94,400	Lung	64,300
Prostate	41,400	Breast	44,300
Colon, rectum	27,400	Colon, rectum	27,500
Pancreas	13,600	Ovary	14,800
Lymphoma	13,250	Pancreas	14,200
Leukemia	11,600	Lymphoma	11,560
Esophagus	8,500	Leukemia	9,400
Liver	8,400	Liver	6,800
Stomach	8,300	Brain	6,100
Bladder	7,800	Uterus	6,000
Kidney	7,300	Stomach	5,700
Brain	7,200	Multiple myeloma	5,100
All sites	**292,300**	**All sites**	**262,440**

US Department of Health and Human Services, Centers for Disease Control and Prevention, National Center for Health Statistics: *Health, United States, 2000 with adolescent health chartbook,* Hyattsville, Md, 2000, National Center for Health Statistics.

Factors Relevant to Prevention
- About 35% of all cancer deaths are likely related to diet (includes obesity).
- Obese patients have increased risk of colorectal, breast, prostate, gallbladder, ovarian, and uterine cancers.
- Foods considered to have protective properties against cancers include the following:
  —Those rich in vitamin A, including dark-green and deep-yellow vegetables and fruits
  —Those rich in vitamin C, including citrus fruits, strawberries, and sweet peppers
  —Cruciferous vegetables, including cabbage, broccoli, Brussels sprouts, and cauliflower
- Smoking accounts for 30% of cancer deaths (lung, bladder, mouth, throat, larynx).
- Alcohol is responsible for about 3% of cancer deaths.
- Diet, smoking, alcohol, and occupational exposure account for more than 73% of all cancer deaths.
- The American Cancer Society (ACS) estimates that if recommended screening programs for early detection and treatment of breast, tongue, colon, rectal, cervical, prostate, and testicular cancers and for melanoma were fully implemented, the 5-year survival rate would rise to 95% and about 115,000 lives would be saved every year.

Colorectal Cancer

Incidence
- Colorectal cancer has the second highest incidence of all cancers.
- Incidence begins to increase after age 40, about doubling every 7 years after age 50.
- About 90% of all colorectal cancers occur in people over age 50.
- Incidence increases in patients with a family history of colorectal cancer.
- Incidence is decreased among patients who regularly use aspirin and other nonsteroidal antiinflammatory drugs and among women who use postmenopausal HRT.

Morbidity and Mortality
Lifetime risk of colorectal cancer is 2.6%.

Factors Relevant to Prevention
- Colorectal cancers develop over 5 to 10 years from benign adenomatous colon polyps.
  —From 20% to 30% of polyps are adenomas.
  —Only 5% to 10% of adenomatous polyps become malignant.
  —Appearance of adenomas begins after age 40 and increases significantly between ages 45 and 50.
- Compared with pathologic findings on colonoscopy, stool guaiac tests for occult blood, taken 3 days in succession, are 52% sensitive for carcinoma, 23% sensitive for polyps greater than 1 cm, and 4.4% sensitive for polyps less than 1 cm.
- Early detection and treatment result in much higher survival rates.
  —Current survival rate is 61%.
  —Survival rates of 80% to 90% are possible with screening for occult blood, sigmoidoscopy, and removal of adenomatous polyps.
- About 20% of colorectal cancers are attributed to a low-fiber diet.
- High-fat diets are also implicated.

Screening Recommendations
- Rectal examinations and six-slide fecal occult blood tests annually after age 40
- Sigmoidoscopy every 3 to 5 years beginning at age 50

Preventive Strategies
- Risk factor analysis includes the following:
  —Age over 50
  —History of adenomas
  —Personal or family history of colorectal cancer or polyps
  —Ulcerative colitis
  —Crohn's disease
  —Personal or family history of genital or breast cancer in women
  —Physical inactivity
- All patients should eat a high-fiber, low-fat diet.

Breast Cancer

Incidence
- Lifetime incidence of breast cancer in women is 1:9.

- Of all new cancers in women, 31% are breast cancer (13% are lung cancer, the second most common cancer in women).
- Incidence increases with age.

Morbidity and Mortality
- Mortality rate has been stable since 1930.
- Breast cancer accounts for 17% of all cancer deaths (25% for lung cancer deaths).
- In situ breast cancer has a cure rate of almost 100%.
- Five-year survival rate for localized breast cancer is 96% (78% in the 1940s).
- Survival rates are currently as follows:
  —5 years: 99%
  —8 years: 83%
  —10 years: 79%

Factors Relevant to Prevention (Table 1-7)
- Risk factors
- Relative risk

Screening Recommendations
- Breast self-examination (BSE) has an average sensitivity of 26% (clinical breast examination, 45%; mammography, 71% to 75%; both clinical breast examination and mammography, 75% to 88%).

TABLE 1-7
Risk Factors for Breast Cancer

Factor	Risk (%)
Family history in first-degree relatives	
One member	1.4-2.8
Two members	4.2-6.8
Nulliparity	1.5-1.9
First child born after age 30	1.9
First menstrual period before age 12	1.2-1.3
Last menstrual period after age 55	1.5-2.0
Atypical hyperplasia on previous biopsy	2.2-5.0
Obesity	1.2
Current oral contraceptive use	1.5
Past oral contraceptive use	1.0
Postmenopausal HRT	1.2-2.1
Alcohol use	
1 drink/day	1.4
2 drinks/day	1.7
3 drinks/day	2.0

From Lewis SM, Heitkemper MM, Dirkin SR: *Medical-surgical nursing,* ed 5, St. Louis, 2000, Mosby, pp 1478-1479.
HRT, Hormone replacement therapy.

- Regular screening mammography results in a 20% to 35% decrease in mortality among women age 50 to 69.
- A 1995 meta-analysis showed a statistically significant reduction (24%) in mortality among women age 40 to 50 who were screened by mammography.
- Biennial mammography plus annual clinical breast examination is as effective as both done annually.
- Official recommendations regarding breast cancer screening differ among the ACS, American Academy of Family Physicians, and U.S. Preventive Health Services Task Force.
- Up-to-date research on the effectiveness of screening methods and scheduling is important to clinicians.

Lung Cancer

Incidence
- Second highest incidence of all cancers for both men and women in the United States
- Most preventable of all cancers

Morbidity and Mortality
- Leading cause of cancer mortality for both men and women
- Five-year survival rate only 13%

Factors Relevant to Prevention
- Small number of cases result from exposure to industrial pollutants.
- About 87% of all lung cancers are attributable to smoking.
- A major public health goal is to reduce environmental tobacco smoke (ETS).
- About 3000 lung cancer deaths annually in nonsmoking adults are attributable to ETS.

Screening Recommendations
Although a chest x-ray film and sputum cytologic examination detect lung cancer at a presymptomatic stage, no definitive data indicate that early detection results in improved prognosis.

Preventive Strategies
People of all ages should be educated about cigarette smoking as the cause of lung cancer with the message, "It's addictive. Don't start. If you have started, stop."

Carcinoma of the Cervix (Cervical Cancer)

Incidence

- Incidence of invasive cervical cancer is decreasing.
- Incidence increases steadily through age 50, then remains stable.
- Worldwide, cervical cancer is the most common malignancy in women.
- In the United States, cervical cancer ranks eighth among cancers in women.

Morbidity and Mortality

- Carcinoma of the cervix results in 4900 deaths each year.
- Patients with a preinvasive lesion of cervical intraepithelial neoplasia (CIN II, or carcinoma in situ) have a 100% cure rate with appropriate treatment.
- Women with localized cancer have a 5-year survival rate of 91%.
- Patients with distant spread have a 4-year survival rate of 30%.
- The overall 5-year survival rate is 68%.
- The mortality rate has declined by 70% in the last 40 years because of early detection with Papanicolaou (Pap) testing.

Factors Relevant to Prevention

- Squamous cell carcinoma of the cervix occurs almost exclusively in women who have had coitus.
- Average time for progression to invasive carcinoma is an additional 10 years.
- CIN may regress spontaneously in 30% to 50% of cases.
- At least 30% of patients with CIN III progress to invasive carcinoma.

Risk Factors

- Early age for first intercourse
- Women who have coitus less than 1 year after menarche are 26 times more likely to develop cervical carcinoma than the general population.
- Multiple sexual partners
- Human immunodeficiency virus (HIV) infection
- Herpes simplex virus infection
- History of condylomas (human papillomavirus [HPV] infection)
- Smoking

- Low socioeconomic status
- No Pap testing
  - From 15% to 20% of American women do not have regular Pap tests, which accounts for the majority of cervical carcinomas.
  - One Pap test is 55% to 80% sensitive (20% to 45% of cases are missed).
  - Specificity in Pap results and effectiveness depend on proper sampling, proper specimen handling, and quality of the laboratory.

Screening Recommendations

- All women should begin having Pap tests when they become sexually active.
- After at least three negative annual Pap tests, the frequency can be reduced to every 3 years among low-risk populations.
- Pap tests can be discontinued in women over age 65 who have had consistently normal examinations.

Preventive Strategies

- Review risk status at each visit, particularly in patients with multiple sexual partners, HPV infection, or other risk factors.
- Advise patients that barrier contraceptives, such as the condom, do not necessarily prevent cancer of the cervix, but they do prevent transmission of sexually transmitted diseases (STDs).

Skin Cancer

Incidence

- About 800,000 cases of basal and squamous cell skin cancer occur annually, with an additional 38,300 cases of malignant melanoma.
- Incidence is twice that of any other cancer.
- Incidence continues to rise dramatically.

Morbidity and Mortality

Of the 9430 deaths annually from skin cancer, 7500 are caused by malignant melanoma.

Risk Factors

- Major risk factor: exposure to ultraviolet (UV) light
- Severe sunburns as a child
- Fair complexion

- Multiple or atypical moles
- Family or personal history of skin cancer
- Inability to tan
- Presence of freckles
- History of treatment with ionizing radiation
- Immunosuppression
- Exposure to coal tar, pitch, arsenic, radium, and creosote

Screening Recommendations
- Skin should be thoroughly examined at regular visits.
- All lesions suspected of being malignant should be biopsied or prophylactically excised and submitted for pathologic examination.

Preventive Strategies
- Counsel all patients, particularly those at risk, about the need to avoid exposure to UV light.
- Advise patients, when in the sun, to wear clothing that covers most of the skin or to apply a sunscreen that has a high sun protection factor (SPF 15 or greater).
- Encourage regular self-examination to check for new skin lesions and to examine older lesions that have changed in appearance (size, color, and texture).

Prostate Cancer

Incidence
- Prostate cancer is the most common non-cutaneous cancer in men.
- Risk increases with age, beginning at age 50.
- About 317,100 new cases occurred in 1996.
- Black men have the highest incidence of prostate cancer in the world, 37% higher than white men.
- Population studies indicate that the consumption of high levels of dietary fat may be implicated in an increased incidence of prostate cancer.

Prevalence
- Prevalence increases with age.
- Studies have shown microscopic evidence of prostate cancer in 30% of autopsies of men age 30 to 49.
- Estimated prevalence among men over age 80 ranges up to 100%.

Morbidity and Mortality
Morbidity is associated with metastases that result in bone pain and urinary tract obstruction.

Factors Relevant to Prevention
- Only a small number of men with microscopic evidence of prostate cancer have clinical evidence of disease.
- According to many specialists, if all men lived to old-old age, 100% would develop prostate cancer.

Screening Recommendations
- Principal screening tests are digital rectal examination (DRE); serum tumor markers, such as the prostate-specific antigen (PSA); and transrectal ultrasound.
- None of these tests prolongs life, and the sensitivity and specificity are difficult to calculate.
- Routine screening for prostate cancer is not recommended on a population basis.
- Clinicians should counsel all men over 50 about the availability, risks, and benefits of PSA testing.

Osteoporosis

Incidence
- Hip fractures related to osteoporosis occur in 1.3 million persons every year.
- Fractures of the hip, vertebrae, and distal forearm occur in about 50% of postmenopausal women.
- Degree of osteoporosis depends on peak bone density at ages 20 to 30 and the rate of bone loss after age 30.

Prevalence
- An estimated 15 to 20 million Americans have osteoporosis.
- All patients with osteoporosis are at high risk for fractures.

Cost to Society
Direct and indirect costs of caring for patients with fractures related to osteoporosis are about $8 billion annually.

Morbidity and Mortality
- Between 12% and 20% of hip fractures lead to death.

- About 50% of hip fractures result in significant disability.

Factors Relevant to Prevention

- Beginning at menopause, bone loss in women increases by 2% to 3% a year, then gradually returns to premenopausal rates of loss.
- Men follow the same sequence, but their bone loss is about 66% of that in women.
- Before age 30, adequate intake of calcium affects the peak bone mass (Table 1-8).
- After age 30, adequate intake of calcium slows the rate of bone loss slightly.
- Both men and women require 1 g of elemental calcium daily to maintain a zero calcium balance.
- In postmenopausal women who are not receiving estrogen replacement therapy (ERT), even increasing calcium intake to 1.5 g/day does not maintain zero calcium balance.
- Women of all ages have an 80% prevalence of inadequate calcium intake.
- ERT is the best method to prevent accelerated bone loss and reduce risk of fractures by 25% to 50%.
- Discontinuing ERT results in a return to accelerated bone loss.
- Regular weight-bearing exercise also helps to maximize peak bone mass and slow bone loss.
- Gains in lumbar bone mass are seen in postmenopausal women who follow a weight-bearing exercise program.

Risk Factors

- Family history of osteoporosis
- Advancing age
- Female gender
- Caucasian or Asian race
- Early menopause (including surgical)
- Underweight
- Cigarette smoking
- History of dietary calcium deficiency
- Hypogonadism (men)
- Sedentary lifestyle
- Hyperthyroidism
- Subtotal gastrectomy
- Hemiplegia
- COPD
- Glucocorticoid medications
- Anticonvulsant medications

Polymyalgia Rheumatica

- Many women develop polymyalgia rheumatica after age 45.
- Treatment consists of corticosteroids.
- Two to 3 years after beginning prednisone, the woman may no longer have polymyalgia rheumatica but will be disabled by vertebral disease.

Protective Factors

- Obesity, with its associated increased endogenous estrogen levels
- Thiazide diuretics, which decrease calcium excretion

Screening Recommendations

- No specific screening tests are available.
- Effectiveness of densitometry is uncertain.

Preventive Strategies

- All women should be advised to take in 1000 mg of dietary calcium every day.
- Postmenopausal women not receiving ERT should increase intake to 1500 mg plus supplemental vitamin D (400 to 800 mg).
- Those who cannot meet the recommended level of dietary calcium should receive supplemental calcium.
- Risk status should be determined at menarche and monitored regularly.
- At menopause, women should be reevaluated for risk factors and considered for ERT.

TABLE 1-8
Nutritional Sources of Calcium

Source	Serving Size	Amount of Calcium (mg)
Milk	1 cup	300
Cheese (low fat)	1 oz	185
Yogurt (nonfat)	1 cup	450
Yogurt (whole milk)	1 cup	275
Cottage cheese (1%)	½ cup	70
Dark leafy greens	½ cup	150-180
Other vegetables	½ cup	30-100
Fruits	1 serving	<25

From Lewis SM, Heitkemper MM, Dirkin SR: *Medical-surgical nursing,* ed 5, St. Louis, 2000, Mosby, p 1276.

- All women should be advised to continue or begin weight-bearing exercises, 50 to 60 minutes three times per week.

Sexually Transmitted Diseases

Incidence
- Peak incidence of STDs occurs in teenagers and young adults.
- Teenagers account for 2.5 million cases.
- In 1994, 20,627 cases of syphilis were reported.
- Incidence of STDs has decreased since 1990, after two decades of increased incidence.
- Incidence of gonorrhea has decreased from a peak in 1974 to 420,000 cases in 1994, with 60% in people under age 25.
- Actual incidence of STDs may be twice the reported figures.
- Estimated annual incidence of chlamydia infection is 4 million cases, costing $2.4 billion.
- About 120,000 infants every year are infected with chlamydia at birth.
- About 500,000 new cases of genital herpes occur each year.
- STDs cluster in large urban areas, particularly in poor, minority communities and in rural southeastern states.

Prevalence
- Because of the prolonged length of infection, the two most prevalent STDs are herpes simplex virus (HSV) and human papillomavirus (HPV).
- Cumulative prevalence of genital HSV infection alone is 20 million cases.
- Most cases of chlamydial infection are asymptomatic, but an estimated 5% of the general population is affected.

Cost to Society
For pelvic inflammatory disease (PID) alone, the cost per year is $2.6 billion.

Morbidity and Mortality
- More than 200,000 women every year, 20% of whom have PID, become involuntarily infertile.
- About 50% of all ectopic pregnancies are a result of PID.
- More than 20% of women with only one episode of PID develop chronic pelvic pain.

Factors Relevant to Prevention
- All STDs have a high asymptomatic carrier rate, making prevention of transmission difficult.
- Most significant risk factor is multiple sexual partners.
- Only abstinence, monogamy, or condom use dramatically affects the risk.

Screening Recommendations
- No screening tests are recommended for the general population.
- Routine serologic tests for syphilis should be done on all pregnant women and persons at high risk for infection.
- High-risk groups should also have a screening gonorrhea culture and direct fluorescent antibody test or enzyme-linked immunosorbent assay (ELISA) for chlamydia at routine pelvic examinations.
- Persons with multiple sexual partners should be examined every year.
- All sexually active adolescent women should be screened for chlamydia infection.
- High-risk women should be screened for gonorrhea during pregnancy.
- Screening asymptomatic patients for HSV is not recommended.

Preventive Strategies
- Education about STDs should begin before the start of sexual activity.
- Clinicians should maintain a high index of suspicion for all STDs because of the extremely high rates of asymptomatic and minimally symptomatic patients.
- In high-risk populations, even with few or no symptoms, most experts recommend presumptive treatment of chlamydia.

Human Immunodeficiency Virus Infection

Incidence
- The number of new cases of acquired immunodeficiency syndrome (AIDS) is rapidly increasing among women.
- The estimated number of new cases in the United States ranges from 40,000 to 80,000 annually.

Prevalence
- The Centers for Disease Control and Prevention (CDC) estimates that 600,000 to

1.2 million persons in the United States are currently infected with HIV.

- Within 10 years of infection, 50% of individuals develop AIDS and another 40% develop associated clinical illnesses.
- The number of AIDS cases was estimated at 130,000 to 205,000 in 1995.

Cost to Society
Cost of treatment alone has increased from $2.2 billion in 1988 to $13 billion in 1992 and $15 billion in 1995.

Morbidity and Mortality
- Worldwide, an estimated 2.6 million deaths resulted from AIDS in 1999.
- Of the total 476,899 patients reported to the CDC through June 1995, 62% have died.
- HIV is the leading cause of death in men age 25 to 44 and is among the top 10 causes of death for men and women age 1 to 44.

Factors Relevant to Prevention
Groups with the highest incidence of HIV include hemophiliacs, homosexual men, intravenous drug users, those with multiple sexual partners, patients who received multiple blood transfusions after 1977 and before blood screening in 1985, patients with other STDs, and infants born to infected mothers.

Screening Recommendations
- All patients should be screened for risk status by means of a careful sexual and drug use history.
- Frequency of screening depends on the population of the area.
- Patients in high-risk groups should be encouraged to be tested for HIV antibodies.
- Early detection of HIV infection is important in curtailing its spread, particularly from mother to child.
- Treatment during pregnancy decreases vertical transmission to the infant.

Preventive Strategies
- Broad dissemination of educational information is imperative.
- The best prevention is to avoid exposure to HIV-infected individuals.

- Younger teenagers in particular need to understand the great risks of having unprotected sex and sharing needles.
- At-risk women of childbearing age should be strongly counseled to have annual HIV antibody screening.
- Women found to be HIV positive should be counseled not to conceive.
- Clinicians should take precautions to guard against inadvertent transmission in the clinic and to protect health care workers from infection.

BIBLIOGRAPHY

American Cancer Society: *Cancer facts and figures: 1996*, Atlanta, 1996, American Cancer Society.

American College of Cardiology/American Heart Association Practice Guidelines: http://www.acc.org/clinical/guidelines/index.html.

Carpenter CCJ, Fischl MA, Hammer SM, et al: Antiretroviral therapy for HIV infection in 1997: updated recommendations of the International AIDS Society—USA Panel, *JAMA* 227(24):1962-1969, 1997.

Edelman CL, Mandle CL: *Health promotion throughout the lifespan*, ed 3, St Louis, 1994, Mosby.

Expert Panel on the Detection, Evaluation, and Treatment of High Blood Cholesterol in Adults: Summary of the second report of the National Cholesterol Education Program (NCEP). Adult Treatment Panel II, *JAMA* 269:3015-3023, 1993.

He J, Vupputuri S, Allen K, et al: Passive smoking and the risk of coronary heart disease: a meta-analysis of epidemiologic studies, *N Engl J Med* 340:920-926, 1999.

HSTAT: Health Services/Technology Assessment Text: http://text.nlm.nih.gov/ftrs/gateway.

Jekel JF, Elmore JG, Katz DL: *Epidemiology, biostatistics, and preventive medicine*, Philadelphia, 1996, WB Saunders.

Klaus BD, Godesky MJ: Clinical implications of alcoholism in patients with HIV/AIDS, *Nurse Pract* 22(10):101-104, 1997.

Klaus BD, Godesky MJ: Drug interactions and protease inhibitor therapy in the treatment of HIV/AIDS, *Nurse Pract* 23(2):102-106, 1998.

McPhee SJ, Schroeder SA: General approach to the patient: health maintenance and disease prevention. In Tierney LM, McPhee SJ, Papadakis MA, editors: *Current medical diagnosis and treatment 2000*, New York, 2000, Lange Medical Books/McGraw-Hill.

Morse RM, Heffron WA: Disease prevention. In Rakel RE, editor: *Essentials of family practice*, Philadelphia, 1998, WB Saunders.

Murray RB, Zenter JP: *Health assessment and promotion strategies through the life span*, ed 6, Stamford, Conn., 1997, Appleton & Lange.

Smart CR, Hendrick RE, Rutledge JH, Smith RA: Benefit of mammography screening in women ages 40-49 years: current evidence from randomized control trials, *Cancer* 75:2788, 1995.

Smith A: New MI treatment guidelines reflect current findings, *Clinician Rev* 9(10):79-84, 1999.

Tucker KL, Hannan MT, Chen H, et al: Potassium, magnesium, and fruit and vegetable intakes are associated with greater bone density in elderly men and women, *Am J Clin Nutr* 89:727-730, 1999.

US Preventive Services Task Force: *Guide to clinical preventive services*, Alexandria, Va., 1996, International Medical Publishing.

REVIEW QUESTIONS

1. Most health promotion and disease prevention occurs in the:
   a. Patient's home
   b. School health class
   c. Primary care setting
   d. Hospital setting

2. One of the goals related to health promotion is to:
   a. Assess genetic factors that influence health
   b. Monitor the patient's blood pressure on a regular basis
   c. Take blood samples for laboratory analysis
   d. Determine the cause of the patient's recent mood swings

3. The definition of primary care includes all the following **except:**
   a. First-contact care
   b. Episodic care
   c. Comprehensive care
   d. Care provided over time

4. Primary care is provided for:
   a. Only the patient
   b. Only the patient and spouse
   c. The patient and family
   d. The patient, family, and community

5. Health promotion incorporates all the following **except:**
   a. Identification of health risk
   b. Plan to reduce health risks
   c. Screening for possible health problems
   d. Caring for patients with terminal illnesses

6. Patients with no symptoms of disease but with risk factors for a particular disease or diseases receive:
   a. Tertiary prevention
   b. Secondary prevention
   c. Primary prevention
   d. Risk reduction

7. Risk factors that cannot be changed include all of the following **except:**
   a. Age
   b. Obesity
   c. Genetic makeup
   d. Gender

8. Obstacles that prevent patients from receiving comprehensive health care include all of the following **except:**
   a. Lack of personal, family, and community resources
   b. Time constraints, particularly with regard to school or work hours of patients and providers
   c. Patients' lack of knowledge about the benefits of preventing disease
   d. Availability of educational materials regarding risk reduction and disease prevention

9. Questions about screening tests include all the following **except:**
   a. Will the patient benefit if the test indicates a particular disease?
   b. Does the screening test ensure that appropriate treatment is available?
   c. Is the screening test accurate?
   d. Does the screening test have adverse effects?

10. The leading cause of death in the United States is:
    a. Lung cancer
    b. Heart disease
    c. Emphysema (COPD)
    d. Motor vehicle accidents

11. Many of the most significant and specific causes of death are preventable and include all of the following **except:**
    a. Tobacco use
    b. Diet patterns
    c. Microbes
    d. Sexual behavior

12. The presenting event for patients with coronary heart disease may be:
    a. Fainting
    b. Acute pain
    c. Headache
    d. Sudden death

13. Which one of the following measures should **not** be included as a prevention strategy for heart disease?
    a. Acquisition of information to construct a family history, indicating known causes of death
    b. Program of exercise that includes aerobic exercises, brisk walking for 30 minutes, and other types of exercise done at least 3 days per week all year

c. Low-fat, low-cholesterol, preferably high-fiber diet
d. Assessment of cardiac function biennially or annually

14. The low-density lipoprotein level considered ideal is:
    a. <160 mg/dl
    b. <165 mg/dl
    c. <170 mg/dl
    d. <200 mg/dl

15. Which one of the following does **not** need to be eliminated to reduce intake of fat and cholesterol?
    a. Cheese
    b. Whole milk
    c. Egg whites
    d. Hot dogs, bacon, liver

16. The estimated number of stroke survivors in the United States currently is:
    a. 500,000
    b. 1 million
    c. 2.5 million
    d. 3.8 million

17. The annual cost to society of cerebrovascular accident is estimated to be:
    a. $500 million
    b. $1 billion
    c. $15 billion
    d. $23 billion

18. The major risk factor for stroke is:
    a. Transient ischemic attacks
    b. Hypertension
    c. Occasional blurred vision
    d. Loss of sensation in one part of the body

19. The estimated number of Americans who are addicted to alcohol, drugs, or both is:
    a. 3 million
    b. 5 million
    c. 10 million
    d. 18 million

20. Persons who are dependent on alcohol have an overall risk of death that is _____% above normal.
    a. 50
    b. 100
    c. 200
    d. 250

2

Health Care Policy and Professional Issues

HEALTH CARE POLICY

Health care policy is an area of growing importance to health professionals. Policy encompasses (1) the choices that a society, segment of society, or organization makes regarding its goals and priorities and (2) the ways it will allocate its resources. Policy reflects the values of those setting the policy.

Public policies are formed by governmental bodies, such as legislation passed by the U.S. Congress and the regulations written from that legislation. Public policy is a purposive course of governmental action to deal with an issue of public concern. Public policy regarding tobacco, for example, includes a law that bans the selling of cigarettes within a specified radius of a school.

Social policies are usually directives that promote the welfare of the public, such as a local ordinance that sets age limits on those who purchase tobacco or alcohol. Such policies promote the welfare of children.

Health policies include directives that promote the health of citizens. The federal government, for example, could decide to pay for smoking prevention programs for those in the military and their families. State governments might require this coverage by companies providing Medicaid managed care.

Institutional policies govern workplaces, reflect the institution's goals and operations, and set policies and work requirements for employees (e.g., hours, salary levels). Under institutional policy an organization can institute a no-smoking policy that prohibits employees from smoking anywhere in the building or on the premises.

Organizational policies pertain to the rules governing and official positions taken by organizations, such as state nurses' associations or specialty nursing organizations.

All policies are generated by politics and reflect societal values, beliefs, and attitudes.

Policy formulation occurs in the following ways:
1. Enactment of legislation and its accompanying rules and regulations, which have the weight of law
2. Administrative decisions in interagency and intraagency activities, including interpretive guidelines for rules and regulations
3. Judicial decisions that interpret the law

POLITICS

Politics means "influencing." The Prussian chancellor Otto von Bismarck defined politics as "the art of the impossible." Influencing others is usually a long and difficult process, requiring multiple strategies to make others believe in and support a position or viewpoint. Politics arise in regard to allocation of scarce resources, when particular groups or organizations compete for these scarce resources and use persuasive measures to influence these decisions.

One example of "politicking" occurred when a coalition of women's organizations, scientists, and legislators informed the public that most of the federally funded research in the United States focused primarily on men. The knowledge gained from one-gender research about cardiac disease, for example, would probably not be applicable to women, as has since been found, when research began to include women as subjects in the study of heart disease. Women exhibit symptoms of heart disease that are different from those of men. Women react differently to cardiac drugs than do men. However, these changes were the result of many people who worked together to bring about changes in policy that mandated that women be included in research studies about particular diseases. Many other examples show the effects of politics in bringing about legislative changes.

Only recently have health professionals recognized that they can—and *need* to—have a voice in health care policy. To exercise the freedom to affect policy, however, particularly public policy, a person needs to understand the terms used, the boundaries of available actions, and the extent of both personal and group/organizational power in effecting change. Experts believe that policy is not made by the President or by Congress, but by groups and organizations devoted to particular causes and philosophies that require federal or state support. For example, many groups and organizations address only environmental problems and issues. These groups confer, develop new methods to improve the environment, then present their ideas and strategies to members of Congress through letters, telegrams, meetings, advertisements, and other measures so that eventually, action will be taken to improve environmental conditions.

Official government policies reflect the beliefs of the administration in power and provide direction for the philosophy and mission of government organizations. Specific policies undergird the "shoulds" and "should nots" of agencies. Agency policies can be broad and general, such as those that formulate the relationship of a particular agency to other government groups. Other policies may be in the form of specific announcements, as in operational procedures, which usually are narrow and direct. State boards of nursing, for example, are government agencies created by legislatures to protect the public through regulation of nursing practice. Procedure manuals in hospitals detail precise steps to be followed under specified circumstances and guide nurses' actions in carrying out particular nursing tasks.

Both specific and general policies are developed as guidelines for employees' behaviors within an organization. The terms *policies* and *procedures* are frequently used interchangeably, but policies are generally broader.

Laws represent types of policy. Legal directives guide public and private behavior, and laws serve to define action that reflects the will of society or some part of society. Such laws are developed at the local, state, federal, and international levels and are primary factors in guiding the conduct of individuals and groups. Lawmaking comes under the purview of the legislative branch of government in the United States, although executive orders and judicial interpretations of the law have the "force of law." The President, by executive order, can nullify previous laws or portions of laws for the common good.

Judicial interpretation can occur in the following three ways:

1. Courts may interpret the meaning of laws that are written in broad terms and are somewhat vague, and courts may be asked to rule on areas in which the law is unclear or controversial.
2. Courts can determine how some laws are to be applied.
3. Courts can declare a law made by Congress or the states to be unconstitutional, thus nullifying the statutes entirely.

Courts are idealized as being above the political activity that surrounds the federal or state legislature and are considered beyond the influence of politically powerful interest groups.

POLICY DEVELOPMENT

In general the process of policymaking involves four major stages, as follows:

1. Setting the agenda
2. Developing legislation and related regulations
3. Implementing the program to carry out the policy
4. Evaluating the program and its effectiveness in carrying out the policy

These stages are addressed sequentially, but as the policy process proceeds, it is frequently neither sequential nor logical. For example, defining the problem, which occurs during the agenda-setting stage, often changes during the legislative process; the scope of the problem may be expanded or narrowed. The design of the program may be altered during implementation. During the evaluation (final) stage, more important problems may be discovered that demand resolution and that must go through the same process on the national agenda as potential new policies.

Setting an agenda involves (1) identifying a particular societal or other problem that affects most or all of the citizens and (2) bringing it to the attention of government. Legislating policy and developing the law's regulations (how the law will be implemented) constitute the formal response of government to the request for policy changes or to a new policy. Governmental responses are political; the decisions about who, what, when, and how are made within a framework of power, influence, and negotiation. A program is set up to achieve the policy's goals. Evaluation determines how effectively the program has achieved the stated goals. Based on evaluation, the program may be modified to be more effective or discontinued because it did not achieve its stated goals.

Throughout the process of policy development, both formal and informal interactions occur among active participants in the process, within and outside the government. Participants may include private citizens, legislators, bureaucrats, lobbyists, or institutional groups (e.g., courts, political parties, special interest groups).

Nursing Profession

The nursing profession itself constitutes a special interest group. Therefore all professional nurses should be knowledgeable about governmental, legislative, and policy processes so that the profession can have a voice in influencing policies that affect its practice or interests.

Victor Fuchs, a nursing advocate and noted economist at the Stanford University School of Medicine's Department of Health Research and Policy, believes that nurses as a group have not been as involved as they should be in formulating health care policies. When nurses speak on health policies, however, he finds it difficult to distinguish between patient advocacy and advocacy for their own interests; these two are often separate agendas that run parallel. For example, nurses may ask for more nurses per specific patient numbers, then request shorter working hours. Nurses have not taken a major stance that was contrary to or did not focus on the interests of the nursing profession. Fuchs believes that nurses need to take a broader view of health care and health care policy and that people need to think about health and medical care from an economic perspective.

Fuchs also believes that major changes in health policy do not depend on health and medical care but on society. The United States will not have national health insurance unless, Fuchs says, "the external circumstances make it politically viable and politically attractive, which means a depression, a war, or large-scale civil unrest [revolution]." Choices will increase within the framework of a managed care environment, however, with more research-based outcomes using newer technologies to assess health status and its changes.

Nurses were "at the table" during President Clinton's efforts to reform health care. He believed that the United States was ready to make changes and that Congress would enact new laws and policies regarding health care delivery. As Dr. Fuchs said, however, "The country wasn't ready for health care reform because everything has to be up in the air and uncertain to disrupt one-seventh of the nation's economy"—the cost of health care.

Circumstances were also unfavorable for massive changes in the health care system. In the current anti-egalitarian trend, people are moving away from the idea that everyone should receive the same amount of medical care and moving toward the concept that some people are willing and able to buy more health care and thus will receive more. The 1990s represented a decade of peace and prosperity during which the standard of living for most people increased by variable degrees. Medical care is directed more toward quality of life than extension of life. Individuals generally do not change their lifestyle, and thus improve their health, by stopping smoking, greatly reducing fat in their diets, and exercising regularly. Fuchs believes that individuals should accept greater personal responsibility for their health to decrease those diseases that occur later in life because of smoking, alcohol and drug abuse, and unhealthy diets; emphysema, liver disease, kidney disease, and other conditions require long-term, expensive treatment. Also, quality of life can be applied to housing, transportation, sufficient food, and work, areas where equality does not exist.

Nurses and the nursing profession are at the center of many health-related issues. Professional nurses should be in the forefront of those who formulate and decide on health care issues. Theoretically, nurses have the knowledge and the power to influence health policy and to provide expertise in the design, implementation, and evaluation of health care programs. The input of nurses, however, should be based on a broad perspective, not solely on the promotion of nursing issues.

The many roles of advanced practice nurses as providers of direct care, researchers, consultants, educators, administrators, consumer advocates, and political activists reveal the expanding character of professional nurses. Actions that initiate policy changes—setting agendas and developing, implementing, and evaluating programs to carry out the agendas—mandate changes that will affect health care policy for the decades ahead. Foresight, in addition to working toward achieving sound health care policies, makes the difference in people's lives.

STRATEGIES FOR DEVELOPING HEALTH CARE POLICY

For too long, nurses have been focused interiorly, on their own issues, circumstances, and wishes, perhaps because, for many years, women and nurses were "ordered to care" and not much else. Their opinions were not sought, and even nursing administrators were not allowed in the "inner sanctum" of male dominance in hospitals or other health care organizations. With advanced education, additional knowledge, and greater appreciation of how to influence public policy, professional nurses have taken a more active part in legislation and governmental procedures in the last decade.

Part of nurses' education should be to work together as a united group, putting aside internal issues and focusing on society's needs. Nurses must learn more about how to debate all sides of particular issues, from all perspectives—private citizen, legislator, health professional, and patient. Practicing the art of debate regarding how to challenge, contest, dispute, argue, and settle issues should be an integral part of education, particularly at the master's level. If all 2.9 million nurses in the United States were to become a unified organization who addressed health care policies as a single group, their power would be over-

whelming. Nurses have fragmented into separate, smaller groups, however, who argue rather than putting their skills, knowledge, and power into speaking out publicly with one purpose: to make health care better and more available to all people. Health care for all may not result in equality of care, but health care can be improved for all.

A strong, unified professional organization is needed to make nurses' power and influence felt at the highest levels. Only a small percentage of nurses are members of the American Nurses' Association (ANA). Changes in membership cost may help to encourage all nurses to join, with fees based on level of education or income. Some measure should allow all registered nurses (RNs) to join the ANA and actively participate in its work and political arm. Mistakes were made in the past regarding the level of education required to be "professional RNs" versus "technical RNs" and to be certified as nurse practitioners (NPs). These internal actions affected the attitudes of nurses who had been passed over when education became the focal point.

Much of nursing's lack of a "single voice" has thus centered on internal struggles, many of which have been settled. Educational levels of RNs remain (associate degree, baccalaureate degree), but diploma schools of nursing largely have been closed or united with community colleges' or 4-year colleges' nursing programs. These actions are past history, however, with their effects mostly forgotten as older nurses have left or retired from nursing. More recently, controversy arose because of the national recognition granted to nurse practitioners as advanced practice nurses. Other groups (e.g., clinical nurse specialists, nurse-midwives, nurse anesthetists) thought that they, too, should be included under this umbrella title and receive the same respect accorded NPs. This issue was resolved at a national conference of nursing faculty and administrators in the late 1980s. The group, consisting mainly of master's-prepared clinical nurse specialists and faculty from schools of nursing, voted to include all master's-prepared specialist nurses under the designation of "advanced practice nurses."

The nursing profession has reached a plateau; most nurses agree that the bachelor-of-science (BS) degree in nursing is appropriate, and many associate-degree nurses are continuing in programs to earn the BS degree. Specialization in advanced practice is at the master's-degree level, but less than 1% of RNs have earned doctoral degrees. Advanced practice nurses have knowledge and skills in managing change, conflict resolution, communication, negotiation, group process, and inpatient care in specialized areas such as gerontologic, acute, primary, and pediatric care. These nurses are able to advocate for and develop health care policy.

As they begin this new millennium, nurses must work together to achieve U.S. health care goals for diverse ethnic and cultural groups. The United States espouses diversity and pluralistic approaches to problem solving. Despite many health policy changes (primarily cost-cutting measures) since the 1980s, no clear vision shows how health care services will be organized and delivered in the future. To a large extent, insurers have become health planners and health providers, providers are becoming insurers, pharmaceutical companies and suppliers manage disease states, and hospitals are seen as cost centers, with many merging or closing. Health care education and delivery are moving to the Internet, where consumers can find information about how best to treat their health problems.

Payment methods are changing rapidly, with some people predicting a three-tiered system in the future based on the individual's and family's ability to pay for insurance, with rationing at the lower two tiers of the system. Corporate leaders advocate capitated managed care as being a less costly method of providing health insurance coverage to workers; politicians also advocate this method for Medicare and Medicaid populations. Managed care is a strategy for rationing care for those in the middle tier. In the top tier, wealthy Americans will continue to have open-ended access to health care services and freedom to choose their providers.

Some experts predict that the current state of chaos will evolve into new organized delivery systems, with varying types of ownership and diverse alliances among hospitals, physicians, and insurers that will be designed to capture a large market share and that will provide cost-effective care to defined populations.

ORGANIZED, INTEGRATED SYSTEMS

Characteristics of organized, integrated systems include the following:
- A continuum of care that includes primary, acute, and long-term care
- Willingness to assume financial risk
- Clinical and financial outcomes data based on meticulous research methods
- Both horizontal and vertical integration of services
- Integration of medical and surgical services
- Integration of a large array of clinical services in all local markets

Health care professionals (insurers, providers, administrators) must be willing to work together to provide care that is appropriate, available, necessary, and cost-effective to large groups of people from all economic and cultural levels. These types of systems will require the development of (1) structures of political accountability in each community and (2) governance structures that will encourage coordination and sound decision making about allocation of resources at the local level. The key factors necessary to develop these integrated systems include the following:
- Organizational culture
- Improved integrated information systems
- Internal incentives
- Total quality management
- Physician leadership
- Increased growth of group practices

Others hope that the current chaos will evolve into a single-payer system with significant government regulation to ensure a level playing field for all Americans. People who advocate for this approach do not view markets as being able to work effectively and efficiently to provide health care services. These groups view health care as a *right* that should be provided in a way similar to that of other developed countries, such as Canada and the United Kingdom, with "international standards" of health care delivery, as follows:
- Universal coverage of the total population
- Comprehensive principal benefits
- Payment (contributions) based on income rather than individual insurance purchases
- Cost control by means of administrative mechanisms, such as binding fee schedules, global budgets, and limitations on system capacity

Change probably will be influenced even more by informed consumers who will exert their power over corporate and government payers, politicians, insurers, and health care providers. Educational strategies must be developed to educate the public about accountability, self-responsibility in maintaining one's own health, and informed decision making about purchasing the means to improve one's health care.

The current system of health care is still based on episodic care (rather than continuous care) that aims at preventing illness, treating illness in its earliest stages, and providing long-term care for those with terminal or end-of-life health problems. An episodic approach to health care does not work and is extremely expensive. Incremental approaches also do not work. The entire health care system needs to be restructured, perhaps geographically, by creating local areas and determining the health care needs in that population; recruiting or stationing appropriate numbers of health care providers in each local area, with adequate and expert administrative and financial managers; and making allocations based on the needs in these individual regions.

Health care providers can help create a national system of health care delivery by developing a workable system that adequately reimburses providers, eliminates the "middle-man insurance marketers," and provides continuous appropriate care for all the people in each geographic area, with payment based on income, age, and ability to pay. Outcome data would be meticulously collected on every person within the geographic area to determine the effectiveness of care. Cost analyses would determine cost of care per individual based on number, acuity, and duration of health problems.

The main obstacle to such a global plan of health care is the capitalistic perspective, in which everyone expects to become rich and to compete for individual status in terms of accruement of wealth, rather than to be satisfied with income that is equitable but not excessive for the level of health care provided. In other words, the element of greed must be accounted for in the United States along with limited resources. In addition to health care, all people should have adequate housing, food, and safety.

POLICY ANALYSIS

Policy analysis is the systematic description and explanation of the causes and consequences of government action and inaction and is not restricted to goal-oriented actions. Representatives from many disciplines are engaged in research on governmental policies in terms of system outputs. The newest addition to university curricula about policy is the study of policy science theory and methodology.

Policy analysis is conducted primarily in universities and policy research organizations, which use principles and analytic tools from other disciplines (e.g., economics, probability theory, statistics) in conjunction with legislatures, governmental agencies, and related organizations. Roles of analysts include the academically based "objective technician," the politically oriented "issue advocate" who promotes societal welfare, and the "client advocate," whose goal is to develop the best case for the employer (e.g., lobbyists). Nurses usually function as issue advocates.

Policy analysis is undergirded by a problem-solving approach, in which (1) a definition or description of the problem is developed, with its specific objectives; (2) alternative strategies for resolving issues are identified; (3) ramifications (e.g., project size, costs, time) of each strategy are considered; (4) evaluation criteria are developed according to the strategy selected; and (5) recommendations are made regarding optimal solutions.

POWER IN POLITICAL ANALYSIS

Power is recognized as one of the most complex sociologic and political concepts to define and measure. The term is used freely by many in all arenas of both public and private organizations and groups, often with individuals not understanding its meaning within particular contexts. Max Weber's definition is often used: "Power . . . is the probability that one actor within a social relationship will be in a position to carry out his own will despite resistance, regardless of the basis on which this probability rests." Power may be a means to an end or an end in itself, as shown in wars, coups d'etat, and political arenas. Power is usually a major issue among stakeholders within a particular organization or those involved in a particular contest. *Stakeholders* are those individuals or groups who have influence over the issue or who could be mobilized to become involved in the contest. Recruiting stakeholders is an aim for all factions interested in winning a particular argument or contest, such as union members fighting for higher wages.

In 1959, French and Raven developed a typology of sources of power. In 1979, policy experts Hersey, Blanchard, and Natemeyer expanded this and identified the following seven sources of power:

1. *Coercive power* is rooted in real or perceived fear of one person by another.
2. *Reward power* is based on the perception of the potential for rewards or favors by honoring the wishes of a powerful person or group.
3. *Legitimate (positional) power* is associated with position in organizations, not personal qualities.
4. *Expert power* is based on special knowledge, talents, or skills, as contrasted with positional power.
5. *Referent power* emanates from admiration, charisma, or shared beliefs and mutual identification among people with similar backgrounds.
6. *Information power* is present when one individual or group has or is believed to have special and specific information that other individuals or groups want to obtain.
7. *Connection power* is based on the assumption that particular individuals or groups have privileged connections with powerful individuals or organizations.

These power types are helpful in understanding the dynamics of power in organizations or political groups in all settings: work, community, organizations, and government.

ETHICAL ISSUES IN POLICY AND POLITICS

Policymakers and politicians face ethical issues every day. Ethical issues usually involve the following:

- Personal conduct: is it right and good?
- Conduct toward others: is it fair, equal, and honest?
- Responsibilities and obligations: are they carried out with integrity and to the very best of one's ability?
- Conduct when conflict arises with respect to others' values, beliefs, questions about economics, or cultural biases and values: are the issues confronted with good judgment and fairness and dealt with sensitively and comprehensively to resolve conflicts so that everyone wins in some way?

One's own ethical principles must be known, understood, and internally affirmed before engaging in political activities. Having a firm basis for right conduct and judicious actions is necessary at any time and particularly with controversial issues.

INVOLVEMENT IN ORGANIZATIONS

Organizational membership is a vital part of one's personal and professional life. In all disciplines, membership in one's professional association is an essential part of career growth and advancement in the profession. For nurses, membership in the ANA is basic to professional life. Often it is difficult to see what professional associations do for the individual member, but the individual must look at what the association accomplishes *for the nursing profession*. Professional associations should **not** be involved in supporting particular persons running for local or national offices. Associations can openly and publicly encourage their members to be involved in supporting their choice of candidates, but it is not appropriate for associations to support particular candidates. Doing so can damage the association politically and economically, as it did in past years when the ANA expressed its support for a U.S. presidential candidate, and the other candidate won. If the person endorsed by the association wins, rewards or recognition may occur, but risks are involved.

Political action committees (PACs) engage exclusively in political activity. The ANA-PAC was initially known as the Nurses' Coalition for Action in Politics when it was established in 1974. In 1985 the ANA House of Delegates voted to change the name to ANA-PAC to affirm the link to the ANA.

PROFESSIONAL ISSUES IN NURSING

Despite the resolution of many professional issues that dominated the early years of NPs, such as acceptance by both nursing and medical groups and becoming part of the health care mainstream, other issues have surfaced more recently, including quality of education and practice, numbers of NP graduates, reimbursement, and "telehealth" and interstate licensure.

Quality of Nurse Practitioner Faculty and Graduates

With the growing number of NP programs, many specialty areas are concerned about NP faculty being fully qualified and competent and graduates being adequately prepared, in both theory and clinical practice, to care for diverse populations with many different, variably severe illnesses.

Recently, NPs have become more involved as triage nurses using telephone and telehealth communications. Triaging patients requires particular knowledge and skills, whether or not the nurse provides hands-on care. Initial diagnosis is crucial to treatment, prognosis, and recovery of the patient. The same applies to all NPs practicing in the various specialties, with patients and their families, as members of interdisciplinary teams.

Numbers of Nurse Practitioners

Concern surrounds the increasing numbers of NPs and their place in the health care system regarding competition for patients and reimbursement. Will the market become overloaded, thus decreasing the marketability of all NPs? If 20% of the total number of practicing NPs are graduating every year, the total will soon come up against a crowded market. Many schools have pushed this issue aside as not being relevant. More attention needs to be focused on this potential problem before the profession becomes saturated and before NPs must compete actively for patients and salaries.

The 44 million uninsured persons in the United States (35% Latinos, 25% blacks, 20% whites), will eventually require various forms of health care. Where will payment for these services come from? Uninsured persons are primarily young people in low-paying jobs. Employers do not offer health insurance, and health insurance premiums are too expensive. This growing problem over the last 30 years will soon become one of the most serious social problems in the United States. The situation is worse despite efforts to solve the problem and despite annual U.S. expenditures of $1.1 trillion for health care. The problem will only worsen as the number of people receiving Medicaid and Medicare benefits (now 70 million) increases because of the aging population. This older population mainly includes divorced or widowed older women who have lost health insurance once provided through their husbands' employers. As single women age and some buy individual health insurance, the insurers raise premiums by as much as 20% to 25%, almost every year. Within a few years these individual buyers of health insurance will be paying twice or three times the initial cost. Lack of access to preventive or diagnostic services compounds the problem and results in late-stage diagnosis and early deaths from treatable conditions. People who do not have or cannot afford health insurance or health care are treated as second-class citizens, regardless of their background and former earning capacity. Many are too proud to seek care at clinics or emergency rooms and die of acute conditions such as pneumonia or ruptured appendix. The U.S. health care industry continues to brush these issues aside, as if, by ignoring them, they will disappear completely. Such magical thinking will never solve problems.

Reimbursement

Reimbursement issues continue to be a concern to NPs themselves and may become a greater problem with the changing economics of health care delivery. This concern relates to both the increasing rate of immigration to the United States of Latinos and other groups, who swell the ranks of low-paid workers who cannot afford health insurance, and the possible oversupply of health care professionals. Those on the lower rungs of practice (i.e., nurses, NPs, specialist nurses) will earn considerably less than those on the higher rungs (i.e., physicians, physician specialists, physician assistants).

These concerns will be addressed only when the following actions occur:

- Enough middle-class and upper-class people are personally outraged by poor access to health care and say to their legislators, "This is no longer tolerable. Too many people cannot afford to receive health insurance or health care of any kind, at any level."

- Health-related disasters occur, such as a major epidemic with great mortality, or many deaths result from little or no health care.
- Some person (leader) takes steps to make health care available to all, even at only a minimal level, to identify early disease or to prevent epidemics through adequate immunization programs.

According to James Tallon, president of the United Hospital Fund of New York and chairman of the Kaiser Commission on Medicaid and the Uninsured, "We are just on the edge of believing that it is acceptable and expected that certain groups will be uninsured. And that is the beginning of the end."

Currently it is pointless to accuse providers who were once overpaid, at massive duplication of technology even among neighboring hospitals, and condemn other decisions that prevented equitable health care and reasonable rather than excessive profits. In addition, racial and cultural discrimination, disregard for poor people, and lack of care for immigrants have made the current situation almost irreparable. In recent years the chief financial officers (CFOs) of health care organizations and facilities have garnered the highest profits, often in the millions of dollars, while the real workers (i.e., health care providers) have earned only a fraction of these amounts. Administrators, CFOs, clinicians, and other providers must unite and lobby for a comprehensive strategy that will meet the health care needs of all U.S. citizens. Health care costs must be lowered by regulating and rationing care for all people, from the very rich to the very poor, to prevent catastrophic changes in all facets of life and possible revolution.

Nurses represent the largest number of health care providers in the United States. Nurses are trusted by more people and can wield greater influence based on their knowledge of health care than any other provider group. Politicians pay attention to numbers. If the nursing profession could gather all its members and demand changes that will result in adequate health care for all people at the lowest cost, the effort, although not agreeable to many, would be acceptable to most.

Telehealth and Interstate Licensure

Nurse practitioners are now becoming increasingly involved in providing clinical services via telehealth, especially for people in rural areas who have limited access to health care providers. Several of the NP professional organizations are also actively involved in helping to resolve these issues. The 1997 Comprehensive Telehealth Act, sponsored by Senator Kent Conrad (D-ND) and passed by the 105th Congress, listed NPs as both "referring" and "consulting" clinicians eligible for Medicare reimbursement. This bill also proposed that the Secretary of Health and Human Services "look into easing the licensing burdens of telehealth practitioners who are now forced to be licensed in every state in which they administer telehealth services, and are now required to pay the licensing fee in every state in which they interact with patients."

Some of the nursing professions have discussed national licensure for all nurses, but the circumstances differ from state to state, and no conclusions have yet been reached.

In 1999 the 106th Congress introduced three bills that address Medicare reimbursement, as follows:

- S. 770 Comprehensive Telehealth Act of 1999, sponsored by Senator Conrad
- H.R. 1344 Triple-A Rural Health Improvement Act of 1999, sponsored by Representative Jim Nussle (R-IA)
- S. 980 Promoting Health in Rural Areas Act of 1999, sponsored by Senator Max Baucus (D-MT)

These three bills propose that the federal government preempt the licensing of health professionals by state, which would greatly facilitate clinicians' ability to provide care by telehealth to larger groups of patients over a wider geographic area.

In addition, the 1997 Telemedicine Report to Congress devoted a chapter to legal issues such as telehealth licensure and made several recommendations to Congress. The National Council of State Boards of Nursing (NCSBN) has been an active member in activities with respect to clinical services across state lines. Information about the NCSBN's activities and the NCSBN's Advanced Practice Registered Nurse (APRN) Task Force's work on "Uniform APRN Licensure/Authority to Practice Requirements" can be followed at http://www.ncsbn.org. These concerns have become national issues and require resolution through the federal government and other national resources.

BIBLIOGRAPHY

Axt L: Pennsylvania rules to permit triage, *Clinician News* 4(5):36, 2000.

Brown C: Ethics, policy, and practice: interview with Emily Friedman, *Image J Nurs Sch* 31(3):259-262, 1999.

Christoffel KK: Public health advocacy: process and product, *Am J Public Health* 90(5):722-726, 2000.

Curtis BT, Lumpkin B: Political action committees. In Mason DJ, Leavitt JK, editors: *Policy and politics in nursing and health care,* ed 3, Philadelphia, 1998, Saunders.

Hanley BE: Policy development and analysis. In Mason DJ, Leavitt JK, editors: *Policy and politics in nursing and health care,* ed 3, Philadelphia, 1998, Saunders.

Heinrich J: Organization and delivery of health care in the United States: the health care system that isn't. In Mason DJ, Leavitt JK, editors: *Policy and politics in nursing and health care,* ed 3, Philadelphia, 1998, Saunders.

Helmuth L: NIH, under pressure, boosts minority health research, *Science* 288(5466):596-597, 2000.

Herrick T: NPs raise the volume on impanelment discrimination, *Clinician News* 4(5):1, 4, 6, 2000.

Leavitt JK, Mason DJ: Policy and politics: a framework for action. In Mason DJ, Leavitt JK, editors: *Policy and politics in nursing and health care,* ed 3, Philadelphia, 1998, Saunders.

Milstead JA: *Health policy and politics: a nurse's guide,* Gaithersburg, Md, 1999, Aspen.

Shepard PM: E-medicine, *Clinician News* 4(5):13-14, 30, 2000.

Skaggs BJ, deVries CM: You and your professional organization. In Mason DJ, Leavitt JK, editors: *Policy and politics in nursing and health care,* ed 3, Philadelphia, 1998, Saunders.

Spetz J: Victor Fuchs on health care, ethics, and the role of nurses, *Image J Nurs Sch* 31(3):255-258, 1999.

Telehealth and state licensure, *Nurse Pract* 24(8):12-13, 1999 (letters).

REVIEW QUESTIONS

1. Policy is concerned with all the following **except:**
   a. Priorities and goals
   b. Selection of public officials
   c. Allocation of resources
   d. Values

2. Public policy is formed by local, state, and federal governments regarding issues that include all the following **except:**
   a. Safety
   b. Gun control
   c. Restrictions regarding sale of liquor or tobacco to minors
   d. Placement of warning signs for drivers

3. Social policy is closely related to (and sometimes the same as) public policy and includes all the following **except:**
   a. Building permits
   b. Setting age limits on those who can buy tobacco or alcohol
   c. School lunches
   d. Speed limits

4. Institutional policies include all the following **except:**
   a. Goals
   b. Operational methodology
   c. Retirement age of employees
   d. Smoke-free environment in the building and surrounding property

5. State nurses' associations develop official positions and recommendations under:
   a. Public policy
   b. Social policy
   c. Organizational policy
   d. Institutional policy

6. All policies are generated by:
   a. Governmental groups
   b. Organizational officials
   c. Politics
   d. Public demand

7. *Politics* means:
   a. Consensus
   b. Influence
   c. Directing
   d. Power struggles

8. The four stages of policymaking include all the following **except:**
   a. Agenda setting
   b. Writing legislation and regulations
   c. Developing strategies
   d. Evaluating the effects of the law and regulations

9. Policy analysis is concerned with:
   a. Evaluation of each policy as it is developed and implemented
   b. Goals and priorities of the policy
   c. Systematic description and explanation of the causes and consequences of governmental action and inaction
   d. System outputs from governmental policies

10. Victor Fuchs says that major health policy changes occur based on:
    a. What is happening in health care
    b. What is advocated by physician groups
    c. What is happening in society
    d. Special interest groups

11. Nurses' influence can be wielded successfully because of their:
    a. Level of education
    b. Knowledge of health and health care
    c. Knowledge of people's needs
    d. Numbers

12. Health care professionals, including insurers, providers, and administrators, must be willing to work together to provide care that requires all the following **except:**
    a. Appropriateness
    b. Availability
    c. High technology
    d. Cost-effectiveness

13. The U.S. health care system will likely change as the result of:
    a. Economic status of the United States
    b. Growing number of older people requiring care
    c. Changing ethnic and cultural characteristics of the U.S. population
    d. Informed consumers

14. The U.S. health care system needs to be reorganized and administered on a:
    a. Local level
    b. State level
    c. National level
    d. Geographic level

15. The most critical professional issue now facing educators and nurse practitioners is:
    a. Quality of care given by nurse practitioners
    b. Number of nurse practitioners being graduated each year
    c. Reimbursement for nurse practitioner services
    d. Nursing leadership

16. The greatest change occurring in the U.S. population is:
    a. Greater number of older persons
    b. Increasing percentage of immigrant populations
    c. Increasing cost of care
    d. Cost of therapeutic drugs

17. In U.S. rural areas, reimbursement to health care providers comes primarily from:
    a. Individual payers
    b. Medicare
    c. Medicaid
    d. Supplemental health insurance

18. In largely rural states in the western United States, health care is provided via telehealth. By means of the Internet, physicians and nurses can provide services to those far from cities and without readily accessible health care. The major need of these providers is for:
    a. Greater knowledge of indigenous diseases
    b. Greater ability to diagnose and treat rapidly
    c. Greater capability to meet needs of people in more than one state
    d. Improved language skills to communicate with Native Americans, Latinos, and Asians

19. The bills recently introduced in the U.S. Senate and House of Representatives have been sponsored by senators or representatives from:
    a. Large, rural states
    b. California
    c. Washington and Oregon
    d. The Southwest

20. Nurses as a group are capable of making significant changes in the current health care system by:
    a. Becoming organized at the local, state, and national levels
    b. Becoming active members of nursing associations
    c. Becoming active in nursing's political action committees
    d. All the above

3

Legal and Ethical Issues

LEGAL ISSUES
Nurse Practice Acts

Each state has enacted professional practice acts for physicians, nurses, nurse-midwives, physician assistants, dentists, and other providers through statutory law. These practice acts are based on the police power that the federal government grants each state to protect the safety of its citizens. The acts vary from state to state, but all address their profession as follows:

- Describe how to obtain a license and enter practice in the particular state.
- Define the educational requirements for entry into practice.
- Describe the selection process for members of the state board and the categories of membership.
- Identify situations that are grounds for disciplinary action (i.e., circumstances in which a license can be suspended or revoked).
- Identify the process for disciplinary actions, including diversionary techniques.
- Outline the appeal process if the individual professional believes that the disciplinary actions taken by the board are not fair or valid.
  Some boards outline the scope of practice allowable within the state.

Tort Law

A *tort* is a civil (not criminal) wrong, other than breach of contract, in which the law provides a remedy by allowing the injured person to seek damages. Negligence and professional negligence come under this type of law.

Negligence is conduct that falls below the standards established by law for the protection of others against unreasonable risk of harm. Negligence is currently the predominant cause

of action for accidental injury in the United States.

Professional negligence refers to the conduct of professionals (e.g., physicians, nurses, dentists, lawyers) that falls below a professional standard of due care.

- *Acts of omission* are those actions that the health professional has **not** done, usually because of oversight; however, acts of omission are not considered to be accidental because they come under professional responsibilities.
- *Acts of commission* are those actions that the health professional **does,** that are alleged to be more or less harmful to the patient, but that are not done willfully with intent to harm.

Liability is responsibility for a possible or actual loss, penalty, evil, expense, or burden for which law or justice requires that the individual do something for, pay, or otherwise compensate the victim. The *rule of personal liability* holds that everyone is responsible for his or her own behavior, including negligent behavior.

The law **does not** require the nurse to protect against every possible harm to the patient. The law **does** require that the nurse carry out care in accordance with what other reasonably prudent nurses would do in the same or similar circumstances.

- Nurses should know the standards of care applicable in all states as well as in their state.
- The American Nurses' Association (ANA) publishes standards of care for all types of nursing specialties in all settings.
- Nurses should know the standards of care that are required in their health care facility; these are generally included in the "policies and procedures" manual.

Complete nursing documentation, including date and time, is essential for all nursing actions performed, particularly in a court of law.

- "If it's not documented, it wasn't done." This rule undergirds all nursing care in all circumstances.
- Sentences need not be complete, as long as the meaning is clear about who, what, when, and where.

Intentional Torts

Intentional torts are civil wrongs that are considered to be done deliberately by the defendant. Although some acts may appear to be caused by oversight rather than deliberate action, they are not considered accidents because they relate to specific rights and responsibilities. Intentional torts related to health care institutions and professionals include assault, battery, false imprisonment, and conversions of property.

Assault is the threat of touching another person, although actual contact is not required to bring a charge of assault. The damage or harm experienced by the victim involves fear, anxiety, or dread.

Battery is actual contact with the person, without that person's consent, and includes touching the body, clothing, or any object (e.g., purse) that is attached to the person. The victim need not be conscious of the tort of battery; the person's personal integrity has been violated.

False imprisonment is restriction of a person's movements against the person's will, for any length of time and with no means of escape. The victim must be aware of the restraint applied. In health care settings, physical restraints of any kind may be interpreted as false imprisonment, as may hospitalization against the patient's wishes. Recent changes by the Joint Commission on the Accreditation of Healthcare Organizations (JCAHO) indicate that no type of restraint is permitted.

A nurse may act in a way that could be interpreted by a patient as *intent to inflict emotional distress.* For example, a nurse who takes away a patient's call bell may cause severe distress.

Conversion of property is the intent to interfere with the property of another by stealing, transferring, or disposing of it, without the person's consent. A family member may try to take the property of another by claiming to hold the power of attorney.

Defamation

Defamation may indicate *libel* (written) or *slander* (spoken), either of which can result in a decrease or loss of respect for the victim's reputation, veracity, or loyalty. Defamation requires the following:

- There must be a communication (publication) about the person to a third party.
- The communication must be harmful to the person's reputation.
- The result must be that others' regard for the person is decreased or that others avoid associating with the person.

Only a living person may be defamed. Defamation is a personal matter; stating that "All nurses are incompetent" is not actionable. To be acceptable in court as defamation, the communication (publication) needs to have been made with malice (the person stated it, knowing it to be false or totally disregarding its truth or falsity). A person whose reputation has been harmed can claim damages of considerable magnitude and variety.

Confidentiality

This tort protects the strict confidentiality of patients in sharing private information with health care providers. Health care professionals should not reveal any patient information among themselves or to others, except as it relates to therapeutic treatment of the patient. For example, a physician should not tell colleagues that a patient is homosexual if this personal disclosure has no connection to the patient's plan of care and if it may change providers' attitudes toward the patient.

In treating patients with mental health problems or those with chemical dependency, federal and state laws prohibit disclosure of such information to anyone, without the patient's consent.

Invasion of Privacy

This tort protects the individual's right to be free from unreasonable intrusions into private affairs; this is the right "to be left alone." For example, a nurse should not photograph a procedure being performed on a patient and then show it without first obtaining the patient's written consent. A more common error is for a nurse to inspect a patient's belongings without consent.

Sexual Harassment

Sexual harassment encompasses unwelcome sexual advances, requests for sexual favors, and other oral or physical conduct or written communication of an intimidating, hostile, or offensive nature or action taken in retaliation for reporting such behavior, regardless of where such conduct might occur. Sexual harassment involving patients or personnel is a problem in many facilities, as follows:

- It affects about 42% of women in all occupational settings.
- Men also report incidents of sexual harassment.
- Often the harassed person is too intimidated or too fearful of losing rights or care to mention the incident.
- Persons of all ages are harassed, including older women in nursing homes.
  Laws exist to protect sexually harassed persons.

Good Samaritan Law

The Good Samaritan Law is enacted by each state to protect and encourage health care professionals to provide care in emergency situations. This law provides immunity from civil liability when a person provides assistance in an emergency. The following conditions apply under this law:

- Care must be provided in good faith.
- Care must be gratuitous (no compensation).
- A higher standard of care may be required because of the caregiver's higher level of education and experience.
- The nurse is expected to provide care at the level of care provided by any nurse in similar circumstances.
- Statutes do not cover a person who is soliciting business or representing an agency.
- Statutes do not cover the care rendered in an emergency department situation.
- Care provided should not be willfully or wantonly negligent.

Litigation

Lawsuits against nurses most often involve the following:

- Medication errors
- Failure to monitor, report, and obtain needed medical assistance for a patient whose condition is changing
- Failure to challenge an inappropriate order

- Failure to report a lack of qualifications to provide nursing care for a particular group of patients, when asked to "float" to another unit
- Delegating nursing tasks to unlicensed health care workers

When delegating, the registered nurse (RN) must document the following:

- The task was properly assigned to an unlicensed health care worker who was competent to perform the work safely.
- Adequate supervision was provided to the worker.
- The RN provided appropriate follow-up and evaluation of the work.

The RN must know what tasks can be appropriately delegated to unlicensed personnel.

Nursing Students

- RNs who are faculty or preceptors for nursing students should not assign students to provide nursing that is beyond the students' present level of preparation.
- Students are held to the standard of an RN for the tasks they perform.
- Students must be instructed on the first day that they are expected (1) to communicate frequently with the faculty member or preceptor, (2) to ask questions freely, and (3) not to perform any task for which they are unqualified or have had too little experience.
- Clinical faculty or preceptors are supervising six to eight students or more and may not be immediately available to answer questions when they arise. The student should wait until the supervisor is free before acting.

Impaired Nurses

Impaired nurses are unable to function effectively because of substance abuse. This is a growing concern because of its impact on patient safety. Special programs within professional organizations can assist nurses to become free of drugs or alcohol and return to active practice.

Reimbursement

Third-party reimbursement for advanced practice nurses has created mixed reactions among health professionals because of increased competition for scarce health insurance dollars and "turf battles" about who is in charge of the patient's care. In some instances, other health care workers whose services can be reimbursed have been hired to do tasks that nurses can do equally well or better.

Quality Assurance and Peer Review

The mechanisms of quality assurance and peer review are used to evaluate and maintain a predetermined level of quality care. Often, physicians and nurses form a combined peer review group to evaluate performance and decide on changes in current practices to increase quality (efficiency, effectiveness) of care.

Rights Involving Death and Dying

- Physician-assisted suicide has just been disallowed by the U.S. Supreme Court, which stated that a difference exists between allowing a person to die by removing life supports and causing a person to die by active means.
- Many physicians and others who care for people during terminal illnesses favor making decisions strictly on an individual basis because of the wide variations among patients and their needs at this stage.
- No agreement exists on a definition of parameters that constitute death.
- Physicians and others have often disregarded patients' and families' wishes related to "do not resuscitate" (DNR) orders.

Advanced Directives: Living Will and Durable Power of Attorney

- These mechanisms provide for implementation of the Patient Self-Determination Act, passed by Congress in 1990, which requires hospitals to inform patients regarding advanced directives. In some states, all patients admitted to hospitals are required to complete the advanced directives form.
- The *living will* enables the person to provide explicit directions regarding what measures to use or not to use during a terminal illness, in relation to life-support equipment and procedures.
- The *durable power of attorney* (DPA) differs from the usual power of attorney in that the DPA does not become effective until patients cannot make decisions for themselves, thus enabling the DPA to act on behalf of patients, whose wishes are in writing and known. The DPA is especially important in

states where living wills are considered advisory and can be ignored.

Credentials

Credentials are the documented qualifications that an individual earns in attaining competency (at the minimal level) and proficiency (at advanced levels). Credentials can be diplomas, certificates, or awards that document the educational and experiential (clinical) preparation that the person has completed.

Licensure

Licensure is a process by which a governmental agency (i.e., state board of nursing) grants permission to an individual to practice nursing. The agency is responsible for the licensing and registration process, developed early in the 1900s as a way of protecting the public's welfare by ensuring that only nurses who had successfully completed a program in a recognized school of nursing could be licensed and registered to practice. Previously, anyone claiming to be qualified could practice nursing.

Licensure is a legal requirement for nurses to practice. Students need a diploma, associate degree, or baccalaureate degree to sit for the National Council Licensure Examination for Registered Nurses (NCLEX-RN).

Accreditation

Accreditation is a process by which a nongovernmental agency or organization approves and grants status to institutions or programs (not individuals) that meet predetermined standards or outcomes. Seeking accreditation is a voluntary process. Hospitals and other health care facilities are accredited by the JCAHO. Accreditation occurs both initially, when the hospital has just opened, and periodically, every 3 to 5 years.

Nursing programs have been accredited by the National League for Nursing (NLN) since 1949. The American Association of Colleges of Nursing (AACN) and the NLN have assumed collaborative responsibility for accreditation of all nursing education programs by establishing joint agreements regarding the standards and requirements to be met by institutions applying for initial or renewal accreditation. Currently, the NLN accreditation process requires that the school prepare a detailed self-study report according to written criteria, which is sent to the board of review. The board then assigns two or three NLN representatives, selected from faculty experienced and knowledgeable regarding the level of nursing education offered by the particular school. The NLN evaluators prepare a detailed report of their findings. The board votes (1) to accredit fully for 8 years, (2) to accredit with recommendations for a specified number of years and earlier than the usual reevaluation of the nursing program, or (3) to defer accrediting the program until specific deficits are fulfilled.

Nursing programs and schools voluntarily seek NLN accreditation to show that their program has been evaluated and meets established standards for educating and preparing students to become licensed as RNs.

Certification

Certification is a voluntary process by which a nongovernmental agency or association certifies that an individual licensed to practice a profession has met certain predetermined standards specified by that profession for specialty practice. The nursing license is recognized as indicating minimum competency; the certification credential indicates preparation beyond the minimum level, usually in a specific area of nursing, such as the following:

- The American Association of Nurse Anesthetists certifies nurses prepared to practice as certified nurse anesthetists (CNAs); certification is required for all nurse anesthetists to enable them to practice. In addition, certification must be renewed periodically to continue to practice. The required level of educational preparation is moving toward the master's degree.
- The American Nurses Credentialing Center (ANCC) certifies RNs in a variety of specialty areas. For all areas a bachelor-of-science-in-nursing (BSN) degree is required; for certification in advanced practice specialties (nurse practitioner, clinical nurse specialist) a master's degree is required.
- The American College of Nurse-Midwives (ACNM) certifies nurses prepared to practice as nurse-midwives. The ACNM does not require a master's degree for certification, but the educational preparation must have occurred within an ACNM-approved program.

ETHICAL ISSUES

Because of the complexity of the current health care field and the extensive interaction among technologic, economic, and moral areas, health professionals need to know about legal and ethical ramifications of practice. Ethics has once more become the foundation that enables the nurse to practice with full knowledge of the legal and ethical implications associated with health care delivery, now in the twenty-first century. A major factor in health care delivery has been the implementation of managed care in the 1990s, first in California and then in the other states.

Interpretation of ethical situations is grounded in ethical theories, moral principles, moral reasoning, and caring. These provide a base from which to consider ethics, ethical decisions, and responsible behavior in relation to the role of health professional. Decades of philosophic, theoretic, empirical, and clinical work on ethics in nursing are coalescing into a new model of ethics that may inform and transform nursing and health care. The structures of the relationships among ethics, law, and nursing practice are fluid and dynamic.

Moral Principles

Moral principles serve as a foundation for moral conduct and as reference points for ethical decision making in health care. Although opinions vary as to the number of moral principles, the following four are accepted as basic principles:

1. Respect for autonomy
2. Nonmaleficence
3. Beneficence
4. Justice

Other basic moral principles are fidelity (keeping promises, or the duty to be faithful to commitments), veracity (telling the truth), confidentiality, and privacy. These can be considered as subprinciples under the first four.

Moral reasoning is the interpretive process that helps to connect one's moral values with one's ethical choices. It is the analytic process whereby one examines the salient features in an ethical situation and makes a judgment or chooses a course of action that is congruent with one's moral beliefs and values. Moral values do not remain static; they change with maturity.

Respect for autonomy refers to individual freedom of choice or liberty, although it is not an "all-or-nothing" entity. Most experts agree that there are levels or gradations of autonomy. In health care, autonomy is the patient's right to self-determination without outside control.

Nonmaleficence states that one should do no harm. Determining what is harmful is one of the most difficult problems in clinical practice.

Beneficence entails the obligation to (1) prevent harm, (2) remove harm, and (3) do good. Some experts believe that the principle of beneficence incorporates the concept of nonmaleficence. The concepts that should be balanced under beneficence are risks, harms, benefits, and effectiveness. For nurses, beneficence is the duty to actively do good for patients. The determination of what is "good" for a particular patient must be defined by the patient, the patient's family, the health care team, clergy, and others who may be relevant to the decision (e.g., lawyer).

Justice refers to fairness and "receiving one's due." *Distributive justice* addresses the allocation and distribution of scarce benefits when there is competition for them. Justice is the duty to treat all patients fairly, without regard to age, socioeconomic status, or other variables.

Current thinking favors autonomy and nonmaleficence as preeminent for health care, since they emphasize respect for person and avoidance of harm. No universal agreement, however, exists. Ethical decisions can be based on *deontologic* precepts, which are derived from Judeo-Christian traditions ("all life is worthy of respect"); on *teleologic* theory ("that which causes a good outcome is a good action"); or on *situational ethics* ("decisions made in one situation cannot be generalized to another situation"; i.e., all decisions are separate and based on the particular situation, making decisions different for every case). The basic premises on which nurses must base behaviors are incorporated into the International Council of Nurses' Code for Nurses.

Many issues have inherent conflicts that produce divided opinions about what is right and what is wrong in particular cases. Issues surrounding abortion, for example, include the following questions:

- When does life begin?
- Does the fetus have rights?
- Is abortion ever morally justified?

Euthanasia also raises complex questions, as follows:

- Is euthanasia ever morally justified?
- Is providing futile care contradictory to the patient's rights?

Questions on reproductive issues depend on the specific circumstances and include the following:

- Is artificial insemination ethical?
- What are the rights of individuals involved in surrogate motherhood?
- Is it ethical to use fetal tissue in laboratory experimentation?
- Is in vitro fertilization appropriate and ethical?
- How should the information about genetic defects be used prenatally?

The controversial issue of physician-assisted suicide was struck down by the U.S. Supreme Court in June 1997.

No individual is capable of making or should make a final decision about any of these questions. Most large health care facilities, churches, private organizations, and academic groups study ethical issues. Consulting with biologic scientists, health care professionals, clergy, patients, and families, they try to arrive at a decision that is reasonable, just, inevitable, and satisfactory to all parties. External factors (e.g., scarce resources, rationing of health care, managed care restrictions) may play a larger role in these decisions in the future.

Ethical Theories

Three categories of theories related to ethics are virtue, consequentialist, and deontologic; all have historically provided the foundation for ethics in relation to nursing. Ethical theories help to answer the question, "What ultimately determines ethical behavior?"

- Is it *good outcome* (consequentialism)?
- Is it *good intent* (nonconsequentialism)?

Deontology is a *nonconsequentialist* theory of ethical inquiry. It views actions as right or wrong not because of their consequences or the good that is derived, but because of their characteristic of making things **right,** by means of the following:

- Fidelity to promises
- Truthfulness
- Justice

The theory of deontology stresses that an individual's actions must be guided by rules and motivated by the intention of doing one's **duty.** Consequences are irrelevant.

Consequentialism includes theories with the belief that **good** is defined by the consequences of an action. In *utilitarianism,* as espoused by John Stuart Mill (1806-1873), actions that result in the most good are most useful. The greatest good for the greatest number of people is the collective good, not that of the individual. The problem is, Who defines "good"?

Rules of conduct may develop from the following bases:
- Divine revelation
- Intuition/instinct
- Common sense
- Social contracts

Regardless of the base for behaviors, the individual must freely choose what is right or wrong in any given situation. The problem is, Who decides what rules to follow? This question often leads to conflicting opinions.

Contextual Reasoning

This way of considering ethical aspects focuses only on the presenting situation. Contextual reasoning is favored by many ethicists for the following reasons:
- It is built on the specific causes of ethical and moral conflict.
- It rejects adherence to absolute principles and a search for clear-cut answers.
- It is rooted in tradition (what has gone before), not on pure reason or moral intuition; this is similar to the use of precedents in law.
- *Casuists* reject the concept of universal principles as being too vague and too inflexible for the infinite variety of situations that can occur.

Contextualism

Contextualism holds that, while maintaining objectivity about the patient's situation, nurses perform appropriate ethical actions that depend on the following three factors:
- The relationship of the agreement that nursing roles create between nurse and patient, similar to the physician-patient relationship
- The specific aspects of the patient's situation
- The knowledge and abilities that the nurse brings to decisions and actions

With contextualism, more experience and knowledge regarding the nursing role create greater awareness of what the nurse is doing and why, as follows:
- The more a nurse takes her profession seriously, the more she enlarges or revises her ethical obligation as dictated by traditional ethical beliefs; her view is broadened and encompasses more than traditional ethical theories and beliefs have to offer.
- The nurse must know and appreciate ethical theory, even if it has little influence in guiding actions and decisions.

The nurse considers all aspects of the situation.
- The nurse's level of *awareness* in a particular situation helps determine how to act effectively for **this** patient in **this** situation.
- It is appropriate for nurses to have an emotional reaction to every clinical dilemma (i.e., "This situation is unique and important and requires all my knowledge and expertise to guide my decisions and actions").

Ethics Committees

Ethics committees provide the following services:
- Review or write institutional policies based on ethical considerations.
- Deliberate about complex cases and, when appropriate, make recommendations to the proper parties.
- Educate staff and community.

Members of ethics committees usually include the following:
- Physician(s)
- Nurse(s)
- Administrator(s)
- Clergy
- Members of community (not health professionals)

Ethics and Health Care

Domains
- Business ethics
- Medical ethics
- Educational ethics
- Writing/publishing ethics

Levels of Ethical Action and Decision Making
- Micro (individual)
- Meso (institutional)
- Macro (government/societal)
- Mega (global)

Managed Care

Managed care usually involves institutional ethics (e.g., health maintenance organization, HMO), business/financial ethics, and biomedical ethics. Physicians and nurses have a primary obligation to the patient and a secondary obligation to the institution and society not to waste scarce resources.

A typical question is, What antibiotic should be prescribed? For example, antibiotic A costs $2, and antibiotic B costs $50 but is not on the HMO's list of approved drugs. Which one is better if both seem similar?

Managed care has resulted in legal changes in the physician-patient relationship, which was initially built on a contractual basis. Because of particular court decisions (e.g., what medical procedures can be used in specific cases), the courts are moving toward making managed care a consumer buyer-seller (fiduciary) relationship. This is based on the courts of equity, which require that all parties act in good conscience, even to the point of not asserting their legal rights. In some cases the courts ask that patients put their utmost trust and confidence in physicians when patients are often in the most vulnerable situation (i.e., no one fully understands the situation, and it is difficult to make decisions).

The doctrine of *informed consent* has been expanded under managed care. This area is highly controversial because it involves deciding what information to disclose to a patient when no treatment is or will be made available (e.g., transplants, new treatments). Do patients need to be told that they are not receiving state-of-the-art treatment? The dilemma is the need to inform all patients to the same degree in all similar circumstances.

Common Ethical Situations

Adequate Assessment and Testing

The patient, a known alcoholic, comes to the clinic because of "chest pain on the side." The nurse practitioner (NP), a recent graduate of an adult NP program, examines the patient, listens to breath sounds, and uses percussion to determine lung expansion on inspiration. The NP sees that the patient had a chest x-ray film on the previous visit 3 months earlier, which was normal. Further questioning indicates that the patient had a fall the previous week, when the pain apparently began. The NP notes that the patient has a slight cough. The history and physical examination do not indicate a particular disease or infection. The NP writes a prescription for an analgesic and instructs the patient to return if the pain persists.

The patient returns 3 weeks later with the same symptoms. A chest film shows a moderate pleural effusion at the base of the right lung. How could the nurse's assessment have been improved on the previous visit?

This is a typical case of not always knowing how many tests to order. Despite a negative (normal) chest film 3 months earlier, it would have been useful to order a repeat radiograph to rule out causes of chest pain, such as a fractured rib or, in this case, a developing pleural effusion that signaled tuberculosis (TB).

Accurate diagnosis was delayed, and the patient was admitted to the hospital for treatment of both the pleural effusion (aspiration) and the TB (medications). He was hospitalized for 3 months. On discharge his condition was good; he had not been drinking while hospitalized, and he received excellent care and three or four meals a day.

The NP omitted an important part of assessment and diagnostic testing at her initial assessment, when the patient complained of chest pain. Accurate diagnosis and therapy were delayed unnecessarily. Information provided by the patient indicated that the chest pain related to a fall, which skewed the NP's judgment about the probable cause of symptoms.

This new NP learned a valuable lesson early in practice: assess thoroughly and use critical thinking and appropriate judgment in diagnosing and treating patients.

Patients' Right to Information

A patient wants to know his blood pressure reading, and the NP responds, "It's fine." The patient wants the specific numbers, however, and when the NP leaves momentarily, he obtains the information from his chart, which had been left on the table. The NP returns, sees the patient examining his chart, and tells him to stop. The NP does provide his blood pressure measurement, however, and the patient is satisfied.

The NP recognized the error in not responding immediately to the patient's request to know his blood pressure. Patients have a legal and ethical right to know information about themselves, and health care professionals have the responsibility of providing this information when asked. Other critical information, such as telling the patient that he has not responded to treatment for cancer and that surgery is the next alternative, should be provided by the physician, who will also explain more about the surgical procedure. In hospital and other settings, NPs must know the limits of their responsibilities and must distinguish between information they can divulge to the patient and information the physician should divulge.

BIBLIOGRAPHY

Bayer R: Health policy and ethics forum: whither occupational health and safety? *Am J Public Health* 90(4):532, 2000.

Birkholz G: Malpractice data from the national Practitioner Data Bank, *Nurse Pract* 20(3):32-35, 1995.

Brent NJ: *Nurses and the law,* Philadelphia, 1997, Saunders.

Edgar H: Homicide prosecutions and progress toward workplace safety, *Am J Public Health* 90(4):533-534, 2000.

Gonzalez RI, Gooden MB, Porter CP: Eliminating racial and ethnic disparities in health care, *Am J Nurs* 100(3):56-58, 2000.

Hall JK: *Nursing ethics and law,* Philadelphia, 1996, Saunders.

Medicare and Medicaid programs; hospital conditions of participation: patients' rights, *Federal Register* 64:36069-36089; *Clinician Rev* 9(9):118, 121, 1999.

Peters S: Too much information? Washington debates medical errors reporting, *Am J Nurse Pract* 4(3):30, 2000.

Starr DS: Tips for everyday clinical practice: handling patient complaints, *Clin Advisor* 80, September 1999.

REVIEW QUESTIONS

1. Which statement best defines ethics?
   a. Set of beliefs about the profession of nursing
   b. Moral philosophy that guides professional practice
   c. Decisions made in the best interest of all persons
   d. Individual's perspective on issues that affect nursing

2. Priority ranking of a person's values is called:
   a. Veracity review
   b. Personal value system
   c. Values accounting
   d. Behavioral guides

3. A nurse faced with incompetent practice in a colleague is probably basing thinking on the ethical principles of:
   a. Fidelity
   b. Veracity
   c. Beneficence
   d. Justice

4. When asked by a patient's wife regarding a diagnosis of AIDS, the nurse is guided by the ethical principle of:
   a. Veracity
   b. Justice
   c. Autonomy
   d. Beneficence

5. Which precept states that it is best to provide the greatest good for the greatest number?
   a. Deontology
   b. Veracity
   c. Fidelity
   d. Utilitarianism

6. Which ethical dilemma involving the use of technology has captured the public's interest?
   a. Societal mandate to reduce costs of health care
   b. Increased life expectancy
   c. Widespread computerization of medical records
   d. Maintaining unresponsive patients on life-support systems

7. When nurses' personal values are in conflict with professional values, nurses must make decisions that lead to all the following results **except:**
   a. Arriving at the optimum outcome for the patient
   b. Demonstrating accountability for care provided
   c. Providing care within the individual's level of knowledge
   d. Having primary concern for their own well-being

8. Decisions regarding which patients will receive a donor organ involve the ethical principles of:
   a. Beneficence
   b. Veracity
   c. Justice
   d. Autonomy

9. Which factor has the most impact regarding the ethical dilemma, "Is health care a right or a privilege"?
   a. High-tech versus high-touch care
   b. Computerization of medical records
   c. Escalating health care costs
   d. Hiring of unlicensed persons to provide nursing care

10. The use of advance directives relates to which ethical principle?
    a. Justice
    b. Autonomy
    c. Beneficence
    d. Veracity
11. Which description best defines malpractice?
    a. Principles based on society's moral code
    b. Members of society deciding what "ought" to be done
    c. Negligence in providing professional services by licensed persons
    d. Legal term that concerns a person who fails to do what a reasonably prudent person with the same skill and level of knowledge would do in the same or similar circumstances
12. State boards of nursing have the authority to:
    a. License nurses and stipulate practice guidelines for advanced practice nurses (e.g., nurse practitioners, nurse-midwives, clinical nurse specialists)
    b. Enact statutes
    c. Set payment mechanisms for nurses
    d. Send nurses to jail
13. Which elements are required to prove malpractice?
    a. Duty of care, breach of duty, injury, proximate cause
    b. Patient self-determination, prudent behavior, inaccurate assessment, legal authority
    c. Standards, consent, battery, disciplinary action
    d. Standards, delegation, failing to carry out a medical order, injury
14. A nurse reports a medication error in which a patient was given a wrong medication but had no ill effects. What necessary element is lacking to prove malpractice?
    a. Breach of duty
    b. Duty of care
    c. Injury
    d. Standard of care
15. A patient has a central venous line, and the dressing needs to be changed using sterile technique. The registered nurse in charge delegates the responsibility of changing the dressing to an unlicensed assistive person. The unlicensed assistive person does not know sterile technique and contaminates the area, and the patient develops an infection. Which of the following statements is **true**?
    a. The unlicensed assistive person is guilty of malpractice.
    b. The hospital is not responsible for the actions of its employees.
    c. No great harm came to the patient, so a malpractice suit cannot be brought.
    d. The nurse is responsible for the outcomes of all tasks delegated.
16. Civil law is concerned with:
    a. Protection of individual rights
    b. Decision making based on the nursing process
    c. Negligence and malpractice torts
    d. Guilt related to criminal behavior
17. Which strategy can a nurse use to prevent being named in malpractice suits?
    a. Request supervision for all care provided
    b. Refuse to sign name in patients' records
    c. Maintain good relationships with patients and families
    d. Have malpractice insurance
18. Criminal law applies to acts that:
    a. Violate civil law
    b. Threaten society
    c. Are known as torts
    d. Protect the consumer
19. Licensure is defined as:
    a. A legal permit to protect the public from unsafe and incompetent health care practitioners
    b. Having responsibility for one's own actions
    c. A voluntary process of evaluation and credentialing showing that preset standards and criteria have been met
    d. A type of voluntary credentialing that recognizes an individual's knowledge and skills in a particular area of practice
20. Which term is used when a patient agrees to have a procedure done, after the physician explains the procedure's risks and benefits?
    a. Standard of care
    b. Informed consent
    c. Statute
    d. Response

4

Respiratory Disorders

DIAGNOSTIC TESTS

Arterial blood gases (ABGs) are measured to assess the adequacy of ventilation and oxygenation and the acid-base status. Oxygen saturation of hemoglobin is normally 95% or higher. The partial pressure of arterial oxygen (Pao$_2$), normally 80 to 100 mm Hg, is increased in patients with hyperventilation and decreased in patients with cardiac decompensation, chronic obstructive pulmonary disease (COPD), and particular neuromuscular disorders. Partial pressure of carbon dioxide (Paco$_2$), normally 38 to 45 mm Hg, may be higher in patients with emphysema, obstructive lung disease, and reduced function of the respiratory center and lower in those who are pregnant and in the presence of pulmonary emboli and anxiety. Normal pH of arterial blood is 7.40, ranging between 7.35 and 7.45. Box 4-1 lists abbreviations and definitions used in pulmonary function.

Bronchoscopy allows visualization of the trachea, bronchi, and some bronchioles for diagnosis of tumors, trauma, and hemorrhage; to obtain brushings for cytologic examination; and to remove foreign bodies from the bronchi.

Chest x-ray examination is used to diagnose pneumonia, pneumothorax, tuberculosis, rib fractures, and degenerative changes in the spine or shoulder girdles.

A *computed tomography (CT) scan* shows discrete cross-sectional structural layers and aids in diagnosis of lung and pancreatic tumors, emboli, and aortic calcification or dissection.

Magnetic resonance imaging (MRI) shows cross-sectional layers of anatomic structures by means of magnetic energy exposure, revealing tumors, vascular abnormalities, and infections.

Pulmonary angiography (arteriography) is the gold standard to diagnose pulmonary emboli as small as 3 mm in diameter.

Pulmonary function tests (PFTs) determine the capacity of the lungs to exchange oxygen and carbon dioxide efficiently. One kind of respiratory function test measures ventilation (the ability of the bellows action of the chest and lungs to move gas in and out of alveoli). Another kind of PFT measures the diffusion of gas across the alveolar capillary membrane and the perfusion of the lungs by blood. Efficient gas exchange in the lungs requires a balanced ventilation-perfusion ratio (V/P), so that areas receiving ventilation are well perfused and areas receiving blood flow are capable of ventilation.

Spirometry evaluates the air capacity of the lungs by means of a spirometer, which measures and records the volume of inhaled and exhaled air; this information is needed to assess pulmonary function (Table 4-1).

A *V/P scan* shows movement or the lack of movement of air in the lungs and the blood supply to specific lung areas. A normal V/P scan shows even distribution of radiotracer throughout both lungs, ruling out significant pulmonary emboli and the need for additional diagnostic tests. A high probability scan shows multiple segment or larger defects with normal ventilation in at least one area of abnormal perfusion (V/P mismatch). If neither of the aforementioned results is noted, the V/P scan is considered nondiagnostic and further studies are required (Tables 4-2 and 4-3).

BOX 4-1
Abbreviations Used in Pulmonary Function

A-aDO$_2$	Alveolar-arterial PO$_2$ difference (gradient)	PAO$_2$	Partial pressure of alveolar O$_2$
DLCO	Diffusing capacity for carbon monoxide (mL/min/mm Hg)	PaCO$_2$	Partial pressure of arterial CO$_2$
		PaO$_2$	Partial pressure of arterial O$_2$
ERV	Expiratory reserve volume	PB	Barometric pressure
FEF$_{25\%-75\%}$	Mean forced expiratory flow during the middle of FVC	PCO$_2$	Partial pressure of CO$_2$
		PETCO$_2$	Partial pressure of end tidal CO$_2$
FEV$_1$(L)	Forced expiratory volume in 1 sec, in liters	PIO$_2$	Partial pressure of inspired O$_2$
FEV$_1$, 96FVC	Forced expiratory volume in 1 sec as percentage of FC	PO$_2$	Partial pressure of O$_2$
		PV	Partial pressure of mixed venous (pulmonary arterial) blood
FIO$_2$	Percentage of inspired O$_2$		
FRC	Functional residual capacity	PVO$_2$	Partial pressure of mixed venous O$_2$
FVC	Forced vital capacity	PVCO$_2$	Partial pressure of mixed venous CO$_2$
[H$^+$]	Hydrogen ion concentration (nanomole/L)	Q	Perfusion (L/min)
IC	Inspiratory capacity	Raw	Airway resistance
IRV	Inspiratory reserve volume	RV	Residual volume
MEF 50% FVC	Mid-expiratory flow at 50% of FVC	TLC	Total lung capacity
		V	Ventilation (L/min)
MEP	Maximal expiratory pressure (cm H$_2$O)	VA	Alveolar ventilation (L/min)
MIF 50% FVC	Mid-inspiratory flow at 50% of FVC	VC	Vital capacity
		VCO$_2$	CO$_2$ production (L/min)
MIP	Maximal inspiratory pressure (cm H$_2$O)	VD	Dead space volume
MVV	Maximal voluntary ventilation	VO$_2$	O$_2$ consumption (L/min)
PAaCO$_2$	Partial pressure of alveolar CO$_2$	VT	Tidal volume

TABLE 4-1
Spirometric Measurements

Measurement	Definition	Utility
Forced vital capacity (FVC)	Total volume of air that can be forcefully exhaled from the lungs after maximal inspiration	Good indicator of patient effort
Forced expiratory volume in one second (FEV$_1$)	Volume of air expelled in the first second of the FVC test	Measures both large and small airway function
Forced expiratory flow rate from 25% to 75% of the FVC (FEF$_{25\%-75\%}$)	Maximal mid-expiratory rate	Measures small airway function
Peak expiratory flow rate (PEFR)	Maximal flow rate (liters) achieved in the FVC test	Correlates well with the FEV$_1$
FEV$_1$/FVC Ratio	FEV$_1$ divided by FVC	80% is considered normal

TABLE 4-2
Lung Volumes

Lung Volume	Definition
Total lung capacity (TLC)	Volume of air in the lungs after a maximal inspiration
Functional residual capacity (FRC)	Volume of air in the lungs at the end of expiration
Residual volume (RV)	Volume of air remaining in the lungs after maximal expiration

TABLE 4-3
Obstructive and Restrictive Lung Diseases

Type of Disease	Definition
Obstructive	Characterized by obstruction to airflow: COPD, asthma, chronic bronchitis
Restrictive	Characterized by decreased lung volumes, but without airflow obstruction: Interstitial lung disease, expiratory muscle weakness, stiff (noncompliant) chest wall, spinal deformity

OBSTRUCTIVE PULMONARY DISORDERS

Obstructive pulmonary disorders are characterized by increased resistance to airflow resulting from airway obstruction or narrowing.

Chronic Obstructive Pulmonary Disease or Emphysema

Definition
- COPD is characterized by chronic bronchitis or emphysema and airflow obstruction that is generally progressive, may be accompanied by airway hyperreactivity, and may be partially reversible.
- Emphysema is classified according to the portion of the acinus (respiratory tissue distal to a single terminal bronchiole) affected by mild disease.
  —Panacinar emphysema (PAE) affects all of the acini.
  —Centrilobular emphysema (CLE) begins in the respiratory bronchiole and spreads

peripherally; it is the most common form of emphysema in smokers and affects upper and posterior portions of the lungs more severely than the bases.
- COPD (emphysema, bronchitis) and asthma are physiologically different, and each has a specific biophysiologic makeup, but there is some similarity in symptoms.

Risk Factors
- Cigarette smoking (the most common single causative factor, which also interacts with every other risk factor)
- Inhalation of environmental lung irritants; chronic exposure to inorganic and organic dusts and toxic gases
- Occupational exposure to grains; chemicals, such as toluene diisocyanate; or dust (e.g., cotton mills)
- Secondhand smoke exposure
- Familial alpha$_1$-antitrypsin deficiency
- Poor socioeconomic status (inverse relationship between income and smoking behavior)
- Intravenous drug use
- Talcosis (i.e., exposure to talcum powder dust)

Etiology
- One or more of the risk factors, or others elicited by patient's history

Incidence
- About 14 million people in the United States are affected, and about 90,000 deaths each year are attributed to COPD and asthma combined.

Pathogenesis
- Gross changes from chronic bronchitis include erythematous, edematous mucosa with copious mucous airway secretions and possibly pus.
- Histologic changes not specific to COPD occur in the airways of longtime cigarette smokers.
  —The submucosal glands are enlarged, and their ducts dilated.
  —Focally, areas of squamous metaplasia replace pseudostratified columnar epithelium.

—Neutrophils and lymphocytes infiltrate the mucous membranes but are sparse.

—Airway smooth muscle may be hypertrophied.

—The terminal and respiratory bronchioles have varying degrees of secretory obstruction, goblet cell metaplasia, inflammation with a predominance of macrophages, increased smooth muscle, and distortion due to fibrosis and loss of alveolar attachments.

—At autopsy, emphysematous lungs are grossly overdistended and do not collapse when the thorax is opened. Bullae may be present on the lung surfaces. Respiratory airspaces do not appear enlarged or destroyed on the cut surface of freshly sectioned lungs, which must be fixed in inflation to make these signal changes evident.

- Mild bronchiolitis, the earliest lesion described in smokers, does not obstruct airflow until the lesion increases in severity and is accompanied by terminal bronchiolitis.
- Emphysema becomes evident about the same time as terminal bronchiolitis; both steadily increase in severity as COPD progresses.
- In patients with emphysema, elastin fibers in the lung parenchyma are ruptured and frayed.
- In the elastase-antielastase hypothesis, emphysema results when elastic fibers are digested by unopposed neutrophil elastase, which is normally opposed by alpha$_1$-antitrypsin. Premature onset of emphysema is common among patients with homozygous alpha$_1$-antitrypsin deficiency.
- The number of neutrophils that can be lavaged from the lungs is about five times higher in smokers than in nonsmokers, although the proportion of neutrophils is similar (1% to 3%).

Diagnosis

Signs and Symptoms (Table 4-4)
- History of cigarette smoking
- Cough, pronounced in the morning on arising
- Shortness of breath and wheezing
- Sputum production
- Dyspnea (a classic symptom), leading to inability to perform activities of daily living (ADL)

- Easy fatigability
- Weakness
- Frequent or recurrent respiratory infections
- Cachectic appearance: with pink skin color (adequate oxygenation)
- In severe cases, hemoptysis, persistent chest pain, and blue-purple complexion, indicating chronic hypoxemia
- Edematous lower extremities from right-sided heart failure (cor pulmonale)
- Skeletal deformity: kyphoscoliosis and "barrel chest"
- Use of accessory muscles of neck and pursed-lip breathing
- Breath sounds are decreased and diminished throughout the lungs
- History and physical examination
  —Diagnosis is made by history and confirmed by physical findings.
  —Physical examination should focus on the respiratory and cardiovascular systems, with particular attention given to the abdomen.
- Chest x-ray examination shows overexpansion of lungs, an enlarged heart, decreased peripheral markings, a flattened diaphragm, and apical bullae.
- PFTs (Table 4-5)
  —Lung volumes and spirometry to demonstrate respiratory function.
- Simple spirometry:
  —Forced vital capacity (FVC) and forced expiratory volume in 1 second (FEV_1) are decreased.
  —FEV_1/FVC ratio less than 65% indicates COPD.
- Lung volumes
  —Increased residual volume (RV), functional residual capacity (FRC), and total lung capacity (TLC) are common as a result of loss of elastic recoil of the lungs.
  —Vital capacity is frequently decreased but may be near normal.
  —Electrocardiography (ECG) assesses concomitant cor pulmonale.
  —ABGs are as follows: PO_2 low 70s; PCO_2 low to normal.
  —Oxygen saturation is adequate.
  —Polycythemia and eosinophilia, as evidenced by a complete blood cell count (CBC), could indicate acute infection.

TABLE 4-4
Signs and Symptoms in Advanced COPD

Diagnosis/Therapy	Emphysema Predominant	Bronchitis Predominant
History, physical	Major complaint: dyspnea, Major complaint: chronic cough, often severe. Age: >50. Cough: rare, with scant, clear, mucoid sputum. Recent weight loss, thin, appear ill, use accessory muscles to breathe. Normal breath sounds. No ankle edema.	Major complaint: chronic cough, with mucopurulent sputum, frequent chest infections. Age: late 30s-40s. Often overweight, cyanotic, but breathe easily at rest. Chest is noisy, crackles and wheezes usually present. Most have ankle edema.
Laboratory studies	Hgb usually normal (12-15 g/dl); PaO_2 normal or slightly reduced (65-75 mm Hg); SaO_2 normal or mildly reduced (35-40 mm Hg). Chest x-ray: hyperinflation with flattened diaphragms; vascular markings are diminished, mostly at apices.	Hgb usually increased (15-18 g/dl); PaO_2 reduced (45-60 mm Hg); $PaCO_2$ mildly to markedly elevated (50-60 mm Hg). Chest x-ray: increased interstitial markings ("dirty lungs"), mostly at bases; diaphragms not flattened.
Pulmonary function tests	Airflow obstruction throughout. Total lung capacity increased, often greatly. DL_{CO} reduced. Static lung compliance increased.	Airflow obstruction throughout. Total lung capacity usually normal, may be mildly increased. DL_{CO} normal. Static lung compliance normal.
SPECIAL EVALUATIONS		
V/Q matching	Increased ventilation to high V/Q areas, i.e., high dead space.	Increased perfusion to low V/Q areas
Hemodynamics	Cardiac output normal to slightly low. Pulmonary artery pressures mildly elevated and increase with exercise.	Cardiac output normal. Pulmonary artery pressures elevated, often greatly, and worsen with exercise.
Nocturnal ventilation	Mild-to-moderate degree of oxyhemoglobin desaturation, not usually associated with obstructive sleep apnea.	Severe oxyhemoglobin desaturation, often associated with obstructive sleep apnea.
Exercise ventilation	Increased minute ventilation for level of oxygen consumption. PaO_2 tends to fall; $PaCO_2$ falls slightly.	Decreased minute ventilation for level of oxygen consumption. PaO_2 may rise; $PaCO_2$ may rise significantly.

TABLE 4-5
Selected Pulmonary Function Tests

Test	Definition
TESTS DERIVED FROM SPIROMETRY	
Forced vital capacity (FVC)	The volume of gas that can be forcefully expelled after maximal inspiration
Forced expiratory volume in 1 sec (FEV_1)	The volume of gas expelled in the first second of the FVC maneuver
Forced expiratory flow from 25% to 75% of the forced vital capacity ($FEF_{25\%-75\%}$)	The maximal midexpiratory airflow capacity rate
Peak expiratory flow rate (PEFR)	The maximal airflow rate achieved in the FVC maneuver
Maximum voluntary ventilation (MVV)	The maximum volume of gas that can be breathed in 1 min (usually measured for 15 seconds, multiplied by 4)
LUNG VOLUMES	
Slow vital capacity (SVC)	The volume of gas that can be slowly exhaled after maximal inspiration
Total lung capacity (TLC)	The volume of gas in the lungs after a maximal inspiration
Functional residual capacity (FRC)	The volume of gas remaining in the lungs at the end of a normal tidal expiration
Residual volume (RV)	The volume of gas remaining in the lungs after maximal expiration
Expiratory reserve volume (ERV)	The volume of gas representing the difference between functional residual capacity and residual volume

From Chesnutt MS, Prendergast TJ: Lung. In Tierney LM, McPhee SJ, Papadakis MA, eds: *Current medical diagnosis & treatment 2000,* New York, 2000, Lange Medical Books/McGraw-Hill, p 269.

—Sputum examination detects chronic colonization of *Streptococcus pneumoniae* or *Haemophilus influenzae.*

—Sputum culture is necessary only when pneumonia is suspected.

Differential Diagnosis
- Bronchial asthma
- Bronchiectasis (recurrent pneumonia, hemoptysis, digital clubbing, and abnormal x-ray examination findings)
- Cystic fibrosis
- Bronchopulmonary mycosis
- Central airway obstruction

Complications
- Acute bronchitis
- Pneumonia
- Pulmonary embolization
- Left ventricular failure (may worsen otherwise stable COPD)
- Pulmonary hypertension
- Cor pulmonale
- Chronic respiratory failure
- Spontaneous pneumothorax (in a small number of those with emphysema)
- Hemoptysis (may result from chronic bronchitis or may indicate bronchogenic carcinoma)

Prevention
- Eliminate chronic exposure to tobacco smoke.
- Smoking cessation: slows the decline in FEV_1 in those who are age 40 to 60, with mild airway obstruction.
- Vaccination against pneumococcal and influenza infections is beneficial but does not alter the course of COPD.

Treatment
- Management of COPD in the ambulatory setting includes specific, symptomatic, and secondary therapy.
- Treatment depends on severity
  —Stage I: FEV_1 ≥50%
  —Stage II: FEV_1 35% to 49%
  —Stage III: FEV_1 <35%

Specific Therapy
- Suggest avoidance of environmental irritants.

- Give an influenza vaccine annually (risk of serious complications from influenza is greater in these patients).
- Give an initial pneumococcal vaccine, and repeat after 6 years.
- Recommend smoking cessation. After smokers stop smoking, the FEV_1 increases slightly for a few years, then follows a path similar to that of nonsmokers. Cough and sputum expectoration diminish over a few months; sputum may be more viscid. However, lost lung function is not regained. Cessation delays the onset of exertional dyspnea and decreases the risk of dying of COPD.
- Give supplemental oxygen for patients with resting hypoxemia.
  —This is the only therapy documented as altering the natural history of COPD.

Symptomatic Therapy
Anticholinergic drugs
- Ipratropium bromide is superior to sympathomimetic aerosols in achieving bronchodilation in patients with moderate to severe COPD.
  —It has a slower onset but a longer duration of action than sympathomimetic agents in those with stable COPD.
  —Combined with other bronchodilators, it enhances and prolongs bronchodilation.
  —Side effects are minimal.
  —Benefits are lost when drug is discontinued.
  —The usual dosage is 2 to 4 inhalations (18 micrograms each) q6h.
  —It may also be given in a nebulizer (solution of 0.02%).
- Beta$_2$-agonists are given via a metered-dose inhaler. Patients with the greatest bronchodilator responses have the lowest annual decline in FEV_1 and the highest 5-year survival rate. Inhalation results in more rapid onset of action and greater bronchodilation with fewer side effects (e.g., skeletal muscle tremor).
  —Metaproterenol
  —Albuterol
  —Terbutaline
  —Pirbuterol
- The preferred administration mode is the metered-dose inhaler.
  —Patients should be taught to inhale the aerosol slowly, starting at the resting end-

expiratory position, with a brief breath-hold at the end of a full inhalation.

—Patients with poor coordination should inhale the aerosol after it is delivered into a small chamber (spacer).

Theophylline
- Theophylline is a third-line agent, after ipratropium and sympathomimetic agents.
- It is used in patients who do not respond to inhaled bronchodilators or in those with sleep-related disturbances.
- Theophylline improves muscle performance by decreasing smooth muscle spasm.
- It improves dyspnea, exercise performance, and pulmonary function.
- Sustained-release theophylline improves oxyhemoglobin saturation during sleep.

Corticosteroids
- Corticosteroids do not benefit most patients with chronic stable COPD.
- Those on oral corticosteroids had a 20% increase in FEV_1, but this was only 10% better than those who received a placebo.
- A trial of oral corticosteroids (e.g., prednisone 0.5 mg/kg for 2 to 4 weeks) can be given to evaluate effects by means of spirometry.

Antibiotics
- Antibiotics may be necessary to treat infections.
  —Trimethoprim-sulfamethoxazole (TMP-SMX) 160 mg/800 mg twice a day
  —Amoxicillin or amoxicillin-clavulanate 500 mg q8h
  —Tetracycline 250 mg qid

Therapy for Thinning and Mobilization of Secretions
- Patients should maintain good hydration.
- Steam inhalation, especially in early morning
- Postural drainage
- Controlled coughing—2 to 3 successive coughs after deep inhalation

Secondary Therapy
- Improving the health of the whole person is the goal.
- Institute oxygen therapy.
  —A 24-hour regimen is better than a 12-hour nocturnal regimen.
  —Long-term oxygen therapy should be given to those patients who meet certain criteria with regard to PaO_2 and arterial saturation.

—Encourage the patient to exercise to capacity.
- Proper nutrition is necessary to avert weight loss.
- Optimal hydration must be maintained.
- Lung transplantation may be necessary.
- Lung volume reduction surgery is a new, experimental procedure that relieves dyspnea and improves exercise tolerance in those with advanced diffuse emphysema and lung hyperinflation.
- Pulmonary rehabilitation programs should be begun.
- Alpha$_1$-antitrypsin deficiency must be treated.

Prognosis
- Prognosis for patients with clinically significant COPD is poor.
- The median survival time is about 4 years.
- The most important predictive factor is the degree of pulmonary dysfunction as measured by FEV_1 at the time the patient is first examined.

Patient/Family Education
- Patients and family members should be strongly encouraged to stop smoking.
  —Simply telling people to quit has a 5% success rate.
  —In a group of smokers given behavior modification instruction and nicotine gum, a 22% sustained abstinence at 5 years was reported.
  —The nicotine transdermal patch increases cessation rates in motivated smokers.
  —Early reports regarding those who use bupropion are promising.
- Instruct in effective controlled coughing and postural drainage techniques.
- Emphasize the importance of avoiding others who may have an upper respiratory tract infection (URI).
- Instruct patient regarding medications, including the reasons for prescribing, action, side effects, dosage, and times for administration.
- Explain the nature of the condition, its cause or causes, and its effects on the body; emphasize that therapy is effective in alleviating symptoms.
- Provide information about resources available locally and nationally.

- List symptoms or changes in breathing that should be reported to the health care provider without delay.
- Instruct the patient regarding the use, care, and cleaning of oxygen equipment.
- Emphasize that no damaged electrical wires or smokers should be allowed near oxygen because of the danger of explosion and fire.

Follow-up/Referral

- Patients with COPD are followed closely initially, while diagnostic testing and drug therapy evaluation continue.
- In those with severe COPD, weekly visits by a nurse are needed to maintain close monitoring of oxygen use, symptoms, and sleep problems.

Asthma

Table 4-6 provides a severity classification of asthma.

- Asthma is a chronic inflammatory disorder of the airways characterized by the following:
  —Airway inflammation
  —Airway hyperreactivity to a wide variety of stimuli
  —Airway obstruction (increased resistance) that is usually reversible in response to treatment or spontaneously
- Asthma is regarded as a subacute inflammatory disorder of the airways.

Epidemiology

- Data show that there has been a linear increase in asthma worldwide.
- Asthma affects more than 12 million people in the United States (5% of the population).
- Between 1982 and 1992, prevalence increased from 34.7 to 49.4 per 1000 persons.
- In this same 10-year period, the death rate increased 40%, from 13.4 to 18.8 per million, and the death rate was five times higher for blacks than for whites.
- Asthma is the leading cause of hospitalization among children and the leading cause for school absenteeism.
- In the United States, about 5000 deaths per year are attributed to asthma.

Risk Factors

- Not all risk factors for asthma are known.
- Genetic factors play a role. The strongest predisposing factor identified for the development of asthma is atopy, an inherited tendency to experience immediate allergic reactions (e.g., asthma, atopic dermatitis, vasomotor rhinitis) because of the presence of an antibody (atopic reagin) in the skin or bloodstream.
- Exposure to environmental pollutants increases risk for asthma.
- Blacks are at higher risk.

TABLE 4-6
Classification of Asthma Severity

Classification	Symptoms	Nighttime Sxs	Lung Function
Mild intermittent	Symptoms ≤2 times/week. Asymptomatic and normal PEF between exacerbations. Exacerbations brief (few hours to few days); intensity may vary.	≤2 times/month	FEV_1 or PEF ≥80% predicted; PEF variability <20%
Mild persistent	Symptoms ≥2 times/week but <1 time/day. Exacerbations may affect activity.	>2 times/month	FEV_1 or PEF >80% predicted; PEF variability >30%
Moderate persistent	Daily symptoms. Daily use of inhaled short-acting β₂-agonist. Exacerbations affect activity. Exacerbations ≥2 times/week, may last days.	>1 time/week	FEV_1 or PEF >60% to <80% predicted; PEF variability >30%
Severe persistent	Continual symptoms. Limited physical activity. Frequent exacerbations.	Frequent	FEV_1 or PEF ≤60% predicted; PEF variability >30%

From National Asthma Education and Prevention Program: Expert Panel Report 2: Guidelines for the Diagnosis and Management of Asthma. National Institutes of Health Pub No 97-4051, Bethesda, MD, 1997.

- Susceptibility to stimuli that cause asthma attacks places an individual at higher risk.
- Persons in lower socioeconomic levels are at higher risk.
- Poor nutrition places an individual at higher risk.

Etiology (See Previous Discussion of Risk Factors)

- Exposure to inhaled allergens (e.g., house dust mites, cockroaches, cats, seasonal pollens)
- Exercise
- Upper respiratory infection
- Rhinitis
- Sinusitis
- Postnasal drip
- Aspiration
- Gastroesophageal reflux
- Weather changes
- Stress
- Exposure to environmental tobacco smoke
- Particular drugs (e.g., aspirin; nonsteroidal, antiinflammatory drugs)
- Exposure to occupational allergens
- Uncompensated congestive heart failure (precipitates bronchospasm known as *cardiac asthma*)

Pathogenesis

- Denudation of airway epithelium
- Airway edema
- Collagen deposition beneath the basement membrane
- Inflammatory cell infiltration with neutrophils, eosinophils, and lymphocytes, especially T lymphocytes
- Hypertrophy of bronchial smooth muscle and mucous glands (may result in plugging of small airways with thick mucus)
- Inflammation of the airways contributes to airway hyperresponsiveness, airflow limitation, respiratory symptoms (e.g., recurrent episodes of wheezing, breathlessness, tightness in the chest, and cough, particularly during the night and early morning), and chronicity of the disease.
- Bronchospasm due to smooth muscle contraction used to be considered the major contributor to airway obstruction; now, inflammatory disease of the airways is known to have a critical role, particularly in chronic asthma.

- Even in mild asthma, there is an inflammatory response involving infiltration, particularly with activated eosinophils and mast cells, and epithelial cell desquamation.
- Mast cells are important in the acute response to inhaled allergens and perhaps in exercise, but do not play a major role in the pathogenesis of chronic inflammation.
- The number of eosinophils in peripheral blood and airway secretions correlates closely with the degree of bronchial hyperresponsiveness.
  —All asthmatics with active disease have hyperresponsive (hyperreactive) airways, seen in an exaggerated bronchoconstrictor response to many different stimuli; the degree of hyperresponsiveness is linked to extent of inflammation, and both correlate with severity of the disorder and the need for drug therapy.
  - T-cell activation of the allergic response is an important factor in the inflammation that is characteristic of asthma; T cells and their secretory products (cytokines) perpetuate airway inflammation.

Diagnosis (See Table 4-6)

Signs and Symptoms

- Episodic or chronic symptoms of airflow obstruction, including cough, breathlessness, wheezing, chest tightness
- Symptoms are often worse at night or in the early morning.
- Prolonged expiration and diffuse wheezes on physical examination
- Limitation of airflow, based on pulmonary function testing or positive bronchial provocation challenge
- Complete or partial reversibility of airflow obstruction, either spontaneously or after bronchodilator therapy

Physical Findings

- Nasal mucosal swelling ⎫
- Increased nasal secretions ⎬ seen in patients with allergic asthma
- Nasal polyps ⎭
- Hunched shoulders
- Use of accessory muscles of respiration
- Wheezing during normal breathing ⎫ indicates presence
- Prolonged forced expiratory phase ⎬ of airflow obstruction

- In severe asthma, airflow may be too limited to produce wheezing; the only diagnostic evidence on auscultation may be reduced breath sounds throughout, with prolonged expiration.

Diagnostic Tests
- ABGs, blood pH—in mild asthma, ABGs may be normal, but respiratory alkalosis and increased alveolar-arterial oxygen difference (A-a DO_2) are often present; in severe exacerbations, hypoxemia develops and the $PaCO_2$ returns to normal.
- Increased $PaCO_2$ and respiratory acidosis usually indicate respiratory failure and the need for mechanical ventilation.
- Pulmonary function tests provide baseline data regarding the degree of airway obstruction, disturbance in gas exchange, and the airways' response to inhaled allergens; measure response to drugs; and monitor patients over the long term.
- Peak expiratory flow (PEF) meters are hand-held devices designed to monitor PEF at home.
  - Their use is limited by wide variability in PEF reference values and the lack of normative brand-specific reference values.
  - PEF measurements can be compared in a patient who uses the same PEF meter consistently.
  - PEF is usually lowest when the patient first awakens and highest several hours before the midpoint of the day (diurnal variation).
  - PEF values vary with gender, age, height.
  - PEF values less than 22 L/min indicate airflow obstruction.
- Static lung volumes and capacities
- Dynamic lung volumes and capacities, including exercise testing
- Eosinophil count
- Sputum examination
- Chest x-ray—not necessary unless pneumonia or complications of asthma are suspected; radiograph shows only hyperinflation; may show bronchial wall thickening, diminished peripheral lung vascular shadows.
- Allergen identification is often useful in patients with persistent asthma.
- Other tests (e.g., for gastroesophageal reflux disease [GERD] or paranasal sinus disease) may be helpful in those with relevant symptoms, or those with refractory asthma.

Differential Diagnosis
- Chronic obstructive pulmonary disease
- Heart failure
- Small pulmonary emboli
- Bronchial obstruction secondary to malignancy, aortic aneurysm, endobronchial tuberculosis (TB), or sarcoidosis

Complications
- Exhaustion from effort to breathe
- Airway infection
- Cor pulmonale
- Tussive syncope
- Pneumothorax—rarely
- Acute hypercapnic and hypoxic respiratory failure occurs in acute disease.

Prognosis
- Variable, depending on the severity of disease, age at onset, frequency of attacks, appropriate ongoing treatment, and other factors

Table 4-7 lists drug therapy for mild-to-moderate asthma.

Patient/Family Education
- Use a detailed written treatment plan based on signs and symptoms or expiratory flow rates, with explanations as necessary.
- Explain the nature of the disease to the extent possible.
- List symptoms that accompany an acute attack.
- List measures to take early in the attacks to minimize their severity and shorten the duration of symptoms.
- Instruct the patient regarding the need to recognize patterns of symptoms that might indicate inadequate control or the need for additional therapy.
- Instruct the patient regarding contributors to asthma attacks: dust mites, molds, cockroaches, animal dander, other potential allergens.
- Inform the patient and family about when to take the patient to a hospital emergency room or when to call 911 for assistance.

TABLE 4-7
Managing Patients with Asthma*

Patient Status	Quick Relief	Long-term Control
Mild intermittent	Short-acting bronchodilator: inhaled β_2-agonists. Intensity of therapy depends on severity of exacerbation. If need for this medication becomes more than twice a week, may need to begin long-term control therapy.	No daily therapy needed.
Mild persistent	Short-acting bronchodilator: inhaled β_2-agonists as needed for symptoms. Treatment depends on degree of symptoms. If need for more frequent use increases, may require long-term control Rx.	One daily medication: antiinflammatory: inhaled corticosteroid (low dose) or cromolyn or nedocromil.
Moderate persistent	Short-acting bronchodilator: inhaled β_2-agonists as needed to relieve symptoms; increasing need indicates long-term control is required.	Daily medication: antiinflammatory: inhaled corticosteroid (low-medium dose) and a long-acting bronchodilator: long-acting inhaled β_2-agonists, sustained-release theophylline or long-acting β_2-agonist tablets. If needed: antiinflammatory: inhaled corticosteroid (medium-high dose) *and* long-acting bronchodilator: long-acting inhaled β_2-agonists, sustained-release theophylline or long-acting β_2-agonist tablets.
Severe persistent	Short-acting bronchodilator: inhaled β_2-agonists as needed for symptoms. Increasing use indicates need for additional long-term control.	Daily medication: antiinflammatory: inhaled corticosteroid (medium dose) and long-acting bronchodilator: long-acting inhaled β_2-agonists, sustained-release theophylline; or long-acting β_2-agonist tablets *and* corticosteroid tablets or syrup (2 mg/kg/d, usually not to exceed 60 mg/d).

From Tierney LM, McPhee SJ, Papadakis MA: *Current medical diagnosis & treatment*, ed 39, New York, 2000, Lange Medical Books/McGraw-Hill, p 277.
*Continual patient education throughout, according to patient status and need for new or changed medication, beginning with basic facts about the disease, inhaler/inhalation chamber technique, actions of medications, self-care and care plans, environmental control measures to take.

- Emphasize the importance of close contact with the physician or nurse practitioner at all times; have telephone numbers at hand.

Follow-up/Referral
- Regularly scheduled office visits, at least every 6 months or more often as indicated by the patient's response to therapy and/or need for more frequent monitoring, are essential for periodic assessment and ongoing monitoring of the patient's condition to determine therapeutic goals, appropriate pharmacologic therapy, and the level of the patient's understanding and compliance.
- Give an annual influenza vaccination (verify that patient is not egg-sensitive).
- Give a pneumococcal vaccination q6yrs.

- Spirometry should be performed at the initial assessment and at least every year or two after that.

RESTRICTIVE LUNG DISORDERS

Restrictive lung disorders are characterized by decreased compliance of the lungs, chest wall, or both. Extrapulmonary conditions involve the central nervous system, neuromuscular system (e.g., amyotrophic lateral sclerosis [ALS] [Lou Gehrig disease], myasthenia gravis). Intrapulmonary restrictive lung disease involves the pleura or the lung tissue (e.g., TB, cancer).

Acute Bronchitis
Definition
- Acute bronchitis or tracheobronchitis is usually a self-limited, secondary infection of the

trachea and bronchi that may develop as a result of an upper respiratory infection with common viruses or *Mycoplasma pneumoniae.*

Risk Factors
- Recent upper respiratory infection
- Exposure to organisms that cause acute bronchitis
- Debilitated condition
- Patients with chronic lung or heart disease
- Older age
- Exposure to airborne irritants and allergens
- Incompetent glottic function, such as in the elderly or alcoholic patient, resulting in aspiration of upper airway secretions

Etiology
- Comes after or occurs with an acute upper respiratory infection
- Rhinovirus and coronavirus have high prevalence and are commonly implicated as causes of acute bronchitis.
- Secondary bacterial infection
- *M. pneumoniae,* influenza, and adenovirus tend to cause a more severe bronchitis, with fever and substernal pain.
- Acute irritative bronchitis may be caused by various mineral and vegetable dusts; fumes from strong acids; ammonia; certain volatile organic solvents, such as chlorine, hydrogen sulfide, sulfur dioxide, or bromine; environmental irritants, such as ozone and nitrogen dioxide; and tobacco smoke.
- In cough-variant asthma, the degree of bronchoconstriction is not enough to cause wheezing. It may be caused by allergen inhalation in an atopic person or chronic exposure to an irritant in a person with relatively mild airway hyperreactivity; treatment is the same as for asthma.

Pathogenesis
- Hyperemia of the mucous membranes is the earliest sign.
- There may be desquamation, edema, leukocytic infiltration of the submucosa, and production of sticky or mucopurulent exudate.
- The protective functions of bronchial cilia, phagocytes, and lymphatics are disturbed, and bacteria may invade the normally sterile bronchi, resulting in accumulation of cellular debris and mucopurulent exudate.
- Cough is essential to eliminate bronchial secretions.
- Airway obstruction may result from edema of the bronchial walls, retained secretions, and spasm of bronchial muscles in some patients.

Diagnosis
Signs and Symptoms
- Mild bronchitis
  —Symptoms begin 1 to 2 weeks after an acute URI.
  —Cough
  —Sputum production, variable presence
  —No fever
  —Adventitious breath sounds
- Severe bronchitis
  —Persistent cough
  —Sputum production
  —Fever
  —Burning substernal chest pain
  —Myalgias
  —Wheezing and diffuse crackles may be present.

Diagnostic Tests
Acute bronchitis is a diagnosis of exclusion.
- Perform a chest x-ray to rule out pneumonia.
- Sputum examination and cultures are not helpful.
- White blood cell count may be normal to slightly elevated.

Differential Diagnosis
- Pertussis is increasing among adults, with rates exceeding 20% in those with a cough lasting longer than 2 weeks in urban areas.
  —The diagnosis of pertussis is made by taking a nasopharyngeal culture on special media for *Bordetella,* combined with patient's history and symptoms.
  —Diagnosis by a single antibody test in acute serum is used to detect sporadic cases.
  —The treatment for pertussis is as follows.
   ~ Give a 14-day course of erythromycin 40 to 50 mg/kg per day (max. 2 g/day), in two doses.

~ Give TMP/SMX to patients allergic to erythromycin.
- Upper respiratory infection
- Pneumonia
- Acute asthma attack
- Allergic reaction
- Chronic bronchitis
- Chronic aspiration
- Influenza

Treatment
- For cough only (no fever, myalgias, malaise, or chest pain): codeine sulfate 15 to 30 mg q4-6h
- Antibiotic therapy
  —Empiric use of antibiotics is not supported by the literature.
  —For culture-proven *M. pneumoniae* infection, give a 2-week course of erythromycin, tetracycline, or clarithromycin.
- Inhaled bronchodilator
  —Albuterol may be used for wheezing or chest tightness.
- Symptomatic therapy
  —For cough suppression, treat with dextromethorphan or codeine if necessary.
  —Instruct the patient to use analgesics such as acetaminophen for fever and myalgias.
  —Have the patient maintain adequate hydration.
  —The patient should avoid inhaled steam and cool mists, as these may contaminate airways with gram-negative aerobic bacteria.
  —Evidence is lacking that expectorants alter the clinical course.

Prognosis
- With appropriate therapy, the prognosis is excellent.

Patient/Family Education
- Strongly encourage smoking cessation.
  —In 50% of those who stop smoking, the chronic cough resolves completely within 1 month.
- The patient should avoid lung irritants and environmental pollutants.
- Emphasize the importance of drinking plenty of fluids, at least 1 to 2 quarts per day.
- Provide information about all medications, reasons for prescribing, dose, schedule, side effects, and the importance of taking all medications as prescribed.
- Instruct regarding use of bronchodilators, and inform the patient about the danger of overuse.
- List symptoms that may signal complications and thus the need to call the physician or nurse practitioner.

Follow-up/Referral
- The patient should be seen within 1 week to assess response to therapy.
- If symptoms worsen or if the patient fails to show improvement in 2 days, further evaluation is necessary.
- Referral to a specialist in pulmonary diseases may be required.

Pneumonia

Definition
Pneumonia is an acute infection of the lower respiratory tract (terminal bronchioles and alveolar sacs). Every year in the United States, about 3 million people develop pneumonia, and between 40,000 and 70,000 die. It ranks fifth among all disease categories as a cause of death, and it is the most common lethal nosocomial (hospital-acquired) infection.
- Pneumonia is classified in the following ways:
  —Community-acquired pneumonia results from exposure outside the hospital environment.
  —Nosocomial pneumonia develops at least 46 hours after admission to a hospital or other health care facility.
  —Aspiration pneumonia is caused by the inhalation of oropharyngeal secretions during vomiting or with altered gag reflex, and glottis dysfunction.
  —Opportunistic pneumonia is seen in immunocompromised patients, such as those with HIV infection, organ transplantation, or neoplasms, and those receiving cytotoxic chemotherapy.

Risk Factors
- Advanced age
- Decreased immune response

- Altered level of consciousness; potential for aspiration
- Pain, causing decreased inspiratory effort
- Weakness, causing decreased cough and loss of sigh mechanism
- Alcohol abuse
- HIV infection
- Sickle cell disease
- Splenectomy
- Hematologic disorders
- Underlying COPD
- Endotracheal intubation
- Malnutrition

Etiology

Pneumonia has many causative organisms.
- Bacteria
  - *Streptococcus pneumoniae*
  - *Staphylococcus aureus*
  - Group A β-hemolytic Streptococcus
  - *Haemophilus influenzae*
  - *Escherichia coli*
  - *Klebsiella pneumoniae*
  - *Pseudomonas* species
- Viruses
  - Adenovirus
  - Herpes simplex
  - Cytomegalovirus
  - Respiratory syncytial virus
- Mycoplasma
  - *Mycoplasma pneumoniae*
  - *Chlamydia pneumoniae*
- Fungi
  - *Histoplasma capsulatum*
  - *Cryptococcus neoformans*
  - *Aspergillus* species
  - *Candida* species
- Protozoa
  - *Pneumocystis carinii* pneumonia (PCP)
- Rickettsiae
  - *Coxiella burnetii* (Q fever)
- Inhalation of causative organisms in the air
- Aspiration of pharyngeal secretions
- Hematogenous dissemination from distal foci
- From a contiguous site (e.g., acute bronchitis, empyema, subphrenic abscess)

Pathogenesis

- Bacteria lodge in the bronchioles, where they proliferate and initiate an inflammatory process in alveolar spaces, resulting in the production of a protein-rich fluid that acts as a culture medium for the growth of organisms and as a means of spreading the infection to other segments of the lungs.
- The infection nearly always proceeds in stages.
  - The earliest stage is congestion, characterized by serous exudate, vascular engorgement, and rapid proliferation of organisms.
  - The next stage is red hepatization, so named because the consolidation in the lungs make them appear liver-like. In this stage, the air spaces are filled with polymorphonuclear cells, and vascular congestion continues with extravasation of RBCs into the air spaces.
  - The next stage is gray hepatization, which involves the accumulated fibrin from the inflammatory process, including the disintegration of WBCs and RBCs, and congestion in the air spaces from the exudate
  - The final stage is resolution, during which the exudate is resorbed.

Diagnosis

Signs and Symptoms
- Acute pneumonia
  - Abrupt onset with shaking chills
  - Acutely ill appearance
  - Fever 102° F to 105° F (39° C to 40.5° C)
  - Productive cough
  - Rusty-colored (blood-streaked) sputum
  - Dyspnea
  - Pleuritic chest pain, often with a pleural friction rub
  - Cyanosis
  - Confusion/lethargy in the elderly (may be the first sign of infection)
  - Older persons are more likely to develop concomitant UTI and bacteremia.
  - Altered breath sounds: coarse inspiratory wheezing, bronchial breath sounds that are diminished over the area(s) of consolidation
  - Percussion dullness, increased tactile fremitus, whispered pectoriloquy
- Viral pneumonia
  - Clinical manifestations vary from mild upper respiratory symptoms to severe

pneumonia; incubation period is about 2 days after exposure.

—Fever up to 105° F (40.5° C)
—Malaise and prostration
—Headache and retroorbital pain
—Myalgias
—Chills, suggesting secondary bacterial infection
—Dry, hacking cough
—Sputum is scant or slightly bloody
—Marked dyspnea
—Pleuritic chest pain (less common than in bacterial pneumonia)
—Cyanosis—heliotrope (reddish purple) due to replication of virus in the lungs
—Scattered crackles and moist wheezes
—May be complicated by secondary bacterial infection of the ears, sinuses, throat, and/or lungs

Diagnostic Tests

- Gram's stain of sputum: staphylococci, gram-negative rods, other organisms
- Sputum culture: usually positive in bacterial pneumonia, negative in viral pneumonia
- Blood cultures: up to 50% of pneumococcal pneumonias show bacteremia
- CBC with differential: bacterial pneumonia is almost always associated with leukocytosis and shift to the left; viral, rickettsial, and fungal pneumonias are associated with leukopenia
- Chest x-ray: necessary to confirm diagnosis; most patients have an infiltration at the time of presentation or within 24 hours of the onset of symptoms; findings are less reliable in dehydrated patients
- Arterial blood gases or oxygen saturation: hypoxemia of 60 mm Hg on room air is a poor prognostic indicator
- CT scan: tomography is more sensitive than chest x-ray in complicated pneumonia such as lung abscess, interstitial disease, and cavitary tuberculosis
- Serologic HIV test with informed consent: recommended by the Centers for Disease Control and Prevention for hospitalized patients between the ages of 15 and 54 who are treated in facilities in which the prevalence of AIDS is 1/1000 hospital discharges

- CD4 cell count: <200 mm³ indicates advanced HIV infection when informed consent for HIV test cannot be obtained
- Between 30% and 50% of patients have no identifiable pathogen despite a clinical picture of bacterial pneumonia.
- The most reliable sources of specimens on which to base diagnosis are those taken from normally sterile sites: blood or pleural fluid from patients with empyema.
- Special culture techniques, stains, serologic assays, or lung biopsies are required to identify mycobacteria, chlamydia, anaerobic bacteria, viruses, fungi, legionellae, rickettsiae, and parasites.

Treatment

- Recommend using respiratory support, including oxygen if indicated.
- Antibiotics are selected on the basis of Gram's stain results.
- For penicillin-sensitive strains of S. *pneumoniae*, penicillin G is the preferred agent.
- For patients who are not severely ill, use penicillin G or V 250 to 500 mg PO q6h.
- For parenteral therapy of uncomplicated pneumococcal pneumonia, use aqueous penicillin G 500,000 to 2 million units IV q4-6h.
  —About 25% of strains of S. *pneumoniae* are resistant to penicillin.
  —Most resistant strains respond to high doses of penicillin, cefotaxime, or ceftriaxone.
- The newer quinolones (levofloxacin, sparfloxacin, grepafloxacin, and trovafloxacin) are preferred therapy for penicillin-resistant strains and for patients who are sensitive to penicillin.
- Vancomycin, the only drug with consistent activity, is active against all strains of S. *pneumoniae* and is often preferred for severely ill patients in areas with high rates of resistance.
- Oral antibiotics include erythromycin or clindamycin 300 mg q6h.
- Parenteral therapy includes cefotaxime 1 to 2 g IV q6h, ceftriaxone 1 to 2 g IV q12h, cefazolin 500 mg IV q8h, erythromycin 500 mg IV q6-8h.
  —Most third-generation cephalosporins, other than cefotaxime and ceftizoxime,

are essentially inactive against *S. pneumoniae.*

Supportive Therapy
- Bed rest
- Fluids
- Analgesics for pleuritic pain
- Oxygen for patients with cyanosis, significant hypoxemia, severe dyspnea, circulatory disturbances, or delirium

Prognosis
- Although morbidity and mortality from pneumococcal pneumonia have decreased significantly since the advent of penicillin, the infection accounts for 85% of all lethal cases of community-acquired pneumonia.
- Overall mortality rate is about 10%.
- Treatment has little effect on mortality in the first 5 days of illness.
- Factors that may predict a poor prognosis include the following:
  - Age extremes (younger than 1 year, older than 60 years)
  - Positive blood cultures
  - Involvement of more than 1 lobe
  - A peripheral WBC $<5000/\mu l$
  - The presence of other problems: cirrhosis, heart failure, neoplastic disease, immunosuppression, agammaglobulinemia, actual or functional asplenia, uremia, systolic hypotension, diabetes mellitus
  - Involvement of certain serotypes (3 and 8)
  - Development of extrapulmonary complications (e.g., meningitis, endocarditis)
  - Male gender
  - Altered mental status
  - Tachypnea
  - Absence of pleuritic chest pain
- In patients with no improvement on therapy, look for one or more of the following:
  - Far-advanced disease (most common)
  - Wrong etiologic diagnosis
  - Adverse drug reaction
  - Superinfection
  - Inadequate host defenses due to associated conditions
  - Noncompliance with pharmacologic regimen
  - Resistance to antibiotics

  - Complications (e.g., empyema; metastatic foci of infection, which is systemic infection)

Prevention
- The polyvalent pneumococcal vaccine, which contains polysaccharide antigens of 23 strains of *S. pneumoniae,* prevents or lessens the severity of most pneumococcal infections in immunocompetent patients.
- It should be given particularly to those more than 65 years old and those with any chronic disease that may increase the risk of community-acquired pneumonia.
- Revaccination every 6 years is recommended.
- The vaccine can be given to hospitalized patients; vaccines against pneumonia and influenza can be given simultaneously, immediately after an episode of pneumonia.

Patient/Family Education
- Explain the nature and cause of the infection, the course of treatment, and the importance of adherence to pharmacologic therapy (reason for taking, dose, schedule), and of realizing that full recovery may take weeks to months.
- Instruct about the importance of rest, sufficient fluid intake, and nutritious diet.
- List symptoms that signal the need for calling the nurse practitioner: worsening symptoms, new symptoms, increased difficulty in breathing, blood in sputum, chest pain, recurrence of fever.

Follow-up/Referral
- Telephone contact with patient 24 hours after the initial visit is usually necessary.
- Symptoms of pneumococcal pneumonia usually abate after 48 to 72 hours from the start of therapy; the time of response is somewhat longer with other pathogens and compromised host defenses.
- If significant clinical improvement has not occurred within 4 days, the patient should be reevaluated.
- Resolution of the infiltrate may take several weeks, particularly in patients with severe disease, empyema, bacteremia, or preexisting chronic lung disease (e.g., COPD).

- Persistent infiltration 6 weeks or more after therapy may indicate underlying bronchogenic neoplasm or TB.
- After clinical resolution of pneumonia, a chest x-ray exam is recommended to exclude persistent lung abnormalities suggestive of endobronchial obstruction.
- A follow-up at 2 weeks for younger patients and 8 weeks for older patients is necessary.

Pneumonia from Other Causes

Staphylococcal Pneumonia

- Staphylococcal pneumonia accounts for about 2% of community-acquired pneumonias and 10% to 15% of nosocomial pneumonias.
- Those most at risk are infants and older persons.
- The course of staphylococcal pneumonia can sometimes be fulminant; most patients do not appear very ill; the course may be indolent.
- The signs and symptoms are about the same as for pneumococcal pneumonia.
  - Differing features include recurrent rigors, tissue necrosis with abscess formation, pneumatoceles (common in infants and children), empyema, and a fulminant course with marked prostration.

Diagnosis
- Look for the appearance of *S. aureus* in sputum and blood cultures.
- A chest x-ray resembles bronchopneumonia, with or without abscess formation or pleural effusion.
- Lobar consolidation is uncommon.
- Pneumatoceles strongly indicate staphylococcus.

Prognosis and Treatment
- The mortality rate is 30% to 40%, due to the serious associated conditions present.
- A fulminant lethal course occurs in previously healthy adults who develop the pneumonia following influenza.
- Most strains of *S. aureus* produce penicillinase and methicillin, which cause resistance to antibiotics, and resistance is increasing.

- Preferred therapy is oxacillin or nafcillin 2 g IV q4-6h (or) alternatively, a cephalosporin—cephalothin or cefamandole 2 g IV q4-6h.
- Clindamycin 600 mg IV q6-8h is active against 90% to 95% of strains.
- Vancomycin 1 g IV q12h should be used for methicillin-resistant strains.

Streptococcal Pneumonia

- Lancefield group A β-hemolytic streptococci are a relatively rare cause of pneumonia; the largest epidemics occurred among recruits during WWI, with only sporadic cases since then.

Pneumonia Caused by Gram-negative Bacilli

- Gram-negative bacilli account for less than 2% of community-acquired pneumonias, but account for most nosocomial pneumonias, some of which are fatal.

Etiology
- The most important pathogen is *Klebsiella pneumoniae*, which causes Friedlander's pneumonia.
- Other organisms include *Pseudomonas aeruginosa, Escherichia coli, Enterobacter* spp., *Proteus* spp., *Serratia marcescens*, and *Acinetobacter* spp.
- *P. aeruginosa* is the most common pathogen in patients with cystic fibrosis; neutropenia; and advanced AIDS, bronchiectasis, and pneumonias acquired in intensive care units.

Signs and Symptoms
- Patients have a bronchopneumonia similar to other bacterial lung infections, but with a high mortality (see later section on prognosis).
- All the organisms may cause abscess formation.
- Friedlander's pneumonia frequently affects the upper lobes and produces sputum that looks like currant jelly, tissue necrosis with early abscess formation, and a fulminant course.

Diagnosis
- Gram's stain of sputum shows many gram-negative bacilli, but distinguishing them

morphologically is impossible; sputum cultures are not helpful for the same reason.
- Cultures of blood, pleural fluid, or a transtracheal aspirate obtained before treatment is begun confirm the diagnosis.

Prognosis and Treatment
- The mortality rate for gram-negative bacillary pneumonia is about 25% to 50%, even when antibiotics are given.
- Cephalosporin (cefotaxime 2 g IV 16h (or) ceftazidime 2 g IV q8h) is the preferred therapy.
- Other effective drugs include imipenem 1 g IV bid (or) ciprofloxacin 500 to 750 mg po bid given alone or combined with an aminoglycoside: gentamicin or tobramycin 1.7 mg/kg IV q8h (or) 5 to 6 mg/kg once/day.
- The aminoglycosides should not be used alone.

Pneumonia of Legionnaires' Disease
- An outbreak among members of the American Legion in Philadelphia in 1976 led to the discovery of the bacterium *Legionella pneumophila.*
- Retrospective studies then show cases of legionellosis as early as 1943, and other organisms have been classified in the genus.
- Currently, over 30 proposed species of Legionella exist; at least 19 species have been linked to pneumonia, the most common being *L. pneumophila* (85% to 90% of cases), followed by *L. micdadei* (5% to 10%), and then *L. bozemanii* and *L. dumoffii*, all morphologically similar.
- The diseases that these organisms cause are asymptomatic seroconversion; a self-limited, flu-like illness without pneumonia often called Pontiac fever; legionnaires' disease, the most serious and most commonly recognized form, characterized by pneumonia; and rare localized soft tissue infections.
- Risk factors include smoking, alcohol abuse, and immunosuppression, especially from corticosteroids.

Occurrence
- Legionnaires' disease accounts for 1% to 8% of community-acquired pneumonias that

result in hospitalization, and about 4% of lethal nosocomial pneumonias.
- Cases appear sporadically, often in late summer and early fall.
- Transmission between persons has not been shown.
- *L. pneumophila* outbreaks tend to occur in buildings (e.g., hotels, hospitals) or where water supplies have been contaminated and the aerosolized organisms are spread from evaporative condensers of air conditioning systems or contaminated showerheads.
- Legionnaires' disease can occur in any age, but most patients are middle-aged men.

Prognosis and Treatment
- Mortality is greater than 15%, even with treatment; response in all patients is slow; recovery takes weeks to months, and x-ray abnormalities persist for more than 1 month.
- Erythromycin 1 g IV q6h is the preferred drug.
- Those with less serious illness can be given erythromycin 500 mg PO qid (or) ciprofloxacin 750 mg PO bid (or) azithromycin 500 mg followed by 250 mg once daily.
- Seriously ill patients can be given erythromycin with rifampin 300 mg bid PO or IV for at least 3 weeks to prevent relapses.

Mycoplasmal Pneumonia
- *Mycoplasma pneumoniae* is the most common pathogen of lung infections in those aged 5 to 35 years.
- The incubation period is 10 to 14 days.
- Epidemics occur in closed populations such as schools, the military, and families.

Pathogenesis
- The organism attaches to and destroys ciliated epithelial cells of the respiratory tract mucosa, producing interstitial pneumonitis, bronchitis, and bronchiolitis.

Signs and Symptoms
- Initially, flu-like symptoms occur with malaise, sore throat, and dry cough, which gradually become more severe.
- Acute symptoms last for 1 to 2 weeks, followed by gradual recovery, although malaise and fatigue may persist for several weeks.

- Physical examination findings tend to be minimal compared with patients' complaints and x-ray changes.
- A maculopapular rash occurs in 10% to 20% of patients.

Course
- The disease is usually relatively mild, with spontaneous recovery.
- Other cases are severe, sometimes causing adult respiratory distress syndrome, with extrapulmonary complications (e.g., hemolytic anemia, thromboembolism, polyarthritis, neurologic syndromes such as myelitis, peripheral neuropathy, or cerebellar ataxia).

Viral Pneumonia
- Among adults, the viruses that most commonly cause pneumonia are influenza A and B; more rarely, other causative organisms include adenovirus, varicella-zoster virus, Epstein-Barr virus, coxsackievirus, and Hantavirus.
- Among older patients, important pathogens to look for include influenza, parainfluenza, and respiratory syncytial viruses.
- Patients with compromised cell-mediated immunity often develop pulmonary infections from latent viruses, especially cytomegalovirus (CMV).
- Most viral infections result from exposure to infected persons who are shedding the specific virus.

Pathogenesis
- Viruses invade the bronchiolar epithelium, causing bronchiolitis; the infection may extend to the pulmonary interstitium and alveoli, resulting in pneumonia.
- Affected areas are congested and hemorrhagic at times; a severe inflammatory reaction develops composed of mononuclear cells.
- Alveoli may contain fibrin, mononuclear cells, and occasionally neutrophils.
- In severe cases, there may be hyaline membranes.
- Characteristic viral inclusions may occur with adenovirus, CMV, respiratory syncytial virus, or varicella-zoster virus.

Diagnosis
- Signs and symptoms include bronchitis, bronchiolitis, pneumonia, headache, fever, myalgia, a cough that produces mucupurulent sputum.
- Diagnostic tests that can be used are as follows.
  —Chest x-ray: interstitial pneumonia or peribronchial thickening
  —Lobar consolidation and pleural effusions are not common but may occur with bacterial superinfection.
  —WBC: often low, but may be normal or moderately elevated in superinfection
  —Sputum smears: few bacteria with dominance of monocytes, with no evidence of bacterial pathogens
  —Definitive diagnosis of viral pneumonia is achieved through recovery of the virus from throat washings or tissue, typical inclusions in cytopathology or biopsy specimens, or serologic assays.
  —Most hospital laboratories do not have facilities for viral culture.

Treatment
- Treatment is based on pathogen.
  —For adults, use acyclovir 5 to 10 mg/kg q8h.
  —For CMV pneumonia, use ganciclovir 5 mg/kg IV bid and immune globulin (IV immune globulin or CMV immune globulin in organ transplant patients); this therapy has not been shown to be helpful in AIDS patients.
  —Some patients, especially those with influenza, develop superimposed bacterial infections that require antibiotics (organisms: *Streptococcus pneumoniae*, *Staphylococcus aureus*; more infrequently: *Haemophilus influenzae*, group A β-hemolytic streptococci and *Neisseria meningitidis*).

Prognosis
- The prognosis is variable, depending on the causative organism, the age of the patient, and associated diseases.

Pneumonia Caused by *Pneumocystis carinii*
- *P. carinii* is now considered a fungus rather than a protozoan.

- It causes disease only when defenses are compromised, most often when there are defects in cell-mediated immunity as in hematologic malignancies, lymphoproliferative diseases, cancer chemotherapy, and AIDS.
- About 30% of patients with HIV infection have *P. carinii* pneumonia as the initial AIDS-defining diagnosis.
- More than 80% of AIDS patients have this infection at some time if prophylaxis is not given.
- HIV-infected patients become vulnerable to *P. carinii* pneumonia when the CD4 helper cell count is <200/μl.

Diagnosis
- Signs and symptoms
  —Fever is present.
  —Dyspnea may occur.
  —A dry, nonproductive cough may occur acutely within several days, or subacutely over several weeks.
  —A chest x-ray exam characteristically shows diffuse, bilateral perihilar infiltrates, but 20% to 30% of patients have normal chest x-rays.
  —Arterial blood gases show hypoxemia and an increase in the alveolar-arterial oxygen gradient.
  —Pulmonary function tests show altered diffusing capacity.
  —A definitive diagnosis requires histopathologic demonstration of the organism with methenamine silver, Giemsa, Wright-Giemsa, modified Grocott, Weigert-Gram, or monoclonal antibody stain.
  —Sputum specimens are obtained by expectoration or bronchoscopy; the average sensitivity is 60% for expectoration and 90% to 95% for bronchoscopy with alveolar lavage.

Treatment
- TMP-SMX 20 mg/kg/day (trimethoprim) in four doses IV or PO for 21 days is the preferred regimen.
- Treatment can begin immediately without a definitive diagnosis since cysts persist for weeks.
  —Side effects include skin rash, neutropenia, fever.

- An alternative therapy is pentamidine 3 to 4 mg/kg IV once daily; atovaquone 750 mg PO bid; trimethoprim 20 mg/kg/day with dapsone 100 mg/day PO; maquine base 15 mg/day PO. All regimens are given for 21 days.
  —Pentamidine can have serious side effects, including renal failure, hepatotoxicity, hypoglycemia, leukopenia, fever, rash, or gastric intolerance.
- Corticosteroids are advocated for those with PaO_2 <70 mm Hg: prednisone 40 mg bid for 5 days, 20 mg bid for next 5 days, then 20 mg/day for duration of treatment. Corticosteroids reduce hypoxemia, the need for intubation, and late fibrosis.
- Supportive measures include using oxygen therapy, sometimes requiring postivie end-expiratory pressure to maintain PaO_2 $\geq$60 mm Hg.

Prognosis
- Overall mortality in hospitalized patients is 15% to 20%.
- Prognosis depends on the status of the patient initially, the severity of the infection, the organism, and response to therapy.

Tuberculosis

Definition
TB is an infectious disease caused by the acid-fast bacillus *Mycobacterium tuberculosis*, *M. bovis*, or *M. africanum*. *M. tuberculosis* can affect the lungs and also the gastrointestinal (GI) tract, bones, joints, the nervous system, lymph nodes, and skin.
- The disease is characterized by the formation of tubercles, fibrosis, and cavities in the lungs.
- Patients with TB, either presumed or confirmed, should be treated by a physician who is highly experienced in managing this condition.

Risk Factors
- Exposure can be through inhalation of organisms dispersed as droplet nuclei from a person with pulmonary TB whose sputum smear is positive; the organism may float in the air for several hours, increasing the chance of spread.
- Persons more than 70 years old are at greater risk.
- TB is twice as prevalent in blacks as in whites in all age groups.

- Although specific immunologic defense against TB occurs only after infection, considerable innate defense is usually present against initial infection; therefore, health care personnel can work closely with TB patients for years without a conversion of the tuberculin skin test. However, blacks are less resistant to initial infection than whites.
- In HIV-infected persons, the incidence has increased alarmingly, particularly among blacks and Hispanic IV drug users—most often, urban men 25 to 44 years old.
- Recently, signs of a potentially very dangerous epidemic of TB have appeared, with incidence in New York increasing 30% between 1992 and 1993, with a likely development of organisms resistant to all first-line drugs.

Etiology
- Active TB is due both to recrudescence of formant TB infection and to newly acquired infection.

Pathogenesis
- The stages of TB are primary or initial infection, latent or dormant infection, and recrudescent or adult-type TB.
- An estimated 90% to 95% of primary TB infections are not recognized, producing only a positive skin test and a latent or dormant infection (Table 4-8).
  —Primary TB infection can become active at any age, producing clinical TB in any or-

gan, most often in the apical area of the lung, but also in the kidney, long bones, vertebrae, lymph nodes, and other sites.
- Activation usually occurs within 1 to 2 years of initial infection, but it may occur after years or decades, after onset of diabetes mellitus, during periods of stress, after treatment with corticosteroids or other immunosuppressants, in adolescence, or in later life (>70 years of age), but especially following HIV infection. Subtotal gastrectomy and silicosis also predispose persons to development of active TB.
- The initial infection leaves nodular scars in the apices of one or both lungs, called *Simon foci,* which are the most common seeds for later active TB.
- The frequency of activation is unaffected by calcified scars of primary infection (*Ghon foci*) or by residual calcified hilar lymph nodes.

Prophylaxis
- Chemoprophylaxis is indicated primarily in those whose tuberculin skin test converted from negative to positive within 2 years.
- Those benefiting most from prophylaxis are small children, older children, and those younger than 25 years old, who are most likely to develop clinical TB.
- In older persons, prophylaxis is indicated only when conversion of the tuberculin skin test is definite (i.e., an increase of ≥15 mm from a previous negative reaction).

TABLE 4-8
Classification of Positive Skin Test Reactions*

Reaction Size	Group
≥5 mm	Persons with HIV infection or those at risk for HIV infection. Close contacts of individuals with tuberculosis. Persons with chest x-rays consistent with old healed tuberculosis.
≥10 mm	Persons from countries with a high incidence of tuberculosis: Asia, Africa, and Latin America. Intravenous drug users. Medically underserved, low-income populations, including blacks, Hispanics, and Native Americans. Long-term residents of correctional institutions, nursing homes, and mental institutions. Persons with the following medical conditions that increase the risk of tuberculosis: gastrectomy, being ≥10% below ideal body weight, jejunoileal bypass, diabetes mellitus, silicosis, chronic renal failure, corticosteroid or other immunosuppressive therapy, leukemia, lymphoma, and other malignancies.
≥15 mm	Other high-risk populations. All other persons.

From Recommendations of the American Thoracic Society: American Review of Respiratory Diseases 142:725, 1990.
*A Mantoux skin test reaction is considered positive if the transverse diameter of the indurated area reaches the size required for the specific group. All other reactions are considered negative.

- Prophylaxis is strongly recommended in HIV-infected persons whose tuberculin reaction is at least 10 mm, because the protective effect of T-cell immunity is lost; in children younger than 4 years old who have close contact with a person whose sputum smear is positive for acid-fast bacilli; and those in whom the infection may progress rapidly, resulting in serious disease before the test becomes positive.
- Chemoprophylaxis consists of isoniazid 300 mg/day for 6 to 9 months for adults, unless resistance is suspected; for children, the dosage is 10 mg/kg/day, up to 300 mg, given as a single morning dose.
  —In infected children and in older-age tuberculin converters, isoniazid therapy has been shown to be 98.5% effective in preventing development of clinical TB.
- Patients with clinical TB become noninfectious within 10 to 14 days after onset of therapy.

Diagnosis

Signs and Symptoms

- Patients with pulmonary TB are often asymptomatic, sometimes only stating that they don't feel well, even though a chest x-ray shows distinct abnormalities.
- A cough is the most common symptom, but it may be ascribed to smoking, recent cold, or influenza. At first, the cough produces some sputum that may be yellow or greenish, usually on arising, becoming more productive as the disease progresses.
- Patients may have night sweats.
- Dyspnea from a spontaneous pneumothorax or pleural effusion may occur.
- Hemoptysis does not usually occur until the disease is in an advanced stage.

Diagnostic Tests

- Chest x-ray exam: multinodular infiltrate above or behind the clavicle (most common location) indicates recrudescence of old TB infection.
- Sputum culture: AFB organisms are a strong indication of TB, but definitive diagnosis can be made only with polymerase chain reaction (PCR) identification of *M. tuberculosis*, which takes 3 weeks or longer.

- Fiberoptic bronchoscopy: done usually in patients who cannot produce sputum.
- Transbronchial biopsy: performed on infiltrative lesions, with the specimen submitted for culture, histologic evaluation, and PCR.
- Gastric washings: have been largely replaced by bronchial washings and biopsy, and especially post-bronchoscopy sputum.
- Tuberculin skin test: although far from definitive, it is an essential part of diagnosis.

All patients with a presumptive or confirmed diagnosis of TB must be reported promptly to the appropriate local health department.

Differential Diagnosis

- Other mycobacterial or granulomatous infections
- Pneumonia
- Neoplasm, especially lymphoma, primary lung cancer
- Hematogenous or lymphogenous metastases
- Sarcoidosis
- Lung abscess
- Collagen vascular or vasculitic disease

Course of Disease

- The course varies depending on multiple factors: size of inoculum, virulence of organism, competence of host defense, presence of other diseases (e.g., diabetes, HIV infection).
- The course is usually more rapid among blacks and Native Americans than among whites.
- TB in older adults, particularly from a long-dormant infection, can go undiagnosed for months or even years.
- When pulmonary TB occurs in a nursing home, infection may spread quickly among the other residents.
- Miliary TB and TB meningitis, once thought to be common in children, are found more often among older people today.

Treatment (Tables 4-9 and 4-10)

- The two drugs most often given simultaneously are isoniazid (INH) and rifampin (RMP); others include ethambutol (EMB), pyrazinamide (PZA), and streptomycin (SM) in doses appropriate for age and weight of patient.

TABLE 4-9 Drugs for Treating Mycobacterial Disease in Adults	
Drug	**Daily Dose and Route**
FIRST-LINE AGENTS	
Isoniazid	300 mg PO or IM
Rifampin	600 mg PO or IV
Ethambutol	15-25 mg/kg PO
Pyrazinamide	25 mg/kg PO
Streptomycin	15 mg/kg IM
SECOND-LINE AGENTS	
Amikacin	15 mg/kg IM
Capreomycin	15 mg/kg IM
Ethionamide	0.5-1 g PO
Cycloserine	0.5-1 g PO
Levofloxacin	500 mg PO twice daily

From Tierney LM, McPhee SJ, Papadakis MA: *Current medical diagnosis & treatment,* ed 39, New York, 2000, Lange Medical Books/ McGraw-Hill, p 1370.

TABLE 4-10 Minimum Recommended Duration of Antituberculous Therapy	
Regimen	**Duration (months)**
Isoniazid + rifampin + pyrazinamide*	6
Isoniazid + rifampin	9
Rifampin + ethambutol + pyrazinamide	6-9
Rifampin + ethambutol	12
Isoniazid + ethambutol	18-24

From Tierney LM, McPhee SJ, Papadakis MA: *Current medical diagnosis & treatment,* ed 39, New York, 2000, Lange Medical Books/ McGraw-Hill, p 1370.
*Pyrazinamide for the first 2 months only.

- When INH and RMP are given together, a susceptible organism has about one chance in 1×10^{12} of surviving and replicating.
- The American Thoracic Society and the Centers for Disease Control and Prevention recommend a regimen of RMP and INH daily for 6 months, with PZA 30 mg/kg/day for the first 2 months.

Prognosis
- Almost all patients with tuberculosis who receive appropriate treatment are cured; relapse rates are less than 5% with current regimens.
- The major cause of treatment failure is noncompliance.
- Most patients treated with the recommended four-drug regimen are culture-negative by 3 months.

Prevention
- Isoniazid 300 mg once daily for 6 to 12 months is about 80% effective in preventing active disease in persons with a positive tuberculin (PPD) skin test.
- A dose of 900 mg twice weekly (directly observed) is as effective.

Patient/Family Education
- Provide information regarding the nature and cause of the disease and how it is transmitted.
- Emphasize need for prolonged (months) treatment, even after patient feels well.
- Instruct patient and family about all prescribed drugs, including the reason for taking, dosage, schedule, action, and side effects.
- Emphasize the importance of reporting new or worsening symptoms, such as hemoptysis, chest pain, dyspnea, hearing loss, vertigo.
- Instruct patient about adequate food and fluid intake.
- Evaluate cultural and socioeconomic factors that may affect compliance.

Follow-up/Referral
- Follow-up monthly during treatment, with liver function tests, sputum smear, and culture.
- Evaluate patient regarding side effects of medications at each visit.
- Patients with a history of tuberculosis are followed annually for several years after therapy is concluded to ensure against recurrence of infection.

Lung Cancer
- Most lung cancer patients are treated by pulmonary oncology specialists; however, in the primary care setting, the nurse practitioner can often identify early symptoms and refer the patient for early diagnosis and treatment.

Definition
- Tumors of the lungs may be benign or malignant, primary tumors, or metastases from

primary cancers of other organs. Primary lung tumors include bronchogenic carcinoma (the most common type of lung cancer), bronchial carcinoid, and a number of uncommon types.

Classification

- About 90% of malignant cancers belong to one of the four major cell types of bronchogenic carcinoma (i.e., primary malignant tumors of the airway epithelium).
  —Squamous cell carcinoma and adenocarcinoma are the most common types of bronchogenic carcinoma. Each type accounts for 30% to 35% of primary tumors.
  —Small cell carcinoma accounts for 20% to 25% of primary tumors, and large cell carcinoma accounts for 15%.
- Other malignant epithelial tumors include adenosquamous carcinoma, carcinoid tumor, bronchial gland carcinomas, and other rare tumors.

Characteristics of Squamous Cell Carcinoma

- Squamous cell carcinoma tends to originate in the central bronchi as an intraluminal neoplasm, which makes it easier to diagnose at an early stage of development.
- It tends to metastasize to regional lymph nodes.
- About 10% of these tumors cavitate.

Characteristics of Small-Cell Carcinoma

- Small-cell carcinoma develops in the central part of the bronchi.
- It narrows bronchi by extrinsic compression.
- Widespread metastases are common.

Characteristics of Adenocarcinoma and Large-Cell Carcinoma

- These two types are similar in their clinical presentation.
- They develop in the periphery of the lungs and are therefore not easily diagnosed early by means of sputum examination.
- Typically, both metastasize to distant organs.
- Bronchioloalveolar cell carcinoma, a subtype of adenocarcinoma, is a low-grade carcinoma that is present in about 2% of cases of bronchogenic carcinoma.
  —This type presents as single or multiple pulmonary nodules or as an alveolar infiltrate.

Risk Factors

- Cigarette smoking is the most significant cause of lung cancer in both men and women.
- Secondhand smoke
- Age between 50 and 70; fewer than 5% of lung cancer patients are younger than 40 years of age
- Ionizing radiation (indoor radon gas, therapeutic radiation)
- Asbestos
- Heavy metals (nickel, chromium)
- Industrial carcinogens (chloromethyl ether)
- Air pollution (e.g., coke oven emissions)
- Scars on the lungs
- Genetic factors
- COPD

Epidemiology

- About 400,000 deaths a year occur in the United States because of tobacco exposure.
- Lung cancer accounts for 32% of cancer deaths in men and 25% of cancer deaths in women; the rate for women is rising sharply each year.
- Bronchogenic carcinoma accounts for more than 90% of lung cancer in men and more than 80% of cases in women.
- About 87% of all lung cancers are attributable to tobacco exposure.

Pathogenesis

- All of the carcinomas develop within lung tissue or associated airways, gradually impinging on space and causing obstruction and other symptoms.

Diagnosis

Signs and Symptoms

- Only 10% to 25% of patients are asymptomatic at the time of diagnosis.
- Symptomatic lung cancer is usually advanced and not resectable.
- Initial symptoms are nonspecific.
  —Cough
  —Weight loss
  —Dyspnea
  —Chest pain
  —Hemoptysis
- Physical findings may be completely absent.
- Central tumors that obstruct segmental, lobar, or main stem bronchi may cause atelectasis and postobstructive pneumonitis.

- Peripheral tumors may cause no abnormal physical findings.
- Extension of the tumor to the pleural surface may cause pleural effusion.
- Clubbing, hepatomegaly, and lymphadenopathy are present in about 20% of patients.
- Superior vena cava syndrome, Horner's syndrome (miosis, ptosis, enophthalmos, and loss of sweating on the affected side), Pancoast's syndrome (neurovascular complication of superior pulmonary sulcus tumor), recurrent laryngeal nerve palsy with hoarseness, phrenic nerve palsy with hemidiaphragm paralysis, and skin metastases are each seen in fewer than 5% of cases.
- Paraneoplastic syndromes (extrapulmonary organ dysfunction not related to effects of the primary carcinoma or its metastases) occur in 15% to 20% of patients (Table 4-11).
  —Manifestations of paraneoplastic syndromes may precede, coincide with, or come after the diagnosis of lung cancer.
  —Diagnosing these syndromes is important because treatment of the associated symptoms may improve the patient's well-being even though the primary tumor is not curable. Sometimes, resection of part or all of the tumor results in immediate resolution of these syndromes.
- Tumor secretory products are associated with lung cancer.

Diagnostic Tests
- Laboratory
  —Cytologic examination of expectorated sputum provides definitive diagnosis in up to 80% of centrally located tumors but less than 20% in cases of peripheral nodules.
  —Examination of pleural fluid shows cytologic evidence for cancer in 40% to 50% of patients with malignant pleural effusion from lung cancer.
  —Pleural biopsy demonstrates histologic evidence of cancer in about 55% of patients.
    ~ Biopsy and cytologic study of pleural fluid combined establish a diagnosis in about 80% of patients with malignant pleural effusion.
  —Tissue for histologic confirmation of lung cancer can be obtained through various methods: bronchoscopy, percutaneous needle aspirate, mediastinoscopy, lymph node biopsy or biopsy of metastatic sites (e.g., skin), and thoracotomy.

TABLE 4-11
Paraneoplastic Syndromes in Lung Cancer

Classification	Syndrome	Common Histologic Type of Cancer
Endocrine and metabolic	Cushing's syndrome	Small cell
	Inappropriate secretion of antidiuretic hormone (SIADH)	Small cell
	Hypercalcemia	Squamous cell
	Gynecomastia	Large cell
Connective tissue and osseous	Clubbing and hypertrophic pulmonary osteoarthropathy	Squamous cell, adenocarcinoma, large cell
Neuromuscular	Peripheral neuropathy (sensory, sensorimotor)	Small cell
	Subacute cerebellar degeneration	Small cell
	Myasthenia (Eaton-Lambert syndrome)	Small cell
	Dermatomyositis	All
Cardiovascular	Thrombophlebitis	Adenocarcinoma
	Nonbacterial verrucous (marantic) endocarditis	
Hematologic	Anemia	All
	Disseminated intravascular coagulation	
	Eosinophilia	
	Thrombocytosis	
Cutaneous	Acanthosis nigricans	All
	Erythema gyratum repens	

From Tierney LM, McPhee SJ, Papadakis MA: *Current medical diagnosis & treatment*, ed 39, New York, 2000, Lange Medical Books/McGraw-Hill, p 1370.

- Imaging
  —Chest radiography shows abnormal findings in nearly all patients with lung cancer.
    ~ Comparison of old and current chest radiographs is particularly helpful.
    ~ Findings are usually nonspecific: hilar masses or enlargement, peripheral masses, atelectasis, infiltrates, cavitation, and pleural effusions.
    ~ Squamous cell and small cell carinomas usually produce a hilar mass, mediastinal widening, and cavitation.
    ~ Peripheral masses are generally adenocarcinomas.
  —CT scans, MRI, and ultrasound are useful in some patients. All depend on initial detection of a suspicious lesion on chest x-ray.
- Special examinations
  —Staging of lung cancer is done with the TNM international staging system: T = primary tumor, N = nodal involvement, and M = distant metastases.
    ~ Small cell carcinoma is not evaluated by this method, but staged as limited or extensive.

Treatment

- Surgery—only about 25% of patients are candidates for surgery, and many of these are found to have nonresectable disease at the time of surgery.
- Chemotherapy—combination chemotherapy is the treatment of choice for small cell carcinoma, resulting in considerable improvement in median survival. Single-agent chemotherapy has no proven value.
- Radiation therapy is used to palliate symptoms (e.g., cough, hemoptysis, pain).
- Photoresection with the Nd:YAG laser is sometimes performed to relieve obstruction in bronchi, improve dyspnea, and control hemoptysis.

Prognosis

- The overall 5-year survival rate for lung cancer is 10% to 15%.
- The overall 5-year survival rate after "curative" resection of squamous cell carcinoma is 35% to 40%, compared with 25% for adenocarcinoma and large cell carcinoma.

- Patients with small cell carcinoma rarely live for 5 years after the diagnosis is made, regardless of therapy.

Patient/Family Education
- Discourage smoking by patient, family members, and visitors to improve breathing function and prevent development of lung cancer in others.
- Discuss with the patient and family treatment modalities and possible side effects such as stomatitis, alopecia, anorexia, weight loss, nausea, or edema.
- Instruct the patient and others to avoid environmental pollutants.
- Encourage adequate intake of fluids and high-calorie, high-protein foods.
- Introduce the concepts of advanced directives and living wills.
- Encourage an annual chest x-ray for those at high risk of developing lung cancer.
  —A smoking history of more than 40 packs per year
  —COPD
  —Interstitial lung disease
  —Chronic exposure to secondhand smoke
  —Exposure to industrial pollutants (e.g., asbestos, uranium)

Follow-up/Referral
- Encourage the patient to use community and family resources to maintain quality of life and comfort (e.g., American Cancer Society).
- Follow-up should be geared to monitoring symptoms of worsening disease, side effects, and treatable complications.

BIBLIOGRAPHY

Asthma Module: http://www.vh.org/Providers/Textbooks/DiffuseLung/DiffuseLung.html

Barnes PJ: Mechanisms in COPD: differences from asthma, *Chest* 117(2) Suppl.:10S-14S, 2000.

Barr LF: Lung cancer. In Barker LR, Burton JR, Zieve PD, *Principles of ambulatory medicine*, ed 5, Baltimore, 1999, Williams & Wilkins.

Beers MH, Berkow R: Pulmonary disorders. In *The Merck manual of diagnosis and therapy*, ed 17, Whitehouse Station, NJ, 1999, Merck Research Laboratories.

Biskupic J: FDA can't regulate tobacco, Supreme Court rules 5 to 4. In *The Washington Post*, p A1, A20, March 22, 2000.

Chesnutt MS, Prendergast TJ: Lung. In Tierney LM, McPhee SJ, Papadakis MA: *Current medical diagnosis & treatment 2000*, ed 39, New York, 2000, Lange Medical Books/McGraw-Hill.

Creer TL, Winder JA, Tinkelman D: Guidelines for the diagnosis and management of asthma: accepting the challenge, *Journal of Asthma* 36(5):391-407, 1999.

Dean NC, Silver MP, Bateman KA: Frequency of subspecialty physician care of elderly patients with community-acquired pneumonia, *Chest* 117(2):393-397, 2000.

Emphysema and Other Obstructive Lung Diseases Module: http://www.vh.org/Providers/Textbooks/DiffuseLung/Text/Emphysema.html

Hurd S: The impact of COPD on lung health worldwide: epidemiology and incidence, *Chest* 117(2) Suppl.:1S-4S, 2000.

Jablonski RA: Discovery asthma in the older adult, *The Nurse Practitioner* 25(3):14, 24-25, 29-32, 35-36, 39-41, 2000.

Lung Tumors 3-D Visualization and Measurements: http://everest.radiology.uiowa.edu/DPI/nlm/apps/lngtumor/lngtumor.html

Phipps WJ: Management of persons with problems of the lower airway. In *Medical-surgical nursing: concepts & clinical practice*, ed 6, St. Louis, 1999, Mosby.

Pulmonary Edema Module: http://www.vh.org/Providers/Textbooks/DiffuseLung/Text/Edema.html

Shannon MT, Wilson BA, Stang CL: *Health professionals' drug guide 2000*. Stamford, CT, 2000, Appleton & Lange.

Stach SL: Improving self-care in adults with asthma using peak expiratory flow rate home monitoring, *Journal of the American Academy of Nurse Practitioners* 12(2):59-73, 2000.

Strauss GM, Gleason RE, Sugarbaker DJ: Screening for lung cancer: another look: a different view, *Chest* 111:754, 1997.

The Nurse Practitioner Journal: http://www.tnpj.com

Weiland J: The differential diagnosis of COPD and asthma, *The Journal of COPD Management* 1(1):10-15, 2000.

White P, Georas SN: Common pulmonary problems: Cough, chest pain, dyspnea, and abnormal chest x-ray. In Barker LR, Burton JR, Zieve PD: *Principles of ambulatory medicine*, ed 5, Baltimore, 1999, Williams & Wilkins.

Wise RA, Liu MC: Obstructive airways diseases: asthma and chronic obstructive pulmonary disease. In Barker LR, Burton JR, Zieve PD: *Principles of ambulatory medicine*, ed 5, Baltimore, 1999, Williams & Wilkins.

REVIEW QUESTIONS

1. Studies regarding causes of obstructive pulmonary emphysema show that chronic obstructive pulmonary disease usually:
   a. Is caused by bronchial asthma
   b. Is characterized by chronic bronchitis or emphysema
   c. Is caused by destruction of elastic tissue
   d. Is followed by the development of pulmonary carcinoma

2. Treatment of severe or prolonged attacks of asthma that require hospitalization does NOT include:
   a. Sedatives
   b. Theophylline
   c. Sympathomimetic amines
   d. Corticosteroids

3. The best test to rule out pulmonary emboli is:
   a. Forced vital capacity (FVC)
   b. Forced expiratory volume in one second (FEV_1)
   c. Ventilation/perfusion scan
   d. Peak expiratory flow rate

4. The test to measure Functional Residual Capacity shows:
   a. The volume of air in the lungs after maximal inspiration
   b. The volume of air in the lungs at the end of expiration
   c. The volume of air remaining in the lungs after maximal expiration
   d. The volume of air in the lungs with normal inspiration

5. The most significant symptom experienced by patients with pulmonary edema is:
   a. Dyspnea
   b. Syncope
   c. Substernal pressure
   d. Palpitations

6. Symptoms/signs of chronic obstructive pulmonary disease associated with emphysema usually include:
   a. Decreased total lung capacity
   b. Early cor pulmonale   *Chr. Bronchitis*
   c. Low or normal arterial P_{CO_2}
   d. Normal diffusing capacity

7. Treatment of chronic airway obstructive lung disease includes primarily:
   a. Bronchodilators such as ipratropium bromide (Atrovent) and β_2-agonists (metaproterenol [Alupent], albuterol [Proventil])
   b. IV aminophylline
   c. Long-term corticosteroids
   d. Antibiotics for infection

8. The number of deaths each year from asthma in the United States is:
   a. 1500
   b. 2000
   c. 3500
   d. 5000

9. The patient with asthma who comes into contact with a triggering agent generally experiences:
   a. An immediate allergic reaction
   b. A response that fluctuates over a 30-minute period
   c. A delayed response that occurs an hour after the contact
   d. A seizure as response

10. A 25-year-old man comes to the emergency room complaining of rust-colored sputum and fever for two days accompanied by chills. Physical examination shows dullness and moist wheezes in the left lower chest. The most likely diagnosis is:
    a. Tuberculosis
    b. Pulmonary edema
    c. Left lower lobe atelectasis
    d. Left lower lobe pneumonia

11. The statement that best describes squamous cell carcinoma is:
    a. It probably makes up 55% of all lung cancers.
    b. It originates in the central bronchi, making it easier to diagnose early.
    c. Patients are likely to be female.
    d. It does not metastasize to regional lymph nodes.

12. Both acute and chronic asthma are characterized primarily by:
    a. Airway obstruction
    b. Airway inflammation
    c. Thinning of the epithelial basement membrane
    d. Diminution of bronchial smooth muscle

13. In severe asthma, airflow may be quite limited, and findings on auscultation of the lungs include primarily:
    a. Pronounced wheezing
    b. Markedly increased breath sounds
    c. Markedly decreased breath sounds throughout
    d. Shortened expirations

14. Most viral pneumonias are characterized by:
    a. Low-grade fever
    b. Productive cough
    c. Fever up to 105° F (40.5° C)
    d. Few systemic symptoms

15. Tuberculosis, an infection caused by *Mycobacterium tuberculosis*, is transmitted among people primarily
    a. By ingestion via the gastrointestinal tract
    b. Through a break in the skin
    c. By airborne droplets from infected persons
    d. By contact with an infected person's body fluids

16. Primary tuberculosis is undetected in _____ _____% of cases. In these persons, the tuberculin skin test becomes positive, and the infection becomes latent or dormant.
    a. 25% to 30%
    b. 50% to 55%
    c. 75% to 80%
    d. 90% to 95%

17. The initial tuberculosis infection can leave nodular scars in the apices of the lungs. These nodules are called:
    a. Calcified Gord's foci
    b. Simon's foci
    c. Residual lesions
    d. Apical foci

18. The most high-risk group of people for the development of tuberculosis is:
    a. People in prisons
    b. IV drug users
    c. HIV-infected persons
    d. Homeless persons

19. The most common symptom in patients with TB is:
    a. Dyspnea
    b. Development of a "barrel" chest
    c. Cough
    d. Pulmonary cavities

20. Factors that may predict a poor prognosis for those with community-acquired pneumonia include all of the following EXCEPT:
    a. Young age (15 to 40 years old)
    b. Involvement of more than one lobe
    c. Male gender
    d. Absence of pleuritic chest pain

21. The number of people affected by chronic obstructive pulmonary disease in the United States is estimated to be:
    a. 6 million
    b. 10 million
    c. 14 million
    d. 18 million

22. An FEV_1/FVC ratio of less than 65% indicates
    a. Asthma
    b. Cavitary tuberculosis
    c. Chronic obstructive pulmonary disease
    d. Advanced lung cancer
23. The pathogenesis of asthma includes which one of the following:
    a. Denudation of airway epithelium
    b. Airway enlargement
    c. Atrophy of bronchial smooth muscle and mucous glands *Hyperplasia*
    d. Decreased numbers of eosinophils in peripheral blood and airway secretions
24. In patients with asthma, mast cells are important in the acute response to inhaled allergens, but they do not play a major role in the pathogenesis of:
    a. Airflow limitation
    b. Respiratory symptoms
    c. Chronic inflammation   *acute response*
    d. Hypertrophy of smooth muscle
25. Peak expiratory flow (PEF) meters are used by asthma patients at home, but their usefulness is limited by all but the following EXCEPT:
    a. The lack of normative brand-specific reference values
    b. PEF values vary with gender, age, and height
    c. The wide variability in PEF reference values
    d. PEF measurements can be compared in a patient who uses the same PEF meter all the time
26. The differential diagnoses of asthma include all of the following EXCEPT:
    a. Large pulmonary emboli
    b. Cardiac failure

c. Chronic obstructive pulmonary disease
d. Aortic aneurysm that is impinging on the bronchial airways

27. The prognosis in patients treated for acute bronchitis is:
    a. Poor
    b. Guarded
    c. Good
    d. Excellent
28. In March 2000 the U.S. Supreme Court ruled that:
    a. The Food and Drug Administration (FDA) can regulate how cigarettes are sold and marketed
    b. The FDA cannot regulate how cigarettes are sold and marketed
    c. The FDA can regulate how cigarettes are marketed
    d. The FDA can regulate how cigarettes are sold
29. About _____% of all lung cancers are attributable to exposure to tobacco.
    a. 56%
    b. 68%
    c. 74%
    d. 87%
30. About ___*400,000*___ deaths occur each year in the United States from tobacco-related causes. Many victims began using tobacco products as children.
    a. 100,000
    b. 200,000
    c. 300,000
    d. 400,000

5

Cardiovascular Disorders

HYPERTENSION

The primary care clinician likely sees more patients with hypertension than with any other disorder, except for upper respiratory infections.

Definition

Hypertension is defined as elevation of the systolic and/or diastolic blood pressure (BP), either primary or secondary (Table 5-1).

- *Isolated systolic hypertension (ISH)* = ≥140 mm Hg systolic, <90 mm Hg diastolic; generally increases with age until at least age 80.
- Data show that 85% to 90% of cases are essential (primary) high blood pressure (HBP); 5% to 10% of cases are secondary to bilateral renal parenchymal disease, and 1% to 2% are due to potentially curable conditions.

Risk Factors

- Age—diastolic BP increases with age until age 55 or 60
- Family history
- Black race
- Cigarette smoking
- High salt intake

Prevalence

- An estimated 50 million people in the United States have hypertension (systolic BP ≥ 140 mm Hg and/or diastolic ≥ 90 mm Hg) (or) are taking hypertensive medication.
  - Of those with hypertension, only about 24% have their BP controlled.
  - About 30% of those with hypertension are not aware that they have HBP.

- The prevalence of HBP is decreasing in the United States, but the reason for this decline is unknown.
- Population prevalence percentages are:
  - White adults—10% to 15%
  - Black adults—20% to 30%; morbidity and mortality rates are higher in blacks
  - Mexican American adults—20% to 25%

Etiology/Cause

- In about 95% of cases, no cause can be established.
- In young people, secondary hypertension due to renal insufficiency, renal artery stenosis, or coarctation of the aorta makes up a greater—but still relatively small—number of cases.

Pathogenesis

- The cause of primary hypertension is not known; its hemodynamic and pathophysiologic abnormalities are not likely to result from a single cause.
  - Heredity is a predisposing factor, but the precise mechanism is not clear.
  - Environmental factors (e.g., sodium intake, obesity, stress) seem to be factors only in people who are genetically susceptible to the disorder.
  - Dahl salt-sensitive rats, which are genetically prone to hypertension when given a high-salt diet, do not excrete water or sodium as rapidly as those from Dahl salt-resistant rats, even before hypertension is present.

TABLE 5-1
Classification of Blood Pressure for Adults

Classification	Systolic (mm Hg)	Diastolic (mm Hg)
Optimal	<120	<80
Normal	<130	<85
High-normal	130-139	85-89
Stage 1 HBP (mild)	140-159	90-99
Stage 2 HBP (moderate)	160-179	100-109
Stage 3 HBP (severe)	≥180	≥110

From Joint National Committee on the Detection, Evaluation, and Treatment of High Blood Pressure: The sixth report of the Joint National Committee on Detection, Evaluation, and Treatment of High Blood Pressure (JNC VI). *Archives of Internal Medicine* 157:2413-2446, 1997.

—The pathogenic mechanisms lead to increased total peripheral vasoconstriction, to increased cardiac output (CO), or to both because BP = CO (flow) times resistance.

—Increased intravascular and extravascular fluid volume are seen by many to be significant factors, fluid increases can raise BP only by increasing CO (increasing venous return to the heart), or by increasing total peripheral resistance (by causing vasoconstriction), or both; however, increased fluid volume often does neither.

• Abnormal sodium (Na) transport across the cell wall due to a defect in or inhibition of the Na-K pump (Na^+, K^+-ATPase), or due to increased permeability to Na^+, as has been described in some cases of hypertension; the result is increased intracellular Na, which makes the cell more sensitive to sympathetic stimulation.

—Because Ca follows Na, it is thought that the accumulation of intracellular Ca (and not NA by itself) is responsible for the increased sensitivity.

—ATPase may cause norepinephrine to be pumped back into the sympathetic neurons to inactivate this neurotransmitter; the inhibition of this mechanism could likely enhance the effect of norepinephrine.

—Defects in sodium transport have been described in normotensive children of hypertensive parents.

• Stimulation of the sympathetic nervous system

—It raises BP, which is usually higher in hypertensive or prehypertensive persons than in normotensive persons.

↑ SNS

—It is not clear whether this hyperresponsiveness occurs in the sympathetic nervous system, or in the myocardium and vascular smooth muscle that it innervates, but it can often be detected before sustained hypertension develops.

—A high resting pulse rate can be a manifestation of increased sympathetic nervous activity, which is a widely accepted predictor of hypertension development.

↑ P @ rest

—Some hypertensive patients have a higher than normal circulating plasma catecholamine level at rest, especially early in the clinical development of hypertension.

—In those with HBP, the baroreflexes seem to sustain, not counteract, HBP, a phenomenon known as "resetting the barostats," which could also be a result of hypertension rather than a cause.

—Some hypertensive patients have defective storage of norepinephrine, thereby permitting more to circulate.

• The renin-angiotensin system

—The juxtaglomerular apparatus helps regulate volume and pressure.

—Renin, a proteolytic enzyme formed in the granules of the juxtaglomerular apparatus cells, catalyzes conversion of the protein angiotensinogen I, a decapeptide; this inactive product is cleaved by a converting enzyme, primarily in the lung but also in the kidney and brain, to an octapeptide (angiotensin II), a potent vasoconstrictor that also stimulates release of aldosterone.

Renin
↓
Ag I
↓
Ag II

—Another substance found in the circulation is the des-ASP heptapeptide (angiotensin III), which is as active as angiotensin II in stimulating aldosterone release but has much less pressor activity.

—Renin secretion is controlled by at least four mechanisms that are not mutually exclusive:

~ A renal vascular receptor responds to changes in tension in the afferent arteriolar wall.

~ A macula densa receptor detects changes in the delivery rate or concentration of NaCl in the distal tubule.

~ Circulating angiotensin has a negative feedback effect on renin secretion.

~ The sympathetic nervous system stimulates renin secretion via the renal nerve mediated by beta receptors.

—Plasma renin activity (PRA) is usually normal in patients with primary HBP, but is suppressed in about 25% and elevated in about 15%.

~ HBP is more often accompanied by low renin levels in blacks and in older persons.

~ The accelerated (malignant) phase of hypertension is often accompanied by elevated PRA.

—Although angiotensin is generally accepted as being responsible for renovascular hypertension, at least in the early phase, there is no consensus about the role of the renin-angiotensin-aldosterone system in patients with primary HBP, even in those with high PRA.

• The mosaic theory

—States that multiple factors sustain elevated BP even though only one was initially responsible (e.g., the interaction between the sympathetic nervous system and the renin-angiotensin-aldosterone system):

~ Sympathetic innervation of the juxtaglomerular apparatus in the kidneys releases renin.

~ Angiotensin stimulates autonomic centers in the brain to increase sympathetic discharge.

~ Angiotensin stimulates production of aldosterone, which results in Na retention.

—Hypertension leads to more hypertension.

~ Other mechanisms become involved when HBP due to an identifiable cause

(e.g., catecholamine, renin, and angiotensin from renal artery stenosis; aldosterone from an adrenocortical adenoma) has existed for some time.

~ Smooth muscle cell hypertrophy and hyperplasia in the arterioles from prolonged hypertension reduce the caliber of the lumen, thereby increasing total peripheral resistance (TPR).

~ Trivial shortening of hypertrophied smooth muscle in the thickened wall of an arteriole reduces the radius of an already narrowed lumen to a much greater extent than if the muscle and lumen were normal.

~ This may be why the longer HBP has existed, the less likely surgery for secondary causes will restore BP to normal.

• Deficiency of a vasodilator substance

—Rather than excess of a vasoconstrictor (e.g., angiotensin, norepinephrine), a deficiency of a vasodilator may cause HBP.

~ The kallikrein system, which produces the potent vasodilator bradykinin, is now being studied.

~ Extracts of renal medulla contain vasodilators, including a neutral lipid and a prostaglandin; if these vasodilators were absent because of renal parenchymal disease or bilateral nephrectomy, it would result in elevated BP.

—The endothelium's role in hypertension is also being studied.

• Secondary hypertension

—This type of HBP is associated with renal parenchymal disease (e.g., chronic glomerulonephritis or pyelonephritis, polycystic renal disease, collagen disease of the kidney, obstructive uropathy) or pheochromocytoma, Cushing's syndrome, myxedema, coarctation of the aorta, or renovascular disease.

—Other associations may be oral contraceptive use, alcohol excess, sympathomimetics, corticosteroids, cocaine, or licorice.

—HBP resulting from chronic renal parenchymal disease occurs from a combination of a renin-dependent mechanism and a volume-dependent mechanism.

~ In most cases, increased renin activity cannot be demonstrated in peripheral blood, and meticulous attention to fluid balance usually controls HBP.

Primary Hypertension

Nephrosclerosis

Hallmark

Risk Factors
- Smoking
- Diabetes mellitus
- Age > 60 years
- Gender (men, postmenopausal women)
- Family history of cardiovascular disease: women > 65 years, men > 55 years

Pathology
- No early pathologic changes occur in primary hypertension.
- Later, generalized arteriolar sclerosis develops, especially in the kidney (nephrosclerosis); it is characterized by medial hypertrophy and hyalinization.
  - Nephrosclerosis is the hallmark of primary hypertension.
- Later, left ventricular (LV) hypertrophy and eventually dilation develop gradually.
- Coronary, cerebral, aortic, renal, and peripheral atherosclerosis are more common and more severe in those with hypertension; HBP accelerates atherogenesis.
- Hypertension is a more significant factor for stroke than for atherosclerotic heart disease.
- Tiny Charcot-Bouchard aneurysms, seen in perforating arteries, especially those of the basal ganglia, are frequently seen in people with hypertension, which may be a source of intracerebral hemorrhage.

Hemodynamics
- Not all patients with primary hypertension have normal CO and increased TPR; in the early labile phase of hypertension, CO is increased and TPR is inappropriately normal for the level of CO.
- TPR increases and CO later returns to normal, probably because of autoregulation.
- Patients with high, fixed diastolic pressures often have decreased CO.
- The role of the large veins in the pathophysiology of primary hypertension has not been studied; vasoconstriction early in the disease may contribute to increased CO.
- Plasma volume tends to decrease as BP increases, but some patients have expanded plasma volumes.

- Hemodynamics, plasma volume, and PRA variations are evidence that primary hypertension is more than a single entity, or that different mechanisms are involved in different stages of the disorder.
- Renal blood flow gradually decreases as the diastolic BP increases and arteriolar sclerosis begins.
- Glomerular filtration rate (GFR) remains normal until late in the disease and, as a result, filtration fraction is increased.
- Coronary, cerebral, and muscle blood flow is maintained unless concomitant severe atherosclerosis is present in the vascular beds.
- If heart failure (HF) is not present, CO is normal or increased, and peripheral resistance is generally high in hypertension due to pheochromocytoma, primary aldosteronism, renal artery disease, and renal parenchymal disease.
- Plasma volume is usually high due to primary aldosteronism or renal parenchymal disease, and may be subnormal in pheochromocytoma.

Systolic Hypertension (with Normal Diastolic Pressure)

- This is not a discrete entity; it often results from increased CO or stroke volume (e.g., labile phase of primary hypertension, thyrotoxicosis, arteriovenous fistula, aortic regurgitation).
- In older persons with normal or low CO, it usually reflects inelasticity of the aorta and its major branches (arteriosclerotic hypertension).

Signs and Symptoms
Signs and symptoms depend on the cause of hypertension, its duration and severity, and the degree of its effects on target organs.
- Primary hypertension is asymptomatic until complications develop in target organs (e.g., LV failure, atherosclerotic heart disease, cerebrovascular insufficiency with or without stroke, renal failure).
- A fourth heart sound (S_4) and broad, notched P-wave abnormalities on the electrocardiogram (ECG) are among the earliest signs of hypertensive heart disease.

  S_4 early sign

- Echocardiographic evidence of LV hypertrophy may appear later.
- Chest x-ray is often normal until the late dilated phase of hypertensive heart disease.

- Aortic dissection or leaking aneurysm of the aorta may be the first sign of hypertension or may complicate untreated hypertension.
- Polyuria, nocturia, diminished renal concentrating ability, proteinuria, microhematuria, and nitrogen retention are late manifestations of arteriolar nephrosclerosis.
- Retinal changes may include retinal hemorrhages, exudates, papilledema, and vascular accidents.
  —Stages of hypertensive retinopathy
    ~ Stage I: constriction of retinal arterioles only
    ~ Stage II: constriction and sclerosis of retinal arterioles
    ~ Stage III: hemorrhages and exudates in addition to vascular changes
    ~ Stage IV (malignant hypertension): papilledema

Diagnosis

Signs and Symptoms

- Diagnosis of primary hypertension is made by higher-than-normal systolic or diastolic BP readings (two BP readings, in both arms, on each of 3 days), after ruling out secondary causes of HBP.
  —More readings are often necessary for those in the lower ranges of hypertension and especially for patients with markedly labile hypertension.

Diagnostic Procedures

- History and physical examination
- CBC
- Serum K^+ (hypokalemia is typical of hyperaldosteronism)
- Fasting blood glucose (hyperglycemia is seen in diabetes and pheochromocytoma)
- Plasma lipids (to determine atherosclerosis risk)

- Serum uric acid (elevation is a contraindication for diuretic therapy)
- Urinalysis
- Renal function studies
- Serum amylase, creatinine, K, Na, glucose, total, high density, and low density lipoprotein cholesterol)
- ECG

- The more severe the hypertension, and the younger the patient, the more extensive the evaluation should be.
- Procedures to search for secondary causes (e.g., renal scintigraphy, chest x-ray, screening for pheochromocytoma, and renin-sodium profiling) are not routinely done.

Treatment (Tables 5-2 to 5-4, Box 5-1, and Tables 5-5 and 5-6)

Complications/End Results

Target organ disease (TOD); clinical cardiovascular disease (CCD)

- Heart disease
  —LV hypertrophy
  —Angina or prior myocardial infarction
  —Prior coronary revascularization
  —HF
- Stroke or transient ischemic attacks (TIAs)
- Nephropathy
- Peripheral vascular disease
- Retinopathy

Patient/Family Education

Lifestyle Modifications to Prevent and Treat Hypertension

- Lose weight if needed.
- Limit alcohol intake to ≤ 1 oz of ethanol (24 oz of beer, 10 oz of wine, 2 oz of 100-proof whiskey) per day (less for those with small stature).
- Increase aerobic exercise to 30 to 45 min 5 to 7 days/week.
- Reduce sodium intake to no more than 2.4 g (6 g of NaCl)/day.
- Maintain adequate intake of dietary potassium.
- Maintain adequate intake of dietary calcium and magnesium for health.
- Reduce intake of dietary fat and cholesterol.

Follow-up/Referral (Table 5-7)

Pheochromocytoma

Definition

Pheochromocytoma is a tumor of chromaffin cells that secrete catecholamines, causing hypertension.

(Because this type of tumor occurs only in (1 of 1000 patients with hypertension, its etiology and pathogenesis will not be presented here; the signs and symptoms, however, are included.)

TABLE 5-2
Combination Drugs Used for Arterial Hypertension

Class of Drug	Drugs
Diuretic with β-blocker	Propranolol hydrochloride and hydrochlorothiazide* *HCTZ*
	Metoprolol tartrate and hydrochlorothiazide*
	Atenolol and chlorthalidone*
	Timolol maleate and hydrochlorothiazide*
	Bisoprolol fumarate and hydrochlorothiazide†
Diuretic with ACE inhibitor	Captopril and hydrochlorothiazide*
	Benazepril hydrochloride and hydrochlorothiazide*
	Lisinopril and hydrochlorothiazide*
	Enalapril maleate and hydrochlorothiazide*
ACE inhibitor with calcium blocker	Amlodipine and benazepril hydrochloride*
Angiotensin II receptor blocker with diuretic	Losartan and hydrochlorothiazide*

From Barker LR: Hypertension. In Barker LR, Burton JR, Zieve PD, eds: *Principles of ambulatory medicine*, ed 5, Baltimore, 1999, Williams & Wilkins, pp 844-867.
*Not approved for initial therapy.
†Approved for initial therapy.

TABLE 5-3
β -Blockers Used for Arterial Hypertension

Drug	Trade Name	Usual Daily Dose	Adverse Effects	Comments
Acebutolol*†	Sectral	200-800 mg	Bronchospasm, fatigue,	Contraindicated in pa-
Atenolol*	Tenormin	25-100 mg	insomnia, sexual	tients with asthma,
Betaxolol*	Kerlone	10-20 mg	dysfunction, exacer-	greater than first-
Bisoprolol*	Zebeta	2.5-20 mg	bation of HF, mask-	degree heart block, or
Carteolol†	Cartrol	2.5-10 mg	ing of symptoms	sick sinus syndrome;
Carvedilol†	Coreg	12.5-50 mg‡	of hypoglycemia,	use with caution in
Labetalol†	Normodyne	200-1800 mg‡	triglycerideemia,	HF and insulin-treated
	Trandate	200-1800 mg‡	decreased high den-	diabetics; should not
Metoprolol*	Lopressor	50-300 mg‡	sity lipoprotein cho-	be discontinued
	Toprol XL	50-300 mg‡	lesterol (except for	abruptly in patients
Nadolol	Corgard	40-240 mg	pindolol, acebutolol,	with ischemic heart
Penbutolol†	Levatol	20-40 mg	penbutolol, carteolol,	disease; carvedilol has
Pindolol†	Visken	10-60 mg‡	and labetalol)	been approved for
Propranolol	Inderal	40-320 mg‡		treating CHF
Propranolol, long-acting	Inderal LA	60-320 mg		
Timolol	Blocadren	20-60 mg‡		

From Massie BM: Systemic hypertension. In Tierney LM, McPhee SJ, Papadakis MA, eds: *Current medical diagnosis & treatment 2000,* New York, 2000, Lange Medical Books/McGraw-Hill, pp 454-455.
*Cardioselective.
†Carteolol, penbutolol, and pindolol are partial agonists (intrinsic sympathomimetic activity).
‡Usually given in divided doses bid.

TABLE 5-4

Calcium Blockers Used for Arterial Hypertension

Class	Drug	Trade Name	Usual Dose qd	Adverse Effects	Comments
Benzothiazepine derivatives	Diltiazem, sustained release	Cardizem SR	120-360 mg*	Headache, dizziness, asthenia, flushing, edema, negative inotropic effect	Contraindicated in heart failure due to systolic dysfunction, sick sinus syndrome, or greater than first-degree heart block; may cause liver dysfunction
	Diltiazem, extended release	Cardizem CD	120-360 mg		
		Dilacor XR	120-360 mg		
		Tiazac	120-360 mg		
Diphenyl-alkyamine derivatives	Verapamil	Calan	120-360 mg†	Same as for benzothiazepine derivatives, plus constipation	Same as for benzothiazepine derivatives
		Isoptin	120-360 mg†		
	Verapamil, sustained release	Covera-HS	120-480 mg‡		
		Calan SR	120-480 mg		
		Isoptin SR	120-480 mg		
		Verelan	120-480 mg		
Dihydropyridines	Amlodipine	Norvasc	2.5-10 mg	Dizziness, flushing, headache, weakness, nausea, heartburn, pedal edema, gingival hyperplasia, tachycardia	Contraindicated in CHF, with the possible exception of amlodipine; research has shown an association between short-acting nifedipine therapy and increase in MI
	Felodipine	Plendil	5-20 mg		
	Isradipine	DynaCirc	5-20 mg*		
		DynaCirc CR	5-20 mg		
	Nicardipine	Cardene	60-120 mg†		
	Nicardipine, sustained release	Cardene SR	60-120 mg*		
			30-90 mg		
	Nifedipine, extended release	Procardia XL	30-90 mg		
		Adalat CC			
	Nisoldipine	Sular	10-60 mg		

From Massie BM: Systemic hypertension. In Tierney LM, McPhee SJ, Papadakis MA, eds: *Current medical diagnosis & treatment 2000,* New York, 2000, Lange Medical Books/McGraw-Hill, p 458.
*Usually given in divided doses bid.
†Usually given in divided doses tid.
‡Entire dose is given at bedtime.

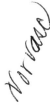

Diagnosis

Signs and Symptoms

- Hypertension is the most dominant sign, which may be paroxysmal (45%) or persistent (50%), but is rarely absent (5%).
- The elevated BP is caused by secretion of one or more of the catecholamine hormones or precursors: norepinephrine, epinephrine, dopamine, or dopa.
- Tachycardia
- Diaphoresis
- Postural hypotension
- Tachypnea
- Flushing
- Cold, clammy skin
- Severe headache
- Angina
- Palpitation
- Nausea and vomiting
- Epigastric pain
- Visual disturbances
- Dyspnea
- Paresthesias
- Constipation
- A sense of impending doom
- Paroxysmal attacks may be precipitated by palpation of the tumor, postural changes, abdominal compression or massage, β-blockers, and micturition, if the tumor is in the bladder.

BOX 5-1
Calcium Blockers

- Calcium blockers are potent peripheral vasodilators; they reduce BP by decreasing TPR.
- Verapamil and diltiazem slow the heart rate, decrease AV conduction, and have a negative inotropic effect on myocardial contractility (similar to β-blockers).
  - Should not be given to patients with > first-degree heart block or LV failure.
- β-Blockers, verapamil, and diltiazem should not be given to patients with LV dysfunction.
- The dihydropyridine derivatives (amlodipine, felodipine, isradipine, nicardipine, nifedipine, nisoldipine) have a less negative inotropic effect than the nondihydropyridines, but can cause reflexive tachycardia in some patients.
- These drugs are more potent peripheral vasodilators than the nondihydropyridines, making them effective in most patients; in long-term therapy, however, their effects do not seem to be more potent than nondihydropyridine calcium blockers.
- As indicated, studies (nonrandomized case-control and cohort) show that short-acting nifedipine was associated with increased rates of MI compared with other classes of drugs; therefore it should not be used to treat hypertension, nor should short-acting diltiazem be used as an antihypertensive; long-acting calcium blockers are preferred.
- Calcium blockers are preferred over β-blockers for hypertensive patients with angina pectoris and bronchospastic disease of Raynaud's disease.

Data from information presented by Gottlieb SH, Calkins H: Arrythmias. In Barker LR, Burton JR, Zieve PD, eds: *Principles of ambulatory medicine,* ed 5, Baltimore, 1999, Williams & Wilkins, pp 768-798, 821-843.

TABLE 5-5
ACE Inhibitors Used for Arterial Hypertension

Drug	Trade Name	Usual Daily Dose	Adverse Effects	Comments
ACE INHIBITORS				
Benazepril	Lotensin	10-40 mg	Rash, cough,	Contraindicated in pregnancy; can cause
Captopril	Capoten	25-300 mg*	angioedema,	reversible acute renal failure in
Enalapril	Vasotec	5-40 mg	hyperkalemia,	patients with bilateral renal arterial
Fosinopril	Monopril	10-60 mg	dysgeusia	stenosis or unilateral stenosis in a solitary kidney; proteinuria may occur,
Lisinopril	Prinivil	5-40 mg		rare at recommended doses; hyper-
	Zestril	5-40 mg		kalemia can occur, especially in those
Moexipril	Univasc	7.5-30 mg*		with renal insufficiency or taking
Quinapril	Accupril	5-80 mg		NSAIDs, potassium-sparing diuretics,
Ramipril	Altace	2.5-10 mg		or potassium supplements; hypotension
Trandolapril	Mavik	1-4 mg		occurs at beginning of therapy, in those with high plasma renin activity or receiving diuretic therapy, or with other causes of hypovolemia
ANGIOTENSIN II RECEPTOR BLOCKERS				
Irbesartan	Avapro	75-300 mg	Dizziness,	Contraindicated in pregnancy; except for
Losartan	Cozaar	25-100 mg	angioedema	proteinuria and neutropenia, these
Valsartan	Diovan	80-320 mg	(rare)	drugs can produce the same adverse effects as ACE inhibitors on renal function, serum potassium, and BP

From Massie BM: Systemic hypertension. In Tierney LM, McPhee SJ, Papadakis MA, eds: *Current medical diagnosis & treatment 2000,* New York, 2000, Lange Medical Books/McGraw-Hill, p 457.
NSAIDs, Nonsteroidal antiinflammatory drugs.
*Usually given in divided doses bid.

TABLE 5-6
Adrenergic Inhibitors Used for Arterial Hypertension

Class	Drug	Trade Name	Usual Dose	Adverse Effects	Comments
Central-acting α-agonists	Clonidine	Catapres	0.1-1.2 mg/day* to	Drowsiness, sedation, dry mouth, fatigue, sexual dysfunction; localized skin reaction to clonidine patch	Rebound hypertension may occur with abrupt discontinuance, especially with prior therapy with high doses or with continuation of concomitant β-blockers; methyldopa may cause liver damage and Coombs'-positive hemolytic anemia; should be used cautiously in older persons because of orthostatic hypotension; interferes with measurements of urinary catecholamine levels by fluorometric methods
	Clonidine transdermal	Catapres TTS	0.1-0.3 mg/wk		
	Guanabenz	Wytensin	4-64 mg/day*		
	Guanfacine	Tenex	1-3 mg/day		
	Methyldopa	Aldomet	500-2000 mg/day*		
α-Adrenergic blockers	Doxazosin	Cardura	1-16 mg/day	"First-dose" syncope, orthostatic hypotension, weakness, palpitations, headache	Use cautiously in older persons because of orthostatic hypotension; relieves symptoms of benign prostatic hypertrophy
	Prazosin	Minipress	2-20 mg/day*		
	Terazosin	Hytrin	1-20 mg/day		
Peripheral-acting adrenergic blockers	Guanadrel sulfate	Hylorel	10-100 mg/day	Diarrhea, sexual dysfunction, orthostatic hypotension guanadrel SO_4, guanethidine; lethargy, nasal congestion, depression, activation of peptic ulcer (rauwolfia alkaloids, reserpine)	Contraindicated in patients with history of depression (reserpine); use cautiously in patients with history of peptic ulcer (reserpine); use cautiously because of orthostatic hypotension (guanadrel SO_4, guanethidine)
	Guanethidine	Ismelin	10-100 mg/day		
	Rauwolfia alkaloids	—	50-100 mg/day		
	Reserpine	—	0.1-0.2 mg/day		

From Massie BM: Systemic hypertension. In Tierney LM, McPhee SJ, Papadakis MA, eds: *Current medical diagnosis & treatment 2000,* New York, 2000, Lange Medical Books/McGraw-Hill, p 460.
*Given in divided doses bid.

TABLE 5-7
Follow-up Guidelines R/T Blood Pressure Readings

Blood Pressure	Systolic	Diastolic	Follow-up Schedule
Normal	<130	<85	Recheck in 2 years
High normal	130-139	85-90	Recheck in 1 year (lifestyle changes)
HYPERTENSION			
Stage 1 (mild)	140-159	90-99	Confirm within 2 months
Stage 2 (moderate)	160-179	100-109	Evaluate/refer within 1 month
Stage 3 (severe	>180	>110	Evaluate/refer within 1 week

From Sixth Report of the Joint National Committee on Detection, Education, and Treatment of High Blood Pressure (JNC VI), *Archives of Internal Medicine* 157:2413, 1997.

- Because of their hyperkinetic states, these patients may appear hyperthyroid, but are euthyroid.

Diagnostic Procedures
- Physical examination is usually normal unless performed during a paroxysmal attack.
- The severity of retinopathy and cardiomegaly is often less than might be expected, related to the degree of hypertension.
- Urinalysis may show that the urinary metabolic products of epinephrine and norepinephrine are the metanephrines: vanillylmandelic acid (VMA) and homovanillic acid (HVA).
- These substances may appear sporadically in persons with pheochromocytoma but are also seen in patients; in coma, dehydration, or extreme stress states; in those being treated with rauwolfia alkaloids, methyldopa, or catecholamines; or after ingestion of foods containing large amounts of vanilla, especially if renal insufficiency is present.

Treatment
- Phentolamine mesylate must be available to terminate any hypertensive crisis.
- Surgical removal of the tumor is the treatment of choice, after the patient has been restored to optimal physical condition by the use of a combination of α- and β-blockers (phenoxybenzamine 40 to 160 mg/day and propranolol 30 to 60 mg/day PO, in divided doses).

Prognosis
- Patients with hypertension who are untreated are at great risk of a disabling or fatal LV failure, myocardial infarction (MI), cerebral hemorrhage or infarction, or renal failure at an early age.
- Hypertension is the most significant risk factor predisposing to stroke (cigarette smoking and hypercholesterolemia are other risk factors), and to coronary atherosclerosis.
- The higher the BP and the more severe the retinal changes, the worse the prognosis.
  - Fewer than 5% of patients with group 4 (malignant) hypertension with papilledema and less than 10% of patients with group 3 changes in the retina survive 1 year without treatment.
- Coronary artery disease is the most common cause of death among treated hypertensive patients.
- Systolic BP is a more significant predictor of fatal and nonfatal cardiovascular events than diastolic BP.
  - In a follow-up of men screened for the Multiple Risk Factor Intervention Trial, overall mortality was related to systolic BP, regardless of diastolic BP.
- In cases of pheochromocytoma, unless the tumor is malignant, the outcome of treatment and surgery is favorable.

Patient/Family Education
- Primary hypertension is a treatable (but not curable) disease.
- Diet, exercise, lowering of serum cholesterol, reduced salt (and perhaps potassium) intake, and weight loss all help to lower BP.
- Patients should be thoroughly knowledgeable about the condition, and how their self-care measures can control BP and help to prolong their lives.
- All medications should be explained as to reason for prescribing, action, dose, and schedule.
  - Emphasize the importance of taking medications according to directions.
  - Provide a list of ways that will help patients remember to take medications on time.

ANGINA PECTORIS
Definition
Angina pectoris is a clinical syndrome due to myocardial ischemia characterized by precordial discomfort or pressure, typically precipitated by exertion and relieved by rest or sublingual nitroglycerine.

Risk Factors
- Hypertension
- History of high blood lipids (increase in concentration of total cholesterol and low-density lipoprotein [LDL], low concentration of high-density lipoproteins [HDL]
- History of atherosclerotic heart disease
- Severe myocardial hypertrophy

- Severe aortic stenosis or insufficiency
- Increased metabolic demands (e.g., hyperthyroidism, anemia, paroxysmal tachycardia with rapid ventricular rates)
- Diabetes mellitus
- Cigarette smoking
- Oral contraceptives
- Personality type
- Sedentary lifestyle
- High-fat diet
- Obesity

Etiology/Cause

- Cause of angina pectoris is usually critical coronary artery obstruction due to atherosclerosis.
- Coronary embolism
- Aortic regurgitation
- Hypertrophic subaortic stenosis (increases cardiac workload)

Pathogenesis

- Patients with a long history of angina are found, at autopsy, to have extensive coronary atherosclerosis and patchy myocardial fibrosis.
- There may be microscopic or gross evidence of old MI.
- Angina occurs when cardiac work and myocardial O_2 demand exceed the ability of the coronary arteries to supply oxygenated blood.
  - Heart rate, systolic tension or arterial pressure, and contractility are the major determinants of myocardial O_2 demand.
  - An increase in any of these factors in a setting of reduced coronary blood flow can induce angina.
    - ~ Exercise in the patient with a critical degree of coronary stenosis induces angina, which is relieved by rest.
- As the myocardium becomes ischemic, coronary sinus blood pH falls, cellular K loss occurs, lactate production replaces lactate use, ECG abnormalities appear, and ventricular performance deteriorates.
- LV diastolic pressure often rises during angina, to levels that induce pulmonary congestion and dyspnea.
- The pain associated with angina is believed to be a direct manifestation of myocardial ischemia and resulting accumulation of hypoxic metabolites.

Diagnosis

Signs and Symptoms

- The characteristics of angina are usually constant for a given patient, so that any change/deterioration in the pattern of symptoms should be considered serious (e.g., increased intensity, decreased threshold of stimulus, longer duration, occurrence when the patient is sedentary or just waking from sleep).
- Angina is most frequently precipitated by physical activity, usually lasts no longer than a few minutes, and subsides with rest.
- Angina discomfort is worse if exercise follows a meal.
- Symptoms are worse during cold weather, when walking into the wind, or on first contact with cold air on leaving a warm room.
- Angina may occur at night, preceded by a dream that is accompanied by striking changes in respiration, heart rate, and BP.
- Angina attacks may occur several times a day or may be occasional episodes, with no symptoms between attacks.
- Attacks may increase (crescendo angina) to a fatal outcome, or may gradually decrease or disappear if adequate collateral coronary circulation develops, if the ischemic area becomes infarcted, or if HF or intermittent claudication supervenes and limits activity.
- Angina may occur at rest (angina decubitus), usually accompanied by moderate increases in heart rate and BP; if the angina is not relieved, the higher BP and increased heart rate may increase unmet myocardial O_2 needs and make MI more likely.
- Often the discomfort associated with angina is not perceived as pain.
  - Patients describe it as an ache, pressure ("it feels like an elephant is standing on my chest"), rapidly becomes a severe, intense, precordial crushing sensation.
  - Discomfort may radiate to the left shoulder and arm; straight through to the back; to the throat, jaws, and teeth; or may be felt in the upper abdomen.
  - Because the discomfort of angina seldom occurs in the area of the cardiac apex, the patient who points to this exact area or describes fleeting, sharp, or hot sensations usually does not have angina.

- Location of the discomfort is variable but most often is substernal.
- During attacks of angina, signs of heart disease may be absent, although during an attack, the heart rate may increase somewhat, BP is often elevated, apical impulse is more diffuse, and heart sounds become more distant.
- Palpation of the precordium may reveal localized systolic bulging or paradoxical movement, reflecting segmental myocardial ischemia and regional dyskinesia.
- In the ischemic episode, the second heart sound may become paradoxical due to prolonged LV ejection.
- A fourth heart sound is common.
- A midsystolic or late-systolic apical murmur (shrill but not loud) may be heard, due to papillary muscle dysfunction secondary to ischemia.

Diagnostic Tests
- The diagnosis is confirmed if reversible ischemic ECG changes are seen during an attack.
  —S-T segment depression
  —ST segment elevation
  —Decreased R-wave height
  —Intraventricular or bundle branch conduction disturbances
  —Dysrhythmias, usually ventricular extrasystoles
- An abnormal resting ECG neither establishes nor refutes the diagnosis.
- A test dose of sublingual nitroglycerin will relieve discomfort in from 1.5 to 3 minutes.
- Between attacks, the ECG and LV function tests are normal in 30% of patients.
- Exercise stress ECG testing: an ischemic ECG response during or after exercise is characterized by a flat or downward-sloping ST segment depression ≥ 0.1 mV (1 mm on the ECG when properly calibrated), lasting ≥0.08 sec.

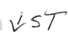

Differential Diagnosis (Table 5-8)

Treatment
- The goal of therapy is to prevent or reduce ischemia and minimize symptoms.
- The underlying cause of the angina must be determined.
- The primary risk factors must be reduced as much as possible.
- Smoking cessation for ≥ 2 years reduces the risk of MI to the level of those who never smoked.
- Hypertension should be treated diligently; even mild hypertension increases cardiac workload.

TABLE 5-8	
Causes of Chest Pain	
Causes	**Examples**
COMMON	
Chest wall	Nonspecific musculoskeletal, costochondritis, Tietze's syndrome
Cardiac	Angina
Pulmonary	Tracheitis, pleurodynia, pneumonia
Gastrointestinal	Esophageal reflux/spasm
Neurologic	Cervical spine disease (radicular)
LESS COMMON	
Chest wall	Herpes zoster, thoracic outlet syndrome, fractured rib, tumor
Cardiac	Dissecting aortic aneurysm, pericarditis
Pulmonary	Pneumothorax, pulmonary hypertension
Gastrointestinal	Peptic ulcer disease, abdominal infection, peritonitis

From White P, Georas SN: Common pulmonary problems: cough, hemoptysis, dyspnea, chest pain, and abnormal chest x-ray. In Barker LR, Burton JR, Zieve PD, eds: *Principles of ambulatory medicine*, ed 5, Baltimore, 1999, Williams & Wilkins, p 668.

- Digitalis sometimes intensifies angina, probably because increased myocardial contractility raises O_2 demand in the presence of fixed coronary blood flow.
- Reduction of total and LDL cholesterol with diet supplemented by drugs if necessary
- An exercise program that emphasizes walking should be introduced.
- Three classes of drugs are usually effective, alone or in combination.
  —Nitrates
  —β-Blockers
    ~ These two classes completely block sympathetic stimulation of the heart and reduce systolic pressure, heart rate, contractility, and CO, which decreases cardiac O_2 demand.
  —Calcium blockers
    ~ These vasodilators are an important part of therapy, particularly regarding angina with hypertension and to counter coronary spasm, if present.
- Antiplatelet drugs are used to oppose platelet aggregation, a major factor in the genesis of MI and unstable angina.
- If these measures do not elicit appropriate patient response, angioplasty and coronary artery bypass surgery must be considered, at which point the patient is referred to cardiac specialists.

Prognosis

- The major adverse outcomes of angina pectoris are unstable angina, MI, recurrent MI, and sudden death due to dysrhythmias.
- Annual mortality is about 1.4% in men with angina and no history of MI, a normal resting ECG, and normal BP.
- Mortality increases to 7.5% if systolic hypertension is present, to 8.4% when the ECG is abnormal, and to 12% if both risk factors are present.
- Lesions of the left main coronary artery or in the proximal anterior descending vessel indicate particularly high risk; although outcome correlates with the number and severity of coronary vessels involved, in stable patients, the prognosis is surprisingly good, even with three-vessel disease, if ventricular function is normal.
- Reduced ventricular function, usually measured by analysis of ejection fraction, adversely influ-

ences prognosis, especially in patients with three-vessel disease.
- Prognosis also correlates with symptoms, and is better in patients with mild or moderate angina (Class I or II) than in those with severe exercise-induced angina (Class III).

Patient/Family Education

- Educate the patient and family, as necessary, regarding cigarette smoking, high-fat diet, high total cholesterol and LDL, low HDL, and how these can be changed.
- Emphasize the importance of exercise, and that tolerance can be increased gradually by small increments every day or week.
- Explain all medications: reasons for giving, action, side effects, and dose and scheduling.
- List signs and symptoms that indicate need to call the clinician immediately.
- Outline a low-fat diet.
- Outline a plan for smoking cessation.

MYOCARDIAL INFARCTION
Definition

Ischemic myocardial necrosis usually results from abrupt reduction in coronary blood flow to a segment of myocardium.

Risk Factors

- History of angina pectoris and undiagnosed atherosclerosis of the coronary arteries.
- Patients who develop angina and MI often have a history of cigarette smoking, high-fat diet, and sedentary lifestyle.

Etiology/Cause

- In over 90% of patients with acute MI, the cause is an acute thrombus, often associated with plaque rupture, which occludes the artery that supplies the damaged area, which was previously partially obstructed by an atherosclerotic plaque.
- Altered platelet function resulting from endothelial changes in the atherosclerotic plaque is assumed to contribute to thrombogenesis.
- Right ventricular infarction usually results from occlusion of the right coronary or a dominant left circumflex artery.
- MI has been reported in patients with coronary spasm and otherwise normal coronary arteries.

- Cocaine causes intense coronary arterial spasm; users of this drug may present with cocaine-induced angina or MI.

Pathogenesis

- MI is predominantly a disease of the LV, but damage may extend to the right ventricle or the atria.
- Some degree of RV dysfunction occurs in about 50% of patients with an inferior-posterior infarction, producing hemodynamic abnormality in 10% to 15% of patients.
- Inferior-posterior infarcts occur as a result of right coronary occlusion or occlusion of a dominant left circumflex artery.
- The extent of myocardial damage correlates with the ability of the heart to continue functioning as a pump.
- Patients who die from cardiogenic shock usually have an infarct, or a combination of scar and new infarct, of ≥ 50% of LV mass.
- Anterior infarcts tend to be larger and have a worse prognosis than inferior-posterior infarcts.
  —These infarcts usually result from occlusion of the left coronary arterial tree, especially the anterior descending artery.
- Transmural infarcts involve the whole thickness of myocardium from epicardium to endocardium.
  —These infarcts are characterized by abnormal Q waves on ECG.
  —Nontransmural or subendocardial infarcts do not extend through the ventricular wall and cause only ST segment and T-wave abnormalities.
  —The depth of transmural necrosis cannot be exactly determined clinically; these are classified by ECG as either Q wave or non-Q wave.
  —The volume of myocardium destroyed can be estimated by the extent and duration of creatine kinase (CK) elevation.

Diagnosis

Signs and Symptoms

- About two thirds of patients experience prodromal symptoms days to weeks before the actual MI occurs.
  —Unstable or crescendo angina
  —Shortness of breath
  —Fatigue

- The first symptom of acute MI usually is deep, substernal, visceral pain described as aching or pressure, often with radiation to the back, jaw, or left neck and arm.
- The pain is similar to that of angina, but is generally more severe, longer lasting, and relieved little if any by rest or nitroglycerin.
- About 20% of MIs are "silent" in that the discomfort is mild, and may go unnoticed by the patient, particularly women.
- In cases of severe MI, the patient may become quite anxious and have a sense of impending doom.
- Nausea and vomiting may occur, especially in inferior MI.
- Related symptoms may be present: those of LV failure, pulmonary edema, shock, or significant dysrhythmias.
- On examination, the patient appears to be in severe pain, is restless and apprehensive, with pale, cool, diaphoretic skin.
- Peripheral or central cyanosis may be present.
- The BP is often variable, and the pulse may be thready.
- Heart sounds are usually somewhat distant.
- An S₄ is virtually always present.
- A soft, blowing systolic murmur may occur, reflecting papillary muscle dysfunction.
- Friction rubs, usually evanescent, are common on the second and third day post-MI, with Q-wave infarcts.

Complications

- Dysrhythmia
- Sinus node disturbances
- Atrial dysrhythmias
- Atrioventricular (AV) block
- Ventricular dysrhythmias
- Heart failure (HF)
- Right ventricular (RV) infarction
- Hypoxemia
- Hypotension
- Cardiogenic shock
- Recurrent ischemia
- Functional papillary muscle insufficiency
- Myocardial rupture
- Pseudoaneurysm
- Ventricular aneurysm
- Ventricular asynergy
- Mural thrombosis

TABLE 5-9

Killip (Clinical) Classification of Heart Failure in Patients with Acute MI

Class	Description	Incidence (%)	Mortality (%)
I	No HF	40	5
II	Mild LV failure	40	20
III	Pulmonary edema	10	40
IV	Cardiogenic shock	10	90

From Camm AJ: Cardiovascular disease. In Kumar P, Clark M, eds: *Clinical medicine*, ed 4, Edinburgh, 1998, WB Saunders, p 696.

- Pericarditis
- Post-MI syndrome (Dressler's syndrome): develops days, weeks, or months after an MI, with fever, pericarditis with friction rub, pericardial effusion, pleurisy, pleural effusions, pulmonary infiltrates, joint pains

Confirmation of Diagnosis
- History
- Initial and serial ECG
- Serial enzyme changes
- In some cases, definitive diagnosis may not be possible.
- ECG findings are the most important evidence of occurrence of MI.
- Blood tests: erythrocyte sedimentation rate (ESR) is elevated after 12 hours; white blood cell count (WBC) is moderately elevated; differential WBC reveals a shift to the left; CK of cardiac muscle (CK-MB) is seen in blood within 6 hours of myocardial necrosis; levels are high for 36 to 48 hours.
- A normal CK-MB for 24 hours virtually rules out MI.
- Myocardial imaging: slow and expensive, and usually only marginally helpful in diagnosis of MI.
- Right heart catheterization: measurement of right heart, pulmonary artery, and wedge pressures using balloon-tipped catheters that float into position (Swan-Ganz) may help in treatment of complications: severe HF, hypoxia, hypotension.

Treatment
- Most patients with acute MI are hospitalized immediately and cared for in intensive care units (ICUs); primary care clinicians are not involved in the treatment of these patients.

- The goals of therapy are to relieve distress, reverse ischemia, limit infarct size, reduce cardiac work, and prevent and treat complications.

Prognosis
- Predictors of 90% of the mortality in patients presenting with acute MI or S-T segment elevation and receiving thrombolytic therapy
  —Older age (31% of total mortality)
  —Lower systolic BP (24%)
  —Killip class 1 (15%) (Table 5-9)
  —Faster heart rate (12%)
  —Anterior location (6%)
- Of those who die, 60% die of primary ventricular failure before reaching the hospital.
- Mortality of those who survive initial hospitalization in the year after acute MI is 8% to 10%.
- Most deaths occur in the first 3 to 4 months.
- Survivors are at high risk if the following are present: continued ventricular dysrhythmia, HF or poor ventricular function, and recurrent ischemia.
- Good exercise performance without ECG abnormalities indicates a favorable prognosis; abnormal exercise performance is related to poor prognosis.

Patient/Family Education
- Preventive measures should be emphasized in patients with angina.
  —Low-fat, low-salt diet
  —Treatment of hypertension or other circulatory problem
  —Box 5-2 shows the plan of care for MI survivors after hospitalization.
  —Frequent evaluation
- If MI occurs
  —Instruct family about what therapy will likely take place.

BOX 5-2

Plan of Care for MI Survivors after Hospitalization

PATIENT EDUCATION (PATIENT AND SPOUSE/ FAMILY MEMBER)

Understands disease process (damage to the heart that heals in a few months, but leaves a scar)

Understands likely prognosis

Understands and follows progressive activity schedule

Understands approximate timetable for return to work

Understands importance of controlling major risk factors (smoking, hypercholesterolemia, hypertension) and takes responsibility for controlling them

Knows how to recognize principal cardiac symptoms (angina, tachycardia, HF, hypotension) and understands how to use sublingual nitroglycerin

Participates in group classes: counseling, exercise, nutrition

Seeks answers to questions specific to himself/herself

MEDICAL MANAGEMENT

Reviews in-hospital course for prognosis characteristics and medications prescribed at discharge

Assesses and reinforces education points listed above

Checks periodically for complications of infarction (angina, CHF, dysrhythmias)

Checks periodically for indicators of stress, anxiety, depression

Checks ECG 2-3 months after discharge

Some patients receive additional education regarding specific drugs, when prescribed: ACE inhibitor, calcium antagonist, aspirin, β-blocker

Referral for physical conditioning

From Vaitkevicius PV, Stewart KJ: Postmyocardial infarction care, cardiac rehabilitation, and physical conditioning. In Barker LR, Burton JR, Zieve PD, eds: *Principles of ambulatory medicine*, ed 5, Baltimore, 1999, Williams & Wilkins, p 750.

—Keep family and patient informed of progress.

—During critical period, allow family to call the ICU at any time.

• On discharge of patient

—Instructions about rest, exercise, medications, and other aspects of care should be typed and given to the family member who will be providing care.

—The American Heart Association provides patient education and information in a booklet, *After a Heart Attack.*

—All information about medications should be written: reason for giving, action, dose and timing of administration, side effects.

—A list of resources, including names of physicians, nurses, dietitians, and physical therapists, should be provided.

—A schedule of return appointments should be given to the family/patient.

HEART DISEASE
Definition

Heart disease is a general classification of various types of heart conditions that include heart block, dysrhythmias, cardiovascular disease, coronary artery disease (angina), MI, heart murmurs, and HF. Angina and MI have been addressed. Additional sections will be devoted to dysrhythmias, murmurs, peripheral vascular disease, and HF.

CARDIAC DYSRHYTHMIAS
Introduction

New information from electrophysiologic studies of dysrhythmias has expanded our knowledge about the mechanisms that cause dysrhythmias to occur: (1) disorders of impulse formation or automaticity, (2) abnormalities of impulse conduction, (3) reentry, and (4) triggered activity.

Altered automaticity is the mechanism for sinus node arrest, premature beats, and automatic rhythms, and is an initiating factor in reentry dysrhythmias.

Abnormalities of impulse conduction occur at the sinus or AV node, in the intraventricular conduction system, and in the atria or ventricles. These result in sinoatrial (SA) exit block, AV block at the node or below, and development of reentry circuits.

Reentry is the mechanism responsible for many dysrhythmias (e.g., premature beats, most paroxysmal supraventricular tachycardias, and atrial flutter). For reentry to occur, there must be an area of unidirectional block with a related delay to allow repeat depolarization at the site of origin. Reentry is confirmed if the dysrhythmia can be terminated by interruption of the circuit by spontaneous or induced premature beat.

Triggered activity occurs when electrical activity persists after repolarization (after depolarization) and reaches the threshold level required to trigger a new depolarization. This is considered to be the mechanism causing ventricular tachycardia in the prolonged QT syndrome, and in some cases of digitalis toxicity.

Anatomy and Physiology

- A cluster of cells (SA node or sinus node), located at the junction of the superior vena cava and the high right atrium, forms the primary electric generator (pacemaker) of the normal heart.
- These cells produce a rhythmic discharge modulated by autonomic innervation and by circulating catecholamines.
- SA node activity is not seen on the surface ECG but occurs 80 to 120 msec before the onset of the P wave, which represents depolarization of atrial myocardial cells.
- Transmission of impulses from the SA node through the atrium to the AV node appears to be through normal, unspecialized myocardial cells; however, a preferential route of conduction is determined by the muscle bundles that form the atrium.
- The atria are electrically insulated from the ventricles, except by the AV node, whose tortuous conduction pathway delays impulse transmission.
- The AV nodal refractory period usually is longer than that of other heart tissue, is heart-rate dependent, and is modulated by autonomic tone and by catecholamines, adjusting to maximize cardiac output for any given heart rate.
- The AV node is on the atrial side of the annulus fibrosus; specialized conduction tissue, the His bundle, runs along the tricuspid valve ring to the valve trigone, penetrating the annulus fibrosus and continuing through the membranous interventricular septum.
- Where the membranous septum becomes muscular septum, the His bundle divides.
  —The right bundle branch continues down to the right ventricular endocardial surface to reach the anterior and apical muscle of the right ventricle.
  —The main left bundle branch crosses the summit of the muscular interventricular septum to emerge on the left side of the heart just below the noncoronary cusp of the aortic valve; the left bundle divides in a variable manner, but functionally gives rise to a left posterior fascicle, which innervates the septum, and a left anterior fascicle.

- The SA node, perhaps the AV node, and most of the specialized conducting tissues are capable of automatic (spontaneous) phase 4 diastolic depolarization.
- The intrinsic pacemaker rate is highest in the SA node, which dominates the lower, slower latent cardiac pacemakers.
- Sinus rhythm varies remarkably on short-term and long-term recordings.
- Respiratory sinus dysrhythmia, mediated by oscillations in vagal tone, is particularly common in young persons.
  —The oscillations are dampened by, but do not completely disappear with, age.
- Exercise and emotion are potent accelerators of sinus rhythm through sympathetic neural and catecholamine drive.
- Resting sinus rates of 60 to 100 beats/min classically represent the limits of normal, but much slower sinus rates occur in young persons, particularly those trained as athletes.
  —Resting heart rates of <60 beats/min (sinus bradycardia) are not pathologic.
- Sinus tachycardia (ST) is the term used for fast (>100 beats/min) rates.
- Normal persons have a marked diurnal variation in heart rate, with lowest rates present just before early morning waking, when sinus acceleration is substantial.
- Absolute regularity of sinus rhythm is pathologic and occurs with autonomic denervation, as in advanced diabetes.
  See Figures 5-1 through 5-10.

Etiology/Pathogenesis

- Bradydysrhythmias arise through abnormalities of intrinsic automatic conduction, primarily within the AV node and the His-Purkinje network.
- Tachydysrhythmias may develop because of altered automaticity, reentry, or triggered automaticity, which have been identified electrophysiologically but can rarely be differentiated clinically.
  —Most clinically significant tachydysrhythmias are probably caused by reentry.
- Some dysrhythmias cause few or no symptoms but are associated with adverse outcomes.
  —Evidence exists that indicates that prognosis is not necessarily improved by suppressing the dysrhythmias.

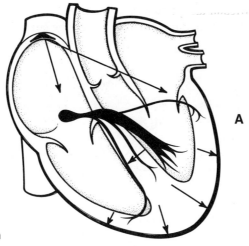

Normal sinus rhythm

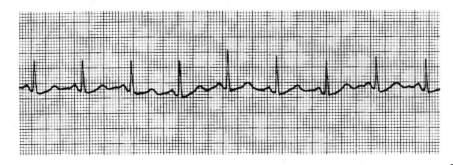

B

- P waves: the P waves are positive (upright) and uniform in lead II. Every P wave is followed by a QRS complex.

- P-R Interval: the normal P-R interval (from the beginning of the P wave to the beginning of the QRS complex) is constant, between 0.12 and 0.2 second.

- QRS complex: the QRS complex duration is 0.1 second or less. Every QRS complex is preceded by a P wave.

- Rhythm: the rhythm is regular.

- Rate: the rate is between 60 and 100 beats/min. It is constant at a given rate, varying less than 10%.

Fig. 5-1   Heart rhythms and dysrhythmias normal sinus rhythm. (**A,** From Conover MB: *Pocket guide to electrocardiography,* ed 4, St. Louis, 1998, Mosby, Inc., p 7; **B,** from Sheehy SB, Lenehan GP: *Manual of emergency care,* ed 5, St. Louis, 1999, Mosby, Inc., p 58.)

- Other dysrhythmias, although symptomatic, are benign.
- The nature and severity of underlying heart disease are usually of greater prognostic significance than the dysrhythmia itself.

Diagnosis

Signs and Symptoms
- Wide variability exists in patient awareness of dysrhythmias, with either palpitations or the more serious symptoms of hemodynamic upset.
- Palpitations (awareness of the heart beating) may be not well tolerated; they are caused by increased force of contraction and/or from disturbance of rhythm.
- Those dysrhythmias that cause hemodynamic upset are usually sustained bradycardias or tachycardias, and may be life threatening, causing dizziness and syncope, which

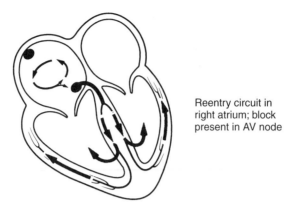

Reentry circuit in right atrium; block present in AV node

Atrial flutter

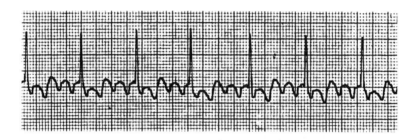

- P wave (F wave): the atrial defections, which often have a "sawtooth" appearance, are known as F (flutter) waves.

- P-R interval: because of the characteristic appearance of the flutter waves, it is often difficult to determine the P-R interval and is therefore not measured.

- QRS complex: the QRS complex duration is 0.1 second or less.

- Rhythm: the rhythm may be regular or irregular, depending on the relationship of atrial to ventricular beats. In this example, the rhythm is regular with a 4:1 conduction ratio (four atrial beats for every ventricular beat).

- Rate: the atrial rate is constant between 250 and 350 beats/minute. The ventricular rate depends on the conduction ratio between the atria and the ventricles.

- ➤ The A-V node protects the ventricles by not allowing every impulse that reaches it to be transmitted to the ventricles. Only one of four impulses is reaching the ventricles, as shown by the 4:1 A-V conduction ratio.

Fig. 5-2 Atrial flutter. (From Sheehy SB, Lenehan GP: *Manual of emergency care,* ed 5, St. Louis, 1999, Mosby, Inc., p 63.)

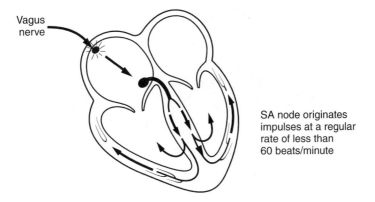

Vagus nerve

SA node originates impulses at a regular rate of less than 60 beats/minute

Sinus bradycardia

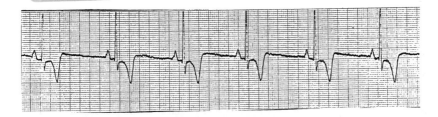

- P wave: the P waves are positive and uniform in lead II. Every P wave is followed by a QRS complex.

- P-R Interval: the P-R interval is normal, between 0.12 and 0.2 second, and is constant from beat to beat.

- QRS complex: the QRS complex duration is 0.1 second or less. Every QRS complex is preceded by a P wave.

- Rhythm: the rhythm is regular.

- Rate: the rate is constant, below 60 beats/minute.

Fig. 5-3   Sinus bradycardia. (From Sheehy SB, Lenehan GP: *Manual of emergency care,* ed 5, St. Louis, 1999, Mosby, Inc., p 60.)

may require that the patient not drive or continue in former occupations (e.g., operating machinery, flying).
— These dysrhythmias require urgent care and often hospitalization.

Diagnostic Tests
- The ECG is the major diagnostic procedure.
  — The surface ECG represents the net electrical forces of myocardial depolarization; although each cardiac cell oscillates over a potential difference of about 90 to 100 mV, ECG signals at the body surface are usually only 1 mV in amplitude.
  — Activation of small structures (e.g., SA node, AV node, His bundle) is not seen.
- The standard 12-lead ECG is crucial for diagnosing various sustained tachycardias; however, it provides only a brief sample of cardiac rhythm, especially when recorded by simultaneous multichannel recorders.
- Ambulatory ECG monitoring is the most powerful method of capturing dysrhythmias and associated events; its value is multiplied

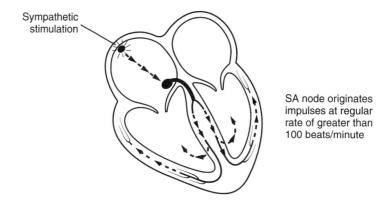

Sinus tachycardia

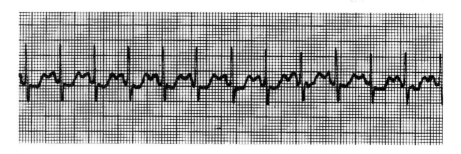

- P wave: the P waves are positive and uniform in lead II. Every P wave is followed by a QRS complex.

- P-R interval: the P-R interval is normal, between 0.12 and 0.2 second, and constant from beat to beat.

- QRS complex: the QRS complex duration is 0.1 second or less. Every QRS complex is preceded by a P wave.

- Rhythm: the rhythm is regular.

- Rate: the rate is constant, above 100 (100-160) beats/minute.

Fig. 5-4 Sinus tachycardia. (From Sheehy SB, Lenehan GP: *Manual of emergency care,* ed 5, St. Louis, 1999, Mosby, Inc., p 59.)

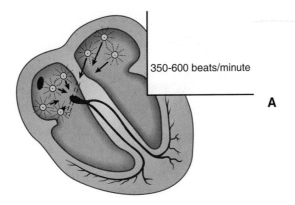

350-600 beats/minute

A

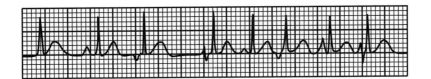

Multifocal atrial tachycardia

- P wave: the P waves vary in configuration, with multiple atrial foci initiating impulses.

- P-R interval: the P-R intervals vary from normal to prolonged. There is no stable relationship between the P waves and the QRS complexes.

- QRS complex: the QRS complex duration is 0.1 second or less.

- Rhythm: the rhythm is irregularly irregular and resembles atrial fibrillation except that P waves are clearly visible.

- Rate: the rate is not constant from beat to beat because of multiple atrial foci, often above 170 beats/minute.

➢ Multifocal (chaotic) atrial tachycardia is sometimes mistaken for atrial fibrillation because the rhythm is also irregularly irregular.

➢ This rhythm is frequently seen in patients with COPD associated with hypoxia. Treatment includes immediate administration of oxygen.

B

Fig. 5-5   Multifocal atrial tachycardia. (**A,** Redrawn from Redman B, Douglas E: Cardiac rhythms of sinus origin. In *Nurse-Beat: Cardiac Nursing Electronic Journal,* Winter 1999-2000, accessed 12/28/2000, http://www.nurse-beat.com/features/0100/sinus.htm; **B,** from Grauer K: *A practical guide to ECG interpretation,* ed 2, St. Louis, 1998, Mosby, Inc., p 48.)

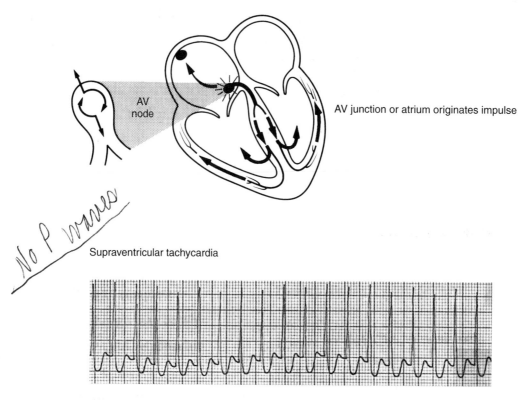

AV junction or atrium originates impulse

No P waves

Supraventricular tachycardia

- P wave: P waves, because of the rate (188 in this example), cannot be clearly enough delineated to establish the diagnosis as sinus, atrial, or junctional tachycardia.

- P-R interval: no P waves are seen; therefore, there is no measurable P-R interval.

- QRS complex: the QRS complex duration is 0.1 second or less.

- Rhythm: the rhythm is regular.

- Rate: the rate is usually above 150 beats/minute.

The normal QRS interval indicates a supraventricular pacemaker.

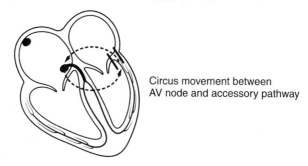

Circus movement between
AV node and accessory pathway

Fig. 5-6   Supraventricular tachycardia. (From Sheehy SB, Lenehan GP: *Manual of emergency care,* ed 5, St. Louis, 1999, Mosby, Inc., p 69.)

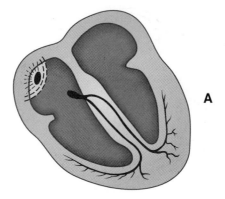

Sinoatrial (S-A) Block

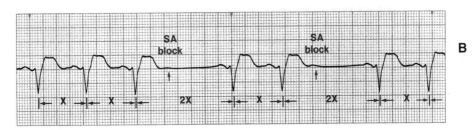

Fig. 5-7   Sinoatriol (SA) block. (**A,** Redrawn from Redman B, Douglas E: Cardiac rhythms of sinus origin. In *Nurse-Beat: Cardiac Nursing Electronic Journal,* Winter 1999-2000, accessed 12/28/2000, http://www.nurse-beat.com/features/0100/sinus.htm; **B,** from Huszar RJ: *Basic dysrhythmias: interpretation and management,* ed 2, St. Louis, 1994, Mosby, Inc., p 129.)

when the patient keeps a written record of symptoms.

—This type of recording is not as useful when dysrhythmias are infrequent.

- Patients with life-threatening dysrhythmias should be monitored in the hospital to avoid a fatal out-of-hospital event.

- History—as in most other conditions, the history usually provides sufficient information on which to base a working diagnosis.

—Patients are usually able to accurately report the fast, completely irregular palpitations of paroxysmal atrial fibrillation (AF), and can tap out accurately the regular tachydysrhythmias to within 10 beats/min.

- On physical examination, it is important to distinguish between brief, episodic dysrhythmias (e.g., ectopic beats, second-degree AV block) and sustained dysrhythmias, the onset and end of the irregular beats, and any other related symptoms.

—Many clinicians (wrongly) believe that a well-tolerated tachydysrhythmia is a supraventricular tachycardia rather than a ventricular tachycardia (VT), and vice versa.

- Palpation of the peripheral pulse, which reflects ventricular activation, and the jugular venous pulse (JVP), which reflects atrial and ventricular activation, is essential for diagnosis and can positively identify VT (if AV dissociation is present) from their sustained regular tachydysrhythmias (e.g., AF, atrial flutter, atrial and ventricular ectopic beats [VEBs], and second-degree and third-degree heart block).

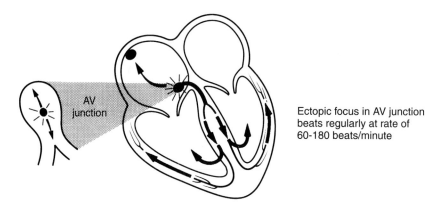

Ectopic focus in AV junction beats regularly at rate of 60-180 beats/minute

Junctional tachycardia

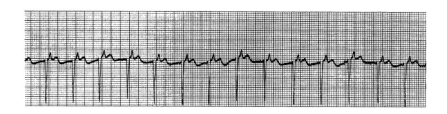

- P wave: when the P waves are present before or after the QRS complexes, they are inverted (negative) in Lead II. Often, no P waves are seen because they are either within the QRS complexes or there has been no atrial depolarization.

- P-R interval: when the inverted P waves are visible before the QRS complexes, the P-R interval is short—0.12 second or less. If the P waves are within or following the QRS complexes, no P-R interval can be measured.

- QRS complex: the QRS complex duration is 0.1 second or less.

- Rhythm: the rhythm is regular.

- Rate: the rate is above 100 (100-170) beats/minute.

When no P waves are present with a dominant junctional pacemaker, two posibilities exist: either the atria and ventricles are depolarized simultaneously **(A)**, or there is retrograde block and the atria are not depolarized **(B)**. Junctional rhythm with a rapid rate is seen in digitalis toxicity and myocardial infarction.

Fig. 5-8 Junctional tachycardia. (From Sheehy SB, Lenehan GP: *Manual of emergency care,* ed 5, St. Louis, 1999, Mosby, Inc., p 67.)

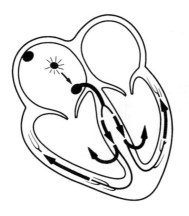

Atrial origin of
abnormal impulse

Premature atrial concept (PAC)

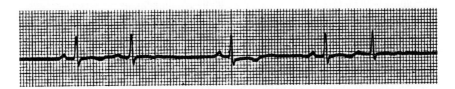

- P wave: the configuration of the P wave of the PAC differs from that of the dominant rhythm. If the PAC is early, the P wave may be completely or partially hidden within the preceding T wave.

- P-R interval: the P-R interval may be normal or prolonged, and often differs from the P-R interval of the dominant rhythm.

- QRS complex: the QRS complex duration is 0.1 second or less.

- Rhythm: the regularity of the basic rhythm is disturbed by the PAC. It may be quite irregular when there are many PACs.

- Rate: the rate depends on the basic rhythm and the number of PACs present.

➤ PACs may herald paroxysms of atrial tachycardia.

Fig. 5-9   Premature atrial concept (PAC). (From Sheehy SB, Lenehan GP: *Manual of emergency care,* ed 5, St. Louis, 1999, Mosby, Inc., p 76.)

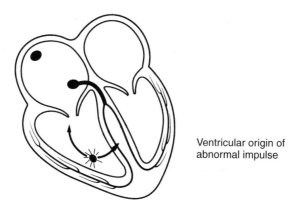

Ventricular origin of
abnormal impulse

Premature ventricular contract (PVC)

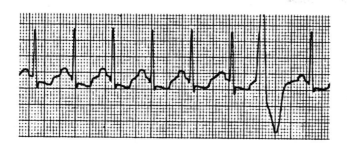

- P wave: the premature ventricular deflection (QRS complex) is not preceded by a P wave.

- P-R interval: there is no measurable P-R interval.

- QRS complex: the QRS complex duration is at least 0.12 second. The QRS complex is often bizarre in appearance compared with the normal QRS complexes.

- Rhythm: the regularity of the basic rhythm is disturbed by the PVC, and may be quite irregular when there are many PVCs.

- Rate: the rate depends on the basic rhythm and the number of PVCs present.

A PVC occurs when an impulse is propagated from a ventricular focus before the next normal beat is due. The QRS complex is usually widened and not preceded by a P wave. Retrograde activation of the atria may occur following a PVC when the ventricular impulse succeeds in penetrating the conduction system all the way to the atria, thus producing a retrograde P wave *(large arrow)*, or the sinus P waves may continue. The ladder diagram shows the origin of the PVC within the ventricles, with retrograde depolarization of the atria.

Fig. 5-10   Premature ventricular contract (PVC). (From Sheehy SB, Lenehan GP: *Manual of emergency care,* ed 5, St. Louis, 1999, Mosby, Inc., p 75.)

TABLE 5-10
Vaughan Williams' Classification of Antidysrhythmic Drugs

Classification	Antidysrhythmic Drugs
Class Ia	Quinidine, procainamide, disopyramide
Class Ib	Lidocaine, mexiletine, tocainide
Class Ic	Flecainide, propafenone
Class II	β-Adrenergic blocking drugs
Class III	Amiodarone, sotalol, bretylium, ibutilide
Class IV	Verapamil, diltiazem
Other	Adenosine, digoxin

From Kumar P, Clark M: Cardiovascular disease. *Clinical medicine*, ed 4, Edinburgh, 1998, WB Saunders, p 670.

Treatment (Table 5-10)

- Reassuring the patient is of great importance because awareness of irregular heart beats can arouse high anxiety.
- Antidysrhythmic drugs are the mainstay of management for significant dysrhythmias (see Table 5-10).
  —No universally effective drug exists; all have safety limitations, and can aggravate or promote dysrhythmias.
  —Drug selection is often trial and error.
  Patients with significant dysrhythmias will be referred to a cardiac specialist, who will prescribe and oversee the therapy for each patient

Class I Drugs

Class I drugs include sodium channel blockers and other older antidysrhythmic drugs (e.g., quinidine).
- Action: all reduce the maximal rate of depolarization of the action potential and thus slow conduction.
- They are effective in suppressing VEBs but, to varying degrees, depress LV performance.
- All have been associated with prodysrhythmias (promoting dysrhythmias).
- Subclassifications
  —Ia: drugs with intermediate onset and end
  —Ib: those with short effects
  —Ic: those with prolonged effects
- Quinidine (class Ia) prolongs action potential and refractoriness (seen on ECG as QT prolongation).
  —It is broad-spectrum and is effective in suppressing VEBs and VT, and in controlling narrow QRS tachycardias, including atrial flutter and atrial fibrillation.
  —Elimination half-life ($t_{1/2}$) is 6 to 7 hours.
  —If an initial test dose is tolerated, the maintenance dose is 200-400 mg PO q4-6h.
  —Dosage is adjusted so that QRS duration is <140 msec, unless there is preexisting bundle branch block and QT is <550 msec.
  —About 30% of patients develop adverse reactions: gastrointestinal (GI) symptoms (diarrhea, colic, flatulence) are most common, and fever, syncope, thrombocytopenia, and liver function abnormalities also occur.
- Procainamide (class Ia) has much less effect than quinidine on refractoriness.
  —The major metabolite, *N*-acetyl procainamide, also has antidysrhythmic effects and contributes to procainamide's efficacy and toxicity.
  —It is given cautiously intravenously (IV), (100 mg over 1 to 2 minutes) repeated q5 minutes to a maximum dose of 600 mg, with monitoring of BP and ECG.
  —Oral procainamide has a short elimination half-life of <4 hours, requiring frequent dosing or using sustained-release forms; the oral dose is 250 to 625 mg q3-4h.
- Disopyramide (class Ia) produces little change in the refractory period.
  —Its elimination half-life is 5 to 7 hours.
  —Oral dose is usually 100 to 150 mg q6h.
- Lidocaine (class Ib) has significant first-pass hepatic metabolism.
  —It produces minimal myocardial depression; it has little effect on the sinus node, atria, or AV node, but has great effect on His-Purkinje and ventricular myocardial tissues.
  —It can suppress the ventricular dysrhythmias that complicate MI (VEBs, VT) and reduce the incidence of primary ventricular fibrillation (VF) when given prophylactically in early acute MI.
  —Asystolic events are increased, indicating SA and AV nodal effects.
  —Elimination half-life is 30 to 60 minutes.
  —Given only IV: 100 mg over 2 minutes, then 50 mg 5 minutes later if the dysrhythmia has not reverted; an infusion of 4 mg/minute (2 mg/minute in patients over age 65) is then

started, which, if continued for >12 hours, may reach toxic levels.

—Adverse effects are neurologic rather than cardiac: tremor, convulsions.

- Phenytoin is listed under various classifications but is probably class Ib.
  - —It was used extensively to manage dysrhythmias, especially for suppressing ventricular dysrhythmias of digitalis toxicity, until newer drugs became available, and digitalis toxicity became less frequent.
  - —Adverse effects include gingival hyperplasia and blood dyscrasias.
- Class Ic drugs are the most powerful antidysrhythmias but have been associated with a significant risk of prodysrhythmias and depression of cardiac contractility.
  - —These effects are not common in hemodynamically normal hearts (e.g., Wolff-Parkinson-White [WPW syndrome] but are significant in those with extensive cardiac damage and subject to life-threatening ventricular tachydysrhythmias.
  - —Class Ic drugs are used in these patients only when the dysrhythmia is nonresponsive to other drugs.
  - —Class Ic drugs are highly effective in medical cardioversion of AF and for prophylaxis of AF attacks; these have become the principal indications for these drugs, and incidence of prodysrhythmia is relatively low.
- Flecainide is a highly effective antidysrhythmic with profound effect on the Na channel, resulting in markedly slowed conduction, but refractoriness is minimally affected.
  - —LV performance may be depressed.
  - —It can control symptomatic VEBs, VT, and the reciprocating tachycardias of WPW syndrome.
  - —Elimination half-life is 12 to 27 hours.
  - —It is given 100 mg PO q8-12h.
  - —It was associated with increased mortality in treating symptomatic and minimally symptomatic VEBs following acute MI.
  - —Although the drug is usually well tolerated, blurred vision and paresthesia are infrequently reported.
  - —QRS prolongation of 25% indicates toxicity.

Class II Drugs

Class II drugs (β-blockers) are probably the most powerful and least toxic, but their antidysrhythmic effects are often overlooked; they prevent VF and raise the threshold to VF.

- In general, class II drugs are well tolerated but may depress LV function, particularly at clinically effective dose levels.
- They are contraindicated in bronchospastic airway disease, and used cautiously in other lung diseases.
- Side effects include GI disturbances, insomnia, nightmares, and lassitude, which is common but usually short-lived.

Class III Drugs

Class III drugs interfere with the K channel to alter the plateau phase of the action potential and increase refractoriness; these drugs can promote dysrhythmias.

- Amiodarone is a powerful antidysrhythmic.
  - —It has few cardiovascular side effects.
  - —Its moderate vasodilator action produces little or no LV depression, and SA node activity is affected very little.
  - —This drug prolongs refractoriness, prolongs the QT interval.
  - —Elimination half-life is >50 days, with substantial delay in onset of action.
  - —Loading doses of 600 to 1200 mg/day PO for 7 to 10 days are usual but with no increase in onset of action.
  - —Maintenance dose is ≤200 mg/day PO.
  - —In cases of life-threatening dysrhythmias, amiodarone has been given IV, 3 to 7.5 mg/kg over 1 hour; with IV use, ECG monitoring is required because of the risk of induced AV block.
  - —Cardiovascular toxicity is rare, but amiodarone is too toxic for long-term use, other than for severe dysrhythmias (e.g., narrow QRS complex dysrhythmias not responsive to other therapy).
  - —Side effects include pulmonary fibrosis from long-term use, photosensitive dermatitis, liver abnormalities, peripheral neuropathy, corneal microdeposits (reversible on stopping the drug), hypothyroidism, which can be treated with thyroid hormone during therapy, and hyperthyroidism, which usually requires stopping amiodarone.
- Racemic (D-L) sotalol has class II and III antidysrhythmic properties, but class III effects (QT prolongation, refractory period change) are de-

tectable; they are largely masked by the drug's β-blocking properties.

—Most class III activity is in the D-isomer.

—Give PO, 80 to 160 mg q12h.

—It depresses LV performance and has been known to promote dysrhythmias.

—Contraindications to β-blockers are applied to racemic.

—In studies of D-sotalol, mortality was increased.

- Ibutilide is a class III drug (prolongs repolarization) that is very different from amiodarone and sotalol.

—Its effect is mediated by activating a slow inward Na current rather than by blocking outward K currents.

—It can terminate acute AF with 40% success and atrial flutter with 65% success.

—It is given over 10 minutes as an infusion of 1 mg for patients weighing 60 kg, or 0.01 mg/kg for patients weighing less.

—It has been associated with torsades de pointes, and patients should be monitored by staff familiar with the treatment for torsades de pointes.

Class IV Drugs

Class IV drugs are calcium blockers (Ca entry blockers). *Procardia   Adalat*

- Nifedipine, like other dihydropyridines, has almost no electrophysiologic effects, but verapamil and diltiazem influence AV nodal electrophysiology and may alter that of Ca-dependent ischemic cells.

- Verapamil acts on the AV node, slowing conduction. *CAl AN*

—It is used to manage narrow QRS tachycardias that involve the AV node.

—These tachycardias are terminated in almost 100% of cases when the drug is given IV, 5 to 15 mg over 10 minutes.

—Given to patients in VT, however, serious adverse reactions can occur, including VF, intractable hypotension, and death; it is contraindicated for broad QRS tachycardias.

—It is given for prophylaxis of dysrhythmias, but its substantial first-pass hepatic metabolism limits its clinical use.

- Diltiazem is similar to verapamil but has a longer half-life, which makes it less acceptable as IV therapy for narrow QRS tachycardia, but

Cardizem

has little or no first-pass hepatic metabolism, which makes it a better choice for chronic dysrhythmia prophylaxis.

Other Drugs

- Digoxin shortens atrial and ventricular refractory periods and prolongs conduction in the AV node.

—Given IV; the digitalizing dose is 1 mg, given slowly, under ECG control, with full resuscitative equipment available.

—The maintenance dose is 0.125 to 0.25 mg/day PO, depending on weight and renal function.

—Digoxin toxicity may be manifested by anorexia, nausea, vomiting, and serious dysrhythmias (VEBs, atrial ectopic beats, sometimes paroxysmal atrial tachycardia with block), or second- or third-degree AV block.

—Digoxin toxicity is treated with digoxin immune Fab, which is safer and more logical than using an antiarrhythmic drug; however, stopping the drug for 48 hours, then starting again at a lower dose is usually successful.

Pacemakers

Pacemakers are used extensively for dysrhythmias.

- Nomenclature for pacemaker generators (usually 4 letters)

—The chamber stimulated: *A*, atrium, *V*, ventricle, *D*, both (dual)

—Chamber where sensing occurs: (A, V, or D)

—Sensory mode: *I*, inhibition by a sensed impulse; *T*, triggering by a sensed impulse; *D*, dual modes of response

—Programmability or rate modulation capacity: *P*, programming for 2 functions; *M*, programming for more than two; *R*, rate modulation

- A pacemaker that senses and paces in both chambers is the most physiologic approach to pacing patients who remain in sinus rhythm.

- Permanent pacemakers are implanted in cases of symptomatic bradydysrhythmias, asymptomatic Mobitz II AV block, and in those with complete heart block.

- Technology has produced more sophisticated pacing methods and most are now able to be programmed to suit patients' needs; low-energy circuitry and better battery designs improved length of operability.

- Screening devices and interference-resistant circuitry also eliminated the risk of automobile distributors, radar antennae, microwave ovens, and airport security detectors interfering with the operation of pacemakers.
- Magnetic resonance imaging (MRI) and operative diathermy may interfere with pacemakers, and cellular phones are a source of electromagnetic emissions, which should be avoided by those who wear pacemakers.
- Pacemakers are made for different kinds of dysrhythmias: antibradycardia pacemakers, antitachycardia pacemakers, implantable cardioverter-defibrillators, and antitachycardia pacing pacemakers.

Other Treatments

- Radiofrequency (RF) ablation can be used on a discrete generator or pathway that causes the dysrhythmia, and which can be destroyed by RF lesions.
  - —AV node ablation (used for ventricular rate control in AF) is possible in >99% of patients.
  - —Cure rates of 85% are reported for cures of atrial flutter.
  - —RF ablation is very safe; deaths (1/2000) occurred primarily through cardiac perforation and tamponade (1/2400).
- Surgery, using an epicardial or endocardial approach, after localizing the accessory pathway by catheter or epicardial mapping, can destroy the pathway, thus eliminating the dysrhythmia, with >95% success rate and an operative mortality of <0.1%.
  - —RF ablation has made conventional surgery for WPW syndrome almost obsolete.

ATRIAL FIBRILLATION
Definition

Alcohol abuse

AF is a rapid, irregular atrial rhythm. It is the most common chronic dysrhythmia.

Risk Factors

- A common dysrhythmia, AF occurs in 5% to 10% of patients over age 65.
- AF can occur in younger patients, usually in a paroxysmal form.
- Other underlying heart disease: rheumatic heart disease, coronary artery disease, hypertension, or hyperthyroidism

- —AF may be the initial presenting sign in thyrotoxicosis.
- Alcohol abuse (binge or chronic heavy drinking); this should be considered in every patient with AF.
- AF sometimes reverts to normal sinus rhythm, but then recurs.

Etiology/Cause

- Multiple reentrant wavelets
- Pericarditis
- Chest trauma or chest surgery
- Pulmonary disease
- Medications such as theophylline and β-adrenergic agonists may cause attacks in people with normal hearts.
- Ingestion of alcohol, either chronically or in binge drinking, can precipitate an attack; even small amounts of alcohol in persons who are predisposed to AF will cause an attack ("holiday heart").

Pathogenesis

- During an attack of AF, the atria are in a seemingly chaotic rapid rhythm.
- The rapid atrial rate is produced by multiple interlacing wavelets of reentrant activity.
- Intraatrial recordings show rates of more than 350 beats/min.
- AF is the only common dysrhythmia in which the ventricular rate is rapid and the rhythm very irregular.
  - —The atrial rate is 400 to 600 beats/min, but most impulses are blocked at the AV node.
  - —The ventricular response is completely irregular, ranging from 80 to 180 beats/min.
  - —Because of the varying stroke volumes resulting from varying periods of diastolic filling, not all ventricular beats produce a palpable peripheral pulse.
  - —The difference between the apical rate and the pulse rate is the "pulse deficit," which is greater when the ventricular rate is high.

Diagnosis

Signs and Symptoms

- Patients are usually aware of the rapid heart rate, sometimes perceived as chest discomfort.
- The hemodynamic consequences of AF may be felt by the patient as weakness, faintness, and breathlessness.
- Most patients appear anxious.

Diagnostic Tests
- ECG shows the pattern typical of AF.

Treatment

- Management of any underlying (causative) disorder (e.g., hyperthyroidism), which when treated is the only cause that abolishes AF
- Other objectives of therapy are to control the ventricular response rate, to restore sinus rhythm, and prevent emboli.
- The ventricular response rate is usually controlled with digoxin, which increases AV conduction delay and block.
- If digoxin alone is not sufficient, a β-blocker or a calcium blocker (e.g., diltiazem, verapamil) is added.
- Short-term control of ventricular rate to prepare for direct current (DC) cardioversion is usually done with a β-blocker or verapamil to avoid digoxin dysrhythmias.
- AF may be converted to sinus rhythm in some patients with class Ia and Ic drugs with amiodarone.
- DC electroversion is the most successful treatment.
- If these measures fail to maintain sinus rhythm, RF ablation will interrupt AV conduction, making it necessary to implant a permanent pacemaker.
- The risk of emboli in AF is greatest with left atrial enlargement and mitral valve abnormalities; however, long-term anticoagulation with warfarin should be considered for all patients with AF.

Prognosis

- Outcome depends on the severity of underlying cardiac disease, and whether sinus rhythm can be maintained over time.
- Dysrhythmias are frequently the cause of sudden death in adults, particularly those who have a history of heart disease and who are older.
- With appropriate treatment at the outset of AF, the patient can have many more years of relatively good health.

Patient/Family Education

(Applicable to all patients with dysrhythmias)
- The patient and family should be kept apprised of the nature of the condition, its treatment, and its usual course, from the beginning.

- The importance of following the cardiologist's directions should be repeated.
- Instructions about rest, diet, taking medications, and return visits should be written and given to the patient at discharge.
- Reassurance of the patient is necessary to allay fears.

ATRIAL FLUTTER *No "P" waves*
Definition

Atrial flutter is a rapid regular atrial rhythm.

Risk Factors

cardiac reason

- Ischemic heart disease
- Rheumatic heart disease
- Congestive cardiomyopathy
- Atrial septal defect
- Mitral valve disease
- Chronic obstructive pulmonary disease (COPD)
- Thyrotoxicosis

Etiology/Cause

- Atrial flutter is caused by a constant well-defined macroreentrant circuit in the right atrium.

Pathogenesis

- Atrial flutter results in atrial rates of about 300 beats/min.
- Usually, there is a 2:1 AV conduction block so that the ventricular response is about 150 beats/min.
- Unlike AF, both the atrial and the ventricular rates are regular.
- Unlike AF, atrial flutter rarely occurs in persons who are otherwise healthy.

Diagnosis

Signs and Symptoms
- Patients are usually aware of a rapid heart rate.
- Sometimes, the flutter waves can be seen in the jugular pulse.
- In some patients, an S_4 is audible, which is not present in AF.
- Patients frequently appear anxious.

Diagnostic Tests
- The ECG pattern commonly shows "sawtooth" flutter waves.
- P waves are absent.

- If the AV node is diseased, higher degrees of AV block are seen, usually a multiple of 2 (4:1, 8:1).

Treatment

- Atrial flutter is often a chronic and very refractory dysrhythmia that is difficult to treat medically.
- If there is no contraindication, electric cardioversion is the treatment of choice if atrial flutter persists, even if there is a high degree of AV block.
- If atrial flutter recurs after cardioversion, antidysrhythmic therapy or catheter ablation of the reentry circuit should be considered.
  - Catheter ablation of atrial flutter is accomplished successfully in more than 90% of patients with few if any complications.
- Atrial flutter is less likely to respond to antidysrhythmic drug therapy.

Prognosis

- Atrial flutter is a condition that is difficult to treat and to maintain sinus rhythm.
- Atrial flutter tends to recur because of the underlying physiologic mechanisms that cause it.
- Paying attention to diet, exercising, being treated for other underlying cardiac conditions, taking medications as prescribed, and keeping appointments for return visits are all necessary for the patient's family and the patient to know.
- Even though all of the known preventive measures are taken to avoid additional attacks, AF is difficult to treat and recurrences can occur suddenly, without warning.

CHAOTIC MULTIFOCAL ATRIAL TACHYCARDIA
Definition

Chaotic multifocal atrial tachycardia is a rapid, irregular atrial rhythm.

Risk Factors

- Severe, chronic lung disease
- Taking theophylline—these dysrhythmias are often a feature of severe chronic lung disease and may be exacerbated by theophylline

Etiology/Cause

- Present like AF, but the tachycardias are not caused by multiple interlacing wavelets of reentry (as in AF), but by focal pacemaker abnormalities

Pathogenesis

- Arise from pacemaker (nodal) abnormalities
- Are often associated with severe chronic lung disease

Diagnosis

- These tachycardias are characterized by varying P-wave morphology (three or more foci) and markedly irregular PP intervals.
- Rate is usually between 100 and 140 beats/min.
- Rapid abnormal P waves precede the QRS complexes.

Treatment

- Treat the underlying lung disease.
- Verapamil 240 to 480 mg PO qid in divided doses

REGULAR NARROW QRS TACHYCARDIAS (SUPRAVENTRICULAR TACHYCARDIAS)
Definition

This is a sustained tachydysrhythmia in which the QRS appears normal and has a duration of 20 msec.

- One of the most common narrow QRS tachycardias is the reciprocating tachycardia of the WPW syndrome.
- Three forms of regular narrow QRS tachycardia are
  - AV nodal reentry tachycardia
    - ~ Intra-AV tachycardia (intranodal)
    - ~ Para-AV tachycardia (paranodal)
  - Nodal reentry tachycardia
  - These are paroxysmal regular tachycardias due to reentry through abnormal pathways within or beside the AV node.
- The abnormal (slow) pathway may not show the decremental conduction properties characteristic of the fast pathway—the AV node.
- The most common ($\geq$95%) is a fast-slow tachycardia, using the AV node for antegrade conduction and the abnormal pathway for retrograde conduction, in which P waves occur almost simultaneous with, and are obscured by, the QRS complex.
- The much less common slow-fast AV nodal reentry tachycardia produces P' waves before

most QRS (RP' > PR), a rhythm that may present in an incessant form.

Diagnosis

Signs and Symptoms

- Tachycardia is usually paroxysmal with sudden onset and may be initiated by a premature atrial ectopic beat with a critical PR interval.
- Rate is usually 160 to 200 beats/min.
- Palpitations are universal, but variably tolerated.

Treatment

- Vagotonic maneuvers (Valsalva's maneuver, carotid sinus massage, ice water diving reflex, swallowing of ice-cold water), particularly if used before the dysrhythmia has stabilized, may terminate the paroxysm.
- If these methods are ineffective, the dysrhythmia sometimes stops during sleep, but most patients feel sick enough to seek medical help.
- Acute attacks respond dramatically to IV verapamil or adenosine.
- If medications fail to halt the dysrhythmia, electric conversion (pacing, low-energy DC shock) is considered next.
- Alternative drug therapy includes digoxin, often given in a high dosage (e.g., 0.375 to 0.5 mg/day) with β-blockers or calcium blockers, or any of these alone, may be effective.
- Most patients with this dysrhythmia are candidates for pathway RF ablation.
  - Most centers report success rates of >95%, with <1% of patients requiring permanent pacemaker implantation for collateral AV nodal because of damage.

RECIPROCATING TACHYCARDIAS

Definition

These tachycardias involve accessory pathways, and are paroxysmal, regular tachycardias. The accessory pathway is a congenital feature, which may not present symptoms until as late as middle-age; it typically presents during the first year of life.

Risk Factors

- Congenital condition
- Exercise
- Family history

Etiology/Cause

- In the most common form, activation is from atria to ventricles through the normal AV node, returning via the accessory pathway to the atria (orthodromic).

Pathogenesis

- A narrow QRS tachycardia results, during which P waves are inscribed after the QRS complex (PR > RP).
- Very rarely, conduction is in the opposite direction, resulting in a broad QRS complex antidromic reciprocating tachycardia.
- In the WPW syndrome, an accessory pathway that links the atria and ventricles, bypassing the AV node, is the structural basis for the dysrhythmia.
  - ECG shows a short PR interval and slurred QRS complex (delta wave).
  - Antegrade conduction over the accessory pathway is necessary to create the short PR interval and the delta wave, but retrograde conduction is important for sustaining orthodromic reciprocating tachycardia.
  - Thus a concealed accessory pathway (normal PR, no delta wave, in sinus rhythm) may support the dysrhythmia.
- In the Lown-Ganong-Levine (LGL) syndrome, the accessory pathway joins the atrium with His bundle tissue, bypassing the AV node.
  - The PR interval is short, as in WPW syndrome, but the QRS complex is normal.
  - Patients with LGL syndrome have the same type of dysrhythmias as those with WPW syndrome; treatment is similar.

Diagnosis

Signs and Symptoms

- Signs and symptoms of reciprocating tachycardia usually appear during the first year of life, in the teens and 20s, or in middle age (45 to 60 years).
- In patients in their teens and 20s, the typical attack occurs suddenly, often associated with exercise.
  - Attacks may last for only a few seconds, or for several hours, but rarely for more than 12 hours.
  - In a healthy, fit person, the tachycardia is well tolerated and there may be few symptoms.
  - More serious is the situation in which disorganization of the tachycardia occurs,

moving to AF, because of rapid and potentially life-threatening ventricular response that may follow, in which the rate can be more than 250 beats/min.

- Patients in middle age who have this congenital condition may develop tachycardia because of an age-related increase in initiating atrial and ventricular premature beats.

Treatment

- An attack will likely respond to vagotonic maneuvers (e.g., Valsalva's, ice-water facial immersion), which slow AV nodal conduction and destabilize the reentry circuit, preferably instituted soon after the onset of the attack.
- If this type of maneuver is not successful, verapamil or adenosine will result in sufficient AV node conduction delay to stop the reentrant activity.
- An alternative is to use class Ia or Ic drugs to slow conduction in the accessory pathway, which may be the weakest link in the reentrant circuit.
  —IV flecainide, propafenone, procainamide, and disopyramide are effective and safe for acute management.
- In practice, when a narrow QRS tachycardia is seen, most patients will be given IV adenosine or verapamil, which terminates the dysrhythmia by briefly blocking or slowing conduction in the AV node, rather than affecting the accessory pathway.

ATRIAL FIBRILLATION AND WOLFF-PARKINSON-WHITE SYNDROME

AF is a medical emergency in the presence of antegrade conduction over an accessory pathway because the normal rate-limiting effects of the AV node are bypassed and excessive ventricular rates may lead to VF.

- Treatment for these patients usually occurs in cardiac ICUs and will not be described in detail here.
- DC conversion is the treatment of choice; medical treatment may cause an increase in the ventricular rate.
  —Drugs, such as verapamil and other calcium blockers, are contraindicated in the treatment of AF associated with the WPW syndrome.

ATRIAL TACHYCARDIA
Definition

A rapid regular atrial rhythm due to intra-atrial reentry or to abnormal automaticity in the atrial walls.

Risk Factors

- Cardiac tumor
- Pericarditis
- Digoxin
- Alcohol
- Toxic gases

Etiology/Cause

- The narrow QRS complex tachycardia arises from an abnormal automatic focus or localized intra-atrial reentry.
- Any of the risk factors listed may cause onset of tachycardia, but many times the cause remains unknown.

Pathogenesis

- Characteristically, the P wave precedes the QRS complex (PO > RP).
- Because the source of the dysrhythmia may be anywhere in the atria, the P-wave vector is inconsistent.

Diagnosis

Signs and Symptoms
- ECG findings (see Etiology/Cause)

Treatment

- If digoxin therapy/toxicity is not the cause of the atrial tachycardia with block (this finding is almost diagnostic of digoxin toxicity), β-blockers or verapamil are the drugs of choice.
- Atrial mapping by catheter can locate the focal generator or at least part of the intraatrial reentry responsible for maintaining the dysrhythmia.
  —RF energy applied at these areas cures most atrial tachycardias.

BROAD QRS COMPLEX DYSRHYTHMIAS
Definition

A broad QRS complex dysrhythmia is a rapid regular ventricular rhythm with QRS duration ≥ 120 msec.

- This category includes VEBs, VT, and torsades de pointes.
- Antidromic reciprocating tachycardia is a broad QRS tachycardia in which conduction from atria to ventricles is by an accessory pathway with retrograde return to the atria via the AV node.

Ventricular Ectopic Beats

Definition

VEBs are premature beats caused by an abnormal electric focus in the ventricles. VEBs may or may not cause symptoms or be of prognostic significance. Although VEBs were once considered always pathologic, 24-hour ECG studies show that they occur in normal persons.

Diagnosis

Signs and Symptoms
- Unless very frequent, isolated VEBs do not cause hemodynamic upset and are usually asymptomatic.
- Symptomatic VEBs are usually perceived as a missed beat, although this sensation is likely related more to the following augmented sinus beat than to the VEB itself.

Treatment
- VEBs are clinically significant when they occur in the presence of aortic stenosis, HF, and late (>2 days) post-MI.
- Outcome depends on the frequency of the VEBs.
  —More than 10/hour is considered a threshold number.
- No research has shown benefits of VEB suppression, even with other cardiac disorders.
- In post-MI patients, mortality is higher in those given antidysrhythmic drugs, particularly flecainide (class Ic) than in those given placebo.

Prognosis
- Outcomes for high-risk post-MI patients, determined by the frequency of VEBs, may be improved by β-blockers and procedures to modify the underlying coronary artery disease (e.g., angioplasty, coronary artery bypass grafting), rather than by giving class I antidysrhythmic drugs.

VENTRICULAR TACHYCARDIA
Definition

VT is a rapid succession of three or more consecutive ventricular beats at a rate of ≥120 beats/min.
- VT may be monomorphic or polymorphic, unsustained or sustained for 30 seconds or requiring resuscitative intervention.
- Short unsustained VT is common in acute MI but is not significant and should not be treated if asymptomatic.
- Sustained VT complicates many heart disorders, particularly late-phase MI, LV cardiomyopathies, and RV dysplasia.

Risk Factors
- Post-MI
- Other cardiac disorders (see Definition)

Etiology/Cause
- Underlying cardiac disease

Pathogenesis
- Unless cardiac disease is present, or the patient is post-MI, often the pathogenesis of VT is unknown.

Diagnosis
Signs and Symptoms
- Any broad-QRS (QRS ≥ 120 msec) tachycardia should be considered VT until proven otherwise.
- ECG findings
  —Independent P-wave activity
  —Fusion or capture beats
  —Uniformity of QRS vectors in the V leads (concordance)
  —A frontal plane QRS negative axis > −30°
- A tachycardia not originating in the ventricles (e.g., narrow-QRS tachycardia) can be conducted aberrantly to produce a broad QRS complex tachycardia.
  —Although rare, this tachycardia is frequently and wrongly diagnosed as VT.
- Treatment occurs in cardiac ICUs.

TORSADES DE POINTES
Definition

Torsades de pointes, a VT, is characterized by a continuously changing QRS vector: "twisting of the points."

Risk Factors

- Congenital long QT syndrome (rare)
  - —Jervell and Lange-Nielsen syndrome—autosomal recessive with associated deafness
  - —Romano-Ward syndrome—autosomal dominant with no deafness
  - —These patients have striking QT abnormalities of both duration and shape.
  - —If torsades de pointes develops in these patients, the outcome is often fatal.
  - —Most recently, the genetic basis of at least three congenital long QT syndromes has been determined: two involve K^+ channels, and the third is a coding abnormality for a sodium channel.
    - ~ Patients with the coding abnormality for a sodium channel may respond to the sodium channel blocker mexiletine; investigations are being conducted.

Etiology/Cause

- In practice, torsades de pointes is provoked by drugs, especially antidysrhythmics that are contraindicated in treatment for the condition.
- Electrolyte imbalance

Pathogenesis

(See Etiology/Cause.)

Diagnosis

- The diagnosis is made by ECG readings: rapid, irregular, sharp complexes that continuously change from an upright to an inverted position.
- Between periods of tachycardia, the ECG shows a prolonged QT interval.
  - —The corrected QT is ≥0.44 sec.

Treatment

- Any electrolyte disturbance is corrected.
- Causative drug(s) are stopped.
- The heart rate is maintained with atrial or ventricular pacing.
- IV isoprenaline may be effective when QT prolongation is acquired.
- β-Blockers or left stellectomy are advised if the QT prolongation is congenital, in which case isoprenaline is contraindicated.

Prognosis

- Variable, depending on origin of the QT prolongation, timing, and accuracy of therapy.

- Sudden death has been reported in association with torsades de pointes.

VENTRICULAR FIBRILLATION
Definition

VF is a rapid irregular ventricular rhythm with essentially zero cardiac output.

Risk Factors

- Recent MI
- Severe underlying coronary disease
- Acute MI with shock, with or without HF
- Myocardial reperfusion after thrombolytic therapy

Etiology/Cause

- VF is usually provoked by a ventricular ectopic beat (VEB), especially in acute myocardial infarction, ventricular tachycardia, or torsades de pointes.
- Multiple interlacing reentrant wavelets of electrical activity

Pathogenesis

- At the cellular level, electric activity may be organized, but the global effect is that no mechanical contraction occurs and there is no effective cardiac output.

Diagnosis

Signs and Symptoms
- VF is diagnosed by ECG readings.
  - —ECG shows shapeless, rapid oscillation, and there is no hint of organized complexes.
- The patient is pulseless and becomes rapidly unconscious; respirations cease.

Treatment

- VF is fatal unless reversed by DC countershock.
- VF rarely reverses spontaneously.
- Electric defibrillation
- VF usually occurs soon after an MI and is treated while the patient is still hospitalized.

Prognosis

- Success rates for DC cardioversion of primary VF are 95%; both short-term and long-term prognoses are excellent.
- Primary VF complicating acute MI cannot be predicted.

—Lidocaine, magnesium, or β-blockers offer some protection from this event, but lidocaine increases the risk of asystole.

- In secondary VF, a success rate of 30% for resuscitation and a hospital mortality rate for resuscitated survivors of 70% indicate its seriousness.
- In VF after myocardial reperfusion, success rates after resuscitation are high.

ASPECTS OF PHYSIOLOGY RELATED TO THE HEART: PRELUDE TO HEART FAILURE

At rest and during exercise, CO, venous return, and distribution of blood flow with O_2 delivery to the tissues are balanced by neurohumoral and intrinsic cardiac factors: preload, the contractile state, afterload, the rate of contraction, substrate availability, and the extent of myocardial damage determine LV performance and myocardial O_2 requirements. The Frank-Starling principle, cardiac reserve, and the oxyhemoglobin dissociation curve play a role.

- *Preload:* (the degree of end-diastolic fiber stretch) reflects the end-diastolic volume, which is influenced by diastolic pressure and the composition of the myocardial wall.
  —The end-diastolic pressure, especially if it is above normal, is a reasonable indication of preload in many conditions.
  —LV dilation, hypertrophy, and changes in myocardial distensibility or compliance modify preload
- *Contractile state:* in isolated cardiac muscle is characterized by the force and velocity of contraction; these are difficult to measure in the intact heart
  —Expressed as the ejection fraction (LV stroke volume/end-diastolic volume)
- *Afterload:* (the force resisting myocardial fiber shortening after stimulation from the relaxed state) is determined by the chamber pressure, volume, and wall thickness at the time of aortic valve opening
  —Clinically, afterload approximates systemic BP at or shortly after aortic valve opening and represents peak systolic wall stress
  —Heart rate and rhythm also influence cardiac performance.
- *Reduced substrate availability:* (e.g., of fatty acid or glucose), especially if O_2 availability is re-

duced, can impair the force of cardiac contraction and myocardial performance
- *Tissue damage:* (acute with MI or chronic with fibrosis due to various diseases) impairs local myocardial performance and imposes an additional burden on viable myocardium
- *Frank-Starling principle:* states that the degree of end-diastolic fiber stretch (preload) within a physiologic range is proportional to the systolic performance of the ensuing ventricular contraction
  —This mechanism operates in HF but, because ventricular function is abnormal, the response is inadequate.
  —If the Frank-Starling curve is depressed, fluid retention, vasoconstriction, and a cascade of neurohumoral responses result in the syndrome of CHF.
  —Over time, LV remodeling (change from the normal ovoid shape) with dilation and hypertrophy further compromise cardiac performance, particularly during physical stress.
  —Dilation and hypertrophy may be accompanied by, or cause, increased diastolic stiffness.
- *Cardiac reserve:* (unused ability of the resting heart to deliver O_2 to the tissues) this is an important part of cardiac function during emotional or physical stress; the mechanisms include increased heart rate, systolic and diastolic volume, stroke volume, and tissue extraction of O_2.
  —In physically fit athletes during maximal exercise, the heart rate may increase from 55 to 70 beats/min at rest to 180 beats/min.
  —CO (stroke volume × heart rate) may increase from its normal resting value of 6 to 25 L/min.
  —O_2 consumption may increase from 250-1500 ml/min, which is not enough to meet tissue metabolic demands; therefore the tissues extract more oxygen and mixed venous blood oxygen falls considerably.
    ~ Increased arteriovenous oxygen difference $(A - VO_2)$ due to lower venous oxygen content is a common adaptive mechanism in HF.
- *The oxyhemoglobin dissociation curve:* influences O_2 availability to the tissues and can provide another reserve mechanism in HF.
  —The position of this curve is often expressed as P_{50} (the partial pressure of O_2 in the blood at 50% oxyhemoglobin saturation).

—An increase in the normal P_{50} (27 ± 2 mm Hg) indicates a rightward shift of the oxyhemoglobin dissociation curve (decreased affinity of hemoglobin [Hb] for O_2).

—For a given PO_2, less O_2 is combined with Hb, and the saturation is lower; at the capillary level, more O_2 is released and available to the tissues.

—Increased hydrogen ion concentration (reduced pH) shifts the curve to the right (Bohr effect), as does increased concentration of 2,3-diphosphoglycerate in red blood cell (RBC) count, which alters the spatial relationships within the Hb molecule.

—Hb characterized by a leftward shifting of the curve has an increased affinity for O_2.

HEART FAILURE
Definition

HF is symptomatic myocardial dysfunction resulting in a characteristic pattern of hemodynamic, renal, and neurohormonal responses.

- No definition of HF is completely satisfactory.
  —HF occurs when, despite normal venous pressures, the heart is unable to maintain sufficient CO to meet the demands of the body.
  —Congestive heart failure (CHF) develops when plasma volume increases and fluid accumulates in the lungs, abdominal organs (particularly the liver), and peripheral tissues.

Risk Factors

- Any factor that increases myocardial work may precipitate or aggravate heart failure.
  —Dysrhythmias
  —Thyrotoxicosis
  —Pregnancy
  —Anemia
  —Endocarditis
  —Pulmonary infection
  —Adjustment of HF therapy

Etiology/Cause

- Myocardial dysfunction (e.g., ischemic heart disease, cardiomyopathy, hypertension)
- Volume overload (e.g., valvular regurgitation—aortic or mitral)
- Obstruction to outflow (e.g., aortic stenosis)

BOX 5-3

Pathophysiologic Changes in Heart Failure

Ventricular dilation
Myocyte hypertrophy
Increased collagen synthesis
Altered myosin gene expression
Altered sarcoplasm Ca^{2+}-ATPase density
Increased ANP secretion
Salt and water retention
Sympathetic stimulation
Peripheral vasoconstriction

Data from Gottlieb SH: Heart failure. In Barker LR, Burton JR, Zieve PD, eds: *Principles of ambulatory medicine*, Baltimore, 1999, Williams & Wilkins, pp 821-843; Massie BM, Amidon TM: Cardiac failure. In Tierney LM, McPhee LM, Papadakis MA, eds: *Current medical diagnosis & treatment 2000*, New York, 2000, Lange Medical Books/McGraw-Hill, pp 416-426.
ANP, Atrial natriuretic peptide.

- Obligatory high output (e.g., anemia, thyrotoxicosis, Paget's disease, beriberi, systemic-to-pulmonary shunts)
- Compromised ventricular filling (e.g., constrictive pericarditis, pericardial tamponade, restrictive cardiomyopathy)
- Altered rhythm (e.g., atrial fibrillation)

Pathogenesis (Box 5-3)

- When the heart fails, considerable changes occur in the heart and peripheral vascular system in response to the hemodynamic changes associated with HF.
- These physiologic changes are compensatory to maintain cardiac output and peripheral perfusion.
- However, as HF progresses, these mechanisms are overwhelmed and become pathophysiologic.
- Development of pathophysiologic peripheral vasoconstriction and sodium retention reflects loss of beneficial compensatory mechanisms and represents cardiac decompensation manifested by the onset of clinical HF.
- Factors involved include: venous return, outflow resistance, contractility of the myocardium, and salt and water retention.

Myocardial Remodeling in Heart Failure

- Myocardial hypertrophy is one of the major adaptations to hemodynamic overload of the left ventricle.

—As cardiac myocytes are terminally differentiated, this occurs by an increase in myocyte size and the growth of nonmyocyte components (e.g., vascular smooth muscle cells and fibroblasts).

—Collagen synthesis may also increase.

- These structural changes result in an increase in myocardial volume and mass, impaired systolic and diastolic function, and impaired coronary blood flow.

Changes in Myocardial Gene Expression

- Hemodynamic overload of the ventricle stimulates changes in cardiac contractile protein gene expression.
- The overall effect is to increase protein synthesis, but many proteins also switch to fetal and neonatal isoforms.

Abnormal Calcium Homeostasis

- Calcium ion flux within myocytes plays a pivotal role in the regulation of contractile function.
  - —Excitation of the myocyte cell membrane causes the rapid entry of calcium into myocytes from the extracellular space via calcium channels.
  - —This triggers the release of *intracellular* calcium from the sarcoplasmic reticulum and initiates contraction.
  - —Relaxation results from the uptake and storage of calcium by the sarcoplasmic reticulum.
- In HF, there is a prolongation of the calcium current in association with prolongation of contraction and relaxation.
  - —One mechanism may be a decrease in sarcolemmal Ca^{2+}-ATPase density.

Apoptosis

- Apoptosis (or "programmed cell death") is the process by which cells self-destruct after the induction of endonucleases that degrade deoxyribonucleic acid (DNA).
  - —It is a normal feature in the developing fetus and in some adult tissues (e.g., thymus).
- Apoptosis has been demonstrated in animal models of ischemic reperfusion, rapid ventricular pacing, mechanical stretch, and pressure overload.

- Preliminary research in humans suggests that apoptosis occurs in patients with idiopathic dilated cardiomyopathy, and it is proposed that the spiral of ventricular dysfunction characteristic of HF may result from the initiation of apoptosis by cytokines, free radicals, and other triggers.

Cardiac Hormones ↗ ANP - c̄ Stretch

- Atrial natriuretic peptide (ANP) is released from atrial myocytes in response to stretch.
- ANP induces diuresis, natriuresis, vasodilation, and suppression of the renin-angiotensin system.
- Levels of circulating ANP are increased in CHF and correlate with functional class, prognosis, and hemodynamic state.
- The renal response to ANP is attenuated in HF, probably secondary to reduced renal perfusion, receptor down-regulation, increased peptide breakdown, renal sympathetic activation, and excessive renin-angiotensin activity.
- The potential therapeutic benefits of the natriuretic peptides have been investigated by the administration of ANP given IV and the inhibition of the enzyme responsible for breakdown of the peptide (neural endopeptidase [NEP]).
  - —Initial results suggest that these drugs might have a therapeutic role in the future.

Endothelial Function in Heart Failure

- The endothelium has a central role in the regulation of vasomotor tone.
- In patients with heart failure, endothelium-dependent vasodilation in peripheral blood vessels is impaired and may be one mechanism of exercise limitation.
- The cause of abnormal endothelial responsiveness is complex but relates to abnormal release of both nitric oxide and vasoconstrictor substances (e.g., endothelin [ET]).
- ET secretion from a variety of tissues is stimulated by many factors: hypoxia, catecholamines, angiotensin II, and stress.
- Although most of the ET produced by the vascular endothelium in response to these

stimuli is secreted abluminally, endothelin is also found circulating in plasma.
- Plasma ET concentration is elevated in patients with HF; the levels correlate with the severity of hemodynamic disturbance.
- Preliminary data indicate that the major source of circulating ET in HF is the pulmonary vascular bed.

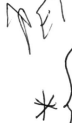

- ET has many actions that potentially contribute to the pathophysiology of heart failure
  —Vasoconstriction
  —Sympathetic stimulation
  —Renin-angiotensin system activation
  —LV hypertrophy
- Research data indicate that the acute intravenous administration of ET antagonists improves hemodynamic abnormalities in patients with congestive cardiac failure, and oral endothelin antagonists are currently being developed.

Diagnosis

- It is useful clinically to divide HF into the syndromes of right, left, and biventricular (congestive) cardiac failure, although it is rare for any part of the heart to fail in isolation.

Right Heart Failure
- Occurs in association with
  —Chronic lung disease (cor pulmonale)
  —Pulmonary embolism or pulmonary hypertension
  —Tricuspid valve disease
  —Pulmonary valve disease
  —Left-to-right shunts (e.g., atrial or ventricular septal defects)
  —Isolated RV cardiomyopathy
  —Mitral valve disease with pulmonary hypertension
- The most frequent cause of right HF is secondary to left HF.

Signs and Symptoms
- Fatigue
- Breathlessness
- Anorexia
- Nausea
- Jugular venous distension ($\pm$ v waves of tricuspid regurgitation)
- Tender smooth hepatic enlargement
- Dependent pitting edema
- Development of free abdominal fluid (ascites)
- Pleural transudates (commonly right-sided)
- Dilation of the right ventricle produces cardiomegaly and may result in functional tricuspid regurgitation.
- Tachycardia and a RV third heart sound (S_3) are usual.

Left Heart Failure S_3 or S_4
- Causes
  —Ischemic heart disease (most common cause)
  —Systemic hypertension (chronic or "malignant")
  —Mitral and aortic valve disease
  —Cardiomyopathies
  —Mitral stenosis causes left atrial hypertension and signs of left HF, but does not itself cause failure of the left ventricle.

Signs and Symptoms
- Fatigue
- Exertional dyspnea
- Orthopnea
- Paroxysmal nocturnal dyspnea
- Physical signs are not prominent until a late stage, or if the ventricular failure is acute.
  —Cardiomegaly is indicated by a displaced and often sustained apical impulse.
  —Auscultation reveals an LV S_3 or S_4 that, with tachycardia, is described as a gallop rhythm.
  —Dilation of the mitral annulus results in functional mitral regurgitation.
  —Crackles are heard at the lung bases.
  —In severe HF, the patient has pulmonary edema.

Biventricular (Congestive) Heart Failure
- Biventricular CHF is used to describe patients in whom right HF is a result of preexisting left HF.
- Physical signs and symptoms are therefore a combination of right and left HF.

Acute Heart Failure
- The rapid onset of acute HF occurs most commonly of acute myocardial infarction when there is extensive loss of ventricular muscle.

- May also occur as a result of rupture of the interventricular septum, producing a ventricular septal defect
- Acute valvular regurgitation also precipitates acute HF.
  - —Acute valvular regurgitation occurs in papillary or chordal rupture, producing mitral regurgitation or sudden aortic valve regurgitation in infective endocarditis.
- Other causes include obstruction of the circulation by acute pulmonary embolus and cardiac tamponade.
  - —In these cases, HF can occur with a relatively normal heart size.

Diagnostic Tests

- A clinical diagnosis of HF should always be confirmed using objective measures of LV structure and function (usually echocardiography).
  - —Two-dimensional and Doppler echocardiography establishes the presence of systolic and/or diastolic impairment of the left or right ventricles and may reveal the etiology (valve disease, regional wall motion abnormalities in ischemic heart disease, cardiomyopathy, amyloid) of intracardiac thrombus.
  - —An ejection fraction of <0.45 is generally accepted as evidence for systolic dysfunction.
- Chest x-ray—to show cardiac size and evidence of ischemia and hypertension
- ECG
- Blood tests
  - —CBC
  - —Liver function tests
  - —Urea
  - —Electrolytes
- Resting and stress radionuclide angiography multiple-gated acquisition scan (MUGA)—ejection fraction, regional wall motion abnormality
- Ambulatory ECG monitoring for 24 to 48 hours—if dysrhythmia is suspected
- Serum ANP levels are over 70% sensitive and specific for detecting LV systolic dysfunction.

Treatment (Box 5-4)
- Goals of therapy
  - —Relieve symptoms
  - —Slow progression of the disorder

BOX 5-4

Treatment of Heart Failure

DRUGS
Diuretics (thiazide or loop)
Angiotensin-converting enzyme (ACE) inhibitors
Digitalis glycosides
Vasodilator combination (hydralazine and nitrate)
β-Adrenoceptor blockers (metoprolol, bisoprolol)
Antidysrhythmics
Anticoagulants
Positive inotropes

DEVICES AND SURGERY
Coronary artery bypass grafting
Pacemaker/implantable cardioverter-defibrillator (ICD)
Heart transplantation
Cardiomyoplasty

Data from Gottlieb SH: Heart failure. In Barker LR, Burton JF, Zieve PD, eds: *Principles of ambulatory medicine*, ed 5, Baltimore, 1999, Williams & Wilkins, pp 821-843; Massie BM, Amidon TM: Cardiac failure. Tierney LM, McPhee SJ, Papadakis MA, eds: *Current medical diagnosis & treatment 2000*, New York, 2000, Lange Medical Books/McGraw Hill, pp 416-426.

  - —Improve prognostic indicators
- Treat any factor that is suspected of aggravating the cardiac failure
  - —Smoking cessation
  - —Alcohol intake reduction or elimination
  - —Effective therapy for hypertension
  - —Effective therapy for hypercholesterolemia
  - —Appropriate drug therapy after MI
- Physical activity
  - —For patients with exacerbation of CHF, bed rest reduces the demands of the heart and is useful for a few days.
  - —Movement of interstitial fluid promotes diuresis, which also aids in minimizing demands of the heart.
  - —However, prolonged bed rest may result in development of deep vein thrombosis, which, while the patient is in bed or reclining in a chair, can be prevented by regularly scheduled leg exercises, low-dose subcutaneous heparin, and elastic support stockings.
  - —Low-level endurance exercise (e.g., 20 to 30 minutes walking three to five times/week or 20 minutes cycling at 70% to 80% of peak heart rate five times/week) is strongly encouraged in patients with compensated HF to reverse "deconditioning" of peripheral muscle metabolism.

—Strenuous isometric activity should be avoided.
- Diet
  —Large meals should be avoided.
  —Weight reduction should be initiated as necessary.
  —Salt restriction is important, although a low-sodium diet is unpalatable and of questionable value.
  —Alcohol has a negatively inotropic effect and patients should abstain.
- Vaccination
  —Recommended that patients with HF be vaccinated against pneumococcal disease and influenza
- Drug therapy
  —Diuretics act by promoting renal excretion of salt and water by blocking tubular reabsorption of sodium and chloride.
  —The resulting loss of fluid reduces ventricular filling pressures (preload), produces consistent hemodynamic and symptomatic benefits, and rapidly relieves dyspnea and peripheral edema.
  —IV loop diuretics (furosemide) relieve pulmonary edema by arteriolar vasodilation, which reduces afterload, an action that is independent of its diuretic action.
- **Any patient with HF or a history of pulmonary edema should receive IV fluids VERY slowly while being monitored carefully.**
  —Too-rapid administration of IV fluids can cause massive CHF because of cardiac overload.
  —Spironolactone is a specific competitive antagonist to aldosterone, which produces a weak diuresis but with a potassium-sparing action.
  - ~ These drugs should be avoided in patients with renal failure and in patients taking angiotensin-converting enzyme (ACE) inhibitors unless there is persistent hypokalemia.
- Vasodilator therapy
  —Diuretics and sodium restriction serve to activate the renin-angiotensin system, promoting formation of angiotensin, a potent vasoconstrictor, which increases afterload.
  —Other neural and hormonal reactions also increase preload and afterload; these compensatory mechanisms are initially beneficial in maintaining blood pressure and redistributing blood flow, but in the later stages of HF they are deleterious and reduce cardiac output.
  —Studies show the value of vasodilator therapy in HF: they improve prognosis and limit the development of progressive HF.
- Arteriolar vasodilators
  —Drugs such as β-adrenergic blockers (e.g., prazosin) and direct smooth-muscle relaxants (e.g., hydralazine) are potent arteriolar vasodilators.
  —Calcium channel blockers also reduce afterload, but first-generation calcium antagonists (diltiazem, nifedipine) may have a detrimental effect on LV function in patients with HF.
  - ~ Research shows that second-generation calcium antagonists (e.g., amlodipine) are safe in heart failure and of possible prognostic benefit in those with non-ischemic etiology; reduced afterload results in increased cardiac output.
- Venodilators
  —Short- and long-acting nitrates (e.g., glyceryl trinitrate and isosorbide mononitrate) act by reducing preload and lowering venous pressure, resulting in reduction in pulmonary and dependent edema.
  —If used for long periods, patients develop tolerance, with loss of efficacy and consequent worsening of HF.
  —Combined therapy with hydralazine and oral nitrates has been shown to improve mortality and exercise performance, and may be useful when ACE inhibitors are contraindicated.
- ACE inhibitors
  —ACE inhibitors lower systemic vascular resistance and venous pressure, and reduce levels of circulating catecholamines, which results in improved myocardial performance.
  —The beneficial hemodynamic effect of these drugs seems to be independent of their inhibition of ACE as they are equally effective when plasma renin activity is normal.
- β-Adrenoceptor blocking agents
  —These drugs symptoms, exercise tolerance, and LV function improve in patients with HF from any cause.

—Carvedolol, a nonselective vasodilator β-blocker with added vasodilator and antioxidant properties, was shown to produce significant improvement in mortality; initially, the ejection fraction may decline, but it usually returns to baseline within a month and then increases after 3 months.

~ Initial doses should be low, and titrated slowly over a period of months rather than days.

—There is no agreement regarding the timing of β-blocker therapy.

- Inotropic agents
  —Digitalis glycosides have been used for many years in patients with HF and AF, but their use in patients with normal sinus rhythm is controversial.
  —Studies show that digoxin improves exercise tolerance, increases LV ejection fraction, and alleviates signs and symptoms of CHF, but some studies show that digoxin may increase mortality in patients with MI.
  —β-Adrenergic agonists
  ~ Dobutamine, dopexamine, and dopamine are examples of IV adrenergic agonists.
  ~ These agents are used in patients with acute LV failure and in those with end-stage HF as a bridge to transplantation.
  ~ Intermittent dobutamine therapy may produce long-lasting improvements in symptoms and exercise tolerance, but at the cost of increased mortality.

- Summary
  —Generally now recognized that all patients with clinical HF should receive therapy with diuretics and an ACE inhibitor
  —Patients with AF should be digitalized, but those in sinus rhythm may also be improved by adding digoxin or a β-blocker.
  —Patients with asymptomatic LV dysfunction are at risk of progressive deterioration and should be treated with prophylactic ACE inhibitor therapy.
  —Patients with ischemic HF and ongoing ischemia, and those intolerant of ACE inhibitors or in whom they are contraindicated (hypotension, renal insufficiency, hyperkalemia), may benefit from nitrate/hydralazine therapy.

- Nonpharmacologic therapy
  —Revascularization: coronary artery disease is the most common cause of HF; the role of revascularization in patients with HF is unclear.
  —Patients with angina and LV dysfunction have a higher mortality from surgery (10% to 20%), but probably have the most to gain with respect to improved symptoms and prognosis.
  —Pacemakers or implantable cardioverter-defibrillators (ICDs) are indicated in patients with SA disease and AV conduction block.
  ~ These devices may have a minor role in patients with prolonged PR intervals, left bundle branch block, and severe mitral regurgitation.
  ~ In patients with a history of sustained VT or VF, ICDs are effective in terminating further episodes of ventricular dysrhythmia; their effectiveness compared with established drug therapy has not been studied.

- Heart transplantation
  —Since the advent of cyclosporine in the late 1970s and improved immunosuppressive regimens, heart transplantation has become the treatment of choice for younger patients with severe intractable HF whose life expectancy without a transplant is less than 6 months.
  —In carefully selected recipients, the 1-year survival is over 80%, and 70% at 5 years.
  —The quality of life is dramatically improved in the majority of patients.

PULMONARY EDEMA
Definition

Acute pulmonary edema is a life-threatening manifestation of acute LV failure secondary to sudden onset of pulmonary venous hypertension.

Risk Factors

- History of heart disease/failure

Etiology/Cause

- Acute myocardial infarction
- Severe ischemia
- Exacerbation of CHF

- Acute volume overload of the left ventricle (valvular regurgitation or ventricular septal defect)
- Mitral stenosis

Pathogenesis

- A sudden rise in LV filling pressure results in rapid movement of plasma fluid through pulmonary capillaries into the interstitial spaces and alveoli.

Diagnosis

Signs and Symptoms

- Patients with acute pulmonary edema present with a characteristic picture
  —Extreme dyspnea
  —Deep cyanosis
  —Tachypnea with peripheral circulatory shutdown
  —Hyperpnea
  —Restlessness
  —Anxiety
  —Feeling of suffocation
  —Thready pulse
  —Pallor
  —Diaphoresis
  —BP is difficult to obtain
  —Labored respirations
  —Crackles are heard over both lung fields, anteriorly and posteriorly.
  —Some patients have marked bronchospasm or wheezing (cardiac asthma).
  —Productive cough with blood-tinged (pink), frothy sputum, which can be copious
  —Summation gallop on auscultation of the heart (merger of S_3 and S_4)
  —Severe hypoxemia
  —CO_2 retention is a late, ominous sign of secondary hypoventilation and requires immediate care.
  —Chest x-ray shows signs of pulmonary vascular redistribution, blurriness of vascular outlines, increased interstitial markings, and the butterfly pattern of distribution of alveolar edema.
  —In cardiogenic pulmonary edema, the pulmonary capillary wedge pressure is always elevated, often over 25 mm Hg.

Treatment

- The patient should be placed in a sitting position with legs dangling over the side of the bed,

which facilitates respiration and reduces venous return.
- Oxygen by mask to obtain an arterial P_{O_2} greater than 60 mm Hg
- Treatment of severe pulmonary edema occurs in ICUs.
- If respiratory distress is severe, endotracheal intubation and mechanical ventilation are necessary.
- Morphine 4 to 8 mg IV (subcutaneous administration is effective in milder cases)
  —Morphine is repeated in 2 to 4 hours.
  —However, morphine can cause CO_2 retention, reducing the ventilatory drive.
- IV diuretic (furosemide 40 mg) or higher dose if patient has been on diuretic therapy
- Sublingual or IV nitrates and phlebotomy of about 500 ml of blood, or plasmapheresis
- ACE inhibitors
- β-Blockers
- Digitalis

Prognosis

- Variable, depending on the severity of cardiac disease, age, response to therapy, and other factors

PERIPHERAL VASCULAR DISEASE

Acute Peripheral Arterial Occlusion

Definition

An acute peripheral arterial occlusion is an occlusion of blood supply to the extremities by atherosclerotic plaques (atheromas), a thrombus, or an embolism.

Risk Factors

- Acute or chronic ischemic heart disease
- History of atherosclerosis
- Hypertension
- Elevated levels of LDL
- Cigarette smoking
- Diabetes mellitus
- Obesity
- Male sex
- Family history of premature atherosclerosis

Etiology/Cause

- Most large arterial emboli originate in the heart, usually (94%) due to atherosclerosis or other heart disease, usually ischemic heart disease.
- AF is frequently present.

- Atherosclerotic plaques from any location in the body

Pathogenesis
- Peripheral arterial occlusion usually causes acute or chronic ischemia in the area.
- Acute ischemia is caused by a ruptured proximal arteriosclerotic plaque.
- Sustained elevation of blood homocysteine predisposes to premature atherosclerosis of the aorta and its branches, the peripheral arteries, the cerebral arteries, and perhaps the coronary arteries, as a result of damage to endothelial cells.

Diagnosis
Signs and Symptoms
- The clinical picture depends on the vessel involved, the extent of obstruction, how rapidly occlusion progresses, and whether collateral blood flow is adequate.

Acute Occlusion
- Sudden onset of severe pain
- Coldness
- Numbness
- Pallor in the area or extremity
- Pulses are absent distal to the obstruction.
- Acute occlusion may result in severe ischemia manifested by sensory and motor loss and, after 6-8 hours, tender induration of muscles on palpation.
- In acute occlusion of the aorta (saddle embolus or thrombosis), all pulses in the lower extremities are absent.
- Most often, acute occlusions occur at bifurcations just distal to the last palpable pulse (e.g., with occlusion at the common femoral bifurcation, the femoral pulse may be palpable; with occlusion at the popliteal bifurcation, the popliteal pulse may be palpable.

Chronic Occlusion
- Symptoms occur relating to the insidious development of tissue ischemia
  - Claudication: pain, ache, cramp, or tired feeling that occurs on walking; most common in the calf but may occur in the foot, thigh, hip, or buttocks
  - Claudication is made worse by walking rapidly or uphill, but is usually relieved by 1- to 5-minute rest (sitting is not necessary).
  - After resting, the person can walk for the same distance again before pain returns.
  - Disease progression is according to the decreasing distance that the person can walk without symptoms.
  - Eventually, ischemic pain can occur at rest and develops in the most distal parts of a limb as a severe, unrelenting pain or ache aggravated by elevation and often preventing sleep.
  - For relief, the patient dangles the foot/feet over the edge of the bed, or sits in a chair with legs dependent.
- If claudication is the only symptom, the limb usually appears normal, but the pulses are diminished or absent.
  - Level of arterial occlusion and the location of intermittent claudication are closely correlated
- In men, impotence may be a symptom of occlusion.
- With extreme ischemia of the lower leg, the foot is painful, cold, and usually numb.
  - In chronic cases, the skin becomes dry and scaly with poor nail and hair growth.
  - As ischemia worsens, ulceration begins, often in the toes or heel, sometimes on the leg, especially after local trauma.
  - Severely ischemic leg may atrophy.
  - Sustained and extensive ischemia leads to necrosis and gangrene.

Diagnostic Tests
- Arterial occlusion can usually be diagnosed clinically, but noninvasive tests confirm the diagnosis.
- Doppler ultrasonography
- BP readings at the ankle and at the brachial artery of the arm
  - In severe arterial insufficiency, the BP reading at the ankle is <50% of the BP in the brachial artery.
- Magnetic resonance angiography provides images similar to contrast angiography and is rapidly replacing contrast angiography.

Differential Diagnosis
- Ischemia with rubor, pain, and swelling of the foot on dependency may mimic cellulitis or venous insufficiency.

Treatment/Prevention/Patient Education

- Tobacco in all forms must be eliminated.
- Patients with intermittent claudication should walk 30 to 60 minutes/day, continuing after rest periods as pain occurs.
- At night, the head of the bed should be elevated 4 to 6 in, which improves perfusion in the lower extremities.
- Vasodilators may be prescribed, although their effectiveness is uncertain.
- Calcium blockers and aspirin (thromboxane inhibitors) are useful in patients with occlusive and vasospastic arterial diseases.
- Pentoxifylline 400 mg tid with meals may help to improve intermittent claudication in some patients by improving blood flow and tissue oxygenation.
  - Side effects of pentoxifylline are mild, and so a trial of ≥ 2 months is warranted to evaluate degree of improvement.
- Prophylactic foot care is mandatory, particularly in those with diabetes.
  - Feet should be inspected daily for cracks, fissures, calluses, corns, and ulcers; any sign of these should be treated by a podiatrist.
  - Feet should be bathed daily in lukewarm water with mild soap, and dried gently but thoroughly.
  - A lubricant such as lanolin should be used if skin is dry or scaly.
  - Bland, nonmedicated foot powders can be used for moist feet.
  - Patients should avoid using adhesive tape, corn plasters, hot water bottles, and heating pads on the feet and legs.
  - Shoes should fit well, with wide toes, without open toes or heels, and be changed frequently.
  - Walking barefoot should be avoided.
- Percutaneous endovascular therapy—new noninvasive treatments now exist that obviate open surgery for occlusion and aneurysm
  - Usually done by interventional radiologists, vascular surgeons, or cardiologists
  - The primary mode is percutaneous transluminal angioplasty (PTA), in which a small high-pressure balloon is used to open an obstructed vessel.
  - Stents, metallic-meshlike tubes, are inserted into the vessel at the site of the obstruction; these are strong and keep the vessel open better than balloons, and recurrence rate of obstruction is less; these work best in large vessels (e.g., iliac and renal).
    - ~ Contraindications to PTA of peripheral arteries are diffuse disease, long occlusions, and severe arterial calcification.
- Surgery may be required for thrombosis at the site of dilation, distal embolization, intimal dissection with occlusion by a flap, and complications due to heparin therapy.
  - Thromboendarterectomy, bypass graft, and resection with graft replacement are examples of surgery performed to avert amputation.
  - If amputation becomes necessary, the choice is below-knee to preserve this joint for maximal prosthesis use.

THROMBOANGIITIS OBLITERANS (BUERGER'S DISEASE)
Definition

Thromboangiitis obliterans (Buerger's disease) is an obliterative disease characterized by inflammatory changes in small- and medium-sized arteries and veins. The number of persons diagnosed is decreasing because of greater understanding and use of newer treatment modalities.

Risk Factors

- Cigarette smoking
- Men, 20 to 40 years of age
- About 5% of cases occur in women.

Etiology/Cause

- The cause is unknown, but the disease has not been documented in nonsmokers, pointing to cigarette smoking as a primary etiologic factor.
- This condition may be a reaction to tobacco in persons with a specific phenotype, because of greater prevalence of HLA-A9 and HLA-B5 in those with the disease.
- The condition may be an autoimmune disorder with cell-mediated sensitivity to types I and III human collagen (constituents of blood vessels).

- This condition does not involve the coronary arteries.

Pathogenesis

- Small- and medium-sized arteries and veins and, often, superficial veins in the extremities
- Proliferation of endothelial cells and infiltration of the intimal layer with lymphocytes are characteristics of the acute lesion, although the internal elastic lamina is intact.
- The thrombus becomes organized and, over time, completely recanalizes.
- Older lesions show periarterial fibrosis that may extend into adjacent veins and nerves.

Diagnosis

Signs and Symptoms

- Signs and symptoms are those of arterial ischemia and of superficial thrombophlebitis.
- History of migratory phlebitis, usually in the superficial veins of the foot or leg, is true of about 40% of patients.
- Onset is gradual, beginning in the most distal vessels of the upper and lower extremities and progressing proximally, ending with distal gangrene.
- The patient complains of coldness, numbness, tingling, or burning before there is objective evidence of disease.
- Raynaud's phenomenon is common.
- Intermittent claudication occurs in the affected leg (rarely in the thigh, arm, or hand).
- Pain is persistent as ischemia worsens.

Diagnostic Tests

- Arteriograms usually show segmental occlusions of distal arteries, especially of hands and feet.
- Collateral circulation forms around occlusions and is often more tortuous than those associated with other occlusive diseases.

Treatment/Prevention/Patient Education

- Treatment goals are to maximize blood supply.
- Eliminate smoking—the acute stage will progress unremittingly if the patient continues to smoke.
- Avoid vasoconstriction from exposure to cold or drugs.
- Avoid thermal, chemical, or mechanical injury (poorly fitting shoes, minor surgery of digits, fungal infections).

- Regular walking exercise for 15 to 30 minutes/day
- Feet should be protected by heel pads or by foam rubber booties.
- Hot water bottles and heating pads should not be used.
- Elevate head of bed 6 to 8 in to improve arterial filling through gravity.
- Pentoxifylline, calcium blockers, and thromboxane inhibitors may be of help.
- Because larger vessels are seldom involved, bypass grafts are not done.

RAYNAUD'S DISEASE/RAYNAUD'S PHENOMENON

Definition

Raynaud's disease is a spasm of arterioles, usually in the digits and occasionally in other areas (nose, tongue) with intermittent pallor or cyanosis.

Risk Factors

- Young women
- Associated connective tissue disorders (e.g., scleroderma, rheumatoid arthritis, lupus)
- Other occlusive diseases
- Thoracic outlet syndrome
- Drug toxicity: ergot, methysergide
- Primary pulmonary hypertension
- Trauma

Etiology/Cause

- The cause of Raynaud's disease is not known with certainty.
- Research regarding prostaglandin, metabolism, microcirculation, and the role of the endothelial cell as possible causes is being conducted.
- In addition to those conditions listed above, Raynaud's disease is also associated with migraine headache and variant angina which, together with pulmonary hypertension, suggest a vasospastic mechanism.

Pathogenesis

- The threshold for the vasospastic response is lowered by local cold or anything that activates sympathetic outflow or releases catecholamines (e.g., emotion).
- Early in the disease, the vessels are normal histologically; as the disease advances, the arterial

intima may thicken and thromboses may form in smaller arteries.

Diagnosis

Signs and Symptoms

- Intermittent blanching or cyanosis of the digits is precipitated by exposure to cold or emotional upset.
- Color changes may occur in phases: pallor, cyanosis, redness—reactive hyperemia; or in two phases—cyanosis and redness.
- Color changes do not occur above the metacarpophalangeal joints, and the thumb is rarely involved.
- In Raynaud's disease, trophic skin changes and gangrene are absent, or affect only minimal areas, and symptoms do not worsen, regardless of the number of years that the disorder has been present.
- In Raynaud's phenomenon, there is a recognizable underlying cause.
  - With scleroderma, there may be tightness or thickening of the skin and telangiectases of the hands, arms, or face.
  - Difficulty swallowing
  - Painful trophic ulcers on the fingertips
  - Symptoms of other systems are present.
  - Wrist pulses are usually present, but Allen's test (usually negative in Raynaud's disease) often shows occlusion of the radial or ulnar arterial branches distal to the wrist.

Treatment/Patient Education

Raynaud's Disease

- When the condition is mild, treatment may be limited to protection of the hands and feet from cold.
- Stop smoking (nicotine is a vasoconstrictor).
- Relaxation or biofeedback techniques may help to reduce the number of vasospastic episodes in some patients.
- Prazosin 1 to 2 mg PO at bedtime (repeated in the morning)
- The calcium blocker nifedipine 10 to 30 mg PO tid
- Pentoxifylline 400 mg bid or tid with meals has been effective.
- Phenoxybenzamine 10 mg PO daily to tid and guanethidine 10 mg PO qid to tid have helped in some cases.

Raynaud's Phenomenon

- Diagnosis and treatment of the underlying disorder
- Phenoxybenzamine 10 mg PO daily to tid may be helpful.
- Antibiotics, analgesics, and sometimes surgery to debride ulcerated fingertips may be necessary.
- Research using prostaglandin (thromboxane) is encouraging.
- In both Raynaud's disease and Raynaud's phenomenon, β-blockers, clonidine, and ergot are contraindicated.

VENOUS THROMBOSIS (THROMBOPHLEBITIS)

"white" platelets

Definition

Venous thrombosis is the presence of a thrombus in a vein.

Risk Factors

- Injury to the endothelium of the vein (from indwelling catheters, injection of irritating substances)
- Malignant tumors with resulting hypercoagulability
- Blood dyscrasias
- Oral contraceptives
- Venous stasis in postpartum and postoperative states
- Prolonged bed rest
- HF
- Stroke
- Prolonged immobilization with legs dependent (as on long air flights)
- Strenuous exercise in an affected extremity

Etiology/Cause

- Most venous thrombi originate in the valve cusps of deep calf veins.
- Tissue thromboplastin is released, forming thrombin and fibrin that trap RBCs and propagate proximally as a red or fibrin thrombus.
  - This is the predominant venous lesion, while the white or platelet thrombus is the principal component of most arterial lesions.

Diagnosis

Signs and Symptoms

- Development of an acute thrombophlebitis can occur over hours to 1 to 2 days.

- The condition is usually self-limited, lasting 1 to 2 weeks, when the acute process abates and pain subsides.
- In superficial thrombophlebitis, a thrombosed superficial vein can be palpated as a linear, indurated cord; a deep vein thrombus cannot be palpated.
- The area may be red, painful, tender to the touch, erythematous, and warm in deep vein thrombosis (DVT), the patient may be asymptomatic, or there may be tenderness, edema, warmth, skin discoloration, and prominent superficial veins, over the area of the DVT.
- DVT often involves the popliteal, femoral, and iliac segments, in which there is pain and a hard cord palpable over the involved vein in the femoral triangle, medial thigh, or popliteal space.
- At least three main veins drain the lower leg, so thrombosis in one does not obstruct venous return, and there are no swelling, cyanosis, or dilated superficial veins.
- The patient complains of soreness or pain on standing and walking, usually relieved by rest with the leg elevated.
- On examination, deep calf tenderness can be elicited, but the pain of DVT is not easily differentiated from muscle pain.
- Chronic venous insufficiency in the leg after DVT is noted as edema and dilated superficial veins, and tiredness in the leg.
  —Symptoms occur during standing or walking, and are relieved by rest and elevation of the affected leg.
- Stasis syndrome occurs if edema is not controlled by an elastic support stocking.
  —Skin pigmentation appears on the medial and sometimes the lateral aspect of the ankle and lower leg.
  —Stasis dermatitis and stasis ulceration may develop in these areas.

Diagnostic Tests
- In 50% of cases, DVT cannot be diagnosed by clinical findings alone.
- The diagnosis is confirmed by noninvasive testing or by venography.
- Duplex ultrasonography is diagnostic in most cases in which thrombus involves the iliac, femoral, or popliteal veins.

Treatment
- Goals of therapy are to prevent pulmonary embolism and chronic venous insufficiency.
- Hospitalization may be required initially, but many patients can be treated at home.
- The foot of the bed is elevated 6 in.
- The patient is heparinized.
- Under these treatments, the patient is allowed bathroom privileges.
- Low-molecular-weight heparin is followed soon by oral warfarin, with the dosage adjusted to achieve an international normalization ratio (INR) between 2 and 3.
  —Length of anticoagulant therapy depends on the patient.
  —DVT subsiding in 3 to 6 days in a young, healthy patient with no risk factors may require only 2 months of therapy.
  —Others who are older, with risk factors and demonstrable pulmonary embolus, may require 6 months of therapy.
  —If the patient has more than 2 episodes of DVT, oral anticoagulant therapy should be continued indefinitely.
- When edema subsides, the patient should be measured for a firm below-knee elastic stocking providing 30 to 40 mm Hg pressure to control edema and prevent chronic venous insufficiency.
- If ulcers develop, treatment is Unna's paste boot or bed rest with elevation and compression dressings, either of which will heal most ulcers.
- Large refractory or recurrent ulcers may have to be excised, the incompetent perforating veins ligated, and the area covered with a split-thickness skin graft.

Prognosis/Patient Education
- DVT is usually benign, but can cause fatal pulmonary emboli or chronic venous insufficiency.
- With appropriate treatment and careful follow-up to confirm that the patient is following directions (not smoking, wearing support stockings of the appropriate size and pressure, and taking the prescribed anticoagulant as directed), the patient can have a successful outcome.

BIBLIOGRAPHY
Barker LR: Hypertension. In Barker LR, Burton JR, Zieve PD, eds: *Principles of ambulatory medicine*, ed 5, Baltimore, 1999, Williams & Wilkins, pp 844-887.

Beers MH, Berkow R: Cardiovascular disorders, peripheral vascular disorders. In Beers MH, Berkow R, eds: *The Merck manual of diagnosis and therapy,* ed 17, Whitehouse Station, NJ, 1999, Merck Research Laboratories, pp 1599-1749, 1784-1798.

Gottlieb SH, Calkins H: Arrhythmias. In Barker LR, Burton JR, Zieve PD, eds: *Principles of ambulatory medicine,* ed 5, Baltimore, 1999, Williams & Wilkins, pp 768-798.

Gottlieb SH: Heart failure. In Barker LR, Burton JR, Zieve PD, eds: *Principles of ambulatory medicine,* ed 5, Baltimore, 1999, Williams & Wilkins, pp 821-843.

Massie BM, Amidon TM: Heart. In Tierney LM, McPhee SJ, Papadakis MA, eds: *Current medical diagnosis & treatment 2000,* New York, 2000, Lange Medical Books/McGraw-Hill, pp 351-443.

Massie BM: Systemic hypertension. In Tierney LM, McPhee SJ, Papadakis MA, eds: *Current medical diagnosis & treatment 2000,* New York, 2000, Lange Medical Books/McGraw-Hill, pp 444-466.

Shannon MT, Wilson A, Stang CL: *Health professionals drug guide 2000,* Stamford, Conn, 2000, Appleton & Lange.

Strobos N: Angina pectoris. In Barker LR, Burton JR, Zieve PD, eds: *Principles of ambulatory medicine,* ed 5, Baltimore, 1999, Williams & Wilkins, pp 719-744.

Tierney LM, Messina LM: Blood vessels & lymphatics. In Tierney LM, McPhee SJ, Papadakis MA, eds: *Current medical diagnosis & treatment 2000,* New York, 2000, Lange Medical Books/McGraw-Hill, pp 467-498.

Vaitkevicius PV, Stewart KJ: Postmyocardial infarction care, cardiac rehabilitation, and physical conditioning. In Barker RL, Burton JR, Zieve PD, eds: *Principles of ambulatory medicine,* ed 5, Baltimore, 1999, Williams & Wilkins, pp 744-767.

World Health Organization, International Society of Hypertension 1999 guidelines for hypertension management. *Clinician Reviews* 9(6):123-126, 1999.

REVIEW QUESTIONS

1. Isolated systolic hypertension, in which the systolic pressure is ≥140 mm Hg, and the diastolic pressure is ≤90 mm Hg, usually increases until at least age _____.
   a. 50
   b. 60
   c. 70
   d. 80

2. The cause of primary hypertension is:
   a. One single factor
   b. More than one factor
   c. Genetic factor
   d. High stress

3. Angiotensin II is a powerful:
   a. Decapeptide
   b. Diuretic
   c. Vasodilator
   d. Vasoconstrictor

4. Plasma renin activity is usually normal in patients with primary hypertension, but is suppressed in about _____% of these patients.
   a. 10%
   b. 15%
   c. 20%
   d. 30%

5. Secondary hypertension is associated with other conditions, frequently:
   a. Renal parenchymal disease
   b. Lung disease
   c. Ascites
   d. Blood dyscrasias

6. In the early labile phase of primary hypertension, cardiac output is:
   a. Normal
   b. Decreased
   c. Increased
   d. Unstable

7. The hallmark of primary hypertension is:
   a. Renal calculi
   b. Atherosclerosis
   c. Increased pulmonary edema
   d. Nephrosclerosis

8. Pheochromocytoma is a tumor of the chromaffin cells that secrete:
   a. Cerebral enzymes
   b. Kidney enzymes
   c. Adrenal enzymes
   d. Catecholamines

9. Angina pectoris is caused by:
   a. Atherosclerosis
   b. Exertion
   c. Hypertension
   d. Coronary artery obstruction

10. The clinician, when seeing a patient for the first time who is complaining of chest pain, must differentiate causes of chest pain. These include:
    a. Costochondritis
    b. Influenza
    c. Pharyngitis
    d. Herpes simplex

11. Myocardial infarction is usually the result of:
    a. Physical exertion
    b. Acute thrombus
    c. Atherosclerosis
    d. Abrupt reduction in coronary blood flow to a segment of the myocardium

12. The cluster of cells in the heart that forms the primary electrical generator (pacemaker) of the normal heart is:
    a. The atrioventricular node
    b. The His bundle
    c. The sinoatrial node
    d. Those at the juncture of the inferior vena cava and the aorta

13. Dysrhythmias are usually caused by one of four mechanisms, which include all of the following except:
    a. Abnormalities of impulse formation
    b. Abnormalities of impulse conduction
    c. Triggered impulses
    d. Reentry

14. Bradydysrhythmias arise from abnormalities of intrinsic automatic conduction, primarily in the:
    a. Sinoatrial node
    b. Right bundle branch
    c. Left bundle branch
    d. Atrioventricular node and the His-Purkinje network

15. Quinidine is one of the drugs classified under:
    a. Class Ia
    b. Class Ib
    c. Class II
    d. Class IV

16. Radiofrequency ablation can be used in _____% of patients with atrial fibrillation:
    a. 30%
    b. 50%
    c. 75%
    d. >99%

17. Reciprocating tachycardias involve:
    a. The sinoatrial node
    b. The atrioventricular node
    c. The His-Purkinje network
    d. Accessory pathways

18. The end-diastolic volume is influenced by and can be predicted by which one of the following?
    a. End-diastolic pressure
    b. Right ventricular dilation
    c. Extent of myocardial damage
    d. Afterload

19. The Frank-Starling principle states that:
    a. Dilation and hypertrophy may be accompanied by, or cause, decreased diastolic rigidity.
    b. Left ventricular remodeling affects cardiac performance.
    c. The degree of end-diastolic stretch (preload) within a physiologic range is proportional to the systolic performance of the ensuing ventricular contraction.
    d. The mechanism does not operate in heart failure.

20. A patient with heart failure or with a history of pulmonary edema should receive IV fluids:
    a. At the usual rate
    b. Faster than the usual rate because of depleted stores
    c. Slower than the usual rate to avoid overload
    d. At the minimal rate only to restore fluids lost in diaphoresis, urinary output, vomiting, and other losses

21. On both short-term and long-term recordings, sinus rhythm was shown to be:
    a. Remarkably stable
    b. Remarkably variable
    c. Remarkably unstable
    d. Remarkably unpredictable

22. The dysrhythmia that typically shows "sawtooth" electrocardiogram waves is:
    a. Atrial fibrillation
    b. Ventricular fibrillation
    c. Atrial flutter
    d. Atrial tachycardia

23. The mainstay of management for significant dysrhythmias is/are:
    a. Pacemakers
    b. Antidysrhythmic drugs
    c. Quinidine
    d. Amiodarone

24. The most common chronic dysrhythmia is:
    a. Sinus node dysrhythmia
    b. Atrioventricular node dysrhythmia
    c. Atrial fibrillation
    d. Ventricular fibrillation

25. Torsades de pointes is:
    a. An atrial tachycardia
    b. A ventricular tachycardia
    c. Characterized by a continually changing P wave pattern
    d. A congenitally long QT syndrome

26. Afterload is determined by all but one of the following. Which one is NOT characteristic of afterload?
    a. Degree of relaxation of the chambers
    b. Pressure within the chamber

c. Volume

d. The thickness of the wall when the aortic valve opens

27. Risk factors for heart failure include all but one of the following. Which one is NOT applicable?

a. Pregnancy

b. Anemia

c. Change in therapy for heart failure

d. Sudden weight gain

28. The most frequent cause of right heart failure is:

a. Chronic lung disease (cor pulmonale)

b. Tricuspid valve disease

c. Left-to-right shunts

d. Left heart failure

15/25 wrong

29. Treatment for deep vein thrombosis includes all but one of the following. The therapy NOT included is:

a. Leg exercises

b. Low-dose subcutaneous heparin

c. Bed rest

d. Elastic support stockings

30. Improvement in myocardial performance as a result of angiotensin-converting enzyme inhibitors is a result of all but one of the following. Which one does NOT improve cardiac performance?

a. Increases systemic vascular resistance

b. Lowers venous pressure

c. Reduces levels of circulating catecholamines

d. Lowers systemic vascular resistance

6

Neurologic Disorders

To establish a diagnosis and decide on treatment, the nurse practitioner must first localize the lesion in the nervous system, and determine the likely cause of the signs and symptoms. In the ambulatory population, evidence of neurologic disease may be minimal or early, and many signs and symptoms likely relate to prior acute neurologic events. Several important considerations should be kept in mind during evaluation of these patients: age, gender, the differences in performance over time, and the difference between the signs and symptoms of upper motor neuron (UMN) and lower motor neuron (LMN) lesions.

- For example, a new-onset central paralysis of an arm in a 20 year old could be multiple sclerosis; in a 60 year old, stroke is far more probable.
- If the pattern is peripheral, traumatic nerve injury is likely in the young, whereas tumor is a more important consideration in older persons (Figs. 6-1 and 6-2).
- Most individual neurologic signs and symptoms are not specific for one functional or anatomic disturbance, or for one cause (e.g., loss of a reflex is not necessarily due to motor nerve damage, a hemiparesis is not necessarily due to cerebrovascular disease, and a resting tremor is not necessarily due to Parkinson's disease).
- The pattern of findings from the history and physical examination is usually quite specific and can be used to develop a working diagnosis.
- Depending on the patient's specific signs and symptoms, the nurse practitioner may need to perform a complete neurologic evaluation; more often, only selected areas of the nervous system will need to be evaluated.

- The performance of patients with supposedly stable cerebral disease often varies a great deal from minute to minute, hour to hour, or day to day.
  —The patient may be able to dress, fix breakfast, and bring in the newspaper one morning, be incapable of the same activities the next day, then perform them without difficulty the following morning.
  —The patient may remember the spouse's name in the morning but not in the evening of the same day.
  —The affect of patients with stroke history varies from depressed to euphoric from hour to hour and day to day.
- Family members, confused and angry because of rapid changes in behavior, may ask whether the disease is getting better or worse, or they may surmise that the patient can perform self-care tasks easily but is simply unwilling to do so sometimes.
  —Both patient and family need reassurance that, just as healthy people have good and bad days, so too do people with neurologic disease, but that their actions are erratic and different from how they were before the onset of disease.

THE PATIENT'S HISTORY
Higher Functions and Consciousness

- Determination of handedness is useful when localizing cortical versus subcortical lesions.
  —Is the patient right-handed or left-handed?
  —Most people are left-hemisphere dominant for language.

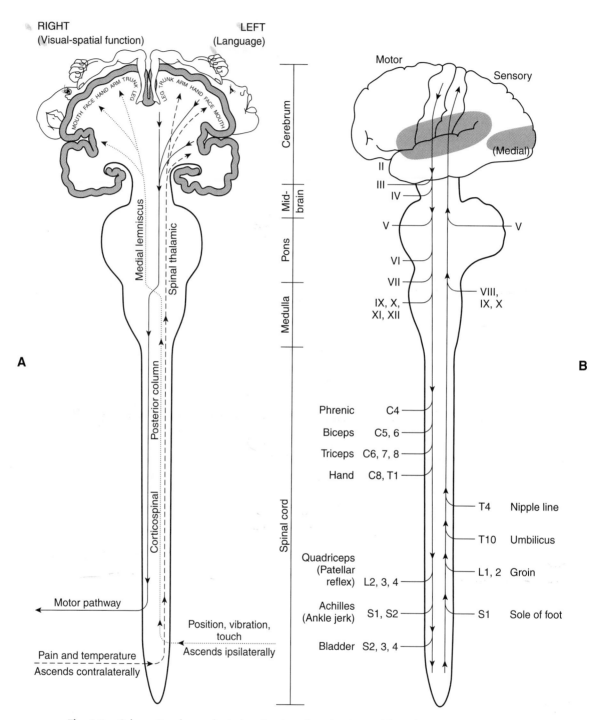

Fig. 6-1 Schematic of neurologic localization. Anterior (**A**) and lateral (**B**) schematics of central nervous system localization. **A,** Upper motor neuron signs ad nonradicular sensory signs can define only the side of the lesion; in general, they do not reveal the level of the lesion. **B,** The presence or absence of other neurologic signs or symptoms can help to specify the level of a localized neurologic problem. (From Haymaker W, Woodhall B: *Peripheral nerve injuries,* ed 2, Philadelphia, 1962, WB Saunders. Courtesy of Barry Gordan, MD, PhD.)

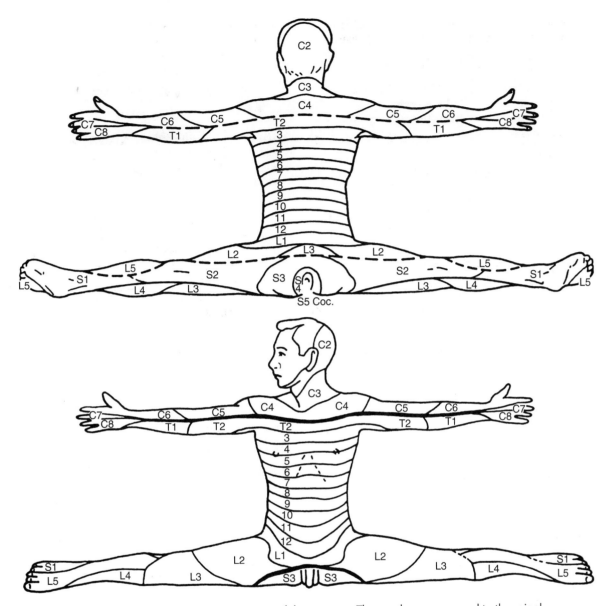

Fig. 6-2   Cutaneous innervation areas of dermatomes. The numbers correspond to the spinal cord level of the dermatome. *C,* cervical; *T,* thoracic; *L,* lumbar; *S,* sacral. (From Haymaker W, Woodhall B: *Peripheral nerve injuries,* ed 2, Philadelphia, 1962, WB Saunders.)

—Some left-handed people are right- or mixed-hemisphere dominant.

—A right-handed patient with right hemiparesis and intact language may have a subcortical lesion.

—A left-handed patient with left hemiparesis and intact language may have a cortical or subcortical lesion.

- Language
  —Has the patient had any problems with thinking or speech? Minor difficulty with finding words is common in normal people, as are brief lapses of memory.
- Memory
  —How is the patient's memory?
  —What kinds of things are forgotten?

—Ask family members: Have any problems with concentration, memory, or general abilities been noticed?

- Acute cerebral function
  —Has the patient ever fainted, lost consciousness, felt dizzy, or had a seizure?
  —Does the patient have frequent or severe headaches? How often?
- Mood
  —How are the patient's spirits?
  —Does the patient feel depressed?
  —Does the patient worry a great deal?
  —How does the patient feel about the future?
  —Does the patient feel self-confident, hopeless, helpless, guilty?
- Hallucinations and delusions
  —Has the patient seen or heard things that are unusual, or things that are not there?
  —Does the patient's imagination seem to play tricks?
  —Does anything feel wrong to the patient?
  —Does the patient perceive that he or she is being controlled by anything or anybody?

THE PATIENT'S NEUROLOGIC EVALUATION

The questions that follow, along with observations made throughout the history and physical examination, are usually sufficient to determine the level of consciousness, language functioning, visual-spatial functioning, level of intelligence, and memory. Systematic mental status examinations are appropriate for patients with psychiatric problems and for those with suspected cognitive impairment.

Cranial Nerves

I: Olfactory
This is not tested during a brief history and physical unless the patient specifically mentions loss of smell or has a history of head trauma with loss of consciousness.

II: Optic
Is vision impaired? Do things seem blurred, or are there patches where it is hard to see? Has vision ever been lost in one eye, or has there been trouble seeing out of one side or in one direction?

- Check vision (with glasses on) using Snellen chart or having the patient read from a newspaper. Test each eye separately. Check fields by confrontation (each eye separately), using finger wiggles. Examine fundi.

III, IV, VI: Oculomotor, Trochear, Abducent
Extraocular movements

- Has there ever been double vision?
- Have the patient move the eyes into all principal positions of gaze (horizontal, vertical, diagonal). Observe for disconjugate movements. Ask about diplopia. Look for nystagmus, lid lag, ptosis. Check pupils for size, symmetry, and reaction to light. Normal pupil size in young people is 3 to 5 mm. A small degree of pupillary asymmetry of 1 mm or less is present in about 5% of the normal population; it may vary from hour to hour, day to day, and it decreases in bright light.

V: Trigeminal
Has there been numbness over the face or difficulty chewing?

- Test corneal reflexes at corresponding points of each eye with a piece of cotton. There is wide variability in sensitivity of the corneas; people who have worn contact lenses have little response. Asymmetry is the most important clue to disease. With a pin, check for symmetry of perception over the forehead, cheek, and chin.

VII: Facial
Has there been any weakness or paralysis of the face?

- Observe for symmetry of nasolabial folds when the face is not moving. Have the patient show teeth, close eyes, frown. Normal people may have a slight degree of resting asymmetry of the face. Both sides should move briskly together on showing teeth, smiling, etc. Lag on one side may be a sign of a slight seventh nerve palsy, central or peripheral.

VIII: Auditory, Vestibular
How is the patient's hearing? Has there been any ringing in the ears or difficulty hearing out of

one side? Any loss of balance, spinning sensations, or dizziness?

IX, X, XII: Glossopharyngeal, Vagal, Hypoglossal

Have there been any problems chewing or swallowing? Does food seem to get caught anywhere? Where? What kinds of food have there been problems with? (Liquids are often the most difficult foods for patients with neurologic problems.)

- Vagal, glossopharyngeal: Inspect uvula for position and for motion by having the patient say "Ahh." Test gag reflex on both sides of the pharynx; look for symmetry of response. Some people have asymmetry of the resting uvula. Bilateral hyperreactions to bilateral absent gag reflex are within the normal range.
- Hypoglossal: Inspect the tongue at rest in the mouth. Have patient protrude it (it should protrude in the midline). Move it to both sides. The tongue normally has small twitches that are not pathologic fasciculations.

XI: Spinal Accessory

Spinal accessory nerve: Test muscles of neck and shoulders. Have patient move head against pressure from your hand, left and right. Have patient shrug (lift shoulders) and retain position against downward pressure from your hand.

Motor

- Has there been any weakness in the arms or legs? Is it there all the time, or does it seem to come and go? Has there been any twitching in the muscles? Where? How often? Any wasting of the muscles? Are there any cramps in the legs? When do cramps occur? Under what circumstances?

Examination for Motor Function

- Look for tremor, other spontaneous movement. Examine for asymmetries of muscle mass; denervation will result in loss of muscle size, with maximum loss reached within 4 months. Disuse over months to years will cause a decrease in muscle mass (e.g., in the legs of patients who are permanently bedridden). Test tone by passively flexing and extending the upper and lower extremities (normal tone is a slight firmness of mus-

cles and slight resistance to passive motion). In *hypotonia*, the muscles are flaccid, without resistance to passive motion; this may indicate LMN or cerebellar disease. *Rigidity* is increased resistance to passive motion throughout the whole range of motion around a joint. With *spasticity* the initial passive motion is easy, but then there is tightening of the muscle (spastic catch), sometimes followed by a sudden release (clasp-knife effect). Spasticity usually affects only one set of muscles around a joint (in the upper extremities, the biceps, forearm pronators, finger flexors; in the lower extremities, the quadriceps, hamstrings, and plantar flexors).

- Test voluntary strength in several major muscle groups. Observe proximal and distal muscles in each extremity; adequate screen is shoulder abduction, elbow extension and flexion, wrist and finger extension, grip strength (clinician uses two fingers), hip flexion (patient sitting), knee extension, and foot dorsiflexion. For relatively precise documentation: 0 = no movement; 1 = flicker; 2 = able to move with gravity eliminated (e.g., lateral motion of arm when recumbent); 3 = able to move against gravity; 4 = able to move against resistance; 5 = normal strength.

Reflexes

- The most important reflexes to test are: biceps (C5-6), triceps (C6-8), patellar (L2-4), Achilles tendon (S1-2), and plantar flexion (L5, S1).
- There is wide variability in reflex response, even in one individual. Symmetry of response between the two sides is important to note.
  —Decreased reflexes: disruption of the sensory or motor nerves of the reflex loop, immediately following a cerebrovascular accident (CVA)
  —Increased reflexes: UMN disease that may be located anywhere between just above the anterior horn cell to the cerebral cortex
  —Babinski sign is dorsiflexion of the big toe after plantar stimulation, with dorsiflexion and spreading of the other toes and dorsiflexion of the foot. The classic Babinski is slow and deliberate, which may be the only indicator of UMN disease.

Gait

- Are there any problems with walking? What kind? Where or when does it happen (e.g., climbing up stairs, walking certain distances)? Is there unsteadiness when erect?

Examination of Gait

- Any tendency for the patient to list or to require support while standing, walking, or sitting should be noted.
- Ask the patient to walk normally, on the heels, and then on the toes.
- Test heel-to-toe (tandem) walking, a test to assess ability to maintain balance on a narrow support base and to show any evidence of ataxia.
- In cerebellar disease, the patient's legs are spread far apart, and there is unsteadiness and lateral swaying. Ask the patient to walk around a chair in both directions, and if ataxia is present, the patient will walk into the chair on the affected side.
- In sensory ataxia (loss of proprioception), the patient is uncertain in moving, with foot slapping because of uncertainty about where the floor is.
- In spastic gait, such as that which occurs in UMN disease, the legs do not flex but circumduct, with foot dragging and diminished arm movement on the affected side.
- In parkinsonian gait, there is loss of swinging in one or both arms; the trunk is bent forward and there is shuffling, rigidity, and festination, in which the upper part of the body goes forward faster than the lower extremities, and the gait accelerates to catch up.
- In LMN paralysis of the pretibial and peroneal muscles, the patient has footdrop, but hip flexion is normal; the patient lifts the foot very high, advances it by swinging it forward, then slaps it down.
- In frontal lobe disease, gait may be wide-based, shuffling, and slow. Turning is slow. However, there is no weakness or loss of sensation.

Fine Motor and Cerebellar Function

- Has there been any shaking or any difficulty in writing, drawing, buttoning, etc?

Examination of Fine Motor and Cerebellar Function

- Ask the patient to touch the thumb to each of the fingers in order. Each hand is tested separately.
- Finger-to-nose-to-finger is tested: the patient touches the examiner's moving finger, then his or her nose, then again the examiner's moving finger. The examiner observes speed, rhythm, intention tremor, and inaccuracy (dysmetria). Tremor from various causes may affect performance.
- Patients are asked to tap each foot separately. Differences in speed, flow of movement, and facility are observed.
  —Normal people have equal ability on both sides and may be better on their dominant side.
  —Repetitive movements that are slow and that require effort, but with no loss of rhythm, are characteristics of UMN lesions.
  —Maintained speed, but with erratic movements and loss of rhythm, indicates cerebellar disease.

Sensation

- Has there been any numbness, tingling, or pain in the arms, legs, or feet? Where? Does position change or any other factor seem to bring it on?

Examination for Sensation

- Testing focuses on symmetry, and differences in proximal and distal perception in all extremities.
- Light touch (posterior columns) does not provide conclusive evidence of abnormality; response can be normal when other sensory abnormalities are found (e.g., pinprick [lateral spinothalamic tract], proprioception/vibration [posterior columns]).
- Vibration is tested with a 128-Hz tuning fork.
- Proprioception is tested by first asking the patient to close his or her eyes. Then the examiner moves the fingers or toes 30 to 45 degrees up or down, and asks the patient to say in which direction the digits have been moved.
- The patient's ability to maintain balance is determined with the Romberg test, which assesses vibration, proprioception, and posterior columns.

—Testing patients who have cerebellar ataxia must be done with caution; test first to see whether they can stand with eyes open and feet together; if they cannot, they have cerebellar ataxia.

—The Romberg test is then performed with the patient standing with feet apart and eyes closed; if posterior columns are intact, the patient may sway very slightly.

—A positive Romberg test is that the patient can maintain balance with feet together and eyes open but loses balance when eyes are closed.

Bladder and Bowel

- Does the patient have any difficulty with constipation or diarrhea? Any uncontrolled urination or stool evacuation? If so, was it associated with the urge to urinate or defecate, or was it spontaneous?
- If a female patient reports problems with urinary incontinence, she may be helped by being taught to use pubococcygeus (Kegel) exercises to strengthen the muscles of the pelvic diaphragm and perineum which, for many patients, results in greater ability to retain urine.

UMN and LMN Disease

- The signs and symptoms of UMN and LMN damage are different.
- UMN lesions affect the pathways that bring a command from the cortex to the anterior horn cell; therefore, UMN function depends on the integrity of the cortex and the corticospinal and corticobulbar tracts.
- LMN lesions affect the final common pathway for muscle movements; LMN function depends on the integrity of the anterior horn cell in the spinal cord and its nerve fiber for carrying impulses to the muscle cells.

UMN Lesions Syndrome

- If the UMN lesion is total, voluntary movements are absent, but involuntary movements may continue (e.g., yawning, laughing, crying, or anger).
- When UMNs are damaged above the crossover of the corticospinal tract in the medulla, motor impairment occurs on the opposite (contralateral) side; if damage occurs below the crossover, motor impairment develops on the same (ipsilateral) side.
- When weakness (paresis) is present, and not paralysis, the lower muscles of the face are weak. Patients have a widened palpebral fissure and difficulty in closing the eyes, but the forehead is spared.
- UMN lesions (e.g., stroke) produce weakness only in voluntary movement, while patients with LMN lesions exhibit the same degree of weakness in both voluntary and involuntary movements.
- In the arm and leg, UMN lesions affect distal muscles much more than proximal muscles.
- UMN lesions are often accompanied by spasticity and hyperreflexia.

LMN Disease

- In LMN, there is peripheral seventh nerve damage, and both the upper and lower facial muscles are affected; at times, mild weakness that produces early Bell's palsy, a LMN lesion, can mimic a UMN pattern.
- Weakness from a permanent LMN lesion is fixed and unchanging.
- Those muscles served by the involved spinal cord segment or peripheral nerve are weak, with none of the widespread effects typical of UMN lesions.
- In LMN lesions, atrophy is apparent within several weeks; in UMN lesions, atrophy is slight and occurs only after several months.
- Muscles are usually flaccid and reflexes may be hypoactive or absent.
- Spinal cord injuries and amyotrophic lateral sclerosis (ALS) result in signs and symptoms of both UMN and LMN lesions.
  - Patients with spinal cord injury have signs of LMN lesion at the level of the injury, caused by localized destruction of the anterior horn cells and their nerve roots. Below the level of injury, there may be a partial or complete UMN syndrome with spasticity, hyperreflexia, and preserved involuntary reflexes.
  - ALS affects both pyramidal tract cells and anterior horn cells, along with LMN-type weakness, fasciculations, and wasting; there is also hyperreflexia and perhaps a Babinski sign.

DIAGNOSTIC TESTS USED FOR NEUROLOGIC DISORDERS

- Routine skull x-rays: lateral, anteroposterior (AP), and inclined AP
  —For suspected skull fracture, metastatic tumor, myeloma, Paget's disease
- Spine x-rays
  —Suspected: cervical spondylitic radiculopathy; cervical or lumbar stenosis, spondylolisthesis, luxation, or subluxation; vertebral fracture; metastatic tumor; other
- Electroencephalography (EEG)
  —Known or suspected seizure disorders, focal brain lesions (e.g., stroke, tumor, abscess), diffuse brain disease (e.g., dementia, delirium, drug effect or withdrawal), sleep disorders
- Lumbar puncture
  —To measure intracranial pressure
  —Suspected: meningitis, chronic infections of the central nervous system (CNS) (e.g., syphilis, acquired immune deficiency syndrome [AIDS], Lyme disease, cryptococcus, tuberculosis [TB]), subarachnoid hemorrhage, demyelinating or inflammatory disease (e.g., multiple sclerosis, Guillain-Barre syndrome), other
- Duplex scan
  —To assess plaque in the common, internal, and external carotid arteries in patients with carotid bruits, transient ischemic attacks (TIAs), stroke
- Doppler examination of the supraorbital carotid
  —The supraorbital is a branch of the internal carotid artery.
  —Supraorbital carotid Doppler is used to confirm suspected significant internal carotid artery stenosis (carotid bifurcation).
- Carotid blood flow in patients with cerebrovascular disease (TIAs, stroke, bruits)
- Transcranial Doppler examination
  —Ultrasound to measure blood velocity in the ophthalmic, middle, anterior, posterior, vertebral, and basilar arteries
- Cerebral angiography (magnetic resonance angiography [MRA])
  —Confirms diagnosis of extracranial and intracranial arterial stenosis, vascular malformations, aneurysms, and vasculitis
- Computed tomography (CT) scans of the head
  —Tumor, ischemic cerebrovascular disease, degenerative disease (e.g., Alzheimer's, Huntington's), hydrocephalus, subdural hematoma, unexplained headaches

- CT scans of the spine
  —Shows both osseous and soft tissues
  —Suspected: disc herniation, spinal dysraphism, facet joint pathology, vertebral fractures
- Magnetic resonance imaging (MRI) of the CNS
  —Early cerebral infarctions, sinusitis, multiple sclerosis, spinal cord abnormalities

All of these procedures and tests have limitations from lesser to greater extent; however, modern technology allows us to visualize CNS structures far better than was true in the past.

FUNCTION AND DYSFUNCTION OF THE CEREBRAL LOBES

- Dysfunction or disease of the cerebral hemispheres may be organic (e.g., of known structural, chemical, or metabolic mechanisms) or nonorganic (unknown cause); the latter includes the major psychoses and many behavioral disorders.
- Organic cerebral dysfunctions may be focal or global in distribution.
- Some disorders, such as apraxia and amnesia, may result from either focal or diffuse brain dysfunction.

Focal Disorders

- Most focal disorders are due to structural abnormalities (e.g., space-occupying lesions [SOLs], stroke, trauma, maldevelopment, scars), and usually affect only the focal functions of the cortex.

Global Disorders

- Global disorders are due to metabolic-chemical disorders or disseminated structural lesions (e.g., diffuse inflammation, vasculopathy, disseminated malignancy).
- Global lesions alter multiple dimensions of cerebral sensory and behavioral function. They often affect subcortical systems, interfering with arousal levels and producing stupor or coma, or with the normal integration of conscious thought, which results in delirium or dementia.

Frontal Lobes

- The frontal lobes influence learned motor activity, and the planning and organizing of expressed behavior.
- The prerolandic-precentral gyrus and the areas just anterior to it (premotor and supplemen-

tary motor areas) on one side of the cerebrum regulate skilled muscular activities on the opposite side of the body.

- The premotor and supplementary cortices also control ipsilateral skilled motor behavior, such as hitting a golf ball.
- Seizures involving the premotor areas characteristically cause adversive movements (i.e., toward the opposite side) of the head, eyes, trunk, and extremities.
- Seizures originating from the precentral gyrus produce classic jacksonian focal motor seizures.
- Behavioral changes produced by injury to the prefrontal area vary according to the lesion's location, size, and rate of development.
  —Unilateral lesions <2 cm in diameter almost never cause symptoms except seizures.
  —Larger lesions, unless they develop rapidly over weeks or months, rather than years, or unless they affect both frontal lobes, may also cause no symptoms.
  —Patients with large basal frontal lesions are apathetic, inattentive to stimuli, indifferent to the implications of their acts, and sometimes are incontinent.
  —Patients with frontal polar or anterior lateral lesions are likely to disregard the consequences of their behavior and tend to be distractible, euphoric, facetious, often vulgar, and indifferent to social niceties.
  —Bilateral acute trauma to prefrontal areas may result in boisterous talkativeness, restlessness, and socially intrusive behavior, often lasting for days or weeks, and usually subsiding spontaneously with resolution of the trauma.

Parietal Lobes

- The postrolandic area of the parietal lobes integrates somesthetic stimuli for recognizing and recalling form, texture, and weight.
- Posterolateral areas provide accurate visual spatial relationships, and integrate the relative perceptions with other sensations to create awareness of trajectories of moving objects and of the position of body parts.
- In the dominant hemisphere, the inferior parietal area transacts mathematic functions, and is closely linked to language recognition and word memory.
- The nondominant parietal lobe integrates the left side of the body with its environment.

- Small lesions of the postcentral cortex cause astereognosis (loss of tactile recognition) in the contralateral hand and body.
- Large interior parietal lesions in the dominant (usually left) hemisphere are often associated with severe aphasia; less damage can cause apraxia, difficulty in calculating, and sometimes right-left disorientation and agraphia.
- Acute injury to the nondominant parietal lobe may remove the patient's awareness of the left side of the body and its environment, and of the serious nature of the injury (anosognosia).
- Some older patients with large right parietal lesions may even deny the existence of the paralysis that affects the left side of the body. Some of these patients lapse into states of global confusion.
- Patients with small lesions become confused when performing learned manual procedures, so that dressing and other familiar, learned activities cannot be performed. This spatial-manual defect is called apraxia.

Temporal Lobes

- The temporal lobes process visual recognition, auditory perception, memory, and emotion.
- Patients with acquired unilateral damage to the right temporal lobe often lose acuity for non-verbal auditory stimuli (e.g., music).
- Left temporal lobe injury interferes severely with recognition, memory, and formation of language.
- Patients with epileptogenic foci in the medial limbic-emotional parts of the temporal lobe often have partial complex seizures, characterized by uncontrollable feelings and abnormal autonomic, cognitive, or emotional functions.
  —Some of these patients may have personality changes such as loss of humor, presence of philosophic religiosity, and obsessiveness; in men, libido may be decreased.

DISORDERS OF CEREBRAL FUNCTION
Aphasia

- Aphasia is a defect or loss of language function in which the comprehension or expression of words, or nonverbal equivalents of words, is impaired, usually as a result of injury to or degeneration of the language centers in the cerebral cortex. This disorder is common in survivors of stroke, but may improve over time.

—Language function resides predominantly in the posterosuperior temporal lobe, the adjacent inferior parietal lobe, the inferolateral frontal lobe, and the subcortical connection between those areas, usually in the left hemisphere, even in left-handed persons.

- Receptive (sensory) aphasias produce dysfunction in comprehending words and in recognizing auditory, visual, or tactile symbols.

  —Subtypes include Wernicke's aphasia: the patient speaks normal words fluently, often including meaningless phonemes, but does not know their meaning or relationships; the result is a jumble of words ("word salad").

  —Alexia is loss of the ability to read words.

- Injury to the inferior frontal gyrus just anterior to the facial and lingual areas of the motor cortex (Broca's area) produces an expressive (motor) aphasia in which the patient's comprehension and ability to conceptualize are relatively preserved, but the ability to form words is impaired.

  —The impairment affects speech (dysphasia) and writing (agraphia, dysgraphia), causing the patient tremendous frustration.

  —Anomia, the inability to name objects, but with retained grammar and syntax, may be receptive or expressive in nature.

  —Prosody, the quality of rhythm and emphasis that adds meaning to speech, is usually influenced by both hemispheres, but sometimes by the nondominant hemisphere alone.

- Brain lesions large enough to impair language function seldom produce pure defects, so that an isolated receptive or expressive aphasia is rare.

- Large frontal-temporal lesions cause global aphasia with severe defects in comprehension and expression.

Apraxia

- Apraxia is the inability to execute purposeful, previously learned motor acts, despite physical ability and willingness to do so.

  —This condition is common in many metabolic and structural diseases that affect the brain diffusely, especially those that impair frontal lobe function.

  —Typically, the patient cannot follow a motor command. Although he understands the words, he cannot recall how to perform learned, complex acts despite his ability to perform the component movements.

  —Selective apraxias with loss of specific movement (e.g., constructional apraxia, which is the inability to draw or build simple forms, or an apraxia for dressing) may accompany dementia and sometimes focal parietal lobe lesions.

  —Most parietal lobe apraxia is related to loss of the area's capacity to recognize spatially executed tasks, even well-learned ones.

- Tests for apraxia include asking the patient to wave goodbye, salute, stop, go, beckon to come near, open a lock with a key, use a screwdriver, use scissors, or take a deep breath and hold it.

Agnosia

- Agnosia is an uncommon neuropsychologic deficit in which an object cannot be identified, despite the ability to identify its tactile or visual elements.

  —Memory that was previously stored in association cortices and related to objects' tactile or visual characteristics is impaired or lost.

  —Affected persons are sometimes able to perceive the general nature of an object, but not the specific object. One might say, "You use it to write with."

- Prosopagnosia is the inability to identify well-known faces, despite being able to identify generic facial features.

- Anosognosia is a severe form of agnosia in which the person loses all memory that a damaged body part (or other object) ever existed.

  —The classic syndrome results from severe damage to the right, nondominant parietal lobe, leaving the bewildered patient unaware that he ever possessed the now paralyzed, desensitized left body parts or the space around them.

  —Clinical testing for agnosia includes asking the patient with left hemiplegia to identify the paralyzed parts of his body or objects located in his left visual field.

HEADACHE AND FACIAL PAIN
Tension Headache

Definition

Tension headache causes pain in the head that is of pressing or tightening character.

- Two subtypes of tension headache are:
  —Episodic: fewer than 180 episodes/year

—Chronic: more than 180 episodes/year, including continuous

Risk Factors
None known

Etiology
- Cause is presumed to be a consequence of psychosocial stress, although the specific stressor cannot always be identified.
- Underlying anxiety or depression may be implicated; the relationship between these possible factors and tension headaches is controversial, in that some specialists consider them to be causes, while others consider them secondary to the headaches.

Pathogenesis
- The precise pathogenesis is unknown.
- Neither increased muscle tension nor precipitating stress is specific to tension headaches.
- Tension and migraine headaches may be different manifestations of the same problem. (See Pathogenesis under Migraine Headaches.)

Diagnosis
- Diagnostic criteria for different types of headache were established by the International Headache Society in 1988.
- Criteria for diagnosing tension headaches:
  —Duration: 30 min to 7 days
  —At least two of the following pain characteristics:
    ~ Pressing/tightening (nonpulsating) quality
    ~ Mild-to-moderate intensity
    ~ Bilateral location
    ~ No aggravation by walking stairs or similar routine physical activity
  —Both of the following:
    ~ No nausea or vomiting (but possible presence of anorexia)
    ~ Photophobia and phonophobia absent, or presence of one but not the other
- Recurrent tension headaches are usually similar in quality and location.
- Patients with chronic tension headaches often have associated depression or anxiety.
  —Some patients with chronic tension headaches state that they have experienced unremitting headache pain for years.

- Physical examination reveals no problems except for neck or scalp muscle tenderness in some patients.

Treatment
- People with intermittent headaches that are not severe usually respond to simple over-the-counter analgesics.
- Patients with continuous daily headaches of months' or years' duration usually have associated depression or anxiety states.
  —The pain is usually relieved only with antidepressants.
- Most patients have tried aspirin or acetaminophen before consulting a primary care provider.
  —A trial of NSAIDs may be helpful.
  —Stronger analgesics include codeine sulfate, propoxyphene (Darvon), and two drugs that contain a combination of analgesics, sedatives, and caffeine:
    ~ Butalbital and caffeine, plus aspirin or acetaminophen, and
    ~ Oxycodone plus aspirin or acetaminophen
  —These drugs can result in dependency; prescription is contingent on a contractual agreement regarding limited use.
- Prophylaxis is warranted for those whose tension headaches are severe or frequent.
  —Tricyclic antidepressants provide the best results (nortriptyline 50-100 mg at bedtime).

Patient and Family Education
- Reassurance and support are essential in the care of patients with tension headaches.
- Explain the nature, possible causes, preventive measures, and methods for relieving headache pain.
- Usually, patients know what activities are best avoided during acute headache episodes; the nurse practitioner may help them to discover other activities that may precipitate or aggravate attacks.
- Often, reduction or elimination of coffee and other foods and drinks that contain caffeine can be helpful, although withdrawal from coffee can induce headache.

Follow-up and Referral
- If there is any question about possible underlying neurologic disease or other poten-

tial cause for headaches, the patient should be referred to the appropriate specialist (e.g., neurologist, neurosurgeon, ophthalmologist, other).

- Many patients can be managed by telephone contact and occasional office visits, depending on the severity and frequency of headaches.

Migraine Headache

Definition

Migraine is defined as a headache that lasts from 4 to 72 hours, builds gradually over minutes to hours, may be lateralized or generalized, throbs, is moderate to severe in intensity, becomes worse with exertion, and is associated with blurred vision, anorexia, nausea, vomiting, or sensitivity to light, sound, and smell.

- Migraines have been related to dilation and excessive pulsation of branches of the external carotid artery. Focal disturbances of neurologic function may precede or accompany the headaches, and these have been attributed to constriction of branches of the internal carotid artery.
- In 1988, the International Headache Society revised the classification of migraine from "common" or "classic" migraine to:
  —Migraine without aura
  —Migraine with aura
- Consensus criteria for migraine without aura:
  1. The patient has had at least five attacks fulfilling 2-4.
  2. Headache attacks last 4 to 72 hours (untreated or unsuccessfully treated).
  3. Headache has at least two of the following characteristics:
     a. Unilateral location
     b. Pulsating quality
     c. Moderate or severe intensity
     d. Aggravation by walking stairs or similar routine physical activity
  4. During headache at least one of the following occurs:
     a. Nausea or vomiting
     b. Photophobia and phonophobia
- Consensus criteria for migraine with aura:
  1. The patient has had at least two attacks fulfilling 2.
  2. At least three of the following four characteristics:
     a. One or more fully reversible aura symptoms indicate focal cerebral cortical or brainstem dysfunction.

b. At least one aura symptom develops gradually over more than 4 minutes, or two or more symptoms occur in succession.
c. No aura symptoms last more than 60 minutes. If more than one aura symptom is present, accepted duration is proportionally increased.
d. Headache follows aura with a free interval of less than 60 minutes. (It may also begin before or simultaneously with the aura.)

- Headaches with aura are subdivided into typical, prolonged, familial, hemiplegic, basilar, aura without headache, and acute onset aura.
- Migraine with typical aura (the most common form with aura) has one of the following types of aura symptoms:
  —Homonymous visual disturbance
  —Unilateral paresthesias or numbness
  —Unilateral weakness
  —Aphasia or unclassifiable speech difficulty
- Fortification hallucinations, which are almost specific for migraine, are slowly enlarging scotomata that are surrounded by luminous angles, and that slowly change shape and appear to move across the visual fields.

Risk Factors

- About 20% to 50% of patients have a family history of migraine, usually in one parent.
- Female sex: about 23 million people in the United States suffer from migraines (18% of women, 6% of men).
- Onset of migraine is usually between 15 and 25 years, although onset can occur at any time throughout the adult life span.

Etiology

- The precise cause of migraine headaches is unknown.

Pathogenesis

- The pathophysiology of migraine headaches is not clearly understood.
- Changes in blood flow in the brain and scalp occur; however, it is not known whether vasodilation and vasoconstriction are a cause or an effect of migraines.
- Cortical spreading depression, defined as fundamental changes in the brain cortex in

which a peak of hyperpolarization is followed by depolarization, may induce neurogenic inflammation with vasodilation, activated white blood cells (WBCs), and permeable capillaries.
- Inflammation results in irritation of perivascular trigeminal sensory fibers.
- A cascade of events then follows, resulting in changes in blood flow and the severe headache.
- Precipitating factors for migraine include:
  —The perimenstrual period, particularly before the onset of bleeding when levels of estradiol are falling
  —Oral contraceptives, particularly off-days, presumably because of falling estrogen levels
  —Menopause when there is frank estrogen deficiency
- Other factors are vasodilators (e.g., nitrates and antihypertensives); alcohol; chocolate; cheese; wines and other foods that contain tyramine; and monosodium glutamate.
- The relationship between diet and migraine remains controversial, and no supportive data have been gathered.
- More recent research suggests that the vascular theory of migraine does not adequately account for many aspects of the migraine syndrome: malaise, autonomic components (e.g., nausea, vomiting, diarrhea, bloating, fluid retention), and the post-headache elation or enhanced sense of well-being that many patients report.
- Other theories regarding pathogenesis include electrical depression, an imbalance in sympathetic nervous system regulation, dysautonomia of the trigeminal nerve, and dysregulation of the ascending brainstem serotonergic system.
- These new considerations of accumulated evidence clearly show that migraine is an organic disease and is not psychologically based.

Diagnosis

Signs and Symptoms (See Classification Criteria)
- A hallmark of migraine is recurrence.
  —The majority of migraine patients have several attacks a year.
  —Some have one or more episodes every week.

- Migraine episodes usually become less frequent and less severe with age.
- A brief prodromal period before the actual onset of migraine may include depression, irritability, restlessness, anorexia, and in some patients (10% to 20%) an aura.
- Migraine is more common than is generally known.
  —Many patients with recurrent moderate-to-severe migraine headaches are misdiagnosed as having tension headaches.
  —Failure of analgesics to alleviate headache in an emotionally healthy patient with recurring headaches justifies a revised diagnosis of migraine.

Differential Diagnosis
- TIAs
  —Headaches occur in 25% of patients with TIAs, but are usually mild.
  —Older patients with suspected migrainous ischemic events, particularly those with migraine equivalents (ischemic symptoms without headache), should be evaluated for TIAs.
- Other cerebrovascular events, particularly in older persons (>50 years)
- Migrainous ischemia, which lasts from 30 minutes to several hours

Treatment
- Migraine headaches cannot be cured, but they can be controlled.
- Avoidance of trigger factors:
  —Nitrates
  —Vasodilators
  —Oral contraceptives
  —Alcohol
  —Irregular sleep habits and sleep deprivation
  —Excess caffeine intake
  —Caffeine withdrawal (should be gradual)
- During an attack, the patient usually feels better lying in a dark room with a cool compress or ice pack on the head.

Pharmacologic Therapy
- Abortive Therapy
  —Acetaminophen, aspirin, or another NSAID is often sufficient for those with mild migraine attacks.
  —Drugs that combine analgesics, barbiturates, or caffeine may effectively relieve pain.

—Ergotamine tartrate, sumatriptan, or an NSAID may be taken at the start of a migraine in a patient who experiences moderate to severe attacks.

  ~ Ergotamine is used because of its vasoconstrictor properties; however, its effectiveness may be due to its serotonin receptor agonist properties.

  ~ Ergotamine is cost-effective and is the first choice among the nonanalgesic agents.

  ~ Ergotamine and sumatriptan are both vasoconstrictors, and therefore should not be taken together.

  ~ Sumatriptan, introduced in 1993, aborts or significantly reduces moderate-to-severe migraine symptoms, even if the headache has been present for several hours.

  ~ Cafergot combines ergotamine tartrate (1 mg) and caffeine (100 mg) is very effective in many patients.

- Prophylactic Therapy (Table 6-1)
  —Drugs that have proved to be effective in migraine prophylaxis include β-blockers, calcium channel blockers, tricyclic antidepressants, and anticonvulsants.
  —Each patient who takes a prophylactic drug is asked to keep a record of the frequency and severity of headaches, and any associated factors or events.

- Patients with intractable migraine headaches are not helped by any known therapy at present and are always referred to a neurologist.

Patient and Family Education

- Patients should be instructed about the nature, cause, signs and symptoms, course, and treatment of migraine headaches.
- Patients should know that there is no known cure for migraine, but that the frequency and severity of attacks can be reduced.
- Written instructions about the use of medications should be clear.
  —For example, ergotamine must be taken at the onset of an attack.
  —Dosage, scheduling, expected action, and side effects for each drug should be provided in writing.
- Patients are instructed about nonpharmacologic therapy (reclining in a darkened room with cold compresses on the head) and any other measure that provides relief.

Follow-up and Referral

- Patients who have migraine are followed by the primary care provider, with consultation of a neurologist and perhaps referral to a neurologist if further evaluation and therapy are needed.

Cluster Headache

Definition

Cluster headache is classified separately from migraine because of its distinct clinical characteristics and different therapy.

- It has been known by other names over the years: Horton's syndrome, histamine headache (a misnomer), and migrainous cranial neuralgia.

Risk Factors

- None known
- No evidence of familial basis

Etiology

- There is no known cause of cluster headaches.
- They occur predominantly in middle-aged men who are thin and who smoke.

TABLE 6-1
Prophylactic Therapy for Migraine

Drug	Dose/Day (mg)
β-BLOCKERS	
Propranolol	80-320
Metoprolol	100-250
Atenolol	50-100
Timolol	10-60
Nadolol	40-240
CALCIUM CHANNEL BLOCKERS	
Verapamil	240-480
TRICYCLIC ANTIDEPRESSANTS	
Amitriptyline	10-150
Nortriptyline	10-150
Doxepin	10-100
ANTICONVULSANTS	
Divalproex	500-1500

From Johnson CJ: Headaches and facial pain. In Barker LR, Burton JR, Zieve PD, eds: *Principles of ambulatory medicine*, ed 5, Baltimore, 1999, Williams & Wilkins, p 1222.

- Onset usually occurs between ages 20 and 50.
- Several triggers are thought to be associated with attacks:
  —Sleep disturbances
  —Alcohol
  —Barometric pressure change

Pathogenesis and Pathophysiology
- The precise pathophysiology of cluster headaches is unknown, but may be similar to that of migraine.

Diagnosis
- The consensus criteria for diagnosing cluster headache, as determined by the International Headache Society in 1988, include:
  1. The patient has had at least five attacks fulfilling 2-4.
  2. A headache causes severe unilateral orbital, supraorbital, or temporal pain that lasts 15 to 180 minutes untreated.
  3. Headache is associated with at least one of the following signs, which must be present on the pain side:
     a. Conjunctival injection
     b. Lacrimation
     c. Nasal congestion
     d. Rhinorrhea
     e. Forehead and facial sweating
     f. Miosis
     g. Ptosis
     h. Eyelid edema
  4. Frequency of attacks varies from one every other day to eight per day.
- Attacks occur in clusters extending over days to weeks, giving the syndrome its name.
- Most cluster episodes last from 4 to 6 weeks, and are followed by long pain-free intervals.
- Intervals between episodes range from 3 months to 5 years, and sometimes longer.
- Most patients have one or two episodes per year.
- Eventually, the problem ceases altogether.
- A typical attack begins with sudden stabbing or burning pain in the eye, orbit, and cheek on one side.
- The pain is usually excruciating.
- Unlike patients with migraine, patients with cluster headaches are usually agitated, and they often pace the floor during the attack.

- The same side is usually involved during a cluster of attacks.
- Attacks may last from a few minutes to 2 hours, but most often 30 to 40 minutes.
- Attacks tend to occur at the same time each day, in the evening just after the patient has gone to bed, or they may awaken the patient from sleep in early morning.
- Nitrates, vasodilators, and alcohol tend to induce attacks.
- Except during an attack, the physical examination of these patients is normal.

Differential Diagnosis
- Tic douloureux
- Acute glaucoma
- Sinusitis
- Peripheral dental abscess
- Atypical facial neuralgia

Treatment
- Abortive
  —Aspirin or acetaminophen, taken immediately, may abort the headache or lessen its effects.
  —If available, 100% oxygen, given for 15 minutes at a flow rate of 7 L/minute, may abort attacks; this may be effective because of its vasoconstrictor effect.
  —Ergotamine, 2 mg given sublingually and repeated twice at 30-minute intervals, is effective in many patients.
  —Subcutaneous sumatriptan is effective in about 75% of attacks.
- Prophylactic
  —Drugs such as β-blockers, verapamil, and tricyclic antidepressants in doses similar to those used in migraine, often prevent attacks.
  —Prednisone 60 to 80 mg/day, tapered over 2 to 4 weeks, decreases the severity and frequency of attacks and shortens the duration of an attack.
  —For patients who have almost daily cluster headaches (chronic paroxysmal hemicrania), lithium carbonate is often effective.

Patient and Family Education
- Instruct the patient and family about the nature of the headaches, signs and symptoms, course, and medications: reason for

taking, dose, schedule, expected effects, and side effects.

Follow-up and Referral
- Follow-up depends on the frequency and severity of attacks.
- If the patient's symptoms are not relieved by the standard regimen, referral to a neurologist is recommended.

Sinus Headache
Definition
Sinus headache is a headache that the patient attributes to sinusitis.

Risk Factors
- History of acute or chronic sinusitis
- Family history of sinusitis

Etiology
- Sinusitis is an uncommon cause of recurrent headaches.
- So-called sinus headaches are diagnosed in terms of other signs and symptoms of sinusitis.

Diagnosis
- Chronic sinusitis often presents diagnostic difficulties, particularly when it involves the sphenoid sinus, which causes a dull boring pain behind the eyes.
- Sinus headache is more likely when there is a history of preceding acute sinusitis.

Treatment, Follow-up, and Referral
- Because sinusitis is not usually the cause of recurrent headaches, referral to an otolaryngologist for evaluation and treatment of sinusitis (either acute or chronic) is recommended.
- If the otolaryngologist does not find evidence sufficient to establish a diagnosis of sinusitis, referral to a neurologist is then recommended.

Giant Cell Arteritis and Polymyalgia Rheumatica (See also Chapter 17)
Definition
- Giant cell arteritis (GCA) is a vasculitis that affects large arteries throughout the body.

- Clinical manifestations are usually caused by involvement of extracranial branches of the carotid artery.
- The most common symptom of GCA is headache.
- GCA is also called temporal arteritis because temporal headaches and a positive temporal artery biopsy are the findings most often associated with the disease.
- Polymyalgia rheumatica (PMR) is a debilitating condition of older people that causes stiffness and aching of the neck and shoulder muscles, and of the pelvic girdle.
- PMR precedes, accompanies, or follows the onset of GCA in about 50% of patients with GCA, although GCA does not occur among patients with PMR in the United States and Europe.

Risk Factors
- Those >50 years of age are at risk.
- Average age of onset is 65 to 70.
- Both are more common in women than in men.
- Neither condition is common in blacks, Latinos, or Asians.
- They are most common in people of northern European descent. In Minnesota, where there is a large northern European population, the incidence of GCA in those over 50 was found to be 17/100,000, and the prevalence was 223/100,000.

Etiology
Unknown

Diagnosis
GCA
- The headache of GCA has no specific features that distinguish it from other headaches.
- It is temporal in over 50% of patients, but it may be occipital, parietal, or holocephalic.
- Patients usually state that the pain is superficial rather than intracranial.
- The pain is made worse by leaning the head against a solid surface or even a hard pillow, or by exposure to cold.
- The headache is described as being worse at night, and building up gradually over several hours.

- Although the headache is not distinguishable from other types of headache, diagnosis is based on other clinical features associated with GCA and PMR.
- Symptoms of pain (claudication) on chewing, swallowing, and arm or tongue motion are highly suggestive of GCA.

PMR

- PMR has an insidious onset.
- Chief complaints are stiffness of the shoulder and pelvic girdle and, less commonly, of the thigh muscles.
- These symptoms cause the patient great difficulty in getting out of bed.
- Associated fever, weight loss, and anorexia are common.
- Examination may reveal some tenderness of the shoulder and neck muscles, but no significant loss of muscle strength.

Treatment (See also GCA and PMR in Chapter 17)

- Both GCA and PMR are thought to be self-limited in most patients, lasting up to 2 years.
- Corticosteroid therapy appears to prevent the most serious complication of GCA, unilateral or bilateral blindness caused by ischemic optic neuropathy. It occurs in 20% to 30% of untreated patients.
- Corticosteroids also seem to relieve symptoms in PMR.

Facial Pain: Tic Douloureux (Idiopathic Trigeminal Neuralgia)

Definition

Tic douloureux is a disorder of the trigeminal (fifth cranial) nerve that results in bouts of excruciating, lancinating pain. Bouts last from seconds to 2 minutes, along the distribution of one or more of the nerve's sensory divisions, most often the maxillary.

Risk Factors

- Tic douloureux is seen almost exclusively in people over age 40.

Etiology and Pathogenesis

- Intracranial arterial and, less often, venous loops that compress the trigeminal nerve root where it enters the brain stem are found

during surgery or autopsy, suggesting that the disorder is a compressive neuropathy.

Diagnosis

Signs and Symptoms

- Pain that is severe, paroxysmal, and lancinating occurs in the structures innervated by the second and third divisions of the trigeminal nerve (lips, gums, cheek, and chin).
- The pain is usually unilateral in a single attack, and remains unilateral in 95% of patients.
- The patient can identify triggers that precipitate pain: points on the face or in the mouth that are touched, a cold wind that flows over the area of the face that is most sensitive to stimuli, or other similar triggers.

Differential Diagnosis

- Multiple sclerosis, acoustic neuroma, aneurysms, and meningiomas can produce pain similar to that of trigeminal neuralgia.

Treatment

- Carbamazepine (Tegretol) 200 mg tablets in two divided doses bid, with breakfast and dinner
  —Dosage is increased every 2 to 3 days to a tid schedule, and up to a total dosage of 300 to 600 mg/day.
  —Side effects are usually minimal: nausea, vomiting, ataxia, vertigo, and transient leukopenia.
  —If leukopenia persists, frequent serial hemograms are performed after 1 and 6 weeks, 3 months, and then periodically.
  —Aplastic anemia is the most serious, but very infrequent, side effect.

Patient and Family Education

- Patients should be informed about possible side effects of carbamazepine, particularly the very low risk of aplastic anemia.
- Instructions regarding dosage and scheduling of medication(s) should be provided in writing.

Follow-up and Referral

- If the patient does not improve with carbamazepine or cannot tolerate the drug, referral to a neurosurgeon is recommended for possible percutaneous radiofrequency treatment of the trigeminal ganglion on the affected side.

SEIZURE DISORDERS
Definition and Classification of Epileptic Seizures (Box 6-1)

- Any paroxysmal disturbance in consciousness, behavior, or motor activity may be termed a spell, fit, or seizure.
- These disturbances are defined as the clinical manifestations of an abnormal, usually brief, excessive or hypersynchronous neuronal discharge in the cerebral cortex or deep limbic structures.

Risk Factors

- Family history of specific seizures
- Vary according to type of seizure (Table 6-2)

Etiology

- Varies according to type of seizure (Table 6-2)
- It is important to emphasize that many partial epilepsies may have secondary generalized seizures, and that the focal onset may be obscured.
  —It is necessary to search for causes of focal seizures even in what appear to be generalized seizures.
- Classification of seizures requires clinical observation.
- Classification of an epilepsy seizure syndrome usually requires clinical, EEG, and imaging data.
- A seizure represents a symptom of cerebral dysfunction, and therefore a primary cause should be sought.
- Epilepsy that derives from definable causes has been termed symptomatic, as opposed to essential or idiopathic seizures.
  —Symptomatic epilepsies frequently arise from identifiable brain lesions (e.g., infections, trauma, tumor, or strokes).
- Patients with idiopathic generalized epilepsies (IGEs) usually have a normal examination, normal screening laboratory tests, an EEG showing a generalized spike-and-wave pattern, and a family history of similar seizures. These patients would not be exhaustively studied for underlying causes.

BOX 6-1
Classification of the Epilepsies

PRIMARY GENERALIZED EPILEPSY (IDIOPATHIC GENERALIZED EPILEPSY [IGE])
Tonic-clonic (grand mal [GTC])
Absence (petit mal)
Myoclonic
Atonic, others

SECONDARY GENERALIZED SEIZURES

PARTIAL (FOCAL) EPILEPSY
With elementary symptomatology
Focal motor
Focal sensory
Vegetative
Psychic
Mixed
With complex symptomatology
Complex partial (psychomotor [CPS])

UNCLASSIFIABLE SEIZURES

From Kaplan PW: Seizure disorders. In Barker LR, Burton JR, Zieve PD, eds: *Principles of ambulatory medicine,* ed 5, Baltimore, 1999, Williams & Wilkins, p 1230.
GTC, Generalized tonic-clonic (seizure); *CPS,* complex partial psychomotor (seizure).

Seizures that Occur for the First Time in an Older Person

- Most seizure disorders begin in the first three decades of life.
- Onset of IGEs almost never occurs after age 30.
- Cerebrovascular disease accounts for 30% to 60% of all new seizures in the elderly population.
- Tumors, the major cause of focal seizures in middle age, have been found to be the cause of 2% to 30% of seizures in elderly patients.
  —Brain tumors in this age group are likely to be malignant.
- In 50% of seizures in older patients, no cause is found.
- When an elderly patient begins having seizures, special effort should go toward finding treatable conditions (e.g., carotid artery stenosis, cardiac arrhythmias, infection, or toxic-metabolic disorders).

Posttraumatic Seizures

- Seizures after head trauma are usually partial (focal) at onset, and secondary general-

TABLE 6-2
Causes* of Seizures with Onset at Various Ages

Adolescence (12-21)	Adult (21-65)	Older (65+)
COMMON CAUSES		
Genetic (g)	Alcohol withdrawal (g)	Cerebrovascular (m)
Mesial temporal sclerosis (f)	Toxins or drugs (g)	Thrombotic
Infection (m)	Drug withdrawal (g)	Embolic
Meningitis	Tumor (f)	Hemorrhagic
Viral encephalitis	Trauma (f)	Cardiac dysrhythmias
TORCH syndrome	Scar	Trauma (f)
Parasites	Subdural hematoma	Tumor (f)
Psychogenic (m)	Mesial temporal sclerosis (f)	Infection (m)
Toxins or drugs (g)	Genetic (g)	Meningitis
	Psychogenic (m)	Viral encephalitis
	Infection (m)	Abscesses
	Meningitis	Syphilis
	Viral encephalitis	Parasites
	Syphilis	
	Parasites	
OCCASIONAL CAUSES		
Metabolic (g)	Metabolic (g)	Alcohol withdrawal (g)
Hypoglycemia	Hypoglycemia	Toxins or drugs (g)
Hyponatremia	Hyponatremia	Drug withdrawal (g)
Hypocalcemia	Hypocalcemia	Hypoxia (g)
Porphyria	Hypomagnesemia	Metabolic (g)
Trauma (f)	Hypoxia (g)	Hypoglycemia
Scar	Cerebrovascular (m)	Hyponatremia
Subdural hematoma	Thrombotic	Hypocalcemia
Tumor (f)	Embolic	
Arteriovenous malformation (f)	Hemorrhagic	
Subarachnoid hemorrhage (m)	Cardiac dysrhythmia	
Eclampsia (m)	Renal failure (g)	
Renal failure (g)	Eclampsia (m)	
RARE CAUSES		
Collagen disease (m)	Collagen disease (m)	Hypertensive encephalopathy
Hepatic failure (g)	Hypertensive	Hyperosmolar (m)
Multiple sclerosis (f)	encephalopathy (m)	Renal failure (g)
	Hyperosmolar (m)	Hepatic failure (g)
	Multiple sclerosis (f)	Degenerative (g)
	Degenerative (m)	Factitious (m)
Idiopathic	Idiopathic	Idiopathic

From Kaplan PW: Seizure disorders. In Barker LR, Burton JR, Zieve PD, eds: *Principles of ambulatory medicine,* ed 5, Baltimore, 1999, Williams & Wilkins, p 1235.
g, Usually generalized; *f,* usually focal; *m,* often mixed; *TORCH,* toxoplasmosis, rubella, cytomegalovirus, herpes simplex.
*Causes listed in order of frequency.

ized seizures often occur after serious head injuries.

- Little risk is associated with seizures after mild head trauma with brief unconsciousness or amnesia, but severe injuries with intracranial hematomas, focal neurologic signs, and unconsciousness for more than 24 hours result in epilepsy in about 10% of patients.
- Moderately severe injuries (skull fractures or unconsciousness for 30 minutes to 24 hours) impose an intermediate risk.

• Injuries over the vertex are more epileptogenic than others.

Prophylactic Therapy
• The value of prophylactic therapy to prevent the onset of posttraumatic seizures has not been determined. While awaiting more data, the following steps are taken.
• Patients with minor scalp lacerations or brief loss of consciousness should not be considered to have a significantly increased risk of epilepsy.
  —A seizure occurring early (within 2 weeks after injury), or while the patient is still in the acute phase of the injury, is not an indication for long-term therapy; however, a second seizure within this time frame could warrant long-term therapy.
• Some patients with brain injuries are usually considered for a 2- to 4-year course of prophylactic phenytoin, particularly following severe, penetrating, or vertex injuries.
• A patient who is experiencing seizures more than 2 weeks after a head injury should be evaluated and managed the same way that one would evaluate and manage a patient with new-onset seizures.
  —In these cases, the seizure should not be construed to be the result of a recent or remote episode of head injury until other treatable causes of seizures have been excluded.

Alcohol-Related Seizures
• Alcohol withdrawal is a common cause of seizures, which occur within the first 48 hours of abstinence, or after marked reduction in alcohol intake following a long period of daily drinking.
  —Most seizures caused by alcohol withdrawal are generalized.
  —In some cases, up to 25% of withdrawal seizures are focal, presumably because of an old cortical scar from trauma, infection, or vascular disease.
• The risk of epilepsy in the alcohol abuser is related to the amount of alcohol consumed, although not being consumed at the time of seizure; the risk is increased in the case of head trauma and intracranial infection in this population.

—If a known alcohol abuser has had a previous withdrawal seizure, then exhibits a typical picture of a generalized seizure without focal features, and has a normal examination and no complications, the evaluation may be limited.
—Often the history is not clear, and findings are equivocal, or the patient has a fever or an elevated leukocyte count. In these circumstances lumbar puncture, EEG, and continued observation are indicated.
—New-onset focal seizures, focal neurologic deficits, fever, neck stiffness, or signs of acute head trauma warrant a CT scan.
• Use of antiepileptic drugs (AEDs) to prevent alcohol withdrawal seizures is controversial.
  —Some experts recommend AEDs for recent seizures or clusters of seizures during alcohol withdrawal, while others say that alcohol withdrawal seizures are self-limited; some studies indicate that treatment is usually ineffective.
  —Patients who are hospitalized for alcohol-related seizures may be given a 5-day course of phenytoin (300 mg/day) to try to prevent seizures and the risks associated with them, such as aspiration pneumonia and falls.
  —Long-term therapy with AEDs is not recommended.
• Seizures may sometimes occur during periods of alcohol consumption, as opposed to periods of alcohol withdrawal.
• Alcohol abusers often abuse other drugs.
  —Concurrent benzodiazepine or barbiturate withdrawal may cause fulminant seizures.

Seizures Associated with Brain Tumors
• Brain tumors do not usually cause epilepsy, although seizures are a common sign of brain tumor.
  —About 33% of intracranial and 50% of intrahemispheric tumors are associated with seizures.
• Current understanding of epilepsy secondary to tumors has changed completely since the advent of CT and MRI.
  —Tumors often cause a single seizure that leads to early investigation and diagnosis with CT or MRI.

—Between 1% and 16% of patients with epilepsy are found to have tumors.

—Young and middle-aged adults with new-onset focal seizures have the greatest chance of having a tumor.

- Seizures may be generalized tonic-clonic or partial.
- Changing and diverse clinical features are highly indicative of neoplasia.
- The most common signs and symptoms of brain tumor are:

—Onset after age 20

—Presence of persistent focal neurologic signs

—Signs of increased intracranial pressure

—Focal unilateral slow waves on the EEG

- Seizure frequency varies according to tumor location and histology.

—Frequent seizures are seen with supratentorial tumors, particularly in the rolandic, temporal, or parietal cortical regions.

—Slow-growing tumors seem to be more epileptogenic.

Seizures in Cardiovascular Disease

- Cerebrovascular disease and epilepsy are the two most common causes of serious neurologic illnesses; they often occur together in the same patient.
- Incidence of early seizures within the first 2 weeks of stroke onset is about 5% in patients with nonembolic stroke.

—Seizures are more likely to be focal (80%) than generalized, and the distribution depends on location of the stroke.

—Only a small percentage of stroke patients develop recurrent seizures: 2.5% of patients with intracranial hemorrhage, and 3% in those with ischemic stroke.

- In ischemic stroke, the highest incidence of seizures is soon after stroke onset.

—Epilepsy is most common (90%) in patients with late-onset (>2 weeks) seizures, but seizures occur in only 33% of those with early-onset seizures.

- Seizures in the elderly raise the suspicion of cerebrovascular disease, and may herald transient ischemia or impending stroke.
- In young people, a seizure may result in a diagnosis of arteriovenous malformation,

aneurysm, collagen vascular disease, or, rarely, cortical thrombophlebitis.

Seizures in Infection

- A seizure is often an early sign of bacterial meningitis, particularly in the very young and very old, who do not exhibit the classic signs and symptoms of meningitis.
- Less fulminant meningitis caused by cryptococcus or tuberculosis causes seizures that recur over weeks or months.
- Viral encephalitis, the childhood exanthems, and the equine viruses also cause seizures in some cases.
- Human immunodeficiency virus (HIV) infection is increasingly of concern as a cause of neurologic and systemic disease.
- Seizures associated with AIDS are usually caused by secondary complications (e.g., cerebral toxoplasmosis or other atypical infections, or by CNS lymphomas).
- Systemic infections may trigger seizures in susceptible patients even though the infection does not involve the CNS.

—When a patient has a seizure and signs of infection, particularly if the seizure is focal or if focal signs are detected on neurologic examination, brain abscess must be ruled out by CT or MRI, usually with contrast.

Diagnosis

- During the examination of a patient with a history of one or more episodes of self-limited disturbance of consciousness or behavior, the most important questions to ask are:

—Did seizures actually occur?

—What type of seizure was it?

—Are there clues in the history, physical, or laboratory tests to indicate a cause for the seizure?

Differential Diagnosis

- These conditions must be evaluated in terms of the patient's age, sex, personal and family history, occupation, and other factors:

—Syncope

—Cerebrovascular disease

—Migraine

—Narcolepsy

—Fluctuating delirium

—Paroxysmal vertigo

—Breath-holding spells
—Episodic movement disorders
—Malingering, factitious illness
—Conversion disorder
—Panic attack
—Hypoglycemia

Diagnostic Tests

- Serum prolactin level may rise two to three times after an epileptic episode, but not in a psychogenic tonic-clonic seizure.
- EEG may show generalized or focal epileptiform activity, or in the absence of such activity may show asymmetries of basic rhythms, focal slow waves, or diffuse slowing, all or any of which may lead to other pertinent testing.
- Cerebrospinal fluid (CSF) is examined for suspected acute or chronic meningitis, subarachnoid hemorrhage, or tumor; and all patients who have seizures of unknown cause warrant CSF examination, to exclude these potentially fatal conditions.
- Cerebral imaging
  —CT head scans are abnormal in 10% of patients with primary generalized seizures.
  —In patients with focal motor or secondary generalized seizures, the CT scan indicated abnormality in 65%.
  —MRI has a higher yield than CT scan, but is not needed for all patients.
- Other diagnostic tests have been largely replaced by newer imaging methods.
  —Skull x-rays
  —Radionuclide brain scan
  —Pneumoencephalography
  —Arteriography
- Newer neurologic tests
  —Imaging of brain metabolism and chemistry by positron emission tomography (PET)
  —Single-photon emission computed tomography (SPECT)
  —Magnetoencephalographic (MEG) recording of brain activity

Treatment

- Epilepsy cannot be cured, except in a few rare instances.
- In 75% of patients, the seizures can be controlled, reducing the number and frequency of seizures.

- Pharmacologic treatment has been much emphasized, but although patients are free of seizures, they may be so toxic from medications as to be essentially unemployable. This situation cannot be regarded as a success.
- Usually, the occurrence of a single seizure does not warrant pharmacologic therapy.
- Patients who have seizures because of alcohol withdrawal, cocaine intake, or tricyclic overdose are treated by removing the precipitating cause.
- A single or early seizures within 2 weeks of a head injury or stroke do not require AED therapy.
- In about one-third of patients who experience a single seizure, the seizure was unprovoked. These patients are willing to take medications over the long term to prevent more seizures and the attendant negative effects on the job, social relations, or the loss of a driver's license.
  —Data show that 16% to 36% of patients who have a first unprovoked seizure will have a recurrence within 1 year.
  —These patients overall have recurrence of seizures within 3 years, and retrospective studies show an even higher recurrence rate.
  —Over a 5-year period, 30% to 80% of patients who have had a single unprovoked seizure will have a recurrence within that time period.
- The recurrence rate is significantly reduced by prescribing AED therapy for patients; recurrence at 1 year was 18% in treated patients, in contrast to 38% in untreated patients.

Guidelines for Treatment of Seizures
(Box 6-2 and Table 6-3)

- A patient having one or more generalized seizures per month is probably being undertreated.
- Dosage should be started at one-quarter or one-half of the anticipated maintenance dose, except for phenytoin and phenobarbital, then increased slightly over several weeks, to prevent early side effects that might discourage the patient from continuing therapy.
  —Because some AEDs remain in the blood for some time, several days to weeks are often required to determine the effects of dosage changes.

- In the past, therapy often consisted of prescribing two drugs to be taken simultaneously (e.g., phenytoin and phenobarbital), but evidence does not support the use of two drugs at the same time, since 90% of new-onset seizures can be controlled with one drug.
- Compliance is a major factor in the success of pharmacologic therapy for epilepsy; therefore, every effort should be made to

simplify the dosage regimen and to select the best-tolerated drug.

- Optimal dosage of an AED will vary considerably among patients; periodic blood levels will help to determine how much medication is circulating.
- The decision regarding how long to maintain treatment with an AED is difficult because seizures remit over time, and absence of seizure activity may occur not because of medications but because of the time factor.
  —About 50% to 66% of patients are entirely seizure free after 2 years of therapy.
  —If an adult patient has no seizures for 5 years on medication, and if treatment is stopped by tapering, the risk of relapse within the next 5 years is 30% to 50%.
  —About 90% of relapses occur within 2 years following discontinuation of the drug.

Prognosis

- Epilepsy cannot be cured; the goal of treatment is to control seizures to the extent possible to allow the person to live normally.

Patient and Family Education

- Patients should be informed about the nature, cause, course, components, and outcome of therapy.

BOX 6-2

Guidelines for AED* Treatment

Make the decision to treat or not to treat.
Select the appropriate drug for the particular type of epilepsy.
Begin drugs slowly and increase levels gradually to avoid toxicity.
Start with one drug, and use it to effect or toxicity before adding another drug.
Choose the simplest regimen possible.
Suspect compliance problems in treatment failure.
Monitor blood levels in problem cases.
Withdraw medications gradually.
Decide how long to treat.

From Kaplan PW: Seizure disorders. In Barker LR, Burton JR, Zieve PD, eds: *Principles of ambulatory medicine,* ed 5, Baltimore, 1999, Williams & Wilkins, p 1240.
*AED, Antiepileptic drug (therapy).

TABLE 6-3

Selected Drugs for Monotherapy According to Seizure Type

Type of Seizure	Drug of Choice	Alternatives
Primary generalized, tonic-clonic	Valproic acid	Carbamazepine (Tegretol) Phenytoin Primidone Phenobarbital
Primary generalized, absence	Ethosuximide Valproic acid	Clonazepam
Primary myoclonic	Valproic acid Clonazepam	Phenytoin Phenobarbital
Partial simple and complex, and secondary generalized epilepsy	Carbamazepine Phenytoin	Valproic acid Phenobarbital Primidone
Mixed forms	Valproic acid Clonazepam	Carbamazepine Phenytoin Phenobarbital

From Kaplan PW: Seizure disorders. In Barker LR, Burton JR, Zieve PD, eds: *Principles of ambulatory medicine,* ed 5, Baltimore, 1999, Williams & Wilkins, p 1240.

- Drug therapy should be emphasized in those patients who require this type of treatment, and compliance is strongly encouraged.
  —Have the patient keep a daily diary that includes the time that the medication was taken, its effects, and any seizures that occur.
  —Such a record may help to emphasize the importance of taking the medication as scheduled to avoid consequences from missed doses.

Follow-up and Referral

- Factors that determine follow-up include frequency of seizures, side effects of medication, and others (e.g., effect of therapy on relationships).
  —Patients who have no seizures for more than a year and have no other problems may be seen once or twice a year.
  —Patients with frequent seizures, who have significant side effects, who have other troublesome problems , or who are being started on a new drug may need to be seen every 2 to 4 weeks.
- Hospitalization or referral of the patient to a neurologist or other specialist may be needed some time during the course of therapy.

PARKINSON'S DISEASE
Definition

- Parkinson's disease is a movement disorder, an idiopathic, slowly progressive CNS disorder characterized by rigidity, resting tremor, and postural instability.

Risk Factors

- Parkinson's disease is the most common neurodegenerative disease of older persons.
- Prevalence increases sharply with age to about 1 in 200 of those over 70 years.
- It affects about 1% of people 65 years of age and older.
- Onset usually occurs after age 40; average age at onset is 57, but it may begin in childhood or adolescence.

Etiology

- The precise cause of Parkinson's disease is unknown, but the fact that it occurs worldwide seems to exclude environmental factors.

- Some studies suggest that the disease is less prevalent in tobacco users than in those who have never smoked.
- Very small doses of the pyridine compound, methylphenyl-tetrahydropyridine (MPTP), cause a severe parkinsonian syndrome, perhaps implicating MPTP-like herbicides as possible etiologic agents.
- Patients who survive encephalitis lethargica, presumed to be a viral disease, develop parkinsonism; however, most neurologists are inclined to think that there is no link between the idiopathic Parkinson's disease and this or any other disease that is caused by any infective agent.
- Although the condition is not inherited, there is occasional clustering in families; it is postulated that a failure of dopamine synthesis, genetically programmed, could be responsible.
- Secondary parkinsonism occurs in some people because of ingestion of antipsycholotic drugs or reserpine, which block dopamine receptors and result in Parkinson's-like symptoms.
- Other causes of secondary Parkinson's disease are carbon monoxide or manganese poisoning, hydrocephalus, structural lesions such as tumors, infarcts that affect the midbrain or basal ganglia, subdural hematoma, and multiple systems atrophy.

Pathogenesis

- In the pars compacta of the substantia nigra, there is a progressive cell degeneration and the appearance of eosinophilic inclusion bodies (Lewy bodies).
- Degeneration also occurs in other brainstem nuclei.
- Biochemically, there is loss of dopamine (and melanin) in the striatum that correlates well with the areas of cell loss, and also with the degree of akinesia.
- However, the underlying cause of the progressive changes in neurotransmitter profile remains unclear.

Natural History

- Parkinson's disease progresses over many years, beginning as a mild inconvenience but slowly overtaking the patient.
  —Remissions do not occur except in rare and short-lived periods of relief, which usually

occur during periods of great emotion, fear, or excitement, when the patient is able to move quickly.

—The rate of progression is variable, with a benign form going over several decades.

—The usual course is 10 to 15 years, with death resulting from bronchopneumonia.

Diagnosis

Signs and Symptoms (Box 6-3)

- The most common symptoms are tremor and slowed movement.
- Patients complain that the limbs feel stiff and ache, and that fine movements are difficult.
- The slowed movement causes the characteristics symptoms of difficulty in rising from a chair or getting into or out of bed.
- The facial expression becomes masklike, which may often lead to initiating diagnostic evaluation for the disease.
- Writing becomes small (micrographia) and spidery, with a tendency to tail off at the end of a line.
- The signs and symptoms are more prominent on one side.

Signs

- Tremor: this is a characteristic 4 to 7 Hz rest tremor, usually decreased by action and increased by emotion; pill-rolling movements between the thumb and forefinger are present.

BOX 6-3

Clinical Features of Parkinsonian Syndrome, Not Idiopathic Parkinson's Disease

Little or no response to L-dopa
Young onset
Early-onset dementia
Rapid progression
Early-onset dysarthria or dysphagia
Prominent and early dysautonomia
Early falling
Impaired ocular motility
Positive family history
LMN, cerebellar, or pyramidal signs

From Reich SG: Common disorders of movement: tremor and Parkinson's disease. In Barker LR, Burton JR, Zieve PD, eds: *Principles of ambulatory medicine*, ed 5, Baltimore, 1999, Williams & Wilkins, p 1279.

- Rigidity: stiffness of the limbs develops that can be felt throughout the range of motion, and is equal in opposing groups of muscles, in contrast to the selective increase in tone seen in spasticity.

  —This "lead pipe–like" rigidity is often more marked on one side, and is present in the neck and axial muscles.

  —The rigidity is often more easily felt when a joint is moved slowly and gently; simultaneous movement of the opposite limb increases the tone of the side being examined.

  —When both rigidity and tremor are present, the smooth plasticity of the increase in tone is broken up into a jerky resistance to passive movement, a phenomenon known as cogwheeling.

- Akinesia: paucity and slowness of movement (bradykinesia) occur; there is difficulty in initiating movement, making normally rapid fine finger movements, such as are used in piano playing or keyboarding, slow and difficult.

  —The immobility of the face gives a masklike facies with the appearance of depression; the smile is gone.

  —The frequency of spontaneous eye blinking is decreased, which produces a serpentine-like state.

- Postural changes: a stoop is characteristic, as is a shuffling gait, with festination and poor arm swing; festination causes the upper part of the body to move forward more quickly than the lower part and legs, so that the patient must use a wall or piece of furniture to stop against to avoid falling forward.

  —Falls are common as the usual corrective righting reflexes fail; patients fall stiffly, like falling trees.

  —The patient sits with the trunk bent forward and motionless, without gestures or animation, although the limbs are tremulous.

- Speech: at first, speech is monotonous, progressing to a characteristic tremulous slurring dysarthria, caused by the combination of akinesia, tremor, and rigidity.

  —Dribbling or drooling is frequent, and dysphagia develops as the disease worsens.

- There is no sensory loss.

BOX 6-4
Differential Diagnosis of Parkinsonism

TOXINS
Manganese
Carbon monoxide
Carbon disulfide
Cyanide
Methanol
MPTP

DRUG-INDUCED
Neuroleptics
Metoclopramide (Reglan)

MULTISYSTEM DEGENERATIVE DISEASES
Progressive supranuclear palsy
Shy-Drager syndrome
Olivopontocerebellar atrophy
Striatonigral degeneration
Amyotrophic lateral sclerosis
Parkinson's disease
Dementia complex of Guam

PRIMARY DEMENTING DISEASES
Alzheimer's disease
Creutzfeldt-Jakob syndrome

HEREDITARY OR FAMILIAL DISEASES
Wilson's disease
Juvenile Huntington's disease
Hallervorden-Spatz syndrome

MULTI-INFARCT STATE

CALCIFICATION OF THE BASAL GANGLIA
Idiopathic
Hypoparathyroidism

POSTENCEPHALITIC

TRAUMA
Dementia pugilistica

From Reich SG: Common disorders of movement: tremor and Parkinson's disease. In Barker LR, Burton JR, Zieve PD, eds: *Principles of ambulatory medicine*, ed 5, Baltimore, 1999, Williams & Wilkins, p 1279.

- The reflexes become brisk, and their asymmetry follows the increase in tone; the plantar responses remain flexor.
- Cognitive function is preserved early in the disease, but dementia sometimes develops in the later stages.
- Gastrointestinal and other symptoms: heartburn, dysphagia, constipation, and weight loss generally occur; urinary difficulties are common, especially in men.
    —The skin is greasy, and sweating is excessive.
- Clinical signs of Parkinsonian syndrome (not idiopathic Parkinson's disease) are listed in Box 6-3.

Differential Diagnosis (Box 6-4)
- No laboratory test exists to confirm Parkinson's disease.
- Diagnosis is made from clinical evidence.

Treatment (Table 6-4)

- Former therapy with anticholinergic drugs did not alter the course of the disease, and frequently caused mental confusion.
- Today, levodopa (L-DOPA) and carbidopa (Sinemet) are used interchangeably.

—Since the hallmark of Parkinson's disease is depletion of dopamine in the striatum, replacement of dopamine is the mainstay of treatment.
  ~ Dopamine does not cross the blood-brain barrier. In its stead, its precursor L-dopa is given, which does cross the blood-brain barrier.
—The combination regimen reduces side effects (e.g., nausea).
—Therapy is begun gradually: co-beneldopa 125 mg, or carbidopa (Sinemet) 110 mg one tablet tid.
  ~ The dosage is increased slowly until adequate improvement has occurred, or until side effects limit further increases in dose.
- Almost all patients eventually require L-dopa therapy.
  —Controversy exists around the optimal time to begin this drug.
  —Those who favor early treatment cite studies that indicate decreased morbidity and mortality.
  —However, the length of time that a patient is on L-dopa may be a risk factor for later motor complications.

TABLE 6-4
Drugs Used for Parkinson's Disease

Drug	Maintenance Dose (mg)
ANTICHOLINERGIC AGENTS	
Trihexyphenidyl (Artane)	2-10
Benztropine mesylate (Cogentin)	0.5-6
DOPAMINERGIC AGENTS	
Carbidopa L-dopa (Sinemet)	400-500 L-dopa
Carbidopa (Sinemet CR)	500-1000 L-dopa
Bromocriptine (Parlodel)	7.5-30
Pergolide (Permax)	1-3
Selegiline (Eldepryl)	10
ANTICHOLINERGIC OR DOPAMINERGIC ACTIVITY	
Amantadine (Symmetrel)	200

From Reich SG: Common disorders of movement: tremor and Parkinson's disease. In Barker LR, Burton JR, Zieve PD, eds: *Principles of ambulatory medicine*, ed 5, Baltimore, 1999, Williams & Wilkins, p 1281.

—The current consensus is that clinical status is determined primarily by disease duration, and that early initiation of L-dopa does not have a major adverse effect on the course of the disease.

- The best course of action is to explain to the patient the options for initial monotherapy.
  —For patients not treated initially with L-dopa, the drug should be added when the disease begins to limit function.
  —Once the patient has responded to L-dopa, the clinician should try to decrease the dosage of other antiparkinsonian medications and, if possible, discontinue them.
  —However, some patients begin to decline when this is attempted, and polypharmacy must be continued.
- As the disease progresses, and as L-dopa alone is insufficient to control the signs and symptoms, a direct-acting dopamine receptor agonist such as bromocriptine or pergolide, or the monoamine oxidase (MAO) inhibitor deprenyl, which prevents catabolism of dopamine, should be added.

Side Effects of L-dopa Therapy

- Nausea and vomiting that occur within one hour of administration are the most common symptoms of excessive dosage.

—Confusion and visual hallucinations also occur with excessive dosage.
—Chorea occurs in acute overdose.

Problems with L-dopa Therapy

- Because of attendant problems with L-dopa therapy, this drug should not be started until necessary.
- In about 50% of patients, the drug becomes ineffective, even with increasing doses, after about 5 years of therapy.
- As the disease progresses, some patients have episodes of severe immobility ("freezing"), which induce falls.
- Response fluctuations also occur, with its effect seemingly turning on and off.
- The duration of action decreases, and dyskinesia becomes prominent toward the end of action of the dose of L-dopa, known as "end-of-dose dyskinesia."
  —The patient then suffers not only from Parkinson's disease itself, but also from a chronic dyskinesia, and severe and sometimes sudden immobility ("on-off syndrome").
- Treatment for these complications includes:
  —Shortening the interval between doses of L-dopa and, perhaps, increasing individual doses may help.
  —Giving selegiline, a type-B MAO inhibitor, which inhibits the catabolism of dopamine in the brain; the drug sometimes smoothes out the response to L-dopa.
    ~ There have been reports about an increased morbidity from cardiovascular disease in patients taking selegiline, but this complication is unproven.
  —Oral dopaminergic agonists are used to add to or replace existing L-dopa therapy.
  —Apomorphine, a dopaminergic agonist that acts directly, given by daily subcutaneous injection, is probably the best method of smoothing out the response fluctuations of L-dopa; a side effect of apomorphine is severe hemolytic anemia.
  —Periods of complete withdrawal of L-dopa ("drug holiday") were advocated in the past. This is no longer recommended because of the common complications that occur when patients deteriorate while off the drug, and the transient nature of the

improvement when carbidopa (Sinemet) was restarted. They require close monitoring, since severe rigidity and akinesia may follow withdrawal of the drug.

New Drug Therapy

- Two newer dopamine agonist drugs that were approved by the FDA in 1997 may preserve L-dopa's effectiveness in the later stages of Parkinson's disease, and may have fewer side effects than bromocriptine and pergolide:
  - Ropinirole
  - Pramipexole
- Two other drugs (catechol-o-methyltransferase inhibitors), which prolong carbidopa/L-dopa activity, but which have not yet been approved, are:
  - Tolcapone
  - Entacapone

Dopaminergic Agonists

- Bromocriptine, lysuride, and pergolide are direct-acting dopamine agonists, which act mainly in D1 and D2 receptors, as well as on receptors D3-5, and are used as alternative or add-on therapy to L-dopa.
  - Other similar drugs are being developed.

Surgical Treatment

- Stereotactic thalamotomy or pallidotomy is a safe, effective treatment for parkinsonian patients with disabling tremor that is unresponsive to medical therapy, or for those with severe fluctuations with dyskinesia or facing waning response to L-dopa.
- In addition to stereotactic surgery for Parkinson's disease, tissue implantation holds promise.
  - Initial apparent success with adrenal-to-caudate implantation resulted in a large number of clinical trials that proved to be disappointing.
  - In place of adrenal transplantation, fetal nigral tissue implantation is being used and its effects studied, the results of which will determine the degree of usefulness of this type of tissue transplantation therapy.

Dementia and Depression in Patients with Parkinson's Disease

- The frequency of dementia in patients with Parkinson's disease varies considerably; a conservative estimate is that dementia occurs in at least 15% to 20% of patients.
  - Although there is a relatively large percentage of patients with Parkinson's disease who develop dementia, it is crucial to acknowledge that dementia is not an inevitable feature.
  - When dementia occurs, patients are troubled with hallucinations, agitation, psychosis, insomnia, or a reversal in the sleep-wake cycle.
  - If these signs and symptoms do not respond to reduction of the dosage of antiparkinsonian medication or administration of a mild sedative, a very low dosage of a neuroleptic may be helpful.
  - Although worsening of parkinsonian signs may occur, the suppression of intolerable behavior usually results in overall improvement in the patient's condition, and eases the caregiver burden.
- Depression is common in Parkinson's disease, and occurs in about 50% of patients.
  - It is not clear whether depression is the result of an intrinsic neurochemical defect or of the patient's response to the disability caused by the disease.
  - A rapid decline in the patient's functional status is often the first sign of depression.
  - Treatment of the depression is to give tricyclic antidepressants or selective serotonin reuptake inhibitors (SSRIs); SSRIs, however, are contraindicated in patients who are taking selegiline.
  - As the depression improves, there is often a concurrent improvement in parkinsonian signs and symptoms.
  - If these drugs (tricyclic antidepressants or SSRIs) are not effective, electroconvulsive therapy is the treatment of choice.

Patient and Family Education

- Explain the nature of Parkinson's disease, particularly the very slow progression, and that with treatment, most patients can remain functional and maintain a normal lifestyle.
- Provide sources of information and support groups, which can be extremely helpful to both the patient and the family. Timing is important because, early in the disease, both patients and families tend to concentrate only on the worst prognosis.
- Explain that the patient's goals of social, professional, and physical involvement in activi-

ties will guide therapy as to when to initiate treatment, and to make changes in the dosing schedule.

- Usual signs and symptoms should be listed, so that both patients and families know what to expect; long-term effects can be addressed later, if necessary.
- Patients and families should realize the importance of continuing physical, social, and professional activities to the degree possible at each stage.
- Additional caregivers may be needed to provide physical care to prevent skin breakdown and the complications of bradykinesia and sedentary living.
- Help is usually needed to keep the patient as mobile as possible, and to provide social and intellectual stimulation.

Follow-up and Referral
- Patients with Parkinson's disease are followed closely for years, often decades.
- Help and support from physicians and nurses are needed at all stages.
- If the patient requires surgery or treatment of depression, referral to a neurosurgeon, neurologist, or psychiatrist may be needed.

DELIRIUM AND DEMENTIA
Delirium
Definition
Delirium is a clinical state characterized by fluctuating disturbances in cognition, mood, attention, arousal, and self-awareness; it arises acutely, either without prior intellectual impairment or superimposed on chronic intellectual impairment.

Risk Factors, Etiology, and Pathogenesis (Box 6-5)
Diagnosis (Box 6-6)
Signs and Symptoms
- Symptoms often fluctuate rapidly, sometimes within minutes, and tend to be worse late in the day (sundown syndrome).
- Clouding of consciousness accompanied by disorientation to time, place, or person
- Lack of ability to focus attention
- Confusion about day-to-day events and daily routines
- Changes in personality and affect
- Irritability
- Inappropriate behavior
- Fearfulness
- Excessive energy
- Frankly psychotic symptoms (e.g., delusions, hallucinations, paranoia)

BOX 6-5
Causes of Delirium

SYSTEMIC INFECTION
Any infection, particularly with high fever (e.g., malaria, septicemia)

METABOLIC DISTURBANCE
Hepatic failure
Renal failure
Disorders of electrolyte balance
Hypoxia

VITAMIN DEFICIENCY
Thiamin (Wernicke-Korsakoff syndrome, beri beri)
Nicotinic acid (pellagra)
Vitamin B_{12}

ENDOCRINE DISEASE
Hypoglycemia
Cushing's syndrome

INTRACRANIAL CAUSES
Trauma
Tumor
Abscess
Subarachnoid hemorrhage
Epilepsy

DRUG INTOXICATION
Anticonvulsant
Anticholinergic
Anxiolytic/hypnotic
Opiates

INDUSTRIAL TOXINS (e.g., DDT, trichloroethylene)

POSTOPERATIVE STATES

From Clarke CRA: Neurological disease. In Kumar P, Clark M, eds: *Clinical medicine,* ed 4, Edinburgh, 1998, WB Saunders, p 1113.
DDT, Dichlorodiphenyltrichloroethane.

BOX 6-6

Diagnostic Criteria for Delirium

- Disturbance of consciousness (e.g., reduced clarity of awareness of the environment), with reduced ability to focus, sustain, or shift attention
- Change in cognition (e.g., memory deficit, disorientation, language disturbance), or development of a perceptual disturbance that is not better accounted for by preexisting, established, or evolving dementia
- Disturbance developing over a short time (usually hours to days), and tending to fluctuate during the course of the day
- For delirium due to a general medical condition:
  —Evidence from the history, physical examination, or laboratory tests that the disturbance is due to the direct physiologic consequences of a general medical condition

- For substance intoxication delirium:
  —Evidence from the history, physical examination, or laboratory tests that either
    ~ Symptoms listed in the first two criteria developed during substance intoxication or
    ~ Drug use is etiologically related to the disturbance
- For substance withdrawal delirium:
  —Evidence from the history, physical examination, or laboratory tests that the symptoms listed in the first two criteria developed during or shortly after a withdrawal syndrome
- For delirium due to multiple etiologies:
  —Evidence from the history, physical examination, or laboratory tests that the delirium has more than one etiology (e.g., more than one general medical condition, a general medical condition plus substance intoxication, or a drug side effect)

Reprinted with permission from the *Diagnostic and statistical manual of mental disorders,* ed 4, Text Revision. Copyright 2000 American Psychiatric Association.

- Quiet, withdrawn, or apathetic behavior in some patients
- Agitation or hyperactivity in others
- Physical restlessness often expressed by pacing
- Expression of contradictory emotions within a short span of time
- Disorganized thinking
- Speech slurred, rapid, use of neologisms, aphasic errors, chaotic patterns
- Distorted patterns of sleeping and eating
- Dizziness in some patients

Diagnostic Tests
- Because delirium can have a grave prognosis, an emergency medical evaluation is imperative.
- Diagnosis is based primarily on the diagnostic criteria (see Box 6-6).
- CBC with differential
- Blood chemistries
- Blood cultures
- VDRL test for syphilis
- Urinalysis and urine culture
- Thyroid function tests
- Vitamin B_{12} levels
- Toxicology screening
- Single CT scan with contrast to detect old or recent infarctions or subdural hematomas

Differential Diagnosis
- Depression
- Functional psychosis (lack of disorientation, memory loss, cognitive impairment, often seen in delirious or intoxicated patients)
- Psychiatric disease
- Alcohol or alcohol withdrawal

Treatment
- The condition is usually reversible if the underlying cause is diagnosed quickly and treated appropriately.
  —Hypoglycemia
  —Infection
  —Electrolyte imbalance
- Despite early diagnosis and treatment, recovery may be slow, particularly in older persons, and may take weeks or months.
- All unnecessary drugs are discontinued.
- Fluids and nutrients are given.
- In patients suspected of alcohol abuse or alcohol withdrawal, thiamin 100 mg IM is given daily for 5 days.
  —Patients suspected of alcohol abuse should be monitored for alcohol withdrawal symptoms.
- Staff and family members should reassure the patient, provide information to maintain orientation, and explain whereabouts

and activities or procedures that are oc-curring.

- Drugs should not be given except to treat in-fection or other underlying conditions.
- Agitation may require therapy to avoid harm to self, family, or staff.
- Restraints are avoided unless absolutely needed to prevent the patient from pulling out the IV or other lines; if used, restraints are released every 2 hours, and discontinued as soon as feasible.
- Medications
  —Haloperidol given PO, IM, or IV, begin-ning with lowest dose of 0.25 to 0.5 mg one to two times/day for up to 4 to 7 days to a maximum of 4 mg/day in two to three divided doses
  —Thioridazine 5 mg PO, increasing gradu-ally to 10 to 25 mg one to two times/day up to 4 to 7 days to a maximum of 400 mg/day in divided doses
  —Newer drugs such as risperidone can be used in place of haloperidol.
  —Short- and intermediate-acting benzo-diazepines (alprazolam, triazolam) can control agitation in the short term, but may worsen confusion.
- All psychoactive drugs are reduced and then stopped as soon as possible to assess recovery.

Patient and Family Education

- Encourage the family to stay with and talk to the patient, which helps to keep the pa-tient oriented to time, place, and person.
- Instruct the patient and family regarding the nature of delirium, its possible causes, treat-ment, and prognosis.
- If patient or family history details are needed, ask family members to fill in gaps.

Follow-up and Referral

- Patients with delirium are usually hos-pitalized until the acute phase passes, and underlying causes are treated and resolved.
- After discharge, patients are followed closely for several weeks, or until it seems clear that the delirium has disappeared and that re-covery is proceeding well.

Dementia
Definition
Dementia is a chronic deterioration of intel-lectual function and other cognitive skills severe enough to interfere with the ability to perform ac-tivities of daily living (ADLs).

Risk Factors
- Dementia can affect persons of any age.
- It is primarily a disease of the elderly, affect-ing about 15% of those over 65, and up to 40% of people over age 80.

Etiology (Table 6-5)
Pathogenesis
- Dementia is characterized by a disturbance of multiple higher cortical functions, in-cluding memory, thinking, orientation, comprehension, calculation, learning capac-ity, language, and judgment.
- Consciousness is not clouded.
- There may be an associated deterioration in emotional control, social behavior, and mo-tivation.
- About 25% of the older population have a psychiatric disability, primarily anxiety and depression.

Diagnosis (Box 6-7)
Dementia of Depression
- This condition was formerly known as pseu-dodementia.
- The term is used to describe patients who at first appear demented, but have depression rather than a neuropathologic disorder.
- These patients regain mental competence when the depression is treated.
- Dementia and depression frequently coexist.
  —In these cases, treating depression is re-quired, but the patient does not fully re-gain normal cognitive functioning.

Diagnosis
- Diagnosis of dementia is based on a com-plete history and mental status examination.
- The American Psychiatric Association (APA) diagnostic criteria for dementia are listed in Box 6-7.
- Depressed patients can be distinguished from patients who have dementia alone, be-cause depressed patients eat little, are con-

TABLE 6-5
Causes of Dementia

Metabolic-Toxic	Structural	Infections
Anoxia	Alzheimer's disease	Bacterial endocarditis
Vitamin B_{12} deficiency	Amyotrophic lateral sclerosis	Brain tumors (selective)
Chronic drug-alcohol nutritional abuse	Brain trauma (acute, severe)	Creutzfeldt-Jakob disease
Folic acid deficiency	Chronic subdural hematoma	Gerstmann-Straussler-Scheinker disease
Hypercalcemia associated with hyperparathyroidism	Dementia pugilistica	HIV-related disorders
Hypoglycemia	Brain tumor	Neurosyphilis (general paresis)
Hypothyroidism	Cerebellar degeneration	Tuberculous and fungal meningitis
Organ system failure	Communicating hydrocephalus	Viral encephalitis
Hepatic encephalopathy	Huntington's disease (chorea)	
Respiratory encephalopathy	Irradiation to frontal lobes	
Uremic encephalopathy	Multiple sclerosis	
Pellagra	Normal-pressure hydrocephalus	
	Parkinson's disease	
	Pick's disease	
	Progressive multifocal leukoencephalopathy	
	Progressive supranuclear palsy	
	Surgery	
	Vascular disease	
	Multi-infarct dementia	
	Wilson's disease	

From Beers MH, Berkow R, eds: Neurologic disorders. *The Merck manual of diagnosis and therapy,* ed 17, Whitehouse Station, NJ, 1999, Merck & Co, Inc, Research Laboratories, p 1393.

BOX 6-7
Diagnostic Criteria for Dementia

DEVELOPMENT OF MULTIPLE COGNITIVE DEFICITS
1. Memory impairment (impaired ability to learn new information or to recall previously learned information)
2. One or more of the following cognitive disturbances:
   a. Aphasia (language disturbance)
   b. Apraxia (impaired ability to carry out motor activities despite intact motor function)
   c. Agnosia (failure to recognize or identify objects despite intact sensory function)
   d. Disturbance in executive functioning (planning, organizing, sequencing, abstracting)

Each of the cognitive deficits described above causes significant impairment of social or occupational functioning and represents a significant decline from a previous level of functioning.

The course is characterized by gradual onset and continuing cognitive decline.

Deficits do not occur exclusively during the course of delirium.

FOR ALZHEIMER'S DISEASE
The cognitive deficits listed in the first criterion (parts 1 and 2) are not due to any of the following:
1. Other CNS conditions that cause progressive deficits in memory and cognition (e.g., cerebrovascular disease, Parkinson's disease, Huntington's disease, subdural hematoma, normal-pressure hydrocephalus, brain tumor)
2. Systemic conditions known to cause dementia (e.g., hypothyroidism, vitamin B_{12} or folic acid deficiency, niacin deficiency, hypercalcemia, neurosyphilis, HIV infection)
3. Substance-induced conditions

FOR VASCULAR DEMENTIA
Focal neurologic signs and symptoms (e.g., exaggeration of deep tendon reflexes, extensor plantar response, pseudobulbar palsy, gait abnormalities, weakness of an extremity) or laboratory evidence indicate cerebrovascular disease (e.g., multiple infarction affecting the cortex and underlying white matter) that is judged to be etiologically related to the disturbance.

FOR DEMENTIA DUE TO OTHER MEDICAL CONDITIONS
Evidence from the history, physical examination, or laboratory tests indicates that the disturbance is the direct physiologic consequence of such conditions as Parkinson's disease, Huntington's disease, Pick's disease, Creutzfeldt-Jakob disease, head trauma, HIV infection, normal-pressure hydrocephalus, hypothyroidism, brain tumor, vitamin B_{12} deficiency, or intracranial radiation.

Reprinted with permission from the *Diagnostic and statistical manual of mental disorders,* ed 4, Text Revision. Copyright 2000 American Psychiatric Association.

stipated, sleep less than normal, and behave best at night.

—Depressed patients respond slowly, but usually accurately.

—They may be semimute, but few are aphasic.

—They rarely forget major current events or matters of great personal importance.

—Severely depressed patients often complain of memory loss that is disproportionate to their examination results.

- Patients with dementia, on the other hand, seldom complain of memory problems.
- As opposed to demented patients, depressed patients have unremarkable neurologic examinations.

Treatment

- Supportive measures are extremely helpful for patients with dementia:

—Frequent orientation reinforcement

—A bright, cheerful, familiar environment

—A minimum of new stimulation

—Regular low-stress activities

—Families that include the patient in all activities, except those that might cause confusion or anxiety

—Sensory stimuli such as a night light, radio, or television

—A safe, secure environment

- Both overstimulation and understimulation should be avoided.

—A signal system should be installed to monitor a patient who wanders.

- Eliminating or limiting drugs with CNS activity will usually improve function.

Depression should be treated with nonanticholinergic antidepressants.

Prognosis

- Although a cure is rarely possible, the health care team can provide help to the family by instructing them about the condition, and that the goal is to prevent complications that may compromise the patient's status.

Patient and Family Education

- The family members should be informed about the nature of dementia, its course, and usual therapy.

- The family needs to know that caring for demented patients is highly stressful, and that working together as a supportive team will help everyone, including the patient and the caregivers.
- Provide a list of support groups and social agencies that can assist in caregiving.
- Issues such as power of attorney, living will, and post-death procedures should be put into writing before the patient becomes incapacitated.

Follow-up and Referral

- These patients are followed primarily at home, through homemaker services, visiting nurse services, social services, and other groups who can be of help.
- Referral to specialists may be needed in cases of falls, if new neurologic signs or symptoms appear, or if psychosis occurs.

ALZHEIMER'S DISEASE
Definition

Alzheimer's disease is a type of dementia characterized by progessive deterioration in memory and cognition. Pathologic changes in the brain include neurofibrillary tangles and β-amyloid plaques in the cerebral cortex and hippocampus.

Risk Factors

- Early-onset forms account for only 2% to 7% of cases, which are usually due to an inherited genetic mutation.
- The common form affects people over 60 years of age.

—The incidence of Alzheimer's disease increases with age.

Etiology

- The cause of Alzheimer's disease is unknown.
- The disease runs in families in about 15% to 20% of cases.
- The remaining cases, so-called sporadic cases, have some genetic determinants.

—At least four distinct genes, located on chromosomes 1, 14, 19, and 21, influence initiation and progression of the disease.

—Chromosome 21 generates the precursor protein for the amyloid protein, which accumulates in the brain of patients with

Alzheimer's disease (as well as with other conditions).

—Chromosome 19 generates apolipoprotein (apo) E alleles 1 to 4 (epsilon1 to epsilon4).

~ The presence of the episilon4 allele increases the risk for Alzheimer's disease in whites.

~ Episilon2 and epsilon4 alleles increase the risk in blacks.

- These findings support the epidemiologic observation that the disease has an autosomal dominant genetic pattern in most early-onset and some late-onset cases, but a variable late-life penetrance.
- Environmental factors are the current focus of active investigation.
  —Unproven speculations include low hormone levels and exposure to metals.

Pathogenesis

- Neurons are lost in the cerebral cortex, hippocampus, and subcortical structures: locus caeruleus, nucleus raphe dorsalis.
  —Selective cell loss occurs in the nucleus basalis of Meynert.
- Cerebral glucose use and perfusion are reduced in some areas of the brain (parietal lobe and temporal cortices in early-stage disease; prefrontal cortex in late-stage disease), as determined by positron emission tomography (PET).
  —Whether this reduction precedes or follows cell death is not known.
  —The microvascular system may also be affected, as seen in congophilic angiopathy.
- Neuritic or senile plaques, composed of neurites, astrocytes, and glial cells around an amyloid core, and neurofibrillary tangles composed of paired helical filaments play a role in the pathogenesis of Alzheimer's disease.
- Senile plaques and neurofibrillary tangles occur with normal aging, but these are much more prevalent in those with Alzheimer's disease.
- Specific protein abnormalities occur:
  —β-amyloid protein is believed to contribute to the pathogenesis of the disease.
    ~ Ongoing research is trying to determine whether amyloid is a toxic cause of cognitive decline, or a biologic reaction and secondary phenomenon.

—Apo E proteins, produced in the brain and liver, influence a number of cerebral processes, including amyloid deposition, cytoskeletal integrity, and efficiency of neuronal repair.

—Apo E's role in Alzheimer's disease is becoming increasingly clear.

~ The protein has three allelic forms, epsilon2, epsilon3, and epsilon4, which results in six genotypes, epsilon2/2, 2/3, 2/4, 3/3, 3/4, and 4/4.

~ The risk of Alzheimer's disease is greatly increased in persons with two epsilon4 alleles, who are more likely to develop the disease between ages 60 and 75.

—Because about 40% of people who reach age 85 develop some form of diagnosable dementia regardless of apo E status, genetic testing is not useful in predicting whether a person will develop Alzheimer's disease in later life.

~ The genetic test is available commercially; its value as an adjunctive diagnostic test, rather than a predictive test, for Alzheimer's disease is being investigated.

- Other proteins are abnormally increased in the brain and appear in the CSF.
  —Whether they are causative or are markers for the disease is not certain.
  —The tau protein (origin is neurofibrillary) has high specificity but low sensitivity for identifying a dementia such as Alzheimer's disease.
  —A slightly different type of tau protein also accumulates in patients with progressive supranuclear palsy.
- Choline acetyltransferase is markedly reduced, which decreases the availability of acetylcholine.
- Somatostatin, corticotropin-releasing factor, and other neurotransmitters are also significantly reduced.

Diagnosis

Signs and Symptoms

- Alzheimer's disease is divided into clinical stages, but the clinical picture in patients varies widely.
  —Progression is not usually as orderly as the following descriptions indicate.
  —The disease progresses gradually, although at times symptoms seem to plateau temporarily.

- The early stage is characterized by loss of recent memory, inability to learn and retain new information, language problems (word finding), mood swings, and personality changes. There may be progressive difficulty in performing ADLs (balancing their checkbook, remembering where they put things). Abstract thinking or proper judgment may be reduced. Patients may respond to loss of control and memory with irritability, hostility, and agitation. Some patients have isolated aphasia or visuospatial difficulties.
  —Although the early stage does not noticeably compromise sociability, family members often report strange behavior and emotional lability.
- During the intermediate stage patients are unable to learn and recall new information; memory for remote events is affected but not fully lost. They may require help with bathing, eating, dressing, or toileting. Behavioral disorganization may be seen in wandering, agitation, hostility, or physical aggressiveness. Patients at this stage have lost all sense of time and place; they often get lost and may not be able to find their own bathroom or bedroom. Although they remain ambulatory, they are at risk for falls or accidents because of confusion.
- Patients in the severe stage are unable to walk or to perform ADLs, and are usually totally incontinent. Recent and remote memory is completely lost. They may be unable to eat or swallow, and are at risk for aspiration pneumonia and malnutrition. Immobility and incontinence place them at risk for pressure sores. Nursing home placement becomes necessary because of their total dependence on others for care. Patients eventually become mute.
- The end stage of Alzheimer's disease is coma and death, usually from infection.
- Alzheimer's disease is usually diagnosed on the basis of clinical findings and ruling out other causes of dementia.
  —A mental status examination is performed; the Folstein Mini-Mental Status Examination is widely used.

Laboratory Tests
- CBC
- Electrolyte panel measurement
- SMA-12/60 (Sequential Multiple Analyzer) tests
- Thyroid function tests
- Folate and vitamin B_{12} levels
- VDRL
- Urinalysis
- ECG
- Chest x-ray
- CT and MRI only to rule out suspected tumor, infarcts, subdural hematoma, and normal-pressure hydrocephalus

Treatment (see Treatment for Dementia)
Prognosis
- Cognitive decline is inevitable; the rate of decline is unpredictable.

Patient and Family Education
- The family should be instructed fully about the disease, its cause, course, treatment, and expected outcome.
- Provide a list of organizations, support groups, and nursing homes that provide care for Alzheimer's patients, and other pertinent information.
- Family members should be encouraged to work together, and to ask for assistance when the caregiver burden becomes onerous.

Follow-up and Referral
- Patients with Alzheimer's disease are followed closely for months or years.
- Referral may be made to specialists as the need arises: a urologist for problems with incontinence, a gastroenterologist for gastrointestinal disturbances, and others. Specialists in urinary incontinence may prove helpful during the early stage of the disease, when the patient is better able to take in, learn, and use new information.

VERTIGO
Definition

Vertigo is an illusion of movement and may be described either as a sensation that the external world is turning around the patient or that the patient is turning in place.

- About 50% of patients who complain of dizziness are actually experiencing vertigo.

Risk Factors

- History of head trauma
- History of taking aminoglycoside medication
- History of acute otitis media

Etiology (Box 6-8)
Pathogenesis

- Lesions at six levels associated with vertigo can be distinguished by signs and symptoms.
  - Within the cerebral cortex: vertigo is sometimes a part of the aura of a partial seizure of temporal lobe origin.
  - Within the pons: transient vertigo occurs in basilar migraine, in syncope, and sometimes in hypoglycemic episodes.
    - ~ Vertigo is also common with brainstem demyelinating or vascular lesions that involve the vestibular nuclei and their connections; a sixth or seventh cranial nerve lesion, an internuclear ophthalmoplegia, or a contralateral hemiparesis help in localization of the lesion.
  - Within the cerebellum: nystagmus (a rhythmic oscillation of the eyes) toward the side of a cerebellar mass (tumor, hemor-rhage, or infarct) develops; ataxia is usually present.
  - At the cerebellopontine angle: sensorineural deafness occurs; sixth, seventh, and fifth cranial nerve lesions develop, followed by cerebellar signs (ipsilateral), and later pyramidal signs (contralateral); nystagmus is often present.
  - Within the petrous temporal bone: a seventh cranial nerve lesion accompanies the eighth cranial nerve symptoms.
  - Within the end organs and semicircular canals: signs and symptoms vary according to cause (see Box 6-8).

Diagnosis

History and Physical Examination

Important questions to ask:

- How often do symptoms occur?
- Are symptoms severe, moderate, or mild? (Those with peripheral lesions often have more severe vertigo.)
- Is there associated nausea or vomiting?
- Are symptoms brought on by noise (Tulio's phenomenon)?

BOX 6-8

Principal Causes of Vertigo

PERIPHERAL CAUSES
Benign positional vertigo
Posttraumatic vertigo
Peripheral vestibulopathy (labyrinthitis, vestibular neuronitis)
Vestibulotoxic drug-induced vertigo (aminoglycosides)
Meniere's syndrome (endolymphatic hydrops)
Inflammatory labyrinthitis (syphilis, vasculitis)
Other focal peripheral disease (acute and chronic otitis media, meningioma, metastatic tumor)

CENTRAL CAUSES
Migraine
Brainstem ischemia and infarction
Cerebellopontine angle tumor (e.g., acoustic neuroma, meningioma, metastatic tumor)
Demyelinating disease (multiple sclerosis, postinfectious demyelination, remote effect of carcinoma)
Cranial neuropathy with focal involvement of the eighth cranial nerve

Intrinsic brainstem lesions (tumor, arteriovenous malformation, trauma)
Other posterior fossa lesions (primarily intrinsic or extra-axial masses of the posterior fossa [e.g., meatoma, metastatic tumor, cerebellar infarction])
Seizure disorder (temporal lobe epilepsy)
Heredofamilial disorders (spinocerebellar degenerations: Friedreich's ataxia, olivopontocerebellar atrophy, others)

SYSTEMIC CAUSES OF VERTIGO AND DIZZINESS
Drugs (anticonvulsants, hypnotics, antihypertensives, alcohol, analgesics, tranquilizers)
Infectious disease (meningitis, systemic infection)
Endocrine disease (diabetes mellitus, hypothyroidism in particular)
Vasculitis (systemic lupus erythematosus, giant cell arteritis, and drug-induced vasculitis)
Other systemic conditions (erythrocytosis, anemia, dysproteinemia, Paget's disease of bone, sarcoidosis, granulomatous disease, systemic toxins)

Adapted from Troost BT: Dizziness and vertigo in vertebrobasilar disease, *Curr Concepts in Cerebrovasc Dis* 14:21, 1979.

- Is there anything that makes symptoms better or worse?
- Does the patient tend to fall? To which side? (Fall is generally toward the side of the canal with the lower function.)
- Is there an associated sensation of tilt or linear movement? (If present, it may be due to a lesion of the otolith.)

The peripheral vestibular structures are closely associated with the peripheral auditory structures, which accounts for possible hearing changes, particularly in the case of Meniere's disease.

Associated Auditory Symptoms

- Is hearing impaired in one or both ears?
- Is tinnitus present (pulsatile or constant)?
- Is there a history of ear infections or draining ears?
- Is there a history of head or neck trauma, recent barotrauma, or recent viral illness?
- Has the patient been exposed to any ototoxic drugs (e.g., aspirin, aminoglycoside, high dosage of loop diuretic)?

Associated Neurologic Symptoms Suggesting Central [C] or Peripheral [P] Causes

- Is diplopia present? [C]
- Is there numbness of the face or extremities? [C]
- Is there weakness in the arms or legs? [C]
- Is there clumsiness in the arms or legs? [C]
- Is there slurring of speech? [C]
- Is there difficulty swallowing? [C]
- Is there blurred vision? [C or P]
- Are there flashing lights? [P]
- Is there an associated headache? [C or P]

The physical examination includes:

- External auditory canal
- Tympanic membrane
- Hearing test
- Observation for nystagmus
- Test for positional vertigo or nystagmus
- Assessment of the vestibulo-ocular reflex (VOR): the head remains stationary while the eyes follow a moving object in cardinal points, forward and backward. When VOR function is lost, images move across the retina when the head moves, which results in visual blurring and image movement.

- Test neurologic and neurovascular areas:
  —Cranial nerves, particularly V, VII
  —Cerebellar
  —Gait
  —Romberg test
  —Motor test

Treatment

- When the working diagnosis is peripheral vertigo of any type, one of the antivertigo antihistamines may relieve symptoms.
  —Meclizine (Antivert, Bonine) 12.5 and 25 mg tablets bid-qid
  —Benzodiazepine (Klonopin) 0.5 mg tablets, 0.25 to 0.5 mg qd-tid
- To relieve symptoms permanently, surgery may be required.
  —Sectioning of the vestibular nerve
  —Repair of an inner ear fistula
  —Labyrinthectomy
- These surgical procedures may result in unilateral deafness.

Patient and Family Education

- Most cases of vertigo are self-limited.
- Medications are prescribed for a short time to relieve associated symptoms.
- The patient is instructed to take the antivertigo medication for 2 to 3 weeks, then discontinue it to assess whether symptoms recur.

Follow-up and Referral

- Patients are followed closely while on medication(s).
- Patients with persistent and disabling vertigo are always referred to an otolaryngologist for further evaluation and treatment.

BIBLIOGRAPHY

Aminoff MJ: Nervous system. In Tierney LM, McPhee SJ, Papadakis MA, eds: *Current medical diagnosis & treatment 2000*, ed 39, New York, 2000, Lange Medical Books/McGraw-Hill.

Barker AS: Help for facial neuralgia sufferers, *The Clinical Advisor* 3(3):64, 2000.

Beers MH, Berkow R: Neurologic disorders. In *The Merck manual of diagnosis and therapy*, ed 17, Whitehouse Station, NJ, 1999, Merck Research Laboratories.

Cattel C, Gambassi G, Sgadari A, et al: Correlates of delayed referral for the diagnosis of dementia in an outpatient population, *J Geront: Med Sci* 55A(2):M98-M102, 2000.

Clarke CRA: Neurological disease. In Kumar P, Clark M: *Clinical medicine*, ed 4, Edinburgh, 1998, WB Saunders.

Clyburn LD, Stones MJ, Hadjisavropoulos T, et al: Predicting caregiver burden and depression in Alzheimer's disease, *J Geront: Soc Sci* 55B(1):S2-S13, 2000.

Frazier LD: Coping with disease-related stressors in Parkinson's disease, *The Gerontologist* 40(1):53-63, 2000.

Health professional drug guide 2000, Stamford, Conn, 2000, Appleton & Lange.

Johnson CJ: Evaluation of the patient with neurologic symptoms; Headaches and facial pain. In Barker LR, Burton JR, Zieve PD, eds: *Principles of ambulatory medicine*, ed 5, Baltimore, 1999, Williams & Wilkins.

Kaplan PW: Seizure disorders. In Barker LR, Burton JR, Zieve PD, eds: *Principles of ambulatory medicine*, ed 5, Baltimore, 1999, Williams & Wilkins.

Knopman D, Donohue JA, Gutterman EM: Patterns of care in the early stages of Alzheimer's disease: impediments to timely diagnosis, *J Am Geriatr Soc* 48(3):300-304, 2000.

Reich SG: Common disorders of movement: tremor and Parkinson's disease. In Barker LR, Burton JR, Zieve PD, eds: *Principles of ambulatory medicine*, ed 5, Baltimore, 1999, Williams & Wilkins.

Shannon MT, Wilson BA, Stang CL: *Health professionals drug guide 2000*, Stamford, Conn, 2000, Appleton & Lange.

Sisson SD, Kramer PD: Dizziness, vertigo, motion sickness, syncope and near syncope, and disequilibrium. In Barker LR, Burton JR, Zieve PD, eds: *Principles of ambulatory medicine*, ed 5, Baltimore, 1999, Williams & Wilkins.

REVIEW QUESTIONS

1. A new-onset central paralysis in a 20-year-old could indicate:
   a. Amyotrophic lateral sclerosis $\not{p}$ 50
   b. Poliomyelitis $<$ 20
   c. Multiple sclerosis
   d. Parkinson's disease $\not{p}$ 40

2. The most important observation to make during the neurologic examination is:
   a. Weakness of muscles or reflexes
   b. Gait disturbances
   c. Slurring of speech
   d. Asymmetry between the right and left sides

3. A positive Babinski is often the only sign of:
   a. A cortical lesion
   b. Upper motor neuron disease
   c. Lower motor neuron disease

4. Festination is defined as:
   a. A parkinsonian characteristic in which the patient, while walking normally, begins to lean forward, with the upper body moving forward faster than the lower trunk and legs, so that the gait becomes faster, to catch up

   b. A tremor that occurs while the patient is at rest and, when the arm is bent at the elbow, it moves in a cogwheel-like fashion
   c. A combination of signs and symptoms that occurs in older persons with Alzheimer's disease, and includes wandering
   d. An abnormal reflex of the biceps and triceps that indicates partial paralysis due to a stroke

5. If a patient is asked to stand with eyes open and feet together, but cannot, the likely diagnosis is: *Have balance*
   a. Alcohol intoxication
   b. Cranial space occupying lesion
   c. Cerebellar ataxia
   d. Cerebral palsy

6. In a lower motor neuron lesion, the peripheral seventh nerve is damaged, which causes:
   a. Paralysis of the lower facial muscles
   b. Paralysis of the upper facial muscles
   c. Paralysis of both the lower and upper facial muscles
   d. Tremor of the tongue

7. Global disorders of the cerebral cortex are due to:
   a. Stroke
   b. Trauma
   c. Space occupying lesions
   d. Diffuse inflammation

8. Patients with large basal frontal lesions exhibit signs such as:
   a. Euphoria
   b. Hyperactivity
   c. Apathy
   d. Use of vulgar language

9. The parietal lobes are dominant in:
   a. Processing visual recognition, auditory perception, memory, and emotion
   b. Spatial relationships, integration of awareness of the trajectories of moving objects, position of body parts, language recognition, and word memory
   c. Perception of nonverbal auditory stimuli (e.g., music)
   d. Processing concepts related to philosophy and religion

10. The most characteristic symptom of tension headache is:
    a. Occipital location
    b. Pain that feels like pressure or a tight band around the head

* *No pulse,   NO N,V*

c. Unilateral pain ~~Bilat~~

d. Presence of both photophobia and phonophobia *absent*

11. Characteristics of migraine headache include all but one of the following. The one sign or symptom that is NOT characteristic of migraine is:
    a. Throbbing
    b. Unilateral pain
    c. Unaffected by walking upstairs or other routine activity
    d. Accompanied by nausea or vomiting

12. Risk factors for migraine headache include all but one of the following. The risk factor that is NOT associated with migraine is:
    a. Onset at age older than 40   *age 10-40*
    b. Family history in 20% to 50% of patients
    c. Female sex: three times more women than men are affected
    d. Onset at any age   *10 - 40 yo's*

13. Giant cell arteritis is characterized by all but one of the following. The characteristic that is NOT associated with giant cell arteritis is:
    a. Vasculitis that affects large arteries throughout the body
    b. Frontal headaches *Temporal*
    c. Carotid arteries are those most commonly affected
    d. Untreated, GCA can cause permanent bilateral blindness

14. The major cause of seizures in older people is largely associated with:
    a. The aging process
    b. Neoplasm
    c. Cerebrovascular disease
    d. Toxic-metabolic disorders

15. One of the primary drugs used in both treatment and prophylaxis of seizures is the antiepileptic drug:
    a. Phenytoin
    b. Aspirin
    c. Acetaminophen
    d. Prednisone

16. Onset of Parkinson's disease occurs:
    a. Between ages 25 and 35
    b. Between ages 35 and 45
    c. Between ages 45 and 65
    d. After age 65

17. The onset of delirium is:
    a. Gradual
    b. Sudden

c. Intermittent

d. Variable

18. Characteristics of dementia are all but one of the following. The one that is NOT associated with dementia is:
    a. Increasing risk of onset with advanced age
    b. Disturbances of multiple higher cortical functions: memory, thinking
    c. Consciousness is clouded   *Delirium*
    d. Disturbance in executive functioning: planning, organizing, abstracting

19. Alzheimer's disease is characterized by all but one of the following. The characteristic NOT associated with Alzheimer's disease is:
    a. The presence of the epsilon4 allele decreases the risk for Alzheimer's disease in the white population.
    b. The disease runs in families in about 15% to 20% of cases.
    c. The disease causes a progressive and inexorable loss of cognitive function that primarily affects older people.
    d. β-Amyloid protein is believed to contribute to the pathogenesis of the disease.   *True*

20. All but one of the following are causes of focal disorders of the cerebral hemispheres. The one that is NOT a cause of a cerebral cortex dysfunction is:
    a. Stroke
    b. Space-occupying lesions
    c. Diffuse inflammation
    d. Maldevelopment

21. Apraxia and amnesia may result from either focal or _____ brain dysfunction.
    a. Cortical
    b. Diffuse
    c. Global
    d. Subcortical

22. Wernicke's aphasia is a subtype of:
    a. Receptive (sensory) aphasia
    b. Alexia
    c. Expressive (motor) aphasia *Brocca's*
    d. Anomia

23. Episodic tension headaches occurrence is:
    a. Fewer than 50 episodes/year
    b. Fewer than 100 episodes/year
    c. Fewer than 140 episodes/year
    d. Fewer than 180 episodes/year

24. Older patients with migraine equivalents (ischemic symptoms without headache) should be evaluated for:
    a. Hypotension
    b. Carotid artery obstruction
    c. Transient ischemic attacks
    d. Aortic valve disease

25. For patients with migraine, ergotamine is used because of its:
    a. Vasodilator properties
    b. Vasoconstrictor properties
    c. Analgesic properties
    d. Antihypertensive properties

26. Cluster headache, a form of migraine, is classified separately from migraine because of its:
    a. Different therapy
    b. Distinctive pathophysiology
    c. Effect on the patient's physical capabilities
    d. Effect on the patient's balance

27. Giant cell arteritis is defined as:
    a. A disease of the small arteries
    b. A disease of the large arteries
    c. A disease of the cranial arteries
    d. A disease of the aorta

28. Polymyalgia rheumatica is defined as:
    a. Arthritis of the joints of the extremities
    b. Arthritis of the spine
    c. Stiffness of the neck and shoulder muscles, and of the pelvic girdle
    d. Arthritis associated with Lyme disease

29. A 56-year-old woman with a history of diabetes mellitus and hypertension comes to the clinic with a complaint of dizziness. The neurologic examination showed that she had postural instability and a tendency to fall forward. Blood pressure (standing) was 100/70 mm Hg, and lying flat was 160/90 mm Hg. Her pulse was 88 beats/minute, regular. Other symptoms included neck and shoulder pain and a "spinning" sensation when standing. The nurse practitioner's first diagnostic test would be:
    a. Discontinue antihypertensive drugs.
    b. Evaluate the vestibular system.
    c. Request an erythrocyte sedimentation rate.
    d. Request a 24-hour monitor for blood pressure reading.

30. The cause of trigeminal neuralgia (tic douloureux) is believed to be:
    a. Compression of the fifth cranial nerve root
    b. A disorder of the fifth cranial nerve from unknown causes
    c. A genetic disorder
    d. Triggers (touch, cold wind, viral infection)

p. 161 - 196

Gastrointestinal Disorders

ABDOMINAL PAIN
Some General Principles Regarding Abdominal Pain

- Abdominal pain is a common complaint in the ambulatory care setting.
- Abdominal pain is described as chronic, either constant or intermittent.
- The clinician needs to consider organic and functional causes, but abdominal pain is more likely to originate in the gastrointestinal (GI) tract than elsewhere.
- Acute pain is usually self-limiting, subsides in 1 to 4 hours, and is usually caused by gastroenteritis (viral) or dietary causes, often excessive, too rich food intake.
- Chronic abdominal pain is most often related to peptic, gallbladder, or diverticular disease; chronic pancreatitis (commonly in alcoholics); or carcinoma (colon or pancreas).
- The patient and the characteristics of the pain are important in assessing abdominal pain:
  - Acute, even severe, pain can be tolerated for short periods if it occurs infrequently and the probable cause is known or suspected.
  - More chronic, less severe pain is often not as well tolerated because it is chronic, and it disturbs the patient's normal activities during the day and sleep at night.
- Individual pain thresholds vary considerably.
  - Pain develops slowly as the tumor grows and the patient becomes less sensitive, compared with severe pain that occurs suddenly and unexpectedly.
  - Organic pain may be reinforced by secondary psychologic gains.

- Older patients with abdominal pain need particular attention.
  - In these patients, even very serious causes of pain may be manifested by quite minimal symptoms.
    - ~ Appendicitis, even a ruptured appendix, may be missed because of few or absent signs and symptoms usually associated with this problem.
  - Pain management can be greatly improved by following some general principles.
  - Assurance that pain can be relieved by medications or surgery is of comfort and helps to increase the level of tolerance to pain.
  - Severe pain often sensitizes a patient to other pain (e.g., lumbar puncture or venipuncture).
  - Reactions to the second cause of pain should not be construed as indicating that the initial pain is insignificant (psychogenic).

Types and Causes of Abdominal Pain

- Abdominal pain can be classified as visceral, parietal, referred, neurogenic, or psychogenic.
- *Visceral pain* occurs because of spasm or stretching of the wall of a hollow viscus.
  - Distention of the capsule or a solid organ (e.g., liver)
  - Inflammation and ischemia or of an abdominal organ or structure
  - Tenderness, including rebound tenderness, is elicited directly over the site of the pain.
  - Small bowel tenderness is usually diffuse rather than localized.

- *Parietal pain* occurs in sites such as the parietal peritoneum, mesentery, and posterior peritoneal covering.
  —These structures are sensitive to distention and inflammation, as are visceral organs and structures.
  —The omentum and anterior abdominal wall are less sensitive.
  —Parietal tenderness is more localized than visceral tenderness (e.g., rebound tenderness is felt over the site of the pain).
  —Peritonitis is a widespread infection or inflammation of the entire abdomen and requires emergency attention.
    ~ Signs of generalized peritonitis include a hard, board-like abdomen and exquisite tenderness.
- *Referred pain* can occur with both visceral and parietal pain.
  —Referral is usually along shared nerve pathways (dermatomes).
  —Gallbladder pain typically radiates to the infrascapular area (the back), and right diaphragmatic pain to the right shoulder.
  —Esophageal pain is easily confused with cardiac ischemic pain (angina).
  —Deep palpation of the primary site may intensify the pain, both locally and at the referred site; palpation at the referred site does not increase pain at the site of origin.
- *Neurogenic pain* (causalgia) is usually felt by the patient as burning that follows the nerve pathway.
  —May be associated with hyperesthesia
  —The spinal root is often involved (e.g., herpes zoster, arthritis, carcinoma).
  —Peripheral neuropathies can also result from surgical trauma and diabetes mellitus.
  —No relationship exists between neurogenic pain and GI functions (eating, defecating).
- *Psychogenic pain* occurs as part of a conversion reaction from psychophysiologic causes, when no organic dysfunction is present (emotions are converted into somatic complaints).
  —Emotional stress can cause painful intestinal spasm in patients with irritable bowel syndrome (IBS).
  —Stress may cause peptic symptoms due to gastric hypersecretion.
- *Metabolic diseases* can also cause abdominal pain (Table 7-1).

—Porphyria, familial Mediterranean fever, or lead poisoning can cause intestinal spasm.
—In hereditary angioneurotic edema, C1 esterase deficiency may cause intestinal swelling, resulting in partial obstruction and pain.
—Hyperparathyroidism can cause peptic ulcer or pancreatitis, both quite painful conditions.
—Hyperlipidemia may cause pancreatitis, but the abdominal pain also occurs in the absence of pancreatic disease.

Diagnosis

- Diagnosis of abdominal pain can be difficult because of the complexity and variety of the organs and structures within the abdominal cavity.
- Identifying the nature of the pain and its location are essential to arriving at a correct diagnosis (Table 7-2).

Physical Examination

- Cold, sweaty, and pale skin indicates possible shock.
- Marbled skin (superficial vessels seen on blanched skin) indicates vasoconstriction, significant hemorrhage, and possible shock.
- Bent-over position while standing or sitting indicates severe abdominal pain (e.g., pancreatitis)
- Pacing and restlessness indicate gallbladder pain and inability to find a pain-free position.
- Inspect abdomen by incident (lateral) lighting to highlight contours of abdomen, masses, pulsations
  —Flank discoloration (Grey-Turner's sign) indicates retroperitoneal hemorrhage.
  —Periumbilical discoloration (Turner's sign, Cullen's sign) indicates intraperitoneal hemorrhage.
- Gallbladder pain worsens on deep inspiration; abdominal guarding is present.
- Auscultation
  —Borborygmus may be audible without a stethoscope.
  —Listen for hypoperistalsis or hyperperistalsis, high tinkles of obstruction.
  —Bruits indicate vascular distortion from aneurysms, compression of blood vessels, or invasion of blood vessels (e.g., invasion of the splenic artery in advanced pancreatic carcinoma).

TABLE 7-1
Causes of Abdominal Pain by Rapidity of Onset

Intestinal Causes	Extraintestinal Causes
SUDDEN ONSET (INSTANTANEOUS)	
Perforated ulcer	Ruptured or dissecting aneurysm
Ruptured abscess or hematoma	Ruptured ectopic pregnancy
Intestinal infarct	Pneumothorax
Ruptured esophagus	Myocardial infarct
	Pulmonary infarct
RAPID ONSET (MINUTES)	
Perforated viscus	Ureteral colic
Strangulated viscus	Renal colic
Volvulus	Ectopic pregnancy
Pancreatitis	Splenic infarct
Biliary colic	
Mesenteric infarct	
Diverticulitis	
Penetrating peptic ulcer	
High intestinal obstruction	
Appendicitis (gradual onset is more common)	
GRADUAL ONSET (HOURS)	
Appendicitis	Cystitis
Strangulated hernia	Pyelitis
Low small intestinal obstruction	Salpingitis
Cholecystitis	Prostatitis
Pancreatitis	Threatened abortion
Gastritis	Urinary retention
Peptic ulcer	Pneumonitis
Colonic diverticulitis	
Meckel's diverticulitis	
Crohn's disease	
Ulcerative colitis	
Mesenteric lymphadenitis	
Abscess	
Intestinal infarct	
Mesenteric cyst	

From Ridge JA, Way LW: Abdominal pain. In Sleisenger MH, Fordtran JS, eds: *Gastrointestinal disease,* ed 5, Philadelphia, 1993, WB Saunders, p 156.

TABLE 7-2
Nature and Location of Abdominal Pain

Organ Involved	Type of Pain	Location of Pain
Esophagus	Burning, constricting	Upper lesions: high substernal Lower lesions: low sternal or referred upward Severe: back
Stomach	Gnawing discomfort, sensation of hunger	Epigastric
Duodenum	Gnawing discomfort, sensation of hunger	Epigastric, left upper quadrant
Small intestine	Aching, cramping, bloating, sharp	Diffuse Periumbilical Terminal ileum: right lower quadrant Lower abdomen
Colon	Aching, cramping, bloating, sharp	Sigmoid: left lower quadrant Rectum: midline, sacrum
Pancreas	Excruciating, constant	Upper abdomen radiating to back
Gallbladder	Severe, later dull ache	Right upper quadrant Radiates to right scapula or interscapular area
Liver	Ache, occasionally sharp	Right lower rib cage Right upper quadrant if liver is enlarged

From Schuster MM: Abdominal pain. In Barker LR, Burton JR, Zieve PD, eds: *Principles of ambulatory medicine,* ed 5, Baltimore, 1999, Williams & Wilkins, p 473.

—Bowel sounds may be diminished or quiet late in mechanical obstruction.

—Elicit a succussion splash: place the stethoscope over the upper gastric area and shake the patient abruptly; a sloshing sound indicates the presence of air and fluid (e.g., delayed gastric emptying).

• Rectal and pelvic examinations aim to locate masses, areas of tenderness, hernias, and genitourinary problems.

Diagnostic Tests
• Complete blood count (CBC)
• Urinalysis
• Test for occult blood
• Chest x-ray
• Plain and upright abdominal x-rays
• Endoscopy by a gastroenterologist
• Proctosigmoidoscopy by a gastroenterologist

Treatment
• Treatment depends on the cause of abdominal pain as determined by the diagnostic procedures.
• Surgery may be required for emergency conditions (e.g., appendicitis, bowel obstruction, or other).

Patient/Family Education
• The patient should be kept informed of procedures, findings, proposed therapy, and description of procedures to be done (e.g., x-rays, endoscopy, surgery).
• When diagnosis is confirmed, the patient should be informed, including the nature of the condition, proposed treatment, usual course of the disease, and expected outcomes.

ESOPHAGEAL DISORDERS
Difficulty Swallowing (Dysphagia)
Definition
Dysphagia includes problems that may occur in any part of the swallowing process, voluntary or involuntary. This symptom is specific and should not be dismissed as an emotional problem.

Risk Factors
• Advanced age
• Tumor of the mouth, throat, or esophagus
• Poor dentition
• Dehydration
• Smoking
• Disturbance of any of the structures involved in swallowing

TABLE 7-3
Types of Dysphagia

Location and Symptoms of Dysphagia	Causes
OROPHARYNGEAL	
Difficulty initiating swallowing, nasal regurgitation, cough, aspiration on swallowing	Structural: web, Zenker's diverticulum, extrinsic compression Muscle: myasthenia, polymyositis, systemic lupus erythematosus Endocrine: thyroid disease Central nervous system: stroke, Parkinson's disease, brainstem tumors
ESOPHAGEAL	
Dysphagia for solids: continuous, intermittent	Carcinoma, stricture Ring, diverticulum, esophagitis
Dysphagia for solids and liquids	Motility disorder: severe narrowing from stricture, esophagitis, tumor

From Katz PO: Disorders of the esophagus: dysphagia, noncardiac chest pain, gastroesophageal reflux disease. In Barker LR, Burton JR, Zieve PD, eds: *Principles of ambulatory medicine*, ed 5, Baltimore, 1999, Williams & Wilkins, p 460.

Etiology/Cause (Table 7-3)

Causes of dysphagia are many because of the highly complex process of swallowing and the different types of structures involved.

- Cancer of the esophagus
- Achalasia
- Diffuse esophageal spasm
- Chronic reflux esophagitis
- Scleroderma of the esophagus
- Esophageal rings and webs
- An anatomic obstruction may be present if the patient complains of difficulty swallowing solid foods (e.g., tumor, stricture, esophageal ring).
- Difficulty swallowing both liquids and solids is more indicative of a disturbance of motility (e.g., achalasia, scleroderma, esophageal spasm).

Pathogenesis

- Numerous underlying factors exist that may cause difficulty swallowing. Several of these problems will be discussed separately below.

Carcinoma of the Esophagus *squamous cell*

Definition

Carcinoma of the esophagus is a malignant tumor that originates in the esophagus; the most common form is squamous cell carcinoma.

Risk Factors

- Both men and women in middle age: forties and fifties
- Cigarette smoking
- Excessive alcohol intake, usually over many years
- Presence of Barrett's esophagus, due to gastroesophageal reflux disease (GERD)

Etiology/Pathogenesis

- Squamous cell and adenocarcinoma are the two most common types of cancer found in the esophagus.

Diagnosis

- Usually the cancer is diagnosed only when symptoms develop; by then the cancer is in an advanced stage, with extension to the regional lymph nodes.
- The history is of gradual development of dysphagia, first for solids, then for both solids and liquids.
- There is a history of gradual weight loss.
- Odynophagia (painful swallowing) may develop.
- Occult blood loss may be detected, but hematemesis usually is not present.

Diagnostic Tests

- Cytologic brushings of the entire esophagus
- Barium swallow to observe for tumor and the degree of obstruction
- Upper endoscopy to establish a histologic diagnosis, which will help to define the most effective therapy
  —A positive tissue diagnosis is made in 95% of patients.

- A computed tomography (CT) scan of the chest to determine whether metastases exist and, if so, where (e.g., lungs, liver)

Treatment
- The treatment for esophageal cancer is usually either surgery or radiation, depending on the cell type and the location of the tumor.
  - Adenocarcinoma is less amenable to radiation therapy.
  - Squamous cell carcinoma responds well to radiation, and this therapy has been shown to be as effective as surgery.
  - Preoperative chemotherapy has been successful recently and should be considered before surgery, even in those with resectable cancer.

Prognosis
- Over 50% of patients with tumor that, preoperatively, was confined to the esophagus were found during surgery to have extensive, incurable disease.
- Regardless of treatment, the prognosis for most patients is poor.
  - Seventy-five percent die within 1 year of diagnosis.
  - Ninety percent die within 5 years of diagnosis.

Patient/Family Education
- The patient and family should be informed about the nature of the condition, while maintaining hope for recovery as well as is possible.
- The important goal of therapy is to maintain an open esophagus, to allow the patient to continue swallowing food, liquids, and saliva.
  - Dilation of the lumen with mercury-weighted rubber dilators, guidewire-assisted polyvinyl dilators, or balloon dilators will usually allow the patient to swallow.
- Palliative care is given to keep the patient as functional as possible.
- Palliative measures are individualized through consultation among physicians, surgeons, oncologists, gastroenterologists, and others.

Achalasia
Definition
Achalasia is an abnormal condition characterized by the inability of a muscle to relax, particularly the lower esophageal sphincter, and complete absence of peristalsis.

Risk Factors
- Both men and women may develop achalasia.
- Peak incidence occurs in those in their forties and fifties.

Etiology
- Some studies show denervation of the esophagus, but the precise cause of the condition is not known.

Pathogenesis
- The pathogenesis is likewise not known.
- Researchers have described abnormalities of the ganglion cells in the distal esophagus (lower esophageal sphincter [LES] zone), in the body of the esophagus, and in the vagal nucleus and its peripheral fibers, but these findings are not consistent.
- Denervation of the esophagus is supported by the exaggerated response of the LES and the body of the esophagus to cholinergic stimulation and to the hormone gastrin.

Diagnosis
Signs and Symptoms
- History of progressive dysphagia for both solids and liquids
- Regurgitation of ingested material
- Pulmonary symptoms (e.g., nocturnal coughing)
- Aspiration pneumonia may be the presenting symptom.
- Substernal chest pain
- A chest x-ray usually shows evidence that the condition exists.
  - The gastric air bubble is absent.
  - An air-fluid level in the dilated esophagus may be seen behind the heart.
- With a very dilated and tortuous esophagus, the mediastinum appears wider than normal.

- Barium esophagram evidence includes
  —Smooth, tapered narrowing of the distal end of the esophagus ("bird beak" or "quill pen" deformity), which fails to open properly
  —Absence of peristalsis
  —Retention of barium and secretions in the more proximal esophagus
- Esophageal manometry usually shows three distinct abnormalities.
  —Absence of peristalsis of the smooth muscle of the esophagus
  —Failure of the LES to relax after a swallow
  —Elevated LES pressure, creating a constant high-pressure zone that obstructs the passage of esophageal contents
  —Manometry may show high-amplitude, simultaneous, repetitive contractions that are not peristalsis; patients with this finding are described as having vigorous achalasia who often experience severe chest pain.

Differential Diagnosis
- Esophageal strictures
- Esophageal carcinomas
- Scleroderma (associated with esophageal motility disturbance)
- Chagas' disease, which may cause megaesophagus and manometric patterns similar to those seen in achalasia
- Idiopathic intestinal pseudoobstruction

Treatment
Treatment is aimed at reducing the pressure gradient between the esophagus and the stomach, resulting in decreased dysphagia.
- Pneumatic dilation, an outpatient procedure that is performed by a gastroenterologist
- Surgery
  —Transection of the circular muscle of the LES zone to the level of the mucosa (Heller's myotomy)
  —Recent experience of injecting botulinum toxin into the LES via endoscopy results in improved esophageal emptying and decreased LES pressure in 70% to 80% of patients.
  —Most patients relapse after 6 months to 1 year, and repeat injection is required.

—The aperistalsis and impaired sphincter relaxation persist after surgery (Heller's myotomy).
- Medical treatment includes nitrates and calcium channel blockers.

Complications
- Some studies indicate that patients with achalasia are at increased risk (incidence of 6% to 29%) for carcinoma of the esophagus.

Prognosis
- Prognosis is variable, depending on the severity of the achalasia, age of the patient, condition of the esophagus, and other factors.
- Beginning with the least invasive treatment first, then proceeding slowly to more intense therapy if the condition warrants it, is the best course.

Patient/Family Education
- Inform the patient and family about the nature of the condition, its relation to symptoms, usual treatment, and outcomes.
- Provide information about a modified diet (e.g., pureed foods) that will minimize dysphagia.

Diffuse Esophageal Spasm
Definition
Diffuse esophageal spasm (DES) is a disorder characterized by intermittent, nonperistaltic esophageal contractions that cause dysphagia and substernal chest pain.

Risk Factors
- None known

Etiology
- Some clinicians believe that this condition has a psychogenic basis.

Pathogenesis
- Contractions of the esophaged sphincters, which are spontaneous, nonperistaltic, and occur simultaneously with contractions (tertiary waves) of the body of the esophagus

Diagnosis

- Because of the location of contractions, their radiation, and their crushing quality, DES is frequently misdiagnosed as ischemic heart disease.
- DES is often goes undiagnosed and is easily confused with other disorders.

Diagnostic Tests

- Barium swallow or videoesophagram may demonstrate the nonperistaltic abnormal contractions that often occur in many normal subjects during barium swallow studies.
- Patients with suspected DES should have esophageal motility studies.

Treatment

- Nitrates (e.g., nitroglycerin, isosorbide)
- Anticholinergics (e.g., dicyclomine [Bentyl])
- Sedatives and antidepressants (e.g., diazepam [Valium], trazodone [Desyrel], doxepin [Sinequan])
- Calcium channel blockers (e.g., nifedipine [Procardia], diltiazem [Cardizem])
- Smooth muscle relaxants (e.g., hydralazine)
- Static dilation by French catheter
- Pneumatic dilation if dysphagia is a prominent symptom

Prognosis

- Prognosis is variable, depending on the degree of contractions and the severity of dysphagia.

Patient/Family Education

- Instruct the patient regarding the nature of the condition, cause if known, treatment, course, and possible outcomes.
- Reassurance of the patient from all health care professionals contacted can be of immense value to these patients.
- Explain all medications, diagnostic procedures, and self-care activities that the patient can carry out to minimize symptoms.
  —Relaxation techniques, biofeedback, and other similar therapies may also provide a great deal of help.

Scleroderma of the Esophagus

Definition

- Scleroderma is a chronically progressive disease for which no specific treatment exists.
- It is characterized by chronic thickening and hardening of the skin caused by new collagen formation, with atrophy of pilosebaceous follicles.
- When the patient has systemic scleroderma, its effects can be seen in the lungs and GI tract by radiography.

Risk Factors

- None known

Etiology

- Eighty percent of patients with scleroderma of the esophagus have the systemic disease.

Pathogenesis

- Unknown
- Several studies have indicated a neural defect rather than a primary myogenic disorder.

Diagnosis

- The major symptoms of esophageal scleroderma are heartburn and dysphagia.
- Symptoms are caused by changes in esophageal motility.
  —LES pressure is very low, which causes gastroesophageal reflux.
  —A gradual decrease in peristaltic waves occurs, culminating in complete aperistalsis in the smooth muscle portion of the esophagus.
  —Refluxed acid remains in the esophagus for longer than normal, eventually causing esophageal stricture from injury and scarring.

Treatment

- Refer patients to a gastroenterologist for further evaluation and therapy.

Esophageal Webs and Rings

Definition

- An esophageal web is a mucosal structure that protrudes into the lumen, usually in the proximal portion.
- The association of iron deficiency anemia with a proximal esophageal web constitutes the Plummer-Vinson syndrome.
- Esophageal rings are located in the distal esophagus and may be either mucosal or muscular.

—Rings exist in about 10% of the population, but do not cause symptoms.

—The ring located just above the gastroesophageal junction is called Schatzki's ring.

Risk Factors
- None known

Etiology
- The cause of webs and rings is unknown.
- They are probably acquired.
- Some evidence indicates that gastroesophageal reflux disease (GERD) is implicated in the development of Schatzki's ring.

Pathogenesis
- Webs and rings cause symptoms when they result in narrowing of the esophageal lumen to less than 13 mm in diameter; patients with esophageal lumen diameters of more than 20 mm do not exhibit symptoms.

Diagnosis
- The typical presenting symptom is intermittent dysphagia for solid foods.
- The patient may be able to point to the area of the ring.
- Sometimes a bolus of food becomes impacted at the site of the ring; the patient regurgitates and then may be able to continue swallowing without difficulty.

Diagnostic Tests
- Barium swallow
- Endoscopy to differentiate rings from annular strictures secondary to reflux esophagitis or carcinoma
- Cine studies to detect webs

Treatment
- Bougienage with a large-caliber dilator often disrupts the lower esophageal ring with complete relief of dysphagia.
  —This procedure may cause discomfort, but causes much less pain than occurs with pneumatic dilation.
  —In anemic patients with webs, treatment of iron deficiency anemia results in rapid regression of the web.

Gastroesophageal Reflux Disease
Definition
- Gastroesophageal reflux occurs when there is a backflow of stomach contents into the esophagus.
- GERD is a chronic disease.

Risk Factors
- Low basal LES pressure
- Episodes of transient LES relaxation not associated with a swallow
- Abnormalities of gastric emptying
- Gastric distention
- Nature and composition of the gastric refluxate (acid, pepsin, and bile)

Etiology
- Any of the listed risk factors can contribute to the development of GERD, but the actual cause of GERD is unknown.

Pathogenesis
- Reflux of acidic stomach contents into the esophagus produces burning pain in the esophagus.
- Repeated episodes of reflux may cause esophagitis, peptic esophageal strictures, or esophageal ulcers.

Diagnosis
- Heartburn is the primary symptom of GERD.
  —About 10% of Americans experience daily heartburn.
  —About 33% of Americans have heartburn at least once a month.
- Chest pain
- Hoarseness
- Cough
- Wheezing

Diagnostic Tests
- A double-contrast barium swallow will show mucosal irregularities.
  —The presence of mucosal irregularities, stricture, and esophageal ulcer indicates an 85% to 95% likelihood of GERD.
  —A normal barium swallow is seen in 50% to 60% of patients who have symptoms of GERD.
- Hiatal hernia is present in 40% to 60% of the general population.

- Endoscopy is used to diagnose and evaluate reflux esophagitis or Barrett's epithelium.
  —If esophagitis is present, the diagnosis of GERD is established with 95% certainty.
- If a stricture is discovered, it should be biopsied to rule out carcinoma.
- If the diagnosis of GERD is in doubt following endoscopy, 24-hour ambulatory pH monitoring of esophageal refluxate should be performed.

Treatment

- GERD is a lifelong disease that requires lifestyle modifications in addition to medical treatment.

- Treatment is divided into phases:
  I. Phase I: modification of lifestyle; successful in 25% of patients
     A. Place 6- to 8-inch blocks under the head of the bed.
     B. The use of more pillows might increase abdominal pressure.
     C. Eliminate certain foods known to be esophageal irritants (e.g., citric juice, coffee, spices).
     D. The patient is instructed not to lie down immediately after eating, but to wait 2 to 3 hours before doing so.
     E. Drugs that decrease LES pressure (e.g., calcium channel blockers, nitrates, sedatives, and theophylline) should be avoided.
     F. Antacids may be taken as needed and are the mainstay for rapid relief of heartburn; duration of action is less than 2 hours.
        1. Gaviscon (2 to 4 tabs 30 minutes after meals and at bedtime) decreases reflux in the upright position and may be superior to other antacids (Maalox TC, Mylanta II).
  II. Phase II: pharmacologic; aimed at decreasing gastric acid secretion (H_2 antagonists or proton pump inhibitors), augmenting LES pressure, and improving esophageal clearance with prokinetic agents (e.g., metoclopramide, cisapride)
     A. Treatment is begun with an H_2 antagonist bid, or a prokinetic agent and continued for 8 to 12 weeks.
        1. Cimetidine 200 mg, ranitidine 75 mg, or nizatidine 75 mg bid

2. Average healing rates are 50% on this regimen.
B. If symptoms do not abate
   1. Add a second drug (e.g., higher dosage H_2 blocker) for another 8 to 12 weeks, or
   2. A proton pump inhibitor can be started.
      a. Omeprazole 20 mg, rabeprazole, or pantoprazole once daily before breakfast results in 95% reduction of gastric acidity over 24 hours.
      b. Studies show that a proton pump inhibitor is the most successful and least costly of these three possible treatment choices.
   3. A second drug can be added.
C. Symptomatic and endoscopic relapse of esophagitis occurs in up to 80% of patients who have been successfully treated.
   1. Most patients require long-term therapy.
      a. H_2-receptor antagonists at full dosage are approved for maintenance therapy; these are effective in maintaining remission in 40% to 60% of patients with nonerosive esophagitis.
      b. Proton pump inhibitors (e.g., omeprazole, lansoprazole) provide the most effective relief of symptoms and are the most effective agents for maintaining remission in up to 80% of patients with erosive esophagitis or Barrett's esophagitis.
III. Phase III: surgery; indicated for 5% to 10% of patients, who have strictures unresponsive to medical therapy, hemorrhage secondary to erosive esophagitis, esophageal ulcers unresponsive to medical therapy, aspiration pneumonia, or reflux-induced hoarseness.

Prognosis

- Prognosis is favorable in patients with all degrees of severity of GERD, but those with the least troublesome symptoms and no complications have the best outcomes.

- New drugs and surgical procedures enable all patients to have minimal symptoms over time.

Patient/Family Education

- As in all other cases of health problems, the patient and family should be instructed about the nature of the condition, its cause if known, treatment, course, and likely outcome.
- All medications and procedures should be explained before they are administered and performed, reasons for their use, medication timing and dosage, effects, and expected outcomes.
- Provide detailed instructions in writing about what the patient and family are to do to prevent symptoms and to promote healing.
  —Stop smoking.
  —Omit foods or beverages that seem to exacerbate the problem.
  —Get information about stress management.

Esophageal Varices

Definition

*Cirrhosis
Alcohol
Ht*

Esophageal varices are dilated submucosal veins that develop in patients with underlying portal hypertension.

- They may result in serious upper GI bleeding.
  —About 50% of patients with cirrhosis have esophageal varices.
  —Only 33% of patients with esophageal varices develop serious bleeding.
  —Bleeding esophageal varices have a higher morbidity and mortality rate than any other source of upper GI bleeding.
  —The mortality rate associated with acute bleeding episodes is 15% to 40%.
  —Over 60% of patients with bleeding esophageal varices die within 5 years.

Risk Factors

- Long-term alcohol abuse
- Cirrhosis of the liver
- Cigarette smoking

Etiology

- The cause of esophageal varices and bleeding is alcohol abuse and associated liver cirrhosis that results in portal hypertension.
- Bleeding occurs when the portosystemic pressure gradient is ≥ 12 mm Hg.

Pathogenesis

- The normal pressure in the portal vein is 5 to 8 mm Hg, with only a small gradient across the liver to the hepatic vein, in which blood is returned to the heart via the inferior vena cava.
- Portal hypertension is classified according to the site of obstruction.
  —*Prehepatic:* due to blockage of the portal vein before the liver
  —*Intrahepatic:* due to distortion of the liver architecture, which can be presinusoidal (e.g., in schistosomiasis) or postsinusoidal (e.g., in cirrhosis)
  —*Posthepatic:* due to venous blockage outside the liver (rare)
- As portal pressure rises above 10 to 12 mm Hg, the compliant venous system dilates, and collaterals occur within the systemic veins.
  —The main sites of the collaterals are
    ~ At the gastroesophageal junction (varices)
    ~ The rectum
    ~ The left renal vein
    ~ The diaphragm
    ~ The retroperitoneum
    ~ The anterior abdominal wall via the umbilical vein
  —The collaterals at the gastroesophageal junction are superficial and tend to rupture.
- Portal vascular resistance is increased in chronic liver disease.
  —Stellate cells are activated and transformed into myofibroblasts.
    ~ In these cells there is *de novo* expression of the specific smooth muscle protein α-actin.
  —Under the influence of mediators (e.g., endothelin, nitric oxide, prostaglandins), the contraction of these activated cells contributes to abnormal blood flow patterns and increased resistance to blood flow.
  —This increased resistance results in portal hypertension and opening of portosystemic anastomoses in both precirrhotic and cirrhotic livers.
  —Patients with cirrhosis have a hyperdynamic circulation, likely due to the release of mediators (e.g., nitric oxide and glucagon), which leads to peripheral and splanchnic vasodilation.

—This effect is followed by plasma volume expansion due to sodium retention, which has a significant effect in maintaining portal hypertension.

- **Bleeding from esophageal varices is an emergency situation and requires immediate action: hospitalization and resuscitation.**

Diagnosis

- Gross bleeding from the mouth and nose is evident, often with vomiting of bright-red blood.
- The patient becomes rapidly shocky, exhibiting falling blood pressure (BP), pallor, weakness, and loss of consciousness.
- Initiate emergency procedures: call 911, transport to nearest emergency room (call ahead to alert the staff).
- Ambulatory care health professionals transfer care of the patient to the emergency team at the hospital.

Treatment

- Prompt replacement of blood volume is essential following insertion of an intravenous line.
- Draw blood for typing and cross-matching, hemoglobin, protime (PT), urea, electrolytes, and liver biochemistry analysis.
- Endoscopy is done to confirm the diagnosis and rule out bleeding from any other sites.
- The varices are injected with a sclerosing agent that may arrest bleeding by producing vessel thrombosis.
- An alternative is to band the varices by mounting a band on the tip of the endoscope, sucking the varix just into the end of the scope, and dislodging the band over the varix using a trip-wire mechanism.
  —This arrests bleeding in 80% of cases and reduces the incidence of early rebleeding.

Complications

- Fifty percent of patients rebleed within 10 days.
- A severe bleed will cause encephalopathy because of the loss of protein in blood, which affects brain structure and function.
- The risk of recurrence is 60% to 80% within 2 years.

- A 20% mortality rate is associated with each episode.

Patient/Family Education

- The cause of esophageal bleeding is the result of portal hypertension, usually caused by cirrhosis of the liver, which in turn is caused by chronic heavy alcohol intake over many years.
- Patients may have gone through many treatment programs to try to stop drinking.
- End-stage liver disease is difficult to manage.
- No alcohol
- Low or no protein diet
- Prevent portosystemic encephalopathy
- Provide supportive care: high carbohydrate diet, limited fluids.

Follow-up/Referral

- After discharge for treatment of bleeding esophageal varices, patients with cirrhosis of the liver need to be seen every 2 to 3 weeks until they are more stable.
- Attention to diet, medications, elimination, skin care, and worsening or new symptoms should be reported immediately.

Esophageal Laceration and Rupture (Mallory-Weiss Syndrome)

Definition

Laceration of the distal esophagus and proximal stomach occurs during vomiting, retching, or hiccuping.

Risk Factors

- Invasive procedures of the esophagus, stomach, or duodenum
- History of chronic heavy drinking
- History of esophageal varices or bleeding

Etiology

- Damage from instrumentation
- Existing intrinsic esophageal disease
- Increased esophageal pressure caused by vomiting or retching
- Boerhaave's syndrome causes spontaneous rupture of the esophagus, and constitutes a catastrophic event with a high mortality rate.
  —Sequelae of Boerhaave's syndrome include mediastinitis and pleural effusion.

[handwritten: Candida Fungal Infection of Esoph]

Pathogenesis

- A cut or tear of esophageal tissue may cause damage to arteriolar walls and become a source of bleeding or hemorrhage.

Diagnosis

- Endoscopy or arteriography confirms the location and severity of the esophageal lesion and the amount of bleeding.
- Such a lesion is not visible on routine x-rays.

Treatment

- Most episodes of bleeding stop spontaneously, but some patients require ligation of the laceration, intra-arterial infusion of vasopressin (Pitressin), or therapeutic embolization into the left gastric artery during angiography to control bleeding.
- Blood transfusion(s) may be needed to replace blood lost during hemorrhage.

Patient/Family Education

- Instruct the patient regarding the nature, probable cause, and treatment of esophageal bleeding or rupture.
  - —Esophageal rupture is an emergency requiring immediate endoscopy, arteriography, or surgery to stop the bleeding and repair the laceration or lesion.
  - —Instruct the patient about self-care to prevent further episodes of bleeding, and to avoid causes of vomiting or retching.

Follow-up/Referral

- During treatment of initial bleeding episode, the patient will likely be placed under the care of a gastroenterologist who, if necessary, would continue caring for the patient following the acute episode.
- Emphasize the need for frequent check-ups to monitor food and alcohol intake, and to check for signs of bleeding (e.g., hemoglobin and hematocrit).

INFECTIOUS ESOPHAGEAL DISORDERS
Fungal Infection

Definition

Mucosal candidiasis involving the esophagus is the most common type of invasive mucosal disease.

Risk Factors

- HIV/AIDS or other systemic disease that causes the patient to be immunocompromised
- Prolonged antibiotic therapy
- Prolonged neutropenia
- Uncontrolled diabetes
- Systemic corticosteroid therapy
- Recent surgery (e.g., solid organ transplants)
- Presence of intravascular catheters (especially in total parenteral nutrition)
- Intravenous drug use

Etiology

- *Candida albicans*, a fungus, is the causative organism.

Pathogenesis

- Invasion of the GI mucosa, particularly in the esophagus, with development of diffuse, linear, yellow-white plaques that adhere to the mucosa

Diagnosis   *[handwritten: Teeth]*

- Some patients are asymptomatic.
- Most patients complain of odynophagia, dysphagia, and chest pain.
- Oral thrush is present in only 75% of patients.
- History of human immunodeficiency virus (HIV)/acquired immunodeficiency syndrome (AIDS)
- Definitive diagnosis is made by endoscopy with biopsy and cytologic brushings.

Treatment

- Depends on the severity of the infection and the physical status of the patient
- Topical agents may be used if the infection is localized in the mouth and throat.
  - —Nystatin 1 to 3 MU "swish and swallow" five times per day
  - —Clotrimazole troches 10 mg dissolved in the mouth five times per day
  - —Systemic agents taken by mouth (e.g., fluconazole)   *[handwritten: Diflucan]*
  - —Intravenous agents (amphotericin B, fluconazole)
- Patients who do not respond to oral therapy are given low-dose amphotericin B 0.3 to 0.5 mg/kg/day intravenously (IV) for 7 days.

Prognosis
- Most patients with infectious esophagitis can be effectively treated with complete symptom resolution.
- Depending on the patient's immune status, relapse of symptoms following therapy may occur, and chronic suppressive therapy may be needed.

Patient/Family Education
- Patients need to be knowledgeable about the cause, transmission, and symptoms of infectious oral and esophageal infections.
- Instruct the patient about preventive measures and symptom recognition in case of recurrence.
- Instruct the patient regarding methods to relieve discomfort (e.g., mouth and throat washes).
- Emphasize the importance of keeping appointments with the nurse practitioner so that therapy can begin as early as possible if the condition recurs.

Follow-up/Referral
- Patient should be contacted every month or so to check on status.
- If it seems necessary, the patient can be scheduled to see the clinician if symptoms are present, or if sexual contact has occurred.

Cytomegalovirus Esophagitis
Diagnosis
- Endoscopy and cytologic brushings will identify the causative organism.
- Symptoms are similar to those of fungal infections.

Treatment
- Ganciclovir 5 mg/kg IV q12h for 3 to 4 weeks is the initial therapy.
  - Neutropenia is a frequent, dose-limiting side effect.
  - If resolution occurs, the drug can be discontinued.
  - If the condition has improved but is not fully resolved, full-dose therapy is continued for another 2 to 3 weeks.
  - In patients with AIDS, ganciclovir 5 mg/kg IV qd is required for suppressive therapy.

- ~ Patients who do not respond to or do not tolerate ganciclovir are treated acutely with foscarnet 90 mg/kg IV q12h for 3 to 4 weeks.
- ~ The principal toxicity in using foscarnet is renal failure.

Herpetic Esophagitis
Definition
Herpetic esophagitis is an infection of the mucosa of the mouth and esophagus.

Risk Factors
- See Fungal Infection section.

Etiology
- The herpes simplex virus is the major cause of herpetic esophagitis.

Pathogenesis
- Oral ulcers may develop in patients infected with the herpes simplex virus.
- Many patients have few symptoms.

Diagnosis
- Direct immunofluorescent antibody slide tests provide rapid, sensitive diagnosis; viral culture may also be used.

Treatment
- In immunocompetent patients, treatment may be symptomatic without need for specific antiviral therapy.
- In immunocompromised patients, oral acyclovir 200 mg PO five times per day or 50 mg/kg IV every 8 to 12 hours for 7 to 10 days
- Those who do not respond to the above therapy require foscarnet 40 mg/kg IV q8h for 21 days.

Prognosis, Patient/Family Education, and Follow-up/Referral
- See Fungal Infection section.

PEPTIC ULCER DISEASE
Definition
A peptic ulcer is an excoriated segment of the GI mucosa, typically in the stomach (gastric ulcer) or in the first few centimeters of the duodenum (duodenal ulcer), that penetrates through the muscularis mucosa.

[handwritten: NSAIDS ↓ Prostaglandin → ↓ Bld flow, ↓ mucus, ↓ HCO_3]

[handwritten: ↓ cell repair]

Risk Factors

- Genetics: duodenal ulcer is three times more common in first-degree relatives than in the general population.
  - Genetic groups at increased risk
    - ~ Pepsinogen I, human leukocyte antigen B5 (HLAB5), and red blood cell acetylcholinesterase
  - In some families, there seems to be an autosomal dominant mode of inheritance, which is not true in other cases.
- Male gender
- History of NSAID use
- Smoking (impairs ulcer healing and increases incidence of recurrence)
- Alcohol ingestion (promotes acid secretion)
- Stress

Etiology *[handwritten: H. PyLori]*

- It is now believed that *Helicobacter pylori* and NSAIDs disrupt the normal mucosal defense and repair, making the mucosa more susceptible to gastric acid damage.
- Diseases associated with peptic ulcer disease
  - B cell mucosa-associated lymphoid tissue (MALT) lymphoma
  - Gastric adenocarcinoma

Pathogenesis

- The mechanisms by which *H. pylori* causes mucosal injury are not clearly understood.
- Theories include the following:
  - Urease produced by the organism catalyzes urea to ammonia, which enables the organism to survive in the acidic environment of the stomach, and may erode the mucous barrier, leading to epithelial damage.
  - Cytotoxins produced by *H. pylori* may also be implicated in epithelial damage.
  - Mucolytic enzymes (e.g., bacterial protease, lipase) seem to be involved in degradation of the mucous layer, making the epithelium more susceptible to acid damage.
  - Cytokines produced in response to inflammation may have a role in mucosal damage and subsequent ulcer formation.
- NSAIDs probably promote mucosal inflammation and ulcer formation through both topical and systemic effects.
  - NSAIDs are weak acids and non-ionized at gastric pH, and they diffuse freely across the mucous barrier into gastric epithelial cells, where H^+ ions are liberated, resulting in cellular damage.
  - NSAIDs also inhibit prostaglandin production, which produces several changes in the gastric microenvironment (e.g., reduced gastric blood flow, reduced mucus and HCO_3 secretion, decreased cell repair and replication), resulting in breakdown of mucosal defense mechanisms.

Diagnosis

The history of symptoms, when they occur, and what relieves them is very helpful in diagnosing peptic ulcer disease.

Signs and Symptoms

- Depend on the location of ulcer(s) and patient's age
- Older people tend to have few, if any, symptoms.
- Pain is the most common symptom, described as gnawing, burning, or a feeling of hunger.
  - Pain may be localized to the epigastrium and is often relieved by food or antacids.
- Symptoms of gastric ulcer do not usually follow a consistent pattern (e.g., eating sometimes exacerbates rather than relieves pain), which is true particularly of pyloric channel ulcers.
  - This type of ulcer may have associated symptoms (e.g., bloating, nausea, vomiting) caused by edema and scarring.
- In duodenal ulcer, pain tends to be consistent. *[handwritten: duodenal]*
  - Pain is absent in the morning upon awaking.
  - Pain appears in midmorning, is relieved by the ingestion of food, but recurs 2 to 3 hours after a meal.
  - Pain that awakens a patient at night is quite common and typical of duodenal ulcer.

Diagnostic Tests

- Endoscopy, cytology, and multiple biopsies are important for distinguishing malignant from benign gastric ulcers.
- Gastrin-secreting malignancy and Zollinger-Ellison syndrome should be considered in a patient with severe ulcer diathesis, especially when ulcers are multiple and located in atypical areas (e.g., postbulbar).

- Fiberoptic endoscopy is the best method for diagnosing and monitoring peptic ulcer disease.
- An alternative to fiberoptic endoscopy is double-contrast barium x-ray.
- Endoscopic examination can identify esophageal ulcers and ulcers located on the posterior wall of the stomach; in addition, it can definitively diagnose *H. pylori* infection.

Treatment

- Currently, therapy is aimed at eradication of *H. pylori* rather than neutralizing or decreasing gastric acidity.
  - Antibiotic therapy is evolving.
  - A single agent should not be used; no single agent can predictably cure *H. pylori*.
  - The combination of bismuth (Pepto-Bismol 2 tablets PO qid), tetracycline 500 mg PO tid, and metronidazole 250 mg PO tid or qid for 2 weeks will cure 80% of infections.
  - A newer combination is as effective and is more conducive to patient compliance: ranitidine bismuth citrate 400 mg PO bid plus clarithromycin 500 mg PO tid for 2 weeks.
  - Proton pump inhibitors suppress *H. pylori* and induce rapid healing of ulcers; triple therapy with proton pump inhibitors has not been approved, but the benefits of these drugs are shorter duration of treatment, twice-daily dosing, excellent tolerability, and very high eradication rates.
  - A three-drug combination, omeprazole 20 mg bid or lansoprazole 15 mg bid, plus clarithromycin 500 mg tid, plus metronidazole 500 mg bid or amoxicillin 1 g tid for 7 to 14 days, can cure infection in about 90% of patients.
- Surgery may be required in cases of perforation, obstruction that does not respond to medical therapy, uncontrolled or recurrent bleeding, suspected malignant gastric ulcer, and symptoms refractory to medical treatment.
  - Weight loss is common after subtotal gastrectomy.
  - Anemia is common usually due to iron deficiency, but sometimes is caused from vitamin B_{12} deficiency due to loss of intrinsic factor or bacterial overgrowth.

  - Dumping syndrome may follow gastric surgical procedures, particularly resections.
    I. Signs and symptoms of early dumping:
       A. Weakness
       B. Dizziness
       C. Sweating
       D. Nausea
       E. Vomiting
       F. Palpitations soon after eating
    II. The cause remains obscure but likely involves autonomic reflexes, intravascular volume contraction, and release of vasoactive peptides from the small intestine.
    III. Treatment: smaller, more frequent meals and decreased carbohydrate intake are usually helpful.

Prognosis

- New research (during the last two decades) has uncovered a definite infective organism, *H. pylori*, as the cause of many gastric and duodenal ulcers that can be treated with specific drugs.
- The focus on acid production and elimination is still part of therapy, but is much less important than before.
- Most patients with peptic ulcer disease can be treated successfully, although recurrences occur after pharmacologic therapy.
- In some instances, surgery is required to treat emergency situations or patients who do not respond to drug therapy, but the need for surgery has declined remarkably in the last 10 years.
- Infectious agents are being identified as the underlying cause of many problems once attributed to other causes (e.g., genetic), including cancer.

Patient/Family Education

- Patients need to be educated about the newer theories of the causes of peptic ulcer disease, and the associated newer treatments.
- Give reassurance that complete resolution of symptoms is possible, although recurrences that are also treatable may occur.
- Explain all procedures, medications, self-care, and preventive measures, and give these directions in writing if possible.
- Medication regimens are becoming more streamlined and effective, helping to ensure patient compliance and early healing.

Follow-up/Referral

- Patients with peptic ulcer disease can usually be treated in the ambulatory care setting, with consultation from the gastroenterologist at frequent intervals.
- After resolution of the current episode, instruct the patient about when to return for check-ups, and to return if symptoms of peptic ulcer recur.

DIARRHEA AND CONSTIPATION
Definitions

- Diarrhea is the increase in frequency, fluid content, or volume of fecal discharge.
- Constipation is difficult or infrequent passage of feces, hardness of stool, or a feeling of incomplete evacuation.

Diarrhea
Risk Factors/Etiology
Osmotic Diarrhea

- Lactose intolerance caused by lactase deficiency
- Use of poorly absorbed salts (e.g., magnesium sulfate, sodium phosphates) as laxatives or antacids.
- Ingestion of large amounts of sugar substitutes (e.g., sorbitol, mannitol) causes osmotic diarrhea as a result of their slow absorption and stimulation of rapid small-bowel motility ("dietetic food" or "chewing gum" diarrhea).
- Eating certain fruits can cause osmotic diarrhea.

Secretory Diarrhea
Secretory diarrhea occurs when the small and large bowel secrete more electrolytes and water than they absorb.

- Bacterial toxins (e.g., cholera)
- Enteropathogenic viruses, bile acids (e.g., after ileal resection)
- Some drugs (e.g., anthraquinone cathartics, castor oil, prostaglandins)
- Peptide hormones (e.g., vasoactive intestinal peptide produced by pancreatic tumors)
- Microscopic colitis (collagenous or lymphocytic colitis) causes 5% of secretory diarrhea.
  —It is 10 times more frequent in women, and usually affects those $\geq$ age 60.

—Symptoms include nausea, vomiting, abdominal pain, flatulence, and weight loss, but many persons are asymptomatic.
—Loperamide is used to control symptoms.
—Histologic changes may resolve with prednisone or sulfasalazine.

Exudative Diarrhea
This type of diarrhea occurs with mucosal diseases (e.g., regional enteritis, ulcerative colitis, tuberculosis, lymphoma, cancer).

- Caused by mucosal inflammation, ulceration, or tumefaction
  —Resultant outpouring of plasma, serum proteins, blood, and mucus increases fecal bulk and fluid content.
  —Involvement of the rectal mucosa may cause urgency and increased stool frequency because the inflamed rectum is more sensitive to distention.

Decreased Absorption Time
Decreased absorption time occurs when chyme is not in contact with an adequate absorptive surface of the GI tract for a long enough time; too much water remains in the feces.

- Factors that decrease contact time are
  —Small- or large-bowel resection
  —Gastric resection
  —Pyloroplasty
  —Vagotomy
  —Surgical bypass of intestinal segments
  —Drugs (e.g., magnesium-containing antacids, laxatives) or humoral agents (e.g., prostaglandins, serotonin) that speed transit by stimulating intestinal smooth muscle

Malabsorption

- Malabsorption produces diarrhea by osmotic or secretory mechanisms.
  —The diarrhea may be osmotic if the unabsorbed material is abundant, water-soluble, and of low molecular weight.
  —Lipids are not osmotic, but some (fatty acids, bile acids) act as secretagogues and cause secretory diarrhea.
- In generalized malabsorption (e.g., tropical sprue) fat malabsorption causes colonic secretion, and carbohydrate malabsorption causes osmotic diarrhea.

- Malabsorption-related diarrhea may develop when the transport of chyme is prolonged, and fecal bacteria proliferate in the small bowel.
  - Factors that decrease transit time and permit bacterial overgrowth include strictured segments, sclerodermatous intestinal disease, and stagnant loops created by surgery.

Paradoxical Diarrhea

Paradoxical diarrhea occurs because of oozing around a fecal impaction in children and in debilitated or demented adults.

Diagnosis

Signs, Symptoms, and History
- Circumstances around onset
- Recent travel
- Food ingested
- Water source
- Medications (prescription and over-the-counter [OTC])
- Duration and severity
- Abdominal pain or vomiting
- Blood in the stool or change in color
- Frequency and timing of bowel movements
- Stool consistency
- Steatorrhea (fatty, greasy, or oily stools with a foul odor)
- Change in weight or appetite
- Rectal urgency or tenesmus

Diagnostic Tests
- Fluid and electrolyte status
- Complete physical examination
- Digital rectal examination
- Proctoscopic and sigmoidoscopic (with biopsy of rectal mucosa) examinations for histologic examination to detect infectious, ulcerative, or collagenous colitis
- Microscopic and macroscopic stool examination: note consistency, volume, presence of blood (apparent or occult), mucus, pus, or excess fat.
  - White blood cells indicating ulceration or bacterial invasion
  - Unabsorbed fat
  - Meat fibers
  - Parasitic infestation (e.g., amebiasis, giardiasis)

  - Stool pH (normal is >6.0) is decreased by bacterial fermentation of unabsorbed carbohydrate and protein in the colon.
  - Alkalinization of the stool will show pink color of phenolphthalein, a commonly abused laxative.
  - With large volume, stool electrolytes can be measured to determine if diarrhea is secretory or osmotic.
- In general, in diseases of the small bowel, stools are voluminous and watery or fatty.
- In colonic diseases, stools are frequent, sometimes small in volume, and may show blood, mucus, or pus, and the patient will have abdominal discomfort.
- In diseases of the rectal mucosa, the rectum may be more sensitive to distention, and diarrhea may be frequent, with small stools.
- Acute diarrhea from dietary indiscretion or acute infection resolves spontaneously.
  - If abdominal pain or fever is present, fecal culture should be done prior to empiric treatment with antibiotics.
- For chronic diarrhea, fecal cultures and microscopy will likely determine whether specific therapy is indicated.
  - Proctoscopy and sigmoidoscopy with biopsies should follow to detect inflammatory causes.

Treatment
- The patient should be referred to a gastroenterologist for treatment.
- The underlying cause of diarrhea (a symptom) should be uncovered.
  - Treatment depends on the type of diarrhea, cause, and symptoms.

Prognosis
- Diagnostic techniques, greater understanding of bowel problems, and better treatment (medications, surgery) all help to shorten the disease process and ensure a favorable outcome.

Patient/Family Education
- Reassure the patient regarding the likelihood of a positive resolution of the problem.
- Explain the nature of the problem, the likely cause, the usual course, and the treatment to be carried out.

—Involving the patient as much as possible in the treatment regimens will help in maintaining a balanced outlook.

- Simple but complete written instructions should be given to the patient at each visit.
  —Questioning patients or asking them to repeat what was told to them will let you know that they understand and can carry out the instructions.

Follow-up/Referral

- Any patient with complex problems with diarrhea or constipation should be referred to a gastroenterologist for complete evaluation, diagnosis, and treatment.
- The specialist will determine the frequency and timing of return visits, and of other follow-up (e.g., telephone calls between visits).

Constipation

Risk Factors

- Older, bedridden, debilitated, or demented patients
- Barium given by mouth or enema

Etiology

- Acute constipation occurs when a change in bowel habits produces infrequent stools or hard stools that are difficult to pass.
  —A sudden change indicates an organic cause (e.g., mechanical bowel obstruction).
  —Adynamic ileus often accompanies acute intra-abdominal disease such as localized peritonitis or diverticulitis.
  —Strong laxatives should be avoided.
  —Acute onset of constipation in a bedridden patient is common.
  —When a change in bowel habits persists for weeks or occurs intermittently with increasing frequency or severity, colonic tumors and other causes of partial obstruction should be suspected.
  —Anal fissures that cause pain or bleeding should be looked for.
  —If no cause is found, treatment should be symptomatic.
- Chronic constipation
  —Normal bowel movements are hampered because the storage, transport, and evacuation mechanisms are disrupted.

—Causes may include systemic disease (e.g., debilitating infections, hypothyroidism, hypercalcemia, uremia, porphyria), but more often the cause is a local neurogenic disorder (e.g., IBS, colonic inertia, Parkinson's disease, cerebral thrombosis, spinal cord injury).

- Many patients become fixated on the bowels: number per day, color and consistency, difficulty of passing stool, etc., and begin to abuse the colon with laxatives, suppositories, and enemas.
  —People with obsessive-compulsive disorders control their anxiety with perfectionist behaviors, their need to rid the body every day of "unclean" wastes.
  —Depression may be associated with failure to defecate every day; in this situation, a circular pattern of behavior can develop, with one causing the other.

Diagnosis

- It is essential to rule out serious bowel disease by appropriate diagnostic techniques and lab studies.
  —CBC
  —Thyroid-stimulating hormone
  —Fasting glucose
  —Electrolytes
  —Colonoscopy for patients with resistant, prolonged, or unusual symptoms
  —Individual psychologic needs must be considered.

Treatment

- The diet should contain enough fiber to ensure adequate stool bulk.
  —Vegetable fiber, which is largely indigestible and unabsorbable, increases stool bulk.
  —Fruits and vegetables are recommended.
  —Cereals containing bran are helpful.
- Laxatives should be selected with care.
  —Contraindications include acute abdominal pain of unknown cause, inflammatory bowel disorders, intestinal obstruction, GI bleeding, and fecal impactions.
- Bulking agents (bran, psyllium, calcium polycarbophil, methylcellulose) provide fiber and are the only laxatives acceptable for long-term use.
  —They normalize both diarrhea and constipation.

- Wetting agents such as detergent laxatives (e.g., docusate) soften stools.
  - Mineral oil softens fecal matter, but it may decrease absorption of fat-soluble vitamins; if used for long periods, it could produce malnutrition, especially in older people.
- Fecal impaction is treated with enemas of warm (43.3° C or 110° F) olive oil, 60 to 120 ml (2 to 4 oz), followed by small enemas (100 ml) of commercially prepared hypertonic solutions.
  - If this treatment fails, manual fragmentation and disimpaction of the mass are necessary.
  - This procedure may be painful, so perirectal and intrarectal application of local anesthetics (e.g., lidocaine 5% ointment) is recommended.
    - ~ Some debilitated patients may require general anesthesia.
- Explanations to patients who are obsessive-compulsive are important, but often it is of little benefit to tell them that their attitude toward defecation is abnormal.
  - The clinician must try to convince patients that daily bowel movements are not essential to good health, that frequent laxatives or enemas (more often than once every 3 days) do not help the bowel to function on its own, and that the way to "cure" stools that are "too thin" or "too green" is not to look at them.

IRRITABLE BOWEL SYNDROME
Definition

Irritable bowel syndrome (IBS) is a motility disorder that involves the entire GI tract, causes recurring upper and lower GI symptoms, and includes variable degrees of abdominal pain, abdominal bloating, and constipation and/or diarrhea.

Risk Factors

- Young age: symptoms usually present during the late teens or early 20s; first-time symptoms rarely appear after age 50.
- Female to male predominance of 2:1

Etiology

- The cause of IBS is unknown.
- Emotional factors, diet, drugs, or hormones may precipitate or aggravate increased GI motility.

Pathogenesis

- Signs and symptoms of IBS seem to be related to exaggeration of normal intestinal motility patterns.
- In normal patients, the dominant type of motor activity is segmenting contractions, which tend to retard the forward movement of intraluminal contents; this impeding activity represents about 90% or more of the wave types recorded.
  - When this type of activity is excessive, constipation ensues.
  - When the activity is markedly diminished, diarrhea occurs; the normal activity is replaced by infrequent mass propulsive movements that may occur five to six times a day during episodes of diarrhea.
- The symptoms of IBS (abdominal pain, constipation, diarrhea) occur because of the quite strong, spastic contractions either of the segmenting (impeding) or propulsive type.
- Motility is influenced by many factors such as meals (e.g., pain, distention, occasional diarrhea), emotionally stressful situations, anxiety, and drugs (e.g., opiates).
  - Symptoms following meals may be related to an exaggeration of the normal biphasic postprandial response, the gastroileocolic response, which consists of an early neurogenic (reflex) component during the first 15 to 30 minutes postprandially, and hormonally stimulated contractions that occur after 40 minutes.
  - The hormonal phase may be initiated by gastrointestinal hormones released during feeding (e.g., cholecystokinin, released as food enters the duodenum).
- Recent research suggests heightened visceral sensory perception as another factor underlying IBS.

Diagnosis

- Usually, patients who present for treatment have had symptoms for months or years.

- Major complaints are pain and altered bowel habits.
- Occurrence of symptoms is variable; in some patients, they are intermittent, with symptom-free periods of days, weeks, or rarely, months; some patients have symptoms every day.
  - Pain is described as crampy, sharp, or burning, relieved by bowel movement.
  - It is important to differentiate patients whose pain causes them to wake up from those whose pain is present after awaking.
  - Pain can occur in any part of the abdomen, but most frequently occurs in the lower abdomen.
  - Some patients report radiation of pain to the lower back and down the legs.
  - When asked to point to the site of pain, most patients use the palm of the hand rather than one finger, and often indicate a broad area by a circular motion.
- Altered bowel habits
  - Usually, patients report alternating diarrhea and constipation, with one predominating.
  - The pattern of bowel changes is consistent in each patient, with variability only in timing and intensity.
  - Most typically, the patient's first stool in the morning is of normal consistency, but is followed rapidly by increasingly loose stools, sometimes associated with flatulence and sometimes precipitated by meals.
    - ~ The patient experiences urgency with each stool, and cramps that may precede the movement are relieved by defecation.
  - Consistency, volume, and shape of stools are variable; formed stools are usually compressed and pencil-shaped; dry, hard pellets may sometimes be passed; fecal incontinence occurs in about 20% of patients.
- Of patients with IBS, 70% have abnormal scores on psychologic tests.
  - The psychologic disturbances most commonly seen in patients with IBS are somatoform disorder, anxiety, depression, and cancerophobia.
  - Depression is often masked, and both patient and clinician overlook it and tend to focus on physical symptoms.
  - Studies show that, of people with IBS, those who seek treatment are those who are more psychologically distressed than those who do not.

Diagnostic Tests
- Physical examination should include observing for signs of hyperthyroidism, masses, adenopathy, partial intestinal obstruction, and abdominal bruits (which might indicate ischemic intestinal angina in older persons).
- Laboratory tests
  - CBC
  - Erythrocyte sedimentation rate (ESR)
  - Three microscopic examinations of stool to rule out blood, ova, and parasites
  - Fiberoptic sigmoidoscopy
  - Barium enema if warranted
  - Small bowel studies may be necessary to rule out Crohn's disease.
- Diagnostic testing should be done early to make certain that serious organic disease is not present.

Differential Diagnosis
- Lactose intolerance
- Travel history to rule out infectious or parasitic diseases
- Hyperthyroidism
- Zollinger-Ellison syndrome
- Medullary carcinoma of the thyroid
- Addison's disease
- Whipple's disease
- HIV infection
- Diverticular disease
- Hyperparathyroidism
- Intestinal obstruction
- Colon cancer

Treatment
- The cause of IBS is unknown; therefore, treatment is symptomatic and relies on education, reassurance, diet, supportive and behavioral therapy, and pharmacotherapy appropriate to both the GI symptoms and any psychologic symptoms.

Prognosis
- Whether treatment changes the prognosis of IBS in not known for certain.
- The more serious the underlying psychologic factors, the longer is the course of IBS, regard-

less of other factors (e.g., symptoms, length of time patient has had the condition).

- Treating patients with IBS requires a clinician who is interested, educated, skilled, and compassionate.

Patient/Family Education

- IBS is a very frustrating condition for both patients and clinicians, largely because of its variability and persistence despite all efforts to treat it.
- Explain in detail the nature of the condition, those factors that may exacerbate symptoms, and those that may relieve symptoms.
- The use and abuse of laxatives and enemas, and the need to confine laxative use to bran and other natural products that contain fiber should be discussed.
- Underlying psychologic factors should be discussed, to face the possibility of the presence of depression, anxiety, high stress, or other problems.
- Because of the prolonged course of IBS, the clinician must be aware of possible addiction to certain drugs, or use of drugs that could exacerbate the condition (e.g., NSAIDs, aspirin).
- Some patients lack a close relative or friend with whom they can talk over problems that produce stress or anxiety; the clinician may need to assume this role, at least from time to time, so a nurturing, supportive patient-clinician relationship is nearly always necessary.

Follow-up/Referral

- Regular, but not necessarily frequent, follow-up visits reassure the patient, whereas as-needed appointments may be perceived by the patient as abandonment or inability of the clinician to offer further help.
- Telephone calls to the patient between visits may provide additional support, but could encourage abuse by those patients who seek secondary gain from being ill.

INFLAMMATORY BOWEL DISEASE: CROHN'S DISEASE AND ULCERATIVE COLITIS

Two major forms of *nonspecific* inflammatory bowel disease are recognized: Crohn's disease, which can affect any part of the GI tract, and ul-

cerative colitis, which affects only the large bowel.

There is overlap between these two conditions in their clinical features and in histologic and radiologic abnormalities; in 10% of cases of colitis a definitive diagnosis of either Crohn's disease or ulcerative colitis is not possible. However, it is necessary to distinguish them because of particular differences in their treatment. It is possible that these two conditions represent two aspects of the same disease.

Epidemiology

- The incidence of Crohn's disease is rising; although it varies from country to country, it affects about 5 to 8/100,000 every year.
- The incidence of ulcerative colitis is stable at 6 to 15/100,000 every year, with a prevalence of 80 to 120/100,000.
  - —The incidence of both is lower in nonwhite races.
  - —Jews are more prone to inflammatory bowel disease than non-Jews; the Ashkenazi Jews have a higher risk than the Sephardic Jews.
- Both conditions can be found worldwide, but are more common in the West.

Pathogenesis

- The etiology of both is unknown, but the racial differences and geographic clustering suggest both genetic and environmental causes.
  - —Familial: both are more common among relatives of patients than in the general population.
  - —Genetic: there are no HLA markers, but HLA-B27 is increased in patients with inflammatory bowel disease and ankylosing spondylitis.
  - —Diet: there is little evidence that supports a dietary factor, although a high sugar intake has been found in patients with Crohn's disease.
  - —Smoking: patients with Crohn's disease are more likely to be tobacco smokers, but conversely there is an increased risk of ulcerative colitis among nonsmokers or ex-smokers.
  - —Infective agent in Crohn's disease: the most attractive hypothesis is that of a transmissible agent; however, no bacterium, virus, or parasite has been definitely identified.
    - ~ Measles virus: a higher than expected rate of Crohn's disease in children born during measles epidemics suggests a role for this

virus, and this also implicates the measles vaccination. In one study, measles-specific DNA fragments were found in Crohn's tissue, but this has not been corroborated.

—Mycobacterium: in cattle and sheep Johne's disease, which is a chronic inflammatory disorder of the distal ileum, is caused by *Mycobacterium paratuberculosis*. Isolation of mycobacterium from Crohn's tissue has been inconsistent, and current evidence is against this being an etiologic agent.

- Multifocal GI infarction due to granulomatous angiitis has been suggested as a primary event in Crohn's disease.
- Inducible nitric acid synthase (INAS) is expressed after activation by bacterial endotoxins or certain pro-inflammatory cytokines. This intramucosal enzyme produces large amounts of nitric oxide intraluminally in an acute attack of colitis. It has antimicrobial properties but could also damage host cells.
- Many immunologic abnormalities have been described in inflammatory bowel disease. It is unclear whether they are the primary or secondary event in the pathogenesis. A suggested mechanism is that a specific or generalized luminal antigen can cause stimulation of immune (antigen-specific) or inflammatory (antigen-nonspecific) responses. It is possible that these responses are abnormal or exaggerated in inflammatory bowel disease.

—Activation of T lymphocytes, tissue macrophages, eosinophils, mast cells, neutrophils, and fibroblasts produces a wide variety of cytokines (e.g., interleukin IL-1, IL-6, TNFs), and chemokines (e.g., eotaxin, macrophage inflammatory protein [MIP]), monocyte chemoattractant protein (MCP), IL-8, eicosanoids (e.g., prostaglandins, thromboxane, LTB4), cell adhesion markers (e.g., E-selectins), endothelial cell leukocyte adhesion molecule (ELAM), and free oxygen radicals all can lead to tissue damage.

- The serum antineutrophil cytoplasmic antibody (ANCA) is increased in ulcerative colitis but not in Crohn's disease; the significance of this is not known.

Pathology

- Crohn's disease is a chronic inflammatory condition that may affect any part of the GI tract from the mouth to the anus.

- It has a particular tendency to affect the terminal ileum and ascending colon (ileocolonic disease).
- Crohn's disease can affect one small area of the gut such as the terminal ileum, or multiple areas with relatively normal bowel in between ("skip lesions").
- It may also involve the whole of the colon ("total colitis") sometimes without bowel involvement.
- Ulcerative colitis can affect the rectum alone (proctitis), can extend proximally to involve the sigmoid and descending colon ("left-sided colitis"), or may involve the whole colon ("total colitis"); in a few patients, there is also inflammation of the distal terminal ileum ("backwash ileitis").

Macroscopic Changes

- In Crohn's disease the involved small bowel is usually thickened and narrowed, with deep ulcers and fissures in the mucosa, producing a cobblestone appearance.
- Fistulas and abscesses may be seen in the colon.
- An early feature is aphthoid ulceration, usually seen at colonoscopy; later, larger and deeper ulcers appear in a patchy distribution, also producing a cobblestone appearance.
- In ulcerative colitis, the mucosa looks reddened, inflamed, and bleeds easily.
- In severe disease there is extensive ulceration, with the adjacent mucosa appearing as inflammatory polyps.
- In fulminant colonic disease of either type, most of the mucosa is lost, leaving a few islands of edematous mucosa (mucosal islands), and toxic dilation occurs.
- On healing, the mucosa returns to normal, but there is usually some residual glandular distortion.

Microscopic Changes

- In Crohn's disease the inflammation extends through all layers (transmural) of the bowel.
- An increase in chronic inflammatory cells and lymphoid hyperplasia is seen.
- In 50% to 60% of patients, granulomas are present (noncaseating epithelioid cells, aggregates with Langhans' giant cells).

- In ulcerative colitis the mucosa shows a chronic inflammatory cell infiltrate in the lamina propria.
- Crypt abscesses and goblet cell depletion are evident.

Diagnosis (Table 7-4)

Crohn's Disease

Signs and Symptoms

- Crohn's disease can appear gradually or acutely.
- Diarrhea is present in 80% of all cases; if the colon is affected, blood is seen.
- Abdominal pain may be colicky or of minimal discomfort.
- Weight loss in 15% of patients
- Malaise
- Lethargy
- Anorexia in 15% of patients
- Nausea
- Vomiting
- Low-grade fever
- Steatorrhea is present in small bowel disease.
- Aphthous ulceration of the mouth is often present.
- Abdominal tenderness and, in some patients, a right iliac fossa mass is palpable; the cause may be inflamed loops of bowel or an abscess.
- Anal examination may reveal edema, tags, fissures, or perianal abscesses, which are very common (80%) in colonic involvement.
- Conditions associated with inflammatory bowel disease include erythema nodosum, arthritis, and iritis.
- Sigmoidoscopy should always be performed for biopsy of mucosa.

—Even with extensive Crohn's disease, the rectum may be spared and be relatively normal, but patchy involvement with an edematous, hemorrhagic mucosa is characteristic.

Ulcerative Colitis

Signs and Symptoms

- Diarrhea with blood and mucus
- Lower abdominal discomfort in some patients
- Malaise
- Lethargy
- Anorexia
- Aphthous ulceration in the mouth
- Ulcerative colitis can be mild, moderate, or severe.
- Ulcerative colitis runs a course of remissions and exacerbations.
- About 10% of patients have persistent, chronic symptoms; others may have only a single attack.
- When ulcerative colitis is confined to the rectum, blood mixed with stool, urgency, and tenesmus are common.
- Normally there are few constitutional symptoms, but frequency of defecation interferes with normal activities to a considerable degree.
- In an acute attack, patients have bloody diarrhea, passing 10 to 20 liquid stools per day.
- Diarrhea also occurs at night, with urgency and incontinence that is severely disabling for patients.
  —Sometimes only blood and mucus are passed.
- Fever, tachycardia, elevated ESR, anemia, and elevated albumin may be present during acute attacks.

TABLE 7-4		
Histologic Comparison of Crohn's Disease and Ulcerative Colitis		
Characteristic	**Crohn's Disease**	**Ulcerative Colitis**
Inflammation	Deep (transmural)	Mucosal
	Patchy	Continuous
Granulomas	++	Rare
Goblet cells	Present	Depleted
Crypt abscesses	+	++

From Kumar P, Clark M: Gastroenterology. In Kumar P, Clark M, eds: *Clinical medicine,* ed 4, Edinburgh, 1998, WB Saunders, p 263.
+, Uncommon; ++, moderate.

- There are no specific physical signs of ulcerative colitis.
- Sigmoidoscopy shows an inflamed, bleeding, friable mucosa.
- Constitutional problems common to both Crohn's disease and ulcerative colitis are arthritis and ankylosing spondylitis, but kidney stones and gallbladder stones are more common in Crohn's disease.
- Colonoscopy is performed in both conditions.
  —In ulcerative colitis, this shows the exact extent of the disease.
- To determine the degree of activity occurring, obtain information from the physical examination, clinical picture, and laboratory tests (e.g., serum albumin, ESR, acute-phase protein).

Differential Diagnosis
- Crohn's disease must be considered in all cases of chronic diarrhea, malabsorption, and malnutrition.
- Both Crohn's disease and ulcerative colitis must be distinguished from amebic and ischemic colitis.
- A rare cause of colitis is Behçet's disease, which also causes orogenital ulcers.
- Collagenous colitis

Treatment
Crohn's Disease
- Symptomatic therapy aims to control diarrhea.
- Antiinflammatory drugs and immunosuppressive drugs are used.
- Anemia is treated with ferrous sulfate 400 mg qd, or folic acid 5 mg qd.
- Severe attacks require corticosteroids 30 to 60 mg qd.
- Increase liquids to treat dehydration.
- Replace electrolytes as needed.
- Elemental diet can induce remission, especially in small bowel disease.
- Surgical management is used only in the event of
  —Failure of medical therapy and when symptoms are producing ill health
  —Complications (e.g., toxic dilation, obstruction)
  —In children, failure to grow

Ulcerative Colitis
- Therapy depends on the severity of the disease.
- Severe attacks require hospitalization and careful monitoring, because the mortality of this condition is still high.
- All patients are given a 5-aminosalicylate acid (5-ASA or mesalamine) compound, which is broken down in the colon by bacteria to release the active agent, 5-ASA.
  —All patients in remission are maintained on a 5-ASA compound for many years.
- Sulfasalazine 3 to 4 g/day, decreasing the dose to 2 g/day as maintenance
- High-dose corticosteroids (e.g., prednisone 60 mg or hydrocortisone 100 mg IV q6h)
- Cyclosporine given intravenously was shown in some studies to induce remission.
- Surgical management
  —Because ulcerative colitis is confined to the colon, colectomy is curative; protocolectomy with an ileostomy is the standard procedure.
    ~ In ulcerative colitis (but not in Crohn's disease), an ileorectal or ileoanal anastomosis is used to avoid ileostomy.
  —The primary indication for surgery is a severe attack that does not respond to medical therapy.

DIVERTICULAR DISEASE OF THE COLON
Definition
Diverticulitis is a disease caused by diverticula, acquired sac-like mucosal projections through the muscular layer of the GI tract that cause symptoms by trapping feces, becoming infected, bleeding, or rupturing.

- Nomenclature of diverticular disease: the distinction between these entities is more than simple semantics; the natural history, pathophysiology, diagnosis, and treatment of these conditions vary, at least to some degree.
  —*Diverticulosis:* the presence of colonic diverticula, without presuming that there are accompanying signs and symptoms
  —*Symptomatic diverticular disease:* diverticulosis with pain and/or altered bowel habits, without diverticular inflammation

—*Diverticulitis:* inflammation of one or more diverticula, usually implying perforation of a diverticulum, and symptoms are almost always present

—*Prediverticular state:* characterized by radiographic, pathologic, and often clinical features of diverticulosis, without formation of diverticula

Risk Factors

- Older age: 20% of men and women > 40 years, 50% > 60 years, and 66% > 85 years have diverticulosis of the colon.
  —Only 5% of people living in the early 1900s had the disease, and the incidence has risen probably because modern milling processes remove 66% of the fiber from flour.
  —Vegetarians have a much lower prevalence of diverticulosis than others.
- Low-fiber diet
- Disordered colonic motility
- Weak colonic wall through which the mucosa herniates to form diverticula
- Loss of muscle mass
- Collagen defects
- Predisposing diseases: scleroderma, Marfan's syndrome, Ehlers-Danlos syndrome, which occur in older people, and which might result in a degenerative process of the colonic muscle and a change in tensile strength of the wall of the colon.

Asymptomatic Diverticulosis

- Many patients in whom diverticulosis was detected on barium enema were asymptomatic.
  —Diverticula were either localized in the sigmoid colon or diffusely spread throughout the colon.
  —The sigmoid colon is involved in 95% of cases.
  —Sigmoid diverticula account for 75% of all colonic disease.
    ~ This may be attributed to the narrow caliber of the sigmoid colon, causing higher intraluminal pressures and therefore a greater risk of herniation.
    ~ The more distal the position in the colon, the higher the prevalence of diverticula, although rectal diverticula rarely occur.

- The natural history of diverticulosis is variable.
  —Symptomatic diverticular disease presents either as painful diverticular disease (75%) or as diverticulitis or hemorrhage (25%).
  —The presence of diverticula precedes the onset of symptoms by several years.

Painful Diverticular Disease

- At some point, most people with diverticular disease develop symptoms.
  —If the symptoms are abdominal pain and alteration in bowel habits, the cause is usually painful diverticular disease.
- The hallmark of this disease is abdominal pain without evidence of an inflammatory process.

Diagnosis

- The abdominal pain is usually characterized as colicky or steady, located in the lower left quadrant, and is usually made worse by meals (likely because of gastrocolic reflex).
- Bowel elimination patterns become irregular in 40% to 63% of cases, with diarrhea, constipation, or both, alternating.
  —These attacks are usually episodic rather than continuous.
- Other symptoms that may occur are nausea, heartburn, and flatulence.
- Physical examination may show tenderness, sometimes significant, in the left lower quadrant.
- A tender sigmoid loop that feels like a sausage may be palpable.
- The complete abdominal exam may be unremarkable.
- Stools are generally negative for occult blood, although rectal bleeding from fissures or hemorrhoids may occur.
- The appearance of fever, leukocytosis, or peritoneal signs indicates more serious diverticular (inflammatory) disease.

Treatment

- High-fiber diet: improves bowel transit and relieves symptoms.
- Anticholinergic or antispasmodic drugs may relieve abdominal pain.
  —Dicyclomine (Bentyl) 10 to 20 mg before meals and at bedtime, or

—Hyoscyamine (Levsin) 0.125 to 0.25 mg q4h as needed

Patient/Family Education

- Instruct the patient that the course of the disease is unpredictable, and attacks will likely be experienced at irregular intervals (months to years) for the rest of his or her life.
- No benefit is derived from taking drugs between attacks, but continuing on a high-fiber diet is recommended.

Diverticulitis

- Diverticulitis increases in incidence with age, the length of time the underlying diverticulosis has been present, and with more numerous diverticula.
- The long-term risk of developing diverticulitis among those with diverticulosis is between 10% and 25%, but probably less in asymptomatic diverticular disease.
- Diverticulitis occurs from perforation of one or more diverticula, usually in the sigmoid colon.
- Causes of perforation include persistently high colonic pressures, or an inflammatory process that weakens the wall of the bowel or diverticulum.
  - The perforation may be evident, with fistula or abscess formation, or microscopic and well confined.
  - Fistulas may form in the bladder, vagina, small bowel, or skin.

Diagnosis

- Diagnosis of acute diverticulitis is based on the clinical picture.
- Cardinal symptoms are abdominal pain and fever.
  - Pain is usually severe, sudden in onset, and persistent, worsening with time and localizing to the left lower quadrant.
- There may be anorexia, nausea, and vomiting.
- Altered bowel habits, particularly constipation, are common.
- Urinary tract symptoms or purulent vaginal discharge may occur because of the spread of inflammation or fistula formation.
- A mass may be palpated in the left lower quadrant on abdominal, pelvic, or rectal examination.
- Occult bleeding occurs in about 25% of patients.

- Leukocytosis is always present.
- Pyuria or hematuria may occur when the bladder or ureter is involved.
- Symptoms of diverticulitis may be diminished in older patients.
  - There may be no pain, fever, or leukocytosis.

Differential Diagnosis

- Painful diverticular disease
- Carcinoma of the colon
- Inflammatory or ischemic bowel disease
- Peritonitis, fever, and leukocytosis point to more serious intra-abdominal problems, which may be diagnosed by endoscopy or barium enema.

Treatment

- Most patients with diverticulitis are hospitalized, placed on bowel and bed rest, and given analgesics, intravenous hydration, and antimicrobial drugs (e.g., clindamycin and gentamicin, or cefotetan) to treat both aerobic and anaerobic organisms.
- About 75% of patients respond to conservative medical therapy, but a surgical consultation should be arranged on admission, in case surgery is needed.
  - The patient's condition usually improves markedly in 3 to 10 days.
- With successful medical management, the patient is discharged to home.
  - The recurrence rate is about 25%, mostly during the first 5 years.
- If the patient fails to respond to conservative management and the acute inflammatory process does not abate, if recurrent attacks of diverticulitis occur, or if obstructive stricture(s) form, surgery is indicated.

Diverticular Bleeding

- The average age of these patients who develop lower GI bleeding because of diverticulosis is 70 years; GI bleeding is the presenting symptom in 16% of patients.
- Most bleeding occurs in patients who are otherwise asymptomatic.
  - In 30% of cases, colonoscopy shows a lesion other than diverticular disease (e.g., cancer or angiodysplasia).
- Diverticular disease is the most common cause of lower GI bleeding in adults, fol-

lowed closely by bleeding from angiodysplasias.
—Both are common in older people.
—Both are usually found in the right colon (66%), even though diverticula occur most frequently in the left colon.
• About 70% of patients (hospitalized) stop bleeding spontaneously.
—The recurrence rate is 20% to 25%, and increases with each bleed.

Patient/Family Education

• Patient and family members should be instructed about signs and symptoms of rebleeding, and that the patient must obtain immediate care at home, in the office, or in the emergency room.
• No evidence exists to show that a high-fiber diet contributes to diverticular perforation or bleeding.
• Patient and family should maintain a diary regarding bowel habits, symptoms, and dietary patterns.

Follow-up/Referral

• Consultation with a gastroenterologist is mandatory for any patient who does not respond to medical management, develops signs of perforation, bleeding, or other symptoms (e.g., fever, increased pain, or signs that an acute abdominal process is occurring).
• If medical management is successful, and the patient is able to resume usual activities with no untoward symptoms, regular checkups (once every 1 to 2 months) should be scheduled to monitor status and evaluate any symptoms that develop.

HEMORRHOIDS
Definition

A complete description and definition of hemorrhoids is not possible because neither the pathogenesis nor the precise cause is known.
• Hemorrhoids are not varicosities of the rectal venous plexus.
• Current thinking is that hemorrhoids are associated with distal displacement of the anal cushions, which are part of the normal anatomy of the anal canal and consist of hemorrhoidal venous and arterial plexuses, smooth muscle, and connective tissue.

—The anal cushions lie under the mucosa.
—These anal cushions allow for the passage of variable-sized stools without disrupting the rectal mucosa.
—The cushions are found in the right anterior, right posterior, and left lateral portions of the anal canal, which are also the common locations of internal hemorrhoids.

Classification of Hemorrhoids

• Small external skin tags that arise from the anal verge
• External hemorrhoids that arise from the inferior hemorrhoidal plexus exterior to the anal verge, and are covered by pain-sensitive skin
• Internal hemorrhoids that arise from the vascular cushions above the anal verge, covered by pain-sensitive mucosa
—First-degree: hemorrhoids that bulge into the lumen of the anal canal and produce bleeding
—Second degree: hemorrhoids that prolapse during defecation but reduce spontaneously
—Third degree: prolapsed hemorrhoids that require manual reduction
—Fourth degree: hemorrhoids that are irreducibly prolapsed
• Thrombosed internal hemorrhoids occur when hemorrhoids prolapse and strangulate, resulting in thrombosis; if swelling continues, gangrene of the hemorrhoids with ulceration occurs, along with local infection or septic phlebitis of the portal venous system.

Prevalence

• Some estimates indicate that hemorrhoids are present in 50% of those over age 50.
• However, in a national health survey only 4.4% of respondents said that they had hemorrhoids.
• Both genders are affected equally, although women develop hemorrhoids at slightly earlier ages, and men more commonly seek treatment.

Diagnosis
Signs and Symptoms
• Asymptomatic hemorrhoids found during a routine examination do not require any treatment.
• External hemorrhoids cause pain, often exquisite, exacerbated by defecation; a tender lump can be felt on examination.
• Bleeding, which is usually mild, can occur.

- Prolapse produces a feeling of fullness in the anal canal, particularly after defecation.
- Fissure may be the major cause of pain associated with hemorrhoids.

Diagnostic Tests and Procedures
- Anoscopy is the definitive diagnostic procedure for internal hemorrhoids.
- Sigmoidoscopy with a flexible fiberoptic sigmoidoscope should be performed on all patients over age 40 with recent onset of bleeding from internal hemorrhoids.

Differential Diagnosis
- Hypertrophied anal papilla
- Rectal prolapse
- Protruding tumors, including anal or rectal carcinoma, or polyps

Treatment
- Without treatment, symptoms resulting from hemorrhoids resolve spontaneously or in response to self-treatment within several days to several weeks, even when thrombosis is present.
- The goal of treatment is to relieve symptoms.
- Most symptoms of hemorrhoids respond to conservative treatment.
- Thrombosed external hemorrhoids require surgical referral.
- Topical preparations such as Anusol-HC or ProctoFoam-HC contain corticosteroids and should not be used longer than 2 to 3 weeks.
- Hemorrhoidectomy is performed for large internal hemorrhoids when conservative treatment has failed.

Patient/Family Education
- Instruct the patient regarding which OTC preparations are best, and indicate the maximum duration of treatment.
- Instruct patients in the use of sitz baths to relieve itching and swelling; they may be used several times a day if necessary.
- NSAIDs may be prescribed for pain relief.
- Give the patient a written list of signs and symptoms that require immediate telephone consultation with the nurse practitioner.

Follow-up/Referral
- Referral to a gastroenterologist surgeon may be required for surgical management.

—Surgical excision of hemorrhoids is performed under local anesthesia in the ambulatory care setting.
—Injection of hemorrhoids with sclerosing agents is performed without anesthesia in the ambulatory setting.
—Rubber band ligation, a simple office procedure, is the usual initial treatment of choice for most symptomatic internal hemorrhoids of all but fourth-degree classification.
—Laser therapy and infrared photocoagulation are available for all but fourth-degree hemorrhoids, but require expensive expertise and equipment.
—The most radical treatment is hemorrhoidectomy, done under regional or general anesthesia in a hospital operating room.

PANCREATITIS
Acute Pancreatitis

Definition
Pancreatitis is inflammation of the pancreas.
- Pancreatitis is classified as either acute or chronic.
  —Acute pancreatitis is an acute inflammation that resolves both clinically and histologically.
  —Chronic pancreatitis is characterized by histologic changes that persist even after the cause has been removed.
  ~ The histologic changes are irreversible and tend to progress, resulting in serious loss of exocrine and endocrine pancreatic function and deterioration of pancreatic structure.

Risk Factors
- Biliary tract disease and alcoholism account for ≥80% of hospital admissions for acute pancreatitis.
- The remaining 20% are caused by drugs (e.g., azathioprine, sulfasalazine, furosemide, valproic acid), and other causes.

Etiology (see Risk Factors section)
- Estrogen use associated with hyperlipidemia
- Infection (e.g., mumps)
- Hypertriglyceridemia
- Endoscopic retrograde cholangiopancreatography

Pancreatitis

Pain thru Back

- Structural abnormalities of the pancreatic duct (e.g., stricture, cancer, pancreas divisum)
- Structural abnormalities of the common bile duct and ampullary region (e.g., common bile duct cyst, sphincter of Oddi stenosis)
- Surgery (particularly stomach and biliary tract, and after coronary artery bypass grafting)
- Vascular disease (e.g., severe hypotension)
- Blunt and penetrating trauma
- Hyperparathyroidism and hypercalcemia
- Renal transplantation
- Hereditary pancreatitis
- Uncertain or unknown causes

Pathogenesis

- In biliary tract disease, attacks of pancreatitis are caused by temporary impaction of a gallstone in the sphincter of Oddi before it passes into the duodenum.
  - The precise pathogenic mechanism is unclear.
  - It is believed that increased ductal pressure triggers pancreatitis.
- Alcohol intake >100 g/day for several years may cause the protein of pancreatic enzymes to precipitate within small pancreatic ductules.
  - In time, protein plugs accumulate, inducing additional histologic abnormalities.
  - After 3 to 5 years, the first clinical episode of pancreatitis occurs, presumably because of premature activation of pancreatic enzymes.
- Edema or necrosis and hemorrhage are prominent gross pathologic changes.
  - Tissue necrosis is caused by activation of several pancreatic enzymes (e.g., trypsin, phospholipase A_2).
- Pancreatic exudate containing toxins and activated pancreatic enzymes permeates the retroperitoneum and at times the peritoneal cavity, inducing a chemical burn and increasing the permeability of blood vessels.
  - This causes extravasation of large amounts of protein-rich fluid from the systemic circulation into "third spaces," producing hypovolemia and shock.

Diagnosis

Signs and Symptoms

- Pancreatic enzymes activate complement and the inflammatory cascade, producing cytokines.

- Patients typically present with fever and an elevated white blood cell (WBC) count, making it difficult to know if the infection is the cause, or if it has developed during the course of pancreatitis.
- Patients have severe abdominal pain that radiates straight through to the back in almost 50% of cases.
  - The severity of the pain usually requires large doses of parenteral narcotics.
  - The pain is steady, boring, and persists for many hours and often several days.
  - Sitting up and leaning forward may reduce the pain; coughing, deep breathing, or vigorous movement often exacerbates it.
- Many patients have nausea and vomiting, resulting in dry heaves.
- The patient appears acutely ill, sweats profusely, and the pulse rate is 100 to 140 beats per minute.
- Respirations are shallow and rapid; BP may be transiently high, or it may be low with significant postural hypotension.
- Temperature may be normal or subnormal.
- Sensorium may be blunted to the point of semicoma.
- Scleral icterus is sometimes present.
- Examination of the lungs may show limited diaphragmatic excursion and evidence of atelectasis.
- Bowel sounds may be hypoactive.
- Cullen's sign (discoloration around the umbilicus) is characteristic of acute pancreatitis; it may also be present in massive abdominal hemorrhage and ruptured ectopic pregnancy.

Diagnostic Tests

- Serum amylase and lipase concentration increase on the first day of acute pancreatitis, and return to normal in 3 to 7 days.
- Supine and upright x-rays of the abdomen may show calculi in the pancreatic ducts (evidence of prior inflammation and therefore chronic pancreatitis).
- Chest x-ray may show atelectasis or pleural effusion, usually left-sided or bilateral, rarely only right-sided.
- Ultrasound may detect gallstones or dilation of the common duct, indicating biliary tract obstruction.

- CT offers better visualization of the pancreas unless the patient is very thin.
- Eighty percent of patients with gallstone pancreatitis pass the stone spontaneously; surgery is indicated for patients who do not improve over 24 hours.
  —Patients who improve usually have an elective laparoscopic cholecystectomy.

Complications
- Death during the first several days of acute pancreatitis is usually due to cardiovascular instability with refractory shock and renal failure or respiratory failure.
- Circulating toxins and enzymes are believed to play a large role in early death.
- Pancreatic infection is usually caused by gram-negative organisms.

Treatment
- In mild edematous pancreatitis, the patient is kept fasting until symptoms of acute inflammation subside, and sufficient fluids are infused to prevent hypovolemia and hypotension.
- Transfer to an intensive care unit is determined on the first day of hospitalization; if hypotension, oliguria, hypoxemia, or hemoconcentration (hematocrit > 50%) is present, the patient is transferred due to severe third space losses.
- Fasting is maintained for up to 4 weeks, and the patient is maintained by parenteral fluids and other methods as needed.
- Pain is controlled with meperidine 50 to 100 mg intramuscularly (IM) q3-4h (morphine is not given because of risk of spasm of the sphincter of Oddi).
- Antibiotic use is controversial; new evidence indicates that prophylaxis with imipenem can prevent infection of sterile pancreatic necrosis, but mortality is unchanged.

Patient/Family Education
- The patient, when coherent and improving, should be instructed about acute pancreatitis and its effects.
- Recovery from such an attack takes weeks to months.
- During recovery, the patient's fluid and nutritional needs must be adequate.

- There is no guarantee that other episodes of acute pancreatic disease will not occur.

Follow-up/Referral
- These patients are carefully followed after discharge, starting at 1-week intervals and increasing the intervals as the patient gets better.

Chronic Pancreatitis
Definition
Chronic pancreatitis is a self-perpetuating disease characterized by pain and ultimately by pancreatic exocrine or endocrine insufficiency.

Risk Factors/Etiology
- Alcoholism (70% to 80% of patients)
  —Risk increases with the duration and amount of alcohol consumed.
  —Only 5% to 10% of heavy drinkers develop pancreatitis.
- Parathyroidism (10% to 15% of these patients develop pancreatitis.)
- Among Asian and African people, tropical pancreatitis, which is related partly to malnutrition, is the most common cause of chronic pancreatitis.
- A stone, stricture, or tumor obstructing the pancreas can lead to obstructive chronic pancreatitis.
- Between 10% and 20% of cases are idiopathic.
- Recently a mutant trypsinogen gene for hereditary pancreatitis, transmitted as an autosomal dominant trait with variable penetrance, has been identified on chromosome 7.

Pathogenesis
- Ethanol is believed to cause secretion of insoluble pancreatic proteins that calcify and occlude the pancreatic duct.
  —Progressive fibrosis and destruction of functioning glandular tissue follow.

Diagnosis
- Persistent or recurrent episodes of epigastric and left upper quadrant pain with referral to the upper left lumbar region are typical.
- Anorexia, nausea, and vomiting frequently accompany the pain.
- Flatulence, constipation, and weight loss are common.

- Abdominal signs during attacks consist mainly of tenderness over the pancreas, mild muscle guarding, and paralytic ileus.
- Attacks may last from a few hours to as long as 2 weeks; pain may become almost continuous.
- Steatorrhea (bulky, foul, fatty stools) may occur late in the course.
- Serum amylase and lipase may be elevated during acute attacks.
- Normal amylase does not exclude the diagnosis.
- Serum alkaline phosphatase and bilirubin may be elevated due to compression of the common duct.
- Glycosuria may be present.
- Excess fecal fat may be seen on chemical analysis of the stool.
- Pancreatic insufficiency may be confirmed by response to therapy with pancreatic enzyme supplements, by a bentiromide (NBT-PABA) test, or by a secretin stimulation test; where tests are available, by decreased fecal chymotrypsin or elastase levels.
- Vitamin B_{12} malabsorption is detectable in 40% of patients, although clinical deficiency of vitamin B_{12} and fat-soluble vitamins is rare.
- X-ray films show calcifications due to pancreatolithiasis in 30% of affected patients.
- Computed tomography (CT) sometimes shows calcifications not seen on x-ray films.
- Endoscopic ultrasonography is showing promise in detecting changes of chronic pancreatitis.
- Endoscopic retrograde cholangiopancreatography is the diagnostic procedure of choice; it is capable of showing dilated ducts, intraductal stones, strictures, or pseudocysts; however, results may be normal in patients with minimal-change pancreatitis.

Treatment
- Coexisting biliary tract disease should be treated surgically.
- A low-fat diet is indicated.
- Alcohol is forbidden.

- Narcotics should be avoided if possible because of the risk of addiction.
- Steatorrhea is treated with pancreatic supplements, selected according to their high lipase activity.
  - Capsules containing 30,000 units of lipase are given before, during, and after meals.
- Concurrent administration of sodium bicarbonate 650 mg before and after meals, H_2-receptor antagonists (e.g., ranitidine 150 mg bid), or a proton pump inhibitor (e.g., omeprazole 20 to 60 mg qd) decrease inactivation of lipase by acid, thereby further decreasing steatorrhea.
- In some cases of alcoholic pancreatitis and in cystic fibrosis, enteric-coated micro-encapsulated preparations may offer benefits.
- Pain secondary to idiopathic chronic pancreatitis may be alleviated in some patients by the use of pancreatic enzymes or octreotide 200 μg subcutaneously (SC) tid.

Surgical and Endoscopic Treatment
- Goals of surgical intervention are to eradicate biliary tract disease, ensure a free flow of bile into the duodenum, and eliminate obstruction of the pancreatic duct.
- Surgery may be needed to drain persistent pseudocysts and to relieve complications.

Prognosis
- Chronic pancreatitis is a serious and debilitating disease.
- The prognosis is best in patients with recurrent acute pancreatitis caused by a remediable condition such as cholelithiasis, choledocholithiasis, stenosis of the sphincter of Oddi, or hyperparathyroidism.
- Treating the hyperlipidemias that frequently accompany the condition may prevent recurrent attacks.
- In alcoholic pancreatitis, pain is most likely to be relieved when a dilated pancreatic duct can be decompressed.
- In patients whose disease is not amenable to decompressive surgery, addiction to narcotics is a frequent outcome of treatment.

Patient/Family Education

- Any form of pancreatitis (acute or chronic) is a serious disease that requires the cooperation and active participation of both patients and family members regarding pain control, diet therapy, unpredictable episodes of attacks, and abstention from alcohol and smoking.
- Managing patients with pancreatitis requires patience, understanding, and compassion.
- Patients with chronic pancreatitis are at risk for suicide; any indications of suicidal intentions should be reported to the clinician immediately.

Follow-up/Referral

- Patients with pancreatitis or any form of pancreatic disease (e.g., cancer) are followed carefully at all stages of treatment, primarily to prevent recurrent attacks, to maintain the patient at optimal functioning, and to keep the patient and family apprised of the most recent research regarding the disease.

Prognosis

- Ranson's 11 prognostic signs are used to estimate the prognosis.
  - If fewer than three signs are positive, the mortality rate is <5%; if three or four are positive, the mortality rate increases to 15 to 20%.
  - The 11 signs are based on blood serum studies (e.g., glucose, lactate dehydrogenase [LDH], aspartate aminotransferase [AST], WBC, calcium, and others).
  - On admission
    - ~ Age > 55 years
    - ~ Serum glucose > 200 mg/100 ml
    - ~ Serum LDH > 350 U/L
    - ~ AST > 250 U/L
    - ~ WBC > 16,000/mm^3
  - Within 48 hours of admission
    - ~ Hematocrit (HCT) decreases > 10%
    - ~ Blood urea nitrogen (BUN) rises > 5 mg/100 ml
    - ~ Serum calcium < 8 mg/100 ml
    - ~ Pao$_2$ < 60 mm Hg
    - ~ Base deficit > 4 mEq/L
    - ~ Estimated fluid sequestration > 6 L

- The mortality rate for severe acute pancreatitis is high, particularly when other body systems are involved (cardiovascular, hepatic, and renal).

BIBLIOGRAPHY

Acute Appendicitis: http://www.brigham.harvard.edu/Cases/bwh/heache/112/full.html

Acute Lower GI Bleeding: http://www.brigham.harvard.edu/Cases/bwh/heache/126/full.html

American Gastroenterological Association: http://www.gastro.org

Anderson KN, Anderson LE, Glanze WD, eds: *Mosby's medical, nursing & allied health dictionary*, St. Louis, 1998, Mosby.

Beers MH, Berkow R: Gastrointestinal disorders. In Beers MH, Berkow R, eds: *The Merck manual of diagnosis and therapy*, Whitehouse Station, NJ, 1999, Merck Research Laboratories, pp 221-343.

Cheskin LJ: Constipation and diarrhea: diverticular disease of the colon. In Barker LR, Burton JR, Zieve PD, eds: *Principles of ambulatory medicine*, ed 5, Baltimore, 1999, Williams & Wilkins, pp 498-514, 521-525.

Clausson JR: Gastroesophageal reflux disease: a rational approach to management, *Clin Rev* 9(6):69-72, 75-77, 80-82, 85-87, 1999.

Colonic Adenocarcinoma: http://www.brigham.harvard.edu/Cases/bwh/heache/85/full.html

Diverticulitis: http://www.brigham.harvard.edu/Cases/bwh/heache/124/full.html

Katz PO: Disorders of the esophagus: dysphagia, noncardiac chest pain, and gastroesophageal reflux, peptic ulcer disease. In Barker LR, Burton JR, Zieve PD, eds: *Principles of ambulatory medicine*, ed 5, Baltimore, 1999, Williams & Wilkins, pp 459-471, 480-491.

Kumar PJ, Clark ML: Gastroenterology. In Kumar PJ, Clark ML, eds: *Clinical medicine*, ed 4, Edinburgh, 1998, WB Saunders, pp 217-287.

McQuaid KR: Alimentary tract. In Tierney LM, McPhee SJ, Papadakis MA, eds: *Current medical diagnosis & treatment 2000*, New York, 2000, Lange Medical Books/McGraw-Hill, pp 553-655.

Photography and Video of the Gastrointestinal Tract: http://www.gastro.com/photo.htm

Schuster MM: Abdominal pain: irritable bowel syndrome. In Barker LR, Burton JR, Zieve PD, eds: *Principles of ambulatory medicine*, ed 5, Baltimore, 1999, Williams & Wilkins, pp 471-480, 514-521.

Shannon MT, Wilson BA, Stang CL: *Health professionals drug guide 2000*, Stamford, Conn, 2000, Appleton & Lange.

Smith GW: Benign conditions of the anus and rectum. In Barker LR, Burton JR, Zieve PD, eds: *Principles of ambulatory medicine*, ed 5, Baltimore, 1999, Williams & Wilkins, pp 1408-1420.

Talley NJ, Vakil N, Ballard ED, et al: Absence of benefits of eradicating *H pylori* in patients with nonulcer dyspepsia, *N Engl J Med* 341(15):1106-1111, 1999.

REVIEW QUESTIONS

1. Which of the following tests is the "gold standard" in the diagnosis of peptic ulcer disease?
   a. Flat and upright abdominal x-rays
   b. Upper endoscopy
   c. Examination of stools for occult blood
   d. Serology for *Helicobacter pylori*

2. Which of the following statements is true regarding the pathogenic role of *H. pylori* in peptic ulcer development?
   a. If one excludes NSAIDs and Zollinger-Ellison syndrome, 100% of duodenal ulcers are caused by *H. pylori*.
   b. More ulcer disease is caused by lifestyle factors such as smoking and alcohol abuse than is caused by infectious organisms.
   c. More gastric ulcers than duodenal ulcers are caused by *H. pylori*.
   d. *H. pylori* has failed to be associated with peptic ulcer disease development in retrospective or prospective research.

3. When empirically treating peptic ulcer disease, it is important to remember that:
   a. A pain relief response to H_2 blockers precludes malignancy as the cause of an ulcer.
   b. All patients require diagnostic studies prior to medical therapy.
   c. A response to treatment does not preclude the possibility of gastric ulcer or carcinoma.
   d. Acid-lowering drugs have been shown to be effective in ridding the gastrointestinal tract of *H. pylori*.

4. Which of the following is the most important modification to include in patient education programs for those with peptic ulcer disease?
   a. Stop smoking.
   b. Avoid aspirin and NSAIDs.
   c. Reduce the intake of alcohol and caffeine.
   d. Eliminate dairy products, such as milk, from the diet.

5. The patient's typical posture in acute pancreatitis is:
   a. Left lateral position with knees flexed
   b. Supine with head elevated to 45 degrees
   c. Prone with head flat
   d. Sitting with upper body bent forward

6. An objective physical finding in patients with acute pancreatitis is:
   a. Cullen's sign
   b. Murphy's sign
   c. McBurney's sign
   d. Homans' sign

7. Which of the following is NOT included in the treatment of acute pancreatitis?
   a. Nothing by mouth
   b. Nasogastric suction to relieve vomiting and abdominal distention
   c. Proton pump inhibitors and H_2 blockers
   d. Total parenteral nutrition may be needed in severe cases when the patient takes nothing by mouth for a longer period.

8. Which analgesic is NOT given to patients with acute pancreatitis?
   a. Codeine
   b. Aspirin
   c. Morphine
   d. Meperidine

9. Which of the following is true regarding the diagnosis of irritable bowel syndrome?
   a. Fever is a predominant sign.
   b. Patients are usually awakened by nocturnal pain.
   c. Crampy pain and constipation are the most common symptoms.
   d. Anorexia and weight loss commonly accompany this disorder.

10. Older patients with abdominal disorders are usually more difficult to diagnose and treat because they usually present with:
    a. Pain so severe that abdominal palpation is not possible
    b. Vague symptoms and often little or no abdominal pain
    c. Higher fever and leukocytosis, and greater degree of dehydration
    d. Increased tendency to bleed, requiring transfusion immediately

11. If acute diverticulitis is suspected, the best and safest diagnostic approach is to order:
    a. Lower endoscopy
    b. Barium enema
    c. Abdominal and pelvic computed tomography with contrast
    d. Flat and upright abdominal x-rays

12. Treatment for gastroesophageal reflux disease occurs in phases. Phase II therapy consists of:
    a. Lifestyle changes
    b. Drug therapy
    c. Maintenance drug therapy
    d. Palliative therapy

13. The direct cause of esophageal varices is:
    a. Alcohol abuse
    b. Cirrhosis of the liver
    c. Portal hypertension
    d. Hepatitis

14. Crohn's disease, one of the two major forms of nonspecific inflammatory bowel disease, affects:
    a. All parts of the gastrointestinal tract (mouth to anus)
    b. Only the rectum
    c. The sigmoid colon
    d. The descending colon

15. When ulcerative colitis is confined to the rectum, which one of the following signs or symptoms is NOT present?
    a. Constipation
    b. Urgency
    c. Tenesmus
    d. Diarrhea

16. Vegetarians are less likely to develop:
    a. Diverticulosis
    b. Crohn's disease
    c. Ulcerative colitis
    d. Irritable bowel syndrome

17. The hallmark of painful diverticular disease is:
    a. An inflammatory process
    b. Constipation
    c. Abdominal pain without evidence of inflammation
    d. Pain that dissipates on eating

18. In which type of pancreatitis are histologic changes irreversible?
    a. Acute pancreatitis
    b. Chronic pancreatitis
    c. Recurrent acute pancreatitis
    d. Pancreatitis due to biliary tract disease

19. Pain can begin suddenly or gradually. The pain of cancer of the colon develops:
    a. Suddenly, in the early stages of the disease
    b. Gradually, in the early stages of the disease
    c. Gradually, in the later stages of the disease
    d. Suddenly, in the later stages of the disease

20. Difficulty swallowing (dysphagia) occurs with many systemic disorders. Which one of the following conditions is associated with difficulty in initiating swallowing?
    a. Ring or diverticulum of the esophagus
    b. Stricture of the esophagus
    c. Myasthenia gravis
    d. Motility disorder

21. Which patients with abdominal pain require detailed evaluation?
    a. Infants and young children
    b. Adolescents
    c. Men ages 35 to 45
    d. Both men and women ages 55 to 80

22. Visceral pain results from:
    a. Tumors of the mesentery
    b. Hyperesthesia
    c. Spasm or stretching of the wall of a hollow viscus
    d. Involvement of the spinal root (e.g., herpes zoster, arthritis)

23. Abdominal pain may be associated with all but one of the following. Which one is NOT a cause of abdominal pain?
    a. Inflammation
    b. Enlarging tumors
    c. Hyperlipidemia
    d. Familial Mediterranean fever

24. Restlessness and pacing often indicate pain from:
    a. Arthritis
    b. Gallbladder
    c. Appendicitis
    d. Kidney stones

25. Achalasia occurs as a result of:
    a. Emotional stress
    b. Inability of a muscle to relax and complete peristalsis
    c. Stretching of a section of the upper gastrointestinal tract
    d. Cancer of the larynx

26. The preferred diagnostic test for diffuse esophageal spasm is:
    a. Barium swallow
    b. Computed tomography scan of the upper gastrointestinal tract
    c. Magnetic resonance imaging of the upper gastrointestinal tract
    d. Videoesophagram

27. One of the risk factors for gastroesophageal reflux disease is:
    a. A low basal lower esophageal sphincter pressure
    b. A high basal lower esophageal sphincter pressure
    c. Decreased peristalsis
    d. Episodes of lower esophageal sphincter contraction

28. The percentage of patients with cirrhosis who have esophageal varices is:
    a. 10%
    b. 20%
    c. 35%
    d. 50%

29. In duodenal ulcer, the pain:
    a. Occurs only at night
    b. Is constant
    c. Is not present in the morning on awakening
    d. Is not relieved by food

30. Hemorrhoids:
    a. Are not varicosities of the rectal venous plexus
    b. Are not associated with anal cushions
    c. Are caused by proximal displacement of anal tissues
    d. Found during a routine examination require immediate treatment

peptic
dug

8

Kidney and Urologic Disorders

197 —
218

THE KIDNEY

- The kidneys' primary functions include the following (Box 8-1):
  —To eliminate fluid waste material from the body
  —To regulate the volume and composition of body fluid

RENAL DISEASE

Signs and symptoms may be discovered incidentally during a routine examination
- Hypertension
- Edema
- Nausea
- Hematuria
  Patient evaluation should include the following:
- Estimate of duration of signs and symptoms
- Determination of whether the disease is acute (hours to days) or chronic, necessary for diagnosis, treatment, and prognosis
  —Acute deterioration of renal function often results in retention of nitrogenous wastes (e.g., urea nitrogen) and creatinine in the blood, which is the condition known as *azotemia*.
    ~ Anemia from low renal erythropoietin production is rare in acute renal failure.
    ~ Normal size kidneys are usually present.
  —Chronic renal failure results from loss of renal function over months or even years.
    ~ Oliguria is unusual in chronic renal insufficiency.
    ~ Small kidneys are more commonly seen with chronic renal failure, although normal size kidneys are most often present.

- Careful urinalysis
  —Midstream clean-catch or catheterized specimen
  —Dipstick examination; if positive, a microscopic examination
    ~ Specific gravity
    ~ pH
    ~ Protein
    ~ Hemoglobin
    ~ Glucose
    ~ Ketones
    ~ Bilirubin
    ~ Nitrites
    ~ Leukocyte esterase
  —Microscopic exam includes the following:
    ~ Crystals
    ~ Cells
    ~ Casts (Table 8-1)
    ~ Organisms
- Assess the glomerular filtration rate (GFR).

BOX 8-1
Functions of the Kidney

EXCRETORY
Excretion of waste products, drugs

REGULATORY
Control body fluid volume and composition

ENDOCRINE
Produce erythropoietin, renin, prostaglandins

METABOLIC
Metabolize vitamin D, small-molecular-weight proteins

TABLE 8-1
Significance of Specific Urinary Casts

Type	Significance
Hyaline casts	Concentrated urine, febrile disease, after strenuous exercise, during diuretic therapy (does not indicate renal disease)
Red blood cell casts	Glomerulonephritis
White blood cell casts	Pyelonephritis, interstitial nephritis (indicates infection or inflammation)
Renal tubular cell casts	Acute tubular necrosis; interstitial nephritis
Coarse, granular casts	Nonspecific; may indicate acute tubular necrosis
Broad, waxy casts	Chronic renal failure (indicates stasis in collecting tubules)

From Watnick S, Morrison G: Kidney. In Tierney LM, McPhee SJ, Papadakis MA, eds: *Current medical diagnosis & treatment 2000,* ed 39, New York, 2000, Lange Medical Books/McGraw-Hill, p 887.

PROTEINURIA
Definition

Proteinuria is a clinical marker indicating that an underlying renal abnormality exists.

- Four major reasons for proteinuria to develop
  - Functional proteinuria from physiologic and psychologic stressors (e.g., acute illness, exercise, emotional stress), or in young people (under age 30), orthostatic proteinuria, in which abnormal amounts of protein are excreted only when the patient is standing
  - Overproduction of circulating, filterable plasma proteins (e.g., Bence Jones proteins associated with multiple myeloma)
  - Glomerular proteinuria is caused by abnormalities in the glomerular basement membrane (GBM) or by changes in the glomerular capillary pressure; all glomerular diseases exhibit some degree of proteinuria.
  - Tubular proteinuria is caused by damaged reabsorption of normally filtered proteins in the proximal tubule (e.g., tubular necrosis, toxic injury, hereditary metabolic disorders such as Wilson's disease and Fanconi's syndrome).
- If the cause of proteinuria is renal or systemic disease, other abnormal measures exist: elevated blood urea nitrogen (BUN) and serum creatinine levels, abnormal urinary sediment, or signs and symptoms such as fever, rash, or vasculitis.
- Dipstick reading depends on many factors.
  - Normal is any measure under 150 mg/24 hour.
  - Whether urine is concentrated or dilute
  - Whether urine is from a 24-hour sample, which is the only reliable way to measure protein in urine
  - Presence of nephrotic syndrome, in which protein excretion is more than 3.5 g/24 hr and has important clinical implications

Treatment

- Underlying disorder, if known, is treated.
- Angiotensin-converting enzyme (ACE) inhibitors are often effective by lowering efferent arteriolar resistance out of proportion to afferent arteriolar resistance, thus reducing glomerular capillary pressure and lowering urinary protein excretion.
  - These are not used in patients whose GFRs are markedly impaired, in whom they may cause renal failure and hyperkalemia.

HEMATURIA

- Hematuria is significant if there are more than three to five red blood cells (RBCs) per high-powered field (HPF).
- A false-positive reading may result from the presence of vitamin C, beets, rhubarb, and myoglobin.
- Transient hematuria, particularly in those under age 40, is not significant.
- Hematuria is due to either renal or extrarenal causes.
- Renal causes account for 10% of cases, and are classified as either glomerular or nonglomerular.
  - Extraglomerular causes
    - ~ Cysts
    - ~ Calculi

TABLE 8-2
Conditions Affecting Serum Creatinine Independent of GFR

Condition	Mechanism
CONDITIONS CAUSING ELEVATION	
Ketoacidosis	Noncreatinine chromogen
Cephalothin, cefoxitin	Noncreatinine chromogen
Other drugs: aspirin, cimetidine, trimethoprim	Inhibition of tubular creatinine secretion
CONDITIONS CAUSING DECREASE	
Advanced age	Physiologic decrease in muscle mass
Cachexia	Pathologic decrease in muscle mass
Liver disease	Decreased hepatic creatine synthesis and cachexia

From Watnick S, Morrison G: Kidney. In Tierney LM, McPhee SJ, Papadakis MA, eds: *Current medical diagnosis & treatment 2000,* ed 39, New York, 2000, Lange Medical Books/McGraw-Hill, p 888.

~ Interstitial nephritis
~ Renal neoplasia
—Glomerular causes
  ~ IgA nephropathy
  ~ Thin GBM disease
  ~ Postinfectious glomerulonephritis
  ~ Membranoproliferative glomerulonephritis (MPGN)
  ~ Systemic nephritic syndromes

ESTIMATION OF GLOMERULAR FILTRATION RATE

• The GFR gives a useful index of overall renal function.
  —The GFR measures the amount of plasma ultrafiltered across the glomerular capillaries and correlates well with the ability of the kidneys to filter fluids and various substances.
    ~ The GFR in normal persons is variable, ranging from 150 to 250 L/24 hour, or 100 to 120 ml/min/1.73 m^2 of body surface area.
    ~ The GFR decreases progressively in both acute and chronic renal diseases.
    ~ A low GFR indicates serious progressive renal disease and diminished total functioning renal mass.
• The GFR can be measured by determining the renal clearance of plasma substances that are not bound to plasma proteins, that are freely filterable across the glomerulus, and that are not selected or reabsorbed along the renal tubules.
  —The formula to determine renal clearance is

$$C = \frac{U \times V}{P}$$

  C = clearance
  U and P = the urine and plasma concentrations of the substance (mg/dl)
  V = urine flow rate (ml/min)
  —In clinical practice, the clearance rate of endogenous creatinine, the creatinine clearance (C_{cr}), is the usual method used for estimating GFR.
• Creatinine is a product of muscle metabolism that is produced at a relatively constant rate and cleared by renal excretion (Table 8-2 and Box 8-2).
  —Creatinine is freely filterable by the glomerulus and not reabsorbed by the renal tubules.
  —With stable renal function, creatinine production and excretion are equal, and plasma creatinine concentrations remain constant.
• Limitations in the creatinine clearance test regarding GFR rate
  —A small amount is normally eliminated by tubular secretion; the amount increases as GFR declines, resulting in overestimation of GFR.
  —In severe renal failure, intestinal microorganisms degrade creatinine.
  —A person's meat intake and muscle mass affect baseline plasma creatinine levels.

BOX 8-2

Conditions Affecting BUN Independently of GFR

INCREASED BUN
Reduced effective circulating blood volume
(prerenal azotemia)
Catabolic states
High-protein diets
Gastrointestinal bleeding
Glucocorticoids
Tetracycline

DECREASED BUN
Liver disease
Malnutrition
Sickle cell anemia

From Watnick S, Morrison G: Kidney. In Tierney LM, McPhee SJ, Papadakis MA, eds: *Current medical diagnosis & treatment 2000,* ed 39, New York, 2000, Lange Medical Books/McGraw-Hill, p 889.

—Drugs (e.g., cimetidine, probenecid, trimethoprim) reduce tubular secretion of creatinine, increasing the renal dysfunction.
—Accurate measurement of creatinine clearance requires a stable plasma concentration over a 24-hour period; during development of and recovery from acute renal failure, the C_{cr} is often not reliable.
• A 24-hour urine collection is necessary for measurement of GFR based on output in urine; Cockcroft and Gault developed a measure of GFR based on plasma creatinine levels, using age, gender, and weight figures in the formula:

$$C_{cr} = \frac{(140 - age) \times weight\ (kg)}{P_{cr} \times 72}$$

—In women, the estimated GFR is 15% less than for men because they have less muscle mass.

IMAGING STUDIES
Radionuclide Studies
• Indicators for renography are
—To measure function and flow
—To determine the contribution of each kidney to overall renal function
—To demonstrate the presence or absence of functioning renal tissue in mass lesions

—To detect obstruction
—To evaluate renovascular disease
• Measure renal function
—Technetium diethylenetriamine pentaacetic acid (^{99m}Tc-DTPA) is freely filtered by the glomerulus and not reabsorbed, and is used to estimate GFR.
—Technetium dimercaptosuccinate (^{99m}Tc-DMSA) is bound to tubules and provides an assessment of functional renal mass.
—Radioiodinated (^{131}I) orthoiodohippurate is secreted into the renal tubules and assesses renal plasma flow (RPF).

Ultrasonography
• Ultrasonography provides noninvasive kidney imaging.
—It identifies the renal cortex, medulla, pyramids, and a distended collection system or ureter.
—It determines kidney size; a kidney less than 9 cm in length indicates significant irreversible renal disease.
—A difference in size of more than 1.5 cm between the two kidneys is seen in unilateral kidney disease.
—It is performed to screen for hydronephrosis, characterize renal mass lesions, screen for autosomal dominant polycystic kidney disease, evaluate the perirenal space, localize the kidney for a percutaneous invasive procedure, and assess post-voiding bladder residual.

Intravenous Urography
• The intravenous pyelogram (IVP) has been for many years the standard imaging procedure for evaluating the urinary tract because it provides an assessment of the kidneys, ureters, and bladder.
—IVP is done to obtain a detailed view of the pelvicaliceal system, assess renal size and shape, detect and localize renal stones, and assess renal function.
~ Ultrasonography has replaced IVP in many clinical situations.
—The dye is filtered and secreted by the renal tubules in normal kidneys, resulting in a nephrogram formed by opacification of the renal parenchyma.

—The density of the nephrogram depends on the GFR.

—The IVP can show differential function between the two kidneys by the rate of appearance of the nephrogram phase.

—The IVP is contraindicated in patients at high risk of developing renal failure.

~ Diabetes mellitus with serum creatinine > 2 mg/dl

~ Severe volume contraction

~ Prerenal azotemia

~ Chronic renal failure with serum creatinine > 5 mg/dl

~ Multiple myeloma

Computed Tomography

- Computed tomography (CT) is required for further investigation of abnormalities detected by ultrasound or IVP.

—Ordinarily the study requires radiographic contrast administration; however, if only demonstration of hemorrhage or calcification is required, no contrast is needed.

—Contrast is filtered by the glomeruli and concentrated in the tubules, which enhances the parenchymal tissue, making abnormalities such as cysts or neoplasms easily identified and allowing good visualization of renal vessels and ureters.

—CT is particularly useful in evaluating solid or cystic lesions in the kidney or the retroperitoneal space, if ultrasound results are less than optimal.

Magnetic Resonance Imaging

- Magnetic resonance imaging (MRI) easily distinguishes the renal cortex from the medulla.

—Loss of corticomedullary function, found in many disorders (e.g., glomerulonephritis, hydronephrosis, renovascular occlusion, renal failure), is evident in MRI.

—For some solid lesions, MRI is superior to CT scan.

—MRI is used in addition, or alternatively, to CT for staging renal cell cancer, and as a substitute for CT in evaluating renal masses, particularly in patients with tumors in whom contrast is contraindicated.

—MRI, in addition, images the adrenal glands very well.

Arteriography and Venography

- These are useful tools to evaluate atherosclerosis or fibrodysplastic stenotic lesions, aneurysms, vasculitis, and renal mass lesions; venography is used to diagnose renal vein thrombosis.

ACUTE RENAL FAILURE
Definition

In acute renal failure the kidneys are unable to excrete wastes, concentrate urine, or conserve electrolytes; acute renal failure is characterized by oliguria and a rapid accumulation of nitrogenous wastes in the blood (azotemia).

Etiology

- The most common cause of acute renal failure is prerenal azotemia due to renal hypoperfusion.
- Hypoperfusion is caused by decreased intravascular volume, change in vascular resistance, and low cardiac output; causes of volume depletion include hemorrhage, gastrointestinal (GI) losses, dehydration, excessive diuresis, extravascular space sequestration, pancreatitis, trauma, burns, toxic injury, pyelonephritis or glomerulonephritis, and lower urinary tract obstruction.
- Low cardiac output is a state of effective hypovolemia that occurs in cardiogenic shock, congestive heart failure, pulmonary embolus, and pericardial tamponade.

Classification

- Acute renal failure is divided into three categories: prerenal azotemia, intrinsic renal failure, and postrenal azotemia.

Diagnosis
Signs and Symptoms
- Sudden increase in BUN or serum creatinine
- Oliguria
- Nausea, vomiting, malaise, altered sensorium, pericardial effusion that may lead to cardiac tamponade, or pericardial friction rub caused by azotemia
- Possible altered fluid homeostasis
- Hypovolemia that may occur in prerenal failure
- Hypervolemia that may occur in intrinsic renal failure or postrenal failure
- Dysrhythmias that occur with hyperkalemia

- Pulmonary crackles resulting from hypervolemia
- Abdominal pain and ileus
- Platelet dysfunction leading to bleeding
- Encephalopathy with asterixis and confusion
- Seizures from fluid and electrolyte abnormalities
- Tetany and perioral paresthesias that may occur from hypocalcemia caused by retention of phosphates

Laboratory Findings
- Elevated BUN and creatinine
- Hyperkalemia due to impaired potassium excretion
- Anion gap metabolic acidosis due to decreased organic acid clearance
- Hyperphosphatemia caused by inability of damaged tubules to secrete phosphorus
- Hypocalcemia occurring with metastatic calcium phosphate deposition
- Anemia
- Impaired erythropoiesis occurring as a result of prolonged acute renal failure

Treatment
Prerenal Azotemia
- Treat the underlying disorder: assess volume status, drug use, cardiac function.
  —Electrolyte imbalances
  —Fluid balance to correct retention or dehydration
  —Determination of cardiac problems that affect total body fluid: cardiac output, tamponade
- Rapid correction of GFR allows full correction of renal function within 1 to 2 days.

Postrenal Azotemia
- Postrenal azotemia is the least common cause of acute renal failure (5% of cases).
  —It occurs when urinary flow from both kidneys is obstructed, caused by lower urinary tract obstruction (ureters, bladder, renal pelvis) or bladder dysfunction.
    ~ Patients may be anuric or polyuric, and complain of lower abdominal pain.

Laboratory Findings
- Laboratory tests may show high urine osmolality, low urine sodium, high BUN:creatinine ratios, low fractional excretion of sodium (FE_{Na}).
  ~ These values are the same as in prerenal azotemia because intrinsic renal failure has not occurred.
  ~ After several days, the urine sodium increases as the kidneys fail and are unable to concentrate the urine.

Intrinsic Renal Failure
- Intrinsic (parenchymal) renal disorders account for 40% to 45% of all cases of acute renal failure.
  —This state is considered after prerenal and postrenal causes have been excluded.
    ~ Primary sites of injury are tubules, interstitium, vasculature, and glomeruli.

Treatment
- Treatment may include dialysis if the intrinsic condition cannot be treated successfully.
  —Life-threatening electrolyte disturbances (e.g., hyperkalemia)
  —Volume overload unresponsive to diuresis
  —Life-threatening acidosis
  —Uremic complications (e.g., encephalopathy, pericarditis, seizures)

Patient/Family Education
- Instruct the patient regarding the nature, cause, usual course, treatment, and expected outcome of treatment.
- Indicate that hospitalization and treatment may be longer than expected, depending on response to therapy.
- Explain the reasons for all medications, procedures, what to expect, and outcomes.
- Before discharge, complete instructions in writing should be given regarding diet, fluid intake, activity, signs and symptoms to watch for that indicate recurrence of renal failure, and telephone numbers to reach the physician, nephrologist, or urologist.

Follow-up/Referral
- Patients with a history of renal failure are followed closely after discharge.
- A nephrologist will have followed the patient while in the hospital and will continue to do so after discharge.
- Return visits are scheduled before discharge.

- Transportation is provided if necessary, to enable the patient to make return visits on schedule.

CHRONIC RENAL FAILURE
Definition
Chronic renal failure (CRF) is the clinical condition resulting from chronic derangement and insufficiency of renal excretory and regulatory function (uremia).

Risk Factors
- Long-standng diabetes mellitus
- History of kidney disease
- Long-standing hypertension

Etiology (Box 8-3)
Pathogenesis
- The functional effects of CRF are
  —Diminished renal reserve
  —Renal insufficiency (failure)
  —Uremia

- The concept of renal functional adaptation underlies the fact that a loss of 75% of renal tissue results in a fall in GFR to only 50% of normal.
- Homeostasis is preserved at the expense of some hormonal adaptations (e.g., secondary hyperparathyroidism, intrarenal changes in glomerulotubular balance).
- Plasma concentration of creatinine and urea, which are highly dependent on glomerular filtration, begins to rise as the GFR declines.
- For substances that are excreted primarily through distal nephron secretion (e.g., potassium), adaptation usually produces a normal plasma concentration until advanced failure occurs.
- Despite a diminishing GFR, sodium and water balance is well maintained by increased fractional excretion of sodium and a normal response to thirst.
- Imbalances may occur if sodium and water are very restricted or if intake is excessive.

BOX 8-3
Major Causes of Chronic Renal Failure

GLOMERULOPATHIES
Primary Glomerular Diseases
IgA nephropathy
Focal glomerulosclerosis
Membranous nephropathy
Membranoproliferative glomerulonephritis
Idiopathic crescentic glomerulonephritis
Glomerulopathies Associated with Systemic Disease
Diabetes mellitus
Postinfectious glomerulonephritis
SLE
Wegener's granulomatosis
Hemolytic-uremic syndrome
Amyloidosis

CHRONIC TUBULOINTERSTITIAL NEPHROPATHIES
Drug-induced hypersensitivity nephritis
Systemic infections
Pyelonephritis (acute bacterial, fungal, viral)
Drug-induced nephrotoxicity
Immunologic reactions
Metabolic diseases
Acute obstructive uropathies
Idiopathic

HEREDITARY NEPHROPATHIES
Polycystic kidney disease
Alport's syndrome
Medullary cystic disease
Nail-patella syndrome

HYPERTENSION
Nephroangiosclerosis
Malignant glomerulosclerosis

RENAL MACROVASCULAR DISEASE
MACROVASCULAR DISEASE (VASCULOPATHY OF RENAL ARTERIES AND VEINS)

OBSTRUCTIVE UROPATHY
Ureteral obstruction (congenital, calculi, malignancies)
Vesicoureteral reflux
Benign prostatic hyperplasia

From Beers MH, Berkow R, eds: Genitourinary disorders. *The Merck manual of diagnosis and therapy,* ed 17, Whitehouse Station, NJ, 1999, Merck & Co, Inc, p 1845.

Diagnosis

Signs and Symptoms

- With mildly diminished renal reserve, patients are asymptomatic and renal dysfunction is detected only by laboratory testing.
- Those with mild to moderate renal insufficiency may have vague symptoms despite elevated BUN and creatinine levels.
- Nocturia occurs due to failure to concentrate the urine during the night.
- Lassitude, fatigue, and decreased mental acuity are often the first signs of uremia.
- Neuromuscular signs include coarse muscular twitches, peripheral neuropathies with sensory and motor phenomena, muscle cramps, and convulsions (usually caused by hypertensive or metabolic encephalopathy).
- Anorexia
- Nausea and vomiting
- Stomatitis
- Unpleasant taste in the mouth
- Malnutrition that causes wasting is frequently present in chronic uremia.
- GI ulcers with bleeding are common.
- More than 80% of patients in advanced CRF have hypertension, a result of hypervolemia and, in some cases, activation of the renin-angiotensin-aldosterone system.
- Hypertension and ischemia result in cardiomyopathy and retention of sodium and water in the kidneys, usually resulting in congestive heart failure and edema (pedal or sacral, depending on position of the patient).
- Pericarditis, often present in chronic uremia, may occur in acute uremia as well.
- Skin color may be yellow-brown.
- Urea may collect in all body fluids, including sweat, and then crystallize on the skin as "uremic frost."
- Pruritus may be a prominent, very uncomfortable, symptom.
- Renal osteodystrophy, which occurs as a result of dialysis in up to 60% of patients, is an abnormal bone mineralization caused by hyperparathyroid function, calcitriol deficiency, or elevated serum phosphorus.
- Abnormal lipid metabolism also occurs with CRF in patients being dialyzed and following renal transplantation.

Diagnostic Tests

- Tests are needed to differentiate between acute, chronic, or acute superimposed on chronic renal failure.
- Progression to CRF is predictable when serum creatinine concentration is > 1.5 to 2 mg/dl.
- Diagnosis becomes more difficult as the patient develops end-stage renal disease.
- Renal biopsy is the definitive diagnostic procedure, but is not done if the patient has small, fibrotic kidneys.
- Urea and creatinine are elevated.
- Plasma sodium concentration may be normal or decreased.
- Serum potassium is normal or perhaps slightly increased, except when potassium-sparing diuretics, ACE inhibitors, β-blockers, or angiotensin receptor blockers are prescribed.
- Other signs that are usually present are abnormal serum calcium, phosphorus, and parathyroid hormone (PTH) levels, vitamin D metabolism, renal osteodystrophy, hypocalcemia, hyperphosphatemia, moderate acidosis, and anemia (normochromic, normocytic). Hematocrit in CRF patients is 20% to 50%, but in patients with polycystic kidney disease it may be 35% to 50%.
- Urinary volume does not respond readily to variable water intake, and urinary osmolality remains close to that of plasma (300 to 320 mOsm/kg).
- Broad, wax-like casts are often present in the urine of patients with advanced renal insufficiency.

Treatment

- Underlying problems that aggravate or cause CRF should be treated specifically: sodium and water depletion, nephrotoxins, heart failure, infection, hypercalcemia, obstruction.
- The progression of CRF does not usually respond to any treatment.
  - If uremia develops, treatment is palliative until decisions are made regarding dialysis or transplantation.
- Nutrition is critical for patients with CRF, especially as it progresses to end-stage renal failure.
  - Sufficient carbohydrate and fat are required to minimize endogenous protein catabolism and prevent ketosis.

—A mixed-protein diet that includes low-quality protein enhances patients' acceptance.

—Daily protein loss must be considered, but decreased protein catabolism and urea generation lessen symptoms such as fatigue, nausea and vomiting, muscle twitching, and confusion; however, there is little to no effect on continued GFR reduction.

—Water-soluble vitamin supplements should be taken daily.

—Sodium intake should not be limited except in cases of hypertension or edema.

—Hyperkalemia is not common, and potassium supplements are usually not needed.

—In early renal failure, dietary phosphorus delays secondary hyperparathyroidism.

—In patients with no signs of hyperparathyroidism, oral calcitriol may be given to prevent hypocalcemia that may occur despite high oral calcium intake.

- Chronic metabolic acidosis can be treated with sodium bicarbonate 2 g/day to decrease symptoms—anorexia, dyspnea, and fatigue—but it is discontinued as symptoms improve.
- Anemia is treated to maintain the hematocrit between 30% and 36%.
- Congestive heart failure, usually due to sodium and water retention, responds to sodium restriction and diuretics.

—Diuretics such as furosemide are effective, even when renal function is markedly reduced.

—If left ventricular function is depressed, angiotensin-converting enzyme (ACE) inhibitors are used.

—If reduction of the extracellular fluid (ECF) does not lower blood pressure (BP), antihypertensive drugs may be used short-term, which may increase azotemia and may require temporary dialysis.

- Pruritus usually responds to ultraviolet phototherapy.
- Activity is not restricted; the patient's level of fatigue maintains it at an acceptable level.

Prognosis

- Prognosis is variable, depending on patient response to therapy and status of the kidneys.
- Generally, patients can be maintained at functional levels for some time.

- End-stage renal disease is fatal, unless the decision is made for long-term dialysis or transplantation.

Patient/Family Education

- The patient and family must be kept informed about the patient's status, therapy in place or under consideration, and prognosis at any particular time.
- Members of the health care team need to be consistent in encouraging the patient to remain interested in his family, his therapy, and his day-to-day triumphs.
- The patient's comfort is paramount, and family members can be instructed about ways to provide comfort measures (e.g., change of position, getting into and out of chair or bed).

GLOMERULONEPHRITIS
Definition

Glomerulonephritis is an inflammation of the glomerulus of the kidney.

Etiology/Classification

- Antineutrophil cytoplasmic antibody (ANCA)–associated: crescentic glomerulonephritis, polyarteritis nodosa, Wegener's granulomatosis
- Antiglomerular basement membrane (anti-GBM) glomerulonephritis: Goodpasture's syndrome
- Immunocomplex: lupus glomerulonephritis, postinfectious glomerulonephritis, cryoglobulinemic glomerulonephritis

Pathophysiology

- Inflammatory glomerular lesions are seen (in order of increasing severity):
  —Mesangio-proliferative
  —Focal and diffuse proliferative
  —Crescentic lesions
- The larger the percentage of glomeruli involved and the more severe the lesions, the more likely it is that the patient will have a poor clinical outcome.
- Immunecomplex deposition occurs when moderate antigen excess over antibody production occurs.
  —Complexes formed with marked antigen excess tend to remain in the circulation.

—Antibody excess with large antigen-antibody aggregates usually causes phagocytosis and clearance of the precipitates by the mononuclear phagocytic system in the liver and spleen.
—Causes include immunoglobulin A (IgA) nephropathy (Berger's disease), peri- or post-infectious glomerulonephritis, lupus nephritis, cryoglobulinemic glomerulonephritis (often associated with hepatitis C virus), and MPGN.

Diagnosis

Signs and Symptoms
- Nephritic syndrome
  —Hypertension
  —Edema
  —Abnormal urinary sediment
- Hematuria, dysmorphic RBCs, RBC casts, mild proteinuria
- Acute renal insufficiency

Laboratory Findings
- Dipstick and microscopic evaluation reveal
  —Hematuria
  —Moderate proteinuria (<2 g/day)
  —Cellular elements (e.g., RBCs, white blood cells [WBCs], casts)
- Twenty-four–hour urine protein excretion and creatinine clearance quantify the amount of proteinuria and document the degree of renal dysfunction.
  —If renal tubules are not affected, the FE_{Na} may be normal.
- Urine and serum protein electrophoresis for multiple myeloma and amyloid, complement levels (C3, C4, CH50), antistreptolysin O (ASO) titer, anti-GBM antibody levels, ANCA titers, antinuclear antibody (ANA) titers, cryoglobulin and hepatitis panels, C3 nephritic factor, renal ultrasound, and renal biopsy

Treatment
- High-dose steroids and cytotoxic agents (e.g., cyclophosphamide)
- Plasma exchange is used in Goodpasture's syndrome.

Patient/Family Education
- The patient should be instructed regarding the nature of the illness, its cause, treatment, and expected outcome.

- All medications and procedures should be explained as needed: rationale, duration of therapy or procedure.
- Before discharge, the patient is instructed regarding diet, activity level, medications, and signs and symptoms to watch for that require immediate attention (e.g., hematuria).

Follow-up/Referral
- Patients with a history of acute renal failure are followed closely every few weeks after discharge to monitor renal function, level of wellness, and medications (schedule, dosage, effects).

GLOMERULAR DISORDERS
Definition
Glomerulopathies are a group of diverse disease processes that affect the glomerulus and include glomerulonephritis.
- The major categories are *inflammatory* (nephritic syndrome) and *hemodynamic* (nephrotic syndrome).
- Acute nephritic syndrome is synonymous with acute glomerulonephritis.
- Nephrotic syndrome consists of symptoms, signs, and laboratory findings due to increased glomerular capillary wall permeability.
- Many systemic diseases can cause nephrotic syndrome (e.g., systemic lupus erythematosus [SLE]), and nephritic syndrome and nephrotic syndrome can occur together.

Nephritic Syndrome
Definition
- Nephretic syndrome is characterized by diffuse inflammatory changes in the glomeruli, manifested by sudden onset of hematuria with RBC casts, mild proteinuria, and sometimes hypertension, edema, and azotemia.

Risk Factors
- Recent infection caused by group A β-hemolytic streptococci such as type 12 (associated with pharyngitis) and type 49 (associated with impetigo).

Etiology
- Any such infection can result in poststreptococcal glomerulonephritis (PSGN).
  —The incidence of PSGN is decreasing in developed countries, but it is common

where epidemics of streptococcal infection occur.

- Acute nephritic syndrome may also occur after viral, parasitic, and fungal infections.
  —The clinical and renal manifestations are similar to those of PSGN.
- A wide spectrum of renal problems may manifest, often mimicking other diseases (e.g., polyarteritis nodosa, renal emboli, drug-induced acute interstitial nephritis).
  —SLE glomerulonephritis may occur, but it is more often associated with nephrotic syndrome.

Pathogenesis

- Lesions are usually confined to the glomeruli, which become hypercellular and thus enlarged; neutrophils or eosinophils and, later, mononuclear cells are involved.
- Epithelial cell hyperplasia is common as an early, short-lived sign.
- Microthrombosis may cause severe damage, resulting in hemodynamic changes and producing oliguria.
  —These changes are often accompanied by epithelial crescents, formed within Bowman's space due to epithelial cell hyperplasia and mediated by growth factors from stimulated macrophages.
- Immunofluorescence microscopy generally shows immunocomplex deposition with IgG and C3 nephritic factor in a granular pattern.
- Electron microscopy shows that these deposits are semilunar or hump-shaped, and located in the subepithelial area.
- The presence of these deposits results in a C-mediated inflammatory reaction that leads to glomerular damage.
- The presumption is that the immune complex contains an antigen related to streptococcal organisms, but no such antigen has been found.

Diagnosis

Signs and Symptoms

- About 50% of patients are seen initially with asymptomatic hematuria, along with mild proteinuria.
- Other patients are found to have full-blown nephritis with gross or microscopic hematuria (cola-colored, brown, smoky, or frankly bloody urine), proteinuria, oliguria, edema, hypertension, and renal insufficiency.
- In 10% of adults, acute nephritic syndrome evolves into rapidly progressive (crescentic) glomerulonephritis (RPGN).
- In patients with remittent disease, renal cellular proliferation disappears after several weeks, but the severity of the inflammatory response varies considerably, and residual sclerosis is common.
- In some cases, the patients never fully recover, but continue to have hematuria or proteinuria for years.

Laboratory Findings

- Protein > 0.5 to 2 g/m^2/day may be excreted.
- Urinary protein/creatinine may be <2 (normal: 0.1 to 0.3).
- Casts containing RBCs and hemoglobin are characteristic; WBCs and granular casts (protein droplets) are common.
- Urinary sediment contains dysmorphic RBCs, WBCs, and renal tubular cells.
- The antibody titer against the causative organism usually rises within 1 to 2 weeks.
  —The increase in antibodies to streptococcal antigenic products is measurable.
  —ASO is the best indicator of upper respiratory infections (URIs).
  —Antihyaluronidase and antideoxyribonuclease B indicate pyoderma.
  —C3 and C4 are usually decreased during the active disease; C levels return to normal in 6 to 8 weeks in PSGN patients, but in almost no patients with MPGN.
  —Cryoglobulinemia persists for several months, but circulating immune complexes are present for only a few weeks.
- Tubular function is often deranged by inflammatory changes in the interstitium, resulting in decreased urinary concentrating capacity, acid excretion, and variable disturbances in nephron solute exchange.
  —With continuing glomerular derangement, the total filtration surface is markedly reduced, GFR declines, and azotemia ensues.
  —GFR is estimated based on serum creatinine concentration or urinary creatinine clearance.

—GFR usually returns to normal within 3 months, but proteinuria often persists for 6 to 12 months, and microscopic hematuria for several years.

- In summary, a history of sore throat, impetigo, or culture-proven streptococcal infection 1 to 6 weeks prior to the onset of the syndrome and an elevated serum titer of antistreptococcal antibodies point to the diagnosis of nephritic syndrome.
  —RBC casts are pathognomonic of any glomerulonephritis, but with history and clinical picture in these cases indicate acute nephritic syndrome.

- Ultrasonography can usually differentiate between acute disease (normal or slightly enlarged kidneys) and exacerbation of chronic disease (small kidneys).

Treatment
- Antibiotic therapy of infections before PSGN develops does not seem to prevent it.
- If a bacterial infection is present, antibiotic therapy should be started.
- Immunosuppressive drugs are not effective.
- Corticosteroids may worsen the disease.
- Protein is restricted if azotemia and metabolic acidosis are present.
- Sodium restriction is appropriate only when circulatory overload, edema, or severe hypertension is present.
- Diuretics (e.g., thiazides, loop diuretics) usually help to manage the expanded ECF volume.
- Hypertension requires aggressive treatment.
- Dialysis may be indicated in severe renal failure.

Prognosis
- Outcome depends on the patient's age, type of infection (sporadic or epidemic), and the stage of renal lesion when the inflammatory stimulus is no longer present.
- Prognosis is good if the initial renal damage is not severe and the source of antigenemia can be reduced or eliminated.
- In most patients, signs and symptoms gradually decrease.
- A marked decline in GFR or development of nephrotic syndrome (in about 30% of patients, particularly those with many subepithelial deposits) with extensive crescent

formation and necrosis indicate a likely rapid progression to end-stage renal failure requiring dialysis or kidney transplantation.

Patient/Family Education
- The complex nature of glomerular diseases makes it difficult to be specific with patients and families regarding nature, course, and outcome of the disease process.
- Reassurance that everything will be done that can be done may be helpful.
- Patients usually respond to encouragement and engendering of a positive state of mind.
- Supportive care and comfort measures are essential elements of therapy.
- Instruct the patient and family about nutritional needs and restrictions, rationale for all dietary requirements, and signs and symptoms to look for that may indicate worsening disease and need for hospitalization.

Nephrotic Syndrome

Definition
Nephrotic syndrome is a predictable complex that results from a severe, prolonged increase in glomerular permeability to protein.

Risk Factors/Etiology
- Primary glomerular diseases (e.g., focal segmental glomerulosclerosis)
- Secondary renal disease (e.g., SLE, diabetes mellitus, amyloidosis, Sjögren's syndrome, Henoch-Schönlein purpura, sarcoidosis, serum sickness)
  —Secondary renal diseases also include drug toxicity, allergenic disorders (insect bites, snake venom), infections (bacterial, viral, protozoal, helminthic), inherited conditions (Alport's syndrome), and others such as toxemia of pregnancy, malignant hypertension, and transplant rejection.

Pathogenesis
- Two mechanisms are believed to account for derangements within the kidneys leading to development of heavy proteinuria (>2 g/m^2/day).
  —The size-selective barrier, which leaks large protein molecules
  —The charge-selective barrier, which fails to retain lower molecular-weight proteins

Diagnosis
Signs and Symptoms
- Frothy urine due to protein content
- Anorexia
- Malaise
- Puffy eyelids
- Retinal sheen
- Abdominal pain
- Wasting of muscles
- Anasarca with ascites
- Pleural effusions
- Focal edema, which may cause difficulty breathing due to pleural effusion or laryngeal edema
- Substernal chest pain from pericardial effusion
- Swollen knees (hydrarthrosis)
- Low, normal, or high BP
  —Variable hypertension, depending on the amount of angiotensin II produced
- Oliguria and acute renal failure may develop due to hypovolemia and decreased renal perfusion.

Laboratory and Physical Findings
- Heavy proteinuria
- Urinary creatinine > 2 g/24 hour
- Hypoalbuminemia
- Urine sediment may contain hyaline, granular, fatty, waxy, and epithelial cell casts.
- Lipiduria is measured by Sudan staining of casts containing lipid granules and other evidence of lipids (fatty droplets).
- Urine potassium is generally high when edema is present.
- Blood studies show that the following are low: levels of β- and γ-globulins, other immunoglobulins, adrenocortical and thyroid hormones, transferrin, ASO protein, and C3.
- Lipemia is shown by increased total cholesterol and triglyceride levels.
  —Lipid levels >10 times normal are associated with severe hypoalbuminemia resulting from increased lipid production and decreased elimination.
- Coagulopathies are common, probably resulting from urinary loss of factors IX and XII, thrombotic factors (urokinase and antithrombin III), and increased serum levels of factor VIII, fibrinogen, and platelets.

Treatment
- Treatment depends on the underlying pathogenetic processes and on the renal pathology.
- Supportive treatment includes a diet that contains about 1 g/kg/d of high-quality biologic protein that is low in saturated fat and cholesterol, but high in fiber; frequent, small meals may be better tolerated.
- Protein restriction is carried out only if the patient is malnourished, or if serum creatinine is elevated and excessive protein intake exacerbates proteinuria.
- Hypolipidemic statin drugs may be ordered to lower cholesterol.
- ACE inhibitors usually reduce proteinuria and lipemia, but may exacerbate hyperkalemia in patients with moderate to severe renal dysfunction.
- Hypovolemia is treated with infusion of plasma or albumin as needed.
- Hypertension is treated with ACE inhibitors and diuretics, or other drugs.
- Thrombosis is common; signs and symptoms of deep vein thrombosis (DVT) or pulmonary emboli should be monitored carefully.
  —Prophylactic anticoagulants may be advisable if serum albumin < 2.5 g/dl.
- Infections may be life-threatening and should be treated aggressively.
  —Elimination of infectious antigens may cure nephrotic syndrome.
- Removal of nephrotoxins may result in remission of nephrotic syndrome (nonsteroidal antiinflammatory drugs [NSAIDs], penicillamine, gold).

Prognosis
- Outcome depends on the underlying cause.
- Remission occurs even after 5 years.
- Prognosis is markedly influenced by infection, hypertension, significant azotemia, hematuria, or thromboses in cerebral, pulmonary, peripheral, or renal veins.

Patient/Family Education
- Instruct the patient and family regarding the nature, cause, course, and treatment of nephrotic syndrome and interactions among diseases (e.g., hypertension, diabetes mellitus).

- List signs and symptoms to look for that indicate worsening of the condition and that indicate the need to contact the clinician right away.
- Write out instructions for diet, medications, fluid requirements, exercise and activity, and information pertinent to the specific patient.

URINARY TRACT DISORDERS
Urinary Tract Infections
Definition
A urinary tract infection (UTI) is an infection of one or more structures in the urinary tract. *Escherichia coli* is the organism most commonly seen in UTIs.

- UTI is a frequent cause for patients to visit ambulatory care settings, and is the most common bacterial infection in all age groups.
- All types of bacterial infections can be identified in UTIs, although the normal urinary tract is sterile and very resistant to bacterial colonization.

Incidence/Risk Factors
- UTIs are more common in male infants than in female infants, perhaps because of the greater frequency of congenital anomalies of the urinary tract in male infants; UTIs in neonates are frequently associated with bacteremia.
- Incidence of bacteriuria in young children is quite low, but it increases to about 5% in girls older than 10 years.
- In patients aged 20 to 50 years, UTIs are about 50 times more frequent in women.
  —History of recent UTI
  —Increased sexual activity
  —Use of spermicide and diaphragm
  —Failure to void after intercourse
- Incidence of UTI increases during pregnancy (4% to 6%).
- Incidence is higher among pregnant women who have sickle cell trait (10% to 15%).
- The much lower incidence of UTI in men is attributed to the long male urethra; absence of colonization by bacteria near the meatus; and an antibacterial factor, prostatic antibacterial factor, present in prostatic fluid and markedly diminished in some men with recurrent prostatic infections.
- The incidence increases in both men and women older than 50 years, but the female:male ratio becomes lower due to increased frequency of prostate disease.

Etiology (Box 8-4)
- About 95% of UTIs occur when bacteria ascend to the bladder from a colonized vaginal introitus and urethra, and up the ureter to the kidney.
- *Escherichia coli* is the most common bacterium and accounts for about 80% of community-acquired infections; *Staphylococcus saprophyticus* organisms account for about 10%.
- In hospitalized patients, *E. coli* is identified in about 50% of UTIs. About 40% of cases are attributed to gram-negative organisms: Klebsiella, Proteus, Enterobacter, Serratia.

BOX 8-4
Urinary Tract Pathogens

BACTERIA
Gram-negative
Escherichia coli
Proteus organisms
Klebsiella organisms
Enterobacter organisms
Pseudomonas organisms
Serratia organisms
Anaerobes
Gram-positive
Enterococci
Staphylococcus aureus
Staphylococcus saprophyticus

OTHER ORGANISMS
Parasites
Echinococcus organisms
Schistosoma haematobium or *S. mansoni*
Protozoa
Trichomonas organisms
Yeasts
Candida organisms
Blastomyces organisms
Coccidioides immitis
Acid-fast organisms
Mycobacterium tuberculosis

From Beers MH, Berkow R, eds: Urinary tract infections. *The Merck manual of diagnosis and therapy*, ed 17, Whitehouse Station, NJ, 1999, Merck & Co, Inc, p 1885.

The remaining 10% are due to gram-positive bacterial cocci: *Enterococcus faecalis,* *S. saprophyticus,* and *Staphylococcus aureus.*

—The nosocomial incidence of bacteremia due to UTI is 73/100,000 patients.

- UTIs in men < 50 years are often due to urologic abnormalities.
- Uncomplicated UTI occurs in younger men who have unprotected anal intercourse, are uncircumcised, have unprotected intercourse with a woman whose vagina is colonized with uropathogens, and in those with acquired immunodeficiency syndrome (AIDS) (CD^{4+} T cell count < 200/μl).
- Complicated UTIs occur where there is urologic impairment due to instrumentation or obstruction (anatomic abnormalities, neurogenic dysfunction, calculi, catheterization).
  - —Obstruction alone does not cause UTI; it predisposes to UTI and makes UTI more difficult to eradicate.
  - —There is little evidence to support the views that the direction of wiping after bowel movements, use of oral contraceptives, or use of tampons plays a role in the pathogenesis of UTIs in women.
- Among nuns, bacteriuria is significantly less frequent (0.4% to 1.6%) in those 15 to 54 years of age as compared with sexually active women.

Pathogenesis

Urethritis

- Bacterial infection of the urethra occurs when organisms that gain access to it acutely or chronically colonize the numerous periurethral glands in the bulbous and pendulous portions of the male urethra, and of the entire female urethra.
  - —The organisms most commonly associated with urethritis are: *Chlamydia trachomatis, Neisseria gonorrhoeae,* and herpes simplex.

Diagnosis, signs, and symptoms

- Gradual onset with mild symptoms
- Men usually have a purulent urethral discharge when *N. gonorrhoeae* is the causative organism; a whitish discharge is seen with other types of organisms.

- The major symptoms in women are frequency, dysuria, and pyuria.
- Pain may be associated with passage of urine across inflamed labia.

Cystitis

- In men, bacterial infection of the bladder is often complicated by and results from ascending infection of the urethra or prostate, or occurs secondary to urethral instrumentation.
- In women, cystitis usually follows sexual intercourse.

Diagnosis, signs, and symptoms

- Onset is often sudden, with frequency, urgency, and burning or painful voiding of small amounts.
- Suprapubic and low back pain are common, along with nocturia.
- The presence of gross hematuria indicates bacterial cystitis.
- Patients with an indwelling catheter, or who have a neurogenic bladder, often have no symptoms relating to the bladder.
- Older patients who develop UTIs are usually asymptomatic.

Differential diagnosis

- In women, other common genital infections that cause dysuria need to be ruled out: vulvovaginitis, sexually transmitted diseases (STDs) (e.g., *C. trachomatis, N. gonorrhoeae,* herpes simplex).

Prostatitis

- Reintroduction of infection into the bladder is usually the cause of chronic bacterial prostate infection.

Diagnosis, signs, and symptoms

- Patients who develop acute prostatitis usually have symptoms of fever, chills, urinary frequency, urgency, perineal and low back pain, symptoms of obstruction to micturition, dysuria, nocturia, and sometimes gross hematuria; the prostate gland is swollen, tender, and indurated.
- Urine culture will usually identify the causative organism since acute prostatitis is usually present in tandem with acute cystitis.
- Chronic prostatitis is less evident; patients usually have recurrent bacteremia, low-grade fever, and back or pelvic pain.

Acute Pyelonephritis

- Acute pyelonephritis is bacterial infection of the kidney parenchyma.
- About 20% of community-acquired bacteremias in women are a result of pyelonephritis; however, pyelonephritis is uncommon in men who have a normal urinary tract; in 30% to 50% of women, pyelonephritis occurs via the ascending pathway despite the direction of urine flow and interference of the vesicoureteral junction.
- Most women who develop pyelonephritis have no functional or anatomic defects of the urinary tract.
- Pyelonephritis is common in girls and in pregnant women following instrumentation or bladder catheterization.
- The kidney is usually enlarged due to inflammatory polymorphonuclear cells and edema.
- Infection is patchy beginning in the pelvis and medulla, and extending to the cortex as an enlarging wedge.
- Chronic inflammatory cells appear within a few days; medullary and subcortical abscesses may develop.
- Papillary necrosis may be present in acute pyelonephritis associated with diabetes mellitus, obstruction, sickle cell disease, or analgesic nephropathy.

Diagnosis, signs and symptoms

- Onset is sudden with chills, fever, flank pain, and nausea and vomiting.
- Symptoms of lower tract UTI are common: frequency, dysuria; costovertebral pain is usually present on the affected side.
- A tender, enlarged kidney may sometimes be palpable.
- Pyuria, leukocytosis, and presence of bacilluria on Gram's stain of urine strongly indicate the diagnosis of acute pyelonephritis.
- WBC casts, when present, are pathognomonic of pyelonephritis, but are also seen in glomerulonephritis and tubulointerstitial nephritis.

Differential diagnosis

- Appendicitis, urolithiasis, and (in women) pelvic inflammatory disease, ectopic pregnancy, and ruptured ovarian cyst

Chronic Pyelonephritis (Chronic Infective Tubulointerstitial Nephritis)

- A chronic, patchy, usually bilateral pyogenic infection results in atrophy and calyceal deformity with overlying parenchymal scarring.
- It occurs in patients treated by dialysis or transplantation, and results in end-stage renal failure in 2% to 3% of these patients.
- Renal scars (known also as reflux nephropathy) are caused by reflux of infected urine up the ureters and into the renal parenchyma via the ducts of Bellini at the papillary tips, then spreading outward along the collecting tubules.
- High-pressure reflux caused by obstruction can result in scars at any age.

Diagnosis, signs, and symptoms

- Symptoms such as flank pain are usually inconsistent and vague.
- The history is of great value in making the diagnosis.

Treatment and Prevention

- In women, voiding after sexual intercourse and not using a diaphragm with spermicide are preventive measures against UTI.
- Low-dose oral antimicrobial drugs as prophylaxis virtually eliminate the incidence of recurrent UTIs.
  —Trimethoprim-sulfamethoxazole 40/200 mg PO daily or three times per week.
  —Fluoroquinolone (e.g., ciprofloxacin, norfloxacin, ofloxacin) or nitrofurantoin (macrocrystals) 50 to 100 mg/day.
- Postcoital trimethoprim-sulfamethoxazole or a fluoroquinolone may be effective.
  —If UTI recurs after 6 months of this regimen, the drugs may be continued for 2 to 3 years.
- This prophylactic regimen is effective in postmenopausal women, also, along with estrogen replacement therapy, which significantly reduces the incidence of recurrent UTIs.
- Treatment for UTIs, urethritis, and cystitis
  —Symptoms may disappear without antimicrobial therapy.
  —Some patients treat themselves with water-loading and do not see a clinician.

- In men, trimethoprim-sulfamethoxazole or a fluoroquinolone is given for 10 to 14 days (shorter courses are associated with recurrent infection).
- In symptomatic women, a 3-day course of trimethoprim-sulfamethoxazole or a fluoroquinolone effectively treats acute cystitis and eliminates potential bacterial pathogens in vaginal and GI reservoirs.
  —Single-dose therapy is not recommended because of the rate of recurrence.
  —A longer course of treatment (7 to 14 days) is recommended for those with history of recent UTI, diabetes mellitus, or with symptoms lasting more than 1 week.
- If pyuria without bacteriuria is present in a sexually active woman, a longer course of a tetracycline or sulfonamide is given, since *C. trachomatis* is presumed to be the causative organism.
- Prostatitis is treated with a 10- to 14-day course of trimethoprim-sulfamethoxazole or a fluoroquinolone, but relapses are common due to poor penetration of most antimicrobials and anatomic abnormalities (e.g., calculi).
- Patients with acute pyelonephritis are treated similarly—14 days with oral trimethoprim-sulfamethoxazole or a fluoroquinolone.
  —If signs of septicemia develop, or if the patient cannot retain oral antimicrobials because of nausea and vomiting, the patient requires hospitalization.
- Chronic pyelonephritis without evident obstruction or recurrent acute episodes has not been proven harmful.
  —Repeated courses of antimicrobials or suppressive therapy are not recommended.
  —Underlying conditions (e.g., hypertension, uremia) must be treated as needed.
  —If obstruction cannot be eliminated, or if recurrent UTI is common, long-term antimicrobial therapy is warranted.

Prognosis
- Because of ease of entry, infections of the urinary tract tend to occur frequently and repeatedly.
- Clear, written instructions about how to avoid infections, and measures of self-care to prevent infection, will help to alleviate recurrent infection and to help patients appreciate that much of the onus for prevention rests with them.
- With appropriate therapy to eliminate causative organisms and prevent the entry of new or different organisms, and with clear preventive measures that patients can carry out for themselves, the prognosis is favorable.

Patient/Family Education
- Instruct the patient regarding the nature, cause, course, and treatment of UTIs and related complications (e.g., pyelonephritis).
- Safe sexual practices are imperative for both sexes.
- Other preventive measures should be explained and written in detail to assist the patient to avoid recurrences and risk of more serious sequelae.
- Patients should be given complete written instructions about medications.
- A written list of signs and symptoms that require contact with the clinician should be given, along with the other written instructions.
- Patients with diabetes mellitus, hypertension, or other systemic disease that might influence or interfere with treatment should be given instructions relevant to their situation.

Benign Prostatic Hyperplasia
Definition
Enlargement of the prostate, benign prostatic hyperplasia (BPH) is the most common benign tumor in men.

Incidence/Risk Factors
- It develops in men over age 50.
- Prevalence increases from 20% in men 41 to 50 years old to 50% in those ages 51 to 60, and to over 90% in men over 80 years old.
  —Age is a risk factor.
- At age 55, 25% of men report obstructive voiding symptoms.
- At age 75, 50% of men report a decrease in the force and caliber of the urinary stream.

- Perhaps genetic factors and racial differences may be risk factors, but none of these data are specific.
  - —Those men under age 60 who undergo surgery may have a heritable form of the condition, probably an autosomal dominant trait.
    - ~ First-degree male relatives carry a risk about fourfold above those without the inherited predisposition.

Etiology

- The etiology is not well understood, but it seems to be multifactorial and under endocrine control.
- Two factors are necessary for the development of BPH.
  - —Dihydrotestosterone (DHT)
  - —Aging: the aging prostate becomes more sensitive to androgens.
    - ~ Prostatic growth in aging dogs appears to be related more to a decrease in cell death than to an increase in cell proliferation.
- Laboratory studies suggest several theories.
  - —Stromal-epithelial interactions (stromal cells may regulate growth of epithelial cells or other stromal cells via a paracrine or autocrine mechanism, by secreting growth factors such as basic fibroblast growth factor or transforming growth factor-β).
  - —As the patient ages, stem cells undergo a block in the maturation process, preventing them from entering into programmed cell death (apoptosis).
  - —The impact of aging in animal studies appears to be mediated via estrogen synergism.
    - ~ Research shows a positive correlation between levels of free testosterone and estrogen, and the volume of the gland.

Pathology

- BPH is a hyperplastic process resulting from an increase in cell numbers.
- As BPH nodules in the transition zone enlarge, they compress the outer zones of the prostate, resulting in the formation of a "surgical capsule." This boundary separates the transition zone from the peripheral zone of the gland, and serves as a cleavage plane for open enucleation of the prostate during simple prostatectomy.

Pathophysiology

- Symptoms relate either to the obstructive component (mechanical obstruction or dynamic obstruction) or to the secondary response of the bladder to the outlet resistance.
- As the prostate enlarges, mechanical obstruction results from intrusion into the urethral lumen or bladder neck, causing a higher bladder outlet resistance, although size of the gland on digital rectal examination (DRE) correlates poorly with symptoms.
- The dynamic obstruction component explains the variability of symptoms.
  - —Prostatic stroma is composed of smooth muscle and collagen, and is rich in adrenergic nerve supply.
  - —The level of autonomic stimulation sets a "tone" to the prostatic urethra.
  - —α-Blocker therapy decreases this tone, resulting in a decrease in outlet resistance.

Diagnosis

Signs and Symptoms

- Obstructive or irritative voiding symptoms
  - —Obstructive symptoms: hesitancy, decreased force and caliber of stream, sensation of incomplete emptying of bladder, double voiding (urinating a second time within 2 hours), straining to urinate, postvoid dribbling
  - —Irritative symptoms: urgency, frequency, nocturia
- Enlarged prostate on rectal examination
- Absence of urinary tract infection, neurologic disorder, stricture disease, prostatic or bladder malignancy
- Size and consistency of the prostate: smooth, firm, elastic enlargement of the prostate
- Induration, if detected, may indicate prostatic cancer, requiring further evaluation.

Laboratory Findings

- Urinalysis to rule out infection or hematuria
- Serum creatinine to assess renal function
- Imaging for those with renal insufficiency (10%)

- Serum prostate specific antigen (PSA) is optional, but is included in the initial evaluation.
  —There is much overlap between PSA levels seen in BPH and in prostate cancer, so its use remains controversial.
- Imaging of the upper urinary tract: IVP or renal ultrasound should be done only when concomitant urinary tract disease or complications from BPH (e.g., hematuria, UTI, renal insufficiency, history of stone disease) are present.
- Cystoscopy is not recommended in determining the need for treatment, but may be used to help determine the surgical approach in patients opting for invasive therapy.

Differential Diagnosis
- Urethral stricture
- Bladder neck contracture
- Bladder stone
- Carcinoma of the prostate
- Irritative symptoms possibly mimicked by UTI
- Neurologic disorders

Treatment
The patient has several treatment options from which to choose.
- Absolute surgical indications
  —Refractory urinary retention (failing at least one attempt at catheter removal)
  —Large bladder diverticula
  —Recurrent urinary infection
  —Recurrent gross hematuria
  —Bladder stones
  —Renal insufficiency
- Watchful waiting

Medical Therapy
- α-Blockers (phenoxybenzamine, prazosin, terazosin, doxazosin, tamsulosin)
- 5α-Reductase inhibitors (finasteride) block the conversion of testosterone to dihydrotestosterone.
- Combination therapy of α-blockers and 5α-reductase inhibitors
- Phytotherapy: use of plants or plant extracts (saw palmetto berry, the bark of *Pygeum africanum*, pollen extract, the roots of *Echinacea purpurea*, others); no research data

support the use or define the effects of this therapy.

Surgical Therapy
- Transurethral resection of the prostate (TURP)
- Transurethral incision of the prostate (TUIP)
- Open simple prostatectomy

Minimally Invasive Surgical Therapy
- Laser therapy
- Transurethral electrovaporization of the prostate
- Hyperthermia
- Transurethral needle ablation of the prostate (TUNA)
- High-intensity focused ultrasound (HIFU)
- Intraurethral stents
- Transurethral balloon dilation of the prostate

Patient/Family Education
- Instruct the patient regarding the nature, cause, most likely course of therapy appropriate to his circumstances, disease state, and expected outcomes.
- If there are choices, each one should be explained in detail, its pros and cons, and its appropriateness for the patient.
  —The best treatment for a particular patient is the one to emphasize.
- Enable the patient to make the decision as independently as possible.

Follow-up/Referral
- The patient is followed closely in "watchful waiting," throughout therapy of the type selected.
- Referral to the most experienced surgeon who specializes in urologic surgery, particularly prostate surgery, is carried out appropriately.
- The medical, surgical, and nursing staffs provide maximum support for the patient throughout the therapeutic process.

BIBLIOGRAPHY
Beers MH, Berkow R: Hepatic and biliary disorders. In Beers MH, Berkow R, eds: *The Merck manual of diagnosis and therapy,* ed 17, Whitehouse Station, NJ, 1999, Merck Research Laboratories, pp 343-407.

Briefel GR: Chronic renal insufficiency. In Barker LR, Burton JR, Zieve PD, eds: *Principles of ambulatory medicine*, ed 5, Baltimore, 1999, Williams & Wilkins, pp 576-603.

Kraus ES: Proteinuria. In Barker LR, Burton JR, Zieve PD, eds: *Principles of ambulatory medicine*, ed 5, Baltimore, 1999, Williams & Wilkins, pp 543-548.

Kumar P, Clark M: Liver, biliary tract, and pancreatic diseases. *Clinical medicine*, ed 4, Edinburgh, 1999, WB Saunders, pp 287-352.

Presti JC, Stoller ML, Carroll PR: Urology. In Tierney LM, McPhee SJ, Papadakis MA, eds: *Current medical diagnosis & treatment 2000*, ed 39, New York, 2000, Lange Medical Books/McGraw-Hill, pp 917-958.

Spector DA: Hematuria. In Barker LR, Burton JR, Zieve PD, eds: *Principles of ambulatory medicine*, ed 5, Baltimore, 1999, Williams & Wilkins, pp 549-553.

Spector DA: Urinary stones. In Barker LR, Burton JR, Zieve PD, eds: *Principles of ambulatory medicine*, ed 5, Baltimore, 1999, Williams & Wilkins, pp 565-575.

Vamos S: Recurrent UTIs after prostate cancer treatment, *Clin Rev* 9(10):105-110, 1999.

Watnick S, Morrison G: Kidney. In Tierney LM, McPhee SJ, Papadakis MA, eds: *Current medical diagnosis & treatment 2000*, ed 39, New York, 2000, Lange Medical Books/McGraw-Hill, pp 886-916.

REVIEW QUESTIONS

1. The kidneys' unique system includes which one of the following:
   a. Ultrafiltration of water
   b. Free ultrafiltration of water and particular compounds from the plasma
   c. Production of non-protein-bound compounds
   d. Selective reabsorption

2. In each kidney there are about _____ nephrons.
   a. 1 million
   b. 3 million
   c. 5 million
   d. 7 million

3. The proposed mechanism of urine concentration is called:
   a. The medullary-tubular system
   b. The countercurrent system
   c. The loop of Henle system
   d. The crosscurrent system

4. A decline in the glomerular filtration rate causes:
   a. Increased concentration of fluid within the kidney
   b. Decreased concentration of fluid within the kidney
   c. Decreased functional ability of the kidney
   d. The kidneys to shut down

5. The kidneys have an enormous reserve of renal excretory capability. The serum urea and creatinine do not rise above the normal range until there is a reduction of _____50-60%_____ in the glomerular filtration rate.
   a. 20% to 30%
   b. 40% to 50%
   c. 50% to 60%
   d. 60% to 70%

6. The best way to monitor glomerular filtration rate status is:
   a. Blood urea nitrogen
   b. Serum creatinine
   c. Protein in the urine
   d. Glomerular filtration rate

7. When is measurement of the glomerular filtration rate necessary? *Baseline*
   a. When serum urea and creatinine are elevated
   b. When the patient becomes oliguric
   c. When serum urea and creatinine are normal
   d. When there is proteinuria present

8. The most widely used method to assess glomerular filtration rate is:
   a. Serum urea
   b. Serum creatinine
   c. Level of proteinuria
   d. Creatinine clearance

9. Decreased erythropoietin secretion by the kidneys results in:
   a. Anemia
   b. Polycythemia
   c. Decrease in white blood cells in the blood
   d. Decrease in platelets in the blood

10. In cases of decreased renal perfusion, the administration of nonsteroidal antiinflammatory drugs causes:
    a. An increase in glomerular filtration rate
    b. A reduction in glomerular filtration rate
    c. No change in glomerular filtration rate
    d. Renal failure

11. One of the most common signs of renal disease is:
    a. Increased serum creatinine
    b. Appearance of protein in the urine
    c. Increased serum urea
    d. Anemia

12. Computed tomography of the abdomen (kidneys, ureters, surrounding tissues) is useful for diagnosing:
    a. Urinary calculi
    b. Renal tumors
    c. Tubular disease
    d. Congenital anomalies

13. Microalbuminuria is an early indicator of:
    a. Diabetes mellitus
    b. Hypertensive renal disease
    c. Renal artery stenosis
    d. Diabetic glomerular disease

14. Four types of urinary stones (calculi) are formed. They are uric acid, struvite, cystine, and _____.
    a. Cholesterol
    b. Lipid
    c. Calcium oxalate or calcium phosphate
    d. Double phosphate

15. Patients with one urinary calculus require:
    a. Limited evaluation ↗ fluids
    b. Extensive evaluation
    c. Hospitalization
    d. Shock wave lithotripsy

16. The major factor that prevents development of urinary tract infections is:
    a. The small meatus as entry for organisms
    b. The degree of acidity of the urinary tract
    c. The sterility of the urinary tract
    d. For females, wiping from front to back after voiding or defecating

17. Acute renal failure is categorized as all but one of the following:
    a. Prerenal
    b. Postrenal
    c. Renal
    d. Intrinsic

18. The survival rate of patients with acute renal failure is:
    a. 20%
    b. 30%
    c. 50%
    d. 60%

19. The risk factors for chronic renal failure include all but one of the following:
    a. History of pulmonary emboli
    b. Long-standing diabetes mellitus
    c. Long-standing hypertension
    d. History of kidney disease

20. Tests are needed to differentiate between acute, chronic, or acute superimposed on chronic renal failure. Progression to chronic renal failure is predictable when serum creatinine concentration is greater than:
    a. 0.5 mg/dl
    b. 1.0 mg/dl
    c. 1.5 mg/dl
    d. 2.0 mg/dl   ↗ acid ↓ pH

21. Chronic metabolic acidosis is treated with:
    a. Furosemide
    b. Angiotensin converting enzyme inhibitors
    c. Ultraviolet phototherapy
    d. Sodium bicarbonate

22. Glomerulonephritis is classified by all but one of the following. The one that is NOT a classification group for this condition is:
    a. Immunocomplex
    b. Antiglomerular basement membrane
    c. Antinuclear antibody-associated
    d. Antineutrophil cytoplasmic antibody-associated

23. The most severe inflammatory glomerular lesion is:
    a. Crescentic lesions
    b. Mesangio-proliferative lesion
    c. Focal and diffuse proliferative lesion
    d. Concentric lesion

24. Nephritic syndrome is synonymous with:
    a. Nephrotic syndrome
    b. Acute glomerulonephritis
    c. Systemic lupus erythematosus
    d. Uremia

25. Nephritic syndrome causes which one of the following?
    a. Production of an antigen by the immune complex   NO Ag has been found
    b. Shrinkage of the cells of the glomeruli   Hypercell.
    c. Deposition of immunoglobulin M   NOT hyp
    d. Epithelial cell hyperplasia

26. Patients with acute glomerulonephritis usually (50%) present with the following sign or symptom:
    a. Asymptomatic hematuria
    b. Lancing flank pain
    c. Light-colored urine   caka cala calor
    d. Decreased urine output

27. The organism that accounts for about 80% of urinary tract infections is:
    a. *Staphylococcus aureus*
    b. *Trichomonas* organisms

c. *Escherichia coli*
d. *Candida* organisms
28. Pyelonephritis is a bacterial infection of the:
    a. Ureters
    b. Kidney collecting ducts
    c. Kidney parenchyma
    d. Kidney pelvis
29. Benign prostatic hyperplasia occurs most frequently in men:
    a. Over age 30
    b. Over age 40

c. Over age 50
d. Over age 70
30. The cause of benign prostatic hyperplasia is
    a. Endocrine effect *only* + *others*
    b. Multifactorial
    c. Genetic
    d. Programmed cell death ↓ *in cell death*

Hepatic and Biliary Disorders

JAUNDICE (ICTERUS)

↑ Bilirubin Blood & Skin

Definition

Jaundice is a yellow discoloration of the skin, mucous membranes, and sclerae of the eyes.

- Bilirubin is the orange-yellow pigment of bile, formed principally by the breakdown of hemoglobin in red blood cells at the end of their life cycle.
  - Water-soluble unconjugated bilirubin normally travels in the bloodstream to the liver, where it is converted to a water-soluble, conjugated form and excreted into the bile; a healthy person produces about 250 mg of bilirubin daily.
  - The majority of bilirubin is excreted in the stool.
  - Normal levels of bilirubin are 0.1 to 1 mg/dl, or 5.1 to 17 µmol/L.

Etiology

- Greater than normal amounts of bilirubin in the blood and in the skin
- Jaundice is a symptom of many disorders: liver disease, biliary obstruction, hemolytic anemias, Gilbert syndrome, and Crigler-Najjar syndrome.

Diagnosis

Signs and Symptoms

- Yellowish tinge: skin, mucous membranes, sclerae
  - Persons with dark skin sometimes have yellow-tinged sclerae, and in these persons, examination of the hard palate is often the best place to evaluate jaundice.
- Nausea and vomiting
- Abdominal pain
- Dark urine
- Clay-colored stools

Diseases Associated with Jaundice

- Unconjugated hyperbilirubinemia
  - Stool and urine color are normal.
  - Mild jaundice and indirect (unconjugated) hyperbilirubinemia with no bilirubin in the urine
  - Splenomegaly develops in hemolytic disorders other than sickle cell anemia.
- Conjugated hyperbilirubinemia
  - Hereditary cholestatic syndrome (intrahepatic cholestasis)
    ~ Patient may be asymptomatic.
    ~ Intermittent cholestasis may occur, with pruritus, light-colored stools, and malaise.
  - Hepatocellular disease
    ~ Malaise
    ~ Anorexia
    ~ Low-grade fever
    ~ Dark urine
    ~ Jaundice
    ~ Amenorrhea
    ~ Right upper quadrant (RUQ) pain usually occurs.
    ~ Liver is enlarged, tender.
    ~ Telangiectasia
    ~ Palmar erythema
    ~ Ascites
    ~ Gynecomastia
    ~ Sparse body hair
    ~ Fetor hepaticus
    ~ Asterixis may be present.

—Biliary obstruction
- ~ Colicky RUQ pain
- ~ Weight loss
- ~ Jaundice
- ~ Dark urine
- ~ Light-colored stools
- ~ Symptoms may be intermittent depending on cause of the obstruction: stones, carcinoma of the ampulla, or junction of the hepatic ducts.
- ~ Occult blood in stools suggests carcinoma, likely in the ampulla.
- ~ Other indications of carcinoma are: hepatomegaly, visible and palpable gallbladder (Courvoisier's sign), ascites, rectal (Blumer's) shelf, and weight loss.
- ~ Fever and chills are indicative of cholangitis.

Diagnostic Tests (Table 9-1)

- Liver biopsy
- Imaging: computed tomography (CT) scan, ultrasonography, magnetic resonance imaging (MRI) to show hepatomegaly, tumors, changes of portal hypertension
- Endoscopic retrograde cholangiopancreatography (ERCP) or percutaneous transhepatic cholangiography (PTC): show cause, location, and extent of biliary obstruction

VIRAL HEPATITIS
Definition

Viral hepatitis is a viral inflammatory disease of the liver.

Risk Factors

- Unprotected sexual contact
- Blood transfusion—risk is less than 1 per 60,000 units transfused in the United States
- Fecal-oral contamination

Etiology

- Viral hepatitis may be caused by any of the hepatic viruses: A, B, C, or delta; only A does not have a chronic form (Table 9-2).

Diagnosis

Signs and Symptoms
- Sudden or gradual onset
- Myalgia
- Arthralgia
- Easy fatigability
- Upper respiratory infection (URI) symptoms
- Pharyngitis
- Anorexia
- Malaise
- Headache
- Pain over the liver (RUQ)—mild, constant
- Fever

TABLE 9-1
Liver Function Tests*

Tests	Normal Values	Hepatocellular Jaundice	Obstructive Jaundice
Bilirubin			
Direct	0.1-0.3 mg/dl	Increased	Increased
Indirect	0.2-0.7 mg/dl	Increased	Increased
Urine bilirubin	None	Increased	Increased
Serum albumin/			
albumin	3.5-5.5 g/dl	Decreased albumin	Unchanged albumin
Serum protein			
Total protein	6.5-8.4 g/dl		
Alkaline phosphatase	30-115 units/L	Increased (+)	Increased (++++)
Prothrombin time	INR of 1.0-1.4. After vitamin K, 10% increase in 24 hrs	Prolonged in severe damage, and without response to parenteral vitamin K	Prolonged in marked obstruction; responds to parenteral vitamin K
ALT, AST	ALT 5-35 units/L; AST 5-40 units/L	↑ in hepatocellular damage, viral hepatitis	Minimally increased

From Friedman LS: Liver, biliary tract & pancreas. In Tierney LM, McPhee SJ, Papadakis MA, eds: *Current medical diagnosis & treatment 2000,* ed 39, New York, 2000, Lange Medical Books/McGraw-Hill, p 658.
INR, International Normalized Ratio.
*Changes in liver function tests in two types of jaundice.

- Chills—in sudden onset infection
- Jaundice—many patients do not develop clinical jaundice
- Pruritus
- Nausea and vomiting
- Dark urine
- Clay-colored stools
- Diarrhea
- Hepatomegaly—mild, in 50% of patients
- Liver tenderness
- Splenomegaly—15% of patients
- Soft, enlarged lymph nodes
- Toxic signs/symptoms may be minimal to severe.

Laboratory Studies
- White blood cell (WBC) count is normal to low, particularly in preicteric phase.
- Serum analysis—antibody (A + C) or antigen (B + D)
- Increased aspartate transaminase (AST) or alanine aminotransferase (ALT), often markedly elevated
- Increased bilirubin in the blood

- Abnormal coagulation of the blood
- Increased alkaline phosphatase
- Large, atypical lymphocytes (as seen in infectious mononucleosis) may occur.
- Mild proteinuria—common
- Bilirubinuria usually precedes appearance of jaundice.
- Marked prolongation of prothrombin time in severe hepatitis correlates with increased mortality.

Differential Diagnosis
- Infectious mononucleosis
- Cytomegalovirus infection
- Herpes simplex viral infection
- Spirochetal disease (e.g., leptospirosis, secondary syphilis)
- Brucellosis
- Rickettsial diseases (e.g., Q fever)
- Ischemic hepatitis
- Drug-induced liver disease
- Prodromal phase must be distinguished from infections such as influenza, URI, exanthematous diseases.

TABLE 9-2
Characteristics of Hepatitis Viruses

Virus	Incubation	Transmission	Source/Spread	Infectivity
A (HAV)	15-50 days	Fecal-oral route	Poor hygiene, contaminated food, water, shellfish, sexual contact, cross-contamination	2 wks before onset of signs, symptoms till 2 wks after symptoms appear
B (HBV)	45-180 days	Exposure to blood or blood products	Contaminated needles, syringes, blood; sex with infected person(s); carriers	Before and after symptoms appear; 4-6 wks after onset of symptoms
C (HCV)	14-180 days	Exposure to blood or blood products; sex with infected person(s)	Same as HBV	1-2 wks before symptoms; lasts through entire illness; carriers: indefinitely
D (HDV)	Not certain; must occur with HBV	Infection occurs only with HBV	Same as HBV	Blood is infectious in all stages of illness
E (HEV)	15-64 days	Fecal-oral route	Contaminated water, poor sanitation; rare in United States, Canada	Unknown; may be similar to HAV
G (HGV) flavivirus	Unknown	Exposure to contaminated blood, material	IV drug users; hemodialysis patients; hemophiliacs; those with chronic hepatits B or C	Chronic viremia that lasts 10+ yrs

Modified from Lewis SM, Collier IC, Heitkemper MM: *Medical-surgical nursing: assessment and management of clinical problems,* ed 4, St. Louis, 1996, Mosby.

Prevention

- Hand washing after bowel movements is required.
- Hand washing by health care workers who come in contact with contaminated materials, bedding, and clothing is required.
- Careful handling of disposable needles, syringes
- Screening of blood for hepatitis B surface antigen (HbsAg), antihepatitis B core (anti-HBc), and antihepatitis C virus (anti-HCV) has markedly reduced the risk of transfusion-associated hepatitis.
- Testing of pregnant women for hepatitis B core antigen (HbcAg), hepatitis B virus (HBV), hepatitis C virus (HCV)
- Immunoglobulin is given routinely to all *close* personal contacts of patients with hepatitis A.
- Hepatitis B immunoglobulin (HBIG) may provide protection if given in large doses within 7 days of exposure.

Treatment

- Bed rest only as needed in the acute phase of illness.
- Return to normal level of activity during convalescence should be gradual.
- If loss of fluids through vomiting or diarrhea occurs, intravenous (IV) administration of 10% glucose solution is given.
- If patients exhibit signs of encephalopathy or severe coagulopathy, fulminant hepatic failure should be suspected, requiring immediate hospitalization.

Pharmacotherapy

- Small doses of oxazepam are safe, but morphine sulfate should not be given.
- Studies show that corticosteroids are of no benefit in patients with viral hepatitis.
- Interferon-α tends to decrease the risk of chronic hepatitis.

Prognosis

- Clinical recovery within 3 to 16 weeks is usual in most patients.
- Recovery is complete, with residual liver dysfunction persisting somewhat longer in only a few patients.
- Mortality rate for all patients is less than 1%, but the rate is usually higher in older patients.

- Hepatitis A may persist for a year or longer.
- The mortality rate for hepatitis E is higher in pregnant women (10% to 20%).
- Chronic hepatitis, determined by elevated aminotransferase levels for more than 6 months, occurs in only 1% to 2% of immunocompetent adults with hepatitis B, but rises to as much as 90% in immunocompromised adults.
- Over 80% of patients with hepatitis C and 40% of patients with hepatitis B develop chronic hepatitis; these patients are also at risk (3% to 5% per year) of hepatocellular carcinoma.

Patient/Family Education

- Instruct patient about the nature of hepatitis: cause, usual course, treatment, and expected outcome.
- Provide written instructions regarding medication(s) schedule/dosage, self-care at home: level of activity, diet, fluid intake, signs/symptoms to watch for that may indicate worsening disease or recurrence.
- Give name and telephone/e-mail contact information for nurse practitioner and physician, as required.
- If possible, it is useful for the patient to maintain a diary of day-to-day events/changes.

Follow-up/Referral

- Close monitoring of signs and symptoms, relevant laboratory tests, weight, food and fluid intake are needed.
- If patient's signs and symptoms become worse, a hepatologist may be consulted regarding further evaluation and treatment.

CHRONIC HEPATITIS
Definition

Chronic hepatitis is a chronic inflammatory reaction of the liver lasting 3 to 6 months, shown by persistently abnormal serum aminotransferase levels and characteristic histologic findings.

Etiology

- HBV, HCV, hepatitis D virus (HDV), autoimmune hepatitis, and certain medications (e.g., methyldopa and isoniazid), Wilson's disease, and α_1-antiprotease (α_1-antitrypsin) deficiency

Categorization

- Based on etiology, grade of portal, periportal, lobular inflammation (minimal, mild, moderate, severe), and stage of fibrosis (none, mild, moderate, severe cirrhosis)

Diagnosis

Signs and Symptoms

Autoimmune Hepatitis

- Usually occurs in young women but can occur in either gender of any age
- Affected people are often positive for human leukocyte antigen (HLA)-B8 and HLA-DR3; in older persons—HLA-DR4
- Usually gradual onset, but 25% present as an acute attack of hepatitis
- Some patients follow a typical viral illness pattern, such as hepatitis A, Epstein-Barr infection, measles, or exposure to a drug or toxin such as nitrofurantoin.
- Serum bilirubin is usually increased; 20% are anicteric.
- Examination: healthy-appearing young woman, with multiple spider nevi, cutaneous striae, acne, hirsutism, and hepatomegaly; amenorrhea may be the presenting sign

Other Signs and Symptoms

- Arthritis
- Sjögren's syndrome
- Thyroiditis
- Nephritis
- Ulcerative colitis
- Coombs'-positive hemolytic anemia
- In classic type I autoimmune hepatitis, antinuclear antibody (ANA) or smooth muscle antibody (either or both) is detected in serum.
- Serum gamma globulin levels are usually elevated, up to 5 to 6 g/dl; in these patients, the enzyme immunoassay for antibody HCV may be falsely positive.
- Type II, rarely seen in the United States, but more common in Europe, is characterized by circulating antibody to liver-kidney microsomes (anti-LKM1) without antismooth muscle antibody or ANA.
- In up to 13% of patients with autoimmune hepatitis, concurrent primary biliary cirrhosis or primary sclerosing cholangitis is seen.

Chronic Hepatitis B

- Chronic HBV infection is usually seen in males.
- May be a continuum of acute hepatitis, or be diagnosed on evaluation of persistently elevated aminotransferase levels
- Chronic HBV infection affects almost 400 million people worldwide, and 1.25 million Americans.
- Early on, hepatitis B e antigen (HbeAg) and HBV deoxyribonucleic acid (DNA) are present in serum, indicating active viral replications.
- Low-level immunoglobulin M (IgM) anti-HBc is present in about 70% of patients; clinical improvement correlates with disappearance of anti HBeAg and HBV DNA from serum, appearance of anti-HBe, and integration of the HBV genome into the host genome in infected hepatocytes.
  —These patients are still at risk for developing cirrhosis and hepatocellular carcinoma.
- Infection by a precore mutant of HBV or spontaneous mutation of the precore region of the HBV genome during the course of chronic hepatitis caused by wild-type HBV may result in particularly severe chronic hepatitis with rapid progression to cirrhosis, particularly when additional mutations in the core gene of HBV are present.

B + D

Delta Agent in Hepatitis B

- Acute delta infection concurrent with chronic HBV infection may cause severe chronic hepatitis, which may progress rapidly to cirrhosis and may be fatal.
- Diagnosis is confirmed by detection of anti-HDV in serum.

Dx) EIA

Chronic Hepatitis C

- At least 80% of patients with acute hepatitis C develop chronic hepatitis C.
- Chronic HCV is clinically indistinguishable from chronic hepatitis due to other causes, and may be the most common.
- Diagnosis is confirmed by detection of anti-HCV by enzyme immunoassay (EIA).
- In a few cases of suspected chronic hepatitis C in which there is a negative EIA, the diagnosis can be confirmed either by a positive

recombinant immunoblot assay (RIBA) or by detection of HCV ribonucleic acid (RNA) in serum by polymerase chain reaction.

- Progression to cirrhosis occurs in 20% of affected patients after 20 years.
  - At increased risk are men, those who drink more than 50 g of alcohol daily, and perhaps those who acquire HCV infection after age 40.
- Those with hypogammaglobulinemia, with human immunodeficiency virus (HIV) infection and a low CD4 count, or with organ transplants and receiving immunosuppressants seem to progress more rapidly to cirrhosis than those persons with chronic hepatitis C who are immunocompetent.

Treatment

- Bed rest is not necessary.
- Well-balanced diet with adequate fluid intake
  - No diet limitations unless there is a need for sodium or protein restriction, as required in fluid overload or encephalopathy

Autoimmune Hepatitis

- Prednisone 30 mg PO daily with azathioprine or mercaptopurine 50 mg PO—improves symptoms; decreases serum bilirubin, aminotransferase, and gamma globulin levels; reduces hepatic inflammation; these drugs/dosages are generally well tolerated
  - Those symptomatic patients with serum aminotransferase levels 10 times higher than normal (5 times higher if serum globulins are elevated at least twice normal) benefit most from therapy.
  - Patients with moderately elevated enzymes may receive treatment, depending on their clinical situation.
- Complete blood counts should be monitored weekly for the first 8 weeks of therapy, and every month thereafter because of the small risk of bone marrow suppression.
- Prednisone is tapered to 20 mg/day after 1 week, then after 2 or 3 weeks to 15 mg/day; a maintenance dose of 10 mg/day is continued.
  - Biochemical improvement is gradual, with normal serum aminotransferase levels achieved after 6 to 12 months, and histologic resolution of inflammation occurring after 18 to 24 months.

- The response rate to prednisone and azathioprine is 80% to 90%.
  - However, cirrhosis does not reverse with therapy, and may develop even after biochemical and histologic remission occurs.
- After resolution of biochemical and histologic markers, medications may be stopped, but the relapse rate is 50% to 90%.
  - Relapses are treated the same as the first attack, then kept on maintenance of azathioprine up to 2 mg/kg and the lowest dose of prednisone to maintain aminotranferase levels at close to normal.
- Those who do not respond to prednisone and azathioprine may be treated with cyclosporine and methotrexate.
- Liver transplantation may be the only alternative to those who do not respond to more conservative therapy.
  - The disease has been known to recur in a few transplanted livers as immunosuppression is reduced.

Chronic Hepatitis B

- Patients with active viral replication (HBeAg and HBV DNA in serum) and elevated aminotransferase levels may be treated with recombinant human interferon alfa-2b at a dosage of 5 MU/day intramuscularly (IM), or 10 MU 3 times/week IM for 4 months.
  - About 40% of patients respond to therapy; response is more common in those with HBV DNA level under 200 mg/ml and high aminotransferase levels.
  - Over 60% of those who respond may eventually clear HBsAg from their serum and liver and develop anti-HBs in serum, signaling recovery.
- The nucleoside analog lamivudine 100 mg PO daily was recently approved for treatment of chronic hepatitis B.
  - This drug reliably suppresses HBV DNA in serum, improves liver histology in 40% of patients, and results in normal ALT levels and HBeAg seroconversion in 20% of patients after 1 year of therapy.
  - About 15% have a mild relapse during therapy because of mutation in HBV DNA that confers resistance to lamivudine.

—Hepatitis activity often recurs when the drug is discontinued, which may necessitate long-term treatment.

—The drug is well tolerated, even by decompensated cirrhosis, and it may be effective in those with rapidly progressive hepatitis B ("fibrosing cholestatic hepatitis") after organ transplantation.

Chronic Hepatitis C

- Improvement in biochemical, virologic, and histologic parameters is seen when these patients are given
  - Recombinant human interferon alfa-2b or alfa-2a, 3 MU 3 times/week for 24 weeks, and "consensus" interferon, a synthetic recombinant interferon derived by assigning the most commonly observed amino acid at each position of several alpha interferon subtypes at a dosage of 9 mg three times/week.
  - Resulting improvement is seen in
    ~ Return of ALT to normal
    ~ Loss of HCV RNA from serum
    ~ Decrease in hepatic inflammation and, sometimes, regression of fibrosis in up to 50% of patients
- Factors that indicate an increased chance of response to treatment
  - Absence of cirrhosis on liver biopsy
  - Low serum HCV RNA levels
  - Infection by genotypes of HCV other than 1a and 1b
- Discontinuation of therapy after 24 weeks results in only 30% to 50% of patients maintaining the improvement.
  - Prolonged therapy of 12 to 18 months increases the duration of remission, and this length of treatment is recommended.
- Higher doses of interferon alfa-2b (e.g., 6 MU three times/week) increase toxicity and do not appear to increase the rate of sustained response.
  - A slow-release, long-acting "pegylated" formulation of interferon taken only once a week is currently in clinical trials.
- The nucleoside analog ribavirin 1000 to 1200 mg/day in two divided doses has been approved for previously untreated patients or those who relapse after an initial response to interferon-α alone, with higher

sustained response rates in 40% to 50%, respectively, in these two groups after combination therapy.

- Interferon-α may be beneficial in treating patients with cryoglobulinemia associated with chronic hepatitis C.
  - A sustained response is unlikely in patients with chronic hepatitis C who have persistently normal serum aminotransferase levels, making them chronic carriers.
- Side effects of interferon, a costly treatment, include flu-like symptoms that occur in almost all patients, and more serious but less common effects such as irritability and depression, thyroid dysfunction, and bone marrow suppression.

Prognosis

- The course of hepatitis is variable and unpredictable.
- Untreated autoimmune hepatitis has a mortality rate at 5 years of 50%, which decreases significantly with treatment.
- Sequelae of chronic hepatitis secondary to hepatitis B include cirrhosis, liver failure, and hepatocellular carcinoma.
  - An estimated 40% to 50% of patients with chronic hepatitis B and cirrhosis die within 5 years after the onset of symptoms, with some improvement with interferon therapy in those who respond.
- Chronic hepatitis C is a slowly progressive, usually subclinical disease that may result in cirrhosis or hepatocellular carcinoma after decades.
  - It is anticipated that the mortality rates among patients with hepatitis C due to cirrhosis or hepatocellular carcinoma will triple in the next two decades.
- Recent studies, however, show that therapy with interferon improves survival and quality of life, is cost-effective, and may reduce the risk of hepatocellular carcinoma in those who respond to treatment.

Patient/Family Education

- Instruct regarding the nature, signs and symptoms, course, and treatment of chronic hepatitis, according to the individual's needs based on the type of hepatitis present.

- Provide written instructions about medications: reason for, dosage, scheduling, and side effects, as appropriate.
- Write out those signs and symptoms, or changes in status, that require immediate attention from the nurse practitioner and/or physician.
- Write out telephone numbers for emergency help.
- Instruct about level of activity, diet, fluid intake, and other aspects of care as needed.

Follow-up/Referral

- Patients with chronic hepatitis, whether active or in remission, are followed closely every 1 to 3 months, as needed, to ensure that appropriate serum levels of aminotransferase are maintained, and that the patient's condition is stable.
- For many patients, consultation with a hepatologist can be quite helpful in guiding therapy.

ALCOHOLIC HEPATITIS
Definition

This condition is characterized by acute or chronic inflammation and parenchymal necrosis of the liver induced by alcohol.

Prevalence

- Alcoholic hepatitis is the most common precursor of cirrhosis in the United States.
- Cirrhosis is among the most common causes of death of adults in America.
- Alcoholic cirrhosis occurs in 8% to 15% of those who consume over 50 g of alcohol (4 oz of 100-proof whiskey, 15 oz of wine, or four 12-oz cans of beer) daily for over 10 years.

Risk Factors

- Adults over age 35
- Gender—women are more susceptible to cirrhosis than men, owing to lower gastric mucosal alcohol dehydrogenase levels.
- Intake of alcohol in amounts equal to or more than those listed above for at least 10 years
- Family history of alcoholism, particularly in first-degree relatives
- Genetic factors also are usually considered to play a role in who becomes an alcoholic, and who then develops cirrhosis.

Diagnosis

- Liver biopsy is the only way to confirm the diagnosis of cirrhosis because other tests of alcoholic hepatitis are applicable to liver disease from causes other than alcohol.

Signs and Symptoms

- Variable, from the asymptomatic person with an enlarged liver to one critically ill who may die suddenly
- Recent episode of heavy drinking
- Anorexia
- Nausea and vomiting
- Hepatomegaly
- Jaundice

Laboratory Findings

- Anemia—usually macrocytic
- Leukopenia—in some patients; disappears when alcohol consumption stops
- Thrombocytopenia—10% of patients, due to a direct toxic effect of alcohol on production of megakaryocytes, or to hypersplenism
- AST is usually elevated, but usually not above 300 units/L; AST is invariably greater than ALT, sometimes by a factor of 2 or more.
- Serum bilirubin is increased in at least 60% of patients; readings above 10 mg/dl and prolonged prothrombin time greater than 6 seconds above normal indicate severe alcoholic hepatitis, with a mortality rate of up to 50%.
- Serum γ-glutamyl transpeptidase (GGTP), mean corpuscular volume, and carbohydrate-deficient transferrin may be elevated; the sensitivity rate of these tests is 70% or less.
- Serum albumin is lower than normal.
- The gamma globulin level is elevated in 50% to 75% of persons with alcoholic hepatitis, even those with no cirrhosis.
- Liver biopsy is required to confirm diagnosis; it also shows macrovesicular fat, polymorphonuclear neutrophil leukocyte (PMN) infiltration with hepatic necrosis, Mallory bodies (alcoholic hyaline), and micronodular cirrhosis if present.
- Ultrasound may be helpful in ruling out biliary obstruction and to assess for subclinical ascites.
- CT scan with IV contrast or MRI may be helpful in selected cases to evaluate collat-

eral vessels, space-occupying lesions (SOLs), or pancreatic disease.

Differential Diagnosis
- Cholecystitis
- Cholelithiasis
- Trauma from drugs (e.g., amiodarone)

Complications
- Ascites may develop in persons with alcoholic hepatitis; usually resolves as hepatitis improves; diuretics are not indicated.
- Bleeding due to coagulopathy
- Deteriorating clinical picture, worsening abdominal pain may be mistaken for an acute abdomen; abdominal laparotomy done based on mistaken diagnosis carries a high postoperative mortality rate

Treatment
General
- Abstinence from alcohol is essential.
- Sufficient carbohydrates and calories are needed to reduce endogenous protein catabolism and promote gluconeogenesis to prevent hypoglycemia; 40 kcal/kg with 1.5-2 g/kg protein improves survival in patients with malnutrition.
  —Use of liquid formulas rich in branched-chain amino acids is not more effective than less expensive means of supplying adequate nourishment.
- Supplemental vitamins (e.g., folic acid, thiamin) are required.

Pharmacologic
- Corticosteroids: methylprednisolone 32 mg/day for 1 month (or equivalent) has been shown to be of benefit in patients with alcoholic hepatitis and either encephalopathy or a greatly elevated bilirubin concentration and prolonged prothrombin time (based on the calculation of prothrombin time minus the control [normal] prothrombin time, times 4.6 plus the total bilirubin in mg/dl is greater than 32)

Prognosis
Short-term
- If the prothrombin time is short enough (<3 seconds above control) to allow liver biopsy without risk, the 1-year mortality rate is 7%, increasing to 18% if there is progressive prolongation of the prothrombin time during hospitalization.
- Patients whose prothrombin time is too long to permit liver biopsy have a 42% mortality rate at 1 year.
- Other unfavorable prognostic factors include serum bilirubin greater than 10 mg/dl, hepatic encephalopathy, and azotemia.

Long-term
- In the United States, the 3-year mortality rate of those who recover from acute alcoholic hepatitis is 10 times greater than normal persons, controlled for age.
- Persons in whom histologic evidence shows severe disease continue to have excessive mortality rates after 3 years; in those whose liver biopsies show only mild alcoholic hepatitis, mortality rates are not increased after 3 years.
- Other unfavorable prognostic indicators are associated with those persons who develop complications of portal hypertension (ascites, variceal bleeding, hepatorenal syndrome), coagulopathy, and severe jaundice after recovery from alcoholic hepatitis.
- Mortality rates continue to climb in those who cannot abstain from alcohol.
  —Liver transplantation is contraindicated in those who cannot abstain for a minimum of 6 months before surgery.

Patient/Family Education
- Psychologic support is necessary for both patient and family members throughout treatment.
- The person addicted to alcohol has many psychologic problems, including extremely low self-esteem, tendency to continually deny a problem, fear of dying, and anxiety about abstinence from alcohol and of withdrawal (delirium tremens).
- Health professionals and others should show compassion and understanding, yet maintain firmly the need for the person to stop drinking.
- Family members need to understand the entire picture (signs, symptoms, consequences of not adhering to treatment or to cessation of drinking), mortality rates, and the patient's unfavorable prognostic conditions if present.

—However, family members also need to be compassionate and to provide the necessary support to enable the patient to change behavior patterns.

- Any improvement should be explained to the patient and family, to encourage continued adherence to treatment and the benefits of even short-term cessation from drinking.
- Diet (high calorie, high protein) should be written out for the family, and financial advice given if needed to provide patient-nourishing meals after discharge (e.g., social service, food stamps, other).
- Physical care of the patient postdischarge should be written for family who will be caring for the patient at home: skin care, monitoring of urine output and episodes of constipation or diarrhea, requiring extra fluid intake.
- Write out information about signs and symptoms of encephalopathy, impending delirium tremens, and other indications of need for emergency care.

Follow-up/Referral

- Patients are followed closely at home by visiting nurses, frequent telephone contact, and return visits to the office or clinic.
- Consultation and counseling provided by a psychiatrist or psychologist who specializes in alcohol addiction may be crucial to the patient's recovery and long-term abstinence from alcohol.

CIRRHOSIS
Definition

Hematemesis / ↑ Varice

Cirrosis is a chronic degenerative disease of the liver in which the lobes are covered with fibrous tissue, the parenchyma degenerates, and the lobules are infiltrated with fat.

Prevalence

- Cirrhosis is the eleventh leading cause of death in the United States; mortality rate is about 9.2 per 100,000 per year.

Etiology

- Determining the cause of cirrhosis is essential for both therapeutic and prognostic rationale.

Pathophysiology

- The clinical picture/signs and symptoms are a result of hepatic cell dysfunction, portosystemic shunting, and portal hypertension.
- All functions of the liver deteriorate, depending on the severity of cirrhosis.
- Gluconeogenesis, detoxification of drugs and alcohol, bilirubin metabolism, vitamin absorption, gastrointestinal function, hormonal metabolism, and others
- Blood flow through the liver is obstructed, resulting in back pressure that causes portal hypertension and esophageal varices.
- Histologic classification divides the severity of cirrhosis into three areas.
  —Micronodular cirrhosis, seen in typical alcoholic liver disease (Laënnec's cirrhosis), in which the regenerating nodules are no larger than the original lobules (about 1 mm or less in diameter)
  —Macronodular cirrhosis, characterized by larger lobules, often measuring several centimeters in diameter and that may contain central veins
    ~ This level corresponds to postnecrotic (posthepatic) cirrhosis; does not necessarily follow episodes of massive necrosis and stromal collapse.

Diagnosis
Signs and Symptoms

- Onset of symptoms, often after a long asymptomatic stage, is usually gradual, sometimes sudden.
- Hematemesis is the presenting sign in 15% to 25% of patients.
- Fever, often present on admission, indicating associated alcoholic hepatitis
- Splenomegaly—present in 35% to 50% of patients
- Weakness
- Fatigability
- Disturbed sleep
- Muscle cramps
- Weight loss
- Anorexia—occurs in advanced cirrhosis, often extreme
- Nausea, vomiting
- Abdominal pain—due either to hepatic enlargement with stretching of Glisson's capsule or to ascites

- Loss of libido, amenorrhea, impotence, sterility, gynecomastia in men
- Hepatomegaly—in 70% of patients: palpable, especially the left lobe; firm but not hard, with a blunt or nodular edge
- Skin manifestations—spider nevi on upper body above breasts, palmar erythema
- Mouth—glossitis, cheilosis—due to vitamin deficiencies
- Jaundice is usually not an early sign, is mild at first, more severe later
- Pleural effusion, ascites, peripheral edema, and ecchymosis are later signs.
- Encephalopathy is characterized by day-night reversal, asterixis, dysarthria, delirium, drowsiness, then coma.

Laboratory Tests
- Liver biopsy as indicated
- Abdominal paracentesis for cell count, culture, albumin level/serum-ascites albumin gradient (>1.1 indicates portal hypertension)

Differential Diagnosis
- After alcohol, the most common causes of cirrhosis are chronic hepatitis C and B.
- "Bronzing" of skin due to hemochromatosis
- Arthritis
- Heart failure
- Diabetes mellitus
- Wilson's disease
- Primary biliary cirrhosis—primarily in women
- Secondary biliary cirrhosis—from chronic biliary obstruction due to stone, stricture, or neoplasm
- Congestive heart failure and constrictive pericarditis may result in hepatic fibrosis ("cardiac cirrhosis") with ascites, which may be mistaken for alcoholic cirrhosis.

Complications
- Upper gastrointestinal (GI) bleeding due to varices, portal hypertensive gastropathy, gastroduodenal ulcer
- Bleeding may be massive, resulting in fatal exsanguination or portosystemic encephalopathy.
- Hepatic Kupffer's cell (reticuloendothelial) dysfunction and decreased opsonic activity may result in increased risk of systemic infection.

- Cardiomyopathy, due to impaired β-adrenergic receptors or altered hemodynamics from portal hypertension

Treatment
General
- Abstinence from alcohol
- Adequate diet—calories and protein up to 100 g/day, but no more than 60-80 g/day if hepatic encephalopathy is present; sodium restriction if fluid retention is present
- Vitamin supplements daily

Complications
- Ascites and edema
  —Treated with diuretics (see Procedures section), paracentesis, transjugular intrahepatic portosystemic shunts (TIPS) (see Procedures section)
- Spontaneous bacterial peritonitis
- Hepatorenal syndrome
- Hepatic encephalopathy
- Anemia
- Tendency to hemorrhage
  —Esophageal varices tear or rupture
- Hepatopulmonary syndrome: triad of chronic liver disease, increased alveolar-arterial gradient while patient is breathing room air, and intrapulmonary vascular dilations that cause right-to-left intrapulmonary shunt
  —Complications are treated individually, if and when they occur.

Pharmacologic
- Spironolactone for those who do not respond to salt restriction, starting with 100 mg/day, increasing by 100 mg every 3 to 5 days to a maximum single daily dose of 400 mg

Procedures
- Paracentesis—for patients with massive ascites and respiratory compromise, refractory to diuretics or diuretic side effects—4 to 6 L may be withdrawn at one time to provide temporary relief
  —Concomitant IV albumin 10 g/L of ascitic fluid removed, to preserve intravascular volume.
  —Large-volume paracentesis can be done daily until ascites is relatively resolved; may decrease the need for hospitalization.
  —Diuretics should be continued if possible to prevent recurrent ascites.

- TIPS—for variceal bleeding and refractory ascites; this procedure is now preferred to that of peritoneovenous shunts, which were done more often in the past and have a high risk for complications (e.g., disseminated intravascular coagulation—65% of patients, with 25% symptomatic, 5% severe); bacterial infections in 4% to 8%; congestive heart failure in 2% to 4%; variceal bleeding from sudden expansion of intravascular volume
- Liver transplantation—indicated only in selected cases of irreversible, progressive chronic liver disease, fulminant hepatic failure, certain metabolic diseases that result from liver defect
  —5-year survival in over 80% of patients with liver transplant
  —Absolute contraindications
    ~ Sepsis
    ~ Malignancy
    ~ Advanced cardiopulmonary disease
    ~ HIV infection
    ~ Lack of patient understanding

Prognosis

- Prognosis of cirrhosis has changed very little over time.
- Unfavorable factors affecting survival
  —Inability to stop drinking alcohol
  —Hematemesis
  —Jaundice
  —Ascites
  —Patients with severe hepatic dysfunction (serum albumin < 3 g/dl, bilirubin 3 mg/dl, ascites, encephalopathy, cachexia, upper GI bleeding)—only 50% survive 6 months

Patient/Family Education

- Patient and family need to understand the nature, cause, complications, course, and treatment of cirrhosis.
- Absolute cessation of alcohol intake needs to be repeated continually.
- Prognosis is difficult to determine for individuals at the start of therapy; depends on factors and events may occur that are largely unpredictable
- As indicated earlier, compassionate understanding of the patient's situation and history are important to avoid further damage to the patient's ego.

Follow-up/Referral

- Patients are followed closely, every month or so, to monitor alcohol intake, physical status—prone to respiratory problems such as pleural effusions, tuberculosis (TB), HIV, bacterial infections, anemia
- At each visit/contact, the patient needs encouragement, support to increase self-esteem as much as possible, gentle reprimand if alcohol intake is too great, provision of aids to stop drinking such as avoiding bars/pubs, limiting time with friends who drink a lot, eating instead of drinking alcohol

PRIMARY BILIARY CIRRHOSIS
Definition

Primary biliary cirrhosis (PBC) is a chronic, progressive, inflammatory disease of the liver.

Etiology/Pathophysiology

- The cause is unknown, although it is classified with autoimmune disorders.
- Autoimmune destruction of intrahepatic bile ducts and cholestasis

Risk Factors

- Gender: women
- Age: 40 to 60 years

Diagnosis
Signs and Symptoms

- Many patients are asymptomatic for years.
- Onset of signs/symptoms is insidious, usually heralded by pruritus.
- As the disease progresses, physical examination reveals hepatosplenomegaly.
- Xanthomatous lesions may appear on the skin, tendons, and around the eyelids.
- Jaundice and portal hypertension are late findings.

Laboratory Findings

- Early in the disease, blood counts are normal.
- Liver function tests indicate cholestasis with elevation of alkaline phosphatase; cholesterol, especially high-density lipoprotein (HDL); in later phases, bilirubin is detected.
- Antimitochondrial antibodies, directed against pyruvate dehydrogenase or other

2-oxo-acid enzymes in mitochondria, are present in 95% of patients.

—Patients with a clinical and histologic picture of primary biliary cirrhosis but no mitochondrial antibodies are diagnosed as "autoimmune cholangitis."

- Serum IgM levels are elevated.
- In advanced disease, adverse prognostic indicators include older age, high serum bilirubin, edema, low albumin, prolonged prothrombin time, and variceal hemorrhage due to portal hypertension.

Differential Diagnosis

- Chronic biliary tract obstruction due to stone or stricture
- Carcinoma of the bile ducts
- Primary sclerosing cholangitis
- Sarcoidosis
- Drug toxicity (e.g., chlorpromazine)
- Chronic hepatitis

Treatment

- No cure exists for PBC.
- Treatment is symptomatic.
  —Ursodeoxycholic acid 10 to 15 mg/kg/day in one or two doses is the preferred medical therapy.
    ~ Patient response shows that this drug slows progression of PBCs improves long-term survival, reduces the risk of esophageal varices, and delays the need for liver transplantation.
  —Colchicine 0.6 mg bid and methotrexate 15 mg/week reduce elevated serum levels of alkaline phosphatase and bilirubin in some patients.
  —Penicillamine, corticosteroids, and azathioprine are of no benefit in PBC, according to research studies.
  —Cholestyramine 4 g or colestipol 5 g in water or juice tid may ease the discomfort of pruritus.
  —Rifampin 150 to 300 mg PO bid is helpful in some patients.
  —Opioid antagonists such as naloxone 0.2 µg/kg/minute IV or naltrexone 50 mg/day PO show promise in treating pruritus.
  —Vitamin A, K, and D deficiencies may occur if steatorrhea is present, and may be made worse if cholestyramine or colestipol is taken.

    ~ Replacement dosages of vitamins are individually determined.
  —Calcium supplement of 500 mg tid may prevent osteomalacia; its benefit in preventing osteoporosis is not clear.
    ~ Some research data indicate that bisphosphonates and estrogen may be helpful in treating osteoporosis.
- Liver transplantation in advanced PBC has a 1-year survival rate of 85% to 90%.

Patient/Family Education

- Both patient and family should be informed about the nature of the disease, its course, signs and symptoms, and that it is not curable, but that, if necessary, liver transplantation can prolong life.
- Instruct regarding all medications prescribed, reason for taking, action, and side effects if any.
- Provide helpful suggestions about minimizing pruritus because this is often the most troublesome symptom (e.g., baths containing sodium bicarbonate, lotion for the skin, cool compresses—whatever works best).
- If the time comes when liver transplantation becomes necessary, the patient and family need thoughtful preparation and full knowledge about the procedure and its consequences (e.g., the hopeful prognosis regarding prolonged survival).

Follow-up/Referral

- These patients, once symptoms develop, are followed closely by the nurse practitioner in consultation with a nephrologist, to keep abreast of new therapy.
- Counseling may be helpful to both patient and family at particular stages of the disease, as when symptoms worsen or when pharmacologic therapy does not seem to be helping.

WILSON'S DISEASE
Definition

Wilson's disease is a condition known as *hepatolenticular degeneration*, a rare autosomal recessive disorder that usually occurs between the ages of 10 and 40.

Etiology/Pathophysiology

- The genetic defect is localized to chromosome 13 and affects a copper-transporting adenosine triphosphatase (ATP7B) in the liver.

—Over 50 different mutations in the gene have been identified, making routine genetic diagnosis unlikely.

- The major physiologic aberration is excessive absorption of copper from the small intestine and decreased excretion of copper by the liver, resulting in increased tissue deposition, particularly in the liver, brain, cornea, and kidneys.
- Recognizing the condition is important because it may masquerade as chronic hepatitis, psychiatric disorders, or neurologic disease.
- The condition is reversible, if treated early to prevent neurologic or hepatic damage.

Diagnosis

Signs and Symptoms

- Usually presents as liver disease in adolescents and as neuropsychiatric disease in young adults.
  - There is great variability in how the condition presents in individuals.
- Wilson's disease should be considered in any child or young adult with hepatitis, splenomegaly with hypersplenism, hemolytic anemia, portal hypertension, and neurologic or psychiatric abnormalities.
  - Hepatic involvement may range from elevated liver function tests to cirrhosis and portal hypertension.
  - Neurologic manifestations are related to basal ganglia dysfunction, with signs of rigidity or parkinsonian tremor.
- Renal calculi, the Franconi defect, renal tubular acidosis, and hypoparathyroidism may occur in patients with Wilson's disease.

Laboratory Findings

- The pathognomonic sign of the condition is the brownish or gray-green Kayser-Fleischer ring, seen in Descemet's membrane in the cornea close to the endothelial surface.
  - The ring is seen best in the superior and inferior poles of the cornea.
  - Slit-lamp examination is usually required to confirm the diagnosis, although the ring may be seen by the examiner with only an ophthalmoscope light.
- Diagnosis is based on increased urinary copper excretion > 100 µg in 24 hours, or low serum ceruloplasmin levels < 20 µg/dl and elevated hepatic copper concentration > 250 µg/g of dry liver.

Treatment

- Restriction of dietary copper (shellfish, organ foods, legumes are all rich in copper)
- Oral penicillamine 0.75 to 2 g/day in divided doses is the drug of choice, which results in urinary excretion of chelated copper.
- Pyridoxine 50 mg/week is given because penicillamine is an antimetabolite of this vitamin.
- Alternative therapy if penicillamine is not tolerated is trientine 250 to 500 mg tid.
- Oral zinc acetate 50 mg tid promotes fecal copper excretion and may be given as maintenance therapy after decoppering with a chelating agent.
- Treatment is continued indefinitely.
- Liver transplantation is indicated for fulminant hepatitis, end-stage cirrhosis, and for some patients with intractable neurologic disease.

Prognosis

- Good, if patient is treated before liver or brain damage occurs

Patient/Family Education

- Patient and family should be instructed about the nature, cause, course, complications, treatment, and expected outcome.
- Both should know that treatment is continued indefinitely.

Follow-up/Referral

- Family members, particularly siblings, should be screened with serum ceruloplasmin, liver function tests, and slit-lamp examination.

DISORDERS OF THE BILIARY TRACT
(TABLE 9-3)
Acute Cholecystitis

Definition

Acute cholecystitis is an acute inflammation of the gallbladder that may become chronic.

Etiology

- The cause is usually a gallstone that cannot pass through the cystic duct.
- An acute attack may be precipitated by a large or fatty meal.

Diagnosis

Signs and Symptoms

- Definite localized pain and tenderness in the right hypochondrium with radiation

TABLE 9-3
Diseases of the Biliary Tract

Disorder	Clinical Features	Laboratory Findings	Diagnosis	Treatment
Gallstones	Asymptomatic	Normal	Ultrasound	None
Cholesterolosis of gallbladder	Biliary colic	Normal	Ultrasound	Laparoscopic cholecystectomy
Adenomyomatosis	May cause biliary colic	Normal	Oral cholecystography	None
Porcelain gallbladder	Usually asymptomatic, high risk of gallbladder disease	Normal	X-ray or CT	Laparoscopic cholecystectomy
Acute cholecystitis	Epigastric or RUQ pain, nausea, vomiting, fever, Murphy's sign	Leukocytosis	Ultrasound, HIDA scan	Antibiotics, laparoscopic cholecystectomy
Chronic cholecystitis	Biliary colic, constant epigastric or RUQ pain, nausea	Normal	Ultrasound (stones), oral cholecystography (non-functioning gallbladder)	Laparoscopic cholecystectomy
Choledocho-lithiasis	Asymptomatic or biliary colic, jaundice, fever, gallstone pancreatitis	Cholestatic liver function tests; leukocytosis, positive blood cultures in cholangitis; elevated amylase and lipase in pancreatitis	Ultrasound (dilated ducts), ERCP	Endoscopic sphincterotomy and stone extraction; antibiotics for cholangitis

From Friedman LS: Liver, biliary tract & pancreas. In Tierney LM, McPhee SJ, Papadakis MA, eds: *Current medical diagnosis & treatment 2000*, ed 39, New York, 2000, Lange Medical Books/McGraw Hill, p 684.

around to the infrascapular area strongly favors the diagnosis of acute cholecystitis.

- The acute attack is characterized by sudden severe, persistent pain that is usually localized in the right hypochondrium, or perhaps the epigastrium.
  - —In uncomplicated cases, the pain subsides within 12 to 18 hours.
  - —Vomiting occurs in about 75% of patients, with variable relief.
  - —RUQ tenderness is almost always present, usually associated with muscle guarding and rebound pain.
  - —The gallbladder is palpable in about 15% of patients.
  - —Jaundice occurs in about 25% of patients and, if persistent or worsening, usually indicates choledocholithiasis.
  - —Fever is common because of the inflammation.

Laboratory Findings
- WBC count is high—12,000 to 15,000/μl
- Total serum bilirubin of 1 to 4 mg/dl is usually seen, even in the absence of common duct obstruction.
- Serum aminotransferase and alkaline phosphatase are usually elevated; aminotransferase may be as high as 300 units/ml or more when associated with ascending cholangitis.
- Serum amylase may be elevated.

Imaging
- X-rays of the abdomen may show radiopaque gallstones in 15% of cases.
- ^{99m}Tc hepatobiliary imaging, using iminodiacetic acid compounds (HIDA scan), shows an obstructed cystic duct, the usual cause of cholecystitis in most patients.
  - —This test has a 98% sensitivity and 81% specificity for acute cholecystitis.

- RUQ ultrasound may show the presence of gallstones but is not specific for acute cholecystitis.
- *Chronic cholecystitis,* the more common condition, develops gradually and is characterized by somewhat milder symptoms.

Differential Diagnosis
- Perforated peptic ulcer
- Acute pancreatitis
- Appendicitis
- Perforated colon carcinoma
- Diverticulum of the hepatic flexure
- Pleurisy on the right side
- Liver abscess
- Hepatitis
- Pneumonia

Complications
- Gangrene of the gallbladder
- Cholangitis—presents with Charcot's triad of signs and symptoms: fever, chills, RUQ pain, jaundice; 95% of patients with this clinical picture will have common duct stones, but only a small proportion of patients with acute cholecystitis have common duct stones
- Chronic cholecystitis—usually develops after repeated episodes of acute cholecystitis, chronic irritation of the walls of the gallbladder from stones; calculi are usually present; the villi of the gallbladder may enlarge and appear as "strawberry gallbladder"

Treatment
Conservative Regimen
- Acute cholecystitis will usually subside by withholding of food, IV alimentation, analgesics, and antibiotics.
  - Meperidine (Demerol) is preferable to morphine because of less risk of spasm of Oddi's sphincter.
- Because of the high risk of recurrence (10% within 1 month, 30% within a year), laparoscopic cholecystectomy is generally performed after 2-3 days of hospitalization, which allows the inflammation to subside under conservative therapy.
  - Patients are usually discharged home 2 days after the procedure, and they are allowed to return to work within 7 days.

  - Cholecystectomy is mandatory if there is evidence of gangrene, abscess formation, or perforation.
- For high-risk patients (older persons, those with diabetes) ultrasound-guided aspiration of the gallbladder (percutaneous cholecystostomy) may postpone or avoid the need for surgery.

Prognosis
- Overall mortality rate of cholecystectomy is <1%, with complete resolution of symptoms.
- In the elderly, hepatobiliary tract surgery is a more formidable procedure with a mortality rate of 10% to 15%.

Patient/Family Education
- The patient and family should be instructed about the nature of the problem, its cause, treatment, and expected outcome.
- The patient is usually brought to the hospital emergency room because of an acute attack of cholecystitis, and is unprepared for the suddenness and pain of gallbladder disease, if he or she has not had a prior attack.
  - He or she will be likely be fearful, confused, in pain, requiring comforting words and reassurance, along with relief of pain.
- Hospitalization and conservative treatment are usual, with the probability of cholecystectomy by laparoscope within a few days of admission.
- Knowing what is happening will greatly relieve both patient and family members.

Follow-up/Referral
- On admission, a gastroenterologist should be brought in to review the case and perform the surgery.
- The patient will be followed postoperatively by the nurse practitioner in consultation with the gastroenterologist, who will have provided the patient with detailed instructions about postoperative care regarding diet, activity, return visits, and any other information that is necessary.
- The nurse practitioner can help to allay the patient's fears about walking/activity and care of the operative incision.

Cholelithiasis

Definition

Cholelithiasis is the presence of gallstones in the gallbladder and occurs in about 20% of the population over age 40—about 20 million people.

Risk Factors

- Older age
- Gender: women are affected more than men.
- Obesity
- Rapid weight loss increases the risk of gallstone formation.
- Cirrhosis of the liver
- Sickle cell disease—in 30% of these persons, due to hemolysis
- Crohn's disease—incidence is high among this group due to disruption of bile salt resorption with associated decreased solubility of bile.
- Native Americans have a high rate of cholesterol cholelithiasis, likely because of genetic predisposition for their development; 75% of Pima women over age 25 have gallstones.

Prevention

- A low-carbohydrate diet and increased physical activity likely help to prevent gallstones.

Pathophysiology

- Gallstones are classified by chemical composition.
  - Stones containing mainly cholesterol
  - Stones containing mainly calcium bilirubinate
    - ~ In Europe and the United States, this type makes up less than 20% of gallstones.
    - ~ In Japan, this type comprises 30% to 40% of stones.
- Three compounds make up 80% to 95% of the total solids dissolved in bile.
  - Conjugated bile salts
  - Lecithin
  - Cholesterol

Diagnosis

Signs and Symptoms

- Patients with gallstones are often asymptomatic; the stones are discovered incidentally when radiographic studies are done for other reasons, or during surgery or autopsy.
- Symptoms of biliary colic usually develop in 10% to 25% of patients within 10 years.

Treatment

- Laparoscopic cholecystectomy is the treatment of choice for patients with symptomatic gallbladder disease.
- Chenodeoxycholic and ursodeoxycholic acids are bile salts given PO to selected patients who reject surgery for up to 2 years to dissolve cholesterol stones.
  - Dose is 7 mg/kg/day of each, or 8 to 13 mg/kg of ursodeoxycholic acid in divided doses each day.
  - These drugs are more effective in patients whose gallbladder is functioning well despite stones.
  - In 50% of patients, gallstones recur within 5 years after therapy is stopped.
- Lithotripsy, once used for both gallstones and kidney stones, is not generally used in the United States at present.

Complications

- If symptoms persist after removal of the gallbladder, the cause may be a wrong diagnosis, functional bowel disorder, technical error, recurrent common bile duct stone, or spasm of Oddi's sphincter.

Patient/Family Education

- The patient and family need to be instructed regarding the nature of the disorder, its cause, treatment, and expected outcome.
  - Drawings or photographs may help the patient to visualize the presence of gallstones and the location of the gallbladder in the abdomen.
- The procedure for cholecystectomy (usually laparoscopic now) is explained to the patient before its scheduled time.
- The patient is given written instructions about care at home at the time of discharge, as to diet, activity, when they may return to work.

Follow-up/Referral

- Patients are followed for up to a month after discharge, until uncomplicated recovery is assured and the patient is comfortable and active.

- Ways to prevent gallstones are explained (e.g., low-carbohydrate diet, increased physical exercise).

BIBLIOGRAPHY

Anderson KN, Anderson LE, Glanze WD, eds: *Mosby's medical, nursing, & allied health dictionary,* ed 5, St. Louis, 1998, Mosby.

Friedman LS: Liver, biliary tract, & pancreas. In Tierney LM, McPhee SJ, Papadakis MA, eds: *Current medical diagnosis & treatment 2000,* ed 39, New York, 2000, Lange Medical Books/McGraw-Hill, pp 656-707.

Mezey E, Bender JS: Diseases of the biliary tract. In Barker LR, Burton JR, Zieve PD, eds: *Principles of ambulatory medicine,* ed 5, Baltimore, 1999, Williams & Wilkins, pp 1391-1400.

Shannon MT, Wilson BA, Stang CL: *Health professionals drug guide 2000,* Stamford, Conn, 2000, Appleton & Lange.

Shovein JT, Damazo RJ, Hyams I: Hepatitis A—How benign is it? *Am J Nurs* 100(3):43-48, 2000.

REVIEW QUESTIONS

1. Jaundice is best observed in:
   a. The skin
   b. The mucous membranes
   c. The hard palate
   d. The sclerae
2. A healthy person produces about _____ of bilirubin daily. *250 mg*
   a. 50 mg
   b. 150 mg
   c. 200 mg
   d. 250 mg
3. One of the major signs of _____ is splenomegaly. *C Hemolytic d/o*
   a. Sjögren's syndrome
   b. Sickle cell anemia *Not c̄*
   c. Hemolytic disorders
   d. HIV infection
4. In patients with obstructive jaundice, the alkaline phosphatase is:
   a. Normal
   b. Decreased
   c. Increased
   d. Greatly increased
5. The incubation period of viral hepatitis caused by hepatic virus A is:
   a. 14 to 180 days
   b. 45 to 180 days
   c. 15 to 50 days
   d. 15 to 64 days

   d No carrier state & does not lead to chronic Hep

6. A major sign of viral hepatitis is:
   a. Clay-colored stools
   b. Generalized rash *No*
   c. Light-colored urine *dark*
   d. Hard, enlarged lymph nodes *soft*
7. One of the disorders in the differential diagnosis of viral hepatitis, seen primarily in adolescents and young adults, is:
   a. Herpes simplex viral infection
   b. Mumps
   c. Infectious mononucleosis
   d. Secondary syphilis
8. Chronic hepatitis is that which lasts:
   a. At least 1 month
   b. 3 to 6 months
   c. 6 to 9 months
   d. 9 to 12 months
9. The best treatment for chronic hepatitis C is recombinant human interferon alfa-2b or alfa-2a, along with:
   a. "Consensus" interferon
   b. Lamivudine *B*
   c. Corticosteroids *auto Immune Hep*
   d. Bed rest *Not necessary*
10. Continuation of therapy for chronic hepatitis C is recommended for:
    a. 24 days
    b. 3 months
    c. 6 to 9 months
    d. 12 to 18 months
11. Alcoholic hepatitis is characterized by:
    a. Small, nodular liver
    b. Parenchymal necrosis of the liver
    c. Increased serum albumin
    d. Decreased aspartate transaminase
12. In the United States, the 3-year mortality rate among those who recover from acute alcoholic hepatitis is _____ *10* times greater than for normal persons.
    a. Two
    b. Five
    c. Eight
    d. Ten
13. Cirrhosis is characterized by:
    a. Fibrous covering of lobes
    b. White, nodular liver
    c. Necrosis of hepatic arterial system
    d. Greatly shrunken liver, normal in appearance

    ✱ {alcoholic Hyaline & Mallory bodies}

14. After alcohol, the most common cause of cirrhosis is:
    a. Resistant tuberculosis
    b. Chronic hepatitis B and C
    c. Bilirubinemia
    d. Wilson's disease

15. Esophageal varices are caused by:
    a. Hepatic inflammation
    b. Bilirubinemia
    c. Portal hypertension
    d. Hepatic encephalopathy

16. The maximum dosage of spironolactone for patients with cirrhosis who do not respond to salt restriction is:
    a. 100 mg/day
    b. 200 mg/day
    c. 400 mg/day *ascites*
    d. 500 mg/day

17. Liver transplantation is recommended for:
    a. Very few patients with cirrhosis
    b. Selected patients with cirrhosis
    c. About 75% of patients with cirrhosis
    d. Almost all patients with cirrhosis

18. The percentage of patients with severe hepatic dysfunction from cirrhosis (serum albumin < 3 g/dl, bilirubin > 3 mg/dl, ascites, encephalopathy, cachexia, upper gastrointestinal bleeding) who survive 6 months is:
    a. 10%
    b. 20%
    c. 35%
    d. 50%

19. Primary biliary cirrhosis is a/an _____ disease of the liver.
    a. Noninflammatory *Inflammatory*
    b. Autoimmune *Destruction of duct*
    c. Contagious
    d. Oncologic

20. The major symptom in primary biliary cirrhosis is:
    a. Nausea
    b. Diarrhea and constipation
    c. Pruritus *↑ toxins*
    d. Right upper quadrant pain for many years

21. One of the most significant laboratory findings that should lead to a work-up and diagnosis of primary biliary cirrhosis is:
    a. Marked hyperbilirubinemia
    b. Greatly increased alkaline phosphatase level

22. The major physiologic aberration in Wilson's disease is:
    a. Increased excretion of copper by the liver ↓
    b. Excessive absorption of copper from the small intestine
    c. Deposition of copper in the long bones, large joints, and pelvis *liver, brain, cornea d*
    d. Excretion of copper in the urine, giving a dark color *DX >100 μg/24° kidneys*

23. The most common cause of acute cholecystitis is:
    a. An obstructed cystic duct ← *thru cystic duct*
    b. An obstructed common bile duct
    c. Cholelithiasis *#1 Answer*
    d. Only cholesterol gallstones

24. The typical pain in acute cholecystitis occurs:
    a. In the epigastric area
    b. In the right hypochondrial area
    c. In the right hypochondrium with radiation to the infrascapular area *p̄ fatty meal*
    d. In the right upper quadrant, resembling appendicitis

25. The most reliable imaging procedure to diagnose acute cholecystitis is:
    a. Plain x-rays of the abdomen *15%*
    b. Magnetic resonance imaging of the abdomen
    c. HIDA scan *98% sensitivity*
    d. Right upper quadrant ultrasound

26. Chronic cholecystitis is:
    a. Very rare
    b. Less common than acute cholecystitis *more comm*
    c. Slightly more common than acute cholecystitis
    d. Far more common than acute cholecystitis

27. One of the complications of chronic cholecystitis is:
    a. "Strawberry gallbladder"
    b. Cholangitis, with Charcot's triad of symptoms
    c. Gangrene of the gallbladder
    d. All of the above

28. Gallstones are present, often without symptoms, in about _____ of the population.
    a. 5% (5 million people)
    b. 10% (10 million people)

Petechiae (21 c.)
d. Enlarged, tender liver

c. 15% (15 million people)
d. 20% (20 million people)

29. Gallstones are classified by chemical composition such as:
    a. Calcium oxylate *Bilirubinate*
    b. Calcium pyruvate
    c. Cholesterol *& Ca Bilirubinate*
    d. Lecithin

— part of

Low CHO diet
for gallstone

30. Cholecystectomy is the treatment of choice for:
    a. Patients with asymptomatic cholelithiasis
    b. Patients with symptomatic cholelithiasis
    c. Patients with a small number of stones
    d. Patients with stones composed of calcium bilirubinate

Endocrine Disorders

HORMONES

Hormones are composed of various chemical structures: polypeptide, glycoprotein, steroid, or amine.

Hormonal Activity

- Effects of hormonal activity occur when hormones interact with receptors
  - On the cell surface (catecholamines and peptide hormones)
  - Inside the cell (thyroid and steroid hormones)

Endocrine Disorders

- Result from an excess or deficiency of hormonal effects

Transport of Hormones

- Most classical hormones are secreted into the systemic circulation in which they travel to distant sites, where they affect the body in distinctive ways.
- Hypothalamic releasing hormones are released into the pituitary portal system, resulting in much higher concentrations of the releasing hormones in the pituitary than in the systemic circulation.
- Many hormones are bound to proteins within the circulation (Table 10-1).
  - Generally, only the free (unbound) hormone is available to tissues (biologically active).
  - Binding of hormones to proteins buffers against rapid changes in plasma levels of the hormone.
    - ~ Some binding protein interactions may be involved in active regulation of hormone action.
      - – Binding proteins are often altered in disease states.

Hormone Control and Feedback

- Most hormone systems are controlled by feedback (e.g., hypothalamic-pituitary-thyroid axis) (Table 10-2 and Fig. 10-1), occurring in steps.
  - Thyrotrophin releasing hormone (TRH) is secreted in the hypothalamus, then travels via the portal system to the pituitary, where it stimulates the thyrotrophs to produce thyroid-stimulating hormone (TSH).
  - TSH is secreted into the systemic circulation, where it stimulates increased thyroidal iodine uptake and thyroxine (T_4) and triiodothyronine (T_3) synthesis and release.
  - Serum levels of T_3 and T_4 are increased by TSH; conversion of T_4 to T_3 (the more active hormone) in peripheral tissues is stimulated by TSH.
  - T_3 and T_4 then enter cells, where they bind to nuclear receptors and stimulate increased metabolic and cellular activity.
  - Blood levels of T_3 and T_4 are sensed by receptors in the pituitary and perhaps the hypothalamus; if these levels rise above normal, TRH and TSH production is suppressed, resulting in reduced T_3 and T_4 secretion.
  - Peripheral levels of T_3 and T_4 fall to normal.
- This is the negative feedback system, which refers to the effect of T_3 and T_4 on the pituitary and hypothalamus; it is the most common mechanism for regulating circulating hormone levels.
- Positive feedback systems regulate the normal menstrual cycle.

Biologic Rhythms

- The most important rhythms are circadian and menstrual.

TABLE 10-1
Plasma Hormones with Important Binding Proteins

Hormone	Binding Protein(s)
T_4	Thyroxine-binding globulin (TBG)
	Thyroxine-binding prealbumin (TBPA)
	Albumin
T_3 (less bound than T_4)	Thyroxine-binding globulin (TBG)
	Albumin
Cortisol	Cortisol-binding globulin (CBG)
Testosterone, estradiol	Sex hormone-binding globulin (SHBG)
IGF-I	IGF-binding proteins (mainly IGF-BP3)

From Drury PL, Howlett TA: Endocrinology. In Kumar P, Clark M, eds: *Clinical medicine,* ed 4, Edinburgh, 1998, WB Saunders, p 896.

TABLE 10-2
Characteristics of Several Different Hormone Systems

Characteristic	Peptides and Catecholamines	Steroids and Thyroid Hormones
Protein binding	No	Yes
Changes in plasma concentrations	Rapid changes	Slow fluctuations
Plasma half-life	Short (seconds to minutes)	Long (minutes to days)
Type of receptors	Cell membrane	Intracellular
Mechanism	Activate preformed enzymes	Stimulate protein synthesis
Secretion	Secretory granules	Direct passage rapidly
	Constitutive + bursts	Related to secretion rate
Speed of effect	Rapid (seconds to minutes)	Slow (hours to days)

From Drury PL, Howlett TA: Endocrinology. In Kumar P, Clark M, eds: *Clinical medicine,* ed 4, Edinburgh, 1998, WB Saunders, p 897.

Other Factors that Regulate Hormones

- Stress—stress-related hormones are: catecholamines, prolactin, growth hormone (GH), adrenocorticotropic hormone (ACTH), cortisol.
- Sleep
- Eating and fasting
  —Insulin secretion is increased and growth hormone is decreased after eating.

Testing Endocrine Function

- Hormones are tested in blood and plasma.
  —Basal levels: from random samples such as for thyroid hormones
- 24-Hour urine collections—used to measure some hormones, but this method is not as reliable as measuring levels in blood or plasma.
- Immunometric type endocrine assays are being used now.

ENDOCRINE DISORDERS

The most common endocrine disorders, except for diabetes mellitus (DM), are

- Thyroid disorders: thyrotoxicosis, primary hypothyroidism, and goiter; four to eight new patients/provider/year
- Subfertility: affects 5% to 10% of all couples, often involves an endocrine component; most disorders are now treatable.
- Menstrual disorders or hirsutism in young women, often associated with polycystic ovary syndrome.
- Osteoporosis: mainly postmenopausal women

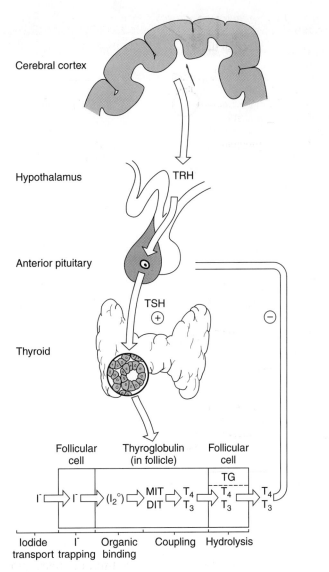

Cerebral cortex

Hypothalamus   TRH

Anterior pituitary

TSH
⊕   ⊖

Thyroid

Follicular   Thyroglobulin   Follicular
cell   (in follicle)   cell

| | | | | TG | |
| I⁻ | I⁻ | (I₂°) | MIT DIT | T₄ T₃ | T₄ T₃ | T₄ T₃ |

Iodide   I⁻   Organic   Coupling   Hydrolysis
transport trapping binding

Fig. 10-1   Synthesis and secretion of thyroid hormones. The box indicates steps that occur within the thyroid gland. Thyroid function is regulated by the hypothalamic-pituitary axis. *TRH,* Thyrotropin-releasing hormone; *TSH,* thyroid-stimulating hormone (thyrotropin); *MIT,* monoiodotyrosine; *DIT,* diiodotyrosine; *TG,* thyroglobulin; *T₃,* triiodothyronine; *T₄,* thyroxine; *I₂°,* iodine; *I⁻,* iodide. (Modified from Ezrin C, Godden J, Volpé R, et al, eds: *Systematic endocrinology,* New York, 1973, Harper & Row.)

- Primary hyperparathyroidism: affects about 0.1% of the population
- Children with short stature or delayed puberty

History of the Diagnosis of Endocrine Disorders (Box 10-1)

A number of drugs may induce endocrine disease or cause signs and symptoms that mimic endocrine disease (Table 10-3).

Autoimmune Diseases

- Organ-specific autoimmune diseases have now been identified for every major endocrine organ (Table 10-4).
  - Characterized by the presence of specific antibodies in the serum, often present for years before clinical symptoms become apparent—conditions more common in women

BOX 10-1
Components of the Patient History in Endocrine Disorders

PAST HISTORY
Previous history of endocrine disease
Previous pregnancies (ease of conception, postpartum hemorrhage)
Relevant surgery (e.g., thyroidectomy, orchidectomy)
Radiation (e.g., to thyroid, neck, gonads)
Drug exposure (e.g., chemotherapy, sex hormones, oral contraceptives)
Childhood developmental milestones and rate of growth

FAMILY HISTORY
Autoimmune disease
Endocrine disease
Essential hypertension
Diabetes

FAMILY MEMBERS
Height
Weight
Body habitus
Hair growth pattern (e.g., baldness, body hair)
Age and sexual development at puberty

SOCIAL HISTORY
Detailed records of alcohol intake, particularly associated with subfertility, obesity
Drug abuse, particularly cannabis use and subfertility
Details regarding occupation, access or exposure to drugs or chemicals
Diet, particularly with regard to salt, licorice, iodine

From Drury PL, Howlett TA: Endocrinology. In Kumar P, Clark M, eds: *Clinical medicine,* ed 4, Edinburgh, 1998, WB Saunders, p 901.

TABLE 10-3
Drugs Associated with Endocrine Disorders

Drug	Effect
(Those that induce endocrine disease)	Increase prolactin, causing galactorrhea
Chlorpromazine	
Metoclopramide (dopamine agonists)	
Estrogens	
Iodine	Hyperthyroidism
Amiodarone*	
Chlorpropamide	Inappropriate ADH secretion
Ketoconazole	Hypoadrenalism
Metyrapone, aminoglutethimide	
DRUGS SIMULATING ENDOCRINE DISEASE	
Sympathomimetics	Mimic thyrotoxicosis or pheochromocytoma
Amphetamines	
Licorice	Increase mineralocorticoid activity; mimic aldosteronism
Carbenoxolone	
Purgatives	Hypokalemia
Diuretics	Secondary aldosteronism
ACE inhibitors	Hypoaldosteronism
DRUGS AFFECTING HORMONE-BINDING PROTEINS	
Anticonvulsants	Bind to TBG—decrease total T_4
Estrogens	Raise TBG and CBG—increase total T_4, cortisol
EXOGENOUS HORMONES OR STIMULATING AGENTS	
Use, abuse, or misuse, by patient or doctor, of the following:	
Steroids	Cushing's syndrome
	Diabetes
Thyroxine	Thyrotoxicosis factitia
Vitamin D preparations	Hypercalcemia
Milk and alkali preparations	
Insulin	Hypoglycemia
Sulfonylureas	

From Drury PL, Howlett TA: Endocrinology. In Kumar P, Clark M, eds: *Clinical medicine,* ed 4, Edinburgh, 1998, WB Saunders, p 902.
ACE, Angiotensin converting enzyme; *TBG,* thyroxine-binding globulin; *CBG,* cortisol-binding globulin.
*Amiodarone may cause both hypothyroidism and hyperthyroidism.

TABLE 10-4
Types of Autoimmune Diseases

Occurrence	Disorder	Mechanism/Evidence
Common	Hashimoto's thyroiditis	Cell-mediated and humoral thyroid cytotoxicity
	SLE	Circulating and locally generalized immunocomplexes
	Goodpasture's syndrome	Antibasement membrane antibody
	Pemphigus	Epidermal acantholytic antibody
	Receptor autoimmunity	
	Graves' disease	TSH receptor antibody (stimulatory)
	Myasthenia gravis	Acetylcholine receptor antibody
	Insulin resistance	Insulin receptor antibody
	Autoimmune hemolytic anemia	Phagocytosis of antibody-sensitized RBCs
	Autoimmune thrombocytopenic purpura	Phagocytosis of antibody-sensitized platelets
Less common	RA	Immunocomplexes in joints
	Scleroderma with anticollagen antibodies	Nucleolar and other nuclear antibodies
	Mixed connective tissue disease	Antibody to extractable nuclear antigen (ribonucleoprotein)
	Polymyositis	Nonhistone ANA
	Idiopathic Addison's disease	Humoral and (?) cell-mediated adrenal cytotoxicity
	Infertility (some persons)	Antispermatozoal antibodies
	Glomerulonephritis	Glomerular basement membrane antibody, or immune complexes
	Bullous pemphigoid	IgG and complement in basement membrane
	Sjögren's syndrome	Multiple tissue antibodies, a specific nonhistone anti-SS-B antibody
	DM (some)	Cell-mediated and humoral islet cell antibodies
Not common	Chronic active hepatitis	Smooth muscle antibody
	Primary biliary cirrhosis	Mitochondrial antibody
	Other endocrine gland failure	Specific tissue antibodies in some cases
	Vitiligo	Melanocyte antibody
	Vasculitis	Ig and complement in vessel walls, low serum component in some cases
	Post-MI, cardiotomy syndrome	Myocardial antibody
	Urticaria, atopic dermatitis, asthma (some cases)	IgG and IgM antibodies to IgE
	Other inflammatory, granulomatous, degenerative, and atrophic disorders	No reasonable alternative explanation

From Beers MH, Berkow R, eds: Immunology, allergic disorders. *The Merck manual of diagnosis and therapy,* ed 17, Whitehouse Station, NJ, 1999, Merck & Co, Inc, p 1062.
SLE, Systemic lupus erythematosus; *RBCs,* red blood cells; *RA,* rheumatoid arthritis; *ANA,* antinuclear antibody; *Ig,* immunoglobulin; *TSH,* thyroid-stimulating hormone; *MI,* myocardial infarction.

—Have a strong genetic component, often with identical-twin concordance rate of 50%, and human leukocyte antigen (HLA) associations (Box 10-2)

Signs and Symptoms (Box 10-3)
• Many endocrine symptoms are vague and diffuse, with a broad range of differential diagnoses.

• Erectile dysfunction (ED) and decreased libido in men
  —Causes
    ~ Psychogenic factors
    ~ Endocrine
    ~ Vascular
    ~ Neurologic

CENTRAL CONTROL OF ENDOCRINE FUNCTION

- The pituitary gland (hypophysis) is no longer considered the "master gland."
- The **hypothalamus** is the final common pathway that receives input from virtually all other areas of the central nervous system (CNS) and directs input to the pituitary (Table 10-5).
  —The hypothalamus has many centers.
  —Its essential functions
    ~ Appetite
    ~ Thirst
    ~ Body heat regulation
    ~ Sleeping/waking
    ~ Influences circadian rhythm, menstrual cycles, and responses to stress, mood, and exercise
    ~ Can alter pituitary hormone secretion
    ~ Modulates activities of the anterior and posterior lobes of the pituitary gland
- Synthetic hypothalamic hormones and their antagonists are available now, for testing aspects of endocrine function and for treatment.
- Most hormones produced by the hypothalamus and the pituitary are secreted in a pulsatile fashion, with brief periods of inactivity and activity.
- Some hormones (e.g., ACTH, GH, and prolactin) have definite circadian or diurnal

---

BOX 10-2

Drugs that Cause Impotence

Alcohol	Leuprolide
Amphetamines	Marijuana
Antihistamines	Methadone
Barbiturates	Methyldopa
β-Blockers	Metoclopramide
Butyrophenones	Monoamine oxidase inhibitors
Carbamazepine	Narcotics
Cimetidine	Phenothiazines
Clonidine	Sedatives
Cocaine	Spironolactone
Guanethidine	Thiazides
Ketoconazole	Tricyclic antidepressants

From Fitzgerald PA: Endocrinology. In Tierney LM, McPhee SJ, Papadakis MA, eds: *Current medical diagnosis & treatment 2000*, ed 39, New York, 2000, Lange Medical Books/McGraw-Hill, p 1082.

BOX 10-3

Common Presenting Signs/Symptoms in Endocrine Disorders

BODY SIZE AND SHAPE
Short stature
Tall stature
Excessive weight or weight gain
Loss of weight

"METABOLIC" EFFECTS
Fatigue
Weakness
Increased appetite
Decreased appetite
Polydipsia/thirst
Polyuria/nocturia
Tremor
Palpitations
Anxiety

LOCAL EFFECTS
Swelling in the neck (goiter)
Carpal tunnel syndrome
Bone or muscle pain
Protrusion of the eyes
Visual loss (acuity or fields)
Headache

REPRODUCTION/SEX
Loss or absence of libido
Erectile dysfunction
Oligomenorrhea/amenorrhea
Subfertility
Galactorrhea
Gynecomastia
Delayed puberty
Precocious puberty

SKIN
Hirsutism
Hair thinning
Pigmentation
Dry skin
Excess sweating

From Drury PL, Howlett TA: Endocrinology. In Kumar P, Clark M, eds: *Clinical medicine*, ed 4, Edinburgh, 1998, WB Saunders, p 901.

rhythms with increased secretion during specific hours of the day.

- Other hormones (luteinizing hormone [LH] and follicle-stimulating hormone [FSH] during the menstrual cycle) have month-long rhythms with superimposed circadian rhythms.
- **TRH** stimulates synthesis and secretion of **TSH** and **prolactin.**
  - **Dopamine** is the major regulator of prolactin and inhibits its synthesis and release.
  - Under specific conditions, dopamine can also inhibit LH, FSH, and TSH release.
- **Gonadotropin-releasing hormone (GnRH),** known as **luteinizing hormone–releasing hormone (LH-RH),** stimulates secretion of both LH and FSH.
- **Somatostatin** exerts negative control over both GH and TSH synthesis and secretion.
  - Somatostatin can also inhibit secretion of insulin.
- GH release is stimulated by **growth hormone–releasing hormone** (GH-RH), and inhibited by somatostatin.
  - The rate of GH production depends on the relative strength of these two stimuli.
- **Corticotropin-releasing hormone** stimulates the release of ACTH from the pituitary.
- **ACTH** is also called corticotropin.
- The pituitary glycoprotein hormones include TSH, LH, and FSH, as well as the placental hormone **human chorionic gonadotropin.**

- TSH regulates the structure and function of the thyroid gland, and stimulates synthesis and release of thyroid hormones.
- TSH synthesis and secretion are controlled by the hypothalamic hormone TRH and by suppression of feedback action of circulating thyroid hormone.
- LH and FSH are stimulated by hypothalamic neurohormone GnRH (LH-RH).
  - LH and FSH are essential in women to stimulate ovarian follicular development and ovulation.
- In men, FSH acts on Sertoli's cells and is necessary for spermatogenesis.
  - LH acts on Leydig's cells of the testis to stimulate testosterone biosynthesis.
- **Human GH** is similar in structure to the placental hormone **human chorionic somatomammotropin.**
  - GH-RH is the major stimulator, and somatostatin the major inhibitor, of synthesis and secretion of GH.
  - GH stimulates somatic growth and regulates metabolism.

PITUITARY HORMONES (BOX 10-4)
Posterior Pituitary Function

- The posterior pituitary secretes **antidiuretic hormone** (ADH, **vasopressin**) and **oxytocin.**
  - The major action of ADH is to promote water conservation by the kidney.

TABLE 10-5
Hypothalamic Neurohormones and Their Effects

Neurohormone	Hormones Affected	Effects
TRH	TSH, PRL	Stimulate both
GnRH	LH, FSH, PRL	Stimulate* (LH, FSH) Stimulate (PRL) (?)
Dopamine	PRL, LH, FSH, TSH	Inhibit all 4
CRH	ACTH	Stimulate
GH-RH	GH	Stimulate
Somatostatin	GH, TSH	Inhibit both

From Beers MH, Berkow R, eds: Immunology, allergic disorders. *The Merck manual of diagnosis and therapy,* ed 17, Whitehouse Station, NJ, 1999, Merck & Co, Inc, p 66.
PRL, Prolactin; *CRH,* corticotropin-releasing hormone.
*LH and FSH are stimulated under physiologic conditions when administered exogenously in intermittent pulses.

BOX 10-4
Pituitary Hormones

ANTERIOR PITUITARY
GH*
Prolactin (PRL)
ACTH
TSH
LH†
FSH

POSTERIOR PITUITARY
Arginine vasopressin (AVP)‡
Oxytocin

From Fitzgerald PA: Endocrinology. In Tierney LM, McPhee SJ, Papadakis MA, eds: *Current medical diagnosis & treatment 2000,* ed 39, New York, 2000, Lange Medical Books/McGraw-Hill, p 1083.
*GH resembles human placental lactogen (HPL).
†LH resembles human chorionic gonadotropin (HCG).
‡AVP is identical with ADH.

~ ADH, like aldosterone, maintains fluid homeostasis, and vascular and cellular hydration.

~ The primary stimulus for ADH release is increased osmotic pressure of body water, sensed by osmoreceptors in the hypothalamus.

~ Secondary stimuli are baroreceptors in the left atrium, pulmonary veins, carotid sinus, and aortic arch that sense volume depletion.

• Diabetes insipidus (DI) is the result of either lack of ADH (central DI) or the inability of the kidney to respond to ADH (nephrogenic DI [NDI]).

PITUITARY DISORDERS
Hypopituitarism

Definition

Hypopituitarism includes endocrine deficiencies due to partial or complete loss of anterior lobe pituitary function.

Risk Factors/Etiology (Table 10-6)
Diagnosis
Signs and Symptoms

• Patients with hypopituitarism may have single or multiple hormonal deficiencies.
• Relate to the underlying cause and to the specific hormones that are missing
• Onset is either sudden or insidious.
• Gonadotropins are lost first, then GH, followed by TSH and ACTH.
• ADH deficiency is rare in primary pituitary disease, but common in stalk and hypothalamic diseases.
• All target glands cease functioning when all related hormones are decreased or absent, causing panhypopituitarism.
• Decrease or lack of LH and FSH in women causes amenorrhea, regression of secondary sexual characteristics, and infertility.
• Lack of gonadotropins in men usually results in erectile dysfunction, testicular atrophy, regression of secondary sexual characteristics, and decreased spermatogenesis with resulting infertility.

TABLE 10-6
Causes of Hypopituitarism

CAUSES AFFECTING THE PITUITARY GLAND (PRIMARY HYPOPITUITARISM)

Pituitary tumors
  Adenomas
  Craniopharyngiomas
Infarction or ischemic necrosis of the pituitary
  Shock, especially postpartum (Sheehan's syndrome), in diabetes mellitus or in sickle cell anemia
  Vascular thrombosis or aneurysms, especially of the internal carotid artery
  Hemorrhagic infarction (pituitary apoplexy)
Inflammatory processes
  Meningitis (tubercular, other bacterial, fungal, malarial)

Pituitary abscesses
Sarcoidosis
Infiltrative disorders
  Langerhans' cell-type histiocytosis (Hand-Schüller-Christian disease)
  Hemochromatosis
Idiopathic isolated or multiple pituitary hormone deficiencies
Iatrogenic
  Irradiation
  Surgical extirpation
Autoimmune dysfunction of the pituitary (lymphocytic hypophysis)

CAUSES PRIMARILY AFFECTING THE HYPOTHALAMUS (SECONDARY HYPOPITUITARISM)

Hypothalamic tumors
  Pinealomas
    Meningiomas
    Ependymomas
      Metastatic neoplasms

Inflammatory processes (e.g., sarcoidosis)
Trauma (sometimes associated with basal skull fracture)
Isolated or multiple neurohormone
  Deficiencies of the hypothalamus
Surgical transection of the pituitary stalk

From Beers MH, Berkow R, eds: Immunology, allergic disorders. *The Merck manual of diagnosis and therapy,* ed 17, Whitehouse Station, NJ, 1999, Merck & Co, Inc, p 70.

- GH deficiency is usually not clinically detectable in adults.
- Decreased ACTH causes hypoadrenalism and associated fatigue, hypotension, and intolerance to stress and infection.
  - —In addition, persons with ACTH deficiency do not have the hyperpigmentation characteristic of primary adrenal failure.
- Sheehan's syndrome occurs in women, causing delay or absence of lactation after birth from pituitary necrosis due to hypovolemia and shock that may have occurred in the peripartum period.
  - —The patient may experience fatigue and loss of pubic and axillary hair.
- Pituitary apoplexy is a symptom caused by hemorrhagic infarction of either a normal pituitary gland or more often a tumor.
  - —Symptoms may include severe headache, stiff neck, fever, and disturbances in vision.
- Varying degrees of hypopituitarism may develop suddenly; the patient may present in vascular collapse due to deficient ACTH and cortisol secretion.
  - —Usually, the cerebrospinal fluid (CSF) has blood in it, and a magnetic resonance imaging (MRI) scan will document hemorrhage.
- **The definite diagnosis of hypopituitarism must be made before having the patient receive hormone replacement therapy.**
- Required to confirm diagnosis are accurate test data relating to structural abnormalities of the pituitary gland, or evidence of hormonal deficits that indicate loss of function of the pituitary gland.
  - —*Tumors:* skull x-rays of the sella turcica and visual field testing provide signs/symptoms of tumor.
  - —*Pituitary adenomas* are detected by high-resolution computed tomography (CT) or MRI with contrast media as required.
  - —Positron emission tomography (PET) is available in specialized centers.
  - —Cerebral angiography is used only when other radiographic tests indicate the possibility of perisellar vascular anomalies or aneurysms.

- Evaluation of thyroid hormones provides an estimate of thyroid function: T_4, T_3, and TSH levels are measured by radioimmunoassay.
  - —All levels will likely be low; an elevated TSH indicates a primary abnormality of the thyroid gland.
- The **insulin tolerance test** is the best method to evaluate ACTH, GH, and prolactin reserves; however, this test is contraindicated in the elderly, those with DM or with severe panhypopituitarism, or when ischemic heart disease or epilepsy is present.
  - —This test alone will not differentiate between primary (Addison's disease) and secondary (hypopituitary) adrenal insufficiency.
- Evaluation of GH is usually not done in adults because the deficiency, if present, is not treated unless short stature is present and epiphyseal closure has not occurred.
- Evaluation of LH and FSH levels is helpful in diagnosing hypopituitarism in postmenopausal women who are not taking exogenous estrogens, and in whom circulating gonadotropin concentrations are normally high (30 MU/ml).

Differential Diagnosis
- Panhypopituitarism must be differentiated from a number of other disorders: anorexia nervosa, chronic liver disease, myotonia dystrophica, and polyglandular autoimmune disease.
- Serum ACTH and TSH are not elevated in hypopituitarism, ruling out primary adrenal or thyroid deficiency.
- Glucocorticoids or megestrol treatment suppress endogenous ACTH and cortisol secretion, which are reversible with discontinuation of the drug.
- Severe illness causes functional suppression of TSH and T_4.
  - —Hyperthyroxinemia reversibly suppresses TSH.

Complications
- Complications may develop from space-occupying lesions, or from surgery or radiation therapy (small vessel ischemia, strokes, second tumors).

- Visual field impairment may occur.
- Hypothalamic damage may result in morbid obesity and in cognitive and emotional problems.
- Patients with untreated hypoadrenalism coupled with stressful illness may develop fever and die in shock and coma.
- Some adults with GH deficiency have increased cardiovascular morbidity.
- Hemorrhage may occur in large pituitary tumors resulting in rapid loss of vision, headache, and acute pituitary failure (pituitary apoplexy), which require emergency decompression of the sella.

Treatment

- The goal of therapy is to replace those hormones missing because of hypofunctioning of the target glands (Table 10-7).
- Underlying causes of hormone deficiencies such as tumors must be treated separately, as well as replacement of hormones.
  —Surgical treatment of tumors of the pituitary or other glands remains somewhat controversial, depending on the location, size, and effects on the body by the tumor.

Prognosis

- Treatment of hormonal deficiencies is generally quite favorable, even when surgery may be required to excise tumors or other procedures.

- Hormone replacement therapy may need to continue for some time after surgery to correct the problem in the gland; continuance is needed to allow time for resolution of the underlying problem and for normal functioning of the gland(s) and hormones to take place.

Patient/Family Education

- As in all other problems, the patient and family should be instructed regarding the nature, cause, course, treatment, and expected outcome.
- If patients have a reasonably accurate picture of the problem and the time required for resolution, they are more likely to be cooperative and optimistic.
- Written instructions are given when the patient is on hormone replacement therapy as to dose, time, and anticipated duration of treatment.
- Signs or symptoms that should not appear or be present should be written, so that the patient can immediately contact the clinician for advice and help in correcting the problem.

Follow-up/Referral

- The patient has been followed closely by an endocrinologist from the beginning and will continue for months to years after therapy/surgery.

TABLE 10-7
Replacement Therapy for Hypopituitarism

Axis	Usual Replacement Therapies
Gonadal	
Male	Testosterone IM or PO, as patch or implant
Female	Cyclical estrogen/progestogen PO or as patch/implant
Fertility	HCG plus FSH (purified or recombinant) to produce testicular development, spermatogenesis, or ovulation
	Pulsatile LH-RH is also used
Breast (Prolactin inhibition)	Dopamine agonist as replacement inhibition (e.g., bromocriptine 3-15 mg/day)
Growth	Recombinant human GH to achieve normal growth in children
	Same therapy for adults where GH affects muscle mass and well-being
Thyroid	Thyroxine 100-150 μg/day
Adrenal	Hydrocortisone 15-40 mg/day (divided doses) or prednisolone 5-10 mg/day
Thirst	Desmopressin (DDAVP) 10-20 μg qd-tid by nasal spray or PO 100-200 μg tid

From Drury PL, Howlett TA: Endocrinology. In Kumar P, Clark M, eds: *Clinical medicine,* ed 4, Edinburgh, 1998, WB Saunders, p 909.
HCG, Human chorionic gonadotropin.

- Some patients have diminished psychosocial functioning, due to suboptimal hormone replacement, or brain dysfunction due to underlying disease, radiation therapy, or surgery.
- Patients may have a normal life span if they receive optimal replacement therapy, and if the underlying hypopituitarism is not progressive.
- Continued monitoring is necessary for many patients.

Hyperpituitarism

Definition

Hyperpituitarism is the hypersecretion of anterior pituitary hormones.
- GH, resulting in acromegaly, gigantism
- Prolactin, resulting in galactorrhea
- ACTH, resulting in pituitary-type Cushing's syndrome

Etiology/Cause

- Syndromes of excessive secretion of GH, also known as hypersomatotropism, are almost always due to adenoma of the somatotrophs.

Pathogenesis

- Many GH-secreting adenomas contain a mutant form of the G_s protein, a stimulatory regulator of adenylate cyclase.
- Mutations of the G_s protein in the somatotrophs bypass the need for GH-RH to stimulate GH secretion.
- A few cases of ectopic GH-RH-producing tumors in the pancreas and lung have also been reported.

Diagnosis

Signs and Symptoms

- GH excess can begin at any age but most often starts in those between the ages of 30 and 60.
- When GH hypersecretion begins after the epiphyses have closed, the earliest clinical sign is coarsening of the facial features and soft tissue swelling of the hands and feet.
- Increased size of the arms and legs (acral parts) led to the term acromegaly.
- Coarse body hair increases.
- Skin becomes thicker and darker.

- Size and activity of sebaceous and sweat glands increase, resulting in excessive perspiration and an offensive body odor.
- Growth of the mandible results in protrusion of the jaw and malocclusion of teeth.
- Proliferation of cartilage tissue of the larynx results in a deep, husky voice.
- In persons with long-standing acromegaly, costal growth occurs, resulting in a barrel chest.
- Joint symptoms are common, and crippling degenerative arthritis may ensue.
- Peripheral neuropathies are common due to compression of nerves by adjacent fibrous tissue and endoneural fibrous proliferation.
- Headaches occur frequently due to the pituitary tumor.
- Bitemporal hemianopia may develop due to a suprasellar extension that compresses the optic chiasm.
- Heart, kidneys, spleen, liver, thyroid, parathyroid glands, and pancreas all become larger than normal.
- Cardiac disease occurs in about 30% of patients, which doubles the risk of death from heart disease.
- Hypertension develops in about 30% of patients.
- Likelihood of malignancy increases twofold to threefold.
- Impaired glucose tolerance occurs in about 50% of cases of acromegaly or gigantism.
- Clinically significant DM occurs in about 10% of patients.
- In women, galactorrhea may occur due to hyperprolactinemia.
  —Lactation occurs frequently in cases of GH excess alone because GH is a potent lactogenic hormone.
- Sexual immaturity is common in gigantism, with about 30% of men developing erectile dysfunction, and almost all women experience irregular menses or amenorrhea.

Diagnostic Tests

- Skull x-rays show cortical thickening, enlargement of the frontal sinuses, and enlargement and erosion of the sella turcica.
- X-rays of the hands show tufting of the terminal phalanges and soft tissue thickening.
- Glucose tolerance is often abnormal.

- Serum phosphate levels are usually elevated due to GH's tendency to increase tubular re-absorption of phosphate, resulting in hyper-phosphatemia.
- Plasma levels of GH as measured by radioimmunoassay are usually elevated.
  - This testing is the simplest method to assess GH hypersecretion.
  - These tests are also important in monitoring response to therapy.
- Fasting blood samples to diagnose acromegaly
  - Response to a glucose load is the standard for diagnosing acromegaly.
- Plasma insulin-like growth factor I (IGF-I), also known as somatomedin-C, is measured in all patients suspected of having acromegaly, whose levels of IGF-I may show a threefold to tenfold increase.
- If no tumor is apparent on CT or MRI, excessive secretion of pituitary GH may be due to a tumor that is producing excessive amounts of GH-RH; elevated plasma levels of GH-RH confirm this diagnosis.

Treatment

- Ablative therapy by surgery or radiation is usually indicated.
- Transsphenoidal resection of the tumor is preferred now, depending on individual endocrinologists and hospitals.
- After surgery, the GH levels after a glucose tolerance test fall to <2 ng/ml, which indicates cure; if the levels are 10 ng/ml, further therapy is needed.
- Medical therapy bromocriptine mesylate up to 15 mg/day PO in divided doses often effectively lower GH levels in some patients
- For those patients in whom surgery, irradiation, or bromocriptine has been ineffective, a long-acting somatostatin analog, octreotide, is given subcutaneously.

Galactorrhea

Definition

Galactorrhea is lactation in men or in women who are not breast-feeding an infant.

Etiology/Cause

- In both men and women, prolactinomas are the most common secretory tumors of the pituitary that produce excessive amounts of prolactin.
- Most tumors in women are microadenomas less than 10 mm in diameter.
  - A small percentage are macroadenomas, which are larger than 10 mm in diameter at the time of diagnosis.
  - Ingestion of particular drugs may also cause hyperprolactinemia and galactorrhea (Box 10-5).

Diagnosis

Signs and Symptoms

- Amenorrhea occurs along with galactorrhea in women; three syndromes of the galactorrhea/amenorrhea syndrome have been reported.
  - Persistent galactorrhea/amenorrhea after pregnancy (Chiari-Frommel syndrome)
  - Galactorrhea/amenorrhea not associated with pregnancy (Ahumada del Castillo syndrome)
  - Galactorrhea/amenorrhea caused by chromophobe adenoma of the pituitary (Forbes-Albright syndrome)
- Headaches and visual disturbances are common complaints in men with prolactin-secreting pituitary tumors.
- Loss of libido and potency occur in about 65% of men.
- Women with galactorrhea/amenorrhea often have symptoms of estrogen deficiency (e.g., hot flashes, dyspareunia).
  - Estrogen levels are often normal.
  - Signs of androgen excess are seen in some hyperprolactinemic women.

Diagnostic Tests

- Basal prolactin levels usually correlate with the size of the pituitary tumor.
- Serum gonadotropin and estradiol levels may be low to normal.
- Absence of elevated TSH rules out primary hypothyroidism.
- High-resolution CT and MRI identify microadenomas.
- Visual field examination is indicated in all patients with macroadenomas and in patients who elect medical treatment or surveillance only.

BOX 10-5
Causes of Hyperprolactinemia

PHYSIOLOGIC
Nipple stimulation in men and women
Pregnancy
Postpartum period
Stress
Food ingestion
Sexual intercourse in some women
Sleep
Hypoglycemia
Early infancy (birth to 3 mos)

PATHOLOGIC
Hypothalamic disorders
Hypothalamic tumors
Nontumor hypothalamic infiltration
  Sarcoidosis
  Langerhans' cell-type histiocytosis
    (Hand-Schüller-Christian disease)
Postencephalitis
Idiopathic galactorrhea (likely an abnormality in
  dopamine secretion)
Head trauma
Prolactin-secreting pituitary tumors
Surgical pituitary stalk section or lesions
Empty sella syndrome
Acromegaly

PATHOLOGIC—cont'd
Cushing's disease
Primary hypothyroidism
Chronic renal failure
Liver disease
Ectopic production of prolactin bronchogenic carcino-
  ma (small cell undifferentiated, not squamous cell)
Hypernephroma
Chest wall lesions
  Surgical scars
  Trauma
  Neoplasms of the chest wall
  Herpes zoster

PHARMACOLOGIC
Psychoactive drugs
  Phenothiazines
  Tricyclic antidepressants
  Butyrophenones (haloperidol)
  Benzamides (metoclopramide)
Antihypertensive drugs
  Reserpine
  α-Methyldopa
  Calcium channel blockers
Oral contraceptives
TRH

From Rebar RW: Practical evaluation of hormonal status. In Yen SSC, Jaffe RB, eds: *Reproductive endocrinology: physiology, pathophysiology, and clinical management,* Philadelphia, 1978, WB Saunders, p 493.

Differential Diagnosis
- Acromegaly (pituitary tumors often co-secrete prolactin and GH)
- Hypothyroidism
- Cirrhosis
- Renal failure
- Systemic lupus erythematosus
- Hypothalamic disease
- Nipple piercing, augmentation mammoplasty, and mastectomy may stimulate prolactin secretion.
- Drugs: phenothiazine derivatives, cimetidine, tricyclic antidepressants, oral contraceptives

Treatment
- Treatment depends on cause (e.g., hypothyroidism is corrected with T_4).
- Dopamine agonists are the treatment of choice for patients with macroprolactinomas and those with hyperprolactinemia who wish to restore normal sexual function and fertility.
  —Cabergoline 0.25 mg PO once/week × 1 week, then 0.25 mg twice/week for 1 week, then 0.5 mg twice/week; dosage is increased every month, based on prolactin levels, to maximum of 1.5 mg twice/week.
  —Alternative drugs are bromocriptine 1.25-20 mg/day PO; pergolide 0.125-2 mg/day PO; quinagolide (Norprolac) 0.075 mg/day PO is a nonergot-derived dopamine agonist not currently available in the United States.
- Treatment of some patients is controversial.
  —Patients with prolactin levels < 100 mg/ml and with normal CT and MRI scans are treated with bromocriptine or kept under observation.

- Bromocriptine is used to treat patients without evidence of tumors because those with hyperprolactinemia and women with estrogen deficiency are at greater risk of developing osteoporosis.
- Bromocriptine is recommended for women who are considering pregnancy and those with excessive galactorrhea.
- Periodic evaluation of basal prolactin levels and radiographic evaluation of the sella turcica are indicated for monitoring purposes.
- Patients with macroadenomas should be treated with bromocriptine only after comprehensive testing of pituitary function and consultation with an endocrinologist, neurosurgeon, and radiologist.
- A major problem with irradiation is that hypopituitarism frequently occurs several years after therapy; therefore this treatment is not used except for patients who have not responded to any other therapy.

Patient/Family Education

- The nature, cause, usual course, and treatment of the condition should be explained to the patient and family members.
- Instruct about medications and treatment choices, if any (e.g., surgery, irradiation), depending on the disease.

Follow-up/Referral

- At least annual evaluation of endocrine function and of the sella turcica is indicated for the remainder of the patient's life after treatment for macroadenoma.

POSTERIOR LOBE PITUITARY DISORDERS
Diabetes Insipidus

Definition

DI is a temporary or chronic disorder of the neurohypophyseal system due to deficiency of vasopressin (ADH), characterized by excretion of excessive amounts of very dilute but otherwise normal urine and by excessive thirst.

- Two causes of diabetes insipidus are possible.
  - Central or vasopressin (ADH)-sensitive DI (discussed here)
  - NDI, in which the kidneys are ADH-resistant

Etiology/Cause

- All of the pathologic lesions associated with DI involve the supraoptic and paraventricular nuclei of the hypothalamus or a large portion of the pituitary stalk.

Pathogenesis

- Simple destruction of the posterior lobe of the pituitary leads to temporary, unsustained DI.
- The posterior lobe is the primary site for ADH storage and release.
- ADH is synthesized within the hypothalamus.
  - Newly synthesized ADH can be released into the circulation as long as the hypothalamic nuclei and part of the neurohypophyseal tract are intact.
- DI may be *primary*, caused by a marked decrease in the hypothalamic nuclei of the neurohypophyseal system, or *secondary (acquired)*, caused by a variety of pathologic lesions.
  - Hypophysectomy
  - Cranial injuries, particularly basal skull fractures
  - Suprasellar and intrasellar neoplasms, either primary or metastatic
  - Langerhans' cell–type histiocytosis (Hand-Schüller-Christian disease)
  - Granulomas
  - Vascular lesions (thrombosis, aneurysm)
  - Infections (encephalitis, meningitis)
- Genetic abnormalities of the vasopressin gene on chromosome 20 are the cause of autosomal dominant forms of primary DI, but many cases of primary DI are idiopathic.

Diagnosis
Signs and Symptoms

- Onset of DI may be abrupt or insidious, and can occur at any age.
- Polydipsia and polyuria are the only signs of primary DI.
- In secondary (acquired) forms of DI, symptoms and signs include those of the associated lesions, as well as those of DI.
- Tremendous quantities of fluid may be ingested and equally large volumes (3 to 30 L/

day) of very dilute urine (specific gravity < 1.005; osmolality < 200 mOsm/L) are excreted.

- Nocturia is nearly always present in DI and in NDI.
- Hypovolemia and dehydration can develop rapidly if urinary losses are not continuously replaced.

Diagnostic Tests

- DI must be differentiated from other causes of polyuria (e.g., decreased synthesis of ADH, decreased release of ADH, osmotic diuresis as in DM, and drugs such as lithium or demeclocycline.
- The water deprivation test is the simplest and most reliable method to diagnose DI but *is performed only when the patient is under continual observation.*
  - —Patients with DI are usually unable to concentrate urine to greater than the plasma osmolality, nor increase their urine osmolality more than 50% after vasopressin.
  - —Patients with NDI are unable to concentrate urine to greater than the plasma osmolality and show no additional response to vasopressin administration.
- Hypertonic saline infusion has been used to test for DI, but can be dangerous in patients unable to tolerate a saline load (e.g., those with heart disease).
- Measuring the circulating ADH concentrations by radioimmunoassay is the most direct method to diagnose DI, but the test is difficult to perform and is not routinely available. In addition, water deprivation is so accurate that direct measurement of ADH is unnecessary.

Differential Diagnosis

- Compulsive (psychogenic) water drinking
  - —This condition may be difficult to distinguish from actual DI.
  - —These patients excrete up to 6 L of fluid/day and are often emotionally disturbed.
  - —They usually do not have nocturia, and thirst does not awaken them at night.
  - —Polydipsia results in increased water intake and suppression of endogenous ADH, which results in polyuria.

- —Chronic water intake decreases medullary tonicity in the kidneys, resulting in resistance to ADH.
- —Response to water deprivation may approach that of patients with partial DI, and show no further response to exogenous vasopressin after water deprivation.
- —If ingestion of large quantities of water continues, it can result in life-threatening hyponatremia.
- —With water restricted to 2 L/day, normal concentrating ability returns, but may take several weeks.

Treatment

- Central DI is treated by hormone replacement therapy, but this should follow treatment of the underlying organic cause of the DI.
- *If appropriate treatment is not provided, permanent renal damage can result.*
- Aqueous vasopressin is given subcutaneously (SC) or intramuscularly (IM), 5-10 U to provide an antidiuretic response that lasts about 6 hours or less.
  - —This drug is not used for long-term therapy but can be used initially in patients who are unconscious or in those undergoing surgical treatment.
- Synthetic vasopressin can be given qid as a nasal spray, with dosage and schedule tailored to each patient.
- Desmopressin acetate, 1-deamino-8-D-arginine vasopressin (DDAVP), provides prolonged antidiuretic activity that lasts 12-24 hours in most patients, and may be given intranasally, SC, or intravenously (IV).
  - —Variation among individuals is great, so specific length of activity must be established for every individual, and morning and evening doses are adjusted separately.
  - —Overdosage can result in fluid retention and decreased plasma osmolality; furosemide is given to counteract retention and induce diuresis.
  - —Headache is a frequent side effect, but reducing the dosage usually resolves the problem.

Patient/Family Education

- As in other conditions, the patient and family need to understand the basic problem, its nature, course, effects, signs and symptoms, and treatment.

- Written instructions should accompany all medications.
- Written signs and symptoms that indicate either the need for emergency treatment or an appointment with the clinician should be given to the patient.

Follow-up/Referral

- These patients should be followed every 1-2 months for at least a year to determine that the condition is completely resolved.

THYROID DISORDERS
Definition

Thyroid disorders include euthyroid goiter, euthyroid sick syndrome, hyperthyroidism, hypothyroidism, thyroiditis, and thyroid cancers.

- Thyroid hormones have two major physiologic effects.
  - —Increase protein synthesis in almost every body tissue.
  - —T_3 increases oxygen consumption primarily in tissues responsible for basal oxygen consumption (e.g., heart, liver, kidney, and skeletal muscle).

Euthyroid Goiter
Definition

Euthyroid goiter is an enlargement of the thyroid gland but without clinical or laboratory evidence of thyroid dysfunction unless the cause is iodine deficiency, which results in endemic (colloid) goiter. Euthyroid goiter is the most common cause of thyroid enlargement and is noted most frequently at puberty, during pregnancy, and at menopause.

Etiology/Cause

- Intrinsic thyroid hormone production defects
- Ingestion of food that contains antithyroid substances that inhibit hormone synthesis, particularly in iodine-deficient countries
- Many drugs (e.g., aminosalicylic acid, lithium, and iodine in large doses) may decrease synthesis of thyroid hormone.

Diagnosis
Signs and Symptoms

- Diagnosis depends on the presence of a soft, symmetric, smooth goiter.
- Radioactive iodine uptake may be normal or high, and thyroid scan is usually normal.
- Thyroid function tests are usually normal.
- Later, multiple nodules and cysts may develop.
- Thyroid antibodies are measured to rule out Hashimoto's thyroiditis as a cause of euthyroid goiter.

Treatment

- In iodine-deficient countries, iodine supplements in iodized salt, oral or intramuscular administration of iodized oil annually, and iodination of water, crops, or animal fodder
- In some cases, suppression of the hypothalamic-pituitary axis with thyroid hormone blocks TSH stimulation because TSH plays a major role in goiter formation.
- Surgical excision of the goiter may be necessary in some cases.

Patient/Family Education

- In many cases, euthyroid goiter poses no danger to health and, unless cosmetically undesirable or an obstacle to breathing or swallowing, can remain in place.
- In older persons, treatment with thyroxine is not recommended because these goiters rarely decrease in size and may harbor areas of autonomy that may result in thyrotoxicosis factitia.

Follow-up/Referral

- Patients are followed on the same schedule as those with no major health problems, to monitor goiter size and patient comfort.
- If changes occur that suggest need for consultation, an endocrinologist is consulted.

Hyperthyroidism
Definition

Hyperthyroidism is a clinical condition encompassing several specific diseases, characterized by hypermetabolism and elevated serum levels of free thyroid hormones, also known as thyrotoxicosis. Affects 2% to 5% of women at some time,

---

BOX 10-6
Causes of Hyperthyroidism

COMMON
Graves' disease (autoimmune)
Solitary toxic nodule/adenoma
Toxic multinodular goiter
Thyrotoxicosis factitia (secret T_4 consumption)
Exogenous iodine
Drugs—amiodarone
Metastatic differentiated thyroid carcinoma
TSH-secreting tumors (e.g., pituitary)

COMMON—cont'd
HCG-producing tumors
Hyperfunctioning ovarian teratoma

UNCOMMON
Acute thyroiditis
  Viral
  Autoimmune
  Postirradiation

From Drury PL, Howlett TA: Endocrinology. In Kumar P, Clark M, eds: *Clinical medicine*, ed 4, Edinburgh, 1998, WB Saunders, p 937.
HCG, Human chorionic gonadotropin.

---

primarily those between the ages of 20 and 40 years. Gender ratio is 5:1.

Etiology/Cause

- Hyperthyroidism results from increased synthesis and secretion of thyroid hormones (T_4 and T_3) by the thyroid gland because of thyroid gland stimulators in the blood, or autonomous thyroid hyperfunction (Box 10-6).
- Excessive release of thyroid hormone from the thyroid gland into the peripheral circulation without increased synthesis of hormones
- The conscious or accidental ingestion of excess quantities of thyroid hormone (thyrotoxicosis factitia)

Graves' Disease

Definition
Graves' disease is the most common cause of hyperthyroidism, is an autoimmune disease, and has a chronic course with remissions and relapses; over time, these patients may become hypothyroid.

- De Quervain's thyroiditis is transient hyperthyroidism from an acute inflammatory process, probably viral in origin.
  - Besides toxicosis, there is usually fever, malaise, and pain in the neck with tachycardia and local thyroid tenderness.
  - Thyroid function tests show initial hyperthyroidism; also, elevated erythrocyte sedimentation rate (ESR) and thyroid uptake scan indicate suppression of up-

take in the acute phase; hypothyroidism, usually transient, may follow in several weeks.
  - Treatment in the acute phase is aspirin, and prednisolone only in acute, severely symptomatic, patients.

Etiology/Cause

- The etiology of Graves' disease is an antibody against the thyroid TSH receptor, resulting in continuous stimulation of the gland to synthesize and secrete excess quantities of T_4 and T_3.
- Graves' disease is sometimes associated with other autoimmune diseases (e.g., insulin-dependent DM, vitiligo, premature graying of hair, pernicious anemia, collagen diseases, polyglandular deficiency syndrome, and myasthenia gravis).

Pathogenesis

- The pathogenesis of infiltrative ophthalmopathy, seen in Graves' disease, is not well understood.
  - It is most frequently seen in active hyperthyroidism.
  - It may occur before the onset of hyperthyroidism or 15 to 20 years after the disease has resolved.
  - Ophthalmopathy improves or worsens independent of the clinical course of hyperthyroidism.
  - The ophthalmopathy may result from immunoglobulins directed to specific anti-

---

BOX 10-7

Signs and Symptoms of Hyperthyroidism

SYMPTOMS	SIGNS
Weight loss	Irritability
Increased appetite	Psychosis
Irritability/behavior change	**Hyperkinesis**
Restlessness	Tremor
Malaise	Systolic hypertension
Muscle weakness	Cardiac failure†
Tremor	**Tachycardia or atrial fibrillation†**
Choreoathetosis	**Warm, vasodilated peripheries**
Breathlessness	Onycholysis
Palpitation	Palmar erythema
Heat intolerance	Thyroid acropachy*
Vomiting	**Pretibial myxedema***
Diarrhea	**Exophthalmus**
Eye complaints*	Lid lag
Goiter	Conjunctival edema
Oligomenorrhea	Ophthalmoplegia
Loss of libido	**Proximal myopathy**
Gynecomastia	

(handwritten: skin oily)

From Drury PL, Howlett TA: Endocrinology. In Kumar P, Clark M, eds: *Clinical medicine*, ed 4, Edinburgh, 1998, WB Saunders, p 937.
Bold, Most characteristic signs.
*Only in Graves' disease.
†Presenting signs in older persons.

gens in the extraocular muscles and orbital fibroblasts.

—The antibodies are distinct from those that initiate Graves' disease–type hyperthyroidism.

Diagnosis

Signs and Symptoms (Box 10-7)

- In older persons, in so-called apathetic thyrotoxicosis, there may be very few signs, and the clinical picture may appear more like hypothyroidism.
  —A high degree of clinical suspicion is essential.

Diagnostic Tests

- Serum TSH is suppressed in hyperthyroidism.
- Serum T_3 or T_4
- Thyroglobulin antibodies are present in most cases of Graves' disease.

Thyroid Storm

Definition

Thyroid storm is characterized by the abrupt onset of more exaggerated symptoms of hyperthyroidism.

- **Thyroid storm is a life-threatening emergency requiring immediate, specific treatment.**
- Occurs as a result of untreated or inadequately treated hyperthyroidism
- May be precipitated by infection, trauma, a surgical procedure, embolism, diabetic acidosis, or toxemia of pregnancy
- Fever
- Marked weakness
- Muscle wasting
- Extreme restlessness with wide emotional swings
- Confusion, psychosis, and sometimes coma
- Hepatomegaly with mild jaundice
- Cardiovascular collapse and shock

Differential Diagnosis

- Although hyperthyroidism is often clinically evident, treatment should never be instituted without biochemical confirmation.
- Anxiety states

Treatment

- Three therapies are available:
  —Radioiodine
  —Antithyroid drugs *(handwritten: I 2 THIOURACIL)*
  —Surgery
- Therapy often depends on patient preference and local expertise.
  —Patient preference, with informed discussion of the alternatives and long-term sequelae, is given great weight.
- Where radioiodine or surgery is selected, patients need to be rendered euthyroid with antithyroid drugs prior to definitive treatment.
- Most patients with hyperthyroidism (90%) have a diffuse goiter.
  —Those patients with large single or multinodular goiters are unlikely to remit after a course of antithyroid drugs.
  —Those with severe biochemical hyperthyroidism are also less likely to respond.
- Iodine is usually not used in routine treatment of hyperthyroidism.
- Iodine is used in emergency treatment of thyroid storm and in patients before undergoing subtotal thyroidectomy.
  —Usual dose is 2 to 3 drops of a saturated potassium iodide solution PO tid or qid,

---

BOX 10-8

Causes of Hypothyroidism

PRIMARY
Congenital
Agenesis
Ectopic thyroid remnants
Defects of Hormone Synthesis
Iodine deficiency
Dyshormonogenesis
Antithyroid drugs
Other drugs (e.g., lithium, amiodarone, interferon)
Autoimmune
Atrophine thyroiditis
Hashimoto's thyroiditis
Infective
Postsubacute thyroiditis

Postsurgery
Postirradiation
Radioactive iodine therapy
External neck irradiation
Infiltration
Tumor
Peripheral Resistance to Thyroid Hormone

SECONDARY
Hypopituitarism
Isolated TSH deficiency

From Drury PL, Howlett TA: Endocrinology. In Kumar P, Clark M, eds: *Clinical medicine*, ed 4, Edinburgh, 1998, WB Saunders, p 932.

300 to 600 mg/day (or) 0.5 g sodium iodide in 1 L 0.9% sodium chloride solution given IV slowly q12h.

- Complications from iodine therapy include
  —Inflammation of the salivary glands, conjunctivitis, and skin rashes
  —Induces transient hyperthyroidism (Jod-Basedow disease) in patients with nontoxic goiters
- Sodium ipodate and iopanoic acid provide excess iodine and are potent inhibitors of the conversion of T_4 to T_3.
  —Combining these agents with dexamethasone, which is also a potent inhibitor of T_4 to T_3 conversion, relieves the symptoms of hyperthyroidism and restores the serum T_3 concentration to normal within a week.
- Radioiodine (^{131}I) is the most common form of therapy in the United States for patients with hyperthyroidism.
  —It is recommended as the treatment of choice for Graves' disease and for toxic nodular goiter in all patients, including children.
  —Ideal dosage is difficult to determine, and response of the gland is unpredictable.
  —If enough radioiodine is given to produce euthyroidism, almost 25% of patients become hypothyroid 1 year later, and the incidence increases every year; however, if lower doses are used, there is recurrence of hyperthyroidism.

Patient/Family Education
- Explain the nature, cause, signs and symptoms, course, and usual therapy of hyperthyroidism.
- Patients usually have a fluctuating course with alternate relapses and remissions, with about 40% having only a single episode, with many patients becoming hypothyroid over time.
- Instruct about medications, actions, side effects, and signs/symptoms to look for that signal the need to contact the clinician.

Follow-up/Referral
- Patients with a history of hyperthyroidism, who have been successfully treated, are evaluated on at least an annual basis.
- Consultation with an endocrinologist is recommended for patients who may be exhibiting signs of recurrence of hyperthyroidism.

Hypothyroidism (Myxedema)

Definition
Hypothyroidism is the condition that occurs as a result of deficiency of thyroid hormone.

Etiology/Cause and Pathogenesis (Box 10-8)
- Primary hypothyroidism, the most common form, is considered to be an autoimmune disease, often occurring as a result of Hashimoto's thyroiditis, and frequently

associated with a firm goiter or, later in the disease process, with a shrunken, fibrotic thyroid gland with little or no function.

- The second most common form is posttherapeutic hypothyroidism, particularly after radioactive iodine therapy or surgery.
- Mild hypothyroidism is common in older women.
- Secondary hypothyroidism occurs as a result of failure of the hypothalamic-pituitary axis due to insufficient TSH secretion from the hypothalamus or lack of TSH secretion from the pituitary.

Diagnosis
Signs and Symptoms (Box 10-9)
Diagnostic Tests
- Serum TSH is the evaluation of choice; TSH level confirms hypothyroidism.
- A low total or free serum T_4 level confirms the hypothyroid state and is particularly important if there is any evidence of hypothalamic and pituitary disease, when TSH may be low or normal.
- Thyroid and other organ-specific antibodies may be present.
- Other abnormalities may include
  —Anemia: normochromic, normocytic; may be macrocytic in cases of pernicious anemia or microcytic in women due to menorrhagia
  —Increased aspartate transferase levels, from muscles or liver
  —Hypercholesterolemia
  —Hyponatremia due to increase in ADH and impaired free water clearance

Differential Diagnosis
- Hypothyroidism must be considered in the following clinical situations:
  —Unexplained menstrual disorders
  —Myalgias
  —Weight change
  —Hyperlipidemia
  —Anemia
  —Unexplained heart failure that does not respond to digitalis or diuretics
  —Ascites
  —Pernicious anemia
  —Depression or psychosis

Complications
- Coronary artery disease and congestive heart failure—may be precipitated by too vigorous thyroid therapy
- Increased susceptibility to infection
- Megacolon occurs in some patients with long-standing hypothyroidism.
- Organic psychoses with paranoid delusions ("myxedema madness")
- Untreated hypothyroidism in a pregnant woman often results in miscarriage.
- "Myxedema coma" may occur in patients with severe hypothyroidism, with hypothermia, hypoventilation, hyponatremia, hypoxia, hypercapnia, and hypotension.
  —Convulsions and abnormal CNS signs may occur.
  —This condition is often precipitated by underlying infection: cardiac, respiratory, CNS; exposure to cold; drug use.

BOX 10-9
Signs and Symptoms of Hypothyroidism

SYMPTOMS	SIGNS
Fatigue/malaise	**Mental slowness**
Weight gain	Psychosis/dementia
Anorexia	Ataxia
Cold intolerance	Poverty of movement
Poor memory	Deafness
Change in appearance	"Peaches and cream" skin
Depression	**Dry, thin hair**
Psychosis	Loss of eyebrows
Coma	Hypertension
Deafness	Hypothermia
Poor libido	Heart failure
Goiter	**Bradycardia**
Puffy eyes	**Pericardial effusion**
Dry, brittle, unmanageable hair	Cold peripheries
	Carpal tunnel syndrome
	Edema
Dry, coarse skin	Large tongue
Arthralgia	Periorbital edema
Myalgia	Deep voice
Constipation	Goiter
Menorrhagia or oligomenorrhea in women	Dry skin
	Mild obesity
	Myotonia
Symptoms of other autoimmune disease may be present	Muscle hypertrophy
	Proximal myopathy
	Slow-to-relax reflexes
	Anemia

From Drury PL, Howlett TA: Endocrinology. In Kumar P, Clark M, eds: *Clinical medicine*, ed 4, Edinburgh, 1998, WB Saunders, p 933.
Bold, Most significant diagnostic signs.

Treatment

- Replacement therapy with T_4 is given for life.
  - The starting dose depends on the severity of the deficiency, and the age and fitness of the patient, particularly regarding cardiac status.
  - In young, healthy individuals, 100 μg/day is appropriate; 50 μg/day is appropriate for the small, old, or frail person.
  - Those with ischemic heart disease are started at even lower doses, particularly when the hypothyroidism is severe and of long standing; dosage for these patients begins at 25 μg/day, and the patient is monitored by electrocardiograms (ECGs). If angina does not occur, the dosage is increased at 3- to 4-week intervals.
- Effectiveness of replacement therapy is monitored by thyroid function tests (TSH and perhaps T_4) at least 6 weeks on a stable dose, with the goal of restoring TSH to within normal limits.

Prognosis

- Most patients exhibit increased serum T_4 levels within 1 to 2 weeks, and near-maximum levels within 1 month.
- With appropriate, early treatment, patients show striking changes in appearance and cognitive function within a few weeks.
- Recovery is return to normal state, but relapses may occur if there is disruption in therapy.
- Hypothyroidism caused by interferon-α resolves within 17 months of stopping the drug in 50% of patients.
- Overmedication with thyroid hormone can result in bone demineralization.

Patient/Family Education

- Instruct the patient carefully regarding the plan of care and how the appropriate dosage will be determined.
- Explain the monitoring method, and that scheduling of appointments will depend on thyroid function tests.
- The better informed the patient is regarding the possibly erratic scheduling of appointments and tests, the more cooperative the patient will be.

Follow-up/Referral

- Ideally, the patient will have been followed closely by both the primary care provider and an endocrinologist throughout.
- Decisions about replacement drug, dosage, and criteria for monitoring should be known and agreed on by health care providers and patient/family.
- Initially, until the patient's response to therapy is evident and appropriate, the appointments occur every 3 to 4 weeks, or as needed by the individual patient.

ADRENAL DISORDERS: THE GLUCOCORTICOID AXIS

The adrenal glands, weighing only 8 to 10 g together, have an outer cortex with three zones (reticularis, fasciculata, and glomerulosa) that produce steroids, and an inner medulla that synthesizes, stores, and secretes catecholamines.

The adrenal steroids are classified according to their major physiologic effects:

- *Glucocorticoids* are so named because of their effects on carbohydrate metabolism (Box 10-10).
- Glucocorticoid production by the adrenal is under hypothalamic-pituitary control. In response to circadian rhythm, stress, and other stimuli, corticotrophin releasing factors (CRF: the major components are corticotrophin releasing hormone and vasopressin) are secreted in the hypothalamus. CRFs travel down the portal system to stimulate ACTH release from the anterior pituitary corticotrophs. Circulating

---

BOX 10-10

Major Actions of Glucocorticoids

INCREASED OR STIMULATED	DECREASED OR INHIBITED
Gluconeogenesis	Protein synthesis
Glycogen deposition	Host response to infection
Protein catabolism	Lymphocyte transformation
Fat deposition	Delayed hypersensitivity
Sodium retention	Circulating lymphocytes
Potassium loss	Circulating eosinophils
Free water clearance	
Uric acid production	
Circulating neutrophils	

From Drury PL, Howlett TA: Endocrinology. In Kumar P, Clark M, eds: *Clinical medicine,* ed 4, Edinburgh, 1998, WB Saunders, p 942.

ACTH stimulates cortisol production in the adrenal. The cortisol secreted (or any other synthetic corticosteroid administered to the patient) causes negative feedback to the hypothalamus and the pituitary to inhibit further CRF/ACTH release. The set-point of the system varies throughout the day according to the circadian rhythm, and is usually overridden by severe stress.

After adrenalectomy or other adrenal damage (e.g., Addison's disease), cortisol secretion is absent or reduced, and ACTH levels will rise.

Glucocorticoid Abnormalities

ACTH and cortisol are released episodically, and in response to stress. In taking a blood sample, the following precautions should be followed:

- Sampling time should be recorded accurately. Usually basal levels are obtained between 8 and 9 AM near the peak of the circadian variation.
- Stress should be minimized.
- Sampling should be delayed for 48 hours after admission if Cushing's syndrome is suspected.
  Mineralocorticoids' secretion is controlled mainly by the renin-angiotensin system. They affect primarily the extracellular balance of sodium and potassium in the distal tubule of the kidney. Aldosterone is the main mineralocorticoid in humans (about 50%), corticosterone contributes to a small degree. The weak activity of the mineralocorticoid cortisol is important because it is present in considerable excess; however, the mineralocorticoid receptor in the kidney is protected from this excess by the intrarenal conversion of cortisol to the inactive cortisone by the enzyme 11β-hydroxysteroid dehydrogenase. Aldosterone is produced only in the zona glomerulosa.

Androgens are secreted in relatively large quantities, but most have only weak intrinsic androgenic activity until metabolized peripherally to testosterone or dihydrotestosterone.

Primary Hypoadrenalism: Addison's Disease

Definition
Adrenocortical hypofunction may be primary (Addison's disease) or secondary. Addison's disease may be acute (adrenal crisis) or chronic.

Etiology/Cause/Incidence
- In this uncommon condition, there is destruction of the entire adrenal cortex, causing reduced production of glucocorticoid, mineralocorticoid, and sex steroid.
  - This decreased production is different from hypothalamic-pituitary disease, in which mineralocorticoid secretion remains largely intact, being predominantly stimulated by angiotensin II.
  - Adrenal sex steroid producton is also largely independent of pituitary action; in Addison's disease, reduced cortisol levels result, through negative feedback, to increased CRF and ACTH production; ACTH is directly responsible for the hyperpigmentation characteristic of Addison's disease.
- Acute adrenal insufficiency is an emergency caused by decreased cortisol.
- Adrenal crisis may occur in the following situations:
  - After stress (e.g., trauma, surgery, infection, prolonged fasting in a patient with latent insufficiency)
  - After sudden withdrawal of adrenocortical hormone in a patient with chronic insufficiency or with temporary insufficiency due to suppression by exogenous glucocorticoids
  - After bilateral adrenalectomy or removal of a functioning adrenal tumor that had suppressed the other adrenal
  - After sudden destruction of the pituitary gland (pituitary necrosis), or when thyroid is given to a patient with hypoadrenalism
  - After injury to both adrenals by trauma, hemorrhage, anticoagulation therapy, thrombosis, infection, or rarely metastatic carcinoma
- Of cases of Addison's disease in the United States, about 70% are due to idiopathic atrophy of the adrenal cortex, probably caused by autoimmune processes.
- The other 30% are due to destruction of the adrenal gland by granuloma (e.g., tuberculosis [TB], which is becoming increasingly common, particularly in developing countries).
  - Other causes include tumor, amyloidosis, or inflammatory necrosis; and antifungal drugs, such as ketoconazole, which block steroid synthesis.
  - Autoimmune adrenalitis results from the destruction of the adrenal cortex by organ-specific autoantibodies.

—Associations with other autoimmune syndromes exist in the polyglandular autoimmune syndromes Types I and II (e.g., type I DM, pernicious anemia, thyroiditis, hypoparathyroidism, premature ovarian failure).

- The incidence of Addison's disease in the general population is about 4/100,000, in all age groups, about equally in both genders, and frequently becomes clinically apparent during metabolic stress or trauma.

Pathogenesis

- The major hormones produced by the adrenal cortex are cortisol (hydrocortisone), aldosterone, and dehydroepiandrosterone (DHEA).
- Adults secrete about 20 mg of cortisol, 2 mg of corticosterone, which acts similarly to cortisol, and 0.2 mg of aldosterone daily.
- Although relatively large amounts of androgens (mainly DHEA and androstenedione) are produced by the adrenal cortex, their primary physiologic activity occurs after conversion to testosterone and dihydrotestosterone.
- In Addison's disease, there is increased excretion of sodium and decreased excretion of potassium, mainly in the urine, which is isotonic, and also in sweat, saliva, and the gastrointestinal (GI) tract.
- Low blood concentrations of sodium and chloride and a high concentration of serum K result.
- Inability to concentrate the urine, together with changes in electrolyte balance, produces severe dehydration, plasma hypertonicity, acidosis, decreased circulatory volume, hypotension, and circulatory collapse.
- Cortisol deficiency contributes to hypotension and produces disturbances in carbohydrate, fat, and protein metabolism and severe insulin sensitivity.
- In the absence of cortisol, insufficient carbohydrate is formed from protein; hypoglycemia and decreased liver glycogen occur.
- These changes cause weakness, partly because of deficient neuromuscular function.
- Resistance to infection, trauma, and other stress-causing events is diminished due to decreased adrenal output.

- Myocardial weakness and dehydration cause reduced cardiac output, and circulatory failure can ensue.
- Decreased cortisol blood levels cause increased pituitary ACTH production and increased blood levels of β-lipotropin, which stimulates melanocytes and results in hyperpigmentation of skin and mucous membranes, which are characteristics of Addison's disease.

Diagnosis

Signs and Symptoms

- Weakness ⎫
- Fatigue ⎬ early symptoms
- Headache
- Nausea and vomiting
- Abdominal pain
- Fever
- Orthostatic hypotension is due to hypovolemia and sodium loss, and is present in 80% to 90% of cases, although supine blood pressure is normal; the cause is mineralocorticoid deficiency.
- Increased pigmentation is seen in darkening of both exposed and unexposed areas of the body, particularly on pressure points (e.g., bony prominences, scars, skinfolds, extensor surfaces).
- Black freckles are commonly seen on the forehead, face, neck, and shoulders, with areas of vitiligo, and bluish-black discolorations of the areolae and the mucous membranes of the lips, mouth, rectum, and vagina.
- Anorexia
- Diarrhea
- Decreased tolerance to cold
- Hypometabolism
- Dizziness
- Syncope
- ECG may show decreased voltage and prolonged P-R and Q-T intervals.
- The electroencephalogram (EEG) shows a generalized slowing of the rhythm.
- The gradual onset and vague nature of early symptoms often result in an incorrect initial diagnosis of neurosis.
- In the later stages of Addison's disease, symptoms are weight loss, dehydration, hypotension, and small heart size.
- **Adrenal crisis** is characterized by profound asthenia; severe pain in the abdomen, lower

back, or legs; peripheral vascular collapse and then renal shutdown with azotemia.
- Body temperature may be subnormal, although severe hyperthermia due to infection often occurs.
  - Adrenal crisis may be precipitated by acute infection and septicemia, trauma, operative procedures, and sodium loss due to excessive sweating during hot weather.

Diagnostic Tests

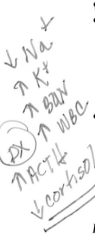

- Eosinophil count may be high.
- Abnormal serum electrolyte levels: low sodium < 130 mEq/L; high K (5 mEq/L); low HCO_3 (15 to 20 mEq/L); and high blood urea nitrogen (BUN)
  - These findings, together with the typical clinical picture, suggest Addison's disease.
- Adrenal insufficiency can be diagnosed by failure to increase plasma cortisol levels or urinary-free cortisol excretion on giving ACTH.
  - An elevated plasma ACTH level and a low plasma cortisol level are diagnostic.

Differential Diagnosis

- Shock (e.g., septic, hemorrhagic, cardiogenic)
- Hyperkalemia is seen in GI bleeding, rhabdomyolysis, hyperkalemic paralysis, and certain drugs (e.g., ACE inhibitors, spironolactone).
- Hyponatremia is seen in hypothyroidism, diuretic use, heart failure, cirrhosis, vomiting, diarrhea, severe illness, and major surgery.
- Acute abdomen with neutrophilia is usually present.
  - Eosinophilia and lymphocytosis are characteristics of adrenal insufficiency.

Treatment

- Acute phase
  - Draw blood sample for cortisol determination.
  - Treat with hydrocortisone 100 to 300 mg IV, and saline *immediately*, without waiting for results.
  - Then give hydrocortisone phosphate or hydrocortisone sodium succinate 100 mg IV immediately; continue IV infusions of 50 to 100 mg q6h for 24 hours.

  - Give same amount q8h on the second day, then adjust dosage in terms of clinical picture.
  - Give broad-spectrum antibiotics because bacterial infection often precipitates acute adrenal crisis.
  - Treat hypoglycemia vigorously.
  - Monitor serum electrolytes, BUN, creatinine.
- Convalescent phase
  - Give oral hydrocortisone 10 to 20 mg q6h, then reduce dosage to maintenance level as indicated.
  - Hydrocortisone twice daily (AM: 10 to 20 mg; PM: 5 to 10 mg)
    - ~ As the dosage of this drug is decreased, add fludrocortisone acetate 0.05 to 0.2 mg daily
- Once the crisis is over, the patient must be evaluated thoroughly to assess the degree of permanent adrenal insufficiency and to establish the cause if possible.

Prognosis

- Rapid treatment will usually reverse signs and symptoms.
- Acute adrenal crisis is often not recognized and not treated because of signs and symptoms similar to other conditions.
- Lack of treatment results in shock that is unresponsive to volume replacement and vasopressin, with imminent death.

Patient/Family Education

- Provide written instructions regarding medications, with dosages, schedules, and actions.
- Write out signs and symptoms of overdose or underdose.
- List situations in which additional dosage may be necessary: infection, surgery, injury, and emotional stress.
- Provide information about preventing infections (e.g., hand washing, personal hygiene, and using clean utensils).
- Emphasize the need for lifelong replacement therapy.

Follow-up/Referral

- Patients with Addison's disease require lifelong monitoring under the supervision of an endocrinologist and primary care physician.

- The nurse practitioner usually follows patients who are stable, with no complications (e.g., infection, emotional crisis).

Cushing's Syndrome

Definition

Cushing's syndrome is the clinical state of increased free circulating glucocorticoid, which occurs most often after the therapeutic administration of synthetic steroids; all spontaneous forms of Cushing's syndromes are rare.

Etiology/Cause/Pathogenesis

- Cushing's syndrome is generally divided into two groups (Box 10-11).
  - Increased circulating ACTH from the pituitary (65% of cases), known as Cushing's disease, or from an "ectopic," nonpituitary, ACTH-producing tumor elsewhere in the body (10%), results in glucocorticoid excess.
  - A primary excess of endogenous (25% of spontaneous cases) or exogenous glucocorticoid hormone alone, with subsequent (physiologic) suppression of ACTH

Diagnosis

- Two parts make up the diagnosis: making a definitive diagnosis and determining, by differential diagnosis, the cause.

Signs and Symptoms (Box 10-12)
Diagnostic Tests

- *24-hour urinary free cortisol measurements:* repeated normal values, corrected for body mass, make a diagnosis of Cushing's syndrome very unlikely.
- *48-hour low-dose dexamethasone test:* healthy persons suppress plasma cortisol to <50 nmol L^{-1}, while those with Cushing's syndrome do not show complete suppression of plasma or urinary cortisol, although levels may decline markedly in a few patients; the overnight dexamethasone test is somewhat simpler, but has a higher false-positive rate.
- *Circadian rhythm:* after 48 hours as an inpatient, the technician takes blood samples at 9 AM and 12 AM, without advance notice to the patient, to measure cortisol; normal persons show a pronounced circadian variation, while those with Cushing's syndrome have high midnight cortisol levels (100 nmol L^{-1}), but the cortisol level at 9 AM may be normal.
- If the suspicion of Cushing's syndrome remains after these preliminary tests, which may be ambiguous to some degree, then specialist evaluation is required.
  - Additional tests may include insulin stress test, desmopressin stimulation test, and CRF tests.

BOX 10-11
Causes of Cushing's Syndrome

ACTH-DEPENDENT DISEASE
Pituitary-dependent (Cushing's disease)
Ectopic ACTH-producing tumors
ACTH administration

NON-ACTH-DEPENDENT CAUSES
Adrenal adenomas
Adrenal carcinomas
Glucocorticoid administration

OTHER
Alcohol-induced pseudo-Cushing's syndrome

From Drury PL, Howlett TA: Endocrinology. In Kumar P, Clark M, eds: *Clinical medicine,* ed 4, Edinburgh, 1998, WB Saunders, p 946.

BOX 10-12
Signs and Symptoms of Cushing's Syndrome

SYMPTOMS	SIGNS
Weight gain (central)	Depression/psychosis
Change of appearance	Acne, hirsutism
Depression	**Thin skin**
Psychosis	**Bruising**
Insomnia	**Hypertension**
Amenorrhea/ oligomenorrhea	Rib fractures
	Osteoporosis
Poor libido	**Pathologic fractures**
Thin skin/easy bruising	Poor wound healing
Muscular weakness	Proximal muscle wasting
Growth arrest in children	**Proximal myopathy**
	Edema of lower legs
Back pain	Frontal balding (female)
Polyuria/polydipsia	Moon face
Old photographs may be helpful in identifying changes	**Plethora**
	"Buffalo hump"
	Kyphosis
	Centripetal obesity
	Pigmentation
	Striae (purple)
	Glycosuria

From Drury PL, Howlett TA: Endocrinology. In Kumar P, Clark M, eds: *Clinical medicine,* ed 4, Edinburgh, 1998, WB Saunders, p 947.
Bold, Most significant diagnostic signs.

Differential Diagnosis

- Alcoholic patients may have hypercortisolism and clinical manifestations of Cushing's syndrome.
- Depressed patients may have hypercortisolism that may be almost impossible to biochemically distinguish from Cushing's syndrome, but without clinical signs/symptoms of Cushing's syndrome.
- Cushing's syndrome can be misdiagnosed as anorexia nervosa (and vice versa) due to muscle wasting and very high urine-free cortisol levels that are present in both conditions, particularly anorexia.
- In pregnancy, urine-free cortisol is increased, but 17-hydroxycorticosteroids remain normal, and diurnal variation of serum cortisol is normal.
- Adrenal CT or MRI scan: adrenal adenomas or carcinomas that cause Cushing's syndrome are relatively large and therefore detectable by CT
- Pituitary MRI: not as definitive as adrenal scan because a pituitary adenoma may be seen, but in a large percentage of cases, is not visible; only a small number of tumors of significant size are detectable by pituitary CT
- Plasma potassium levels: all diuretics are stopped; hypokalemia is common with ectopic ACTH secretion
- High-dose dexamethasone test: if significant cortisol suppression does not occur, an ectopic source of ACTH or an adrenal tumor may be the cause
  - Patients with severe obesity often have an abnormal dexamethasone suppression test, but free cortisol in urine is usually normal, as is diurnal variation of serum cortisol.
  - Certain drugs (e.g., phenytoin, phenobarbital, primidone) accelerate the metabolism of dexamethasone, which causes a "false-positive" dexamethasone suppression test.
  - Estrogens (given during pregnancy, as oral contraceptives, or in hormone replacement therapy (HRT) may also cause lack of dexamethasone suppressibility).
- Patients with familial cortisol resistance have hyperandrogenism, hypertension, and hypercortisolism without having Cushing's syndrome.

- Plasma ACTH levels: low (<10 mg L^{-1}) or undetectable ACTH levels on two or more tests indicate non-ACTH-dependent disease
- CRF test: an unusually strong ACTH and cortisol response to exogenous CRF, with or without vasopressin, suggests pituitary-dependent Cushing's syndrome because ectopic sources rarely respond
- Chest x-ray: a mandatory test to show carcinoma of the bronchus or a bronchial carcinoid, although lesions may be quite small; if ectopic ACTH is suspected, whole-lung and mediastinal CT scanning is indicated
- Other more specialized tests may be undertaken to detect ectopic sources of ACTH.

Treatment

- The choice of treatment depends on the cause.
- The best treatment for patients with pituitary adenoma is selective transsphenoidal resection of the tumor; afterward, the rest of the pituitary usually returns to normal function, although the normal corticotrophs are suppressed and require 6 to 36 months to recover normal function.
  - Hydrocortisone therapy is necessary during the recovery period.
- Those who are not surgical candidates are given a ketoconazole trial.
- In doses of 200 mg q6h; liver enzymes must be monitored for progressive elevation
- Plasma cortisol should be monitored, with the goal of reducing the average level during the day to 150 to 300 nmol L^{-1}, which is equal to normal levels.
- External pituitary irradiation alone is effective in only 50% to 60% of patients and is not helpful to those who are unwilling, or unfit, to have surgery.
- Medical treatment to reduce ACTH with bromocriptine or cyproheptadine is rarely effective.
- Bilateral adrenalectomy is an option of last resort, but is an effective last resort, if all other treatment options fail to control the condition; some centers are performing this by laparoscopy.

Prognosis

- Untreated Cushing's syndrome has a very bad prognosis, with death from hyperten-

BOX 10-13

Common Therapeutic Uses of Glucocorticoids

RESPIRATORY DISEASE
Asthma
COPD
Sarcoidosis
Hay fever (topical)

CARDIAC DISEASE
Postmyocardial infarction syndrome

RENAL DISEASE
Nephrotic syndrome (some cases)
Glomerulonephritides (some cases)

GASTROINTESTINAL DISEASE
Ulcerative colitis
Crohn's disease
Autoimmune hepatitis

OBSTETRICS
Prevention/treatment of ARDs

RHEUMATOLOGIC DISEASE
Systemic lupus erythematosus
Polymyalgia rheumatica
Temporal arteritis
Juvenile chronic arthritis
Vasculitides

NEUROLOGIC DISEASE
Cerebral edema

SKIN DISEASE
Pemphigus, eczema

TUMORS
Hodgkin's lymphoma
Other lymphomas

TRANSPLANTATION
Immunosuppression

From Drury PL, Howlett TA: Endocrinology. In Kumar P, Clark M, eds: *Clinical medicine,* ed 4, Edinburgh, 1998, WB Saunders, p 949.
COPD, Chronic obstructive pulmonary disease; *ARDs,* acute respiratory disease.

sion, myocardial infarction, infection, or heart failure usually ensuing.

- Cortisol hypersecretion should be controlled before surgery or radiotherapy in any case because considerable morbidity and mortality are associated with surgery performed on patients who have not been treated; abdominal surgery is particularly risky.

Uses and Problems Associated with Therapeutic Steroid Therapy

- Other than therapeutic replacement for endocrine deficiency states, synthetic glucocorticoids are widely used for many nonendocrine conditions (Box 10-13).
- Short-term use (e.g., for acute asthma) has only a small risk of significant side effects, except for the suppression of immune responses.
- Long-term therapy with glucocorticoids has greater risks; therapy should be confined to
  —Three weeks or less
  —Prednisone 10 mg/day or less will not cause suppression of the adrenal axis.
- Long-term therapy with synthetic or natural steroids will, in most patients, mimic en-

dogenous Cushing's syndrome; however, symptoms and signs such as hirsutism, acne, hypertension, and severe sodium retention do not occur because synthetic steroids have low androgenic and mineralocorticoid activity.
- Excessive doses of steroids may be absorbed from skin if strong dermatologic preparations are used (Box 10-14).
- Inhaled steroids rarely cause Cushing's syndrome, although they may cause adrenal suppression.

Patient/Family Education

- Instruct the patient and family about the nature, cause, usual course, treatment, and probable outcomes.
- Explain medications, tests, and surgery before events so that the patient is fully cooperative.
- Instruct regarding the plan of care so that the patient knows what to expect.
- Instruct, orally and in writing, regarding important points to be carried out by the patient after discharge (e.g., medications, return visit schedule, exercise, and diet).

BOX 10-14

Adverse Effects of Corticosteroid Therapy

PHYSIOLOGIC
Adrenal and/or pituitary suppression

PATHOLOGIC
Cardiovascular
Hypertension
Gastrointestinal
Peptic ulcer exacerbation (likely)
Pancreatitis
Renal
Polyuria
Nocturia
Nervous System
Depression
Euphoria
Psychosis
Insomnia

ENDOCRINE
Weight gain
Glycosuria
Impaired growth
Amenorrhea

BONE AND MUSCLE
Osteoporosis
Proximal myopathy
Aseptic necrosis of the hip
Pathologic fractures

SKIN
Easy bruising
Thinning

EYES
Cataracts (also, inhaled drug)

IMMUNE SYSTEM
Septicemia
Reactivation of TB
Skin infections (e.g., fungi)

From Drury PL, Howlett TA: Endocrinology. In Kumar P, Clark M, eds: *Clinical medicine*, ed 4, Edinburgh, 1998, WB Saunders, p 950.

Follow-up/Referral
- Patients with Cushing's syndrome or related problem should be followed closely, with regular consultation with the endocrinologist.
- After surgery, the patient is seen every 2 to 3 weeks for 2 to 3 months, then less often if recovery is occurring on schedule and if laboratory data show significant improvement.
- Provide a list of signs and symptoms so that the patient will know when to call the clinician.
- Provide special instructions to family members regarding signs and symptoms to watch for, in case of emergency.

DISORDERS OF CALCIUM METABOLISM
Hypocalcemia
Definition
Hypocalcemia is a decrease in the total plasma calcium concentration below 8.8 mg/dl (2.20 mmol/L) in the presence of normal plasma protein concentration.

Etiology/Cause (Box 10-15)
Pathogenesis
- Hypocalcemia may be due to deficiencies of calcium homeostatic mechanisms, secondary to high phosphate levels or other causes (see Box 10-15). All forms of hypoparathyroidism, except transient surgical effects, are uncommon.
- The DiGeorge syndrome is a familial condition in which the hypoparathyroidism is associated with intellectual impairment, cataracts, and calcified basal ganglia, and at times, with specific autoimmune disease.
- Pseudohypoparathyroidism is a syndrome of end-organ resistance to parathyroid hormone (PTH) due to a defective postreceptor mechanism; its features are short stature, short metacarpals, and intellectual deficit; it is a rare disorder of genetic origin (X-linked dominant trait).
  —The combination of hypocalcemia, elevated level of parathyroid hormone, and typical skeletal abnormalities is virtually diagnostic.

BOX 10-15
Causes of Hypocalcemia

INCREASED PHOSPHATE LEVELS
Chronic renal failure (common)
Phosphate therapy

HYPOPARATHYROIDISM
Surgical—after neck exploration
   (thyroidectomy, parathyroidectomy: common)
Congenital deficiency (DiGeorge syndrome)
Idiopathic hypoparathyroidism (rare)
Severe hypomagnesemia

VITAMIN D DEFICIENCY
Osteomalacia
Vitamin D resistance

RESISTANCE TO PTH
Pseudohypoparathyroidism

DRUGS
Calcitonin
Bisphosphonates

OTHER CAUSES
Acute pancreatitis (very common)
Citrated blood in massive transfusion (not uncommon)

From Drury PL, Shipley M: Rheumatology and bone disease. In Kumar P, Clark M, eds: *Clinical medicine*, ed 4, Edinburgh, 1998, WB Saunders, p 513.

*[handwritten: Chvostek's sign - Tap face → twitchy
Trousseau sign - cuff → tetany - 3 mins]*

Diagnosis

Signs and Symptoms
- Hypoparathyroidism presents with neuro-muscular irritability and neuropsychiatric manifestations.
- Paresthesia, circumoral numbness, cramps, anxiety, and tetany may be present.
- Signs of hypocalcemia are
  —Chvostek's sign: gentle tapping over the facial nerve causes twitching of the facial muscles.
  —Trousseau's sign: inflation of the sphygmomanometer cuff above systolic pressure for 3 minutes induces tetanic spasm of the fingers and wrist.
  —Severe hypocalcemia may cause papilledema and a prolonged Q-T interval.

Diagnostic Tests
- Serum calcium below 8.5 mg/dl indicates hypocalcemia.
- Serum and urine creatinine to evaluate renal status
- Serum PTH levels may be inappropriately low or absent.
- 25-hydroxyvitamin D serum level is low in vitamin D deficiency.
- X-rays of metacarpals may show fourth metacarpals, which occur in pseudohypoparathyroidism.

Treatment
- Urgency of treatment depends on the severity of the symptoms and the degree of hypocalcemia.
  —If symptoms are severe, accompanied by signs of tetany, IV calcium gluconate is given 10 ml initially, then 10 to 40 ml of 10% calcium gluconate in 1 L of 150 mmol L^{-1} saline over 4 to 8 hours.
  —Oral calcium supplements 2 to 10 g daily (40 to 200 mmol calcium) are rarely sufficient alone.
- α-Hydroxylated derivatives of vitamin D are preferred for their shorter half-life, particularly in renal disease, since the others require renal hydroxylation.
  —Daily maintenance dose is 0.25 to 2 μg for alfacalcidol (1 α-OH-D_3); throughout treatment, plasma calcium is monitored frequently to detect hypercalcemia.

Patient/Family Education
- The nature, cause, signs and symptoms, need for continued calcium/vitamin D therapy, and consequences if these are not taken as prescribed should be explained to both patient and family.
- Signs and symptoms of hypercalcemia should be given to the patient in writing,

to prevent this condition—treatment of hypocalcemia is generally life-long.

- Calcium intake and serum levels of calcium and vitamin D are monitored frequently to ensure against hypercalcemia.
- Compliance is often problematic and must be encouraged frequently.

Follow-up/Referral
- Frequent visits at first, to ensure patient compliance in taking oral calcium tablets and vitamin D supplements.

Hypercalcemia

Definition
This condition is characterized by an increase in total plasma calcium concentration above 10.4 mg/dl (2.60 mmol/L).

Etiology/Cause (Box 10-16)
- Hyperparathyroidism and malignancies are by far the most common causes of hypercalcemia (90% of cases).
- Hyperparathyroidism may be primary, secondary, or tertiary.
  - —Primary hyperparathyroidism is caused by single (80%) parathyroid adenomas

or by diffuse hyperplasia of all glands (15% to 20%).
- Parathyroid carcinoma is rare (<1%) but causes severe hypercalcemia.
- The precise cause of primary hyperparathyroidism is not clear, although it seems that adenomas are monoclonal and also possibly hyperplasia.
- Chromosomal rearrangements in the 5' regulatory region of the PTH gene have been identified as one cause, and there are suggestions that inactivation of some tumor suppressor genes at a variety of sites may be involved.
- Secondary hyperparathyroidism is physiologic compensatory hypertrophy of all parathyroids due to hypocalcemia such as occurs in renal failure or vitamin D deficiency.
  - —PTH levels are elevated, but calcium levels are low or normal, and PTH falls to normal after correction of the cause of hypocalcemia where this is possible.
- Tertiary hyperparathyroidism is the development of apparently autonomous parathyroid hyperplasia after longstanding secondary hyperparathyroidism, often occurring in renal failure; plasma calcium and phosphate

---

BOX 10-16
Causes of Hypercalcemia

EXCESSIVE PTH SECRETION
Primary hyperparathyroidism (most common by far), adenoma, hyperplasia, or carcinoma
Tertiary hyperparathyroidism
Ectopic PTH secretion (very rare)

EXCESS ACTION OF VITAMIN D
Iatrogenic or self-administered excess
Granulomatous diseases (e.g., sarcoidosis, TB)
Lymphoma

EXCESSIVE CALCIUM INTAKE
"Milk-alkali" syndrome

MALIGNANT DISEASE
(SECOND MOST COMMON CAUSE)
Secondary deposits in bone
Production of osteoclastic factors by tumors
PTH-related protein secretion
Myeloma

DRUGS
Thiazide diuretics
Vitamin D analogs
Lithium (chronic use)
Vitamin A

OTHER CAUSES
Long-term immobility
Familial hypocalciuric hypercalcemia

OTHER ENDOCRINE DISEASES
Thyrotoxicosis
Addison's disease

From Drury PL, Shipley M: Rheumatology and bone disease. In Kumar P, Clark M, eds: *Clinical medicine*, ed 4, Edinburgh, 1998, WB Saunders, p 513.

are both elevated, phosphate often very much elevated, making parathyroidectomy necessary at this point.

Diagnosis

Signs and Symptoms

- Fatigue, malaise, depression
- *Renal:* there may be renal colic from stones, polyuria, or nocturia, hematuria, and hypertension; polyuria results from the effect of hypercalcemia on renal tubules, reducing their concentrating ability—a mild form of nephrogenic diabetes insipidus; only 20% to 40% show any renal involvement, and primary hyperparathyroidism (HPT) is present in about 5% of stone formers
- *Bones:* bone pain is present; hyperparathyroidism primarily affects cortical bone, and bone cysts and locally destructive "brown tumors" occur, but only in advanced disease; only 5% to 10% of all cases have definite bony lesions
- *Abdomen:* there may be abdominal pain, at times due to peptic ulceration
- *Chondrocalcinosis* and *ectopic calcification:* these occur infrequently in some patients
- *Corneal calcification:* this is a marker of longstanding hypercalcemia but causes no symptoms.
- There may be symptoms from one or more underlying causes.
  - Malignant disease is usually advanced by the time hypercalcemia is diagnosed, with bony metastases.
  - The most common primary tumors are bronchus, breast, myeloma, esophagus, thyroid, prostate, lymphoma, and renal cell carcinoma.
- Severe hypercalcemia is usually associated with carcinoma, hyperparathyroidism, renal failure, or vitamin D therapy.

Diagnostic Tests

- Biochemistry
  - Several fasting serum calcium and phosphate samples
  - *The hallmarks of primary hyperparathyroidism are hypercalcemia and hypophosphatemia.*
- There may be mild hyperchloremic acidosis.
- Renal function is usually normal but baseline data are required.

- In patients with sarcoidosis, vitamin D–mediated hypercalcemia, and some malignancies, hydrocortisone 40 mg tid for 10 days suppresses plasma calcium.
- Protein electrophoresis is done to exclude myeloma.
- Serum TSH and T_3 are done to exclude thyrotoxicosis.
- Abdominal x-rays may show renal calculi or nephrocalcinosis.
- High-definition hand x-rays may show subperiosteal erosions in the middle or terminal phalanges.
- Preoperative imaging is done only for patients with a history of previous parathyroid surgery; methods include the following:
  - Ultrasound, although insensitive to small tumors, is simple and safe.
  - High-resolution CT scan or MRI (the most sensitive method)
  - Radioisotope subtraction scanning: a picture of the parathyroid tissue derived from the difference in uptake beween [201]Th (taken up by thyroid and parathyroid) and [99m]Tc (by thyroid only)

Treatment

- Emergency treatment for severe hypercalcemia
  - Rehydration is essential: usually at least 4 to 6 L of saline first day, 3 to 4 L for several days after; central venous pressure (CVP) needs to be monitored to control hydration rate.
  - IV bisphosphonates are the treatment of choice for hypercalcemia due to malignancy.
    - ~ Pamidronate 15 to 60 mg IV in 0.9% saline or dextrose over 2 to 8 hours or, if not as urgent, over 2 to 4 days
  - Prednisone 30 to 60 mg/day is effective in some cases (e.g., myeloma, sarcoidosis, vitamin D excess) but in other cases is ineffective.
  - Calcitonin has a short action time and is used very little now.
- There are no effective medical therapies for primary hyperparathyroidism, but a high fluid intake should be maintained, a high calcium or vitamin D intake avoided, and exercise encouraged.

—New agents that target the calcium-sensing receptors in the kidney may be of value in the future.
- Surgery
  —Indications for surgery in hyperparathyroidism are controversial.
  —Most specialists agree on the following surgeries:
  ~ Patients with renal stones or impaired renal function
  ~ Bone involvement or marked reduction in cortical bone density
  ~ Unequivocal marked hypercalcemia (2.9 to 3.0 mmol L^{-1})
  ~ The rare younger patient, <50 years old
  ~ History of a previous episode of severe acute hypercalcemia

Patient/Family Education
- Instruct regarding the nature, cause, course, treatment, and expected outcomes of therapy.
- If surgery is indicated, prepare the patient and family as fully as possible about preoperative, perioperative, and postoperative treatment and care.
- On discharge, instruct regarding medications, schedule for return visits to the ambulatory care center, and specific directions about diet, fluid intake, medications, and exercise/activity.

Follow-up/Referral
- The patient will have been under the care of an endocrinologist and surgeon, as well as the primary care provider.
- In older patients who are not candidates for surgery, medical management is the recourse.
- Regular measurements of serum and urinary calcium and renal function are done at every visit (initially every month, then longer intervals as appropriate); bone density of cortical bone is measured every 2 years.

Diabetes Mellitus

Definition
DM is a syndrome with disordered metabolism and inappropriate hyperglycemia due either to a deficiency of insulin secretion or to a combination of insulin resistance and inadequate insulin secretion to compensate.

Classification/Pathogenesis
Until 1997 the classification and terminology regarding DM were these used according to the National Diabetes Data Group of the National Institutes of Health as established in 1979, which were based on pharmacologic rather than etiologic considerations. In 1997 an international committee of experts in the field recommended a new classification based on etiology, which is more definitive.
- Type 1 diabetes is due to pancreatic islet B cell destruction predominantly by an autoimmune process; these patients are prone to ketoacidosis.
- Type 2 diabetes is more prevalent and results from insulin resistance, mainly caused by visceral obesity, with a defect in compensatory insulin secretion.

Type 1 is a severe form of diabetes; it is a catabolic disorder in which circulating insulin is virtually absent, plasma glucagon is elevated, and the pancreatic B cells fail to respond to all insulinogenic stimuli. This form is associated with ketosis in its untreated state. This type occurs most often in children, but occasionally is found in adults, particularly nonobese and elderly, in whom hyperglycemia first appears.

Incidence/Prevalence (Type 1)
- The highest prevalence of type 1 DM is in Scandinavia, affecting 20% of persons with diabetes.
- In Europe, the prevalence is 15%.
- In the United States, the prevalence of type 1 is 10%.
- An estimated 16 million people in the United States have diabetes, of whom 1.4 million have type 1 DM; the remainder have type 2, although a third group has recently been defined by the American Diabetes Association (ADA), known as "other specific types" and including disorders whose cause is not known (see maturity-onset diabetes of the young [MODY] types later).

Etiology
- Certain HLA are strongly associated with the development of type 1 DM.
  —About 95% of patients have either HLA-DR3 or HLA-DR4, compared with 45% to 50% of white controls.

- HLA-DQ genes are even more specific markers of type 1 susceptibility because a particular variety (HLA-DQw3.2) is found in the DR4 patients with type 1, while a "protective" gene (HLA-DQw3.1) is often present in the DR4 controls.
- Also, about 85% of patients have circulating islet cell antibodies when tested in the first few weeks of their diagnosis, when sensitive immunoassays are used.
- Most of these patients also have detectable antiinsulin antibodies before receiving insulin therapy.
- These immune characteristics indicate that type 1 diabetes results from an infectious or toxic insult to persons whose immune system is genetically predisposed to develop a vigorous autoimmune response either against altered pancreatic B cell antigens or against molecules of the B cell resembling the viral protein (molecular mimicry).
- Extrinsic factors that affect B cell function include damage caused by viruses (e.g., mumps, coxsackie B4 virus), toxic chemical agents, or destructive cytotoxins and antibodies released from sensitized immunocytes.
  - The fact that hyperglycemia is ameliorated in patients who are given cyclosporine soon after onset of type 1 diabetes provides further support to the pathogenetic role of autoimmunity as the cause.

Type 2 diabetes represents a heterogeneous group of DM comprised of milder forms, which occur predominantly in adults (occasionally in children).

- More than 90% of all diabetics in the United States are included under this classification.
- Circulating endogenous insulin is sufficient to prevent ketoacidosis but is inadequate to prevent hyperglycemia when need for glucose increases due to tissue insensitivity.

Etiology
- In most cases of type 2 DM, the cause is unknown.
- Tissue insensitivity to insulin has been noted in most type 2 patients regardless of weight and this has significance for several interrelated factors.

  - A putative (still undefined) genetic factor that is aggravated over time by additional enhancers of insulin resistance (e.g., aging, abdominal viscera obesity)
  - There is an accompanying deficiency in response of the pancreas B cells to glucose.
- Both of these factors (tissue resistance to insulin and impaired B cell response to glucose) seem to be further aggravated by increased hyperglycemia.
  - Both defects are ameliorated by treatment that reduces the hyperglycemia to normal.
- Whereas a genetic marker for type 2 DM has not been identified, it has been noted that there is a concordance of over 70% in monozygotic twins, with one developing type 2 DM within 1 year of type 2 DM in the other twin.
- Obesity plays a role also, although the degree and prevalence of obesity vary among racial groups: Asian people: 30%; among North American, Europeans, and Africans: 60% to 70%; among Pima Indians or Pacific Islanders: 100%.
- Nonobese type 2 patients show an absent or blunted early phase of insulin release in response to glucose, but the response can also be elicited in response to other insulinogenic stimuli (e.g., acute IV administration of sulfonylureas, glucagon, or secretin).
  - Although insulin resistance is detected by special tests, it does not seem to be clinically relevant in the treatment of most of these patients.
  - DM in most of these patients is idiopathic, but increasingly, a variety of etiologic genetic abnormalities are being documented in a subset of these patients who have been reclassified as "other specific types."

MODY is a relatively rare monogenic disorder characterized by noninsulin-dependent diabetes with autosomal dominant inheritance, with onset at age 25 or younger.

- Five types of MODY have been described with single-gene defects in chromosomes 7, 12, 13, 17, and 20.
  - MODY 1 includes 74 members of a pedigree known as the R-W family, who are descendants of a German couple who immigrated to Michigan in 1861, all of

whom have been studied since 1958; members have a genetic defect that is a nonsense mutation called hepatocyte nuclear factor-4α (HNF-4α), found on chromosome 20.
- All five MODY types are somewhat different, but all have a genetic basis for their diabetes.

Etiology
- Hyperglycemia in this nonobese group is due to impaired glucose-induced secretion of insulin.

TABLE 10-8
Clinical Features of Diabetes at Diagnosis

Sign/Symptom	Type 1	Type 2
Polyuria, thirst	++	+
Weakness, fatigue	++	+
Polyphagia with weight loss	++	—
Recurrent blurred vision	+	++
Vulovaginitis or pruritus	+	++
Peripheral neuropathy	+	++
Nocturnal enuresis	++	—
Often asymptomatic	—	++

From Karam JH: Diabetes mellitus & hypoglycemia. In Tierney LM, McPhee SJ, Papadakis MA, eds: *Current medical diagnosis & treatment 2000,* ed 39, New York, 2000, Lange Medical Books/McGraw-Hill, p 1156.
+, Less often; ++, more often.

Diagnosis
Signs and Symptoms (Table 10-8 and Box 10-17)
Laboratory findings
- If the fasting plasma glucose level is over 126 mg/dl on more than one occasion, further evaluation is not required.
- If the plasma glucose is less than 126 mg/dl in suspected cases, a standardized oral glucose tolerance test is done (Table 10-9).
- Glycosylated hemoglobin (hemoglobin A_1 measurements)
  —Glycosylated hemoglobin is abnormally high in diabetics with chronic hyperglycemia; this test reflects their metabolic control.
- Self-monitoring of blood glucose provides an ongoing comparative record of the patient's blood glucose taken at several times during the day.

Differential Diagnosis
- Hyperglycemia secondary to other causes (see Box 10-17)
  —Secondary hyperglycemia is associated with various disorders of insulin target tissues (liver, muscle, adipose tissue).
- Nondiabetic glycosuria—a benign, asymptomatic condition; blood glucose is normal

---

BOX 10-17
Causes of Secondary Diabetes Mellitus

LIVER DISEASE
Cirrhosis

PANCREATIC DISEASE
Cystic fibrosis
Chronic pancreatitis
Malnutrition-related pancreatic disease
Pancreatectomy
Hereditary hemochromatosis
Carcinoma of the pancreas

ENDOCRINE DISEASE
Cushing's syndrome
Acromegaly
Thyrotoxicosis
Pheochromocytoma
Glucagonoma

DRUG-INDUCED DISEASE
Thiazide diuretics
Corticosteroid therapy

INSULIN-RECEPTOR ABNORMALITIES
Congenital lipodystrophy
Acanthosis nigricans

GENETIC SYNDROMES
Friedreich's ataxia
Myotonic dystrophy

From Gale EAM, Anderson JV: Diabetes mellitus and other disorders of metabolism. In Kumar P, Clark M, eds: *Clinical medicine,* ed 4, Edinburgh, 1998, WB Saunders, p 961.

Treatment

- Important factors regarding education of patients with DM
  - —Impact of diet and patterns of eating on diabetes
  - —Implications of having DM on ordinary activities, and the reverse
  - —Ability to recognize the signs of worsening DM
  - —Importance of proper foot care
  - —Clarification of misconceptions about DM
- For patients receiving insulin, these additional factors are important.
  - —Correct administration of insulin
  - —The unique constraints imposed by insulin therapy on dietary management and changes in activity
  - —Ability to recognize the symptoms of hypoglycemia and to adjust insulin dosage during episodes of illness
- Excellent educational materials are now available to health care personnel and patients regarding DM and its management.
- Dietary management is essential to managing DM, and is tailored to each individual's needs and personal food preferences.

TABLE 10-9

Diabetes Expert Committee Criteria for Evaluating the Standard Oral Glucose Tolerance Test

Timing During Test Tolerance	Normal Glucose Tolerance	Impaired Glucose Mellitus	Diabetes Mellitus
Fasting plasma glucose (mg/dl)	<110	110-126	>126
Points between 0 and 120 min (mg/dl)	<200	<200	200 at least once
Two hours after glucose load (mg/dl)	<140	>140, <200	>200

From Karam JH: Diabetes mellitus & hypoglycemia. In Tierney LM, McPhee SJ, Papadakis MA, eds: *Current medical diagnosis & treatment 2000*, ed 39, New York, 2000, Lange Medical Books/McGraw-Hill, p 1157.
1. Give 75 g of glucose dissolved in 300 ml of water after an overnight fast to patients who have been receiving at least 150-200 g of carbohydrate daily for 3 days before the test.
2. A fasting plasma glucose > 126 mg/dl is diagnostic of diabetes. However, if the plasma glucose is <126 mg/dl, both of the lower columns must be fulfilled to make the diagnosis of DM.

- The goals of appropriate dietary management are to achieve an acceptable weight, prevent obesity, prevent atherosclerosis, and maintain optimal health.
- Determination of caloric needs varies considerably among individuals, and is based on several factors: present weight and current level of activity.
- Required calories are about 40 kcal/kg or 20 kcal/lb per day for adults with normal activity patterns.
  - ~ A person of 70 kg may require 2800 kcal, whereas lean men who perform ordinary activities may require as many as 3000 to 3500 kcal/day.
  - ~ Caloric requirements are often underestimated; clinicians commonly prescribe 1800-kcal diet for maintenance, even if this level is grossly inadequate for an individual's actual caloric needs.
- Patients who receive insulin have special problems in that they require rigid patterns of food intake.
  - —For patients with type 1 DM, the composition of the diet is less important than the distribution of the amount of food at each meal, day-to-day.
  - —The ADA exchange diet plan is helpful to many patients.
  - —Special dietetic foods are generally expensive and unnecessary.
- General recommendations regarding exercise for people with DM must be given with caution; walking and cycling are probably the best forms of exercise.
  - —The pattern of glycemic response to exercise varies.

Insulin or Oral Hypoglycemic Agents

- An acute episode of ketoacidosis in a type 1 DM patient may be the springboard that initiates insulin dependence.
  - —Insulin dependence is usually absolute and permanent.
  - —In the past, nonobese adults were considered to have type 2 DM when first diagnosed because they had not developed ketoacidosis at the time of diagnosis.
  - —The presence of type 1 diabetes is suspected on the basis of (1) lack of obesity, (2) lack of response to sulfonylurea, and

(3) a low level of insulin C-peptide (a marker for endogenous insulin secretion).

- For type 2 DM patients, the first approach is weight reduction in the obese, noninsulin-dependent person.
- Most patients with symptomatic type 2 diabetes are treated with oral hypoglycemic drugs initially, although some require insulin from the outset.
- The general rule followed by the ADA, the American Medical Association Council on Drugs, and the Food and Drug Administration (FDA) is that oral agents should be limited to patients with symptomatic type 2 diabetes that cannot be controlled by diet alone (within 3-4 months), and in whom adding insulin is impractical or not acceptable.
- The indications for use of insulin in patients with asymptomatic type 2 diabetes are not clear.
  —Insulin is indicated in those patients with type 2 diabetes whose prostaglandin (PG) cannot be controlled by diet or by diet plus oral agents.
- From research data gathered over some years regarding the effects of maintaining PG at normal levels, evidence was clear that in all patients with diabetes, achieving normal levels of blood glucose greatly reduced morbidity and mortality.

Insulin Therapy
- Three major characteristics distinguish the various preparations of insulin: (1) onset and duration of action; (2) purity, which relates to cost, insulin allergy (rare), and insulin resistance; and (3) species of origin, which also affects cost.

Rapid-acting insulin
- Regular insulin (crystalline zinc insulin)—the completely dissolved (clear) preparation that has been in use for many years, particularly in administering it intravenously to treat hospitalized patients who have ketoacidosis.
  —Onset of action of Regular insulin (SC) is 20 minutes, with peak action at 2 to 4 hours and duration of action 4 to 6 hours.
- Insulin lispro, an amino-acid-modified recombinant human insulin, is a recent addition.

—Its onset of action is somewhat faster than Regular insulin and it has a slightly shorter duration of action.

Neutral Protamine Hagedorn (NPH) insulin
- This is a standardized crystalline suspension prepared from Regular insulin, and protamine zinc insulin (PZI).
- NPH insulin is the most commonly used intermediate-acting insulin in the United States.
  —NPH actually has a fairly rapid onset of action and a duration of action that begins to diminish after about 12 hours but may last for up to 20 hours.
  —The combination of NPH and PZI was intended to incorporate the short-acting NPH component to provide insulin effect during the day when meals are elevating blood glucose, and the long-acting PZI component to provide the insulin effect through the night.
  —For most patients, the combined effects are inadequate, although many clinicians still prescribe NPH as a single dose daily, but this practice has been discontinued for a long time in Europe.
  —Increasingly, NPH is being used in combination with sulfonylureas.
  —Mixtures of NPH and Regular insulin (70:30) are now on the market, and are used primarily to control postprandial increase in blood glucose.

The Lente insulin series
- This insulin series was developed to avoid the use of protamine.
- Controlled addition of zinc was done to prepare an amorphous, rapidly absorbed, and rapid-acting material (Semilente insulin) and another crystalline product with slower absorption and longer action.
- In some parts of the United States and in Europe, Lente insulins are used almost exclusively.
- Semilente insulin is similar to Regular insulin in onset and duration of action, but its effects are slightly slower in onset and more prolonged.
  —The major uses of Semilente are in mixtures with Ultralente and as a supplementary dose in conventional therapy regimens.

—Semilente is used very little in the United States.

- Ultralente has a duration of action of more than 24 hours.
  - —Infrequently, it may be used alone.
  - —Its major use is as the long-acting component in the mixture known as Lente insulin.
  - —Ultralente insulin has recently become the backbone of intensified conventional therapy.
  - —The prolonged effect of Ultralente insulin provides the background activity equivalent to the basal infusion rate of an insulin pump.

Mixtures of insulins

- The ideal goal of insulin therapy is a single injection once a day (Table 10-10).
  - —To achieve this goal, insulin effect must be prolonged sufficiently to produce normoglycemia in the morning and at the same time provide adequate daytime control of the increases of blood glucose that occur postprandially.
  - —The action of NPH is generally too short to achieve this goal.
  - —Lente, although a better choice, is often unsatisfactory.
  - —To achieve round-the-clock control of blood glucose, the various insulins are mixed to capitalize on the actions of each.
  - —Too often, however, the combination of different insulins does not provide the precise actions desired for every patient.
  - —In the United States, most diabetologists use NPH and, if needed, prescribe another dose before dinner or at bedtime, a regimen known as a split-dose program.

Oral Hypoglycemics

- Since their introduction about 40 years ago, oral hypoglycemics remain the most widely prescribed drugs for the treatment of hypoglycemia (Table 10-11).
  - —The sulfonylureas are the primary oral hypoglycemic drugs; their action stimulates the pancreas to secrete more insulin.
  - —In 1994 the FDA approved drugs from the biguanide group metformin (Glucophage), which lowers blood glucose and spares insulin.

- —In 1997 the thiazolidine-diones, insulin potentiators, were introduced; troglitazone lowers hyperglycemia and hypertriglyceridemia without associated weight gain or drug-induced hypoglycemia.
- —In 1998 the FDA approved **repaglinide,** which represents a fifth class of oral antihyperglycemic agents that stimulate insulin release despite the absence of a sulfonylurea component in their structure.

TABLE 10-10
Insulins Available in the United States as of June 1997

Trade Name	Form
RAPID-ACTING (REGULAR)	
Humulin R	Human (rDNA)
Humalog (Lispro)	Human (rDNA; modified)
Novolin R	Human
Velosulin human	Human
Pork Regular Iletin II	Pork
Regular Purified Pork	Pork
Regular insulin	Pork
Regular Iletin I	Beef and Pork
Novolin R Penfill (regular)	Human
INTERMEDIATE-ACTING (NPH OR LENTE)	
Humulin L (Lente)	Human (rDNA)
Humulin N (NPH)	Human
Novolin L (Lente)	Human
Novolin N (NPH)	Human (rDNA)
Novolin N Penfill (NPH)	Human (rDNA)
Lente Insulin	Beef
Lente Iletin II	Pork
Pork NPH Iletin II	Pork
NPN-N	Pork
Lente	Pork
Lente Iletin I	Beef and pork
NPH Iletin I	Beef/pork
NPH Insulin	Beef
LONG-ACTING (INSULIN ZINC SUSPENSION)	
Ultralente U	Beef
Humulin U (ultralente)	Human
MIXTURES (NPH/REGULAR)	
Novolin 70:30	Human
Novolin 70:30, Penfill	Human
Humulin 70:30	Human (rDNA)
Humulin 50:50	Human (rDNA)

Modified from Gregerman RI: Diabetes mellitus. In Barker LR, Burton JR, Zieve PD, *Principles of ambulatory medicine*, ed 5, Baltimore, 1999, Williams & Wilkins, p 1036.
rDNA, Recombinant deoxyribonucleic acid.

TABLE 10-11
Oral Hypoglycemic Drugs

Name	Trade Name	Daily Dose (# of doses)	Length of Action (hrs)
SULFONYLUREAS			
Tolbutamide	Orinase	1-3 g (2-3)	12
Chlorpropamide	Diabinese	0.1-0.5 g (1)	24-72
Tolazamide	Tolinase	0.25-1.0 g (1-2)	12-24
Glyburide	Micronase, Diabeta	1.25-20 mg (1-2)	16-24
	Glynase PresTab	0.75-12 mg	
Glipizide	Glucotrol, Glucotrol XL	2.5-40 mg (1-2)	12-24
Glimeparide	Amaryl	1-8 mg (1)	24
Metformin	Glucophage	1000-3000 mg (2)	24
Acarbose	Precose	75-300 mg (3)	NA
Troglitazone	Rezulin	200-600 mg (1)	24
Repaglinide	Prandin	4 mg (2)	3

Modified from Gregerman RI: Diabetes mellitus. In Barker LR, Burton JR, Zieve PD, *Principles of ambulatory medicine,* ed 5, Baltimore, 1999, Williams & Wilkins, p 1047.
NA, Not applicable.

Complications of Diabetes Mellitus
- Diabetic cataracts
- Diabetic retinopathy
- Glaucoma
- Diabetic nephropathy
- Gangrene of the feet
- Diabetic neuropathy
- Chronic skin infections
- Erectile dysfunction
- The clinician must be alert to the potential development of any one or more of the complications and provide treatment as required.

Patient/Family Education
- Patient and family education remains one of the most essential aspects of treatment for the diabetic patient.
- Explain the nature, cause, signs and symptoms, course, and treatment of DM, according to the type that the patient has.
- Changes in perspective about diabetes over the last several years need to be made clear to the patient, who may have read books or articles about DM from the "old" perspective.
- Teach the patient about self-administration of insulin or oral agents, as prescribed, and the importance of taking medications exactly as prescribed, in the appropriate dose.

BOX 10-18
Regular Checks for Patients with Diabetes

CHECKED AT EACH VISIT
Review of self-monitoring results and current treatment
Discuss targets and change where necessary
Discuss any general or specific problems
Continue patient education

CHECKED AT LEAST ONCE A YEAR
Biochemical assessment of metabolic control (e.g., glycosylated Hb test)
Measure body weight
Measure blood pressure
Measure plasma lipids (except in extreme old age)
Measure visual acuity
Examine state of retina (ophthalmoscope or retinal photo)
Test urine for proteinuria
Test blood for renal function (creatinine)
Check condition of feet, pulses, and neurology
Review cardiovascular risk factors
Review self-monitoring and injection techniques
Review eating habits

From Gale EAM, Anderson JV: Diabetes mellitus and other disorders of metabolism. In Kumar P, Clark M, eds: *Clinical medicine,* ed 4, Edinburgh, 1998, WB Saunders, p 974.

- If the patient will be taking insulin, instruct regarding SC injections and injection sites for insulin (e.g., abdomen, thighs).
- Provide exact information about side effects of the prescribed medication(s).

- All instructions should be written as well as oral.
- List signs and symptoms to watch for in both hyperglycemia and hypoglycemia, and actions to take in each case.
- Provide detailed written instructions about care of the feet.

Follow-up/Referral

- After initial evaluation and testing, most patients with diabetes can be managed by the primary care provider, with consultation of the internist or endocrinologist.
- Frequent visits are important, particularly after initial diagnosis, to ascertain whether the patient is following instructions regarding medications, diet, exercise, and foot care (Box 10-18).
- The clinician should be vigilant regarding new signs and symptoms that may indicate complications or reactions to medications.

BIBLIOGRAPHY

American Diabetes Association: http://www/diabetes.org/default.htm; http://www.diabetes.com/ada.html

Beers MH, Berkow R: Endocrine and metabolic disorders. In Beers MH, Berkow R, eds: *The Merck manual of diagnosis and therapy,* ed 17, Whitehouse Station, NJ, 1999, Merck Research Laboratories, pp 63-220.

Busby-Whitehead MJ, Blackman MR: Clinical implications of abnormal lipoprotein metabolism. In Barker LR, Burton JR, Zieve PD, eds: *Principles of ambulatory medicine,* ed 5, Baltimore, 1999, Williams & Wilkins, pp 1122-1149.

Drury PL, Howlett TA: Endocrinology. In Kumar P, Clark M, eds: *Clinical medicine,* ed 4, Edinburgh, 1998, WB Saunders, pp 895-958.

Drury PL, Shipley M: Rheumatology and bone disease. In Kumar P, Clark M, eds: *Clinical medicine,* ed 4, Edinburgh, 1998, WB Saunders, pp 513-516.

Fitzgerald PA: Endocrinology. In Tierney LM, McPhee SJ, Papadakis MA, eds: *Current medical diagnosis & treatment 2000,* New York, 2000, Lange Medical Books/McGraw-Hill, pp 1079-1151.

Gale EAM, Anderson JV: Diabetes mellitus and other disorders of metabolism. In Kumar P, Clark M, eds: *Clinical medicine,* ed 4, Edinburgh, 1998, WB Saunders, pp 959-1006.

Gregerman RI: Diabetes mellitus; thyroid disorders; selected endocrine problems: disorders of pituitary, adrenal, and parathyroid glands; pharmacologic use of steroids; hypocalcemia and hypercalcemia; water metabolism; hypoglycemia; and hormone use of unproven value. In Barker LR, Burton JR, Zieve PD, eds: *Principles of ambulatory medicine,* ed 5, Baltimore, 1999, Williams & Wilkins, pp 1023-1121.

Karam JH: Diabetes mellitus & hypoglycemia. In Tierney LM, McPhee SJ, Papadakis MA, eds: *Current medical diagnosis & treatment 2000,* ed 39, New York, 2000, Lange Medical Books/McGraw-Hill, pp 1152-1197.

Juvenile Diabetes Foundation: http://www.jdf.org/index.html

Managing Your Diabetes: http://diabetes.lilly.com

Shannon MT, Wilson BA, Stang CL: *Health professionals drug guide 2000,* Stamford, Conn, 2000, Appleton & Lange.

REVIEW QUESTIONS

1. The pituitary gland was at one time considered to be the "master gland." The gland that is now recognized as the "master gland" is the:
   a. Parathyroid gland
   b. Hypothalamus gland
   c. Thyroid gland
   d. The pancreas's islets of Langerhan

2. Hormones are of various chemical structures, which include all but one of the following. The one that is NOT a hormonal structure is:
   a. Peptide
   b. Polypeptide
   c. Glycoprotein
   d. Steroid
   e. Amine

3. Although most classical hormones are secreted into the systemic circulation, from which they travel to distant sites to affect the body, each in its distinctive way, hypothalamic releasing hormones are released into the:
   a. Coronary artery circulation
   b. Hepatic circulation
   c. Kidney circulation
   d. Pituitary portal system

4. Hormones that are biologically active are those that are:
   a. Bound to proteins
   b. Free (unbound to proteins)
   c. Bound to high-affinity proteins
   d. Bound to low-affinity proteins

5. When they reach their target tissue/organ, hormones bind to specific receptors:
   a. On the inner layer of the cell
   b. On the nuclear membrane
   c. On the surface of the cell
   d. In the cytoplasm

6. The most common endocrine disease is:
   a. Thyroid disorder, either hypothyroidism or hyperthyroidism
   b. Diabetes mellitus
   c. Osteoporosis
   d. Addison's disease

7. Drugs that can simulate endocrine disorders include all but one of the following:
   a. Licorice
   b. Diuretics
   c. Amiodarone
   d. Antibiotics

8. Clinical syndromes that result from autoimmune diseases that affect all of the endocrine glands include all but one of the following. The one disorder that is NOT a result of autoimmune disease is:
   a. Acromegaly
   b. Pernicious anemia
   c. Addison's disease
   d. Graves' disease

9. Hypopituitarism and the resulting decrease or absence of specific hormones include all but one of the following. The one hormone that is NOT affected is:
   a. Gonadotropins
   b. Growth hormone
   c. Antidiuretic hormone
   d. Sleep/wake cycles

10. Diabetes insipidus is caused by a deficiency of:
    a. Angiotensin II
    b. Insulin
    c. Vasopressin
    d. Melatonin

11. Causes of polyuria, other than diabetes insipidus, include all but one of the following. The one that is NOT a cause of polyuria is:
    a. Osmotic diuresis
    b. Decreased synthesis of antidiuretic hormone
    c. Lithium
    d. Increased synthesis of thyroid-stimulating hormone

12. Primary hypothyroidism is considered to be:
    a. An autoimmune disease
    b. Caused by thyroid-stimulating hormone deficiency
    c. Caused by increased thyroid hormone
    d. A result of vitamin D excess

13. One of the major physiologic effects of thyroid hormones is:
    a. Decreases oxygen consumption
    b. Increases protein synthesis in almost every body tissue
    c. Increases red blood cells
    d. Increases number of alveoli

14. Hyperthyroidism is also known as:
    a. Thyroid storm
    b. Thyroid crisis
    c. Thyrotoxicosis
    d. Euthyroid disease

15. Graves' disease:
    a. Is the most common cause of hypothyroidism
    b. Is an autoimmune disease
    c. Is caused by an antibody against the follicle-stimulating hormone receptor
    d. Runs an acute course with little variation

16. The most common form of hypothyroidism is:
    a. Primary
    b. Secondary
    c. Multifactorial
    d. Idiopathic

17. One of the complications of aggressive thyroid therapy for hypothyroidism is:
    a. Increased susceptibility to cognitive dysfunction
    b. Congestive heart failure
    c. Myxedema coma
    d. Megacolon

18. The adrenal glands' three zones produce:
    a. Catecholamines
    b. Corticotrophin releasing factors
    c. Adrenocorticotropic hormone
    d. Steroids

19. After adrenalectomy, cortisol secretion is:
    a. Increased
    b. Decreased
    c. Unchanged
    d. Variable

20. In Addison's disease there is:
    a. Destruction of the entire adrenal cortex
    b. Increased production of glucocorticoid
    c. Increased production of mineralocorticoid
    d. Increased production of sex steroid

21. The hallmark of primary hyperparathyroidism is:
    a. Hypocalcemia and hyperphosphatemia
    b. Hyperchloremia
    c. Hypercalcemia
    d. Hypercalcemia and hypophosphatemia

22. Cushing's syndrome:
    a. Most often occurs as a primary disease
    b. Is characterized by decreased circulating adrenocorticotropic hormone

  c. Occurs as a result of administration of synthetic steroids

  d. Is caused by a hypothalamic adenoma

23. Repeated normal values of free cortisol in 24-hour urine collections make the diagnosis of Cushing's syndrome:

  a. Highly unlikely

  b. Probable

  c. Suspicious

  d. Very likely

24. The new classification of diabetes mellitus is different from the old system, which was based on insulin dependence. The new classification is based on:

  a. Degree of hypoglycemia at time of diagnosis

  b. Extent of damage to the eyes and kidneys at time of diagnosis

  c. Etiology of the disease

  d. Renal function tests

25. The major consumer of glucose in the body is:

  a. The heart

  b. The endocrine system

  c. The bones and muscles

  d. The brain

26. Patients with type 2 diabetes mellitus:

  a. Are dependent on insulin

  b. Are prone to ketoacidosis

  c. Have hyperinsulinemia

  d. Are generally hypoglycemic

27. The factors related to onset of type 2 diabetes mellitus include all but one of the following. The one NOT characteristic of type 2 diabetes mellitus is:

  a. Excessive calorie intake

  b. Obesity in 60% to 90% of patients

  c. Genetic cause

  d. Involvement of environmental factors

28. Corticosteroid therapy:

  a. Can affect every body system

  b. Affects only the hormonal system

  c. Suppresses the immune response only

  d. Consisting of 10 mg/day of prednisone or less will suppress the adrenal axis

29. Signs and symptoms of the DiGeorge syndrome result from:

  a. Hyperparathyroidism

  b. Hyperthyroidism

  c. Hypoparathyroidism

  d. Hypothyroidism

30. One of the drugs that may cause hypercalcemia is:

  a. Amiodarone

  b. Lithium

  c. Licorice

  d. Loop diuretics

11

Acid-Base, Fluid,
and Electrolyte Disorders

- In healthy persons, the volume and biochemical composition of extracellular and intracellular fluid compartments remain remarkably constant.
- Many disease states cause changes in control either of extracellular fluid (ECF) *volume,* or of the *electrolyte composition* of ECF.
- It is essential for the nurse practitioner to understand these abnormalities to effectively manage these clinical disorders.

DISTRIBUTION AND COMPOSITION OF BODY WATER

- In healthy persons, the total body water constitutes 50% to 60% of lean body weight in men, and 45% to 50% in women.
- In a 70-kg male, total body water is about 42 L, contained in three major compartments
  - —The intracellular fluid (28 L, about 35% of lean body weight)
  - —The interstitial fluid that bathes the cells (9.4 L, about 12%)
  - —Plasma (4.6 L, about 4% to 5%)
- Small amounts of water are contained in bone, dense connective tissue, and epithelial secretions such as digestive secretions and cerebrospinal fluid.
- Intracellular and interstitial fluids are separated by the cell membrane.
- The interstitial fluid and plasma are separated by the capillary wall.

- When no solute is present, water molecules move randomly and in equal numbers in either direction across a permeable membrane.
- If solutes are added to one side of the membrane, the intermolecular cohesive forces reduce the activity of the water molecules.
  - —Therefore water tends to stay in the solute-containing compartment because there is less free diffusion across the membrane.
  - —This ability to hold water in the compartment can be measured as the osmotic pressure.

OSMOTIC PRESSURE

- Osmotic pressure is the primary determinant of the distribution of water between the three major compartments.
- The concentrations of the major solutes that is mainly limited to that compartment, and therefore determines its osmotic pressure (Table 11-1).
  - —K^+ salts in the intracellular fluid (most of the cell Mg^{2+} is bound and osmotically inactive)
  - —Na^+ salts in the interstitial fluid and proteins in the plasma
- Regulation of the plasma volume is a little more complicated because of the tendency of the plasma proteins to hold water in the vascular space by an osmotic effect, which is partly counterbalanced by the hydrostatic pressure in the capillary that is generated by cardiac contraction.

TABLE 11-1

Electrolyte Composition of Intracellular and Extracellular Fluids

Electrolyte	Compartments (Fluids in mmol per L)		
	Plasma Fluid	Interstitial Fluid	Intracellular
Na^+	142	144	10
K^+	4	4	160
Ca^{2+}	2.5	2.5	1.5
Mg^{2+}	1	0.5	13
Cl^-	102	114	2
HCO_3^-	26	30	8
PO_4^{2-}	1	1	57
SO_4^{2-}	0.5	0.5	10
Organic acid	3	4	3
Protein	16	0	55

From Yaquub M: Water, electrolytes, and acid-base homeostasis. In Kumar P, Clark M, eds: *Clinical medicine*, ed 4, Edinburgh, 1998, WB Saunders, p 598.

- A characteristic of an osmotically active solute is that it cannot freely leave its compartment.
- For example, the capillary wall is relatively impermeable to plasma proteins.
  —The cell membrane is "impermeable" to Na^+ and K^+ because the Na^+,K^+-ATPase pump largely restricts Na^+ to the ECF and K^+ to the intracellular fluid.
- By contrast, Na^+ freely crosses the capillary wall and achieves similar concentrations in the interstitium and plasma; therefore it does not contribute to fluid distributions between these compartments.
- Similarly, urea crosses both the capillary wall and the cell membrane and is osmotically inactive.
  —Therefore the retention of urea in renal failure does not alter the distribution of the total body water.
- The conclusion to be drawn from these observations is that body Na^+ stores are the primary determinant of the ECF volume.
  —The extracellular volume (and therefore tissue perfusion) are maintained by appropriate alterations in Na^+ excretion.
  —For example, if Na^+ intake is increased, the extra Na^+ will initially be added to the ECF.
  —The associated increase in extracellular osmolality will cause water to move out of the cells, leading to extracellular volume expansion.

—Balance is restored by excretion of the excess Na^+ in the urine.

DISTRIBUTION OF DIFFERENT KINDS OF REPLACEMENT FLUIDS

- One L of water given intravenously (IV) as 5% dextrose is distributed equally into all compartments.
- One L of 0.9% saline remains in the extracellular compartment.
  —This is therefore the correct treatment for extracellular water depletion—sodium keeps the water in this compartment.
- Adding 1 L of colloid with its high oncotic pressure stays in the vascular compartment and is the treatment for hypovolemia.

REGULATION OF EXTRACELLULAR VOLUME

- Extracellular volume is determined by the sodium concentration.
- Regulation of extracellular volume depends on a tight control of sodium balance, which is exerted by normal kidneys.
  —Renal Na^+ excretion varies directly with the effective circulating volume.
  —In a 70-kg man, plasma fluid constitutes one third of extracellular volume (4.6 L), of which 85% (3.9 L) is on the venous side and only 15% (0.7 L) is in the arterial circulation.
- The unifying hypothesis of extracellular volume regulation in health and disease proposed by Schrier states that the fullness of the arterial vascular compartment (or the so-called effective arterial blood volume [EABV]) is the primary determinant of renal sodium and water excretion.
- Therefore effective arterial blood volume constitutes effective circulatory volume for the purposes of body fluid homeostasis.
- The fullness of the arterial compartment depends on a normal ratio between cardiac output and peripheral arterial resistance.
- Therefore diminished EABV is initiated by a fall in cardiac output or a fall in peripheral arterial resistance (an increase in the holding capacity of the arterial vascular tree).
- When the effective arterial volume is expanded, the urinary Na^+ excretion is increased and can exceed 100 mmol/L.

TABLE 11-2

Mechanisms of Sodium Transport in the Nephron Segments

Tubule Segment	Filtered Na$^+$ Reabsorbed (%)	Major Mechanisms of Luminal Na$^+$ Entry	Major Factors Regulating Transport
Proximal tubule	60-70	Na$^+$-H$^+$ exchange and cotransport of Na$^+$ with glucose, phosphate, and other organic solutes	Angiotensin Noradrenaline
Loop of Henle	20-25	Na$^+$-K$^+$-2Cl$^-$ cotransport	Flow dependent, pressure natriuresis mediated by nitric oxide
Distal tubule	5	Na$^+$-Cl$^-$ cotransport	Flow dependent
Collecting tubules	4	Na$^+$ channels	Aldosterone Atrial natriuretic peptide

From Yaquub M: Water, electrolytes, and acid-base homeostasis. In Kumar P, Clark M, eds: *Clinical medicine*, ed 4, Edinburgh, 1998, WB Saunders, p 601.

- In contrast, the urine can be rendered virtually free of Na$^+$ in the presence of volume depletion and normal renal function.
- Changes in Na$^+$ excretion can be caused by changes both in the filtered load, determined primarily by the glomerular filtration rate (GFR), and in tubular reabsorption, which is affected by multiple factors.
- Changes in tubular reabsorption are usually the main adaptive response to fluctuations in the effective circulating volume. Table 11-2 shows the sites and determinants of segmental Na$^+$ reabsorption.
  - Although the loop of Henle and the distal tubule make an important overall contribution to net Na$^+$ handling, transport in these segments varies primarily with the amount of Na$^+$ delivered—reabsorption is flow-dependent.
  - By comparison, the neurohumoral regulation of Na$^+$ reabsorption to meet body needs occurs mainly in the proximal and collecting tubules.

NEUROHUMORAL REGULATION OF EXTRACELLULAR VOLUME

- Neurohumoral regulation is mediated by volume receptors that sense changes in the effective circulatory volume rather than alterations in the sodium concentrations.
  - These receptors are distributed in both the cardiovascular and renal tissues.
  - *Extrarenal receptors:* are located in the vascular tree in the left atrium and major thoracic veins, and in the carotid sinus body and aortic arch; they respond to a slight reduction in effective circulating volume and cause increased sympathetic nerve activity and a rise in catecholamines; receptors in the cardiac atria control the release of a powerful natriuretic hormone, atrial natriuretic peptide (ANP), from granules located in the atrial walls.
  - *Intrarenal receptors:* are located in the walls of the afferent glomerular arterioles; they respond, via the juxtaglomerular apparatus, to changes in renal perfusion, and control the activity of the renin-angiotensin-aldosterone system; also, sodium concentration in the distal tubule and sympathetic nerve activity change renin release from the juxtaglomerular cells; prostaglandins I$_2$ and E$_2$ are generated within the kidney in response to angiotensin II, acting to maintain GFR, and sodium and water excretion, modulating the sodium-retaining effect of this hormone.
- The receptors distributed in the thoracic tissues (cardiac atria, right ventricle, thoracic veins, pulmonary vessels) are low-pressure volume receptors and are likely of some importance in the volume regulatory system.
- However, there is much evidence that high-pressure arterial receptors (carotid, aortic arch, juxtaglomerular apparatus) predominate over low-pressure volume receptors to regulate volume.

- Probably aldosterone and perhaps atrial natriuretic peptide (or related peptides such as urodilatin) are responsible for day-to-day variations in Na^+ excretion, by means of their ability to augment and diminish Na^+ reabsorption in the collecting tubules.
  - For example, a salt load results in an increase in the effective circulatory and extracellular volume, raising both renal perfusion pressure and atrial and arterial filling pressure.
  - The increased renal perfusion pressure reduces the secretion of renin, and thus that of angiotensin II and aldosterone.
  - The rise in atrial and arterial filling pressure increases the release of ANP; these actions combine to reduce Na^+ reabsorption in the collecting duct, thus promoting excretion of excess Na^+.
- By contrast, in patients on low-sodium intake or in those who become volume-depleted because of vomiting and diarrhea, the ensuing decrease in effective volume enhances the activity of the renin-angiotensin-aldosterone system and reduces the secretion of ANP.
  - The end result is enhanced Na^+ reabsorption in the collecting tubules, which likely accounts for the fall in Na^+ excretion that follows, which thus results in an increase in the extracellular volume to normal.
- With more marked hypovolemia, a decrease in GFR and an increase in proximal and thin ascending limb Na^+ reabsorption also contribute to Na^+ retention.
  - This occurs as the result of enhanced sympathetic nerves acting directly on the kidneys, and indirectly by stimulating the secretion of renin/angiotensin II and nonosmotic release of antidiuretic hormone (ADH).
- The pressure natriuresis phenomenon is likely the final defense against changes in the effective circulating volume.
- Marked persistent hypovolemia results in systemic hypotension and increased salt and water reabsorption in the proximal tubules and ascending limb of Henle.
  - This process may be mediated by changes in renal interstitial hydrostatic pressure and local prostaglandin and nitric oxide production.
- Sodium and water are retained despite increased extracellular volume in edematous conditions such as cardiac failure, hepatic cirrhosis, and hypoalbuminemia.
  - Here, the principal mediator of salt and water retention is the concept of arterial underfilling due either to reduced cardiac output or diminished peripheral arterial resistance.
  - In these settings, arterial underfilling results in reduction of pressure or stretch (i.e., "unloading" of arterial volume receptors), resulting in the same combination of factors as before: activation of the sympathetic nervous system, activation of the renin-angiotensin-aldosterone system, and nonosmotic release of ADH.
  - These neurohumoral mediators promote salt and water retention in the face of increased extracellular volume.
- The common nature of the degree of arterial fullness and neurohumoral pathway in regulating extracellular volume in both health and disease forms the basis of Schrier's unifying hypothesis of volume homeostasis (Fig. 11-1).

REGULATION OF WATER EXCRETION

- Body water homeostasis is maintained by thirst and the urine concentrating and diluting functions of the kidney.
  - These are controlled by intracellular osmoreceptors, primarily in the hypothalamus, to some extent by volume receptors in capacitance vessels close to the heart, and via the renin-angiotensin system.
- Of these, the major (and best understood) control is via *osmoreceptors*.
  - Changes in the plasma Na^+ concentration and osmolality are sensed by the osmoreceptors, which influence both thirst and the release of ADH (also known as vasopressin) from the supraoptic and paraventricular nuclei.
- ADH plays a central role in urinary concentration by increasing the water permeability of the normally impermeable cortical and medullary collecting tubules.
  - This ability of ADH to increase urine osmolality relates indirectly to transport in the ascending limb of the loop of Henle, which reabsorbs NaCl without water.
  - This process is the first step in the countercurrent mechanism and has two effects:

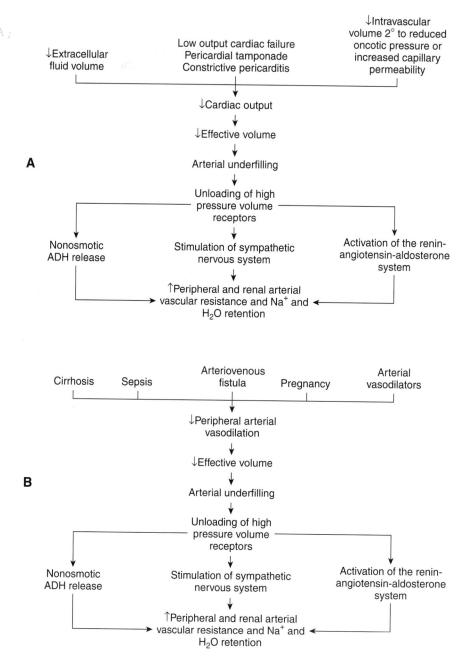

Fig. 11-1 A, Sequence of events in decreased cardiac output and renal sodium and water retention. **B,** Events of arterial vasodilation causing retention of renal sodium and water. (Modified from Schrier RW: *Renal and electrolyte disorders,* New York, 1997, Lippincott-Raven, pp 1-240.)

(1) it makes the tubular fluid dilute, and (2) it makes the medullary interstitium concentrated.

- If ADH is absent, little water is reabsorbed in the collecting tubules, and a dilute urine is excreted.
- The presence of ADH promotes water reabsorption in the collecting tubules down the favorable osmotic gradient between the tubular fluid and the more concentrated interstitium.
  —This process results in an increase in urine osmolality and a decrease in urine volume.
- The cortical collecting tubule has two cell types, each of which has very different functions.
  —*Principal cells* (65%): have sodium and potassium channels in the apical membrane and, as in all sodium-reabsorbing cells, Na^+,K^+-ATPase pumps in the basolateral membrane.
  —The ADH-induced increase in collecting tubule water permeability occurs primarily in these cells.
  —ADH acts on V2 (vasopressin) receptors located on the basolateral surface of principal cells, resulting in the activation of adenyl cyclase; this begins a sequence of events in which a protein kinase is activated, resulting in preformed cytoplasmic vesicles that contain unique water channels, called aquaporins that move toward and are then inserted into the luminal membrane.
  —Water channels span the luminal membrane and permit water movements into the cells down to a favorable osmotic gradient; the water is then rapidly returned to the systemic circulation across the basolateral membrane.
  —When the ADH effect has worn off, the water channels aggregate within clathrin-coated pits, from which they are removed from the luminal membrane by endocytosis, and returned to the cytoplasm.
  —A defect in any part of this process (e.g., attachment of ADH to its receptor, or in the function of the water channel) can cause resistance to the action of ADH and an increase in urine output; this disorder is called *nephrogenic diabetes insipidus.*
  —ADH, in addition to influencing the rate of water excretion, has a central role in osmoregulation because its release is directly affected by the plasma osmolality.
  —At a plasma osmolality of <275 mOsm/kg, which represents a plasma sodium concentration of less than 135 to 137 mmol/L, there is essentially no circulating ADH; as the plasma osmolality rises above this threshold, the secretion of ADH increases progressively.
  —*Intercalated cells:* do not transport NaCl because they have a lower level of Na^+,K^+-ATPase activity; these cells likely have an important role in hydrogen and bicarbonate handling, and in potassium reabsorption in states of potassium depletion.
- Two examples illustrate the basic mechanisms of osmoregulation, which is so efficient that the plasma Na^+ concentration is normally maintained within 1% to 2% of its baseline value.
  —Ingestion of a water load results in an initial reduction in the plasma osmolality, thus diminishing the release of ADH.
  —The ensuing reduction in water reabsorption in the collecting tubules allows the excess water to be excreted in a dilute urine.
  —In contrast, water loss that results from sweating is followed by, in sequence, a rise in both plasma osmolality and ADH secretion, enhanced water reabsorption, and the appropriate excretion of a small volume of concentrated urine.
  —This renal effect of ADH minimizes further water loss but does not replace the existing water deficit.
  —Therefore optimal osmoregulation requires an increase in water intake, mediated by a concurrent stimulation of thirst.
  —The importance of thirst can be illustrated by studies in patients with central diabetes insipidus, who are deficient in ADH.
  —These patients often complain of marked polyuria, caused by the decline in water reabsorption in the collecting tubules, but they do not typically become hyponatremic because urinary water loss is offset by the thirst mechanism.

OSMOREGULATION VERSUS VOLUME REGULATION

- A common misconception is that regulation of plasma Na^+ concentration is closely correlated with the regulation of Na^+ excretion, but it is related to volume regulation, which has different sensors and effectors (volume receptors) from those involved in water balance and osmoregulation (osmoreceptors).

—These two pathways should be considered separately when evaluating patients; a water load, for example, is rapidly excreted in 4 to 6 hours by inhibition of ADH release.

—This process is normally so efficient that volume regulation is not affected and there is no change in ANP release or in the activity of the renin-angiotensin-aldosterone system.

—A dilute urine is excreted, and there is little change in the excretion of Na^+; in contrast, giving isotonic saline causes an increase in volume but no change in plasma osmolality.

—Here, ANP secretion is increased, aldosterone secretion is reduced, and ADH secretion does not change.

—The end result is the appropriate excretion of the excess Na^+ in a relatively iso-osmotic urine.

- In some cases, both volume and osmolality are changed, and both pathways are activated.

—For example, if a person with normal renal function eats salted potato chips and peanuts without drinking any water, the excess Na^+ will increase plasma osmolality, leading to osmotic water movement out of the cells and increased extracellular volume.

—Increase in osmolality stimulates both ADH release and thirst; hypervolemia enhances the secretion of ANP and suppresses secretion of aldosterone.

~ The end result is increased excretion of Na^+ without water.

- The principle of separate volume and osmoregulatory pathways is also apparent in the syndrome of inappropriate ADH secretion (SIADH).

—Patients with SIADH have impaired water excretion and hyponatremia caused by the persistent presence of ADH, but the release of ANP and aldosterone is not impaired, and Na^+ handling remains intact.

—These clinical cases in which hyponatremia must be corrected require restriction of water intake.

- Evidence shows that ADH is also secreted by nonosmotic stimuli, such as stress (e.g., surgery, trauma), significantly reduced effective circulatory volume (e.g., cardiac failure, hepatic cirrhosis), psychiatric disturbances, and nausea, regardless of plasma osmolality.

—This is mediated by the effects of sympathetic overactivity on supraoptic and paraventricular nuclei.

—In addition to water retention, ADH release in these conditions promotes vasoconstriction due to the activation of V1 (vasopressin) receptors distributed in the vascular tissue.

REGULATION OF CELL VOLUME

- All cells must maintain a constant volume, despite extracellular and intracellular osmotic fluctuations.
- Most cells respond to shrinkage or swelling by activating specific metabolic or membrane-transport processes that return cell volume to its normal resting state.
- Within minutes after exposure to hypotonic solutions and the resulting cell swelling, a common feature of many cells is the increase in plasma membrane potassium and chloride conductance.
- Although extrusion of intracellular potassium is a major factor in a regulatory volume decrease, the role of chloride efflux itself is modest because the intracellular chloride concentration is relatively low.
- Other cellular osmolytes, such as taurine and other amino acids, are transported out of the cell to achieve a regulatory volume decrease.
- In contrast, these regulatory mechanisms are operative in reverse to protect cell volume under hypertonic conditions, as is the case in the renal medulla.
- Tubular cells at the tip of renal papillae that are constantly exposed to hypertonic extracellular milieux maintain their cell volume by actively taking up smaller molecules such as betaine, sorbitol, and glycerophosphocholine.

—These changes are mediated by the transcription of a specific enzyme or transporter gene.

- Researchers in biology and physiology are now studying the limitations or alterations of these adaptive responses in various disease states.

CLINICAL USE OF DIURETICS
Loop Diuretics

- These potent diuretics are used in treating any cause of systemic extracellular volume overload.

—They stimulate excretion of both sodium chloride and water, and are helpful in stimulating water excretion in states of relative water overload.

—They also act by causing increased venous capacitance, which leads to rapid clinical improvement in patients with left ventricular failure.

- Undesirable effects of loop diuretics include the following:
  —Urate retention, which can cause gout
  —Hypokalemia
  —Hypomagnesemia
  —Decreased glucose tolerance
  —Allergic tubulointerstitial nephritis and other allergic reactions
  —Myalgia: particularly bumetanide
  —Ototoxicity due to an action on sodium pump activity in the inner ear, particularly with furosemide
  —Interference with excretion of lithium, which can cause toxicity

Thiazide Diuretics

- These are not as potent as loop diuretics, but are widely used in treating essential hypertension.
- Actions include the following:
  —Reduction of peripheral vascular resistance by mechanisms that are not fully understood but that do not appear to depend on their diuretic action.
  —Reduced calcium excretion, which is helpful in patients with idiopathic hypercalciuria but may cause hypercalcemia.
- Undesirable effects include the following:
  —Greater urate retention, glucose intolerance, and hypokalemia
  —Interference with water excretion; may cause hyponatremia, particularly if combined with amiloride or triamterene; this effect is clinically useful in patients with diabetes insipidus

Potassium-Sparing Diuretics

- These are relatively weak and are usually used in combination with thiazides or loop diuretics to prevent potassium depletion.
- Two types are used widely.
  —Spironolactone, an aldosterone antagonist, competes with aldosterone in the collecting ducts, thus reducing sodium absorption.

—Amiloride and triamterene inhibit sodium uptake in collecting duct epithelial cells and reduce renal potassium excretion.

Effects of Renal Function

- All diuretics may increase plasma urea concentration by increasing urea reabsorption in the medulla.
- Thiazides may also promote protein breakdown.
- In some situations, diuretics may also decrease GFR.
- Other effects
  —Excessive diuresis may cause volume depletion and prerenal failure.
  —Diuretics may cause allergic tubulointerstitial nephritis.

INCREASED EXTRACELLULAR VOLUME
Definition

Increased extracellular volume is an increase in the ECF volume caused by a net increase in total body. Sodium content associated with edema formation.

Risk Factors

- This condition occurs in many diseases.
- Physical signs depend on the distribution of excess volume on whether the increase is local or systemic.
- According to Starling's hypothesis, distribution depends on
  —Venous tone, which determines the capacitance of the blood compartment and therefore the hydrostatic pressure
  —Oncotic pressure, which depends mainly on serum albumin
  —Lymphatic drainage
- Depending on these factors, fluid accumulation can occur in expansion of interstitial volume, blood volume, or both.

Signs and Symptoms

- Peripheral edema results from expansion of the extracellular volume by at least 2 L (15%).
  —The ankles are usually the first part to be affected, although the ankles may be spared in patients with lipodermatosclerosis, where the skin is attached and cannot expand to accommodate the added fluid.

- Edema may be present in the face, particularly in the morning.
- In bedridden patients, edema occurs in the sacral area.
- Expansion of the interstitial volume may cause pulmonary edema, pleural effusion, pericardial effusion, and ascites.
- Expansion of the blood volume causes elevated jugular venous pressure, cardiomegaly, additional heart sounds, and increased arterial blood pressure in certain circumstances.

Etiology/Cause

- Extracellular volume expansion is caused by *sodium chloride retention.*
  - Increased salt intake does not normally cause volume expansion because of rapid homeostatic mechanisms that increase salt excretion.
  - However, a rapid IV solution of a large volume of saline will cause volume expansion.
  - Therefore most causes of extracellular volume expansion are related to renal sodium chloride retention.

Heart Failure

- Reduction in cardiac output and the consequent fall in effective circulatory volume and arterial filling lead to activation of the renin-angiotensin-aldosterone system, nonosmotic release of ADH, and increased activity of the renal sympathetic nerves via volume receptors and baroreceptors.
- Enhanced sympathetic activity also indirectly augments ADH and renin-angiotensin-aldosterone response.
- The cumulative effects of these mediators result in increased peripheral and renal resistance, and water and sodium retention.
- These events cause extracellular volume expansion and increased venous pressure, resulting in the formation of edema.

Hypoalbuminemia

- In this condition, the major mechanism is loss of plasma oncotic pressure that leads to loss of water from the vascular space to the interstitial space.
  - Reduction in effective circulatory volume and the resulting fall in cardiac output

and arterial filling cause a sequence of events such as occurs in cardiac failure.
  - This sequence of events results in extracellular volume expansion and increased venous pressure that causes edema formation.
  - Other factors may be involved (e.g., some evidence shows that the nephrotic syndrome itself changes renal sodium handling).

Hepatic Cirrhosis

- The mechanism involved here is also complex, and involves peripheral vasodilation, perhaps due to increased nitric oxide generation that causes reduced effective volume and arterial filling.
  - These factors lead to an activation of a chain of events common to cardiac failure, hypoalbuminemia, and other conditions with marked peripheral vasodilation.
  - The cumulative effect of these mediators results in increased peripheral and renal resistance and water and sodium retention, which causes edema to form.

Sodium Retention

- Decreased GFR reduces the renal capacity to excrete sodium.
- This may be acute, as in the acute nephritic syndrome, or may occur as part of the presentation of chronic renal failure.
  - In end-stage renal failure, extracellular volume is controlled by the balance between salt intake and its removal by dialysis.
- Mild sodium retention can be caused by estrogens that have a weak aldosterone-like effect; this produces the weight gain in the premenstrual phase that so many women experience.
- Other drugs may cause renal sodium retention, particularly in patients whose renal function is already impaired.
  - *Mineralocorticoids and licorice:* licorice potentiates the sodium-retaining action of cortisol; both have aldosterone-like actions.
  - *Nonsteroidal antiinflammatory drugs (NSAIDs)* cause sodium retention in the presence of activation of the renin-an-

giotensin-aldosterone system by heart failure, cirrhosis, and renal artery stenosis.

- Significant amounts of sodium and water may accumulate in the body without clinically obvious edema or evidence of increased venous pressure.
  —Several liters may accumulate in the pleural space or as ascites; these spaces are then referred to as "third spaces."
  —Bone also may act as a pool for sodium and water.

Other Causes of Edema

- Beginning insulin therapy for type 1 diabetes and refeeding after malnutrition are both associated with the development of transient edema; the mechanism is complex.
- Edema may be caused by increased capillary pressure due to relaxation of precapillary arterioles, such as peripheral edema from dihydropyridine calcium-channel blockers (e.g., nifedipine).
- Edema may be caused by increased interstitial oncotic pressure due to increased capillary permeability to proteins that may occur in the rare complement-deficiency syndrome; with therapeutic use of interleukin-2 in cancer chemotherapy; or in ovarian hyperstimulation syndrome.
- Local effects (e.g., premenstrual syndrome [PMS], thrombosis, superior vena cava obstruction) may also cause edema that disappears when the central problem is treated.

Treatment

- The underlying cause(s) must be treated first: heart failure, elimination of drugs such as NSAIDs, left ventricular dysfunction, myocardial ischemia, and cardiac dysrhythmias.
- Use of digitalis, inotropic agents, and afterload reduction to improve cardiac function can decrease or eliminate the need for diuretics by improving Na delivery to the kidneys and thus decreasing renal Na conservation.
- Sodium restriction has only a limited role but is helpful in patients who are resistant to diuretics.
- Techniques that increase venous return stimulate salt and water excretion by affecting cardiac output and ANP release.

—Compression support hose help to mobilize edema in heart failure and are essential in the treatment of venous valve disease of the lower legs.

- The mainstay of therapy is the use of diuretic agents, which increase sodium, chloride, and water excretion in the kidney.

Patient/Family Education

- Instruct the patient and family about the nature of the condition, its cause, the proposed therapy, and expected outcomes.
- Often, both patient and family members can be helpful in assisting the patient to reduce fluid intake by mouth or in reporting new symptoms.

Follow-up/Referral

- Patients are followed for several weeks or months, depending on response to therapy and status of underlying conditions.
- In addition to the primary care clinician, follow-up is continued with consultation of the appropriate specialists such as cardiologist, urologist, or other.

DECREASED EXTRACELLULAR VOLUME
Definition

Decreased extracellular volume is a decrease in the ECF compartment volume caused by a net decrease in total body sodium content.

Risk Factors

- Patients with a history of inadequate fluid intake
- Vomiting
- Diarrhea
- Nasogastric suction
- Ileostomy
- Colostomy
- Diuretic therapy
- Symptoms of diabetes mellitus
- Renal or adrenal disease

Etiology/Cause (Box 11-1)
Pathogenesis

- Losses of Na from the body are always combined with water losses.

BOX 11-1

Principal Causes of Extracellular Fluid Volume Depletion

EXTRARENAL

GI: vomiting, diarrhea, nasogastric suction
Skin: sweating
Dialysis: hemodialysis, peritoneal dialysis
Third-space losses: intestinal lumen, intraperitoneal, retroperitoneal
Burns, trauma

RENAL/ADRENAL

Chronic renal failure; salt-wasting renal disease (medullary cystic disease, interstitial nephritis, some cases of pyelonephritis and myeloma)
Acute renal failure: diuretic phase of recovery
Diuretics
Diabetes mellitus with ketoacidosis or extreme glucosuria
Bartter's syndrome
Adrenal disease: Addison's disease (glucocorticoid deficiency), hypoaldosteronism

From Beers MH, Berkow R, eds: Water, electrolyte, mineral, and acid-base metabolism. *The Merck manual of diagnosis and therapy,* ed 17, Whitehouse Station, NJ, 1999, Merck & Co, Inc, p 124.

- The end result of Na depletion therefore is ECF volume depletion.
- Any change in plasma Na concentration (increase, decrease, stays the same) with volume depletion depends on the route of volume loss (e.g., gastrointestinal [GI], renal) and the type of replacement fluid ingested by or given to the person.
- Other factors may also affect the Na concentration in volume depletion, including ADH secretion or impaired solute delivery to the distal tubule, resulting in water retention.

Diagnosis

Signs and Symptoms (see Risk Factors)

- In mild ECF volume depletion, the only signs may be diminished skin turgor and intraocular tension.
- Orthostatic hypotension (decrease of systolic pressure > 10 mm Hg on standing)
- Tachycardia
- Low central venous pressure (CVP)
- Severe ECF depletion can result in disorientation and overt shock.

- Normal kidneys respond to volume depletion by conserving Na.
  —When volume depletion is severe enough to cause decreased urine volume, the urine Na concentration is usually <10 to 15 mEq/L and urine osmolality is usually increased.
- If metabolic alkalosis is present in addition to volume depletion, the urine Na concentration may be high and therefore misleading as a measure of volume status.
  —In this case, a low urine chloride concentration (<10 mEq/L) is more reliable to indicate ECF volume depletion.
- If the Na losses are due to renal disease, diuretics, or adrenal insufficiency, the urine Na concentration is usually >20 mEq/L.
- Significant ECF volume depletion also frequently results in mild-to-moderate increases in blood urea nitrogen (BUN) and plasma creatinine levels (prerenal azotemia; BUN:creatinine ratio > 20:1).

Treatment

- Mild-to-moderate ECF volume depletion may be corrected by increased oral intake of Na and water, if the patient is conscious and does not have GI dysfunction.
- The underlying cause of volume depletion must be treated (e.g., by discontinuing diuretics or treating diarrhea, ketoacidosis, Addison's disease).
- When volume depletion is severe and accompanied by hypotension or when oral fluid administration is not feasible, IV saline is the fluid of choice, using appropriate precautions.
- When renal excretion of water is normal, Na and water deficits can be safely replaced with 0.9% saline.
- If a disturbance in water metabolism exists, replacement fluids are modified.

Patient/Family Education

- Instruct the patient and family as fully as possible about the condition, its cause, proposed treatment, and expected outcomes.
- Often, family members and the patient can be involved in giving oral fluids or reporting new symptoms.
- Provide reassurance to both the patient and the family.

- Indicate the approximate length of time it will take to restore the patient to homeostasis.

Follow-up/Referral

- Patients with ECF volume depletion may be followed for variable lengths of time, depending on the status of the patient with respect to age and general health, the cause of the volume depletion, and the underlying conditions.

ACID-BASE DISORDERS
Hyponatremia

Definition

Hyponatremia is a decrease in the plasma sodium concentration below 136 mEq/L caused by an excess of water relative to solute.

Risk Factors

- Hyponatremia is the most common electrolyte disorder, occurring in up to 1% of all patients admitted to the hospital.
- Hyponatremia has been reported in over 50% of hospitalized patients with acquired immunodeficiency syndrome (AIDS).
- Mineralocorticoid deficiency
- Osmotic diuresis
- Salt-losing nephropathy

Etiology/Cause (Box 11-2)

- Hypovolemic hyponatremia can result from both extrarenal and renal fluid losses.
  —GI (diarrhea)
  —Third space
- Remarkably large volumes of fluid can be sequestered in pancreatitis, peritonitis, and small-bowel obstruction, or lost in severe, large body surface area (BSA) burns.

Pathogenesis

- Hyponatremia is associated with many conditions, both renal and extrarenal.
- Patients with ongoing renal fluid losses are distinguished from those with extrarenal fluid losses by an inappropriately high urine Na concentration (20 mEq/L).
  —One exception is metabolic alkalosis that often occurs with protracted vomiting, where large amounts of bicarbonate are spilled in the urine, obligating the excretion of Na to maintain electrical neutrality.

BOX 11-2
Principal Causes of Hyponatremia

Hyponatremia with hypovolemia (decreased TBW and Na; relatively greater decrease of Na)
Extrarenal losses
  GI: vomiting, diarrhea
  Third-space losses
    Pancreatitis
    Peritonitis
    Small-bowel obstruction
    Rhabdomyolysis
    Burns
Renal losses
  Diuretics
  Osmotic diuresis (glucose, urea, mannitol)
  Mineralocorticoid deficiency
  Salt-losing nephropathies
Hyponatremia with euvolemia (increased TBW; near normal total body Na)
Diuretics
Hypothyroidism
Glucocorticoid deficiency
States that increase release of ADH (postoperative narcotics, pain, emotional stress)
Syndrome of inappropriate ADH secretion
Primary polydipsia
Hyponatremia with hypervolemia (increased total body Na; relatively greater increase in TBW)
Extrarenal disorders
  Congestive heart failure
  Hepatic cirrhosis
Renal disorders
  Nephrotic syndrome
  Acute renal failure
  Chronic renal failure

From Beers MH, Berkow R, eds: Water, electrolyte, mineral, and acid-base metabolism. *The Merck manual of diagnosis and therapy,* ed 17, Whitehouse Station, NJ, 1999, Merck & Co, Inc, p 127.

  —In metabolic alkalosis, urine Cl concentration frequently differentiates renal from extrarenal sources of volume depletion.

Hypovolemic Hyponatremia

- This condition is characterized by deficiencies in both water and Na, although proportionately more Na than water is lost.
- Hyponatremia can occur when fluid losses, such as those that occur with protracted vomiting, severe diarrhea, or sequestration of fluids in a third space, are replaced with ingestion of free water or treated with hypotonic IV fluid.

- Significant ECF fluid losses also result in the nonosmotic release of ADH, causing water retention by the kidneys and maintenance or further worsening of hyponatremia.
- The normal renal response to volume loss is Na conservation.
  —In extrarenal causes of hypovolemia, a urine Na concentration of <10 mEq/L is frequently seen.

Euvolemic Hyponatremia
- Occurs when total body water (TBW) is increased and there is no significant change in total body Na content.
- Primary polydipsia can cause hyponatremia only when water intake overwhelms the kidney's ability to excrete water.
  —Normal kidneys can excrete up to 25 L/day, so water intake would have to be excessively large, or renal failure would have to coexist.
- Dilutional hyponatremia may occur from excessive water intake without Na retention in the presence of renal failure, Addison's disease, myxedema, or nonosmotic ADH; secretion in cases of stress, postoperative states, or drugs such as chlorpropamide or tolbutamide, opioids, barbiturates, vincristine, clofibrate, and carbamazepine.

Hypovolemic Hyponatremia
- This condition is characterized by an increase in both total body Na content and TBW.
- Causes include heart failure and hepatic cirrhosis but rarely in nephrotic syndrome.
- In these cases, a decrease in effective circulating volume causes the release of ADH and angiotensin II.
  —Hyponatremia results from the antidiuretic effect of ADH on the kidneys, and the direct impairment of renal water excretion by angiotensin.
  —Decreased GFR and stimulation of thirst by angiotensin II also potentiate the development of hyponatremia.
- Added to hyponatremia and edema, low Na concentration (<10 mEq/L) and a high urine osmolality (relative to plasma) occur in the absence of diuretics.

Effects on the Central Nervous System
- In experimental studies, brain cellular water content is elevated in both acute and chronic hyponatremia.
  —As a result of decreased brain cell electrolyte content, the increase in brain water content in chronic hyponatremia is less than would be expected from the degree of plasma osmolality.
  —Therefore symptoms of central nervous system (CNS) dysfunction are more common, and mortality significantly greater, in acute hyponatremia than in chronic hyponatremia.

Syndrome of Inappropriate ADH Secretion
Definition
Syndrome of inappropriate ADH secretion (SIADH) is less than maximally dilute urine in the presence of plasma hypoosmolality and hyponatremia.

Risk Factors
- Unknown, if any

Etiology/Cause
- Listed are some of the causes of inappropriate ADH secretion, but the actual cause of most of these disorders is not known.
- Sustained ADH release
- Level of plasma osmolality
- Osmotic threshold for ADH release is subnormally low (a reset osmostat).
- In some patients, ADH is not suppressed in the presence of low plasma osmolality.

Pathogenesis
- Whereas SIADH is classically attributed to sustained ADH release, several abnormal patterns of ADH release have been identified by ADH radioimmunoassay.
  —In some patients, ADH secretion is erratic and apparently independent of osmotic control.
  —In others, ADH levels vary appropriately with plasma osmolality, but the osmotic threshold for ADH release is abnormally low (a reset osmostat).
  —A small group of patients appear to have a constant low level release of ADH; within

the normal range of plasma osmolality, ADH release is appropriate, but when the plasma becomes hypoosmotic, ADH release is not suppressed.

—Another small group of patients are unable to maximally dilute the urine or excrete a water load but have normal ADH release; these patients have a syndrome of inappropriate antidiuresis rather than SIADH, and may be distinguished only by assay of plasma ADH levels.

Diagnosis

Signs and Symptoms

- Symptoms of hyponatremia occur when the effective plasma osmolality falls to ≤240 mOsm/kg, regardless of the underlying cause.
- The rate of the decrease may be as important as the absolute magnitude of the decrease.
- Manifestations of hyponatremia can be subtle and are primarily mental changes: altered personality, lethargy, confusion.
- As the plasma Na falls below 115 mEq/L, stupor, neuromuscular hyperexcitability, convulsions, prolonged coma, and death can occur.
- Cerebral edema, cerebellar tonsil herniation, and demyelinating lesions (pontine and extrapontine) may occur.
- Neuropathologic changes of *central pontine myelinolysis* associated with hyponatremia have been observed, mainly in patients with alcoholism, malnutrition, or other chronic debilitating illnesses.
- Recent research data indicate that cycling premenopausal women may be especially susceptible to severe cerebral edema in association with acute hyponatremia, perhaps due to inhibition of brain Na^+,K^+-ATPase by estrogen and progesterone, and resultant decreased solute extrusion from brain cells.
  —Reported sequelae include hypothalamic and posterior pituitary infarction and brainstem herniation in severe cases.

Prognosis

- Mortality is significantly greater in acute hyponatremia than in chronic hyponatemia because of effects on the CNS.

- The presence of debilitating diseases appears to influence survival in patients with hyponatremia: alcoholism, hepatic cirrhosis, heart failure, or malignancy.

Treatment

- Treatment of mild, asymptomatic hyponatremia (i.e., plasma Na > 120 mEq/L) is clear, especially if the underlying cause can be identified and eliminated (e.g., diuretic-induced hyponatremia).
  —Stop the diuretic.
  —Replace Na and K as needed.
- The simultaneous presence of hyponatremia, hyperkalemia, and hypotension should suggest adrenal insufficiency, and may require IV glucocorticoid (100 to 200 mg hydrocortisone in 1 L of 5% dextrose and 0.9% saline given over 4 hours).
- When adrenal function is normal and hyponatremia is associated with ECF volume depletion and hypotension, giving IV 0.9% saline usually corrects both the hyponatremia and the hypotension.
  —If the underlying disorder responds slowly or if hyponatremia is marked (plasma Na <120 mEq/L), water restriction by mouth of between 500 and 1000 ml/24 hours is highly effective.
- Patients with dilutional hyponatremia associated with ECF volume expansion due to renal Na retention (e.g., heart failure, cirrhosis, or nephrotic syndrome) have few symptoms caused by hyponatremia.
  —Water restriction along with treatment of the underlying condition is usually successful.
  —Captopril, an angiotensin converting enzyme (ACE) inhibitor, with a loop diuretic is sufficient to correct refractory hyponatremia in patients with heart failure.
- Captopril or other ACE inhibitors may be effective in volume-expansion states characterized by increased activity of the renin-angiotensin-aldosterone axis, as in nephrotic syndrome.
- If SIADH is present, severe water restriction of 25% to 50% of maintenance is required; lasting correction depends on successful treatment of the underlying disease.

- Treatment of hyponatremia is more controversial when symptoms of severe water intoxication (i.e., seizures) are present, or when hyponatremia is severe (plasma Na < 115 mEq/L) and effective osmolality is <230 mOsm/kg.
  —Controversy centers around the pace and extent of hyponatremia correction.
  —A patient with severe but asymptomatic hyponatremia usually responds to stringent water restriction alone, but others recommend administration of hypertonic (3%) saline containing 513 mEq sodium/L; this therapy is recommended by all for patients with severe, symptomatic hyponatremia (i.e., generalized seizures).
  —However, hypertonic saline should be used with great caution in all patients, because of the possibility of precipitating neurologic problems such as central pontine myelinolysis, which can also occur when hyponatremia is corrected too rapidly.

Patient/Family Education
- The patient and family members should be instructed regarding the nature, cause, course, treatment, and expected outcomes of therapy.
- Both patient and family can be helpful in overseeing water restriction, if that is ordered, and in observing new symptoms or changes in the patient's condition.
- Health care professionals should reassure the patient and family that recovery is the goal, depending on other coexisting conditions (e.g., cirrhosis).

Follow-up/Referral
- Throughout the patient's illness, both the clinician and specialists (urologist, neurologist) manage the patient's treatment.
- After discharge, the clinician follows the patient closely for several weeks to make certain that hyponatremia or neurologic symptoms do not occur/recur.

Hypernatremia
Definition
Hypernatremia is an elevation in the plasma sodium concentration above 145 mEq/L caused by a deficit of water relative to solute. Less common than hyponatremia, hypernatremia is one of the most serious electrolyte disorders in adult patients, with reported mortality of 40% to 60%. Na is the major determinant of ECF osmolality; hypernatremia implies hyperosmolality of the ECF compartment, which results in movement of water out of the intracellular space until cellular tonicity increases to that of the ECF.

Risk Factors
- History of vomiting, diarrhea
- History of renal disease
- History of taking loop diuretics
- Burns
- Excessive sweating
- Receiving total parenteral nutrition

Etiology/Cause (Box 11-3)
Pathogenesis
- Hypernatremia is usually caused by excessive loss of water from the body that is not adequately replaced.
- The patient may have an impaired thirst mechanism.
- The severity of the underlying disease that usually results in an inability to drink is considered to be partly responsible for the high mortality seen in hypernatremia.
- Either hyponatremia or hypernatremia can occur with severe volume loss, depending on the relative amounts of salt and water lost, and the amount of water drunk before the patient is seen.
- Renal causes of hypernatremia and volume depletion include treatment with loop diuretics, which inhibit Na reabsorption in the concentrating portion of the nephron and can increase water clearance.
- Osmotic diuresis can also cause impaired renal concentrating ability because a hypertonic substance present in the tubular lumen of the distal nephron (e.g., glycerol, mannitol, and sometimes urea) can cause osmotic diuresis with resulting hypernatremia.
- The most common cause of hypernatremia due to osmotic diuresis is hyperglycemia occurring in nonketotic hyperglycemic-hyperosmolar coma in diabetic patients.
  —Glucose does not penetrate cells in the absence of insulin, and therefore the hyperglycemia further dehydrates the ICF.

BOX 11-3

Principal Causes of Hypernatremia

Hypernatremia with hypovolemia (decreased TBW and Na; relatively greater decrease in TBW)
  Extrarenal losses
    GI: vomiting, diarrhea
    Skin: burns, excessive sweating
  Renal losses
    Loop diuretics
    Osmotic diuresis (glucose, urea, mannitol)
    Intrinsic renal disease
Hypernatremia with euvolemia (decreased TBW; near-normal total body Na)
  Extrarenal losses
    Respiratory; tachypnea
    Skin: fever, excessive sweating
  Renal losses
    Central diabetes insipidus
    Nephrogenic diabetes insipidus

Other
  Inability to access water
  Primary hypodipsia
  Reset osmostat
Hypernatremia with hypervolemia (increased Na; normal or increased TBW)
  Hypertonic fluid administration (hypertonic saline, $NaHCO_3$, total parenteral nutrition)
  Mineralocorticoid excess
    Iatrogenic
    Adrenal tumors secreting deoxycorticosterone
    Congenital adrenal hyperplasia (caused by 11-hydroxylase defect)

From Beers MH, Berkow R, eds: Water, electrolyte, mineral, and acid-base metabolism. *The Merck manual of diagnosis and therapy,* ed 17, Whitehouse Station, NJ, 1999, Merck & Co, Inc, p 131.

- Intrinsic renal disease, such as chronic renal insufficiency, can also prevent a maximally concentrated urine and predispose to hypernatremia.
- When a water deficit exists, hypernatremia occurs without disturbance in Na balance.
- Excessive sweating causes water loss, which results in some Na loss, but sweat is hypotonic, and hypernatremia can result before significant hypovolemia occurs.
- Pituitary or central diabetes insipidus is a defect in the production or release of ADH by the posterior pituitary.
  —These patients, and those with diabetes insipidus, cannot excrete a concentrated urine.
  —The thirst mechanism is intact, but hypernatremia can develop when the patient does not have access to water.
  —The concentrating defect in central diabetes insipidus responds well to exogenous ADH in the form of vasopressin, 1-desamino-8-D-arginine, or other preparations containing ADH.
- Hypernatremia is especially common in the elderly for various reasons: unable to access water, impaired thirst, impaired renal concentrating ability, and increased insensible water losses.
  —In younger people, ADH release is enhanced in response to osmotic stimuli but is decreased in the elderly in response to changes in volume and pressure.

Diagnosis

Signs and Symptoms
- Thirst is the most prominent symptom in hypernatremia.
- Older patients or those who are semiconscious or completely unconscious cannot communicate their thirst.
- CNS symptoms result from brain cell shrinkage: confusion, neuromuscular excitability, seizures, or coma may occur.
- Postmortem findings in patients who die from hypernatremia include cerebrovascular damage with subcortical or subarachnoid hemorrhage and venous thromboses.

Diagnostic Tests
- A water deprivation test can distinguish among several polyuric states.
  —However, because this test can cause dangerous hyperosmolality, the test can be done only under the closest monitoring of electrolyte concentrations, blood and urine osmolality, and volume status.
  —When the maximum urinary osmolality has been reached, 5 U of aqueous vasopressin is given subcutaneously (SC), and urine osmolality is measured after 1 hour.

—The normal response to water deprivation is elevation of urine osmolality to >800 mOsm/L with little or no further increase with vasopressin.

Prognosis

- Mortality from acute hypernatremia is significantly greater than that from chronic hypernatremia, largely because the body can adapt to slower changes; however, overall mortality is high because of CNS hyperosmolality and the severity of underlying disease, which often prevents patients from expressing thirst.

Treatment

- Water replacement is the primary goal of therapy.
  —Response is better in those patients who can take water by mouth.
- For patients unable to drink, IV hydration with 5% dextrose and water (D/W) is begun, but too-rapid administration can lead to glycosuria, which increases salt-free water excretion and increased hypertonicity.
- If patients are severely ill and perhaps in shock, colloid and 0.9% saline are required to increase volume before giving hypotonic saline or free water to correct the hypernatremia.

Patient/Family Education

- Many people find it difficult to understand health problems related to disturbances in electrolyte and water imbalance.
  —Instructions to the patient and family about the condition should be presented in the simplest terms.
- Depending on the patient's age, disease status, and degree of hypernatremia, reassurance regarding recovery can be provided.
- Often, family members can observe for changes in the patient, and feel useful in knowing what to look for and reporting any changes immediately to the staff.
- Frequent communication with the family regarding the patient's status is always welcome.

Follow-up/Referral

- These patients are often followed closely for several weeks or months after recovery from the more acute episode, to monitor Na and

water volume to maintain a correct balance of each.
- Consultation with specialists may also continue: neurologist, nephrologist, or cardiologist as required, until the patient's condition is stable for some time.

DISORDERS OF POTASSIUM METABOLISM
Hypokalemia
Definition
Hypokalemia is a decrease in the serum potassium concentration below 3.5 mEq/L caused by a deficit in total body potassium stores or abnormal movement of potassium into cells.

Risk Factors
- Chronic low intake of dietary potassium
- Excessive loss of potassium (in water) through the kidneys or from the GI tract (vomiting, diarrhea)
- History of chronic laxative abuse
- Clay pica

Etiology/Cause (see also Risk factors)
- Diuretics are by far the most commonly used drugs that cause hypokalemia previous surgery such as bowel diversion.
- Gastric suction for patients undergoing abdominal surgery or other reason
- GI losses may be more severe when simultaneous loss occurs through the kidneys, or in the presence of metabolic alkalosis and stimulation of aldosterone due to volume depletion.
- Total parenteral nutrition can cause transcellular shift of K into cells when glycogenesis is an underlying cause.
- Disease states can cause hypokalemia.
  —Cushing's syndrome
  —Thyrotoxicosis
  —Primary hyperaldosteronism
  —Congenital adrenal hyperplasia
  —Liddle's syndrome is a rare autosomal dominant disorder characterized by severe hypertension and hypokalemia.
  —Bartter's syndrome is an uncommon disorder of uncertain cause characterized by renal K and Na wasting, excessive production of renin and aldosterone, and normotension.

Diagnosis

Signs and Symptoms

- Diagnosis of hypokalemia is made on the basis of plasma or serum K level < 3.5 mEq/L.
- Severe hypokalemia (plasma K < 3 mEq/L) may cause muscle weakness and lead to paralysis and respiratory failure.
- Other types of muscular dysfunction that can occur include muscle cramping, fasciculations, paralytic ileus, hypoventilation, hypotension, tetany, and rhabdomyolysis.
- Persistent hypokalemia can cause impaired renal concentrating ability, which leads to polyuria with secondary polydipsia.
- Metabolic alkalosis is often present, although hypokalemia can also occur with metabolic acidosis.
- Usually, GFR, water, and Na balance are not affected by hypokalemia.
- A state similar to nephrogenic diabetes insipidus can occur with severe K depletion.
- Cardiac effects of hypokalemia are usually minimal until plasma K levels are <3 mEq/L, when hypokalemia may cause premature ventricular and atrial contractions, ventricular and atrial tachycardias, and second- or third-degree atrioventricular block.
- Patients with preexisting heart disease and those receiving digitalis are at risk for cardiac conduction abnormalities, even from relatively mild hypokalemia.
- Usual ECG changes include ST segment depression, increased U-wave amplitude, and T-wave amplitude less than U-wave amplitude (in the same lead).

Treatment

- Routine K replacement is not necessary in most patients receiving diuretics.
- However, preventing hypokalemia is important, particularly in patients also receiving digitalis, in patients with asthma who are receiving β_2-agonists, and in noninsulin-dependent diabetic patients.
  - For these patients, the lowest effective dose of diuretic is prescribed, dietary Na intake is restricted to <2 g/day, and plasma K is monitored frequently after beginning treatment.
  - Once stable K concentration is achieved, monitoring of plasma K can be less frequent, unless medications change or symptoms occur.
- Supplemental K is available in several forms.
  - Liquid potassium chloride is not well tolerated in doses > 25 to 50 mEq because of bitter taste.
  - Enteric-coated K preparations may lead to small bowel ulceration.
  - Wax-impregnated potassium chloride preparations seem to be safe and well tolerated.
  - GI bleeding may be less common with microencapsulated KCl preparations.
- When hypokalemia is severe, symptomatic, or unresponsive to oral therapy, IV potassium is given.
  - Rate of response is limited because of the lag in K deposition in the cells.
  - Even when hypokalemia is severe, it is rarely necessary to give more than 80 to 100 mEq of K in excess of continuing losses in a 24-hour period.
  - Modern, accurate IV infusion pumps decrease the risk of giving highly concentrated KCl solutions, but IV solutions should not exceed 60 mEq/L, and infusion rates should not exceed 10 mEq/hour.
- When hypomagnesemia is present along with hypokalemia, it is usually required to correct the magnesium deficiency to stop renal K wasting and to facilitate K repletion.

Patient/Family Education

- The nature, cause, course, treatment, and expected outcomes of the potassium deficit state should be explained to the patient and the family as clearly as possible.
- A list of potassium-rich foods should be given to the patient.
- A potassium replacement preparation may be needed.
- Write out the signs and symptoms of potassium deficit, and when to call the nurse practitioner.
- The patient should be monitored fairly frequently after diagnosis of potassium deficiency.
- The patient should be made aware of the signs and symptoms of hyperkalemia as well, in case potassium intake exceeds normal losses.

Follow-up/Referral
- Patients are followed every 2 to 4 weeks for a time, until the K level remains stable as seen in several plasma tests.
- Referral to a specialist is usually not necessary unless the patient has underlying medical problems such as diabetes or cardiac disease.

Hyperkalemia
Definition
Hyperkalemia is an increase in the serum potassium concentration above 5.5 mEq/L (plasma potassium above 5.0) caused by an excess in total body potassium stores or abnormal movement of potassium out of cells.

Risk Factors
- The kidneys normally excrete excess K; if hyperkalemia is persistent, renal excretion of potassium may be the underlying problem.
- Metabolic acidosis may lead to transcellular movement of K out of cells.
- Hyperglycemia in the presence of insulin deficiency
- Moderately strenuous exercise, particularly in patients receiving β-blockers
- Digitalis toxicity
- Acute tumor lysis
- Acute intravascular hemolysis
- Acute renal failure with associated oliguria
- Burns
- Internal bleeding
- Adrenal insufficiency (seen often in those with AIDS)
- Certain drugs (e.g., ACE inhibitors, K-sparing diuretics, β-blockers, NSAIDs, cyclosporine, lithium, heparin, trimethoprim)

Etiology/Cause (see also Risk Factors)
- Hyperkalemic familial periodic paralysis is a rare inherited disorder characterized by episodic hyperkalemia due to sudden movement of K out of cells, usually precipitated by exercise.

Diagnosis
Signs and Symptoms
- Usually asymptomatic until cardiac toxicity occurs
  —ECG changes include shortening of the Q-T interval; tall, symmetric, peaked T waves.

—Progressive hyperkalemia results in nodal and ventricular dysrhythmias, widening of the QRS complex, prolongation of the P-R interval, and disappearance of the P wave; later, the QRS complex degenerates into a sine wave pattern, and ventricular asystole or fibrillation follows.

Treatment
- Mild hyperkalemia (plasma K < 6 mEq/L) often responds to decreased K intake and stopping drugs such as K-sparing diuretics, β-blockers, NSAIDs, or ACE inhibitors.
- Adding a loop diuretic can enhance K excretion from the kidneys.
- A plasma K level of 6 mEq/L requires more aggressive therapy, as do patients with acute or chronic renal failure, particularly if hypercatabolism or tissue injury is present, and have a plasma K level of ≥5 mEq/L.
- If there are no ECG abnormalities and plasma K is <6 mEq/L, sodium polystyrene sulfonate in sorbitol is given—15 to 30 g in 30 to 70 ml of 70% sorbitol orally (PO) q4-6h.
  —Na polystyrene sulfonate acts as a cation exchange resin and removes K via the GI mucosa; about 1 mEq of K is removed per g of resin.
  —Patients not able to take this medication by mouth may be given it via retention enema.
- In emergency situations such as cardiac toxicity, the following steps are taken:
  —IV: 10% calcium gluconate, 10 to 20 ml, or 5 to 10 ml of 22% calcium gluceptate) within 5 to 10 minutes
    ~ If the ECG is only a sine wave, the calcium gluconate can be given rapidly (5 to 10 ml in 2 minutes).
  —IV push: 5 to 10 U Regular insulin followed immediately by rapid infusion of 50 ml of 50% glucose, then by 10% D/W at 50 ml/hour to prevent hypoglycemia; the effect on K occurs within 15 minutes.
  —Inhalation of a high-dose β-agonist (e.g., albuterol 10 to 20 mg over 10 minutes (5 mg/ml concentration); onset of action is within 30 minutes, lasting 2 to 4 hours

Patient/Family Education
- Instruct the patient and family regarding the nature, cause, course, treatment, and expected outcomes of therapy.

- In emergency treatment, provide frequent communication regarding the status of the patient, and reassurance about the outcome.
- Precise signs and symptoms of both hypokalemia and hyperkalemia are given in writing to the patient, along with a list of foods/beverages to be avoided to prevent the condition.

Follow-up/Referral

- After recovery from the acute stage of hyperkalemia, the patient is followed in the office or clinic often during the first several weeks by measuring plasma K.
- During follow-up, it is possible to explain in more detail about electrolyte imbalance and what is expected of the patient and family.

DISORDERS OF CALCIUM METABOLISM

Hypocalcemia

Definition

Hypocalcemia is a decrease in total plasma calcium concentration below 8.8 mg/dl (2.20 mmol/L) in the presence of normal plasma protein concentration.

Risk Factors

- Hypoparathyroidism: deficiency in or absence of parathyroid hormone (PTH)
- Idiopathic hypoparathyroidism
- Pseudohypoparathyroidism
- Vitamin D deficiency
- Renal tubular disease
- Renal failure
- Magnesium depletion
- Acute pancreatitis
- Hypoproteinemia
- Enhanced bone formation with inadequate Ca intake
- Septic shock
- Hyperphosphatemia
- Drugs: phenytoin, phenobarbital, rifampin, blood transfusion with blood treated with citrate, radiocontrast agents that contain the divalent ion chelating agent ethylenediaminetetraacetate

Etiology/Cause (see also Risk Factors)

- Hypoparathyroidism: symptoms include cataracts, basal ganglia calcification, chronic candidiasis

Pathogenesis

- Any of the conditions or drugs listed under the Risk Factors section may be involved in causing hypocalcemia.

Diagnosis

Signs and Symptoms

- Clinical signs of hypocalcemia are due to disturbance in cellular membrane potential.
- Symptoms usually stem from neuromuscular irritability.
  —Muscle cramps involving the back and legs
- Slowly developing hypocalcemia may produce mild, insidious encephalopathy, and should be suspected in any patient with unexplained dementia, depression, or psychosis.
- In prolonged hypocalcemia, papilledema may occur, and cataracts may develop after prolonged hypocalcemia.
- Severe hypocalcemia (plasma Ca < 7 mg/dl [<1.75 mmol/L] can cause tetany, laryngospasm, or generalized seizures.
- Tetany results from severe hypocalcemia or from reduction in the ionized fraction of plasma Ca without marked hypocalcemia, which occurs in severe alkalosis.
  —Two characteristic signs of tetany are **Chvostek's sign** and **Trousseau's sign.**
    ~ Chvostek's sign is an involuntary twitching of the facial muscles elicited by a light tapping of the facial nerve just anterior to the exterior auditory meatus; this is present in 10% of healthy people but often absent in chronic hypocalcemia.
    ~ Trousseau's sign is the precipitation of carpopedal spasm by reduction of the blood supply to the hand with a tourniquet or blood pressure (BP) cuff applied to the forearm and inflated to 20 mm Hg above systolic BP and maintained for 3 minutes.
- This sign also occurs in alkalosis, in hypomagnesemia, and in about 6% of people without known electrolyte disturbance.
- Dysrhythmias or heart block may occur in patients with severe hypocalcemia; the ECG shows prolongation of the Q-T and S-T intervals; changes in repolarization, such as T-wave peaking or inversion, may also be seen.

- Other signs and symptoms of hypocalemia
  —Dry, scaly skin
  —Brittle nails
  —Coarse hair
  —Candida infections (associated more with idiopathic hypoparathyroidism)
- Cataracts that occur with long-standing hypocalcemia are not reversible by correction of the plasma Ca.

Diagnostic Tests

- Hypocalcemia is diagnosed by a total plasma Ca level <8.8 mg/dl (<2.20 mmol/L).
- When tetany is present, total plasma Ca is usually ≤7 mg/dl (≤1.75 mmol/L).
- PTH deficiency is characterized by low plasma Ca, high plasma PO_4, and normal alkaline phosphatase.
- Hypocalcemia is the major stimulus for PTH secretion, and would be expected to be elevated in hypocalcemia; however, in hypoparathyroidism, intact PTH is inappropriately low for the plasma Ca level.
- Type I pseudohypoparathyroidism can be distinguished by the presence of hypocalcemia despite the presence of normal to elevated levels of circulating PTH.
- In osteomalacia or rickets, typical skeletal abnormalities may be present.
  —The plasma PO_4 level is often mildly reduced and alkaline phosphatase is elevated, reflecting increased mobilization of Ca from bone.

Treatment

- Acute severe hypocalcemic tetany is treated initially with IV infusion of Ca salts—calcium gluconate is to be given IV as 10 ml of 10% solution over 10 minutes.
  —Response may be dramatic, but may last only a few hours.
- Repeated infusions or adding a continuous infusion may be needed with 20 to 30 ml of 10% calcium gluconate in 1 L of 5% D/W over 12 to 24 hours.
- Infusion of Ca is hazardous in patients receiving digitalis therapy, and should be given slowly, with continuous ECG monitoring.
- Tissue necrosis can result from IV or intramuscular (IM) injections of Ca.

- In transient hypoparathyroidism after thyroidectomy or partial parathryroidectomy, supplemental Ca may be sufficient to prevent hypocalcemia.
- In chronic hypocalcemia, oral Ca and sometimes vitamin D supplements are usually sufficient.
  —Calcium may be given as calcium gluconate 90 mg elemental calcium per 1 g, or calcium carbonate 400 mg elemental calcium per 1 g.
- In all cases, vitamin D therapy will not be effective without adequate dietary or supplemental calcium (1 to 2 g of elemental calcium/day).

Patient/Family Education

- Hypocalcemia is often a complex disease, so that explanations of the problem may need to be divided into segments for easier assimilation.
- Terms should be spelled out in writing and defined.
- Calcium and vitamin D supplements should be written, with accurate dosages and scheduling.
- Signs and symptoms of both hypocalcemia and hypercalcemia should be written, to alert the patient and family regarding symptoms and when to call the clinician for help.

Follow-up/Referral

- Patients are followed for weeks or months after an acute episode of hypocalcemia to monitor status and to determine whether sufficient calcium is being taken, along with vitamin D.

Hypercalcemia

Definition

Hypercalcemia is an increase in total plasma calcium concentration above 10.4 mg/dl (2.60 mmol/L).

Risk Factors

- Excessive bone resorption

Etiology/Cause (Box 11-4)
Pathogenesis

- Primary hyperparathyroidism is probably the most common cause of hypercalcemia in the general population.

BOX 11-4

Principal Causes of Hypercalcemia

EXCESSIVE BONE RESORPTION
PTH excess; primary hyperparathyroidism, parathyroid carcinoma, familial hypocalciuric hypercalcemia, advanced secondary hyperparathyroidism
Humoral hypercalcemia of malignancy (i.e., hypercalcemia of malignancy in the absence of bone metastases)
Malignancy with bone metastases; particularly carcinoma, leukemia, lymphoma, and multiple myeloma
Hyperthyroidism
Vitamin D toxicity; vitamin A toxicity
Immobilization: particularly in young, growing people or in those with Paget's disease of bone; in elderly with osteoporosis, paraplegics, and quadriplegics

EXCESSIVE GI CALCIUM ABSORPTION AND/OR INTAKE
Milk-alkali syndrome
Vitamin D toxicity
Sarcoidosis and other granulomatous diseases

ELEVATED PLASMA PROTEIN CONCENTRATION
Uncertain mechanism
Myxedema, Addison's disease, postoperative Cushing's disease
Thiazide diuretic treatment
Infantile hypercalcemia

MISCELLANEOUS
Lithium intoxication, theophylline intoxication
Aluminum-induced osteomalacia
Neuroleptic malignant syndrome

ARTIFACTUAL
Prolonged venous stasis while obtaining blood samples
Exposure to blood-contaminated glassware

From Beers MH, Berkow R, eds: Water, electrolyte, mineral, and acid-base metabolism. *The Merck manual of diagnosis and therapy,* ed 17, Whitehouse Station, NJ, 1999, Merck & Co, Inc, p 146.

—The incidence of hyperparathyroidism increases with age and is higher in postmenopausal women.
- The syndrome of familial hypocalciuric hypercalcemia is transmitted as an autosomal dominant trait, characterized by persistent hypercalcemia, often from an early age, elevated levels of PTH, and hypocalciuria.
- Secondary hyperparathyroidism occurs when chronic hypocalcemia, which is caused by conditions such as renal insufficiency or intestinal malabsorption syndromes, stimulates increased secretion of PTH.
- Humoral hypercalcemia of malignancy occurs most often in association with various squamous cell carcinomas, renal cell carcinoma, breast cancer, or ovarian cancer.
  —Assays yield undetectable or markedly suppressed levels of PTH, despite the presence of hypophosphatemia, phosphaturia, and elevated levels of nephrogenous cyclic adenosine monophosphate (cAMP).
- Exogenous vitamin D produces excessive bone resorption and increased intestinal Ca absorption and hypercalciuria.

- Sarcoidosis is associated with hypercalcemia in up to 20% of patients, and hypercalciuria in up to 40% of patients; these increased levels are also seen in other granulomatous diseases: tuberculosis (TB), leprosy, berylliosis, histoplasmosis.
- Immobilization, especially prolonged bed rest, can cause hypercalcemia due to accelerated bone resorption.
- In milk-alkali syndrome, excessive amounts of Ca and absorbable alkali are ingested, resulting in hypercalcemia, renal insufficiency, and metabolic alkalosis.
  —Chronic ingestion of high doses of calcium carbonate, usually to prevent osteoporosis, particularly in conjunction with thiazide diuretic use, has been reported to cause severe hypercalcemia in some patients.

Diagnosis
Signs and Symptoms
- Patients with mild hypercalcemia are often asymptomatic.
  —The condition is often discovered during routine laboratory tests.
- Symptoms include the following:
  —Constipation

—Anorexia

—Vomiting

—Abdominal pain

—Ileus

- Impaired renal concentrating ability causes polyuria, nocturia, and polydipsia.
- Plasma Ca > 12 mg/dl (>3.00 mmol/L) is associated with muscle weakness, emotional lability, confusion, delirium, psychosis, stupor, and coma.
- Kidney stones are common in the presence of hypercalcemia.
- Prolonged severe hypercalcemia may cause renal failure or irreversible kidney damage resulting from deposition of Ca salts in the kidney parenchyma.
- Cardiac symptoms of hypercalcemia include ECG changes: shortened Q-Tc interval and dysrhythmias in patients taking digitalis.
- Secondary hyperparathyroidism is associated with hypercalcemia, in which bone lesions of osteitis fibrosa cystica appear, particularly in long-term dialysis patients.
- Primary hyperparathyroidism is usually characterized by hypercalcemia, hypophosphatemia, and excessive bone resorption; hypercalcemia may be the only presenting sign.
- In the syndrome of familial hypocalciuric hypercalcemia, patients are usually asymptomatic, although severe pancreatitis may sometimes occur.
- The cause of hypercalcemia may be derived from the history and physical examination; x-ray evidence of osteolytic or osteoblastic lesions, or the characteristic lesions of hypoparathyroidism, may more clearly identify the cause.

Diagnostic Tests

- In hyperparathyroidism, the plasma Ca is rarely >12 mg/dl, but the ionized plasma Ca is almost always elevated.
- A low PO_4 level indicates some form of hyperparathyroidism, particularly with an elevated PO_4 clearance (decreased tubular reabsorption of PO_4) and mild hyperchloremia with or without acidosis.
- Differentiation between primary and secondary hyperparathyroidism is often possible by comparing laboratory findings: primary hyperparathyroidism has a high plasma Ca and normal plasma PO_4; if the PO_4 is elevated, secondary hyperparathyroidism is the more likely diagnosis.
- If hyperparathyroidism causes increased bone turnover, plasma alkaline phosphatase is often increased.
- The diagnosis of humoral hypercalcemia of malignancy is usually made by the presence of PTH-related peptide.
- Familial hypocalciuric hypercalcemia has an onset in young people, frequent occurrence of hypermagnesemia, and hypercalcemia without hypercalciuria in other family members.
- The milk-alkali syndrome is diagnosed by the combination of hypercalcemia, metabolic alkalosis, and azotemia with hypocalciuria; when Ca and alkali ingestion ceases, the plasma Ca level rapidly returns to normal, although renal insufficiency can persist if nephrocalcinosis is present.

Treatment

- Treatment of hypercalcemia depends on symptoms, severity of Ca elevation, and the underlying cause.
- If the symptoms are mild and the plasma Ca is <11.5 mg/dl (<2.88 mmol/L), treating only the underlying disease is usually sufficient.
- Therapy to lower plasma Ca is necessary if plasma Ca exceeds 15 mg/dl (3.75 mmol/L).
  - In patients with normal renal function, the treatment of choice is IV saline 0.9% with added KCl, and furosemide to increase renal excretion of Ca by expanding the ECF, with the goal of having the patient achieve a urine volume of at least 3 L/day.
  - For patients with hypercalcemia associated with malignancy, salmon calcitonin 4 to 8 IU/kg SC q12h, and prednisone 30 to 60 mg/day PO in three divided doses usually controls severe hypercalcemia in patients with cancer; (or) plicamycin (mithramycin) 25 µg/kg IV in 50 ml of 5% D/W over 3 to 6 hours is very effective in treating hypercalcemia in patients with malignancy; (or) gallium nitrate infusion

is used if the patient does not respond to other therapy; (or) bisphosphonates are now widely used in conjunction with saline and furosemide to inhibit osteoclasts from resorbing bone.

—In patients with vitamin D toxicity, prednisone 20 to 40 mg/day PO usually controls the hypercalcemia.

—In patients with sarcoidosis, chloroquine phosphate 500 mg/day PO may reduce $1,25(OH)_2D_3$ synthesis and reduce plasma Ca levels.

—In hyperparathyroidism that is symptomatic and progressive, surgery is the treatment of choice; the goal is to remove all excess functioning tissue and all adenomatous glands; to prevent subsequent hyperparathyroidism, a small portion of a normal-looking parathyroid gland may be impanted in the sternocleidomastoid muscle or SC in the forearm; when an experienced surgeon performs the surgery and removes all abnormally functioning parathyroid glands in the neck and mediastinum, the cure rate may be as high as 90%; ^{99m}Tc sestamibi, a new radionuclide agent for parathyroid study, is being increasingly used in surgery because it is more sensitive and specific than previously available agents.

Patient/Family Education

- The complexity of hypercalcemia associated with hyperparathyroidism requires a clear, careful explanation of the nature, cause, course, treatment, and expected outcomes of therapy.
- In many cases, unless severity or complications are factors, conservative therapy to lower plasma Ca levels may be all that is required; the possibility of surgery is not discussed until all other measures have resulted in little or no response.
- The clinician must be able to answer questions and to provide additional information as needed.

Follow-up/Referral

- These patients are followed closely throughout the treatment stage, once the diagnosis has been made.

- The primary care provider is often the connecting link among the specialists who may become involved in treating the patient, and who will follow the patient posttreatment or postsurgery to assess for recurrence of hypercalcemia or symptoms of other problems.

DISORDERS OF PHOSPHATE METABOLISM
Hypophosphatemia

Definition

Hypophosphatemia is a decrease in plasma phosphate concentration below 2.5 mg/dl (0.81 mmol/L).

- Phosphate is one of the most abundant elements in the body.
- Most phosphorus is combined with oxygen as phosphate (PO_4).
- About 85% of the 500 to 700 g of phosphate in the body is found in bone.
- In soft tissues, phosphate is found in the intracellular compartment; it is an integral component of several organic compounds including nucleic acids and the phospholipids of cell membranes.
- Phosphate is also closely involved in aerobic and anaerobic energy metabolism.
- Red blood cell 2,3-diphosphoglycerate (2,3-DPG) plays a crucial role in oxygen delivery to tissues.
- Phosphate depletion can occur in many disease states, and results in conservation of phosphate by the kidneys.
- Phosphate in bone is a reservoir and can buffer changes in plasma and intracellular PO_4.

Risk Factors

- Acute alcoholism
- Diabetic ketoacidosis (recovery phase)
- Severe burns
- Patients on total parenteral nutrition (TPN)
- Patients with severe respiratory alkalosis

Etiology/Cause (see also Risk Factors)

- Clinically significant hypophosphatemia occurs in relatively few settings.
- The most common occurrence is a fall in renal PO_4 reabsorption, but this is not associated with intracellular phosphate depletion.

- Hyperparathyroidism
- Cushing's syndrome
- Hypothyroidism
- Hypomagnesemia
- Hypokalemia
- Theophylline intoxication
- Long-term diuretic administration
- Severe chronic hypophosphatemia is usually caused by a prolonged negative PO_4 balance caused by chronic starvation or malabsorption, particularly when combined with vomiting, copious diarrhea, or chronic ingestion of antacids that contain PO_4-binding aluminum.

Diagnosis
Signs and Symptoms
- Hypophosphatemia is usually asymptomatic.
- When symptoms occur, they are usually anorexia, muscle weakness, and osteomalacia resulting from chronic depletion.
- Hematologic problems associated with profound hypophosphatemia include hemolytic anemia, decreased release of oxygen from hemoglobin, and impaired leukocyte and platelet function.
- In severe hypophosphatemia, progressive encephalopathy, coma, and death may occur if not corrected urgently.

Diagnostic Tests
- The condition may be found serendipitously on routine blood tests.
- Plasma PO_4 levels indicate the presence of depleted phosphate.

Treatment
- Choice of therapy is based on the severity of the hypophosphatemia and the underlying cause(s).
- One L of low-fat or skim milk provides 1 g of PO_4, and may suffice for mild phosphate depletion.
- Stopping problematic drugs (e.g., antacids, diuretics) is required.
- Oral phosphate up to 3 g/day may be given in tablets that contain sodium or potassium phosphate.
- IV phosphate must be given when the plasma PO_4 falls below 0.5 mEq/L (0.16 mmol/L), or when CNS symptoms are present, or when the patient cannot take oral

medications: potassium phosphate 2 mg/kg IV given over 6 hours, although alcoholics may require ≥ 1 g/day.
   —In ketoacidosis, up to 3 g of phosphate may be required in the first 24 hours.
- In patients with impaired renal function, plasma Ca and PO_4 are closely monitored throughout the course of therapy; in these patients, sodium phosphate, rather than potassium phosphate, is preferable.

Patient/Family Education
- Instruct the patient and family regarding the nature, cause, course, treatment, and expected outcomes of hypophosphatemia.
- Explain the rationale for medications, whether PO or IV, and monitoring of plasma PO_4 levels.

Follow-up/Referral
- These patients require relatively frequent follow-up once the acute phase is over and the patient returns home.
- Instruct the patient regarding sources of phosphate (e.g., low-fat or skim milk 1 L a day to provide 1 g of phosphate).
- Visits are less frequent as the patient's condition warrants.

Hyperphosphatemia
Definition
Hyperphosphatemia is an increase in plasma phosphate concentration above 4.5 mg/dl (1.46 mmol/L).

Risk Factors
- Renal insufficiency (GFR < 20 ml/min)
- Excessive use of phosphate-containing enemas
- Excessive oral administration of PO_4

Etiology/Cause (see also Risk Factors)
- Occurs as a result of transcellular shift of phosphate into the extracellular space (e.g., diabetic ketoacidosis, crush injuries, nontraumatic rhabdomyolysis, systemic infections, and tumor lysis syndrome).

Pathogenesis (see also Etiology/Cause)
- Hyperphosphatemia plays a critical role in the development of secondary hyperparathyroidism and renal osteodystrophy in patients receiving chronic dialysis.

Diagnosis

Signs and Symptoms

- Most patients with hyperphosphatemia have no symptoms.
- In patients with chronic renal failure with associated hyperphosphatemia, soft tissue calcifications are commonly seen, particularly if the plasma $Ca \times PO_4$ product exceeds 70 (in mEq/L) for prolonged periods.

Treatment

- Reduced intake of phosphate
  —Avoidance of foods that contain high amounts of phosphate
  —Use of phosphate-binding antacids taken with meals (e.g., calcium carbonate)
- Many causes of hyperphosphatemia are self-limiting.

Patient/Family Education

- Instruct regarding the nature, cause, course, treatment, and expected outcome of therapy.
- Provide a written list of foods that are high in phosphate, which should be avoided.
- Explain the rationale for medications and therapy.

Follow-up/Referral

- Patients are followed closely, particularly those with decreased renal function, which is often a major cause of hyperphosphatemia.
- Monitoring of plasma PO_4 levels on a regular basis is necessary.

DISORDERS OF MAGNESIUM METABOLISM
Hypomagnesemia

Definition

Hypomagnesemia is a plasma concentration of magnesium (Mg) below 1.4 mEq/L (0.70 mml/L).

- Magnesium is the fourth most plentiful cation in the body.
  —A 70-kg adult has about 2000 mEq of Mg.
  —About half that amount is sequestered in bone and is not readily exchangeable with other compartments.
  —The ECF contains only about 1% of total body Mg; the remainder is in the intracellular fluid (ICF) compartment.

- Normal plasma Mg concentration ranges from 1.4 to 2.1 mEq/L (0.70 to 1.05 mmol/L)

Risk Factors

- Multiple metabolic and nutritional disorders

Etiology/Cause

- The most common causes of clinically significant hypomagnesemia are malabsorption syndromes of all types.
  —Elevated fecal Mg likely relates to the level of steatorrhea rather than to deficient bowel absorption per se.
- Protein-calorie malnutrition (e.g., kwashiorkor)
- Parathyroid disease, after removal of parathyroid tumor
- Chronic alcoholism (inadequate intake and excessive renal excretion)
- Inadequate intake of Mg
- Impaired renal or GI absorption
- Prolonged TPN
- Loss of body fluids via gastric suction, severe diarrhea, lactation
- Conditions of abnormal renal conservation of Mg (e.g., hypersecretion of aldosterone, ADH, or thyroid hormone)
- Hypercalcemia
- Diabetic acidosis
- Cisplatin or diuretic therapy

Diagnosis

Signs and Symptoms

- Anorexia
- Nausea and vomiting
- Lethargy
- Weakness
- Personality change
- Chvostek's sign or spontaneous carpopedal spasm
- Tremor and muscle fasciculations
- CNS signs: development of tetany correlates with concomitant hypocalcemia and hypokalemia.
  —Possibly tonic-clonic seizures, particularly in children

Diagnostic Tests

- Unexplained hypocalcemia and hypokalemia should suggest the possibility of Mg depletion.

- Hypomagnesemia is present when Mg depletion is severe.
- Causes of Mg depletion (e.g., alcoholism, steatorrhea) also cause hypocalcemia and hypocalciuria, which would indicate hypomagnesemia.
- Hypokalemia with increased urinary K excretion and metabolic alkalosis may be present.

Treatment

- Magnesium salts is the specific therapy (magnesium sulfate or magnesium chloride) for severe hypomagnesemia, in which deficits of almost 12 to 24 mg/kg may be present.
  —About twice the amount of the estimated deficit should be given to patients with intact renal function because 50% of Mg is excreted in urine.
  —Half the dose is given in the first 24 hours, the remainder over the next 4 days.
- When Mg must be given parenterally, $MgSO_4$ 10% solution is given IV, or a 50% solution is given IM.
- The plasma Mg level is monitored frequently during treatment, particularly if the patient has renal insufficiency.
- Patients with both Mg depletion and hypocalcemia require replacements for both deficits.
- In patients with severe symptomatic hypomagnesemia (e.g., generalized seizures, Mg < 1 mEq/L), 2 to 4 g of $MgSO_4$ may be given IV over 5 to 10 minutes.
  —If seizures persist, the dose can be repeated to a total of 10 g over the following 6 hours.
  —When seizures stop, 10 g in 1 L of 5% D/W can be infused over 24 hours, followed by up to 2.5 g q12hr to replace the deficit in total Mg stores, and prevent further drop in plasma Mg.
- If plasma Mg is <1 mEq/L but symptoms are less severe, $MgSO_4$ is given IV in 5% D/W at a rate of 1 g/hr as slow infusion, for up to 10 hours.
- In less severe cases of hypomagnesemia, gradual repletion is accomplished by smaller parenteral doses over 3 to 5 days until the plasma Mg level is normal.

Patient/Family Education

- Explain the nature of the condition, its cause(s), course, treatment, and expected outcomes.
- Instruct the patient regarding medications ordered and how they will help.
- Give reassurance to both the patient and the family, particularly if the patient is severely ill; seizures are frightening to those who have never seen them.

Follow-up/Referral

- These patients are followed during their routine visits after the acute recovery phase, when visits are more frequent to monitor plasma Mg levels and signs and symptoms that may be present.
- Instruct the patient regarding dietary sources of magnesium to maintain the plasma level within normal ranges; adjustments can be made if necessary.

Hypermagnesemia

Definition

Hypermagnesemia is a plasma magnesia concentration above 2.1 mEq/L (1.05 mmol/L).

Risk Factors

- Ingestion of magnesium-containing antacids or purgatives
- Renal impairment or failure

Etiology/Cause

- The most frequent cause of hypermagnesemia, which is relatively rare, is deficient excretion in the urine because of renal impairment or failure.
- Chronic ingestion of magnesia in laxatives or antacids

Pathogenesis (see Risk Factors and Etiology/Cause)

Diagnosis

Signs and Symptoms

- If plasma concentration of Mg reaches 5 to 10 mEq/L (2.5 to 5 mmol/L), the electrocardiogram (ECG) shows prolongation of the P-R interval, widening of the QRS complex, and increased T-wave amplitude.

- Deep tendon reflexes (DTRs) disappear as the Mg concentration nears 10 mEq/L.
- Hypotension
- Respiratory depression and narcosis occur with increasing hypomagnesemia.
- Cardiac arrest may occur when blood Mg levels exceed 12 to 15 mEq/L (6.0 to 7.5 mmol/L).

Treatment
- In the presence of severe Mg toxicity, circulatory and respiratory support are required, with IV administration of 10 to 20 ml of 10% calcium gluconate.
  —Calcium gluconate often reverses many of the Mg-induced changes, including respiratory depression.
- IV furosemide can increase Mg excretion if renal function is adequate and volume statis is maintained.
- Hemodialysis may be required in severe hypermagnesemia because a large fraction (70%) of blood Mg is ultrafilterable.
- In cases in which hypermagnesemia is associated with hemodynamic compromise and hemodialysis is not feasible, peritoneal dialysis is an option.

Patient/Family Education
- Although rare, hypermagnesemia can be a life-threatening condition, depending on the plasma level and ability of the kidneys to excrete Mg.
- Often, these patients are older and may have other coexisting medical problems (e.g., malignancy, respiratory, or cardiac).
- Explain the nature, cause, course, treatment, and expected outcomes.
- Maintain a positive demeanor but indicate that the patient is severely ill.
- Report immediately to the family any positive responses of the patient to therapy.

Follow-up/Referral
- These patients are followed closely after recovery from the acute episode to make sure that no signs or symptoms of hypermagnesemia recur and to monitor the plasma Mg frequently as essential to knowing the patient's status.

- The patient should be told not to take magnesium-containing laxatives or antacids without specific permission of the clinician, and for only one dose, unless a satisfactory substitute is available.

ACID-BASE METABOLISM
- The blood hydrogen ion (H^+) concentration is maintained within narrow limits.
- Arterial plasma H^+ concentration ranges from 37 to 43 nmol/L (37×10^{-6} to 43×10^{-6} mEq/L).
- Maintaining H^+ within these narrow limits is essential for normal cellular function, because of the high reactivity between H^+ and other compounds, particularly proteins.
- The pH (negative logarithm of H^+ concentration) is a much less cumbersome measure of physiologic H^+ concentration, and is widely used in clinical medicine.
  —The normal arterial blood pH ranges from 7.37 to 7.43.
- Both pulmonary and renal function maintain blood pH within the normal range.
  —Respiratory changes in minute ventilation occur quickly in response to acid-base disturbances and rapidly alter blood pH by changing carbonic acid concentration through changes in blood P_{CO_2}.
  —The kidneys vary the renal excretion of acid or base equivalents and ultimately alter plasma HCO_3^- concentration to alter blood pH.
- Renal adaptations to changes in acid-base balance occur over several days, but respiratory-driven changes occur within minutes to hours.
- Wide fluctuations in H^+ concentration are also prevented by the presence of several pH buffers, which are weak acids that exist in equilibrium with the corresponding base at physiologic pH.
  —Buffers respond to changes in H^+ by shifting the relative concentrations of the buffer and the corresponding base to dampen the change in pH.
  —Phosphates, ammonia, proteins including hemoglobin, and bone all provide pH buffering capacity, but the major pH buffer in the blood, which is the most relevant to clinical acid-base disturbances, is the bicarbonate/carbonate acid system.

TABLE 11-3

Primary Changes and Expected Compensation in Simple Acid-Base Disturbances

Disorder	[H⁺]	pH	[HCO₃⁻]	Pco₂	Compensation
Metabolic acidosis	↑	↓	↓↓	↓	P_{CO_2} (↓) 11 to 13 mm Hg for every 10 mmol (↓↓) in [HCO_3^-]
Metabolic alkalosis	↓	↑	↑↑	↑	P_{CO_2} (↑) 6 to 7 mm Hg for every 10 mmol (↑↑) in [HCO_3^-]
Respiratory acidosis	↑	↓	↑	↑↑	*Acute:* [HCO_3^-] (↑) 1 mmol for every 10 mm Hg (↑↑) in P_{CO_2} *Chronic:* [HCO_3^-] (↑) 3.5 mmol for every 10 mm Hg (↑↑) in P_{CO_2}
Respiratory alkalosis	↓	↑	↓	↓↓	*Acute:* [HCO_3^-] (↑) 2.5 mmol for every 10 mm Hg (↓↓) in P_{CO_2} *Chronic:* [HCO_3^-] (↑) 5 mmol for every 10 mm Hg (↓↓) P_{CO_2}

From Beers MH, Berkow R, eds: Water, electrolyte, mineral, and acid-base metabolism. *The Merck manual of diagnosis and therapy,* ed 17, Whitehouse Station, NJ, 1999, Merck & Co, Inc, p 156.

- The enzyme carbonic anhydrase quickly converts carbonic acid in the blood to CO_2 and water.
  —The partial pressure of CO_2 gas (P_{CO_2}) is easily measured in blood samples and is directly proportional to blood CO_2 content.
    ~ Therefore P_{CO_2} is used to represent the concentration of acid in the system.
- The concentration of base in the system can be directly determined by measuring HCO_3^- concentration.
- Plasma bicarbonate and CO_2 concentrations and pH are chemically related to one another by the Henderson-Hasselbalch equation:

$$pH = 6.1 + \log \frac{HCO_3^-}{0.03 \times P_{CO_2}}$$

in which 6.1 is the pKa (negative logarithm of the acid dissociation constant) for carbonic acid, and 0.03 relates P_{CO_2} to the amount of CO_2 dissolved in plasma.
- Although somewhat cumbersome and difficult to use at the bedside, the Henderson-Hasselbalch equation represents a very important relationship.
  —It predicts the ratio of HCO_3^- to dissolved CO_2, rather than their actual concentrations, and determines blood pH.
- This buffer system is physiologically important because both the pulmonary and renal mechanisms for regulating pH work by adjusting this ratio.
  —The P_{CO_2} can be adjusted quickly by changes in respiratory minute ventilation, whereas plasma (HCO_3^-) can be changed by regulating its excretion by the kidneys.
- Clinical disturbances of acid-base metabolism are defined in terms of the HCO_3^-/CO_2 buffer system.
  —Increases or decreases in HCO_3^- are termed metabolic alkalosis or acidosis, respectively.
- Simple acid-base disturbances include both the primary change and an expected compensation.
  —In metabolic acidosis, there is a primary fall in plasma HCO_3^- concentration and a secondary fall in the P_{CO_2} due to respiratory compensation (Table 11-3).
- Mixed acid-base disturbances are more complex disorders in which two or more primary alterations coexist.
- Compensatory mechanisms also exist in mixed acid-base disturbances.
- Mixed disturbances are usually recognized when either less or more than the predicted compensation for a given primary acid-base disturbance is present.
  —Nomograms permit simultaneous plotting of pH, HCO_3^-, and P_{CO_2} and greatly simplify the recognition of mixed disorders.
  —Measurement of these three factors, and recognition of the underlying disease process, is usually sufficient to accurately solve most clinical acid-base disturbances.
- Treatment must address each of the primary disturbances.

- Acid-base disturbances can significantly affect oxygen transport and tissue oxygenation.
- Acute changes in H^+ concentration rapidly affect the oxyhemoglobin dissociation curve (Bohr effect).
  —Acidemia shifts the curve to the right (decreased affinity of hemoglobin [Hb] for O_2; facilitated release of O_2 to tissues).
  —Alkalemia shifts the curve to the left (increased affinity of Hb for O_2; diminished release of O_2 to tissues).
- However, when acidosis or alkalosis is chronic, these acute effects on Hb-O_2 binding are modified by more slowly developing changes in erythrocyte concentrations of 2,3-diphosphoglycerate (2,3-DPG).
  —Therefore chronic elevations in H^+ ion inhibit 2,3-DPG formation, resulting in increased affinity of Hb for O_2, and chronic depression of H^+ ion increases 2,3-DPG, resulting in diminished affinity of Hb for O_2.
- These rapid changes in oxygen transport and tissue oxygenation may play a role in producing the CNS symptoms of acute alkalemia, although their clinical significance in acidosis is not clear.
- The kidneys have a major role in regulating ECF HCO_3^- concentration.
  —Almost all of the plasma bicarbonate is filtered by the glomerulus.
  —Large amounts of H^+ ions are secreted into the renal proximal tubular lumen in exchange for Na.
  —For each hydrogen ion secreted, one bicarbonate ion is reclaimed to the ECF.
  —Therefore net reabsorption of filtered bicarbonate occurs.
  —Because the pH of the fluid leaving the proximal tubule is about 6.5, most of the filtered bicarbonate is reabsorbed in the proximal tubule.
  —In the distal tubule, hydrogen ion secretion is partially dependent on aldosterone-mediated Na reabsorption.
  —Bicarbonate reabsorption can continue in the distal nephron up a steep gradient as urine pH can be lowered in this segment of the nephron to as low as 4.5 to 5.0.
  —Throughout the nephron, secreted hydrogen ion is buffered by urinary buffers such as PO_3 (titratable acid) and ammonia.
  —Thus filtered bicarbonate can be generated to replace that lost in body buffer reactions.
  —Because filtered Na is reabsorbed either in association with Cl or by cationic exchange with hydrogen ion or, to a lesser extent, K, the total Na reabsorbed equals the sum of the Cl reabsorbed and hydrogen ion secreted.
  —Therefore an inverse relationship exists between Cl reabsorption and hydrogen ion secretion, which is highly dependent on the existing level of Na reabsorption.
- Renal bicarbonate reabsorption is also influenced by body K stores.
  —A general reciprocal relationship exists between intracellular K content and hydrogen ion secretion.
  —Thus K depletion is associated with increased hydrogen ion secretion, and attendant bicarbonate generation, leading to a bicarbonate increase in ECF and metabolic alkalosis.
- Finally, renal bicarbonate reabsorption is influenced by the P_{CO_2} and the state of chloride balance.
  —Increased P_{CO_2} leads to increased bicarbonate reabsorption.
  —Cl depletion leads to increased Na reabsorption and bicarbonate generation by the proximal tubule.
  —Cl depletion usually is synonymous with ECF volume depletion.

Metabolic Acidosis

Definition

Metabolic acidosis is a condition of low arterial pH, reduced plasma HCO_3^- concentration, and usually compensatory alveolar hyperventilation that results in decreased P_{CO_2}.

Risk Factors
- Increased acid production
- Exogenous acid administration

Etiology/Cause (see Risk Factors and Box 11-5)
Pathogenesis
- The accumulation of acid equivalents in the body (increased H^+ ions)
- If the acid load cannot be handled by the respiratory system (increased CO_2 to form bicarbonate), metabolic acidosis (arterial pH ≤ 7.35) results.

BOX 11-5
Principal Causes of Primary Metabolic Acidosis and Metabolic Alkalosis

METABOLIC ACIDOSIS
With elevated anion gap
  Ketoacidosis (diabetes, chronic alcoholism)
  Lactic acidosis
  Renal failure
  Intoxication (ethylene glycol, methanol, paraldehyde, salicylates)
With normal anion gap
  GI alkali loss (diarrhea, ileostomy, colostomy)
  Renal tubular acidosis (types I, II, and IV)
  Interstitial renal disease
  Ureterosigmoidostomy, ureteroileal conduit
  Acetazolamide therapy
  Ingestion of ammonium chloride

METABOLIC ALKALOSIS
Chloride-responsive
  Vomiting or nasogastric drainage
  Surreptitious laxative abuse
  Diuretics
  Posthypercapnic states
Chloride-resistant
  Severe Mg or K deficiency
  Diuretics (thiazides, loop drugs)
  Hypermineralocorticoidism (Cushing's syndrome, primary aldosteronism, renal artery stenosis)
  Glyrrhetinic acid (licorice, chewing tobacco)
  Inherited disorders (Bartter's syndrome, Gitelman's syndrome)

From Beers MH, Berkow R, eds: Water, electrolyte, mineral, and acid-base metabolism. *The Merck manual of diagnosis and therapy*, ed 17, Whitehouse Station, NJ, 1999, Merck & Co, Inc, p 158.

Diagnosis
- Calculating the anion gap is helpful in making a differential diagnosis of metabolic acidosis.
  - The anion gap is estimated by subtracting the sum of the Cl and HCO_3^- concentrations from the plasma Na concentration.
  - Negatively charged plasma proteins account for most of the anion gap; the charges of other plasma cations (K, Ca, Mg) and anions (PO_4, sulfate, organic ions) usually balance out.
  - The accepted range for the anion gap is 12 ± 4 mEq/L; however, this range is based on normal ranges of electrolyte concentrations, as measured by methods used in the 1970s.
  - Most laboratories now use different techniques; the normal range of the anion gap has decreased and may be as low as 5 to 11 mEq/L.
  - Clinicians need to consider particular laboratories' reference range when assessing the anion gap.
- When an acid is added to the ECF, it is rapidly buffered by HCO_3^- according to the following reaction:

$$HA + HCO_3^- \rightarrow H_2CO_3 + A^- \rightarrow CO_2 + H_2O + A^-$$

- When metabolic acidosis is caused by the accumulation of unmeasured anions (e.g., sulfates in renal failure, ketone bodies in diabetic ketoacidosis, or lactate or exogenous toxic agents such as ethylene glycol or salicylates), the anion gap is elevated.
  - If the acid anion is chlorine, hyperchloremic metabolic acidosis will result.
  - Because chlorine is part of the formula for anion gap, hyperchloremic metabolic acidosis does not result in an increased anion gap.
  - Renal or extrarenal losses of HCO_3^- produce hyperchloremic (nonanion gap) metabolic acidosis because renal mechanisms retain chloride in an attempt to preserve ECF volume.
- When an increased anion gap occurs, the presence of one or more substances that usually result in acidosis can be inferred.
  - The most common causes of an increased anion gap metabolic acidosis are listed in Box 11-5.
  - In diabetic ketoacidosis, the absence of insulin (and excess of glucagon) results in metabolic production of the ketoacids—acetoacetic acid, β-hydroxybutyric acid, acetic acid—by the liver.
  - These ketoacids account for the acidosis as well as the unmeasured anion.

—Ketoacidosis also commonly occurs with chronic alcohol ingestion and poor dietary intake due to poor carbohydrate intake and inhibition of gluconeogenesis by alcohol.

—The diagnosis of ketoacidosis is confirmed by the presence of ketoacids in the plasma.

—Ketoacids are usually detected by reaction with nitroprusside.

—Nitroprusside reacts with acetoacetic and acetic acids, but not with β-hydroxybutyric acid.

—In alcoholism, ketoacidosis is caused primarily by β-hydroxybutyric acid.

—In some cases, patients with diabetic ketoacidosis also have an increased proportion of β-hydroxybutyric acid resulting from an increased ratio of reduced to oxidized nicotinamide adenine dinucleotide (NADH/NAD).

—Because the usual methods of measuring ketone bodies do not measure β-dihydroxybutyric acid, the standard nitroprusside test may underestimate the degree of ketosis in these patients.

• Another frequently encountered cause of an increased anion gap metabolic acidosis is lactic acid, which is produced by the anaerobic metabolism of pyruvic acid.

—Low levels of lactic acid are normally produced from glucose via normal glycolytic pathways; but if increased lactate production or decreased use occurs, lactate can accumulate.

—Hypoperfusion of tissue as occurs in shock leads to both increased lactate production and decreased use, and is the most common cause of lactic acidosis.

—Hepatic dysfunction caused by poor hepatic perfusion or hepatocellular damage can also cause lactic acidosis because of diminished conversion of lactate back to glucose.

—Alcoholism can also cause lactate accumulation by a similar mechanism.

—Lactic acidosis occurs in certain malignancies, diabetes mellitus, and AIDS, as well as idiopathically.

• Renal failure is also a cause of increased anion gap metabolic acidosis.

—Various substances accumulate in plasma with decreased renal function, including PO_4, sulfates, urate, and hippurate.

—Because varying degrees of uremia are sometimes present with other forms of increased anion gap metabolic acidosis, an increased anion gap should be ascribed to renal failure only after a comprehensive search for other causes.

—Various overdoses also cause increased anion gap metabolic acidosis: in salicylate, methanol, or ethylene glycol poisoning, interference with normal intermediary metabolism and accumulation of exogenous organic anions cause metabolic acidosis.

—Prompt recognition is crucial to minimize organ damage in these patients; when acidosis is present with a normal anion gap, impaired renal H^+ ion excretion should be suspected.

—Impaired renal acid excretion can be due to intrinsic renal disease, such as renal tubular acidosis (RTA) or interstitial renal disease, or in response to extrarenal volume and HCO_3^- losses, which occur primarily via the GI tract: protracted diarrhea, villous adenoma of the colon, or drainage of biliary, pancreatic, or intestinal fluid.

• In urinary tract diversion (e.g., ureterosigmoidostomy), Cl in the urine is exchanged for HCO_3^- by the colon, and urine ammonium is also absorbed.

—Because of problems associated with ureterosigmoidostomy, it is rarely performed.

—Patients with ureteroileostomy (ileal conduits) or orthotopic bladder construction have fewer problems with metabolic acidosis, particularly if renal function is not impaired.

Signs and Symptoms

• Signs and symptoms of acidosis are often obscured by and difficult to separate from those of underlying disease.

• Mild acidosis may be asymptomatic or just be accompanied by vague symptoms such as lassitude, or nausea and vomiting.

- In severe metabolic acidosis (pH < 7.20, $HCO_3^- < 10$ mEq/L), the most characteristic finding is increased ventilation, part of the respiratory compensatory responses.
  - At first, small increases in depth of inspirations occur; later, increased frequency of respirations with pursed lip breathing can be seen (Kussmaul's respirations).
  - Signs of ECF volume depletion may be present, particularly in patients with diabetic ketoacidosis or GI volume losses.
  - Severe acidosis may cause circulatory shock due to impaired myocardial contractility and peripheral vascular response to catecholamines, followed by progressive obtundation.

Diagnostic Tests

- In metabolic acidosis, the arterial pH is < 7.35 and HCO_3^- is < 21 mEq/L.
  - If pulmonary function is unimpaired, the P_{CO_2} is < 40 mm Hg due to respiratory compensation.
- In simple metabolic acidosis, the P_{CO_2} may fall about 11 to 13 mm Hg for each 10 mEq/L reduction in the plasma HCO_3^-.
  - A greater or less than usual decline in the P_{CO_2} indicates the coexistence of primary respiratory alkalosis or of respiratory acidosis or other primary metabolic disturbance.
- When renal function is normal and volume depletion is absent, the urine pH can fall below 5.5 with severe acidosis.
  - If pH decline is less than maximal, urine pH fall implies kidney dysfunction due to acute or chronic renal insufficiency, tubulointerstitial disease, or renal tubular acidosis.
- In diabetic ketoacidosis, hyperglycemia is almost always present; ketonemia can be documented in most cases by the nitroprusside test, but hydroxybutyric acid is not detected by nitroprusside.
- Ethylene glycol poisoning should be suspected in patients with unexplained acidosis and oxalate crystals in the urine.
  - Very high anion gaps (20 to 40 mEq/L) usually occur in ethylene glycol and methanol poisoning.
  - Both substances can be measured in plasma.

- Salicylate poisoning is characterized by respiratory alkalosis soon after ingestion and by metabolic acidosis later.
- Because volume depletion often accompanies acidosis, mild azotemia (BUN 30 to 60 mg/dl) is often seen.
  - Greater elevations of BUN, particularly in conjunction with hypocalcemia and hyperphosphatemia, suggest renal failure as the cause of acidosis.
  - Hypocalcemia may also occur in cases of septic shock.

Treatment

- Treatment of acidemia with HCO_3^- is often intuitive, but sodium bicarbonate therapy is clearly indicated only in certain circumstances.
  - When metabolic acidosis results from inorganic acids (i.e., hyperchloremic or normal anion gap acidosis), HCO_3^- is required to treat the acid-base disturbance.
  - However, when acidosis results from organic acid accumulation (i.e., increased anion gap acidosis), as in lactic acidosis, ketoacidosis, or the intoxication syndrome from ethylene glycol, methanol, paraldehyde, or salicylates, the administration of HCO_3^- is controversial.
  - **Opponents** of $NaHCO_3$ therapy state that the mortality of each of the conditions is most closely related to the severity of the underlying disease process rather than to the degree of acidemia.
  - Other arguments against the use of alkali therapy are the potential for Na and volume overload, hypokalemia, CNS acidosis, hypercapnia, and alkalosis overshoot.
  - Conversely, acidosis is known to be associated with a variety of detrimental cardiovascular effects, including decreased responsiveness to pressor agents.
  - Acidotic patients are especially vulnerable to further decreases in pH by relatively minor changes in plasma HCO_3^- concentration.
  - **Proponents** of $NaHCO_3$ therapy state that increased anion gap acidosis also frequently occurs in conjunction with renal insufficiency and renal tubular acidosis, conditions in which treatment with $NaHCO_3$ is not controversial.

—Regardless of whether NaHCO$_3$ is given or not given, the underlying disease must be identified and treated.

• Despite arguments for and against the use of NaHCO$_3$, most experts continue to use, with care, IV sodium bicarbonate to treat severe metabolic acidosis (pH < 7.20).
  —The appropriate dosage can be specifically calculated, and hemodialysis may be needed to remedy potentially serious volume overload in patients with renal insufficiency.

• Management of lactic acidosis is mainly supportive, while at the same time trying to discover the reasons behind the development of the condition.

• Treatment of intoxication with methanol or ethylene glycol is a medical emergency because of the toxicity of metabolites of these compounds.
  —Treatment includes IV administration of ethanol to inhibit metabolism and using hemodialysis if renal dysfunction is present.

Patient/Family Education

• As in all other circumstances, the patient and family should be instructed regarding the nature, cause, course, treatment, and expected outcomes of therapy.

• Recovery from the metabolic acidosis is assured, but underlying disease may be the major problem requiring comprehensive assessment and intensive treatment.

Follow-up/Referral

• These patients, depending on underlying disease, are followed for several weeks after treatment for the metabolic acidosis, to ensure that recurrence is not a factor, while treatment for the underling disease continues, perhaps with some alteration due to the recent episode of metabolic acidosis in efforts to prevent its recurrence yet satisfactorily treating the other condition(s) such as diabetes or cardiovascular disease.

Metabolic Alkalosis

Definition

Metabolic alkalosis is a condition of elevated arterial pH, increased plasma HCO$_3^-$ concentration, and usually compensatory alveolar hypoventilation resulting in increased Pco$_2$.

Risk Factors

• Preceding symptoms of metabolic alkalosis, there has been either a loss of ECF or an increase in bicarbonate in the body, or perhaps both.

• Loss of acid-containing gastric contents by vomiting or nasogastric suction

• Excessive loss of acid via feces or urine

• Transcellular movement of H$^+$ ions into alkali gain that can occur with acute or chronic excessive alkali administration, particularly in patients with renal insufficiency or severe volume depletion

• Long-term use of diuretics

Etiology/Cause (see also Risk Factors)

• Sometimes it is difficult to discover the precise cause of metabolic alkalosis.
  —For metabolic alkalosis to develop, however, factors must be present that inhibit renal excretion of HCO$_3^-$ (volume depletion, K deficiency, and/or mineralocorticoid excess are the most common factors that inhibit renal excretion of bicarbonate).

• Regardless of the cause, the kidneys usually quickly correct the alkalosis by rapidly excreting excess HCO$_3^-$.

• Infusion of NaHCO$_3$ can cause metabolic alkalosis, and it usually occurs during cardiopulmonary resuscitation (CPR), or shortly after.

• The milk-alkali syndrome is caused by chronic ingestion of excessive amounts of calcium carbonate.
  —Findings include hypercalcemia, nephrocalcinosis, renal insufficiency, and metabolic alkalosis.

• When hypoventilation (hypercapnia) lasts for more than a few days, renal mechanisms compensate for the respiratory acidosis by retaining HCO$_3^-$.

• When hypercapnia is corrected rapidly, usually by mechanical ventilation in the clinical setting, metabolic alkalosis can result (posthypercapnia metabolic alkalosis), which usually responds to minute ventilation and brings it to a more appropriate level.

• Diuretics are frequently the cause of both Cl$^-$-responsive and Cl$^-$-resistant states.

• Diuretics can cause acute contraction of ECF volume and secondary hypermineralocorticoidism, both of which are responsive to Cl (volume) administration.

—However, a Cl-resistant state can occur with ongoing diuretic therapy due to high urinary Cl losses and concomitant K depletion.

- Severe Mg or K deficiency can cause increased renal H^+ ion excretion and subsequent alkalosis that is unresponsive to volume replacement until electrolyte deficiencies are corrected.

- In states of persistent adrenal steroid excess, alkalosis results from mineralocorticoid-mediated reabsorption of Na in the distal tubule.

—Na reabsorption in the distal tubule results in ECF volume expansion and persistent K and H^+ ion secretion.

- Causes of increased mineralocorticoid activity include primary hyperaldosteronism, Cushing's syndrome, renin-secreting tumors, renal artery stenosis, and inborn adrenal enzymatic defects.

Pathogenesis (see Etiology/Cause)
Diagnosis
Signs and Symptoms

- The most common signs of metabolic alkalosis are irritability and neuromuscular hyperexcitability.

—These signs may be due to hypoxia from a transient shift to the left of the oxyhemoglobin dissociation curve.

- Alkalemia causes increased protein binding of ionized Ca despite unchanged total plasma Ca, in which severe alkalemia may cause the ionized Ca to fall low enough to initiate tetany.

- Because hypokalemia often accompanies metabolic alkalosis, signs of concomitant K depletion (e.g., muscular weakness, cramping, ileus, and polyuria) may be present.

Diagnostic Tests

- Diagnosis of metabolic alkalosis requires measurement of plasma HCO_3^- and arterial pH.

—Arterial pH is 7.45, and HCO_3^- is 40 mEq/L in primary metabolic alkalosis.

—Lower HCO_3^- may occur due to compensation for chronic respiratory acidosis.

- Increased PCO_2 of up to 50 to 60 mm Hg may occur because of compensatory hypoventilation, particularly in patients with mild renal insufficiency.

- In addition to increased plasma HCO_3^-, the electrolyte pattern in metabolic alkalosis may include hypochloridemia, hypokalemia, and sometimes hypomagnesemia.

- When metabolic alkalosis is associated with ECF volume depletion, the urine Cl is almost always low (<10 mEq/L), but urine Na may exceed 20 mEq/L.

- On the other hand, when metabolic alkalosis is associated with primary adrenal steroid excess and volume expansion, there is high urine chloride.

- Urine pH in metabolic alkalosis is alkaline, except in the presence of severe K depletion when paradoxical aciduria can occur.

Treatment

- Mild metabolic alkalosis usually requires no treatment.

- Metabolic alkalosis usually resolves when ECF chloride (and volume) deficits are replaced with oral or IV saline.

- In the posthypercapnic state, persistent metabolic alkalosis responds to Cl administration, usually as K or NaCl solutions.

- NaCl should be given with caution in patients who tend to develop volume overload; KCl is usually the preferred solution.

- In severe K deficiency or in patients with hypermineralocorticoidism, alkalosis is Cl resistant, and cannot be corrected until K is also replaced.

- Specific treatment must be directed at the underlying disease processes.

Patient/Family Education

- Metabolic alkalosis, like other similar problems, is not easily understood by those with no experience in these conditions.

- Clear, simple instructions to the patient and family about the nature, cause, course, treatment, and expected outcomes should be given, and feedback from both as to their level of understanding should be requested.

- Both the patient and family members should be kept apprised of the patient's condition throughout treatment.

- Treatments aimed at underlying disease should be explained and differentiated from therapy directed at the metabolic alkalosis.

Follow-up/Referral

- Comprehensive treatment of the alkalosis and the underlying disease will enable the patient to resume usual activities at home.
- Written instructions about signs and symptoms of metabolic alkalosis should be given to the patient, in case of recurrence, and directions specific to the underlying disease also, to enable the patient to care for himself or herself more efficiently and effectively.
- Office visits are relatively frequent for the first month or two after hospitalization or intensive treatment for the alkalosis, then less frequently as the patient recovers fully.

Respiratory Acidosis

Definition

Respiratory acidosis is a condition of low arterial pH, hypoventilation resulting in an elevated. P_{CO_2}, and usually compensatory increase in plasma HCO_3^- concentration.

Risk Factors

- Depression of the central respiratory center caused by drugs, anesthesia, neurologic disease, or abnormal sensitivity to CO_2; abnormalities of the chest bellows caused by poliomyelitis, myasthenia gravis, Guillain-Barré syndrome, or crush injuries of the thorax; severe reduction of the alveolar surface area for gas exchange caused by conditions characterized by ventilation/perfusion imbalances such as chronic obstructive pulmonary disease (COPD), severe pneumonia, pulmonary edema, asthma, or pneumothorax); and laryngeal or tracheal obstruction.

Etiology/Cause (see Risk Factors)
Pathogenesis

- The blood CO_2 content is a function of rates of CO_2 production and disposal.
- CO_2 production varies with the percentage of calories that are derived from carbohydrates while the rate of alveolar ventilation controls the disposal of CO_2 by the lungs.

- The partial pressure of CO_2 gas (P_{CO_2}) is directly proportional to the total amount of CO_2 contained in a solution of blood.
- Any increase in P_{CO_2} due to increased CO_2 production is rapidly handled by increased alveolar ventilation.
- Similarly, a decrease in alveolar ventilation results in pulmonary CO_2 retention and causes respiratory acidosis.
- Respiratory acidosis is often associated with neurologic changes, which may be exacerbated by the development of CSF or grain intracellular acidosis, concurrent hypoxia, and metabolic alkalosis.

Diagnosis
Signs and Symptoms

- Metabolic encephalopathy with headache and drowsiness that progresses to stupor and coma are the most common characteristics of respiratory acidosis.
  —These signs and symptoms usually develop slowly along with increasing respiratory failure.
  —Sudden, full-blown encephalopathy may be precipitated by sedatives, pulmonary infection, or high fraction of inspired oxygen (F_IO_2) in patients with advanced respiratory insufficiency.
  —The encephalopathy is reversible if hypoxic brain damage has not occurred.
- Asterixis and multifocal myoclonus can occur in conjunction with the neurologic condition.
- Sometimes there is dilation of retinal venules and papilledema caused by increased intracranial pressure.

Diagnostic Tests

- In acute respiratory acidosis, the low pH is due to the acute elevation of P_{CO_2}.
- HCO_3^- may be normal or slightly increased.
- A sudden increase in the P_{CO_2} is associated with an increase in plasma HCO_3^- of about 3 to 4 mEq/L because of cellular buffering.
- When renal compensation is fully developed, as in chronic respiratory acidosis, the fall in pH is blunted due to renal HCO_3^- retention and elevation of plasma HCO_3^-.

Treatment

- Treatment must be directed to correcting the underlying pulmonary disturbance.
- Severe respiratory failure with marked hypoxemia may require mechanically assisted ventilation.
- Sedation (narcotics, hypnotics) should not be given except as necessary to facilitate mechanical ventilation.
- The lowest O_2 concentration needed to raise the Pao_2 to an acceptable level (>50 mm Hg) should be given by mask, beginning with a 24% O_2 concentration.
- The Pco_2 should be closely monitored.
- In patients with chronic respiratory failure who are on a ventilator, the Pco_2 should be lowered gradually, particularly when renal compensation is well established.
- By providing adequate inspired O_2, lowering the Pco_2 slowly, and correcting K and Cl deficits, neurologic complications (e.g., seizures, death) will be prevented.

Patient/Family Education

- Respiratory acidosis is a potentially serious condition that must be corrected carefully and cautiously, particularly when there is concomitant disease of any kind.
- Instruct the patient and family about the nature, cause, course, treatment, and expected outcomes of therapy.
- The patient may need to be in the intensive care unit for a time, and family members need to be kept apprised of the patient's condition as often as appropriate.
- Explanation about why mechanical ventilation is temporarily necessary will allay their fears of life-threatening illness.

Follow-up/Referral

- During the acute phase, specialists will care for the patient: pulmonologist, hematologist, urologist, and whomever else may be needed as consultant in specific circumstances.
- After discharge, the patient can be followed by the clinician.
- Close monitoring of blood gases will be needed for a few weeks, until stability has been completely achieved.
- Treatment of underlying disease is ongoing.

Respiratory Alkalosis

Definition
Respiratory alkalosis is a condition of elevated arterial pH, hyperventilation resulting in a low Pco_2, and usually compensatory decrease in plasma $HCO_3{}^-$.

Risk Factors
- Anxiety that causes hyperventilation
- CNS disorders
- Salicylism
- Hepatic cirrhosis
- Hepatic coma
- Hypoxemia
- Fever
- Pain
- Gram-negative septicemia

Etiology/Cause (see also Risk Factors)
- Hyperventilation that results in excessive loss of CO_2 in expired air causes respiratory alkalosis.

Pathogenesis
- As the Pco_2 and cerebral tissue Pco_2 fall, both plasma and brain pH rise.
- Cerebral vasoconstriction results and may produce cerebral hypoxia and the typical symptoms of hyperventilation.

Diagnosis
Signs and Symptoms
- Both rate and depth of breathing increase markedly, particularly when respiratory alkalosis is caused by cerebral or metabolic disorders.
- The breathing pattern in the anxiety-induced syndrome varies from frequent, deep, sighing respirations to sustained, obviously rapid deep breathing.
- Patients usually are unaware of their breathing pattern.
- Sometimes, the major complaint is an inability to catch one's breath, or to get enough air, despite the fact that unimpaired overbreathing is occurring.
- Tetany, circumoral paresthesias, acroparesthesias, or light-headed syncope may occur.
- Blood lactate and pyruvate levels increase, and ionized Ca falls.

- In all situations, the diagnosis of hyperventilation is confirmed by a low P_{CO_2}.

Diagnostic Tests
- In acute respiratory alkalosis, a rapid fall in P_{CO_2} to 20 to 25 mm Hg is associated with a drop in plasma HCO_3^- of no more than 3 to 4 mEq/L due to cellular buffering.
- In chronic respiratory alkalosis, the plasma HCO_3^- may decline by 4 to 5 mEq/L for each 10 mm Hg reduction in P_{CO_2}.

Treatment
- Reassurance is essential for patients with respiratory alkalosis due to anxiety.
- Rebreathing expired CO_2 from a paper bag is usually helpful.
- An alternative is to instruct the patient to hold the breath as long as possible, and repeat the sequence 6 to 10 times.
- When hyperventilation is due to hypoxemia, oxygen administration and correcting abnormal pulmonary gas exchange are appropriate.
- If the patient has neurologic symptoms, a slow change in P_{CO_2} will prevent serious neurologic complications.

Patient/Family Education
- Reassurance should be given to the family as well as the patient.
- As the patient recovers from the acute hyperventilatory phase and begins to feel better, the family will also be able to see the improvement.
- Instruct the patient and family about the nature, cause, course, treatment, and expected outcome of therapy.

Follow-up/Referral
- After discharge, the patient can be followed by the primary care practitioner.
- The patient may require psychosocial therapy for anxiety, which can be suggested, and a consultant selected with experience in handling anxiety states.
- Long-term cure is attainable, particularly as the patient is able to manage stress and related anxiety episodes.

BIBLIOGRAPHY

Anderson KN, Anderson LE, Glanze WD, eds: *Mosby's medical, nursing, & allied health dictionary*, ed 5, St. Louis, 1998, Mosby-Year Book, Inc.

Beers MH, Berkow R: Water, electrolyte, mineral, and acid-base metabolism. In Beers MH, Berkow R, eds: *The Merck manual of diagnosis and therapy*, ed 17, Whitehouse Station, NJ, 1999, Merck Research Laboratories, pp 120-164.

Gregerman RI: Selected problems: hypocalcemia and hypercalcemia; water metabolism. In Barker LR, Burton JR, Zieve PD, eds: *Principles of ambulatory medicine*, ed 5, Baltimore, 1999, Williams & Wilkins, pp 1108-1115.

Okuda T, Kurokawa K, Papadakis MA: Fluid & electrolyte disorders. In Tierney LM, McPhee SJ, Papadakis MA, eds: *Current medical diagnosis & treatment 2000*, New York, 2000, Lange Medical Books/McGraw-Hill, pp 860-885.

Yaqoob M: Water, electrolytes and acid-base homeostasis. In Kumar P, Clark M, eds: *Clinical medicine*, ed 4, Edinburgh, 1998, WB Saunders, pp 597-624.

REVIEW QUESTIONS

1. In healthy men, the total body water makes up what percentage of lean body weight?
   a. 30%
   b. 45%
   c. 50%
   d. 65%
2. Water molecules move randomly and in equal numbers in either direction across a permeable membrane ONLY when:
   a. The molecular weight of each is the same.
   b. The cell membrane is of large enough size.
   c. No solute is present.
   d. NaCl is present.
3. Water tends to stay in which compartment, and why?
   a. In the compartment with no solutes, which allows for greater diffusion
   b. In the compartment that contains solute, which does not allow free diffusion across the membrane
   c. In the interstitial compartment where there is greater room for movement
   d. In the compartment with the largest amount of magnesium
4. Normally, there tends to be less bicarbonate (HCO_3^-) in which compartment?
   a. Plasma
   b. Interstitial fluid
   c. Intracellular fluid
   d. Extracellular fluid

5. The cell membrane is relatively impermeable to Na and K because:
   a. The sodium-APTase pump restricts Na to only one compartment
   b. The potassium-ATPase pump restricts the movement of K across membranes
   c. The cell membrane is "impermeable" to plasma proteins
   d. The Na^+,K^+-ATPase pump restricts Na to the extracellular fluid, and K to the intracellular fluid

6. One L of water (as 5% dextrose), given IV, is distributed:
   a. Only to the intracellular compartment
   b. Only to the extracellular compartment
   c. To all the compartments equally
   d. Only to the body tissues

7. The biochemist Schrier states that the primary determinant of renal sodium and water excretion is:
   a. The glomerular filtration rate
   b. The effective arterial blood volume
   c. The amount of sodium in the extracellular compartment
   d. The amount of water in the kidneys

8. The neurohumoral regulation of Na reabsorption to meet body needs occurs primarily in which part(s) of the kidney?
   a. The distal tubule
   b. The loop of Henle
   c. Both the distal tubule and the loop of Henle
   d. The proximal and collecting tubules

9. Body water homeostasis is maintained by all but one of the following functions. Which one is NOT a factor in maintaining body water homeostasis?
   a. Vasoconstrictors
   b. Thirst
   c. Urine concentrating function of the kidney
   d. Urine diluting function of the kidney

10. Loop diuretics stimulate the excretion of all but one of the following. Which one is NOT excreted because of loop diuretic stimulation?
    a. NaCl
    b. Water
    c. Urate
    d. Potassium

11. Increased extracellular volume is caused primarily by:
    a. Increased total body water
    b. Increased total body sodium
    c. Increased lymphatic drainage
    d. Increased venous tone

12. Loss of sodium from the body is always combined with:
    a. Potassium retention
    b. Urate retention
    c. Water loss
    d. Extracellular volume expansion

13. Normal kidneys can excrete water up to:
    a. 10 L/day
    b. 15 L/day
    c. 20 L/day
    d. 25 L/day

14. Symptoms of hyponatremia occur when:
    a. The plasma osmolality rises above 300 mOsm/kg of water (normal = 280 to 295 mOsm/kg)
    b. The plasma osmolality falls to ≥240 mOsm/kg
    c. Plasma sodium falls below 120 mEq/L
    d. Plasma chloride fall below 80 mEq/L

15. A major treatment for hyponatremia is:
    a. Restricting water intake to <500 to 1000 L/day
    b. Stopping diuretic therapy
    c. Giving 500 ml of hypertonic saline solution (3%) IV
    d. Stabilizing cardiac output in cases of congestive heart failure

16. Risk factors for the development of hypernatremia include all but one of the following. Which one is NOT a risk factor for hypernatremia?
    a. Vomiting, diarrhea
    b. Loop diuretics
    c. Diabetes mellitus
    d. Mineralocorticoid excess

17. The diagnosis of hypokalemia is made on the basis of:
    a. Muscle weakness
    b. History of loss of body water through excessive vomiting or diarrhea
    c. Presence of metabolic alkalosis
    d. Plasma or serum potassium level of <3.5 mEq/L

18. The cause of symptoms of mild, insidious encephalopathy, dementia, depression, or psychosis may actually be:
    a. Hypokalemia
    b. Hyperkalemia
    c. Hypocalcemia
    d. Hypercalcemia
19. The most common cause of hypercalcemia in the general population is:
    a. Deficient vitamin D
    b. Prolonged strenuous exercise
    c. Primary hyperparathyroidism
    d. Certain granulomatous diseases
20. Metabolic alkalosis usually resolves when:
    a. Extracellular fluid volume is decreased by diuretics and water restriction
    b. Extracellular fluid volume deficit is replaced with ingestion of salt water
    c. Extracellular fluid chloride deficit is replaced with IV saline
    d. Extracellular fluid chloride and volume deficits are replaced with oral or IV saline
21. Mortality is significantly greater in acute hyponatremia than in chronic hyponatremia because of:
    a. Effects on the heart
    b. Effects on the central nervous syndrome
    c. Effects on the lungs
    d. Effects on the liver
22. The most prominent symptom in hypernatremia is:
    a. Profuse diuresis
    b. Headache
    c. Thirst
    d. Nausea
23. Hyperkalemia is usually asymptomatic until:
    a. Cardiac toxicity occurs
    b. Seizures occur
    c. Respiratory failure occurs
    d. Confusion develops

24. In emergency situations involving hyperkalemia:
    a. IV β-blocker is given first
    b. IV furosemide is given first
    c. IV Regular insulin is given first
    d. IV calcium gluconate is given first
25. Two characteristic signs of tetany are:
    a. Horton's and Blastock's signs
    b. Bartholomew's and Macedon's signs
    c. Chvostek's and Trousseau's signs
    d. Pavlov's and Zinnema's signs
26. Symptoms of hypocalcemia usually result from:
    a. Neuromuscular irritability
    b. Cardiomyopathic irritability
    c. Hepatic injury
    d. Muscular rigidity
27. Excessive bone resorption is usually the cause of:
    a. Hypocalcemia
    b. Hypokalemia
    c. Hyperkalemia
    d. Hypercalcemia
28. One of the most abundant elements in the body is:
    a. Calcium
    b. Sodium
    c. Phosphate
    d. Potassium
29. The most common cause of clinically significant hypomagnesemia is:
    a. Malabsorption syndrome
    b. Renal impairment
    c. Deficient excretion of urine
    d. Excessive use of laxatives
30. The Henderson-Hasselbalch equation is used to determine:
    a. Plasma HCO_3^-
    b. Plasma calcium level
    c. Plasma pH
    d. Plasma phosphate level

12

Hematologic Disorders

ANEMIAS
Definition

Anemia means decreased numbers of red blood cells (RBCs) or hemoglobin (Hb) content.

- Hematocrit (HCT) is <41% (Hb < 13.5 g/dl [males])
- HCT is <37% (Hb < 12 g/dl) (females)
- The term anemia is used incorrectly as a diagnosis; however, anemia really refers to a complex of signs and symptoms.
  - The type of anemia defines its pathophysiologic mechanisms and its essential nature, which guides its treatment.

Risk Factors (Box 12-1)
Etiology/Cause (see Box 12-1)
Pathogenesis

- Pathogenesis varies with the cause or type of anemia (Box 12-2).

Iron Deficiency Anemia
Definition

Iron deficiency anemia (IDA) is a chronic anemia characterized by small, pale RBCs and iron depletion.

Incidence
- IDA is the most common cause of anemia worldwide.

Etiology
- The most common cause of IDA, and which must be considered first, is blood loss; in adults, this is almost always the cause.
- Pathognomonic: absent bone marrow iron stores (or)
- Serum ferritin < 12 µg/L

Background Information
- Total body iron ranges between 2 and 4 g.
  - 50 mg/kg (men)
  - 35 mg/kg (women)
- Most (70% to 95%) iron is present in hemoglobin in circulating RBCs.
- One ml of packed RBCs (not whole blood) contains about 1 mg of iron.
- Men: RBC volume is about 30 ml/kg (e.g., a 70-kg man will have about 2100 ml of packed RBCs and therefore 2100 mg of iron in his circulating blood).
- Women: RBC volume is about 27 ml/kg (e.g., a 50-kg woman will have 1350 mg of iron circulating in her RBCs).
- Only 200 to 400 mg of iron is present in myoglobin and nonheme enzymes; the amount of iron in plasma is negligible.
- Other than circulating RBCs, iron is in the storage pool:
  - Iron is deposited either as ferritin or as hemosiderin, located in macrophages.
  - Storage iron varies from 0.5 to 2 g; about 25% of women in the United States have none.
- The average American diet contains 10 to 15 mg of iron/day.
  - About 10% of this is absorbed in the stomach, duodenum, and upper jejunum.
  - Dietary iron present as heme is efficiently absorbed (10% to 20%); less nonheme iron is absorbed because of interference by phosphates, tannins, and other constituents of food.
  - Small amounts of iron (e.g., 1 mg/day) are lost by exfoliation of skin and mucosal cells.

BOX 12-1
Anemias Classified by Cause

BLOOD LOSS
Acute
Chronic

DEFICIENT ERYTHROPOIESIS
Microcytic
Iron deficiency
 Iron-transport deficiency
 Iron utilization
 Iron reutilization
 Thalassemias (see RBC defects under Excessive
  Hemolysis)
Normochromic-normocytic
 Hypoproliferation
  In kidney disease
  In endocrine failure (thyroid, pituitary)
 Aplastic anemia
 Myelophthisis
 Myelodysplasia
Macrocytic
 Vitamin B_{12} deficiency
 Folate deficiency
 Copper deficiency
 Vitamin C deficiency

EXCESSIVE HEMOLYSIS
Extrinsic RBC defects
 Reticuloendothelial hyperactivity with splenomegaly

Extrinsic RBC defects
 Immunologic abnormalities
  Isoimmune (isoagglutinin hemolysis)
  Autoimmune hemolysis
  Warm antibody hemolysis
  Cold antibody hemolysis
 Paroxysmal nocturnal hemoglobinuria
Mechanical injury
 Trauma
 Infection
Intrinsic RBC defects
 Membrane alterations
  Congenital
   Congenital erythropoietic porphyria
   Hereditary elliptocytosis
   Hereditary spherocytosis
  Acquired
   Stomatocytosis
   Hypophosphatemia
Metabolic disorders (inherited enzyme deficiencies)
 Embden-Meyerhof pathway defects
 Hexose monophosphate shunt defects
  (G6PD deficiency)
Hemoglobinopathies
 Sickle cell anemia (Hb S)
 Hb C, sickle cell, and E diseases
 Thalassemias (β, β-δ, α)
 Hb S-β-thalassemia disease

From Beers MH, Berkow R, eds: Hematology and oncology. *The Merck manual of diagnosis and therapy,* ed 17, Whitehouse Station, NJ, 1999, Merck & Co, Inc, p 852.

BOX 12-2
Classification of Anemias by Mean Corpuscular Volume

MICROCYTIC
Iron deficiency
Thalassemia
Anemia of chronic disease

MACROCYTIC
Megaloblastic
 Vitamin B_{12} deficiency
 Folate deficiency

Nonmegaloblastic
 Myelodysplasia, chemotherapy
 Liver disease
 Increased reticulocytosis
 Myxedema

NORMOCYTIC
Can be many causes

From Linker CA: Blood. In Tierney LM, McPhee SJ, Papadakis MA, eds: *Current medical diagnosis & treatment 2000,* ed 39, New York, 2000, Lange Medical Books/McGraw-Hill, p 500.

- No physiologic mechanisms exist in the body to increase normal losses of iron.
- Menstrual blood loss has a major role in iron metabolism.
  —Average monthly loss is about 50 ml (0.7 mg/day).
  —In some women, blood loss may be 5 times the average.
    ~ These women must absorb 3 to 4 mg of iron/day from foods.
    ~ This amount cannot reasonably be absorbed; therefore these women are almost always iron-deficient.
- Pregnancy may also cause imbalances in iron needs/absorbed, when need rises to between 2 and 5 mg/day in both pregnancy and lactation.
  —Iron replacement therapy is usually required.
- Gastrointestinal (GI) blood loss, usually in occult blood, is important to identify and treat.
  —Chronic intake of aspirin may be one cause.
- Chronic hemoglobinuria may cause iron deficiency (more than 1 mg/day of iron may be lost in this way).
- Another common cause is traumatic hemolysis due to an abnormally functioning cardiac valve prosthesis.

Diagnosis

- Not investigating mild anemia is a serious error because evidence of its presence indicates an underlying disorder, and its severity reveals little about its genesis or true clinical significance.

Signs and Symptoms

- Blood loss should be the first consideration.
- The signs and symptoms of anemia reflect cardiovascular-pulmonary compensatory responses to the severity and duration of tissue hypoxia.
  —Severe anemia (Hb < 7 g/dl) will manifest weakness, vertigo, headache, tinnitus, spots before the eyes, fatigability, drowsiness, irritability, and even bizarre behavior.
  —Tachycardia, tachypnea, palpitations (anemia itself)
  —Severe deficiency causes smooth tongue, brittle nails, and cheilosis.

—Dysphagia due to development of esophageal webs (Plummer-Vinson syndrome) may occur.
—Pica may occur, in which patients crave items such as ice chips, laundry starch, and lettuce, which have little if any iron.
—Amenorrhea, loss of libido, jaundice, and splenomegaly can occur.
—Finally, heart failure or shock can result.

Laboratory Findings

- Depletion of iron stores is seen in anemia, with no change in RBC size.
- Serum ferritin becomes abnormally low (<30 μg/L).
- Serum total iron-binding capacity (TIBC) increases.
- As the anemia worsens, serum iron values will fall to less than 30 μg/dl.
- Transferrin saturation will be less than 15%.
- Early on, the mean corpuscular volume (MCV) remains normal, then falls, and the blood smear shows hypochromic, microcytic cells.
  —Anisocytosis develops (variations in RBC size).
  —Poikilocytosis ensues: variation in shape of RBCs.
  —Severe anemia shows a bizarre peripheral blood smear, totally unlike a smear of normal cells: severely hypochromic cells, target cells, pencil-shaped cells.
- The platelet count is normal in mild anemia, but is elevated in more severe anemia.
- Mechanisms of increased destruction (e.g., sequestration by the spleen, antibody-mediated hemolysis, defective RBC membrane function, abnormal Hb) help in the differential diagnosis of hemolytic anemias.

Laboratory Tests

- Complete blood count (CBC)
- RBC counts
  —RBC indices include the following:
    ~ MCV, a direct measure of red cell size; microcytic and macrocytic anemias have very limited differential diagnoses, so by noting the MCV, diagnosis can focus on microcytic or macrocytic anemia.

~ Causes of anemia with low MCV
- Iron deficiency
- Thalassemia
- Anemia of chronic inflammation (occasionally)
- Sideroblastic anemia (congenital, rare)
- Some hemoglobinopathies (e.g., Hb E)
- Aluminum toxicity
~ Mean corpuscular Hb (MCHb)
~ Mean corpuscular Hb concentration (MCHbC)
- Reticulocyte count—best method to assess the response of the bone marrow to anemia
—The normal reticulocyte count is about 1%, which represents the 1% of new cells released into the circulation daily from the bone marrow.
—The normal life span of RBCs is 100 days.
- Serial HCT values over a few days or weeks often provide clues to the mechanism of the anemia.
—Total shutdown of production in the marrow in the absence of bleeding or hemolysis results in a fall in the HCT value of 3 to 4 percentage points/week.
—If the value falls more rapidly, bleeding or hemolysis is occurring.
—Anemia with an appropriate reticulocyte response in the absence of bleeding usually indicates hemolysis.
- RBC fragility (osmotic fragility) shows the percentage of NaCl at which hemolysis begins and the percentage at which the first tube shows complete hemolysis.
- Other laboratory tests are required for specific anemias and bleeding disorders.

Differential Diagnosis
- Anemia of chronic disease
—Normal or increased iron stores in bone marrow
—Normal or elevated ferritin level
—TIBC may be normal or low.
- Thalassemia
—Greater degree of mucocytosis for any level of anemia, than does iron deficiency

—RBCs become abnormal earlier in the development of anemia; many target cells are present at all stages.
- Sideroblastic anemia (less common)

Treatment
- Oral iron
—Ferrous sulfate 325 mg tid: provides 180 mg of iron daily; 10 mg is absorbed (more may be absorbed, depending on the severity of the anemia).
~ Normal response: return of HCT level to 50% of normal within 3 weeks; 100% normal within 2 months.
~ $FeSO_4$ is continued for 3 to 6 months to replenish iron stores.
—Causes of failure to respond to iron therapy
~ Noncompliance
~ Incorrect diagnosis: may be anemia of chronic disease or thalassemia
~ GI blood loss that exceeds the rate of new erythropoiesis
- Parenteral iron
—In cases of intolerance to oral iron, GI disease (e.g., inflammatory bowel disease), continuing blood loss that cannot be corrected
~ Risk of severe hypersensitivity precludes administration of parenteral iron unless it is absolutely required.

Patient/Family Education
- Instruct regarding the nature of the condition, possible/probable cause(s), treatment, expected outcome of therapy
- Be certain to inform the patient/family that oral iron often causes very dark stools and not to panic if that occurs, as it is not significant.
- Emphasize the need to adhere strictly to the daily dosage.

Follow-up/Referral
- It may be necessary to refer the patient to a gastroenterologist or hematologist if anemia continues despite iron therapy, to discover other possible causes.
- Close monitoring during oral iron therapy is essential; response must be carefully noted, and changes/referral made as necessary.

Anemia of Chronic Disease

Definition

This condition was initially ascribed to the presence of chronic disease (e.g., rheumatoid arthritis [RA]), but it can occur transiently with any infection or inflammation.

Incidence

- This is the second most common type of anemia worldwide.

Etiology

- As indicated, this type of anemia can occur with virtually any acute or chronic infection or inflammation.
- Patients undergoing hemodialysis lose both iron and folate.

Pathogenesis

- Three pathophysiologic mechanisms are identified with this anemia.
  —Slightly shortened RBC survival is seen in patients with cancer and chronic infections.
   ~ Cause is not certain, but a 50,000-kilodalton (kD) protein has been found in some cancer patients.
  —Erythropoietin (EPO) production and marrow responsiveness are decreased, causing deficient erythropoiesis.
   ~ Cause: macrophage-derived cytokines (e.g., interleukin-1β, tumor necrosis factor-α, interferon-β) are found in those with inflammatory states, infections, and cancer.
  —Intracellular iron metabolism is impaired.
   ~ In chronic disease, reticulum cells hold iron from senescent RBCs, making iron unavailable for Hb synthesis by the erythron.

Diagnosis

Signs and Symptoms

- Same as for anemia, often not as pronounced
- Should be suspected in anyone with acute infectious or inflammatory disease, as well as those with chronic disease such as RA

Laboratory Findings

- A false diagnosis may be made on the basis of decreased serum iron and percentage saturation, but these findings must be coupled with an increased TIBC to establish a diagnosis of iron deficiency anemia—not anemia of chronic disease.
- Low serum iron
- Low TIBC
- Normal or increased serum ferritin, or normal or increased bone marrow iron stores
- In persons with significant anemia (<60% of baseline), concomitant iron deficiency or folic acid deficiency should be investigated.
- Hct rarely goes below 25%, except in patients with renal failure.
- MCV is normal or slightly decreased.
- Transferrin saturation may be extremely low.

Treatment

- No treatment is needed in most cases.
- For some patients, RBC transfusions are needed to treat symptomatic anemia.
- Purified recombinant erythropoietin is effective in treating anemia of renal failure and other secondary anemias (e.g., anemia related to cancer or inflammatory disorders such as RA).
- In patients with renal failure, adequate intensity of dialysis is necessary to achieve optimal response to erythropoietin.
- Erythropoietin is available as epoetin alfa; it must be injected SC three or more times/week (dose is 10,000 units); it is very expensive and is used only to alleviate anemia in those who are transfusion-dependent or when the quality of life is obviously improved, as indicated by the hematologic response.

Patient/Family Education

- The nature of the anemia, whether symptomatic or not, is explained to the patient, and its likely cause.
- Treatment may not be needed for many patients with acute infection or inflammation, in whom the anemia will correct when the infection or inflammation is treated.
- If concomitant iron or folate deficiency is present, the necessary oral medications are given, with reasons, action, length of therapy, and tests that will confirm efficacy of the therapy.

Follow-up/Referral

- If the patient is discovered to have cancer, he or she will be referred to an oncologist in the appropriate specialty (e.g., gynecology, GI, kidney).
- If an infectious disease specialist is needed, that referral will be made.
- The primary physician and nurse practitioner continue to follow the patient, along with the specialist(s) through treatment and recovery or terminal illness.
- If the patient does become terminally ill, referral to a hospice is suggested to the family and patient.

The Thalassemias

Definition

- These comprise a group of chronic, inherited, microcytic anemias characterized by defective Hb synthesis and ineffective erythropoiesis that are particularly common in persons of Mediterranean, African, or Southeast Asian ancestry.

Incidence

- Thalassemia is among the most common inherited hemolytic disorders among the populations mentioned.
- In blacks, the gene frequency for α-thalassemia is about 25%; the phenotypic (clinical) expression occurs in 10%.

Etiology

- The cause is unbalanced Hb synthesis caused by decreased production of at least one globin polypeptide chain (α, β, γ, δ).
- β-Thalassemia results from decreased production of β-polypeptide chains.
  —It is an autosomal dominant trait.
    ~ Heterozygotes are carriers, and have asymptomatic mild-to-moderate microcytic anemia (thalassemia minor).
    ~ The typical symptoms occur in homozygotes (thalassemia major).
- α-Thalassemia results from decreased production of α-polypeptide chains and has a more complex inheritance pattern because genetic control of α-chain synthesis involves two pairs of structural genes.
  —Heterozygotes for a single-gene defect (α-thalassemia-2 [silent]) are usually free of clinical abnormalities.
  —Heterozygotes for a double-gene defect or homozygotes for a single-gene defect (α-thalassemia-1 [trait]) manifest a clinical picture similar to heterozygotes for β-thalassemia.
  —Inheritance of both a single-gene defect and a double-gene defect more severely impairs α-chain production.
  —α-Chain deficiency results in the formation of tetramers of excess β chains (Hb H) or in infancy γ chains (Bart's Hb).
  —Homozygosity for the double-gene defect is lethal because Hb that lacks α chains does not transport oxygen.

Diagnosis

- Quantitative Hb studies are used for routine clinical diagnosis.

Signs and Symptoms

- Clinical features of thalassemias are similar but vary in severity.
  —β-Thalassemia minor is clinically symptomatic.
  —β-Thalassemia major (Cooley's anemia) presents with symptoms of severe anemia, markedly expanded marrow space, and transfusional and absorptive iron overload.
    ~ Jaundice
    ~ Leg ulcers
    ~ Cholelithiasis (as in sickle cell anemia)
    ~ Splenomegaly is common; the spleen may be huge.
      – If splenic sequestration develops, the survival time of transfused normal RBCs is shortened.
    ~ Bone marrow hyperactivity causes thickening of the cranial bones and malar eminences.
    ~ Long bone involvement makes pathologic fractures common.
    ~ Growth rates are impaired; puberty may be significantly delayed or absent.
    ~ Iron deposits in cardiac muscle may cause dysfunction and heart failure.
    ~ Hepatic siderosis is typical, leading to functional impairment and cirrhosis.
- α-Thalassemia-1 (trait) has a presentation similar to β-thalassemia minor.
- Patients with Hb H disease often have symptomatic hemolytic anemia and splenomegaly.

Laboratory Findings

- Elevation of Hb A_2 is the diagnostic test for β-**thalassemia minor.**
- In β-**thalassemia major,** Hb F is usually increased, sometimes as much as 90%, and Hb A_2 is usually increased to >3%.
- In β-**thalassemia major,** anemia is severe, often with Hb ≤ 6 g/dl.
  - RBC count is elevated.
  - Blood smear is virtually diagnostic, with many nucleated erythroblasts, target cells, small pale RBCs, and punctate and diffuse basophilia.
  - X-ray findings show characteristic chronic marrow hyperactivity.
    - ~ The cortices of the skull and long bones are thinned, and the marrow space is widened.
    - ~ The diploic spaces in the skull may be accentuated, with the trabeculae having a sun-ray appearance.
    - ~ In the long bones, areas of osteoporosis may be seen.
    - ~ The vertebral bodies and skull may have a granular or ground-glass appearance.
    - ~ The phalanges may lose their normal shape, and appear to be rectangular or biconvex.
- In β-**thalassemias,** the percentages of Hb F and Hb A_2 are usually normal.
  - Diagnosis is usually one of exclusion of other causes of microcytic anemia.
- **Hb H disease** is diagnosed by showing the fast-migrating Hb H or Bart's fractions on Hb electrophoresis.
  - Recombinant deoxyribonucleic acid (DNA) gene mapping, particularly the polymerase chain reaction, has become standard for prenatal diagnosis and genetic counseling.
- Serum bilirubin, serum iron, and serum ferritin levels are increased.
- Bone marrow shows marked erythroid hyperplasia.
- In β- or α-**thalassemia minor,** mild-to-moderate microcytic anemia is usual.
  - Serum iron and serum ferritin tests will help to rule out iron deficiency.

Treatment

- Patients with α-thalassemia or β-thalassemia minor are clinically normal and require no treatment.
- Patients with microcytosis should be identified (by Medic-Alert bracelet) so that they will not be subjected to repeated evaluations for iron deficiency and mistakenly given iron supplements.
- Patients with **Hb H disease** should take folate supplements and avoid medicinal iron and oxidative drugs such as sulfonamides.
- Patients with severe thalassemia should be maintained on a regular transfusion schedule and receive folate supplements.
  - Splenectomy is performed if hypersplenism causes a marked increase in the transfusion requirement.
  - Deferoxamine is given as an iron-chelating agent to avoid or postpone hemosiderosis.
    - ~ Oral iron chelators are under clinical investigation and are effective, but toxicity (agranulocytosis) may limit their use indefinitely.
  - Allogeneic bone marrow transplantation (BMT) has been introduced as treatment for β-thalassemia major.
- Children who have not yet experienced iron overload and chronic organ toxicity do well, with long-term survival in more than 80% of cases.

Patient/Family Education

- Patients who develop any of the thalassemia anemias may already be familiar with the diseases, their genetic cause, and their own susceptibility.
- For patients who have no knowledge of the anemia, instruct fully regarding the type of anemia present, its treatment, expected outcome, and prognosis.
- For those with severe thalassemia, the more extensive treatment options (e.g., BMT) should be explained, with specific pros and cons, to help them to make appropriate decisions about their own care.

Follow-up/Referral

- Patients with mild disease do not require treatment but should be advised to wear a Medic-

Alert bracelet to let other clinicians know that they have anemia but do not require further evaluation or iron replacement therapy.

- Patients with severe anemia are followed closely and monitored on a regular basis to determine the course of their disease, to make treatment decisions early so that appropriate arrangement can be made (e.g., for splenectomy, BMT, or other).

VITAMIN DEFICIENCIES
Vitamin B_{12} (Cobalamin) Deficiency
Definition
Decreased intake of vitamin B_{12}, resulting in typical signs and symptoms of the effects of the deficiency on the body (see Diagnosis section).

Sources
- Primarily meats (e.g., beef, pork, organ meats), liver, eggs, milk, milk products.

Functions
- Vitamin B_{12} plays a major role in the following:
  —Maturation of RBCs
  —Neural function
  —DNA synthesis related to folate
  —Synthesis of coenzymes (methylcobalamin, adenosylcobalamin) and methionine

Absorption
- Occurs in the terminal ileum and requires **intrinsic factor,** a secretion of parietal cells of the gastric mucosa, for transport across the intestinal mucosa

Stores
- Liver B_{12} stores are normally sufficient to sustain physiologic needs for 3 to 5 years, in the absence of intrinsic factor, and for 3 to 12 months in the absence of total enterohepatic reabsorption capacity.

Etiology (Table 12-1)
Diagnosis
Signs and Symptoms
- Anemia develops slowly but progressively as B_{12} stores are depleted from the liver.
  —Signs and symptoms usually do not adequately indicate the intensity of the problem because the slow progress allows for physiologic adaptation to occur.
- Splenomegaly and hepatomegaly may be present.
- GI manifestations
  —Glossitis (burning of the tongue) may be an early symptom.
  —Anorexia
  —Intermittent diarrhea and constipation
  —Vague abdominal pain, not localized
  —Significant weight loss is common.
- Neurologic symptoms may be present, even when anemia is not present.
  —Mild-to-moderate weakness
  —Diminished or lost reflexes
  —Loss of peripheral position sense and vibratory sensation (extremities)

TABLE 12-1
Causes of Vitamin B_{12} Deficiency

Cause	Source
Inadequate diet	Veganism, breast-feeding by vegan mothers, chronic alcoholism (rare), fad diets
Inadequate absorption*	Lack of intrinsic factor (pernicious anemia, destruction of gastric mucosa, endocrinopathy); small intestine disorders (celiac disease, sprue, malignancy, drugs), vitamin B_{12} malabsorption, competition for B_{12} from fish tapeworm, blind loop syndrome
Inadequate utilization	Antagonists, enzyme deficiencies, organ disease (liver, kidney, malignancy, malnutrition), transport protein abnormality
Increased requirement	Hyperthyroidism, infancy, parasitic infestation, α-thalassemia
Increased excretion	Inadequate binding in serum, liver disease, kidney disease

From Herbert VD, Colman N: Folic acid and vitamin B_{12}. In Shils ME, Young VR, eds: *Modern nutrition in health and disease,* ed 7, Philadelphia, 1988, Lea & Febiger, pp 388-416.
*Most patients have inadequate absorption.

—Spasticity, positive Babinski's sign, more severe loss of proprioceptive and vibratory sensation (lower extremities), ataxia; all occur in later stage

—Upper extremities become involved later and with less consistency than the legs.

—Yellow-blue color blindness may occur.

—Irritability, depression, paranoia, delirium, confusion, spastic ataxia, postural hypotension; all occur in advanced stage

Laboratory Findings

- Macrocytic anemia with MCV > 100 fL
- Smear shows macro-ovalocytosis, anisocytosis, and poikilocytosis.
  - RBC volume distribution width (RDW) is high.
  - Howell-Jolly bodies (residual fragments of the nucleus) are common.
  - In untreated patients, reticulocytopenia may be present.
  - Hypersegmentation of granulocytes is one of the earliest findings.
  - Neutropenia develops later.
  - Thrombocytopenia is present in about 50% of severe cases.
  - Platelets are often bizarre in size and shape.
- Bone marrow shows erythroid hyperplasia and megaloblastic changes.
- Serum indirect bilirubin may be elevated due to ineffective erythropoiesis and shortened survival time of defective RBCs.
- Lactate dehydrogenase (LDH) is usually very elevated, indicating significant ineffective hemopoiesis and increased hemolysis.
- Serum ferritin is usually increased (>300 ng/ml), consistent with hemolysis.
- Serum vitamin B_{12} < 150 pg/ml indicates with relative certainty B_{12} deficiency.
  - In possible false-negative serum B_{12} lab reports, serum methylmalonic acid assay is the gold standard for diagnosing B_{12} deficiency, especially in older patients.

Differential Diagnosis

- Multisystem disease must be differentiated from compressive cord lesions and multiple sclerosis (neurologic defects allowed to persist for months or years become irreversible).

Further Evaluation

- Once B_{12} deficiency is established, the pathophysiologic mechanism must be identified so that it can be treated.
  - Autoantibodies to gastric parietal cells are identified in 80% to 90% of patients with pernicious anemia; antibodies to intrinsic factor in the serum and achlorhydria (gastric analysis) are seen in most patients with pernicious anemia; achlorhydria is confirmed if pH rises to between 6.8 and 7.2 after giving histamine.
- The Schilling test measures absorption of radioactive B_{12} with and without intrinsic factor.
  - Useful particularly to establish the diagnosis in treated patients who are in remission, or those whose diagnosis is uncertain.
- GI x-rays should be done if a positive diagnosis of pernicious anemia is made because the incidence of gastric cancer is increased in these patients.
  - GI x-rays may also show other causes of megaloblastic anemia (e.g., intestinal diverticula or blind loops—small-bowel patterns that are characteristic of sprue).
  - GI x-rays should be repeated if signs or symptoms develop later: positive test for occult blood in stool, abdominal discomfort.

Treatment

- Calculation of the required amount of B_{12} to be given is problematic.
  - Replacement of liver stores accounts for 3000 to 10,000 µg, during which B_{12} retention decreases.
- Usually, vitamin B_{12} 1000 µg intramuscularly (IM) two to four times/week is given until the hematologic picture returns to near normal, then the same amount is given once a month.
  - Although correction of hematologic parameters occurs within 6 weeks, neural improvement takes up to 18 months.
- **Giving folic acid instead of B_{12} to patients who are B_{12}-deprived is contraindicated because it may cause fulminant neurologic deficit.**
- Oral iron therapy is given before B_{12} therapy if iron deficiency is diagnosed (ab-

sence of stainable iron in bone marrow or other indicators; e.g., serum ferritin < 200 ng/ml).

- B_{12} therapy must be maintained for life, unless the pathophysiologic mechanism for the deficiency is corrected.

Patient/Family Education
- Instruct regarding the nature of the condition and its cause, course, treatment, prognosis, and expected outcome (e.g., lifelong B_{12} therapy).
- Explain all procedures, tests, and medications: reason for, what to expect, what is expected of the patient, outcome.
- Indicate the signs and symptoms that the patient exhibits that mandate therapy, and the duration and effects of therapy.

Follow-up/Referral
- It may be necessary to follow these patients for life, depending on the pathophysiologic cause of the B_{12} deficiency.
- Referral to specialists (e.g., gastroenterologist, hematologist, surgeon) may be necessary as soon as the diagnosis and pathophysiologic mechanism, which direct treatment, are determined.

Anemia Caused by Folate Deficiency

Definition
Folate is critical in the formation of the nervous system during fetal and neonatal periods. Neural tube defects with severe neurologic deficits occur when adequate folate is not ingested during pregnancy.

Etiology (Table 12-2)
Sources of Folate
- Fresh green leafy vegetables
  - —Long cooking destroys folates.
  - —Liver stores provide only a 2- to 4-month supply when intake is low.
  - —Alcohol interferes with folate intermediate metabolism, intestinal absorption, and enterohepatic salvage.
  - —People who are marginally malnourished, who are chronic alcoholics, or who have liver disease are prone to macrocytic anemia from folate deficiency.
- Fruits
- Organ meats
- Liver
- Dried yeast

Functions of Folate
- Maturation of RBCs
- Synthesis of purines, pyrimidines, and methionine
- Conversion of homocysteine to methionine, and of deoxyuridylate to thymidylate, which is a critical step in DNA synthesis.

Diagnosis
- Clinical characteristics are those of anemia.
- Folate deficiency is indistinguishable from B_{12} deficiency regarding peripheral blood and bone marrow pictures.

TABLE 12-2
Causes of Folate Deficiency

Cause	Source
Inadequate intake*	Diet lacking fresh, slightly cooked food; chronic alcoholism; TPN
Inadequate absorption*	Malabsorption syndromes (e.g., celiac disease, sprue), drugs (phenytoin, primidone, barbiturates, cycloserine, oral contraceptives?); folic acid malabsorption (congenital, acquired), blind loop syndrome
Inadequate utilization	Folic acid antagonists (methotrexate, pyrimethamine, triamterene, diamidine compounds, trimethoprim), anticonvulsants?, enzyme deficiency (congenital, acquired), vitamin B_{12} deficiency, alcoholism, scurvy
Increased requirement	Pregnancy, lactation, infancy, malignancy (especially lymphoproliferative), increased hemopoiesis (especially β-thalassemia major), increased metabolism
Increased excretion	Renal dialysis (peritoneal or hemodialysis); vitamin B_{12} dependency?, liver disease

From Herbert VD, Colman N: Folic acid and vitamin B_{12}. In Shils ME, Young VR, eds: *Modern nutrition in health and disease,* ed 7, Philadelphia, 1988, Lea & Febiger, pp 388-416.
TPN, Total parenteral nutrition.
*Inadequate intake and inadequate absorption are the most common causes.

—Megaloblastic anemia
—Megaloblastic changes in mucosa
- No neurologic abnormalities are associated with folate deficiency, as they are with B_{12} deficiency.

Laboratory Findings
- RBC folate level < 150 ng/ml is diagnostic of folate deficiency.
- Megaloblastic anemia is present.
- Serum vitamin B_{12} is normal.

Differential Diagnosis
- Laboratory findings confirm folate deficiency, and rule out vitamin B_{12} deficiency.
- Alcoholic patients may have concomitant anemia of liver disease, with characteristic macrocytic anemia and target cells.
- Patients with human immunodeficiency virus (HIV)-related diseases and treated with zidovudine develop macrocytosis without megaloblastic changes.
- Hypothyroidism is linked with mild macrocytosis and pernicious anemia.

Treatment
- Folate replacement therapy is 1 mg/day PO, which produces rapid improvement and a sense of well-being.
    —Total correction of hematologic abnormalities occurs within 2 months.

Patient/Family Education
- Explain the nature of the deficiency, cause, treatment required, duration, and expected outcomes.
- Instruct regarding dietary sources of folic acid and to not overcook fresh vegetables.

Follow-up/Referral
- The nurse practitioner usually consults with a hematologist during the diagnostic phase of patient evaluation, then follows the patient throughout therapy and final evaluation to ensure that the folate level is normal.
- With adequate education, patients should not develop folate deficiency again.

SICKLE CELL DISEASE
Definition
Sickle cell disease (Hb S) affects about 0.15% of blacks in the United States, and 8% to 13% who carry the sickle cell gene. Sickle cell disease occurs almost exclusively in blacks and is characterized by sickle-shaped RBCs resulting from homozygous inheritance of Hb S.

Risk Factors
- Inherited sickle cell gene
- Black race
- Greek, Italian, Arabian and Indian ancestry, whose members also may have the sickle cell gene or trait

Etiology/Cause
- Hb S results from a mutation in the β-globin chain in Hb that, when oxygen tension is reduced, causes the formation of rigid elongated tactoids that distort RBC shape and increase RBC rigidity.
    —The clumping together of sickled cells leads to tissue ischemia and infarction.

Pathogenesis
- All people (heterozygous for Hb S) with sickle cell trait are well and are not anemic.
    —The peripheral cell appears normal, but sickling is seen if the blood is deoxygenated.
    —Electrophoresis shows 40% Hb S and 60% Hb A; Hb A_2 and Hb F are present in normal concentration.
- Although persons with sickle cell trait lead relatively normal lives, at times clinical events do occur that are attributable to the presence of sickle cell Hb.
    —Splenic infarction at high altitudes (above 10,000 ft) has been reported.
    —Occasionally, infarctions occur in more vital organs during vigorous exercise.
- All persons with sickle cell trait have renal tubular dysfunction resulting in hyposthenuria.
    —Severe hematuria may occur from hypertonicity in the renal medulla, resulting in sickling and leading to ischemia and tubular infarction.
    —Those with sickle cell trait have a higher incidence of renal infections, particularly women during pregnancy.

- It is important to identify people with sickle cell trait so that they may receive genetic counseling.
  —A couple, both heterozygous for Hb S, should be informed that they have a 25% chance of having a child with sickle cell anemia.
  —Prenatal diagnosis of sickle cell anemia by amniocentesis is now possible.

Sickle Cell Anemia

- Sickle cell anemia is present in about 0.15% of the black population.
- The anemia is usually severe, resulting in significant morbidity and a shortened life expectancy.
- One of the most disturbing clinical features of the illness is the occurrence of painful (thrombotic) crises, which are recurrent episodes of severe pain, usually in the limbs and abdomen, caused by sickling-induced ischemia.
- Patients have a lifelong, severe anemia, with HCT values that range from the high teens to the low thirties (average is midtwenties).

Pathogenesis

- The primary mechanism of the anemia is extravascular hemolysis, so that there is a chronic reticulocytosis and a chronic indirect hyperbilirubinemia.
- Patients usually have leukocytosis, the white blood cell (WBC) count rising occasionally as high as 30,000 to 40,000 during a painful crisis.
- A mild thrombocytosis is usually present.
- The peripheral smear shows markedly distorted RBCs, including characteristic sickle cells.
- On electrophoresis, only Hb S with a variable amount of Hb F (no Hb A) is present.
- Multiple, often repetitive, episodes of organ ischemia are caused by sickling.
- Result in a broad spectrum of abnormalities
  —The bones appear abnormal on x-ray, showing old infarctions that mimic changes of osteomyelitis.
  —Medullary spaces are usually widened by the marked compensatory expansion of bone marrow.
  —The spine generally appears distorted.

—Aseptic necrosis of the femoral head is common, and may require joint replacement.
—Splenomegaly usually disappears by age 8 because of repeated infarction of the spleen; adults with sickle cell anemia are essentially autosplenectomized, which contributes to the susceptibility to infections, especially pneumococcal infections.
—Gallstones are common, and these patients frequently develop cholecystitis, which is very difficult to distinguish from intrahepatic cholestasis resulting from sickling in the hepatic sinusoids.
—Over time, patients usually develop cardiomegaly and chronic myocardial disease related to repeated microinfarctions of the heart.
—Murmurs are common and may be erroneously diagnosed as rheumatic or congenital heart disease.
—Venous thromboses and pulmonary embolism are common.
—Cardiovascular accidents (CVAs) are often seen, with associated infarction and intracerebral and subarachnoid hemorrhage.
—Seizures occur in many patients.
—Retinopathy that may result in blindness usually develops because of the blocking of retinal capillaries with subsequent neovascularization; annual examinations by an ophthalmologist are necessary.

Genetic Basis for Sickle Cell Disease

- The genes that code for Hb S and Hb C are alleles.
- The Hb C mutation is common in blacks, with a 2% prevalence.
- This syndrome is similar to that of sickle cell anemia (Hb S) but is not as severe.
- The spleen in 50% of adults with sickle cell disease is palpable, but not in most patients with sickle cell anemia (Hb S).

Treatment

- Treatment is given according to the body system affected, and the manifested signs and symptoms.
  —In painful thrombotic crises, which may last from several hours to several days or

weeks, with high fever and neutrophilia, the patient is usually treated with narcotics and hydration. No specific treatment exists that will shorten the crisis. The possibility of addiction to narcotics is high, and dose and time should be limited as much as possible. If pain is severe and persistent, hospitalization is required.

—Infections are treated immediately and vigorously.

—Hemolytic and aplastic crises occur, but acceleration of hemolysis is not common. If HCT drops below baseline, it is likely because of decreased marrow production, and is much more common in children, sometimes necessitating hospitalization and transfusion. In chronic severe hemolysis, folic acid deficiency usually results, with associated reticulocytopenia and thus more severe anemia. A daily dose of 1 mg of folic acid is needed by most patients.

—When thromboembolization occurs, patients often develop deep vein thrombosis or pulmonary embolism, which are treated with anticoagulants. Venography is avoided because of the possible development of leg ulcers. Distinguishing between pulmonary thrombosis/embolism and pneumonia is important because thromboembolization usually requires hospitalization for evaluation and treatment.

—Leg ulcers are often large and refractory to treatment. Skin grafting helps temporarily, but usually the small benefit does not warrant the time and discomfort involved. Frequent evaluation, elevation of the legs, and support stocking or elastic bandages are used.

—Hematuria is common in patients with sickle cell trait, sickle cell anemia, and sickle cell disease, lasting days to weeks, caused by medullary ischemia. Increased fluids help to maintain a high urine flow and thus prevent formation of clots that could obstruct the urine pathway.

—Priapism is common in Hb S and Hb C disease, often resulting in permanent impotence; if urologic intervention is proposed, it should be done within a few hours of the onset of the problem, and is often only temporarily helpful.

Preventive Measures
- Several large controlled studies show that treating patients with hydroxyurea decreases the incidence of painful crises in some patients with sickle cell anemia, and requires close monitoring by a hematologist throughout therapy; long-term side effects must be considered before beginning treatment with the drug.
- Sickle cell disorders cause lifelong chronic illness and frequent periods of crisis.
  —Pneumococcal vaccine is recommended for all patients.
  —Early signs of infection are treated promptly and vigorously.
- These patients are susceptible to narcotic addiction, and are generally not given to ambulatory patients.
- Folic acid is usually required, 1 mg/daily.
- All patients should be seen at least annually by an ophthalmologist.
- Incentive spirometry has proven to be of benefit for patients with pulmonary complications in pain crises.

Patient/Family Education
- A full explanation of the disease and its variants should be provided, in writing, to patients, including the nature of the condition, signs and symptoms, medical and nursing procedures usually required, and methods of prevention to allay symptoms, prevent infection, and maintain the patient's health at an optimal level.
- Health care professionals assigned to the patient must make themselves available all the time, or provide a backup system that is faultless.
- Sickle cell patients have frequent episodes of serious illness and may become dispirited and disabled to a large extent.
- A high-powered support system must be established early, including parents, the health care team, social workers, visiting nurses, and others involved in the care of the patient.
- Respite care for parents or spouses is often needed and should be provided.

Follow-up/Referral
- Besides the primary care provider, the health care should be continually under the supervision of a hematologist who consistently cares for the patient and is available for consultation whenever needed.
- The nature of sickle cell disease/anemia makes it mandatory that continuous monitoring occur to evaluate the patient's status on a daily or weekly basis, detect early signs of complications, and provide the support needed by the patient and the family.

COAGULATION DISORDERS

Coagulation disorders generate a solid fibrin clot from circulating soluble fibrinogen, which is the body's major defense against loss of blood, particularly from large vessels.
- The best screening tests to detect abnormalities of clotting are the partial thromboplastin time (PTT) and the prothrombin time (PT).
  - These tests measure different phases of the early parts of the coagulation process, but both measure the later phase of the process—the conversion of prothrombin to thrombin and the subsequent conversion of fibrinogen to fibrin.
- Clotting time is not a sensitive test for coagulation disorders.
- Patients who have a deficiency of one or more of the coagulation proteins are more likely to have extensive soft tissue bleeding or major hemorrhage in response to trauma than are patients with disorders of the vasculature or of blood platelets (petechiae are never a sign of abnormal coagulation).
- Hereditary disorders of coagulation are rare; it is unlikely that practitioners will encounter such patients because almost all of them are diagnosed in childhood and are treated by hematologists from the outset.
- Von Willebrand's disease is an inherited abnormality of hemostasis (autosomal dominant) in which there is a reduction in the concentration or structure of a protein, the von Willebrand's factor (VWF).
  - The course of the disease and the extent of laboratory abnormalities vary from one patient to another, but in general the hemorrhagic diathesis is milder than in hemophilia A.

- Acquired disorders of coagulation are more common than are congenital ones.
  - They are usually associated with multiple defects in hemostasis (Box 12-3), such as those seen in patients with disseminated intravascular coagulation (DIC), or in patients taking anticoagulant drugs such as Coumadin.

Acquired Coagulation Disorders
Disseminated Intravascular Coagulation
Definition
DIC is a grave coagulopathy resulting from the overstimulation of clotting and anticlotting processes in response to a disease or injury (e.g., septicemia, acute hypotension, poisonous snakebites, neoplasms, obstetric emergencies, severe trauma, extensive surgery, and hemorrhage). The primary disorder initiates generalized intravascular clotting, which in turn overstimulates fibrinolytic mechanisms; as a result, the initial hypercoagulability is followed by a deficiency in clotting factors with hypocoagulability and hemorrhage.

Risk Factors (see Definition)
Etiology/Cause (see Definition)
Pathogenesis
- DIC results from entrance into or generation within the blood of material with tissue factor activity, initiating coagulation.

BOX 12-3

Advice to Give Patients with a Disorder of Hemostasis

- Take only medication prescribed by the clinician; do not take aspirin or cold remedies; take Tylenol instead of aspirin for pain, colds, and so on.
- Do not drink alcoholic beverages.
- Avoid any activity that might expose you unnecessarily to trauma such as contact sports.
- Wear a bracelet prescribed by the clinician identifying you as a "bleeder" and giving the name of the disorder.
- Call your practitioner
  - If you experience any abnormal bleeding, including excessive menstrual bleeding
  - Before you visit the dentist
  - Before seeing any other clinician
  - If you are hospitalized for any reason without your clinician's knowledge

- DIC usually arises in one of the following four clinical circumstances:
  - Complications of obstetrics: abruptio placentae, saline-induced therapeutic abortion, retained dead fetus syndrome, the initial phase of amniotic fluid embolism—in these conditions, uterine material with tissue factor gains access to the maternal circulation.
  - Infection, particularly gram-negative organisms—gram-negative endotoxin causes generation of tissue factor activity on the plasma membrane of monocytes and endothelial cells.
  - Malignancy, particularly mucin-secreting adenocarcinomas of the pancreas and prostate, and acute promyelocytic leukemia in which hypergranular leukemic cells are thought to release material from their granules with tissue factor activity
  - Shock from any cause, probably because of the generation of tissue factor activity on monocytes and endothelial cells
- Less common causes of DIC are severe head trauma that breaks down the blood-brain barrier and allows exposure of blood to brain tissue with potent tissue factor activity; prostate surgery complications that allow prostatic material with tissue factor activity to enter the circulation; and venomous snake bites in which enzymes that activate factor X or prothrombin, or that directly convert fibrinogen to fibrin, enter the circulation.

Diagnosis

Signs and Symptoms

- Subacute DIC may be associated with thromboembolic complications of hypercoagulability, including venous thrombosis, thrombotic vegetations on the aortic heart valve, and arterial emboli arising from such vegetations; abnormal bleeding is uncommon.
- In acute cases, massive DIC, thrombocytopenia, and depletion of plasma clotting factors create a severe bleeding tendency that is made worse by secondary fibrinolysis (i.e., large amounts of fibrin degradation products form and interfere with platelet function and normal fibrin polymerization).

- When massive DIC is a complication of delivery or surgery that leaves raw surfaces, major hemorrhage results.
- When puncture sites from invasive procedures, such as arterial puncture for blood gas studies, bleed persistently, ecchymoses form at sites of parenteral injections, and serious GI bleeding may occur from erosion of gastric mucosa.
- Acute DIC may cause fibrin deposition in multiple small blood vessels.
- If secondary fibrinolysis fails to lyse the fibrin rapidly, hemorrhagic tissue necrosis may result.
  - The most vulnerable organ is the kidney, where fibrin deposition in the glomerular capillary bed may lead to acute renal failure, which is reversible if the necrosis is confined to the renal tubules (acute renal tubular necrosis) but is irreversible if the glomeruli are destroyed.
- Fibrin deposits in the small vessels of the fingers and toes may result in gangrene and loss of digits, and even limbs.

Laboratory Findings

- Laboratory data correlate with the severity of the disorder.
  - In subacute DIC, when thrombocytopenia is present, normal to slightly prolonged PT, short PTT, normal or moderately reduced fibrinogen level, and an increased level of fibrin degradation products are also present.
  - Acute, massive DIC produces a striking constellation of abnormalities.
    ~ Thrombocytopenia
    ~ A very small clot
    ~ A markedly prolonged PT and PTT because the plasma contains insufficient fibrinogen to trigger the end point of coagulation instruments, and test results are often reported as more than some value (e.g., 200 seconds), which is the interval before the automated instrument shifts to the next sample in the machine
    ~ A markedly reduced plasma fibrinogen concentration
    ~ A positive plasma protamine paracoagulation test for fibrin monomer and a very high level of plasma D-dimer

and fibrin degradation products in the serum

~ Specific clotting factor assays show low levels of multiple clotting factors, particularly factors V and VIII, which are inactivated because activated protein C is generated during DIC.

~ Massive hepatic necrosis can produce laboratory abnormalities resembling acute DIC.

Treatment

- Immediately identify and correct the underlying cause: give broad-spectrum antibiotics in suspected gram-negative infection and evacuate the uterus in abruptio placentae.
- Once the cause of disseminated intravenous coagulation, acquired (DICA) is treated, the DIC itself should subside quickly.
- Replacement therapy may be required: platelet concentrates to correct thrombocytopenia and as a source of factor V in platelets.
- Fresh frozen plasma to increase levels of factor V and other clotting factors and as a source of antithrombin III, which may be depleted secondary to DIC.
- Heparin may be given under specific circumstances.
- **Heparin should never be used in DIC secondary to head injury or when central nervous system (CNS) bleeding for any other reason is suspected.**
- If DIC is associated with malignancy, immediate treatment of the underlying cause is not possible, and use of anticoagulants to prevent DIC is indicated.

Prognosis

- Patients may be acutely ill and in shock from bleeding.
- Recovery time depends on the acuity of the DIC and on the underlying cause.
- Most patients must be hospitalized at the time of onset and treated in the intensive care unit.

Patient/Family Education

- In most instances, DIC occurs so quickly that the clinician cannot take the time to explain to the family what is happening to the patient; as soon as possible, the event can be explained in detail, within the extent of the patient's and family's understanding.
- Treatment of DIC is the essential first step, with treatment of the underlying cause occurring simultaneously or as soon as the patient's condition is stable.

Follow-up/Referral

- Patients are generally hospitalized to treat the acute stage of DIC and to diagnose and treat the cause, which requires variable lengths of time and therapy.
- Stabilized patients are then followed by the practitioner in the outpatient setting.

LEUKEMIAS
Acute Leukemia

Definition
Acute leukemia is a malignancy of the hematopoietic progenitor cell.

Incidence

- Acute lymphoblastic leukemia (ALL) makes up 80% of acute leukemias of childhood, with peak incidence between ages 3 and 7.
  —ALL causes 20% of adult acute leukemias.

Classification

- Acute leukemia is classified as either ALL or acute myelogenous leukemia (AML), also called acute nonlymphocytic leukemia (ANLL).
  —ALL is further classified by immunologic phenotype.
    ~ Common
    ~ Early B lineage
    ~ T cell
  —AML is further classified according to morphology and histochemistry.
    ~ Acute undifferentiated leukemia (M0)
    ~ Acute myeloblastic leukemia (M1)
    ~ Acute myeloblastic leukemia with differentiation (M2)
    ~ Acute promyelocytic leukemia (M3)
    ~ Acute myelomonocytic leukemia (M4)
    ~ Acute monoblastic leukemia (M5)
    ~ Erythroleukemia (M6)
    ~ Megakaryoblastic leukemia (M7)

Etiology

- In most cases, no definitive cause is found.
- Some chemotherapeutic agents, especially procarbazine, melphalan, other alkylating agents, and etoposide, may cause leukemia.
- Leukemias that develop after toxin or chemotherapy exposure often develop from a myelodysplastic prodrome associated with abnormalities in chromosomes 5 and 7.

Pathophysiology

- Malignant cells lose their ability to mature and differentiate.
  —These cells proliferate uncontrollably, replacing normal bone marrow elements.

Diagnosis

Signs and Symptoms

- Most of the clinical findings are due to replacement of normal bone marrow elements by malignant cells.
- Illness of days to weeks is reported by many patients.
- Bleeding due to thrombocytopenia occurs in skin and mucosal surfaces (e.g., bruising, gingivitis, epistaxis, menorrhagia).
- More widespread bleeding occurs in patients with DIC, seen in promyelocytic leukemia and monocytic leukemia.
- Infection results from neutropenia; risk of infection increases as neutrophils fall below $500/\mu l$.
  —Most common pathogens are gram-negative bacteria (e.g., *Escherichia coli*, *Klebsiella* species, *Pseudomonas* species) or fungi (*Candida* and *Aspergillus* species).
  —Infections present as cellulitis, pneumonia, and perirectal abscess.
  —Septicemia in those with severe neutropenia can cause death within a few hours without rapid administration of appropriate antibiotics.
- Gum hyperplasia/hypertrophy
- Bone and joint pain
- On presentation, patients are pale with numerous petechiae and signs of infection (e.g., stomatitis, gum hypertrophy in those with monocytic leukemia).

Laboratory Findings

- Hyperleukocytosis of markedly elevated circulating blasts of more than $200,000/\mu l$.

- The hallmark of acute leukemia is the combination of pancytopenia with circulating blasts.
  —Blasts may not be present in the peripheral smear of up to 10% of patients.
  —Patients with AML may have granules visible in the blast cells.
- Bone marrow is hypercellular, dominated by blasts.
  —An increase of at least 30% of blast cells is required to make a diagnosis of acute leukemia.
- The Auer rod, an eosinophilic needle-like inclusion body in the cytoplasm, is pathognomonic of AML.
- About 95% of patients with ALL show terminal deoxynucleotidyl transferase (TdT).
- Hyperuricemia is often present.
- If DIC is present, fibrinogen level is decreased, prothrombin time is prolonged, and fibrin degradation products or fibrin D-dimers are present.
- Patients with acute lymphoblastic leukemia, particularly T cell, may have a mediastinal mass on chest x-ray.

Differential Diagnosis

- AML must be distinguished from other myeloproliferative disorders, chronic myelogenous leukemia, and myelodysplastic syndromes.
- Acute leukemia resembles a left-shifted bone marrow recovering from a previous toxic insult.
  —If diagnosis is uncertain, a repeat bone marrow study is done in several days to assess whether maturation is occurring.
- ALL is distinguished from other lymphocytic leukemias, lymphomas, and hairy cell leukemia.
  —May also be confused with atypical lymphocytosis of mononucleosis

Treatment

- Younger patients are treated with the goal of cure by steps.
  —Complete remission (normal peripheral blood with resolution of cytopenias)
  —Normal bone marrow with no excess blasts
  —Normal clinical status

- AML is treated first with intensive combination chemotherapy.
  —Daunorubicin and cytarabine
    ~ Effective treatment results in aplasia of bone marrow, which takes 2 to 3 weeks to recover.
  —During this time, intensive supportive care is given.
    ~ Transfusion
    ~ Antibiotic therapy
  —Once complete remission has occurred, postremission therapy is instituted; options are
    ~ Repeated intensive chemotherapy
    ~ High-dose chemoradiotherapy with allogeneic BMT
    ~ High-dose chemotherapy with autologous BMT
- Notable progress has been made in treating acute promyelocytic leukemia (M3):
  —Addition of all-*trans* retinoic acid to initial chemotherapy: improves results of initial treatment and long-term survival
  —Arsenic trioxide can result in remission in patients who have become resistant to other forms of therapy.
- ALL initial treatment
  —Combination chemotherapy with daunorubicin, vincristine, prednisone, asparaginase
  —After complete remission, treatment includes the following:
    ~ CNS prophylaxis to prevent development of meningeal sequestration of leukemic cells.
  —Further treatment is either chemotherapy alone or high-dose chemotherapy plus BMT.

Prognosis
- About 70% to 80% of adults under age 60 with AML achieve complete remission.
  —High-dose postremission chemotherapy (cytarabine) results in cure in 30% to 40%.
- Allogeneic BMT in younger adults with human leukocyte antigen (HLA)-matched siblings is curative in 60% of patients.
- Autologous BMT (new therapy) may cure between 50% and 70% of patients.
- Older adults with AML have complete remission about 50% of the time.

  —Selected patients may be treated with intensive chemotherapy with intent to cure.
- About 90% of adults with ALL achieve complete remission.
  —After postremission chemotherapy, cure occurs in 30% to 50%.
- Children with ALL achieve complete remission in 95% and cure in 60% to 70%.
- If leukemia recurs after initial chemotherapy, BMT is the only curative option.
  —Allogeneic BMT is successful in 30% to 40% of cases for those under age 60.
  —Autologous BMT is curative in 30% to 50% of patients after a second remission is achieved.

Patient/Family Education
- Detailed information is provided about the nature of the type of leukemia, its possible cause, treatment, and expected outcome.
- Each stage of treatment is explained in detail before it is begun.
- Patient and family members require intensive support and encouragement throughout.

Follow-up/Referral
- These patients are often hospitalized for periods of time and followed by specialists in leukemia.
- After remission, patients may be able to be home for brief periods before undergoing second-stage therapy.
- Treatment time is variable, but patients often require care and follow-up for several years.

CHRONIC LEUKEMIA
Chronic Lymphocytic Leukemia

Definition
Chronic lymphocytic leukemia (CLL) is a clonal malignancy of B lymphocytes (rarely T lymphocytes). The disease is usually indolent, with slowly progressive accumulation of long-lived small lymphocytes, which are immunoincompetent and respond poorly to antigenic stimulation.

Risk Factors
- About 75% of cases are diagnosed in patients over 65 years old.
- CLL is twice as common in men.

Etiology/Cause
- The cause of CLL is unknown.
- Some cases appear to be familial.
- CLL is rare in Japan and China and does not appear to increase among Japanese expatriates in the United States, which suggests a genetic factor.

Pathogenesis
- Lymphocyte accumulation probably begins in the bone marrow and spreads to lymph nodes and other lymphoid tissue.
- Splenomegaly may occur.
- Late in the disease, abnormal hematopoiesis results in anemia, neutropenia, thrombocytopenia, and decreased immunoglobulin production.
- Some patients develop hypogammaglobulinemia and impaired antibody response, which may be related to increased T-suppressor cell activity.
- Patients become susceptible to autoimmune diseases characterized by immunohemolytic anemias (usually Coombs' test positive) or thrombocytopenia.

Diagnosis
Signs and Symptoms
- The Rai staging system is used for prognosis.
  - Stage 0: lymphocytosis only
  - Stage I: lymphocytosis plus lymphadenopathy
  - Stage II: organomegaly
  - Stage III: anemia
  - Stage IV: thrombocytopenia
- Onset is usually insidious, but some patients have a rapidly progressive form, with larger, less mature lymphocytes ("prolymphocytic" leukemia).
  - In 5% to 10% of patients, CLL may be complicated by autoimmune hemolytic anemia or autoimmune thrombocytopenia.
  - In 5% of cases, the systemic disease remains stable, but an isolated lymph node will become an aggressive large cell lymphoma **(Richter's syndrome)**.
- The diagnosis is often made from incidental blood tests or during evaluation of asymptomatic lymphadenopathy.

- Symptomatic patients complain of the following:
  - Fatigue
  - Anorexia
  - Weight loss
  - Dyspnea on exertion
  - Sense of abdominal fullness (due to enlarging spleen or palpable nodes)
- Clinical signs and symptoms include the following:
  - Immunosuppression
  - Bone marrow failure
  - Organ infiltration with lymphocytes
  - General lymphadenopathy (80%)
  - Minimal-to-moderate hepatomegaly and splenomegaly (50%)
  - Later, skin pallor occurs due to anemia.
  - Infections: bacterial, viral, and fungal

Laboratory Findings
- The hallmark of CLL is sustained, absolute lymphocytosis ($>5000/\mu l$) and increased lymphocytes ($>30\%$) in the bone marrow.
- At diagnosis, moderate anemia and thrombocytopenia are due to bone marrow infiltration (10%), splenomegaly, or immunohemolytic anemia.

Treatment
- Patients may be asymptomatic for years.
- Therapy is indicated only when active progression or symptoms occur.
- Supportive care
  - Transfusion of packed RBCs for anemia
  - Platelet transfusion for bleeding associated with thrombocytopenia: antimicrobials for bacterial, fungal, or viral infections
  - Herpes zoster (dermatomic)
- Chemotherapy
- Corticosteroids
- Radiotherapy
- Alkylating drugs (e.g., chlorambucil) alone or with corticosteroids are the usual therapy for B-cell CLL
- Fludarabine is more effective
- For hairy cell leukemia
  - Interferon-α (IFN-α)
  - Deoxycoformycin
  - 2-Chlorodeoxyadenosine

- Those with prolymphocytic leukemia and lymphoma leukemia require multidrug chemotherapy; response is only partial.
- Treatment has not been proven to prolong survival.
- *Overtreatment is more dangerous than undertreatment.*

Prognosis
- The median survival of patients with B-cell CLL or its complications is about 10 years.
- A patients in stage 0-II at diagnosis may survive 5 to 20 years without treatment.
- A patient in stage III or IV is more likely to die within 3 to 4 years.
- Progression of bone marrow failure is usually associated with short survival.

Patient/Family Education
- As with other diseases, the patient and family should be instructed about the nature, cause, course, treatment, and expected outcomes of therapy.
- Specific medications and procedures should be explained as to reason for, what to expect, and signs and symptoms that require a call to the clinician.

Follow-up/Referral
- Most symptomatic patients are followed very closely and are frequently hospitalized between remissions or when they develop infections.
- All patients are cared for by a team headed by an oncologist.
- Reassurance and strong support for the patient from both family members and the health care team is essential throughout.

Chronic Myelogenous Leukemia

Definition
Chronic myelogenous leukemia (CML) is a myeloproliferative disorder caused by malignant transformation of a pluripotent stem cell, characterized clinically by striking overproduction of myeloid cells. The disorder formerly known as Philadelphia chromosome-negative CML is now recognized as chronic myelomonocytic leukemia (CMML), a subtype of myelodysplasia.

Risk Factors
- Older age; median age at diagnosis is 42 years

Etiology/Cause
- CML is associated with a characteristic chromosomal abnormality, the Philadelphia chromosome.
  —This chromosome is a reciprocal translocation between the long arms of chromosomes 9 and 22.

Pathogenesis
- A large portion of chromosome 22q is translocated to 9q, and a smaller piece of 9q is moved to 22q.
  —The part of 9q that is translocated contains *abl*, a proto-oncogene and the cellular homolog of the Abelson murine leukemia virus.
  —The *abl* gene goes to a specific site on 22q, the break point cluster (bcr).
  —The fusion gene *bcr-abl* produces a new protein that differs from the normal transcript of the *abl* gene; it has tyrosine kinase activity, which is a characteristic activity of transforming genes.
    ~ The pathogenicity of the *bcr-abl* gene is shown when the gene is introduced into mice models, which then develop leukemia.

Diagnosis
Signs and Symptoms
- Strikingly elevated WBC count
- Markedly left-shifted myeloid series, with a low percentage of promyelocytes and blasts
- Presence of Philadelphia chromosome or *bcr-abl* gene
- At diagnosis, the Philadelphia chromosome-positive clone dominates and often is the only one seen.
- A normal clone is present and is expressed either in vivo after some types of therapy or in vitro in long-term bone marrow cultures.
- Fatigue
- Night sweats
- Low-grade fever due to the hypermetabolic state caused by overproduction of WBCs.
- Sensation of abdominal fullness due to splenomegaly.

- Rarely, a clinical syndrome related to leukostasis occurs in those with a WBC count of 500,000/μl
  - Blurred vision
  - Respiratory distress
  - Priapism
- Enlarged spleen, often markedly enlarged
- Sternal tenderness due to marrow overexpansion
- In rapidly progressive disease
  - Fever, but no infection
  - Bone pain
  - Splenomegaly
- In blast crisis
  - Bleeding
  - Infection due to bone marrow failure

Laboratory Findings

- The hallmark of CML is the markedly elevated WBC count, usually at least 150,000/μl at diagnosis.
- Peripheral blood shows characteristic changes
  - The myeloid series is left-shifted; mature forms dominate and cells present proportionately to their degree of maturation.
  - Blasts are usually <5%.
  - RBC morphology is normal.
  - Platelet count may be normal or elevated, sometimes strikingly high.
- Bone marrow is hypercellular, with left-shifted myelopoiesis.
- The leukocyte alkaline phosphatase score is almost always low, a sign of abnormalities in neutrophils.
- The vitamin B_{12} level is often elevated due to increased secretion of transcobalamin III.
- Uric acid levels may be high.
- The Philadelphia chromosome may be seen in either peripheral blood or bone marrow.
- The *bcr-abl* gene is usually seen in peripheral blood, using molecular techniques with progression to the accelerated and blast phases of disease.
  - Progressive anemia and thrombocytopenia occur.
  - The proportion of blasts in blood and bone marrow increases.
    - ~ The blast phase of CML is diagnosed when blasts make up >30% of bone marrow cells.

Differential Diagnosis

- Reactive leukocytosis associated with infection; in these patients, the WBC count is usually <50,000/μl.
- Myeloproliferative disease, which is characterized by normal HCT, normal RBC morphology, and nucleated RBCs, is rare or absent.

Treatment

- Only rarely when symptoms of extreme hyperleukocytosis occur (priapism, respiratory distress, blurred vision, altered mental state) is treatment instituted with emergency leukophoresis, together with myelosuppressive therapy.
- Recombinant IFN-α has replaced hydroxyurea as the treatment of choice for CML.
  - IFN prolongs the chronic phase of CML and prolongs survival.
  - It is given to all patients who are not going directly to allogeneic BMT.
  - IFN together with low-dose cytarabine is more effective than IFN alone for most patients.
  - The disadvantages of IFN are that it is given SC, is expensive and has side effects (fatigue, myalgias, anorexia) that can impair quality of life.
  - The best results are in giving the full dose of IFN—5×10^6 units/m^2/day for 5 years, then reduced to a lower dose.
    - ~ Many patients cannot tolerate this level of therapy due to side effects.
    - ~ The maximum dose tolerated is determined and continued for at least 9 months.
  - The survival benefit of IFN therapy is limited to those who achieve a cytogenetic response (i.e., the appearance of Philadelphia-negative clones); this takes between 6 and 18 months to assess.
- The only cure is allogeneic BMT.
  - It is available to those <60 years of age who have HLA-matched siblings.
  - About 60% of adults have long-term disease-free survival after BMT.
    - ~ Best results occur when patients have a BMT within 1 year of diagnosis, with 70% to 80% cure rate.

- Young patients with HLA-matched siblings are encouraged to have BMT.
  - If HLA-matched siblings are not available, registered bone marrow donors may be found, but the success rate is not as good as with matched siblings (40% to 60%), which is usually acceptable to those suffering from this fatal disease.
- The blast form of CML is very difficult to treat.
  - Therapy with daunorubicin, vincristine, and prednisone results in remission, usually short, in 70% of cases.

Prognosis
- Median survival is 3 to 4 years.
- Once the disease has reached the accelerated or blast phase, survival is measured in months.
- About 60% of young adults who receive successful allogeneic BMT appear to be cured.
- Patients given IFN-α who achieve a complete cytogenetic response (10%) have an excellent prognosis, with 5-year survival of over 90%.
  - These patients do not do better than those on hydroxyurea.
- Those who achieve a major response (<35% Philadelphia-negative clones) have a 5-year survival rate of over 60%.

LYMPHOMAS
Hodgkin's Disease

Definition
Lymphoma is characterized by localized or disseminated malignant proliferation of tumor cells arising from the lymphoreticular system, primarily involving lymph node tissue and the bone marrow. This group of cancers is also characterized by Reed-Sternberg cells in a reactive cellular background.

Classification
- Hodgkin's disease has four histopathologic subtypes.
  - Lymphocyte-predominant
  - Nodular sclerosis
  - Mixed cellularity
  - Lymphocyte-depleted

Incidence
- A bimodal age distribution occurs, with one peak in those in their twenties and a second peak in those over 50, although the older population may have acquired the disease earlier because most are intermediate-grade non-Hodgkin's lymphomas (NHL).
- In the United States, 6000 to 7000 new cases are diagnosed every year.
- Male/female ratio is 1.4:1

Etiology
- The cause is unknown, but these patients appear to have a genetic susceptibility, seen in twin studies, and environmental associations (e.g., occupation such as woodworkers, Epstein-Barr virus infection, HIV infection).

Diagnosis
Signs and Symptoms
- Painless lymphadenopathy
- Constitutional symptoms
  - Intense pruritus
  - Fever: may be Pel-Ebstein fever with a few days of high fever alternating with a few days to several weeks of normal or subnormal temperature
  - Night sweats
  - Weight loss
- Immediate pain may occur in diseased areas after drinking alcohol, which may lead to early diagnosis.
- Definitive diagnosis is made by lymph node biopsy that shows Reed-Sternberg cells in a characteristic histologic setting.

Laboratory Findings
- Slight-to-moderate polymorphonuclear leukocytosis may be present.
- Lymphocytopenia may occur early and become pronounced in advanced disease.
- Eosinophilia is present in 20% of patients.
- Microcytic anemia occurs in advanced disease due to defective iron reutilization.
  - Low serum iron
  - Low iron-binding capacity
  - Increased bone marrow iron
- Hypersplenism may occur.
- Elevated serum alkaline phosphatase levels may indicate bone marrow or liver involvement, or both.

- Increases in leukocyte alkaline phosphatase, serum haptoglobin, erythrocyte sedimentation rate (ESR), serum copper, and other acute-phase reactants reflect active disease.

Treatment
- Radiation therapy is used initially for those with low-risk stage IA and IIA disease.
- Most patients, including those with stage IIIB and IV disease, are treated with combination chemotherapy using doxorubicin, bleomycin, vincristine, and dacarbazine (ABVD).
    - This is more effective and less toxic than the previous regimen of mechlorethamine, vincristine, procarbazine, and prednisone (MOPP).
    - With ABVD, there is less sterility and less secondary leukemia.
- New, shorter and more intensive regimens show promising results and may replace ABVD in advanced disease.

Prognosis
- Prognosis of patients with stage IA or IIA disease treated by radiotherapy is excellent, with 10-year survival rates greater than 80%.
- Patients with disseminated disease (IIIB, IV) have 5-year survival rates of 50% to 60%.
- Poorer results are true for patients who are older, have bulky disease, and those with lymphocyte depletion or mixed cellularity by histologic examination.
- Those who have recurrence of disease after initial radiotherapy may still be curable with chemotherapy.
    - The treatment of choice in these patients is high-dose chemotherapy with autologous stem cell transplantation, which affords a 35% to 50% chance of cure in patients in whom the disease remains chemotherapy-sensitive.

Patient/Family Education
- Both patient and family members need to understand lymphoma: its cause, course, treatment, and expected outcomes.
- Long-term therapy that often causes unpleasant physical symptoms is difficult for both patients and families.

- Each step in the therapeutic plan should be explained before beginning so that the patient knows what to expect.
- Counseling by an experienced psychologist or psychiatrist may prove beneficial.
- Day-to-day support and encouragement are essential to help the patient through the therapeutic steps.

Follow-up/Referral
- Usually, these patients are followed closely, once the diagnosis is established and symptoms appear.
- Hospitalization may be required from time to time; when the patient is at home, he or she requires gentle and compassionate care from family members.

Non-Hodgkin's Lymphoma
Definition
NHL is a malignant monoclonal proliferation of lymphoid cells in sites of the immune system, including lymph nodes, bone marrow, spleen, liver, and GI tract.

Incidence
- This type of lymphoma occurs more often than Hodgkin's disease.
- In the United States, about 50,000 new cases are diagnosed each year in all age groups.
- Incidence increases with age.
- The course of NHL varies from indolent to rapidly fatal.
- A leukemia-like picture develops in 50% of children and 20% of adults.
- Incidence increases in HIV patients.

Etiology (Box 12-4)
- The cause is unknown, but experimental evidence points to a viral cause for some lymphomas.
- Burkitt's lymphoma, the type most carefully studied to date, has a characteristic cytogenetic abnormality of translocation between the long arms of chromosomes 8 and 14.
    - The proto-oncogene *c-myc* is translocated from its normal position on chromosome 8 to the heavy chain locus on chromosome 14.

BOX 12-4

Classification of Lymphomas

LOW-GRADE
Small lymphocytic
Small lymphocytic, plasmacytoid
Follicular small cleaved cell
Follicular mixed cell

INTERMEDIATE-GRADE
Follicular large cell
Diffuse small cleaved cell
Diffuse mixed cell
Diffuse large cell

HIGH-GRADE
Immunoblastic
Small noncleaved (Burkitt's)
Small noncleaved (non-Burkitt's)
Lymphoblastic
True histiocytic

OTHER
Cutaneous T cell (mycosis fungoides)
Adult T-cell leukemia-lymphoma
Mantle cell
Marginal zone (MALT)
Peripheral T cell
Anaplastic large cell

From Linker CA: Blood. In Tierney LM, McPhee SJ, Papadakis MA, eds: *Current medical diagnosis & treatment 2000,* New York, 2000, Lange Medical Books/McGraw-Hill, p 530.

~ It is likely that overexpression of *c-myc*, in its new anomalous position, is related to malignant transformation.

Diagnosis

Signs and Symptoms
- Indolent lymphoma
  —Often widely disseminated at time of diagnosis, with bone marrow involvement
  —Painless lymphadenopathy, single or multiple
- Intermediate or high-grade
  —Adenopathy
  —Systemic signs/symptoms
    ~ Fever
    ~ Night sweats
    ~ Weight loss
- Burkitt's lymphoma
  —Abdominal pain or fullness (typical predilection)
- Once the diagnosis is established, the patient is staged.
  —Chest x-ray
    ~ May show a mediastinal mass in lymphoblastic lymphoma
  —Computed tomography (CT) scan of abdomen and pelvis
  —Biopsy of bone marrow
  —Lumbar puncture in those with high-risk morphology
    ~ Meninges may be involved, and spinal fluid may contain malignant cells.

Laboratory Findings
- Tissue (lymph node) biopsy establishes the definitive diagnosis.
- Peripheral blood is usually normal.
  —Serum LDH is a useful prognostic marker; now used in risk stratification of treatment.
  —Some patients may present in the "leukemic" phase.
    ~ Differentiating leukemia and lymphoma is of questionable value because the malignant cells have the same characteristics.
- Bone marrow involvement is seen in paratrabecular lymphoid aggregates.

Treatment
- Indolent lymphomas are generally not curable and are treated palliatively.
- Treating patients with lymphoma is difficult because of poor tolerance of aggressive chemotherapy.
  —Myeloid growth factors to reduce neutropenic complications may improve outcomes.
- No treatment is required for asymptomatic patients.
  —Within 1 to 3 years, the disease progresses and requires treatment.
- Combination chemotherapy using ABVD is more effective and less toxic than previous combination drugs; there is less sterility and less secondary leukemia.

- New shorter, more intensive regimens are promising, and may replace ABVD in advanced disease.
- A monoclonal antibody directed against the B-cell surface antigen CD20 (rituximab) is effective in follicular lymphoma that recurs after initial treatment, with response rates of 50% and average duration of response of 1 year.
- Selected younger patients with more aggressive or resistant disease require BMT.
- Those with localized disease are usually given local radiation therapy.
- The cause of low-grade mucosa-associated lymphoid tissue (MALT) lymphomas is now believed to be *Helicobacter pylori* infection; disease confined to the stomach and treated with appropriate antibiotic therapy responds completely.
- Those with intermediate and high-grade lymphomas are treated with curative intent.
  —The mainstay is combination chemotherapy: cyclophosphamide, doxorubicin, vincristine, and prednisone (CHOP).
- Those with high-risk disease are treated more aggressively, with autologous stem cell transplantation; this therapy is preferred for those who relapse after initial chemotherapy.
- Those with special forms of lymphoma (e.g., Burkitt's lymphoma) are treated with intensive regimens tailored to this type.
- The average survival of patients with indolent lymphomas is 6 to 8 years.
- These diseases become refractory to chemotherapy in time, usually when a more aggressive form is developing.

Prognosis
- The International Prognosis Index categorizes those with intermediate grade lymphoma according to risk groups: over age 60, elevated serum LDH, advanced disease (stage III or IV), and poor performance status.
  —With no or 1 risk factor: complete response rates (80%) to standard chemotherapy; most responses are long-term (80%)
  —With 2 risk factors: 70% complete response rate; 70% are long-term

—With 3 or more risk factors: lower response rate and poor survival with standard regimens; more aggressive forms of therapy are needed
  ~ Early high-dose therapy and autologous stem cell transplantation improve the outcome.
- For patients who relapse after initial chemotherapy, treatment and outcomes depend on whether the disease is still sensitive to chemotherapy.
  —If it is, autologous transplantation offers a 50% chance of long-term survival in older patients; the use of myeloid growth factors to reduce neutropenic complications may improve outcomes.

Patient/Family Education
- As with other hematologic diseases, the patient and family need to know the nature, cause, course, treatment, and expected outcomes.
- In many cases, specific information is not possible because of variations in length of treatment, effects of treatment, and factors that affect outcomes such as age, physical status, mental attitude, and degree of available support.
- The important factor is to maintain hope for the patient and family members.

Follow-up/Referral
- Many of these patients, after diagnosis and appearance of signs and symptoms, will need to undergo lengthy treatment, often with remissions and set-backs of various kinds.
- Having at least one stable member of the health care team—the nurse practitioner—to be the "constant" in the patient's life is essential.
- Specialists in hematology, oncology, and lymphoma will be consulted throughout the course of the patient's treatment.

BIBLIOGRAPHY
Beers MH, Berkow R: Hematology. In Beers MH, Burkow R, eds: *The Merck manual of diagnosis and therapy,* ed 17, Whitehouse Station, NJ, 1999, Merck Research Laboratories, p 847.

Linker CA: Blood: Anemias, leukemias, disorders of hemostasis. In Tierney LM, McPhee SJ, Papadakis MA, eds: *Current medical diagnosis & treatment 2000*, New York, 2000, Lange Medical Books/McGraw-Hill, pp 499-552.

Waterbury L: Anemia. In Barker LR, Burton JR, Zieve PD, eds: *Principles of ambulatory medicine*, ed 5, Baltimore, 1999, Williams & Wilkins, pp 619-633.

Waterbury L, Zieve PD: Selected illnesses affecting lymphocytes: mononucleosis, chronic lymphocytic leukemia, and the undiagnosed patient with lymphadenopathy. In Barker LR, Burton JR, Zieve PD, eds: *Principles of ambulatory medicine*, ed 5, Baltimore, 1999, Williams & Wilkins, pp 651-676.

Zieve PD: Disorders of hemostasis. In Barker LR, Burton JR, Zieve PD, eds: *Principles of ambulatory medicine*, ed 5, Baltimore, 1999, Williams & Wilkins, pp 634-641.

Zieve PD, Waterbury L: Thromboembolic disease. In Barker LR, Burton JR, Zieve PD, eds: *Principles of ambulatory medicine*, ed 5, Baltimore, 1999, Williams & Wilkins, pp 642-650.

REVIEW QUESTIONS

1. All but one of the following are classifications of causes of anemias. The one group that is NOT a valid classification is:
   a. Blood loss
   b. Blood dyscrasias
   c. Deficient erythropoiesis
   d. Excessive hemolysis

2. Classification of anemia by mean corpuscular volume includes all but one of the following. Which one is NOT a classification?
   a. Normocytic
   b. Microcytic
   c. Mixed cell size
   d. Macrocytic

3. The most common cause of iron deficiency anemia is:
   a. Low intake of iron
   b. Bone marrow deficit
   c. Decreased iron stores
   d. Blood loss (chronic or acute)

4. Total body iron for women is:
   a. 25 mg/kg
   b. 30 mg/kg
   c. 35 mg/kg
   d. 50 mg/kg

5. Iron is deposited as:
   a. Iron per se
   b. Ferritin
   c. Hemoglobin
   d. Nonheme iron

6. The presence of mild anemia:
   a. Requires no further evaluation
   b. Is encountered frequently in ambulatory patients
   c. Is not related to symptoms of other diseases
   d. Indicates an underlying disorder

7. In iron deficiency anemia, the total iron-binding capacity:
   a. Remains the same
   b. Increases
   c. Decreases
   d. Is unrelated to iron deficiency anemia

8. Anemia of chronic disease is seen in:
   a. Rheumatoid arthritis
   b. Mild skin infections
   c. Gingival inflammation
   d. Chronic diseases only

9. Patients undergoing hemodialysis lose:
   a. Iron
   b. Folate
   c. Both iron and folate
   d. Potassium

10. The thalassemia anemias occur because of:
    a. Defective hemoglobin synthesis
    b. Ineffective erythropoiesis
    c. Loss of hemoglobin due to genetic factors
    d. Both a and b

11. Diagnosis of thalassemia is by:
    a. Quantitative hemoglobin studies
    b. Bone marrow studies
    c. Total iron-binding capacity
    d. Serum ferritin

12. Treatment of α- and β-thalassemia minor is:
    a. Iron replacement therapy
    b. Bone marrow transplantation
    c. Vitamin B_{12} injections every month
    d. Not required; patients are clinically normal

13. Liver vitamin B_{12} stores are sufficient to supply the body's needs for:
    a. 6 to 12 months
    b. 1 to 2 years
    c. 2 to 3 years
    d. 3 to 5 years

14. The usual dose of vitamin B_{12} therapy is:
    a. 250 μg IM every day
    b. 500 μg IM two to four times/week
    c. 1000 μg IM two to four times/week
    d. 1500 μg IM two to four times/week

15. Inadequate amounts of folate ingested during pregnancy result in:
    a. Neural tube defects
    b. Severe vision and hearing deficits
    c. Premature labor
    d. Cardiopulmonary defects

16. Sickle cell disease (Hb S) affects _____%
    of the black population in the United States.
    a. 0.1
    b. 0.15
    c. 0.2
    d. 0.25

17. In a married couple, if both partners have the sickle cell trait, the chance of their offspring having sickle cell disease is:
    a. 10%
    b. 15%
    c. 25%
    d. 50%

18. Patients with sickle cell disease who experience a thrombotic crisis are treated with:
    a. Hydration and narcotics
    b. Hydration alone
    c. Narcotics alone
    d. Blood transfusion

19. Disseminated intravascular coagulation is a very serious coagulopathy caused by overstimulation of:
    a. Clotting processes
    b. Anticlotting processes
    c. Both clotting and anticlotting processes
    d. Platelets

20. Acute leukemia is a malignancy of:
    a. Bone marrow
    b. Hematopoietic progenitor cell
    c. Lymph nodes, spleen, and liver
    d. Gastrointestinal mucosa

21. Most of the clinical findings in patients with leukemia are due to:
    a. Lymphadenopathy
    b. Splenomegaly
    c. Replacement of normal bone marrow by malignant cells
    d. Bleeding due to thrombocytopenia

22. A blast cell is:
    a. Any immature cell (e.g., erythroblast, lymphoblast)
    b. A cell capable of destroying tissue
    c. A cell capable of blastic transformation
    d. A lymphoid cell

23. Most patients with acute leukemia are first treated with:
    a. Combination chemotherapy
    b. Radiation therapy
    c. Bone marrow transplantation
    d. High-dose chemotherapy

24. Chronic lymphocytic leukemia is:
    a. A clonal malignancy of T lymphocytes
    b. A clonal malignancy of B lymphocytes
    c. Usually rapidly progressive
    d. Seen primarily in young people

25. The average survival of patients with chronic lymphocytic leukemia is:
    a. 2 years
    b. 5 years
    c. 7 years
    d. 10 years

26. Chronic myelogenous leukemia is characterized by:
    a. The Philadelphia chromosome
    b. Immunosuppression
    c. Infections—bacterial, viral, fungal
    d. Infiltration of organs with lymphoid cells

27. The hallmark sign in chronic myelogenous leukemia is:
    a. Strikingly elevated lymphoid cells
    b. Strikingly elevated white blood cell count
    c. Strikingly elevated red blood cell count
    d. Splenomegaly and hepatomegaly

28. The only cure for chronic myelogenous leukemia is:
    a. Autologous bone marrow transplantation
    b. Allogeneic bone marrow transplantation
    c. Blood transfusions every week
    d. Interferon therapy

29. The incidence of Hodgkin's disease is characterized by:
    a. Occurring only in young people
    b. Occurring only in those over 70
    c. A bimodal age distribution: those in their twenties and those over 50
    d. Identification of over 20,000 new cases every year

30. Non-Hodgkin's lymphoma is:
    a. A relatively rare disease
    b. Divided into five classifications
    c. Characterized by painless lymphadenopathy
    d. Diagnosed by peripheral blood smear

13

Gynecologic Disorders

GYNECOLOGIC DISORDERS
Premenstrual Syndrome

Definition
Premenstrual syndrome (PMS) is a recurrent, variable cluster of physical and psychologic symptoms that occur during the 7 to 14 days before the onset of menses and abate when menstruation begins.

Incidence
- PMS affects about one third of all premenopausal women between the ages of 25 and 40.
- In about 10% of women, the symptoms are severe.

Diagnosis
Signs and Symptoms
- Not all symptoms occur every month in every patient.
  —Bloating
  —Ankle edema
  —Breast pain
  —Weight gain, or feeling of weight gain
  —Skin disturbances (e.g., flushing, rash, itching)
  —Irritability
  —Aggressiveness
  —Inability to concentrate
  —Depression
  —Food cravings
  —Lethargy
  —Headache
  —Change in libido

Pathogenesis
- Uncertain
  —Psychosocial factors may contribute.

Treatment
- Gonadotropin-releasing hormone (GnRH) agonist therapy, which suppresses ovarian function, results in decreased symptoms.
- Provide reassurance and support.
- Careful evaluation of the patient
- Have the patient keep a personal daily journal for several months to record all signs and symptoms, with precise times and severity on a scale of 1 to 10.
  —If symptoms are present throughout the month, they may indicate depression or some other physical or emotional problem that requires exploration.
- A diet rich in complex carbohydrates is helpful for many patients.
  —Foods high in sugar and alcohol should be avoided to minimize reactive hypoglycemia.
  —Caffeine intake should be reduced when irritability occurs.
- Regular conditioning exercise (e.g., jogging) usually decreases depression and fluid retention, based on several research studies.
- Serotonin reuptake inhibitors (e.g., fluoxetine 20 mg/day) may be helpful in relieving irritability and dysphoria.
- Short-acting benzodiazepines carry the possibility of addiction and are not generally prescribed.

Patient/Family Education

- Understanding, compassion, and emotional support help minimize the patient's anxiety and helplessness.
- Instruct regarding the nature of the condition, its prevalence, possible causes, and current therapy.
- Suggest ways that the patient might implement to minimize symptoms.
  - Analgesics, such as Tylenol
  - Avoid caffeine.
  - Get extra sleep if possible.
  - Wear comfortable, loose clothing.
  - Avoid foods that might contribute to bloating: highly spiced foods, cabbage, onions.
  - Nightly bubble bath in comfortably hot water
  - Muscle relaxation before falling asleep

Follow-up/Referral

- If symptoms are severe or if laboratory findings suggest specific abnormalities, suggest that the patient see a gynecologist who specializes in PMS.
- Provide support and reassurance to both patient and family, acknowledging the troublesome, persistent nature of PMS and difficulty in relieving symptoms.

Abnormal Premenopausal Bleeding

Definition

Abnormal premenopausal bleeding is any bleeding that is excessive, longer periods, and bleeding both during regular menstrual cycles (menorrhagia) and irregular intervals (dysfunctional uterine bleeding [DUB]). Bleeding at the time of ovulation is common, although heavier or irregular intermenstrual bleeding requires further evaluation.

Etiology

- Dysfunctional uterine bleeding is generally caused by overgrowth of endometrium due to estrogen stimulation without adequate progesterone to stabilize growth.

Diagnosis

Signs and Symptoms

- A thorough history is required.
  - Description of the amount of bleeding and length of periods
  - Description of pain at time of or preceding menses
  - Exact date of last menstrual period (LMP)
  - Usual number of pads/tampons used for each period
  - Presence of clots, degree of inconvenience caused by bleeding
  - History of pertinent illnesses
  - List of all medications, including over the counter (OTC), that the patient took during the month
- A careful pelvic examination to check for uterine myomas, adnexal masses or tenderness, infection, and evidence of endometriosis

Laboratory Findings

- Provide instructions regarding taking basal temperatures for a month, indicating days of menstrual period.
- Cervical smears for culture and cytologic studies
- Complete blood count (CBC), erythrocyte sedimentation rate (ESR), blood glucose to rule out anemia, evidence of asymptomatic illness, and diabetes
- Thyroid function tests
- Pregnancy test
- Blood clotting time
- Have the patient return for serum progesterone level 1 week before expected onset of next menstrual cycle
- Endometrial biopsy for analysis regarding secretory activity just before the next menstrual cycle
- Ultrasound may be helpful in evaluating endometrial thickness and to rule out intrauterine or ectopic pregnancy and adnexal masses.
- Endovaginal ultrasound with saline infusion sonohysterography is used to rule out endometrial polyps or subserous myomas.
- Magnetic resonance imaging (MRI) can be used to diagnose submucous myomas and adenomyosis.
- Cervical biopsy and endometrial curettage or aspiration of the endometrium are used to diagnose causes of uterine bleeding such as polyps, tumors, and submucous myomas.
- If cervical cancer is a possibility, multiple quadrant biopsies, or colposcopically di-

rected biopsies, and endocervical curettage are done as a first step.

- Hysteroscopy is done to visualize endometrial polyps, submucous myomas, and exophytic endometrial cancers; it is a helpful test to do before a scheduled dilation and curettage (D & C).

Differential Diagnosis

- The various examinations and laboratory/diagnostic procedures will rule out many causes of uterine bleeding: myomas, polyps, cancer, endometriosis.
- Stress or excessive drug or alcohol use may also cause anovulation and dysfunctional uterine bleeding.

Treatment

- Treat the possible cause or concomitant gynecologic problem(s) such as myomas, infection, pelvic neoplasms, tubal pregnancy, early abortion, or cancer.
- Dysfunctional uterine bleeding is treated with hormones (progestins) that limit and stabilize endometrial growth as the first choice.
- Medical curettage is done with medroxyprogesterone acetate 10 mg/day or norethindrone acetate 5 mg/day.
  —The drug selected is given for 10 to 14 days starting on day 15 of the cycle, after which withdrawal bleeding will occur (curettage).
  —This treatment is repeated for several cycles and may be reinstituted if amenorrhea or dysfunctional bleeding recurs.
- In young women who are actively bleeding, any of the combination oral contraceptives can be given 4 times/day for 1 to 2 days, followed by two pills daily through day 5 and then one pill/day through day 20.
  —After withdrawal bleeding occurs, pills are taken in the usual dosage for three cycles.
- In cases of intractable heavy bleeding, danazol 200 mg qid is sometimes used to create an atrophic endometrium.
  —As an alternative, a GnRH agonist, such as depot leuprolide 3.75 mg intramuscularly (IM) every month, or nafarelin 0.2 to 0.4 mg intranasally twice/day, is used

for up to 6 months to create temporary cessation of menstruation by ovarian suppression.

- Heavy bleeding can also be treated by intravenous (IV) conjugated estrogens 25 mg q4h for three to four doses, followed by oral conjugated estrogens 2.5 mg/day, or ethinyl estradiol 20 g daily for 3 weeks, with added medroxyprogesterone acetate 10 mg/day for the last 10 days of therapy or a combination of oral contraceptives daily for 3 weeks.
  —Any of these methods will thicken the endometrium and control bleeding.
  —In women over age 40, a D & C is done to rule out neoplasm before beginning hormonal therapy.
- If bleeding is not controlled by hormones, D & C is usually indicated to rule out incomplete abortion, polyps, submucous myomas, or endometrial cancer.
- Nonsteroidal antiinflammatory drugs (NSAIDs), such as ibuprofen, naproxen, or mefenamic acid in usual antiinflammatory doses, often reduce blood loss in menorrhagia or that associated with an intrauterine contraceptive device (IUD).

Patient/Family Education

- Provide information regarding the nature of the problem, possible causes, usual treatment, and reassurance that at least one of the conservative forms of therapy usually eliminates the problem.
- Have the patient keep a journal of signs and symptoms that may occur with the therapy decided on, to make sure that the therapy is working and that symptoms are not worsening.
- Discuss level of stress, use of drugs and alcohol, and smoking cessation if appropriate.

Follow-up/Referral

- Patients with DUB can be treated by the nurse practitioner in consultation with a gynecologist.
- At any point in treatment, the patient may be referred for care to the gynecologist, particularly if the patient requires invasive diagnostic procedures or surgery (e.g., D & C).

Postmenopausal Vaginal Bleeding

Definition

Postmenopausal vaginal bleeding is any vaginal bleeding that occurs 6 months or more after cessation of menstrual function.

Etiology

- Atrophic endometrium
- Endometrial proliferation
- Hyperplasia
- Endometrial or cervical cancer
- Administration of estrogens without added progestin
- Atrophic vaginitis
- Trauma
- Endometrial polyps
- Trophic ulcers of the cervix associated with prolapse of the uterus
- Blood dyscrasias

Diagnosis

Signs and Symptoms

- The patient may report a single episode of spotting, or profuse bleeding for days or months.
- Pelvic examination will detect any ulcers, neoplasms, or abrasions that may account for bleeding.

Diagnostic/Laboratory Tests

- Cytologic smears of the cervix and the vaginal pool are taken.
- Vaginal fluid wet mount in saline and potassium hydroxide may show white blood cells (WBCs), infective organisms, or basal epithelial cells showing low estrogen effect.
- Hysteroscopy followed by D & C may be necessary to diagnose endometrial polyps, hyperplasia, or cancer.
- Transvaginal sonography is used to determine endometrial thickness (<5 mm indicates atrophy).

Differential Diagnosis

- Endometrial cancer
- Cervical cancer
- Endometrial hyperplasia
- Endometriosis

Treatment

- Aspiration curettage and polypectomy if polyps are present

- Hormone therapy is given for endometrial hyperplasia.
  - Cyclic progestin (medroxyprogesterone acetate) 10 mg/day × 21 days for 3 months (or)
  - Norethindrone acetate 5 mg/day × 21 days for 3 months
- Repeat D & C or endometrial biopsy is then performed.
  - If tissues are normal and estrogen therapy is reinstated, a progestin is added (see cyclic progestin in Treatment section) for the last 10 to 14 days of each estrogen cycle, followed by 5 days without hormone therapy, to allow the uterine lining to be shed.
  - If D & C shows endometrial hyperplasia with atypical cells, or carcinoma of the endometrium, hysterectomy is necessary.

Patient/Family Education

- Instruct the patient in detail about the role of hormones in reproductive health.
- Provide written instructions about each of the medications prescribed as to reason, action, effects, exact schedule and dosage, and signs and symptoms to look for that warrant a call to the nurse practitioner or physician.
- Ask the patient to keep a daily journal so that exact information can be reported as to timing of menses, signs and symptoms before the period, amount and appearance of menstrual bleeding, and occurrence of bleeding at other times.

Follow-up/Referral

- For most patients, the nurse practitioner can follow with consultation with both the primary care physician and the gynecologist.
- If diagnostic testing shows the need for procedures or surgery, the patient is referred to a gynecologist.

Carcinoma of the Cervix

Definition

Cervical cancer is considered by many experts to be a sexually transmitted disease.

Incidence

- Cancer of the cervix is the third most common gynecologic malignancy.

- It is the eighth most common malignancy among women in the United States.

Risk Factors
- Average age for the development of cervical cancer is about 50.
- Cervical cancer can affect any woman as young as 20.
- About 1% of cervical cancers occur in pregnant or recently pregnant women.
- Risk is inversely related to age at first intercourse.
- Risk is directly related to the lifetime number of sexual partners.
- Risk is increased for sexual partners of men whose previous partners had cervical cancer.
- Human papilloma virus (HPV) infection is closely associated with development of cervical neoplasms and is strongly linked to development of all grades of cervical intraepithelial neoplasia (CIN) and invasive cervical cancer.
- Cigarette smoking poses an increased risk of CIN and cervical cancer.

Pathogenesis
- Precursor cells (cervical dysplasia, CIN) develop into invasive cervical cancer over a number of years.
- CIN grades I, II, and III correspond to mild, moderate, and severe cervical dysplasia.
- CIN III includes severe dysplasia and carcinoma in situ and likely does not regress spontaneously; without treatment, cancer penetrates the basement membrane and becomes invasive cancer.
- Squamous cell cancer accounts for 80% to 85% of all cervical cancers.
- Adenocarcinomas account for most of the remainder—15% to 20%.
- Hematologic spread of invasive cancer is possible.

Diagnosis
Signs and Symptoms
- CIN is usually asymptomatic and is usually discovered because of an abnormal Pap smear.
- Irregular vaginal bleeding, usually postcoital, occurs in early-stage cervical cancer.
- In advanced stages the patient may present with foul-smelling vaginal discharge, abnormal vaginal bleeding, cervical ulceration, back pain, and leg swelling.
- Bladder and rectal fistulas and dysfunction with pain are late symptoms.

Diagnostic Tests
- Over 90% of early asymptomatic CIN can be detected preclinically by cytologic examination of Pap smears obtained directly from the cervix.
  - The false-negative rate is 15% to 40%, depending on the patient population and the laboratory.
- About 50% of patients with cervical cancer have never had a Pap smear or have not had one for over 10 years.
- Colposcopy is used to identify areas that require biopsy and to localize the lesion.
  - Colposcopy-directed biopsy usually provides enough evidence for accurate diagnosis.
  - When cervical cancer is invasive, staging is done based on physical examination, cystoscopy, sigmoidoscopy, IV pyelography, chest x-ray, and skeletal x-rays to determine the extent of metastasis (Table 13-1).

Complications
- Usually associated with metastasis
- Back pain usually indicates neurologic involvement.
- Hemorrhage is the cause of death in 10% to 20% of patients with extensive invasive carcinoma.

Treatment
- Emergency measures for bleeding
  - Vaginal hemorrhage usually is from gross ulceration and cavitation in stage II-IV.
  - Ligation and suturing of the cervix is not generally feasible.
  - Ligation of the uterine or hypogastric arteries may be lifesaving in severe hemorrhage.
  - Monsel's solution and acetone are effective styptics, but delayed sloughing may cause further bleeding.
  - Wet vaginal packing is helpful.
  - Emergency irradiation usually controls bleeding.

TABLE 13-1
Clinical Staging of Cervical Carcinoma

Stage	Description
0	Carcinoma in situ, intraepithelial carcinoma
I	Carcinoma strictly confined to the cervix (extension to the corpus should be disregarded)
IA	Preclinical carcinoma (diagnosed only by microscopy)
IA1	Measured invasion of stroma $\leq$ 3 mm in depth and $\leq$ 7 mm in width
IA2	Measured invasion of stroma > 3 mm and $\leq$ 5 mm in depth and $\leq$ 7 mm in width
IB	Clinical lesions confined to the cervix or preclinical lesions larger than those in stage IA2
IB1	Clinical lesions $\leq$ 4 cm
IB2	Clinical lesions > 4 cm
II	Carcinoma extending beyond the cervix but not to the pelvic wall; carcinoma involving the vagina but not the lower one third
IIA	No obvious parametrial involvement
IIB	Obvious parametrial involvement
III	Carcinoma extending to the pelvic wall, with rectal examination detecting no cancer-free space between the tumor and the pelvic wall; tumor involving the lower one third of the vagina; includes all cases with hydronephrosis or nonfunctioning kidney
IIIA	Extension to the pelvic wall
IIIB	Extension to the pelvic wall and hydronephrosis, nonfunctioning kidney, or both
IV	Carcinoma extending beyond the true pelvis or clinically involving the mucosa of the bladder or rectum (bullous edema does not signify stage IV)
IVA	Spread to adjacent organs
IVB	Spread to distant organs

From Shepherd JH: Staging announcement: Internal Federation of Gynecology and Obstetrics (FIGO) staging of gynecologic cancers: cervical and vulva, *Int J Gynecol Cancer* 5:319, 1995.

Carcinoma in Situ

- For women who have completed childbearing, total hysterectomy is the treatment of choice.
- For those who wish to retain the uterus, alternatives include
  - Cervical conization or ablation of the lesion with cryotherapy or laser
    - ~ Close monitoring by Pap smear every 3 months for 1 year, every 6 months for another year

Invasive Carcinoma

- Microinvasive carcinoma (stage IA) is treated with simple, extrafascial hysterectomy.
  - Stages IB and IIA cancers are treated with either radical hysterectomy or radiation therapy.
  - Stage IIB and III and IV cancers must be treated with radiation therapy.
    - ~ In younger women without contraindications to major surgery, radical surgery results in fewer long-term complications than irradiation and may allow preservation of ovarian function.

Prognosis

- Overall 5-year relative survival rate for carcinoma of the cervix is 68% in white women and 55% in black women in the United States.
- Survival rates are inversely proportional to the stage of cancer:
  - Stage 0 = 99% to 100%
  - Stage IA = 95%
  - Stage IB-IIA = 80% to 90%
  - Stage IIB = 65%
  - Stage III = 40%
  - Stage IV = <20%

Patient/Family Education

- Instruct about the nature of the cancer, its probable cause, treatment, and expected outcome
  - Some patients want to know "up front" about their relative chance of survival; talking first with the family might help health professionals to know how much to tell a particular patient.
    - ~ Ethics committee members usually discuss these types of patients and decide among them, in consultation with the

family, what should be discussed, and when.

—Most psychiatrists stress the fact that patients must not be robbed of hope because it is what patients cling to.

Follow-up/Referral

- These patients are followed closely from the time of diagnosis until full recovery or death.
- Patients are generally relatively young, and require much support and encouragement.
- Patients are usually followed by the nurse practitioner, primary care physician, and oncologic gynecologist, as well as other specialists as needed at particular times.

Endometrial Carcinoma

Definition

Endometrial carcinoma is cancer of the body (corpus) of the uterus.

Incidence

- Adenocarcinoma of the endometrium is the second most common cancer of the female genital tract.
- It is most often found among women ages 50 to 70.

Risk Factors

- Postmenopausal
- History of taking unopposed estrogen in the past
  —Patients' increased risk from estrogen replacement lasts for 10 years or longer after stopping the drug.
- Obesity
- Nulliparity
- Diabetes
- Polycystic ovaries with prolonged anovulation
- Taking tamoxifen to treat breast cancer over extended time

Diagnosis

Signs and Symptoms

- Abnormal bleeding is the presenting sign in 80% of patients.
- The neoplasm may cause obstruction of the cervix with collection of pus (pyometra) or blood (hematometra), causing pain in the lower abdomen and pelvis.

TABLE 13-2
Staging of Endometrial Carcinoma

Stage	Definition
IA	Tumor limited to endometrium
IB	Invasion of $<\frac{1}{2}$ myometrium
IC	Invasion of $>\frac{1}{2}$ myometrium
IIA	Tumor involves only endocervical glands
IIB	Invasion of cervical stroma
IIIA	Invasion of serosa and/or adnexa and/or positive peritoneal cytologic findings
IIIB	Metastases to vagina
IIIC	Metastases to pelvic and/or paraaortic lymph nodes
IVA	Invasion of bladder and/or bowel mucosa
IVB	Distant metastases, including intraabdominal and/or inguinal lymph nodes

From International Federation of Gynecology and Obstetrics (FIGO), 1988.

- Pain does not usually occur until late in the disease, from metastases or infection.

Laboratory Findings

- Pap smears of the cervix sometimes show atypical endometrial cells, but this test is not a sensitive diagnostic test.
- Definitive diagnosis is made by endocervical and endometrial tissue sampling and histologic study.
- Hysteroscopy helps to localize the lesion.
- Vaginal ultrasonography is used to determine the thickness of the endometrium caused by hypertrophy or neoplasm or both.

Prevention

- Immediate endometrial sampling for those patients who report abnormal bleeding or postmenopausal bleeding will show both early changes and actual carcinoma of the endometrium.
- Women who take estrogens, or younger women with prolonged anovulation, are given oral progestins for 13 days at the end of each estrogen cycle to promote periodic shedding of the uterine lining.

Staging

- Examination under anesthesia, endometrial and endocervical sampling, chest x-ray, IV urography, cystoscopy, sigmoidoscopy, transvaginal sonography, and MRI help to determine the extent of cancer and its treatment (Table 13-2).

Treatment
- Total hysterectomy and bilateral salpingo-oophorectomy
- Material from the peritoneum is taken routinely, for cytologic study.
- Initial irradiation or intracavitary radium therapy is indicated if the cancer is poorly differentiated or if the uterus is definitely enlarged in the absence of myomas.
- If invasion is deep into the myometrium, or if sampled preaortic lymph nodes are positive, postoperative irradiation is indicated.
- Palliative treatment of advanced or metastatic endometrial adenocarcinoma is provided by large doses of progestins (e.g., medroxyprogesterone 400 mg IM weekly, or megestrol acetate 80 to 160 mg orally [PO] daily).
- Pain is managed as required with analgesics or opiates.

Prognosis
- Early diagnosis and treatment afford a 5-year survival rate of 80% to 85%.

Patient/Family Education
- Provide reassurance and support to both patient and family throughout.
- Explain all diagnostic procedures, medications, treatments, surgical procedures, and plan of care as it changes over time, with attendant risks if any.
- Make certain that the patient's pain is managed optimally throughout.
- Pay attention to special comforts: shampoo of hair and brushing/combing, teeth cleaning and mouthwash, shower, bath or bed bath, clothing, dressing changes, and other measures to make the patient feel better and look her best.

Follow-up/Referral
- From the time of diagnosis, the patient will be followed by a gynecologist who specializes in oncology, in conjunction with the primary care physician and nurse practitioner.
- Surgery and irradiation are administered appropriately, usually at medical centers with the latest equipment and drugs.

Endometriosis

Definition
Endometriosis is a nonmalignant disorder in which functioning endometrial tissue is present outside the uterine cavity; aberrant cells of the endometrium can be found on the peritoneal or serosal surfaces of abdominal organs, the pelvis, the ovaries, the broad ligament, the posterior cul-de-sac, the uterosacral ligaments and, less commonly, the serosal surfaces of the small and large bowel, ureters, bladder, vagina, surgical scars, pleura, and pericardium, causing abnormal bleeding, pain at various sites where endometrial tissue has implanted, and secondary dysmenorrhea.

Incidence/Prevalence
- Among fertile women, 2% of this population (10% to 15%) experience signs and symptoms of endometriosis, usually concurrently with their menstrual cycles.
  —Prevalence of the condition is 3 to 4 times greater among fertile women than among infertile women.
- The incidence varies but is higher by 6% in first-degree relatives of women with endometriosis than in the general population, suggesting that heredity may be a significant factor.
  —Incidence is higher among women who delay childbearing.
  —Incidence is higher among Asian women.
  —Incidence is higher among those women with müllerian duct anomalies.

Etiology
- Causes, pathogenesis, and natural course are not clearly understood.
- As indicated, genetics may play a role.

Diagnosis (Table 13-3)
- History of pain at various sites relating to menstrual cycle
- Infertility
- Dyspareunia
- Rectal pain and bleeding
- Aching pain tends to be constant, usually starting 2 to 7 days before onset of menses and becoming increasingly severe until the menstrual flow begins to abate.
- Pelvic examination may show tender, indurated nodules in the cul-de-sac, particu-

TABLE 13-3
Stages of Endometriosis

Stage	Extent of Disease	Description
I	Minimal	A few superficial implants
II	Mild	More, slightly deeper implants
III	Moderate	Many deep implants, small endometriomas on one or both ovaries, some filmy adhesions
IV	Severe	Many deep implants, large endometriomas on one or both ovaries, and many dense adhesions, sometimes with the rectum adhering to the back of the uterus

From Beers MH, Berkow R, eds: Gynecology and obstetrics. *The Merck manual of diagnosis and therapy,* ed 17, Whitehouse Station, NJ, 1999, Merck & Co, Inc, p 1961.

larly if the examination occurs just before menstruation.

- Ultrasound may show complex fluid-filled masses that cannot be distinguished from neoplasms.
- MRI is more sensitive and specific in identifying endometrial masses in the adnexae.
- Barium enema may show colonic involvement of endometrial masses.
- Definitive diagnosis is made by laparoscopy or laparotomy and tissue histology.

Differential Diagnosis
- Pelvic inflammatory disease
- Ovarian neoplasms
- Uterine myomas
- Colon cancer (blood in the stool)

Treatment

Medical Treatment
- The goal of treatment is to preserve the patient's ability to bear children, minimize symptoms, and avoid surgery.
- Medications are given to inhibit ovulation for 4 to 9 months, to lower hormone levels to prevent cyclic stimulation of endometriotic implants, and to decrease the size of implants.
  —The GnRH analogs (e.g., nafarelin nasal spray 0.2 to 0.4 mg bid, or long-acting leuprolide acetate 3.75 mg IM every month for 6 months) are given to suppress ovulation.
  —Danazol is given for 6 to 9 months at the lowest dose necessary to suppress menstruation—200 to 400 mg bid; side effects are decreased breast size, weight gain, acne, and hirsutism (androgenic effects).
  —Any of the combination oral contraceptive agents are given, one/day without interruption for 6 to 12 months; breakthrough bleeding is treated with conjugated estrogens 1.25 mg/day for 1 week, or estradiol 2 mg/day for 1 week.
  —Medroxyprogesterone acetate 100 mg IM every 2 weeks $\times$ 4 doses, then 100 mg every 4 weeks; oral estrogen or estradiol valerate 30 mg IM is given for breakthrough bleeding for 6 to 9 months
  —Low-dose oral contraceptives may be given cyclically; prolonged suppression of ovulation often inhibits stimulation of residual endometriosis, when given after one of the therapies previously listed.
  —Analgesics with or without codeine are given during menstrual periods; NSAIDs may be helpful in relieving discomfort.

Surgical Treatment
- The decision regarding surgery depends on the patient's age, her desire to preserve reproductive capacity, and the degree of symptoms.
  —If the woman is under 35, the lesions are resected, adhesions are freed, and the uterus is suspended.
    ~ At least 20% of patients with this treatment can become pregnant.
  —If the woman is over 35, has disabling pain, and both ovaries are involved, the procedure of choice is bilateral salpingo-oophorectomy and hysterectomy.

—Endometrial foci can be treated by laparoscopy with bipolar coagulation or laser vaporization; a meticulous examination of the peritoneum is required to ensure that most implant sites are eliminated.

—Bilateral oophorectomy is curative for patients with severe and extensive disease with pain.

~ After hysterectomy and oophorectomy, hormone replacement therapy is needed.

Prognosis

- With conservative therapy for early or moderately advanced endometriosis, the prognosis for childbearing is good.

Patient/Family Education

- The patient and partner are kept informed of the nature of the condition, its signs and symptoms, course, and treatment to maintain fertility or to eliminate reproductive capacity, depending on age and patient wishes.
- Medications (schedule, dosage), reasons, actions, side effects if any, and expected outcomes are explained in detail, in writing.
- If surgical procedures are to be performed, the patient is instructed about preparation, purpose of the procedure, how long it will take, location (office or hospital operating room), rationale, and expected outcome.

Follow-up/Referral

- These patients are followed for variable lengths of time, depending on extent of endometriosis, therapy, and outcomes.
- While undergoing treatment, the patient is managed by an experienced gynecologist and other specialists as required.
- The time of follow-up continues until the patient is fully recovered, and signs and symptoms have disappeared or abated to a considerable degree.
- In case of recurrence, further treatment may be needed, either conservative or surgical.

Ovarian Tumors

Definition

Ovarian tumors are common; most are benign, but ovarian cancer is the leading cause of death from reproductive tract cancer. The broad range of kinds and patterns of ovarian tumors is due to the complexity of ovarian embryology and differences in origin of tissues.

Incidence

- About 1 in 70 women eventually develops ovarian cancer; 1 of 100 women dies from it.

Risk Factors

- Ovarian cancer occurs primarily in perimenopausal and postmenopausal women.
- Ovarian cancer is more common in industrialized countries, where high-fat diets are more common.
- History of nulliparity, late childbearing, and delayed menopause increase risk.
- Use of oral contraceptives significantly *decreases* risk.
- History (personal or family) of endometrial, breast, or colon cancer increases risk.
- Some (<5%) of ovarian cancer cases are related to an inherited autosomal dominant gene, the *BRCA* gene.
- Women with XY gonadal dysgenesis are predisposed to ovarian malignant germ cell tumors.

Pathology

- At least 80% of malignant ovarian tumors arise from the coelomic epithelium.
  - The most common type is serous cystadenocarcinoma, which accounts for 75% of cases of epithelial ovarian cancer.
  - Others are mucinous, endometrioid, transitional cell, Brenner, clear cell, and unclassified carcinomas.
- The remaining 20% of malignant ovarian tumors that are nonepithelial in origin and malignant tumors in other organs (e.g., breast, gastrointestinal [GI]) that metastasize to the ovaries include the following:
  - Germ cell tumors, which arise from the primary germ cells of the ovary, occur primarily in young women under 30 years of age.
    - ~ Germ cell tumors include dysgerminomas, immature teratomas, endodermal sinus tumors, embryonal carcinomas, choriocarcinoma, and polyembryomas.
  - Stromal malignancies include granulosa-theca cell tumors and Sertoli-Leydig cell tumors.

- Ovarian cancer spreads by direct extension, by intraperitoneal implantation by means of exfoliation of cells into the peritoneal cavity, and by lymphatic dissemination in the pelvis and paraaortic region and less commonly hematogenously to the liver or lungs.

Diagnosis

Signs and Symptoms

- Frequently, women with ovarian tumors, either benign or malignant, are asymptomatic or describe only vague GI symptoms or a feeling of pelvic pressure.
- Those with advanced cancer may have abdominal pain and bloating; a palpable abdominal mass is usually present, with some ascites.

Laboratory Findings

- Elevated serum cancer cell surface antigen 125 (CA125, a glycoprotein found in the serum of patients with ovarian or other glandular cell carcinoma; increasing levels of CA125 indicate continuing tumor growth and may predict a poor prognosis) is greater than 35 units.
  —CA125 is elevated in 80% of women with epithelial ovarian cancer but in only 50% of those with early disease.
  —Premenopausal women with endometriosis or other benign disease may also have elevated serum CA125.
- Imaging
  —Ultrasound is able to differentiate benign ovarian masses that are likely to resolve without treatment from ovarian tumors that may be malignant.
  —Transvaginal sonography (TVS) is helpful in screening high-risk women, but lacks sensitivity for screening low-risk patients.
  —Color Doppler imaging enhances specificity of ultrasound findings.

Differential Diagnosis

- When an ovarian mass is found, it is first classified as functional, benign neoplastic, or potentially malignant.
  —Predictive factors
    ~ Age of patient
    ~ Size of the mass

~ Ultrasound analysis
~ Levels of CA125
~ Symptoms
~ Whether mass is unilateral or bilateral
—An asymptomatic premenopausal woman with a mobile, unilateral, simple cystic mass < 8 to 10 cm can be observed for up to 6 weeks; most such masses resolve spontaneously.
  ~ If the mass is unchanged or larger on repeat examination and TVS, surgical evaluation is required.
—Most ovarian tumors in postmenopausal women require surgical evaluation, except those with an asymptomatic, unilateral simple cyst < 5 cm in diameter and a normal CA125 level, who will be followed closely and evaluated by TVS.
- Laparotomy to explore ovarian tumors is the preferred approach.
  —Laparoscopy may be used in premenopausal women with an ovarian mass small enough to be excised by laparoscopy.
    ~ If cancer is suspected, preoperative evaluation of liver and kidney function, hematologic studies, and chest x-ray are done to determine effects of the tumor.

Treatment

- If ovarian cancer is suspected, exploratory laparotomy is performed by a gynecologic oncologist.
  —Benign masses are removed and unilateral oophorectomy is usually done.
  —For early-stage cancer, therapy is complete surgical staging, then abdominal hysterectomy and bilateral salpingo-oophorectomy with omentectomy and selective lymph node excision.
  —In patients with more advanced disease, aggressive removal of all visible tumor improves survival.
- For all except those with early-stage, low-grade ovarian tumor, chemotherapy after surgery is generally the next step:
  —Combination cisplatin and cyclophosphamide with or without doxorubicin is given.
    ~ Clinical response rates of up to 60% to 70% are reported.

Prognosis

- Diagnosis of ovarian cancer usually occurs in advanced stages when distant metastases have occurred.
  - Overall 5-year survival is about 17% with distant metastases.
  - Overall 5-year survival is about 36% with local metastases.
  - Overall 5-year survival is about 89% for patients with early-stage cancer and no metastases.

Patient/Family Education

- Explain the nature, cause, staging, treatment, and expected outcomes.
- Prognosis can be discussed in general terms, always maintaining patients' hope because individual survival is often unpredictable.
- Provide consistently positive and compassionate care, indicating day-to-day progress, no matter how minimal.

Follow-up/Referral

- Patients are followed closely, before and after surgery or other therapy.
- Family members may be kept more specifically informed than the patient if that seems best, depending on patient requests.
- From the time of diagnosis, patients are usually followed by a gynecologic oncologist.
- Hospice care may be suggested to terminally ill patients or to the family.

Polycystic Ovary (Stein-Leventhal) Syndrome

Definition

Polycystic ovary (Stein-Leventhal) syndrome is an endocrine disturbance characterized by anovulation, amenorrhea, hirsutism, and infertility.

Etiology

- Caused by increased levels of testosterone, estrogen, and luteinizing hormone (LH) and decreased secretion of follicle-stimulating hormone (FSH)
  - The increased level of LH may result from an increased sensitivity of the pituitary to stimulation by releasing hormone or from excessive stimulation by the adrenal gland.

- The condition may also be associated with a variety of problems in the hypothalamic-pituitary-ovarian axis, with extragonadal sources of androgens or with androgen-producing tumors.
- The condition is transmitted as an X-linked dominant or autosomal dominant trait.

Diagnosis

Signs and Symptoms

- Obesity (40% of patients)
- Hirsutism (70%)
- Virilization (20%)
- Amenorrhea (50%)
- Abnormal uterine bleeding (30%)
- Infertility (most)
- Normal menstruation (20%)
- Insulin resistance and hyperinsulinemia when infused with glucose
  - These abnormalities place these patients at increased risk of early-onset type 2 diabetes mellitus.

Pathology

- The affected ovary usually doubles in size and becomes enveloped in a pearly white capsule.
- The increased level of estrogen raises the risk of cancers of the breast and endometrium.

Differential Diagnosis

- Anovulation during the childbearing years may also be caused by
  - Premature menopause (high FSH and LH levels)
  - Rapid weight loss, extreme physical exercise (normal FSH and LH levels for age), or obesity
  - Stopping oral contraceptives (anovulation of 6 months or more may occur)
  - Pituitary adenoma with elevated prolactin (galactorrhea may be present)
  - Hyperthyroidism or hypothyroidism
  - For patients over age 35, screening for an estrogen-stimulated cancer by means of mammography and endometrial aspiration should be performed.

Treatment

- Weight reduction is often beneficial because decreased body fat lowers the conversion of androgens to estrone, thus restoring ovulation.

- Suppression of hormonal stimulation of the ovary, usually by administering female hormones, or resection of part of one or both ovaries
- Treatment is adjusted to the patient's wish to bear children and severity of symptoms.
  —If the patient wishes to become pregnant, clomiphene or other drugs are used to stimulate ovulation.
  —Adding dexamethasone 0.5 mg at bedtime to the clomiphene regimen suppresses adrenocorticotropic hormone (ACTH) and circulating adrenal androgens, thus increasing the likelihood of ovulation and pregnancy.
- Wedge resection of the ovary restores ovulation, but surgery like this is used less often now because of new and effective drugs.
- If the patient does not wish to become pregnant, medroxyprogesterone acetate 10 mg/day for the first 10 days of the month is given, which ensures shedding of the endometrium and prevents hyperplasia.
- If contraception is wished, a low-dose combination oral contraceptive is used, which will also control hirsutism, although treatment must continue for 6 to 12 months before results are seen.
- Hirsutism can be further managed by means of epilation and electrolysis.
  —Spironolactone (aldosterone antagonist) 25 mg bid or tid is also effective for hirsutism.

Patient/Family Education
- Explain the nature, possible causes, treatment, and expected outcome of therapy.
- Give reassurance to the patient that treatments are available.
- List the ways in which the patient can participate in therapy: weight loss, exercise at a reasonable level, or others as appropriate.
- Ask the patient about desire for pregnancy.
- Instruct about all medications and procedures given as to: reason, preparation, precise dose and schedule of drugs, action of drugs, and any major side effects.
- Ask the patient to keep a daily record of signs and symptoms to evaluate drug effectiveness.

Follow-up/Referral
- Patients with polycystic ovary syndrome are usually followed closely by an endocrinologist/gynecologist.
- Drug dosage and scheduling may be adjusted over time, depending on patient response.

Menopausal Syndrome
Definition
Menopausal syndrome is the physiologic cessation of menses due to decreasing ovarian function.
- Menopause is established when menses have not occurred for a year.
  —Any vaginal bleeding in a woman who has not bled for ≥ 6 months requires thorough investigation.
- Premature menopause is ovarian failure of unknown cause that occurs before age 40.
- Artificial menopause may occur because of oophorectomy, chemotherapy, radiation of the pelvis, or any process that impairs ovarian blood supply.

Physiology
- As ovaries age, response to pituitary gonadotropins (FSH and LH) decreases.
  —At first, decreased response results in shorter menstrual cycles, fewer ovulations, decreased progesterone production, and more irregular cycles.
- Eventually, the follicle fails to respond and does not produce estrogen.
  —Without estrogen feedback, circulating levels of FSH and LH increase significantly while circulating levels of estrogen and progesterone are markedly reduced.
  —The androgen androstenedione is reduced by 50%, although testosterone decreases only slightly because the stroma of the postmenopausal ovary continues to secrete substantial amounts, as does the adrenal gland.
  —Androgens are converted to estrogen in the periphery in fat cells and skin, which accounts for most of the circulating estrogen in postmenopausal women.
- Menopause occurs naturally at an average age of 50 to 51 in the United States.
  —Onset of menstruation is influenced by many factors: genetics, state of nutrition, and stress level.

Diagnosis

Signs and Symptoms

- Signs and symptoms range from nonexistent to severe.
  - Hot flashes with sweating are due to vasomotor instability and occur in 50% to 75% of women; duration ranges from more than a year to more than 5 years.
    - ~ Hot flashes coincide with LH pulses, but not every increase in LH produces a hot flash.
    - ~ Women with pituitary failure and do not secrete FSH and LH, do experience hot flashes.
  - Psychologic symptoms
    - ~ Irritability
    - ~ Fatigue
    - ~ Insomnia
    - ~ Inability to concentrate
    - ~ Depression
    - ~ Memory loss
    - ~ Anxiety
    - ~ Nervousness
  - Other
    - ~ Nausea
    - ~ Constipation
    - ~ Diarrhea
    - ~ Arthralgia and myalgia
    - ~ Cold hands and feet
    - ~ Weight gain
- Health problems after menopause
  - Cardiovascular disease becomes more prevalent, including stroke.
  - Osteoporosis due to decreased bone density; risk is higher in the following:
    - ~ Small-boned white women
    - ~ Heavy alcohol drinkers
    - ~ Smokers
    - ~ Women taking corticosteroids
    - ~ Those who are sedentary

Treatment

- Talking with the patient about causes of menopause, and about concerns, fears, and stresses related to the changes occurring at this time of life (e.g., "empty nest," loss of husband), helps to express her feelings and receive support.
- Estrogen and progestin replacement therapy is appropriate for a woman with a uterus.

  - Women who have had a hysterectomy can receive unopposed estrogen safely, with no risk of endometrial cancer.
- For psychologic symptoms, a short course of antidepressants or individual or group counseling may be helpful.

Patient/Family Education

- Provide detailed information about the hormonal changes that occur naturally in women in the perimenopausal period, signs and symptoms, and various therapies to help the individual through the worst of hot flashes, depression, fatigue, and irritability.
- If support groups meet, the patient can be referred to the facilitator or a psychologist who specializes in midlife changes and problems.
- Instruct about the relationship of decreased estrogen to cardiovascular disease and osteoporosis, and about hormone replacement therapy to prevent both.
- Meet with the husband or family members to help the patient accept the ups and downs, both physical and emotional, that may occur with menopause.
- Provide written instructions about hormone replacement therapy, which often causes hot flashes to diminish or stop, and calcium supplements, which prevent severe osteoporosis.
- If the patient smokes or drinks alcohol, encourage her to stop, and replace them with more physical activity and other interests.

Follow-up/Referral

- Patients are followed frequently throughout the perimenopausal and menopausal periods until menses cease and the patient feels comfortable with age-related changes.
- Occasionally, consultation with a psychiatrist or psychologist may be helpful.

CONTRACEPTION
Definition

Contraception is a process or technique for preventing pregnancy by such means as medication, device, or method that blocks or alters one or more of the processes of reproduction so that sexual union can occur without impregnation. Information about all forms of contraception is readily available to those couples who wish to prevent pregnancy and to avoid sexually transmitted diseases (STDs) (e.g., human immunodeficiency virus [HIV]/acquired immunodeficiency syndrome [AIDS]).

Oral Contraceptives

- Oral contraceptives have a theoretic failure rate of less than 0.3% with total adherence to the schedule, and a typical failure rate of 3%.
- The primary action is suppression of ovulation.
- Pills are started on the first or fifth day of the ovarian cycle and taken for 21 days, followed by 7 days of placebo or no medication, continued for every cycle.
  —If a pill is missed, two pills should be taken the next day, plus another method of contraception continued for the remainder of that cycle (e.g., condom or foam).
  —If pills are begun later than the fifth day of the first cycle, a backup method is used for that cycle.
- Low-dose oral contraceptives are *not* contraindicated for women 35 to 50 years of age who are nonsmokers and have no risk factors for cardiovascular disease.

Benefits of Oral Contraceptives
- Menstrual flow is lighter.
- Anemia is less common with lighter flow.
- Dysmenorrhea is relieved for most women.
- Functional ovarian cysts usually disappear, and new cysts do not form.
- Ovulatory pain is relieved.
- Risk of ovarian and endometrial cancer is decreased.
- Risk of salpingitis and ectopic pregnancy may be reduced.
- Acne usually improves.
- Effect on bone mass is beneficial.
- Frequency of development of myomas is lower in long-term users (>4 years).

Selection of Oral Contraceptive
- Any combination containing less than 50 μg of estrogen is suitable for most women.
  —Women taking pills that contain ≥ 50 μg of estrogen should be switched to lower-dose pills (many adverse effects are dose-related).
- Women with acne or hirsutism may be helped by one of the pills containing the newer progestins (e.g., desogestrel, norgestimate), which are least androgenic.

Dosage
- The dose of estrogen in oral contraceptives is four or more times higher than that in estrogen preparations given to menopausal women.
  —More side effects are expected in oral contraceptives.
- Low-dose oral contraceptives most often prescribed in the United States are
  —Loestrin 1/20
  —Lo/Ovral
  —Nordette and Levlen
  —Norinyl 1/35 [N] and Ortho-Novum 1/35 [O]
  —Loestrin 1.5/30
  —Demulen 1/35
  —Brevicon [B], Modicon [M], and Jenest [J]
  —Ovcon 35
  —Ortho-Cept [O] and Desogen [D]
  —Ortho-Cyclen
  —Ortho-Tricyclen
  —Ortho-Novum 7/7/7
  —Tri-Norinyl
  —Triphasil [T] and Tri-Levlen [TL]
  —Micronor [M] and Nor-QD [N]
  —Ovrette
- Cost of these oral contraceptives ranges between $28.04 for a single pill per month and $78.61 for a combination of three pills per month.

Drug Interactions
- Some drugs interact with oral contraceptives, which decreases the effectiveness of the contraception by inducing microsomal enzymes in the liver, increasing sex hormone-binding globulin, and other mechanisms.
  —These drugs include: phenytoin, phenobarbital and other barbiturates, primidone, carbamazepine, and rifampin.
  —Women who take any of these drugs should use a form of contraception other than oral contraceptives (e.g., IUD).

Complications

- The risk of *myocardial infarction* is higher, especially with oral contraceptives that contain ≥50 μg of estrogen (new study shows *insignificant* risk—see bibliography: *BMJ* reference).
- An increased rate of venous *thromboembolism* is seen in women who use oral contraceptives; the risk is low (15/100,000 woman per year), but there is an increased risk for women who use pills that contain progestins (gestodene or desogestrel).
- *Cerebrovascular disease* is increased somewhat with regard to hemorrhagic stroke and subarachnoid hemorrhage; a greater risk of thrombotic stroke is associated with oral contraceptive use.
  —Other risk factors for thrombotic stroke are smoking, hypertension, and age over 35.
- Those who develop symptoms of severe headache, blurred vision, loss of vision, or transient neurologic disorders should stop taking oral contraceptives.
- *Cancer:* cervical dysplasia and cancer have been found in those who have taken oral contraceptives for at least 3 to 4 years.
  —No confirmed association has been found between use of oral contraceptives and breast cancer.
  —Combination oral contraceptives decrease the risk of endometrial carcinoma by 40% after 2 years of use, by 60% after 5 to 11 years of use, and by 80% after >12 years of use.
  —In a few cases, oral contraceptives were associated with benign or malignant hepatic tumors, which may result in rupture of the liver, hemorrhage, and death; risk increases with higher dosage, longer use, and increased age.
- *Metabolic disorders,* such as decreased glucose tolerance, increased triglyceride levels, and diabetes, are associated with oral contraceptive use.
- *Hypertension* sometimes occurs in women who use oral contraceptives; risk increases with age and more years of use.
  —Nonsmoking women under age 40 with well-controlled mild hypertension may continue on the pill.

BOX 13-1

Contraindications to Use of Oral Contraceptives

ABSOLUTE CONTRAINDICATIONS
Pregnancy
Thrombophlebitis or thromboembolic disorders (past or present)
Stroke or coronary artery disease (past or present)
Cancer of the breast (suspected or positive)
Abnormal vaginal bleeding of unknown cause
Estrogen-dependent cancer (suspected or known)
Benign or malignant hepatic tumor (past or present)

RELATIVE CONTRAINDICATIONS
Age > 35 years and heavy smoking (>15 cigarettes/day)
Migraine or recurrent persistent severe headache
Hypertension
Cardiac or renal disease
Diabetes
Gallbladder disease
Cholestasis (during pregnancy)
Hepatitis or infectious mononucleosis
Sickle cell disease (S/S or S/C type)*
Surgery, fracture, or severe trauma
Breast-feeding
Significant depression

From MacKay HT: Gynecology. In Tierney LM, McPhee SJ, Papadakis MA, eds: *Current medical diagnosis & treatment 2000,* New York, 2000, Lange Medical Books/McGraw-Hill, p 748.
*S/S and S/C refer to inheritance patterns.

- *Other:* migraine or vascular headaches occur in some women; if frequent, the pill should be discontinued (Box 13-1).
  —*Amenorrhea:* postpill amenorrhea that may last a year or more, with galactorrhea in some women, may occur; if prolactin levels are elevated, a pituitary prolactinoma may be the cause.

Progestin Minipill

- Oral contraceptives that contain 0.35 mg of norethindrone or 0.075 mg of norgestrel are somewhat less effective than combined oral contraceptives.
  —Failure rates of 1% to 4% are reported.
- These drugs prevent conception by causing thickening of the cervical mucus, making it hostile to sperm, and alteration in transport of ova, which accounts for a higher rate of ectopic pregnancies associated with these

minipills; this effect also decreases pelvic inflammatory infection because the thickened mucus acts as a barrier to organisms.
- Ovulation is inhibited inconsistently.
- The minipill is started on the first day of a menstrual cycle and continued for as long as contraception is desired.
- Low dose and absence of estrogen render the minipill safe during lactation, and may increase the flow of milk.
- It may be preferred by women who want only minimal hormone therapy, and those over age 35.
- The minipill can be used by women with sickle cell disease (both types) and uterine myomas.

Complications and Contraindications
- May cause irregular bleeding (e.g., spotting, prolonged flow, amenorrhea)
- With increase in ectopic pregnancy rate, symptom of abdominal pain should be evaluated thoroughly
- Weight gain and mild headache may occur with minipill use.
- Contraindications listed in Box 13-1 also apply to the minipill.

Contraceptive Injections and Implants (Long-Acting Progestins)

- Progestin (e.g., medroxyprogesterone acetate) 150 mg, given by deep IM injection every 3 months
  - Its effectiveness is 99.7%.
  - Side effects: irregular bleeding, amenorrhea, weight gain, headache; loss of bone minerals may occur
  - Anovulation may be delayed after the last injection.
  - Contraindications are about the same as for the minipill.
- Norplant—a contraceptive implant containing levonorgestrel
  - This system has 6 small Silastic capsules that are inserted subcutaneously (SC) in the inner aspect of the upper arm.
  - Medication is released daily.
  - Contraception is effective for 5 years.
    - ~ In the first year, effectiveness is 99.8%.
    - ~ This level decreases slightly over time.

  - Side effects are irregular bleeding and spotting, amenorrhea, headache, acne, and weight gain.
    - ~ Irregular bleeding is the major reason for removing the implants, done under local anesthesia.
    - ~ Hormone levels drop rapidly after removal of the implants.
  - Contraindications are the same as for the minipill.

Intrauterine Devices

- The IUDs available in the United States now are the Progestasert, which secretes progesterone into the uterus, and the Copper T380A.
  - A few others such as the Lippes Loop are still in use.
  - The failure rate for most IUDs is about 1% to 2%.
  - Contraception is achieved by impaired fertilization due to effects on sperm motility and to abnormal development in the oviduct of any ova that may be fertilized.
  - Progesterone-secreting IUDs must be replaced every year; however, this type causes less cramping and decreased menstrual flow.
  - All-plastic IUDs need not be replaced at specific intervals; some women use them for ≥ 10 years.
  - The copper IUDs must be replaced every 8 years to achieve maximum effectiveness.
- Insertion is performed during or after the menses, at midcycle to prevent implantation, or later in the cycle if the patient is not pregnant.
  - Most gynecologists and obstetricians wait 6 to 8 weeks postpartum to insert an IUD.
  - Inserting an IUD while a woman is breastfeeding creates a higher risk of uterine perforation or embedding of the IUD.
  - Inserting an IUD immediately after an abortion is possible if no sepsis is present and if insertion 4 weeks later, which is most desirable, is not possible.
  - To prevent pelvic inflammation, a single dose of doxycycline 200 mg is given an hour before the IUD is inserted.

Complications (Box 13-2)
- *Pregnancy:* an IUD can be inserted within 5 days after a single episode of unpro-

---

BOX 13-2

Contraindications to IUD Use

ABSOLUTE CONTRAINDICATIONS
Pregnancy
Acute or subacute pelvic inflammatory disease, or purulent cervicitis

RELATIVE CONTRAINDICATIONS
History of pelvic inflammatory disease since the last pregnancy
History of ectopic pregnancy (progestin-containing IUD only)
Multiple sexual partners
Nulliparous woman concerned about future fertility
Lack of available follow-up care
Menorrhagia or severe dysmenorrhea
Cervical or uterine neoplasia
Abnormal size or shape of uterus (e.g., myomas that distort cavity)
Valvular heart disease

---

tected midcycle coitus for postcoital contraception.

— If IUD failure results in a pregnancy, spontaneous abortion is more likely if the IUD in left in place (50%) than if the IUD is removed (25%).

— Spontaneous abortion with an IUD in place carries a high risk of severe sepsis; death can occur quickly.

— Women with an IUD in place who become pregnant should have the IUD removed if the string is visible.

— If the woman wishes an abortion, the IUD can be removed at that time.

— If the woman wishes to maintain the pregnancy, she should be informed about the high risk of sepsis and possibly death.

~ Any fever, myalgia, headache, or nausea requires immediate medical care for possible septic abortion.

— The ratio of ectopic pregnancies to uterine pregnancies is increased among IUD users; the examiner should palpate for adnexal masses in early pregnancy and carefully check the products of conception for placental tissue after abortion.

- *Pelvic infection:* in the first month after insertion of an IUD, there is an increased risk of pelvic infection.

— Infection at the time of insertion is reduced by antibiotic prophylaxis (e.g., doxycycline 200 mg).

— Infection after that time is usually due to sexually transmitted infections.

~ Risk of STDs can be almost totally prevented by limiting IUD use to parous women who have a mutually monogamous relationship.

— IUDs should be discouraged among young nulliparous women because of the increased risk of STDs and resulting threat to fertility.

- *Severe dysmenorrhea or menorrhagia:* IUDs can cause heavy menstrual bleeding, bleeding between periods, and more cramping; women who normally have these problems should probably not use an IUD.

— Progesterone-secreting IUDs may be tried; they cause less bleeding and cramping with menses.

— NSAIDs can be helpful in decreasing bleeding and relieving pain.

- *Partial or complete expulsion:* spontaneous expulsion of an IUD occurs in 10% to 20% of women during the first year after insertion.

— The woman can remove the IUD if it can be seen or felt in the cervical os.

Diaphragm or Cervical Cap

- With contraceptive jelly, the diaphragm is a safe and effective contraceptive.

— The diaphragm has features that are acceptable or not acceptable to women.

— It stretches from behind the cervix to beind the pubic symphysis.

— Failure rates range from 2% to 20%.

— This type has no systemic effects, and provides protection against pelvic infection and cervical dysplasia.

— A disadvantage is that it must be inserted close to the time of coitus, and pressure from the rim may result in cystitis after intercourse.

- The cervical cap with contraceptive jelly is similar to the diaphragm; it fits snugly over the cervix.

— The cap is more difficult to insert and remove than the diaphragm.

— It is used by those who cannot be fitted for a diaphragm because of a relaxed anterior vaginal wall or by those who develop recurrent bladder infections with the diaphragm.

—Risk of toxic shock syndrome is slight, but the risk makes it mandatory that neither diaphragm nor cap be left in place for longer than 12 to 18 hours.

—Neither can be used during menstrual periods.

Foam, Cream, Jelly, and Suppository Methods

- These are available over the counter, are easy to use, and are effective to a degree.
  —Failure rate ranges from 2% to 30%.
  —All contain spermicides nonoxynol-9 or octoxynol-9; both have some antiviral and antibacterial properties.

Condom

- Male condoms of latex or animal membrane provide good protection against pregnancy, equal to that of a diaphragm with spermicidal jelly.
  —When a spermicide (e.g., vaginal foam) is used with the condom, the contraceptive effectiveness is close to that of oral contraceptives.
  —Latex, but not animal membrane, also offers protection against STDs and cervical dysplasia.
  —Those wishing protection against HIV transmission are advised to use latex condoms with spermicide during vaginal or rectal intercourse.
  —Disadvantage of condoms include dulling of sensation and semen spill due to tearing, slipping, or leakage with detumescence of the penis.
- A female condom of polyurethane is available.
  —Its failure rate is about 26%.
  —It is the only woman-controlled contraceptive that provides protection from pregnancy and STDs.

Contraception Based on Fertile Periods— Family Planning

- This method is used by couples who do not wish to use other methods of contraception.
- Intercourse takes place in the postovular phase of the cycle, based on knowledge of fertile periods.

—Highly motivated couples achieve relatively good contraception, but in some, the pregnancy rate may be 20%.

- Methods to detect fertile periods are measured by
  —Increase in clear elastic cervical mucus, brief abdominal midcycle discomfort ("mittelschmerz"), and a sustained rise in basal body temperature about 2 weeks after onset of menstruation.
    ~ Unprotected intercourse is avoided from just after the menstrual period, when fertile mucus is identified, until 48 hrs after ovulation (sustained rise in temperature and disappearance of clear elastic mucus).
  —Calendar method
    ~ Length of the menstrual cycle is observed for at least 8 months.
    ~ The first fertile day is determined by subtracting 18 days from the shortest cycle.
    ~ The last fertile day is identified by subtracting 11 days from the longest cycle.
      – If the cycle runs 24 to 28 days, the fertile period extends from the sixth day of the cycle (24 minus 18) through the seventeenth day (28 minus 11).
  —Basal temperature method
    ~ The safe time for intercourse after ovulation is identified.
    ~ Temperature is taken immediately on waking.
    ~ A slight drop in temperature often occurs 1 to $1\frac{1}{2}$ days before ovulation, and rises about 0.4° C 1 to 2 days after ovulation, and continues for the remainder of the cycle.
    ~ New research indicates that the risk of pregnancy increases starting 5 days before ovulation, peaks on the day of ovulation, and then rapidly decreases to zero by the day after ovulation.

Emergency Contraception

- If unprotected intercourse occurs in midcycle, the following prevent implantation of the fertilized egg, with failure rate < 1.5% if begun within 72 hours after coitus:
  —Ethinyl estradiol 2.5 mg bid for 5 days
  —Ovral (50 µg of ethinyl estradiol with 0.5 mg of norgestrel): two tablets at once, two tablets 12 hours later, or four pills twice, 12

hours apart of Lo/Ovral, Nordette, Levlen, or the yellow pills in the Triphasil or Tri-Levlen regimens

~ Antinausea medication may be needed with these regimens.

~ Bleeding occurs within 3 to 4 weeks.

~ If pregnancy occurs, abortion is recommended because of exposure of the fetus to teratogenic doses of sex hormones.

—Levonorgestrel 0.75 mg given in two doses 12 hours apart, beginning within 72 hours of unprotected intercourse, is more effective, with less nausea and vomiting than experienced with the regimens previously described.

—Mifepristone (RU 486), one dose of 10 mg given within 120 hours after unprotected intercourse, is a highly effective postcoital contraceptive pill with few side effects.

~ This medication is not yet available in the United States.

—IUD insertion within 5 days of one episode of unprotected midcycle coitus also prevents pregnancy.

~ A disadvantage is risk of infection, particularly in case of rape.

• To obtain information about emergency contraception, call 1-888-NOT-2-LATE

Abortion

• Since abortion was legalized in the United States in 1973, maternal mortality rate has significantly decreased; illegal and self-induced abortion has been replaced with newer, safer procedures.

—Legal abortion has a mortality rate of 1:100,000.

~ Morbidity and mortality increase with length of gestation.

—About 90% of abortions are performed before 12 weeks' gestation, and only 3% to 4% after 17 weeks.

—Early abortions are much safer.

—In the first trimester, abortion is performed by vacuum aspiration under local anesthesia.

—In the second trimester, a D & C is done under general or local anesthesia.

—Intraamniotic instillation of hypertonic saline solution or prostaglandins is sometimes used after 18 weeks from the LMP, but is more difficult for the patient.

—Abortions are rarely performed after 20 weeks from the LMP.

Complications

• Retention of products of conception, usually associated with heavy bleeding and infection

—Analysis of the removed tissue can determine presence of ectopic pregnancy signs and symptoms of fever, bleeding, or abdominal pain after abortion should be examined.

—Broad-spectrum antibiotics should be given.

—Reaspiration of the uterus may be needed.

• Emergency care after illegal abortion often requires treatment for hemorrhage, septic shock, or uterine perforation.

—Rh immunoglobulin is given to all Rh-negative women after abortion.

—Contraception should be discussed fully, and contraceptive pills provided.

—For women with a history of pelvic inflammatory infection, prophylactic antibiotics are given.

~ Doxycycline 200 mg PO 1 hour before the procedure (or)

~ Aqueous penicillin G, 1 million units IV 30 minutes before the procedure

~ In the second trimester, cefazolin 1 g IV is given 30 minutes before the procedure.

~ Many clinics prescribe tetracycline 500 mg qid for 5 days after the procedure, for all patients.

Sterilization

• This is the preferred method of contraception for couples who want no more children.

—Because surgical sterilization is permanent, couples should be counseled in detail before sterilization because the procedure is essentially final.

~ Although sterilization is reversible in some patients, it is costly, complicated, and not always successful.

—Vasectomy is safe and simple; the vas deferens is severed and sealed through a scrotal incision under local anesthesia.

—Sterilization of women is performed by laparoscopic bipolar electrocoagulation or plastic ring application on the fallopian tubes, or by minilaparoscopy with Pomeroy tubal resection.

~ Advantages include minimal pain, small incisions, and rapid recovery.

~ Disadvantages of the Pomeroy procedure include more postoperative pain and longer recovery period.

~ The failure rate after tubal sterilization is about 0.5%, which should be discussed with the patient before surgery.

~ Long-term effects include increased risk of menstrual irregularities, but these conclusions are inconsistent.

RAPE

- The nurse practitioner who first sees a rape victim must be empathetic, beginning the encounter with a statement such as, "This is a terrible experience for you to go through. I want to help as much as I can to make it easier."
- The usual procedure is
  —Obtain written consent from the victim, guardian, or next of kin for gynecologic examination and for photographs if they are likely to be useful evidence.
  —Police should be notified; ask for advice about handling, preserving, and transferring evidence.
  —Obtain a detailed history of the event from the victim as to sequence of events, time, place, circumstances, and whether the victim can identify her attacker(s).
  —Do not indicate in any way even a tentative diagnosis, which may be false or incomplete.
  —Note date of LMP, whether she is pregnant, and the time of the most recent intercourse before the assault.
  —Note details such as body orifices penetrated, use of foreign objects, number of attackers.
  —Note the demeanor of the victim: calm, nervous, agitated, confused (drugs or alcohol may be involved).
  —Ask whether the victim came straight to the hospital emergency room, whether she washed herself in any way, or changed clothing.
  —Have the patient undress while standing on a white sheet.
    ~ Hair, dirt, leaves, underclothing, and any torn or stained clothing must be kept as evidence.

—Scrape material from under fingernails and comb pubic hair for evidence.

~ Place all items of evidence in separate bags and label specifically.

—Examine the victim; note any injury, scratch, bruise, or laceration anywhere on the body; injured areas should be photographed.

—Examine her body and genitals with a Wood's light to identify semen, which fluoresces; positive areas should be swabbed with a premoistened swab and air-dried to identify acid phosphatase.

—Colposcopy can identify small areas of injury due to forced entry, particularly the posterior fourchette.

—Pelvic examination is performed gently, with a narrow speculum lubricated with only water; collect material with sterile cotton swabs from vaginal walls and cervix, and make two air-dried smears on a clean glass slide. LABEL ALL SLIDES CAREFULLY.

~ Wet and dry swabs of vaginal secretions should be collected and refrigerated for subsequent acid phosphatase and deoxyribonucleic acid (DNA) analysis.

—Swab the mouth (molars and cheeks) and anus in the same way, if indicated.

~ Place secretions from the vagina, anus, or mouth on slides with a drop of saline, cover with a coverslip, and examine under dry magnification for motile or nonmotile sperm; record percentage of motile forms.

—Order appropriate laboratory tests.

~ Culture of vagina, anus, or mouth, as appropriate, for *Neisseria gonorrhoeae* and chlamydia

~ Pap smear of the cervix, wet mount for *Trichomonas vaginalis,* a baseline pregnancy test, and Venereal Disease Research Laboratory (VDRL) test

~ A confidential test for HIV antibody if desired by the patient, and repeated in 2 to 4 months if results are negative at time of examination

~ Repeat pregnancy test if next period is missed

~ Repeat VDRL in 6 weeks

~ Obtain blood (10 ml with no anticoagulant) and urine (100 ml), particularly if there is a history of forced ingestion of alcohol or injection of drugs.

—All labeled specimens are taken by hand and in person to the clinical pathologist or to the person responsible (not a messenger), with witnesses so as not to breach rules of evidence.

Treatment

- Give analgesics or sedatives as indicated.
- Give tetanus toxoid if deep lacerations contain soil or dirt particles.
- Give ceftriaxone 125 mg IM to prevent gonorrhea.
- Give metronidazole 2 g as a single dose and doxycycline 100 mg bid for 7 days to treat chlamydial infection.
- Prevent pregnancy by one of the methods in the Emergency Contraception section.
- Vaccinate against hepatitis B.
- Ensure that the patient, family, and friends have ongoing psychologic support after discharge.

BIBLIOGRAPHY

Beers MH, Berkow R: Gynecology and obstetrics. In Beers MH, Berkow R, eds: *The Merck manual of diagnosis and therapy,* ed 17, Whitehouse Station NJ, 1999, Merck Research Laboratories, pp 1923-2070.

Cullins VE, Huggins GR: Nonmalignant and vulvovaginal and cervical disorders. In Barker LR, Burton JR, Zieve PD, eds: *Principles of ambulatory medicine,* ed 5, Baltimore, 2000, Williams & Wilkins, pp 1435-1451.

Hutti MH, Hoffman C: Cytologic vaginosis: an overlooked cause of cyclic vaginal itching and burning, *J Amer Acad Nurse Pract* 12(2):55-57, 2000.

Lidegaard O: Oral contraceptives and myocardial infarction: Reassuring new findings (commentary), *BMJ* 318:1585, 1999.

MacKay HT: Gynecology. In Tierney LM, McPhee SJ, Papadakis MA, eds: *Current medical diagnosis & treatment 2000,* New York, 2000, Lange Medical Books/McGraw-Hill, pp 723-757.

Robinson DL, Dollins A, McConlogue-O'Shaughnessy L: Care of the woman before and after an elective abortion, *The American Journal for Nurse Practitioners* 4(3):17-29, 2000.

Schmitt M: Osteoporosis: Focus on fractures, *Patient Care for the Nurse Practitioner* 3(2):61-71, 2000.

Smith JM, Huggins GR: Birth control. In Barker LR, Burton JR, Zieve PD, eds: *Principles of ambulatory medicine,* ed 5, Baltimore, 1999, Williams & Wilkins, pp 1423-1434.

Smith JM, Huggins GR: Early detection of gynecologic malignancy. In Barker LR, Burton JR, Zieve PD, eds: *Principles of ambulatory medicine,* ed 5, Baltimore, 1999, Williams & Wilkins, pp 1452-1458.

Thorogood DN, Faragher B, Dunn N, et al: Oral contraceptives and myocardial infarction: Results of the MICA case-control study, *BMJ* 318:1579-1584, 1999.

1. Premenstrual syndrome affects women primarily between the ages of:
   a. 15 and 25
   b. 25 and 35
   c. 25 and 40
   d. 40 and 50
2. All but one of the following are typical symptoms of premenstrual syndrome. The one that is NOT typical is:
   a. Bloating
   b. Ankle edema
   c. Weight loss
   d. Breast pain
3. The cause of premenstrual syndrome is:
   a. Unknown
   b. Psychosocial factors
   c. Genetics
   d. Stress
4. The cause of dysfunctional uterine bleeding is:
   a. Older age
   b. Estrogen stimulation with inadequate progesterone
   c. Excessive secretion of progesterone
   d. Lack of sufficient endometrial lining
5. Tests usually done for patients with dysfunctional uterine bleeding include all but one of the following. The test NOT usually done is:
   a. Thyroid function tests
   b. Complete blood count
   c. HIV
   d. Coagulation time
6. Other causes of dysfunctional uterine bleeding include all but one of the following. What is NOT considered a cause?
   a. Strenuous exercise
   b. Excessive drug or alcohol use
   c. Myomas
   d. Stress
7. In cases of intractable bleeding, danazol 200 mg qid is sometimes used to create:
   a. Hypertrophic endometrium
   b. Atrophic endometrium
   c. Increased ovarian function
   d. Decreased ovarian function
8. In older women, the test/procedure that is done before beginning hormonal therapy is:
   a. Laparoscopy
   b. Hysterography

c. Endometrial sampling

d. Dilation and curettage

9. Postmenopausal vaginal bleeding is any vaginal bleeding that occurs _____ months after menses have ceased.
   a. 3
   b. 6
   c. 9
   d. 12

10. Carcinoma of the cervix is considered by many experts to be:
    a. Genetically caused
    b. Diagnosed only in older women
    c. A result of repeated trauma
    d. A sexually transmitted disease

11. The risk of cervical cancer is inversely related to:
    a. Age
    b. Age at first intercourse
    c. Age at menarche
    d. Age at first pregnancy

12. Human papilloma virus infection is closely associated with:
    a. Endometrial cancer
    b. Cervical intraepithelial neoplasia
    c. Cervical cancer
    d. Ectopic pregnancy

13. Staging of cervical carcinoma ranges between:
    a. 0 and III
    b. 0 and IIIA
    c. 0 and IIIB
    d. 0 and IVB

14. Emergency treatment for vaginal hemorrhage due to cervical cancer includes all but one of the following. Which one is NOT feasible?
    a. Wet vaginal packing
    b. Emergency irradiation
    c. Ligation and suturing of the cervix
    d. Ligation of the uterine or hypogastric arteries

15. Overall 5-year survival rate for carcinoma of the cervix is 68% in white women and _____ in black women.
    a. 25%
    b. 40%
    c. 50%
    d. 55%

16. Five-year survival rate in patients with stage IV cervical cancer is:
    a. <5%
    b. <10%
    c. <15%
    d. <20%

17. The second most common cancer of the female genital tract is:
    a. Adenocarcinoma of the fallopian tubes
    b. Adenocarcinoma of the endometrium
    c. Adenocarcinoma of the vagina
    d. Adenocarcinoma of the ovaries

18. Patients' increased risk of endometrial cancer from estrogen replacement therapy lasts for _____ after stopping hormone replacement therapy.
    a. 6 months
    b. 12 months
    c. 2 years
    d. 10 years

19. Tests performed in patients with suspected endometrial cancer include all but one of the following. The test NOT usually performed is:
    a. Chest x-ray
    b. Transvaginal sonography
    c. Magnetic resonance imaging of brain
    d. Sigmoidoscopy

20. Early diagnosis and treatment of endometrial cancer results in a 5-year survival rate of:
    a. 35%
    b. 55%
    c. 85%
    d. 95%

21. Endometriosis is a/an _____ disorder.
    a. Malignant
    b. Nonmalignant
    c. Infectious
    d. Genetic

22. In endometriosis, functioning endometrial tissue may be present in all but one of the following. The one area where endometrial tissue is NOT found is:
    a. Bone
    b. Posterior cul-de-sac
    c. Peritoneal or serosal surfaces of abdominal organs
    d. Surgical scars

23. Among fertile women, about _____% experience signs and symptoms of endometriosis.
    a. 5%
    b. 10% to 15%
    c. 20% to 25%
    d. >25%

24. The number of women who eventually develop ovarian cancer is:
    a. 1 in 10
    b. 1 in 30
    c. 1 in 50
    d. 1 in 70

25. Polycystic ovary syndrome is:
    a. A genetic disorder
    b. A hormonal disorder
    c. An endocrine disorder
    d. An age-related disorder

26. Menopause is considered to be established when menses have not occurred for:
    a. 3 months
    b. 6 months
    c. 9 months
    d. 12 months

27. The true failure rate of oral contraceptives is:
    a. 0.3%
    b. 1%
    c. 2%
    d. 3%

28. New evidence from case-controlled studies done in the United Kingdom indicates that risk of myocardial infarction associated with oral contraceptives is:
    a. Not present
    b. Minimally present
    c. Present only when the amount of estrogen is >50 μg
    d. Present only in women over age 35 who take oral contraceptives

29. Failure rates with the progestin minipill are reported as:
    a. <1%
    b. 1% to 2%
    c. 1% to 3%
    d. 1% to 4%

30. The postcoital contraceptive pill mifepristone (RU 486), developed in France, is:
    a. Available only in France
    b. Available only in Europe
    c. Now available in the United States
    d. Not available in the United States

14

Reproductive Disorders

Up to 8 weeks' gestation, both sexes share a common development, each with a primitive genital tract including the wolffian and müllerian ducts, as well as a primary perineum and primitive gonads.

- When a Y chromosome is present, the potential testis develops while the ovary regresses.
- When a Y chromosome is absent, the potential ovary develops and related ducts form a uterus and the upper vagina.

The production of the müllerian inhibitory factor from the early "testis" results in atrophy of the müllerian duct. Under the influence of testosterone and dihydrotestosterone, the wolffian duct differentiates into an epididymis, vas deferens, seminal vesicles, and prostate. Androgens cause transformation of the perineum to include a penis, penile urethra, and scrotum that contains the testes, which descend in response to androgenic stimulation. At birth, testicular volume is 0.5 to 1 ml.

PHYSIOLOGY: MALE

Hormones from the hypothalamic-pituitary-testicular axis control sexual development in the male.

- Pulses of luteinizing hormone–releasing hormone (LH-RH, gonadotropin-releasing hormone [GnRH]) are released from the hypothalamus and stimulate luteinizing hormone (LH) and follicle-stimulating hormone (FSH) release from the pituitary.
- LH stimulates testosterone production from Leydig's cells of the testis.

- Testosterone acts systematically to produce male secondary sexual characteristics, anabolism, and maintenance of libido.
  —Testosterone also acts within the testis to aid in spermatogenesis.
  —Testosterone circulates mostly bound to sex hormone-binding globulin (SHBG).
- FSH stimulates the Sertoli's cells in the seminiferous tubules to produce mature sperm and the feedback glycoprotein hormones, the inhibins (A and B), comprising α and β subunits.
- Testosterone feeds back on the hypothalamus/pituitary to inhibit LH-RH secretion.
- Inhibin causes feedback to the pituitary to decrease FSH secretion.
- Testosterone is necessary for the development of secondary sexual characteristics: growth of pubic, axillary, and facial hair; enlargement of the external genitalia; deepening of the voice; sebum secretion; muscle growth; and frontal balding.

Puberty

- The mechanisms initiating puberty are poorly understood but are thought to result from withdrawal of central inhibition of GnRH release.
  —LH and FSH are low in the prepubertal child.
- In early puberty, FSH begins to increase initially, first in nocturnal pulses, followed by an increase in LH, with a subsequent increase in testosterone levels.
  —Age of development of characteristics of puberty varies considerably among individuals regarding both age, testicular size, and height.

- Pubertal changes begin between ages 10 and 14 years, and are usually complete between the ages of 15 and 17.
  —The genitalia develop, testes enlarge, and the area of pubic hair increases.
  —Rapidity of growth (e.g., height) occurs between 12 and 17 years, during stage 4 of testicular development.
  —Full spermatogenesis occurs relatively late.

Precocious Puberty

- Development of secondary sexual characteristics before the age of 9 years is premature.
  —Idiopathic (true) precocity is very rare in boys but common in girls.
  —With no apparent cause for premature growth of pubic hair and an early growth spurt, these characteristics may be familial and consequently normal.
- Treatment with long-acting LH-RH analogs, which result in suppression of gonadotropin release by means of down-regulation of the receptor and in turn decreased sex hormone production, has been replaced by treatment with cyproterone acetate, an antiandrogen with progestational activity.
- LH-RH analogs are given by nasal spray, subcutaneously (SC), or (preferably) implant.

Other Forms of Precocity

- *Cerebral precocity:* tumors of the hypothalamus and other hypothalamic diseases present in this manner; aggressive exclusion in males is required.
- *Forbes-Albright syndrome:* seen primarily in girls, symptoms/signs are precocity, polyostotic fibrous dysplasia, and pigmentation of skin (café-au-lait)
- *Premature thelarche:* early breast development alone, usually transient, at 2 to 4 years of age; it may regress or continue until puberty
- *Premature adrenarche:* early development of pubic hair with no other changes, usually after age 5 years, and is most common in girls

Delayed Puberty

- About 95% of children have signs of pubertal development by 14 years of age.
- If these characteristics are not evident, evaluation should begin by age 15 years.

- Hypogonadism may be the cause, but most cases are a result of constitutional delay.
  —In constitutional delay, pubertal development, bone age, and stature develop in parallel.
  —Family history may show that other family members experienced the same delayed development.
  —Constitutional delay is quite common in boys but rare in girls.
- Testicular volume > 5 ml indicates the onset of puberty; an earlier sign is increasing serum testosterone.
- Basal LH/FSH levels may identify the site of a defect; LH-RH will show the stage of early puberty.
- If clinical evidence of progression into puberty is present, further evaluation is not necessary.
- If delay is prolonged, and if psychologic problems ensue (e.g., teasing by peers), short-term, low-dose sex hormone therapy may be required, under the supervision of an endocrinologist.

The Aging Male

- In males, aging results in progressive loss of sexual function with decreased morning erections and frequency of intercourse; testicular volume decreases, and gonadotropin levels gradually increase.
- Age of onset of these signs varies considerably.
- If premature hypogonadism is present from any cause, testosterone replacement therapy is given to prevent osteoporosis.
- Agents, such as finasteride inhibit 5α-reductase, is given for benign prostatic hypertrophy (BPH); these agents prevent conversion of testosterone to dihydrotestosterone, which causes local prostatic hyperplasia.
  —Although it is effective, its action is somewhat delayed.

PHYSIOLOGY OF PROLACTIN SECRETION

- Prolactin secretion is controlled by the hypothalamic-pituitary axis.
- Prolactin secretion is inhibited by dopamine.
- Factors that increase prolactin secretion (e.g., thyrotropin-releasing hormone [TRH]) are probably of less importance.
- Prolactin stimulates milk secretion but also decreases gonadal activity.

—It decreases LH-RH pulsatility at the hypothalamic level and to a lesser extent blocks the action of LH on the testis, resulting in hypogonadism.

—This activity is clinically significant.

CLINICAL EVALUATION OF GONADAL FUNCTION

Table 14-1 shows patient history questions to ask and signs of sexual disorders.

Tests of Gonadal Function

- A man having regular satisfactory intercourse or a woman with regular ovulatory cycles is highly unlikely to have significant endocrine disease.
- If symptoms are present, basal measurements of the gonadotropins, estrogen, testosterone, and prolactin levels yield much information.
- *Low testosterone or estradiol with high gonadotropins:* indicates primary gonadal disease
- *Low levels of LH/FSH and of testosterone/estradiol:* infer hypothalamic-pituitary disease
- *Confirmation of normal female reproductive endocrinology:* requires that ovulation be demonstrated, by measuring the luteal phase serum progesterone or by serial ovarian ultrasound in the follicular phase
- *Full demonstration of normal male and female function:* requires a pregnancy
  —The male should have a normal sperm count (20 to 200 $\times$ 10^6/ml), with good motility

(>60% grade I) and few abnormal forms (<20%).

- *Hyperprolactinemia:* confirmed or excluded by direct measurement of two to three samples; levels may increase with stress; ideally, a cannula should be inserted and samples taken through it 30 minutes later.
- *The clomiphene test:* used to examine hypothalamic negative feedback; clomiphene is a competitive estrogen antagonist that binds to but does not activate estrogen receptors, which results in an increase in gonadotropin secretion in the normal person

INFERTILITY

- Primary infertility affects 15% to 20% of married couples.
  —About 35% of cases result from sperm disorders, 20% from ovulatory dysfunction, 30% from tubal dysfunction, 5% from abnormal cervical mucus, and 10% from unidentified factors.
- Based on these figures, it is essential to have simultaneous evaluation of both partners.
- Clinical investigation is warranted after 6 months of unprotected intercourse (some specialists say 1 year).
- In men, a comprehensive history and physical examination are important initially.
  —Endocrinologic profiles and detailed semen analysis provide critical information.
    ~ Oligospermia indicates less than 20 million sperm/ml of ejaculate.
    ~ Azoospermia is the absence of sperm.
  —Spermatogenesis takes about 74 days, making it necessary to review findings over 3 months.
  —The history should include the following:
    ~ Testicular trauma (torsion, cryptorchidism)
    ~ Infections (mumps, orchitis, epididymitis)
    ~ Environmental factors (excessive heat, radiation, chemotherapy)
    ~ Medications (anabolic steroids, cimetidine, spironolactone), which may affect spermatogenesis
    ~ Phenytoin, which may lower FSH
    ~ Sulfasalazine
    ~ Nitrofurantoin, which may affect motility
    ~ Other drugs (alcohol, marijuana)
  —Sexual habits, frequency and timing of intercourse, use of lubricants, and previous fertility experiences also affect fertility.

TABLE 14-1

History Questions to Ask and Signs of Sexual Disorders

The History	Physical Signs
Libido	Evidence of systemic disease
Potency	Frequency of intercourse
Menstruation— relationship to age	Secondary sexual characteristics
Breasts— history of galactorrhea	Genital size (testes, ovaries, uterus)
Hirsutism	Clitoromegaly
	Breast development, gynecomastia
	Galactorrhea
	Extent and distribution of hair

From Drury PL, Howlett TA: Endocrinology. In Kumar P, Clark M, eds: *Clinical medicine,* ed 4, Edinburgh, 1998, WB Saunders, p 915.

- Loss of libido, headaches, or visual disturbances may indicate a pituitary tumor.
- The history may reveal thyroid or liver disease, which may affect spermatogenesis; diabetic neuropathy (retrograde ejaculation) or radical pelvic or retroperitoneal surgery, which may result in absence of seminal emission due to sympathetic nerve damage; or hernia repair, which may cause damage to the vas deferens or to the testicular blood supply.
- The physical examination should focus on signs and symptoms of hypogonadism.
  —Undeveloped secondary sex characteristics
  —Diminished male hair distribution (axillae, body, facial, pubic area)
  —Eunuchoid skeletal proportions (arm span 2 inches > height and upper to lower body ratio < 1.0)
  —Gynecomastia
  —Scrotal contents' testicular size (normal: 4.5 × 2.5 cm, volume 18 ml)
  —Varicoceles evident on standing or with Valsalva's maneuver
  —Palpation of the vas deferens, epididymis, and prostate

Diagnostic Tests: Male

- Semen analysis should be done after 48 to 72 hours of abstinence; the specimen should be analyzed within 1 hour of collection.
  —Abnormal sperm concentrations are <20 million/ml (volumes < 1.5 ml may result in inadequate buffering of the vaginal acidity, and may be due to retrograde ejaculation or androgen insufficiency.
  —Sperm motility is normal if 50% to 60% of cells are motile.
    ~ Abnormal motility may be due to anti-sperm antibodies or infection.
  —Sperm morphology is considered normal if 60% of cells appear normal.
    ~ Abnormal morphology may be due to varicocele, infection, or history of exposure.
- Endocrinologic evaluation is warranted if sperm counts are low or if there is clinical evidence, based on history and physical examination, of signs or symptoms of endocrine disorder.
  —Elevated FSH and LH and low testosterone (hypergonadotropic hypogonadism) are associated with primary testicular failure, which is usually irreversible.

—Low FSH and LH, along with low testosterone, are seen in secondary testicular failure (hypogonadotropic hypogonadism) and may be due to either hypothalamic or pituitary disorders; these defects are often treatable.
—Serum prolactin should be evaluated to rule out pituitary prolactinoma.
—Ultrasound of the scrotum may show subclinical varicocele.
—Vasography may be needed when symptoms indicate ductal obstruction.
—Patients who are azoospermic should have postmasturbation urine samples centrifuged and analyzed for sperm to exclude retrograde ejaculation.
  ~ Patients who are azoospermic with less than 1 ml of ejaculate should have fructose levels in the ejaculate measured; fructose is produced in the seminal vesicles; if absent, it indicates possible obstruction of the ejaculatory ducts.

Diagnostic Tests: Female

- Hysterosalpingography (oil dye) is done within 3 days of the last menstrual period.
  —Will show uterine abnormalities (septa, polyps, submucous myomas) and tubal obstruction
- A repeat x-ray film 24 hours later will confirm tubal patency if there is wide pelvic dispersion of the dye.
  —If the woman has had prior pelvic inflammation, give doxycycline 100 mg bid, begun immediately before and for 7 days after the x-ray study.
- Obstruction of the uterine tubes requires assessment for microsurgery or in vitro fertilization (IVF).
- Infrequent or absent ovulation requires further laboratory evaluation.
  —Elevated FSH and LH levels indicate ovarian failure, resulting in premature menopause.
  —Elevated LH levels with normal FSH levels confirm the presence of polycystic ovaries.
  —Elevation of blood prolactin levels may indicate pituitary microadenoma.
- Major histocompatibility antigen typing of both partners will confirm human leukocyte antigen-B locus homozygosity, found in greater than expected numbers among couples with unexplained infertility.

- Ultrasound monitoring of folliculogenesis may show the occurrence of unruptured luteinized follicles.
- Endometrial biopsy in the luteal phase associated with simultaneous serum progesterone levels will rule out luteal phase deficiency.
- Laparoscopy: about 25% of women whose basic evaluation is normal will have findings on laparoscopy explaining their infertility (e.g., peritubal adhesions, endometriotic implants).

Treatment

Medical Treatment
- Many endocrine abnormalities (e.g., hypothyroidism or hyperthyroidism) are treatable.
- Antibiotic treatment for cervicitis
- Use of condoms for up to 6 months may result in lower antibody levels and improved pregnancy rates for women with abnormal postcoital tests and demonstrated antisperm antibodies that cause sperm agglutination or immobilization.
- Women who do vigorous athletic training often have low sex hormone levels; reduced exercise and some weight gain will likely improve fertility.

Surgical Treatment
- Excision of ovarian tumors or ovarian foci of endometriosis may improve fertility.
- Microsurgical treatment for tubal obstruction caused by salpingitis or tubal ligation will reestablish fertility in a significant number of women.
- Newer surgical techniques for treating cornual or fimbrial block are increasingly successful.
- Peritubal adhesions or endometriotic implants can often be treated via laparoscopy or laparotomy immediately after laparoscopic examination, with written consent for both procedures.

Induction of Ovulation
- Clomiphene citrate—stimulates gonadotropin release, particularly LH, causing plasma estrone (E_1) and estradiol (E_2) to rise, indicating ovarian follicle maturation
  —If E_2 increases sufficiently, an LH surge occurs, triggering ovulation.
    ~ After a normal menstrual period or induction of withdrawal bleeding with progestin, give clomiphene 50 mg orally (PO) daily for 5 days.
    ~ If ovulation does not occur, increase the dose to 100 mg PO daily for 5 days; if ovulation still does not occur, increase the dose to 150, then 200 mg PO daily for 5 days and add chorionic gonadotropin 10,000 units intramuscularly (IM), 7 days after the clomiphene.
    ~ Painful ovarian cyst formation occurs in 8% of patients, warranting discontinuation of treatment.
    ~ Several recent studies have suggested a twofold to threefold increased risk of ovarian cancer when clomiphene is used for more than 1 year.
  —The rate of ovulation after this treatment is 90% if other infertility factors are ruled out; pregnancy rate is high.
    ~ Twins occur in 5% of these patients.
    ~ No increased incidence of congenital anomalies has been reported.
- Bromocriptine—is used only if prolactin levels are elevated and there is no withdrawal bleeding after progesterone administration, in which case clomiphene is used.
  —Bromocriptine should be taken with meals to minimize nausea, diarrhea, dizziness, headache, and fatigue, if these occur.
  —Usual dose is 2.5 mg qd, increased to bid or tid in increments of 1.25 mg.
  —Bromocriptine is discontinued when pregnancy occurs.
- Human menopausal gonadotropin (hMG) is indicated in cases of hypogonadotropism and most other types of anovulation (except ovarian failure).
  —This therapy requires that the patient be under the care of a specialist.
- GnRH is given in cases of hypothalamic amenorrhea that is unresponsive to clomiphene, administered in subcutaneous pulsatile manner.
  —This therapy avoids the dangerous ovarian complications and the 25% incidence of multiple pregnancy associated with hMG, although the overall rate of ovulation and pregnancy is higher with hMG.
- Treatment of inadequate transport of sperm
  —Cervical mucus provides better transport after administration of 0.3 mg of conjugated equine estrogens from days 5 to 15

of the ovarian cycle; ovulation may be delayed.

—Intrauterine insemination of concentrated washed sperm has been used to bypass a poor cervical environment associated with scant or hostile cervical mucus.

~ Sperm must be handled by sterile means, washed in sterile saline or tissue culture solutions, and centrifuged.

~ A small amount of fluid (0.5 ml) containing the sperm is then instilled into the uterus.

- Artificial insemination in azoospermia—donor sperm is used in these cases, usually resulting in pregnancy, assuming female function is normal.

—Both partners must consent to this method.

—Use of frozen sperm is preferable to fresh sperm because frozen sperm can be held pending cultures and blood test results for sexually transmitted diseases, including acquired immunodeficiency syndrome (AIDS).

- Assisted reproductive technologies—in patients with severe endometriosis, oligospermia, and immunologic or unexplained infertility may benefit from the newer techniques for IVF, gamete intrafallopian transfer (GIFT), and zygote intrafallopian transfer (ZIFT).

—These techniques are complex and require a highly experienced team of specialists.

—GIFT involves placing sperm and eggs in the fallopian tubes by laparoscopy or minilaparotomy.

~ Although GIFT is a more invasive procedure than IVF, the success rate is higher—34.4% overall in 1995.

~ The average delivery rate per retrieval using ZIFT was 27.9% in 1995.

MALE REPRODUCTIVE DISORDERS
Hypogonadism

Definition

Hypogonadism is decreased functional activity of the testes, either endocrinologic, gametogonic, or both, that results in retardation of puberty or reproductive insufficiency.

Classification

- *Primary:* primary (hypergonadotropic) hypogonadism—damage to Leydig's cells impairs androgen (testosterone) production and/or damages the seminiferous tubules, resulting in oligospermia or azoospermia and elevated gonadotropins.
- *Secondary:* secondary (hypogonadotropic) hypogonadism—disorders of the hypothalamus or pituitary impair gonadotropin secretion, which may cause erectile dysfunction or infertility.
- *Resistance to androgen action:* response to available androgen is inadequate

Etiology/Cause and Pathogenesis
(Box 14-1)

BOX 14-1
Causes of Male Hypogonadism

REDUCED GONADOTROPINS (HYPOTHALAMIC-PITUITARY DISEASE)
Hypopituitarism
Selective gonadotropic deficiency (Kallmann's syndrome)
Severe systemic illness
Severe underweight

HYPOPROLACTINEMIA

PRIMARY GONADAL DISEASE (CONGENITAL)
Anorchia/Leydig's cell agenesis
Chromosomal abnormality (e.g., Klinefelter's syndrome*)
Enzyme defects
5α-reductase deficiency

PRIMARY GONADAL DISEASE (ACQUIRED)
Testicular torsion
Castration
Local testicular disease
Chemotherapy/radiation toxicity
Renal failure
Cirrhosis/alcohol
Sickle cell disease

ANDROGEN RECEPTOR DEFICIENCY

From Drury PL, Howlett TA: Endocrinology. In Kumar P, Clark M, eds: *Clinical medicine,* ed 4, Edinburgh, 1998, WB Saunders, p 915.
*Klinefelter's syndrome is the most frequent cause of primary hypogonadism.

Primary Hypogonadism: Klinefelter's Syndrome

- This condition is seminiferous tubule dysgenesis associated with the 47,XXY karyotype, in which an extra X chromosome is acquired through maternal (60%) (and to a lesser degree, paternal) meiotic nondisjunction.
- Occurs in about 1/800 live male births.
- The condition involves a sex chromosome abnormality in which there are two or more X chromosomes and one Y, resulting in a phenotypic male.

Diagnosis

Signs and Symptoms (Table 14-2)
- Affected persons tend to be tall, with disproportionately long arms and legs.
- The testes tend to be small and firm.
- About 33% develop gynecomastia.
- Puberty occurs at the normal age, although facial hair growth is light.
- There exists a tendency to learning disabilities; there may be deficits in verbal intelligence quotient (IQ), auditory processing, and reading.
- Variations in signs and symptoms are great.
  - —Many 47,XXY males are normal in appearance and intellect and are discovered only in the evaluation of infertility or in cytogenic surveys of normal populations.
  - —It is likely that all 47,XXY males are sterile.
- There is no increase in homosexuality.
- Testicular development varies from hyalinized nonfunctional tubules to some degree of spermatozoa.
- Urinary excretion of FSH is often increased.
- Gonadotropins are elevated once the normal time of puberty is reached, but testosterone remains in the low-normal to low range.
- *Variants:* mosaicism occurs in about 15% of cases.
  - —Some affected persons have 3, 4, or even 5 X chromosomes along with the Y.
  - —Usually, the greater the number of X chromosomes, the more severe the mental retardation and malformations that occur.

TABLE 14-2
Tests of Gonadal Function

Test	Uses/Comments
MALE	
Basal testosterone	Normal levels exclude hypogonadism
Sperm count	Normal count excludes deficiency
	Motility and abnormal sperm should be noted
FEMALE	
Basal estradiol	Normal levels exclude hypogonadism
Luteal phase progesterone (days 18-24 of cycle)	If >30 nmol/L, suggests ovulation
Ultrasound of uterus	To confirm ovulation
BOTH SEXES	
Basal LH/FSH	Shows state of feedback system for hormone production (LH) and germ cell production (FSH)
HCG test (testosterone or estradiol measured)	Response shows potential of ovary or testis; failure shows primary gonadal disorder
Clomiphene test (LH, FSH measured)	Tests hypothalamic negative feedback system; clomiphene is estrogen antagonist
Postcoital test	Shows state of sperm and sperm-mucus interaction
LH-RH test (rarely used now)	Shows adequacy or inadequacy of LH and FSH stores in pituitary

From Drury PL, Howlett TA: Endocrinology. In Kumar P, Clark M, eds: *Clinical medicine*, ed 4, Edinburgh, 1998, WB Saunders, p 915.

Bilateral Anorchia: Vanishing Testes Syndrome

- It is presumed that the testes were present but were resorbed before birth or soon after birth.
- Normal genitalia and normal wolffian duct structures are present, but the patient lacks müllerian duct structures.
  - —These findings make it apparent that testicular tissue was present during the first 12 weeks of embryogenesis for testicular differentiation to have occurred, and for both testosterone and müllerian-inhibiting factor to have been produced.
- The clinical picture is similar to that of bilateral cryptorchidism, but there is no rise in circulating testosterone after human chorionic gonadotropin (hCG) injections.
- Early correction of cryptorchidism is indicated to try to prevent malignancy or testicular torsion.

Leydig Cell Aplasia

- Congenital absence of Leydig's cells is the cause of male pseudohermaphroditism associated with ambiguous external genitalia.
- Although there is some wolffian duct development, there is not sufficient testosterone production to induce normal male differentiation of the external genitalia.
- Müllerian duct structures are absent because of normal Sertoli's cell production of müllerian-inhibiting hormone.
- Elevated gonadotropins and low testosterone concentrations are seen.
- There is no rise in circulating testosterone after hCG injections.

Noonan Syndrome: Male Turner Syndrome

- May occur randomly, or as an autosomal dominant disorder
- Phenotypic abnormalities include hyperelasticity of the skin, hypertelorism, ptosis, low-set ears, short stature, shortened fourth metacarpals, high-arched palate, and primarily right-sided cardiovascular abnormalities (e.g., pulmonic valve stenosis, atrial septal defect).
- Testes are small or cryptorchid.
- Testosterone may be low, with high gonadotropin levels.
- Almost 80% of males with **myotonic dystrophy** have primary testicular failure, with testic-

ular biopsies that show derangement of spermatogenesis, hyalinization, and fibrosis.
- As with other causes of primary hypogonadism, gonadotropins are elevated, and testosterone levels are low or low-normal.

Adult Seminiferous Tubule Disorders

- Oligospermia or azoospermia associated with infertility may be seen in men who have idiopathic seminiferous tubule failure or who have developed such failure after testicular infections (e.g., mumps, gonorrhea), cryptorchidism, uremia, antineoplastic agents, alcoholism, irradiation, vascular damage, or trauma.
- Semen analysis is abnormal and serum FSH may be elevated, but in the case of mild oligospermia, the levels may be normal.
- Serum testosterone and LH concentrations are usually in the normal range; however, there may be an excessive increase in LH after GnRH stimulation, which suggests mild androgen deficiency.

Test of Seminiferous Tubule Function

- In adolescents or adults, a semen sample collected by masturbation 2 days after abstinence from ejaculation provides an excellent index of seminiferous tubule function.
  - —The volume of normal semen is 1 to 6 ml, $>20 \times 10^6$ sperm/ml, of which 60% are of normal morphology and motility.

Enzymatic Defects

- Defects in all of the enzymatic pathways leading to dihydrotestosterone are known.
- These congenital problems are sometimes associated with congenital adrenal hyperplasia and can cause varying degrees of ambiguity of the external genitalia such as male pseudohermaphroditism.

Secondary Hypogonadism: Panhypopituitarism

- Panhypopituitarism may occur on a congenital or anatomic basis, such as in septo-optic dysplasia or Dandy-Walker malformation, causing deficiency of either hypothalamic-releasing factors or of pituitary hormones.
- Acquired hypopituitarism may be caused by tumors and neoplasia or by their treatment, by vascular disorders, infiltrative disorders (e.g., sar-

coidosis or Langerhans' histiocytosis), infections (e.g., encephalitis or meningitis), and trauma.

- Disorders associated with hypopituitarism usually result in hormone deficiencies, which may be variable and multiple, whether arising from the anterior or posterior pituitary.

Kallmann's Syndrome

- Kallmann's syndrome is characterized by anosmia due to agenesis of the olfactory lobes and hypogonadism secondary to deficiency of hypothalamic GnRH.
- The cause is failure of fetal GnRH neurosecretory neurons to migrate from the olfactory placode to the hypothalamus.
- Inheritance is generally X-linked.
- Other manifestations may include microphallus, cryptorchidism associated with midline defects, and unilateral kidney agenesis.

Signs and Symptoms

- The age of onset of steroid deficiency establishes the clinical presentation.
- During the first trimester of pregnancy, androgen deficiency or defects in androgen action result in inadequate differentiation of the internal wolffian ducts and of the external genitalia.
  —The clinical presentation may range from ambiguity of the external genitalia or male pseudohermaphroditism to fully normal-appearing female external genitalia.
- During childhood, androgen deficiency has few consequences, but if it occurs at the usual time of puberty, secondary sexual development is impaired.
- In adulthood, androgen deficiency has varied manifestations depending on the degree and length of deficiency.
  —Testicular atrophy, decreased libido, potency, and overall strength are often present.
  —Fine wrinkling of the skin around the eyes and lips and sparse body hair may occur with long-standing hypogonadism.
  —Gynecomastia and osteopenia may also develop.

Treatment

- Treatment of the underlying glandular disorder (e.g., hypothalamic, pituitary) is required.

- Adolescents with androgen deficiency are treated with long-acting injectable testosterone enanthate or cypionate, with dose increases over an 18- to 24-month period from 50 mg up to 200 mg q 2 to 4 weeks.
- Adults with androgen deficiency are treated (until male menopause) with 200 mg of injectable testosterone q 2 to 4 weeks or with transdermal testosterone skin patch—2 patches daily unless a major contraindication exists.
  —Potential adverse effects include fluid retention, acne, and sometimes transient gynecomastia.
  —Treatment prevents the risk of osteopenia and vasomotor instability, increases libido, and prevents erectile dysfunction.
- Oral androgens are not used because of their risk of hepatocellular dysfunction or tumor formation.
- Men who want to develop spermatogenesis are treated with menopausal gonadotropins that contain 75 IU each of FSH and LH, one to two vials IM three times a week, with 2000 IU of hCG IM three times/week.
  —This treatment must be given for at least 3 months to affect spermatogenesis.
- Treatment of Kallmann's syndrome with hCG can correct cryptorchidism and establish fertility in adult males.
- Pulsatile GnRH therapy given SC via a portable pump results in endogenous sex steroid secretion, progressive virilization, and fertility.
- In isolated FSH deficiency, epiphyseal closure is usually induced by testosterone by means of its conversion to estrogen by aromatase.

Infertility in Patients with Hypogonadism

Treatment

- Often, a major goal in the treatment of hypogonadal patients is to restore or to improve fertility.
- Patients with hypogonadism may not be infertile, depending on the underlying disorder.
- Infertility that is primarily gonadal is usually resistant to intervention.
- Replacement of testosterone in males suppresses LH and FSH, causing reduced sperm counts and testicular atrophy.

- In patients with central hypogonadism (LH or FSH deficiency), infertility as well as deficient testosterone levels may be treated with gonadotropins.
  —hCG is used for its LH-like activity (human LH is unavailable).
  —Injections of 2000 to 4000 IU of hCG (e.g., Pregnyl, Follutein) three times/week will normalize testosterone levels, usually within a month, and may also stimulate spermatogenesis.
- In patients with primary central failure, agents with both LH- (hCG) and FSH-like activity may be required to initiate spermatogenesis.
  —hCG requires more frequent injections than when giving testosterone, and perhaps should therefore be restricted to those with central hypogonadism who are concerned about fertility.
- Follow-up with treated patients should include questions regarding sexual function and assessment of habitus, beard growth, physical growth, growth of phallus, and extent of deepening of voice.
  —Potency and libido usually return within a few weeks of beginning therapy, but secondary sex characteristics improve gradually over 6 months to a year.
  —Side effects of therapy should be assessed: prostate enlargement, urethral obstruction, gynecomastia.
  —In older patients, a short-acting form of testosterone is best, either via a transdermal system or, for injections, 20 mg of aqueous testosterone propionate (duration, about 3 days). If prostate complications (e.g., acute urethral outlet obstruction) occur, the effect will be short-lived.

Patient/Family Education
- Explain the nature, cause, signs and symptoms, diagnostic tests that will be done, usual course of the disorder, treatment, and follow-up.
- These disorders are not common, and little information is available to the public; the more completely patients understand the underlying problem, the more likely it is that they will participate actively in their own care.

- With most people, there is some hesitation and embarrassment around sexual matters and disorders; health care providers should be sensitive to this and create a trusting, open relationship so that communication becomes easy, or easier.

Follow-up/Referral
- Depending on the nature of the disorder, follow-up, often under the supervision of a specialist in reproductive disorders, may be necessary; sometimes, patients are followed up for months or years.
- If long-term follow-up is anticipated, the patient should know for how long, and what they might do to facilitate their progress.

Erectile Dysfunction
- Many patients with erectile dysfunction have no definable organic cause.
- A detailed history of physical illness, related symptoms, stress, psychologic factors, and drug or alcohol abuse will often help to define possible causes.
- Drugs are often the cause of erectile dysfunction: cannabis, diuretics, metoclopramide, bethanidine/guanethidine, methyldopa, and β-blockers can all produce erectile dysfunction.
- The most recent treatment for erectile dysfunction is sildenafil citrate, a phosphodiesterase inhibitor that increases penile blood flow.
- Specialist advice/treatment is essential.

Gynecomastia
Definition
Gynecomastia is the development of breast tissue in the male.

Diagnosis
- In the adult male, gynecomastia requires a complete assessment to rule out potentially serious underlying such (e.g., bronchial carcinoma, testicular tumor).
- Drugs may cause gynecomastia, especially digoxin and spironolactone.
- Elimination of drugs and significant liver disease leaves no definable cause.

Treatment
- Surgical removal of the superfluous breast tissue is sometimes necessary.

**Patient/Family Education
and Follow-up/Referral**
- See Male Reproductive Disorders section.

PHYSIOLOGY: FEMALE

- In adult women, higher brain centers impose a menstrual cycle of 28 days on the activity of hypothalamic GnRH.
- Pulses of GnRH, at about 2-hour intervals, stimulate release of pituitary LH and FSH.
- LH stimulates ovarian androgen production.
- FSH stimulates follicular development and aromatase activity (an enzyme required to convert ovarian androgen to estrogens).
  - FSH also stimulates inhibin from ovarian stromal cells; in turn, inhibin inhibits FSH release.
- Many follicles are "recruited" for development in early folliculogenesis, but by day 8 to 10, a "leading" follicle is selected for development into a mature graafian follicle.
- Estrogens show a double feedback action on the pituitary, initially inhibiting gonadotropin secretion (*negative* feedback), then later high-level exposure results in increased GnRH secretion and increased LH sensitivity to GnRH (*positive* feedback), leading to the midcycle LH surge and inducing ovulation from the leading follicle.
- The follicle then differentiates into a corpus luteum, which secretes both progesterone and estradiol during the second half of the cycle (luteal phase).
- Estrogen initially, and then progesterone, causes uterine endometrial proliferation to prepare for possible implantation of a fertilized ovum; if implantation does not occur, the corpus luteum regresses, and progesterone secretion and inhibin levels fall so that the endometrium is shed (menstruation) and allows for increased GnRH and FSH secretion.
- If implantation and pregnancy follow, hCG production from the corpus luteum maintains corpus luteum function until 10 to 12 weeks' gestation, at which time the placenta will be making sufficient estrogen and progesterone to support itself and the pregnancy.
- Estrogen circulates, mostly bound to SHBG.
  - Estrogens induce secondary sexual characteristics, development of the breasts and nipples, vaginal and vulval development, pubic hair growth, and growth and maturation of the uterus and fallopian tubes.
  - Estrogen does not increase breast size in other circumstances.

Puberty, Precocious Puberty, and Delayed Puberty (see Physiology: Male, Puberty section)

FEMALE REPRODUCTIVE DISORDERS
(TABLE 14-3)
Hypogonadism

Impaired ovarian function, whether primary or secondary, will lead to both estrogen deficiency and abnormalities of the menstrual cycle. The menstrual cycle is quite sensitive to disruption; cycles become anovulatory and irregular before disappearing altogether. Symptoms will depend on the age at which the failure develops. Therefore before puberty, primary amenorrhea will occur, possibly with delayed puberty. If after puberty, secondary amenorrhea and possibly hypogonadism will result (Table 14-4).

Hirsutism and Polycystic Ovary Syndrome

Definition

Polycystic ovary syndrome (POS), sometimes called hyperandrogenic chronic anovulation, and formerly known as Stein-Leventhal syndrome, is a benign disorder. It is usually characterized by irregular menses, mild obesity, and hirsutism. It usually begins in the pubertal years and worsens over time.

Etiology/Cause
- The cause is usually not known; investigation of possible causes (e.g., neoplasm) is necessary in some cases.

Pathogenesis
- Most patients have abundant cervical mucus on examination.
  - Elevated free estrogens
- Most levels of circulating androgens tend to be mildly elevated.
- The ovaries may be enlarged with smooth, thickened capsules, or may be normal in size.
- Usually, the ovaries contain many 2- to 6-mm follicular cysts; thecal hyperplasia surrounds the granulosa cells.

TABLE 14-3

Differential Diagnosis and Evaluation of Amenorrhea

Diagnosis	Biochemical Markers	Secondary Tests
OVARIAN FAILURE		
Ovarian dysgenesis*	High FSH	Repeat FSH
Premature ovarian failure*	High LH	Karyotype
Steroid biosynthetic defect*	Low estradiol	Laparoscopy/biopsy of ovary
(Ovariectomy)	Normal prolactin	hCG stimulation
(Chemotherapy)		Ultrasound of ovary/uterus
Resistant ovary syndrome		
POS*		
	Normal/high LH	Serum testosterone/androgens; SHBG
	Normal FSH	Ultrasound of ovary
	Normal/SL: high prolactin	Progesterone challenge
	Variable estradiol	Laparoscopy and biopsy of ovary
GONADOTROPIN FAILURE (SEE ALSO HYPOTHALAMIC CAUSES)		
Hypothalamic-pituitary disease*	Low LH	X-ray pituitary fossa
Kallmann's syndrome*	Low FSH	Clomiphene test
Anorexia*	Low estradiol	Possibly LH-RH test
Weight loss*	Normal/low prolactin	Serum thyroxine
General illness*		Pituitary MRI if diagnosis uncertain
POSSIBLE HYPOTHALAMIC CAUSES		
Hypothalamic cause*	Variable LH	Serum thyroxine
Weight gain/loss*	Variable FSH	Serum testosterone, SHBG
Exercise-induced amenorrhea	Normal prolactin	Laparoscopy and biopsy of ovary
Postpill amenorrhea	Low/normal estradiol	Pituitary MRI if diagnosis is uncertain
HYPERPROLACTINEMIA		
Prolactinemia*	High prolactin	Repeat prolactin (if >2000 mU/L, tumor is likely)
Idiopathic hyperprolactinemia*	Normal/low LH	
Hypothyroidism*	Normal/low FSH	Serum thyroxine
POS*	Normal/low estradiol	MRI or CT of pituitary
OTHER ENDOCRINE DISEASE		
Hypothyroidism	Variable LH/FSH/estradiol	Serum thyroxine
Cushing's syndrome	Variable prolactin	Clinically appropriate endocrine and imaging studies
ANDROGEN EXCESS		
Gonadal tumor	High androgen	Androgen measurement (testosterone, androstenedione)
UTERINE/VAGINAL ABNORMALITY		
Imperforate hymen*		Examination under anesthesia
Absent uterus*		Ultrasound of pelvis
Lack of endometrium		Progesterone challenge

From Drury PL, Howlett TA: Endocrinology. In Kumar P, Clark M, eds: *Clinical medicine,* ed 4, Edinburgh, 1998, WB Saunders, p 919.
SL, Serum lipoprotein.
*These conditions may present as primary amenorrhea.

TABLE 14-4
Effects of Estrogen and Symptoms of Estrogen Deficiency

Physiologic Effect	Symptoms of Deficiency
BREAST Development of connective and duct tissue Nipple enlargement and areolar pigmentation	Small, atrophic breasts
PUBIC HAIR Maintenance of female pattern	Thinning and loss of pubic hair
VULVA AND VAGINA Vulval growth Vaginal glandular and epithelial proliferation Vaginal lubrication	Atrophic vulva Atrophic vagina Dry vagina and dyspareunia
UTERUS AND TUBES Myometrial and tubal hypertrophy Endometrial proliferation	Small, atrophic uterus and tubes Amenorrhea
SKELETAL Epiphyseal fusion Maintenance of bone mass	Eunuchoidism (if prepubertal) Osteoporosis

From Drury PL, Howlett TA: Endocrinology. In Kumar P, Clark M, eds: *Clinical medicine*, ed 4, Edinburgh, 1998, WB Saunders, p 917.

- Large cysts containing atretic cells may be present.

Diagnosis
Signs and Symptoms
(see also Pathogenesis)
- Delayed menses may occur.
  - Evaluation should be done if there are no signs of puberty by age 13, if menarche has not occurred by age 16, or if ≥5 years have passed without menarche since the onset of puberty.
  - Women of reproductive age who have had menses should be evaluated if they are amenorrheic for ≥ 3 months, have < 9 menses a year, or are concerned about a change in menstrual pattern.
- A complete history and physical examination are essential.
  - Ask about abnormal growth and development.
  - Ask about family history of genetic anomalies.
  - Ask about diet and exercise, lifestyle, and environmental stresses.

- Evidence of psychologic disturbances should be sought.
- Hormonal alterations of the pubertal process and of secondary sexual characteristics are central to the diagnosis.
- Signs of virilization (masculinization) and hirsutism (hyperandrogenism)
- May be present: temporal balding, voice deepening, increased muscle mass, clitoromegaly, increased libido, and decrease in feminine secondary sexual characteristics (e.g., decreased breast size, vaginal atrophy).
- Extent of pubic hair growth should be noted.
  - It is important not to mistake hypertrichosis (excessive growth of hair on the extremities, head, and back) for true hirsutism and virilization.
- Abnormal genitalia may indicate disorders of sexual differentiation (e.g., male or female pseudohermaphroditism, müllerian duct abnormalities).
- Internal abnormalities may obstruct menstrual flow, causing hematocolpos (accumulation of menstrual blood in the vagina) and hematometra (distention of the uterus).

- Progesterone challenge will help assess the competence of the outflow tract and the level of endogenous estrogens.
  —Medroxyprogesterone acetate 5 to 10 mg/day PO for 5 days, or progesterone 100 to 200 mg IM in oil may be given.
    ~ Bleeding confirms the presence of normal endometrium and of sufficient estrogen to stimulate endometrial growth.
    ~ Women with chronic anovulation bleed, but those with premature ovarian failure do not.
  —Giving active estrogen (e.g., conjugated estrogens 2.5 mg/day for 21 days), plus medroxyprogesterone acetate 5 to 10 days PO for the last 5 days of those days produces bleeding if there is not uterine abnormality.

Diagnostic Tests

- Basal serum levels of FSH, prolactin, and thyroid-stimulating hormone (TSH) should be measured in all women with amenorrhea, to confirm the clinical impression.
  —Prolactin is increased in >30% of amenorrheic women.
    ~ An increased prolactin level should be measured again because it can be increased due to stress, sleep, and ingestion of food.
  —If thyroid function is normal and prolactin is increased, further investigation is warranted to rule out a prolactin-secreting pituitary hormone and other disorders.
  —Increased TSH (>5 MU/L) without increased prolactin indicates primary hypothyroidism.
  —In primary hypothyroidism, increased secretion of TRH stimulates production of prolactin as well as TSH in some women.
  —Increased FSH (>30 IU/L) may indicate ovarian failure.
- Total serum testosterone and dehydroepiandrosterone sulfate (DHEAS) should be measured in hirsute women.
  —Testosterone levels >200 ng/dl suggest an androgen-producing tumor, commonly of ovarian origin.
  —If DHEAS levels are twice as high as the upper limit of normal for the specific laboratory, the patient should be evaluated for an adrenal neoplasm.
  —If neither testosterone nor DHEAS is markedly elevated, extensive testing is unnecessary because serious causes have been eliminated.
- Measuring basal levels of serum LH may help to differentiate polycystic ovary syndrome from hypothalamic or pituitary dysfunction.
  —In POS, circulating LH levels are often increased, thus increasing the ratio of LH to FSH.
  —In hypothalamic or pituitary dysfunction, LH and FSH are normal or decreased.
- X-rays of the sella turcica are indicated for euthyroid women with hyperprolactinemia and for those with low gonadotropin levels, regardless of the prolactin level, to rule out a pituitary neoplasm.
- Computed tomography (CT) or magnetic resonance imaging (MRI) of the sella can determine if the patient has suprasellar extension of a pituitary neoplasm or the empty-sella syndrome, in which the sella turcica is enlarged but contains mainly cerebrospinal fluid (CSF).
- Formal visual field testing is indicated when a pituitary neoplasm is ≥10 mm in diameter on x-ray, or when there is evidence of suprasellar extension.
- Ultrasonography and CT can usually localize an androgen-producing neoplasm before surgical excision.

Treatment

- Treatment depends on the cause.
- No ideal therapy for POS exists.
- Patients may require therapy to induce ovulation if pregnancy is desired, to prevent estrogen-induced endometrial hyperplasia, or to minimize hirsutism and long-term effects of hyperandrogenism (e.g., cardiovascular disease, hypertension).
- For women who have POS and desire pregnancy, clomiphene citrate 50 to 100 mg/day for 5 days is the first choice to induce ovulation because of its simplicity and high success rate (75% ovulation rate, 35% to 40% pregnancy rate).

- For anovulatory women who have POS, are not hirsute, and do not desire pregnancy, an intermittent progestin (e.g., medroxyprogesterone acetate 5 to 10 mg/day PO for 10 to 14 days every 1 to 2 months), or oral contraceptives should be given to reduce the increased risk of endometrial hyperplasia and cancer, and to minimize circulating androgen levels.
- For women who have POS, are hirsute, and do not desire pregnancy, treatment such as bleaching, electrolysis, plucking, waxing, or depilation is suggested because no drug therapy is ideal or completely effective; oral contraceptives are the first line of therapy for mild hirsutism.

Patient/Family Education
- As with all patients, provide information about the nature, cause, signs and symptoms, usual course, and treatment.
- Treatment options should be discussed in detail, and be carried out according to the present and future wishes/desires of the patient regarding pregnancy.
- Written instructions are given with all medications.

Follow-up/Referral
- Depending on diagnosis, treatment, and patient wishes, follow-up may be short- or long-term, often provided by the primary care provider, an endocrinologist, and a gynecologist.

Turner's Syndrome (Bonnevie-Ullrich Syndrome)

Definition
Turner's syndrome (Bonnevie-Ullrich syndrome) is a sex chromosome abnormality in which there is complete or partial absence of one of the two sex chromosomes, producing a phenotypic female.

Incidence
- Turner's syndrome occurs in about 1/4000 live female births.
- About 99% of 45,X conceptions are miscarried.
- Of liveborn infants, 80% with monosomy X have loss of the paternal X.

Pathogenesis
- The chromosomal abnormalities in affected females vary.
- About 50% have a 45,X karyotype.
- Many patients are mosaics (e.g., 45,X/46,XX or 45,X/47,XXX).
- The phenotype varies from a typical Turner's syndrome to normal.
- Sometimes, affected persons have one normal X and one X that has formed a ring chromosome; for this to occur, a piece must be lost from both the short and the long arms of the abnormal X.
- Some affected persons have one normal X and one long arm isochromosome formed by the loss of short arms and development of a chromosome consisting of two long arms of the X chromosome.
  - These persons tend to have many of the phenotypic features of Turner's syndrome; therefore deletion of the short arm of the X chromosome seems to play an important role in producing the phenotype.

Diagnosis
Signs and Symptoms
- Many females with Turner's syndrome are very mildly affected.
- Affected newborns may present with marked dorsal lymphedema of the hands and feet, and with lymphedema or loose folds of skin over the posterior aspect of the neck.
- Signs that may occur include short stature, webbing of the neck, low hairline on the back of the neck, ptosis, a broad chest with widely spaced nipples, multiple pigmented nevi, short fourth metacarpals and metatarsals, prominent finger pads with whorls in the dermatoglyphics on the ends of the fingers, hypoplasia of the nails, coarctation of the aorta, bicuspid aortic valve, and increased carrying angle at the elbow.
- In some persons, telangiectasia occurs in the gastrointestinal (GI) tract, with some intestinal bleeding.
- Mental deficiency is rare, but many have some diminution of certain perceptual abilities and thus score poorly on performance tests and in mathematics, even though they score above average in verbal IQ tests.

- Gonadal dysgenesis with failure to go through puberty, develop breast tissue, or begin menses occurs in 90% of affected persons.
  —The ovaries are replaced by bilateral streaks of fibrous stroma and are usually devoid of developing ova.
  —However, 5% to 10% of affected girls do go through menarche spontaneously.
  —Very rarely, affected women have been fertile and had children.

Diagnostic Tests

- Cytogenic analysis and Y-specific probe studies must be obtained for all persons with gonadal dysgenesis to rule out mosaicism with a Y-bearing cell line (e.g., 45,X/46,XY).
  —These persons are usually phenotypic females who have variable features of Turner's syndrome and are at high risk for gonadal malignancy, especially gonadoblastoma; they should have the gonads removed prophylactically as soon as the diagnosis is made.

Treatment

- Hormone replacement therapy will induce menarche.

Patient/Family Education

- The birth of a baby with Turner's syndrome can be highly traumatic for the parents, as it is for any other anomaly.
- Reassurance is necessary from the beginning, to provide comfort and hope, but always with the caveat that future investigations may show more or fewer associated problems.
- An expert specialist in the field, together with the primary care provider, and social worker to create a strong, long-term team, is ideal.
- The parents should be kept fully informed of new developments, new drugs, and new therapies that will enable the child to be as normal as possible.
- Cognitive testing and complete physical evaluation may not be possible for some months or years, and the parents need to know the length of time that complete evaluation may take.

Follow-up/Referral

- Parents and the affected child are usually followed for years to assess progress in both physical and cognitive functions.
- A major part of long-term follow-up is to provide support to the parents.

BIBLIOGRAPHY

Drury PL, Howlett TA: Endocrinology: Reproduction and sex. In Kumar P, Clark M, eds: *Clinical medicine,* ed 4, Edinburgh, 1998, WB Saunders, pp 910-925.

Harman SM, Blackman MR: Common problems in reproductive endocrinology. In Barker LR, Burton JR, Zieve PD, eds: *Principles of ambulatory medicine,* ed 5, Baltimore, 1999, Williams & Wilkins, pp 1168-1195.

MacKay HT: Infertility. In Tierney LM, McPhee SJ, Papadakis MA, eds: *Current medical diagnosis & treatment 2000,* ed 39, New York, 2000, Lange Medical Books/McGraw-Hill, pp 743-745.

Presti JC, Stoler ML, Carroll PR: Urology: Male infertility. In Tierney LM, McPhee SJ, Papadakis MA, eds: *Current medical diagnosis & treatment 1999,* Stamford, Conn, 1999, Appleton & Lange, pp 913-915.

REVIEW QUESTIONS

1. Endogenous substances cause transformation of the perineum to include a penis, penile urethra, and scrotum that contains testes. These endogenous substances are:
   a. Enzymes
   b. Proteins
   c. Androgens
   d. Glycogens

2. The ducts of the female embryonic genital tract that form the fallopian tubes, uterus, and vagina are the:
   a. Wolffian ducts
   b. Mesonephric ducts
   c. Müllerian ducts
   d. Bartholin ducts

3. All but one of the following are the effects of testosterone. Which one is NOT an effect of testosterone?
   a. Produces male secondary characteristics
   b. Maintains libido
   c. Produces anabolism
   d. Stimulates luteinizing hormone–releasing hormone to be secreted from the hypothalamus/pituitary

4. Precocious puberty is defined as appearance of secondary sex characteristics before the age of:
   a. 7
   b. 8
   c. 9
   d. 10

5. Café-au-lait areas of pigmentation on the skin are characteristic of:
   a. Klinefelter's syndrome
   b. Forbes-Albright syndrome
   c. Turner's syndrome
   d. Dandy-Walker syndrome

6. The causes of male hypogonadism include all but one of the following. The cause NOT associated with male hypogonadism is:
   a. Hyperpituitarism
   b. Chemotherapy/radiation toxicity
   c. Renal failure
   d. Leydig's cell agenesis

7. There is a high probability that all 47,XXY males are:
   a. More likely to be homosexual
   b. Shorter than normal
   c. Sterile
   d. Highly intelligent

8. Normal levels of testosterone exclude:
   a. Hypogonadism
   b. Hypergonadism
   c. Hypopituitarism
   d. Hypothalamic disorder

9. Replacement of testosterone in males has the following effects:
   a. Suppresses luteinizing hormone
   b. Increases follicle-stimulating hormone
   c. Increases sperm counts
   d. Enlargement of testes

10. In females, the 28-day menstrual cycle is imposed by:
    a. The effects of estradiol
    b. The effects of progestin
    c. The gonads
    d. The higher brain centers

11. The number of follicles selected to become a mature graafian follicle, capable of being fertilized, is:
    a. 1
    b. 2
    c. 20
    d. "many"

12. When implantation of the fertilized egg occurs, human chorionic gonadotropin production maintains corpus luteum function until 1 to 12 weeks' gestation, at which time estrogen and progesterone are produced in sufficient amounts by the:
    a. Corpus luteum
    b. Hypothalamic-pituitary axis
    c. Gonads
    d. Placenta

13. Many women who are infertile have a history of:
    a. Pelvic infections
    b. Uterine polyps
    c. Previous induced abortion(s)
    d. Low levels of estradiol

14. All except one of the factors listed are important causes of infertility. The one factor that does NOT affect fertility is:
    a. Amenorrhea/anovulation
    b. Vaginal hypoacidity
    c. Intercourse that does not occur at the time of ovulation
    d. Treated male hypogonadism

15. Women who have antisperm antibodies are instructed to:
    a. Douche with vinegar water bid
    b. Maintain abstinence from sex for 6 months
    c. Use condoms for 6 months
    d. Use a tampon daily, not just during the menstrual period, to decrease the amount of vaginal and cervical mucus

16. Anovulation prevents pregnancy; however, ovulation can be induced by:
    a. Antibiotic treatment
    b. Increased dose of contraceptive for a time
    c. Clomiphene citrate therapy
    d. Hormone replacement therapy

17. The sensitivity of the menstrual cycle to disruptions in, for example, hormone levels is:
    a. Very acute
    b. Moderately acute
    c. Mildly acute
    d. Negligible

18. The Stein-Leventhal syndrome, more commonly known as polycystic ovary syndrome, is a condition that:
    a. Is life-threatening
    b. Leads to ovarian cancer
    c. Is treatable
    d. Is benign

19. Turner's syndrome is caused by:
    a. Excessive levels of hormones during pregnancy
    b. A sex chromosome abnormality
    c. Low levels of progesterone during pregnancy
    d. Gonadoblastoma

20. For maturation, spermatogenesis requires:
    a. 15 days
    b. 24 days
    c. 56 days
    d. 72 days

15

Immunologic Disorders

THE IMMUNE SYSTEM
Definition
The immune system is a network of interacting cellular and soluble components.
- The **function** of the immune system is to distinguish entities within the body as "self" or "nonself" and to eliminate those that are nonself.
- Microorganisms are the principal nonself entities.
  —Others include neoplasms, transplants, and particular foreign substances such as toxins.
- To fulfill its functions, the immune system has evolved two mechanisms:
  —Nonspecific immunity ⎤ These two mecha-
  —Specific immunity ⎦ nisms are linked to and influence each other.

Nonspecific (Innate) Immunity
- This type of immunity
  —Is older phylogenetically
  —Is present at birth
  —Does not require a previous encounter with an offending substance
  —Does not develop memory
- Nonspecific immunity includes the following:
  —Barriers: skin
  —Chemical protection: gastric acid
  —Two cellular components are
    ~ The phagocytic system: its function is to ingest and digest invading microorganisms
      – Neutrophils ⎤ in
      – Monocytes ⎦ blood

– Macrophages in tissues, lungs in alveolar macrophages, Kupffer's cells in liver sinusoids, synovial cells in lining of central nervous system (CNS), mesangial phagocytes in kidneys
    ~ The natural killer (NK) cells: their function is to kill some tumors, microorganisms, and virally infected cells
  —The soluble components are
    ~ Complement proteins
    ~ Acute phase reactants
    ~ Cytokines: nonimmunoglobulin polypeptides secreted by monocytes and lymphocytes in response to interaction with a specific antigen, a nonspecific antigen, or a nonspecific soluble stimulus (endotoxin, other cytokines)

Major Histocompatibility Complex
- The products of the major histocompatibility complex (MHC) are primarily those components that enable the immune system to differentiate self from nonself.
  —MHC genes
    ~ Are on chromosome 6
    ~ Belong to the Ig gene superfamily
    ~ Are subject to recombination
  —**Class I** MHC products consist of human leukocyte antigen (HLA)-A, HLA-B, and HLA-C.
    ~ They are widely distributed.
    ~ They are present on the surface of all nucleated cells and on platelets.
  —**Class II** MHC products consist of HLA-D, HLA-DR, HLA-DP, and HLA-DQ.

389

~ They are less widely distributed.

~ They are present on B cells, macrophages, dendritic cells, Langerhans' cells, and activated (but not resting) T cells.
  - B cells can respond to soluble antigen only when embedded within the MHC.
  - T cells recognize MHC/antigen complex.

~ Antigen-presenting cells (APCs) accomplish antigen processing and linkage of antigen with MHC before they are presented to T cells.
  - APCs are Langerhans' cells, monocytes, macrophages, follicular dendritic cells, and B cells.

~ It appears that antigen, to be processed, must be unfolded, degraded, and fragmented.
  - In exogenous processing, antigen undergoes endocytosis and degradation in lysosomes, is associated with class II MHC products, and is transported to the cell surface.
  - In endogenous processing, antigen is produced intracellularly (e.g., by viral infection) and undergoes degradation outside the lysosomes in organelles known as proteosomes.
  - The resulting peptides are transported to the rough endoplasmic reticulum (RER) by transporter proteins.
  - Once in the RER, the peptides are associated with class I MHC products before transport to the cell surface.

~ It is important to know whether antigen is associated with class I or II MHC because the CD4 and CD8 molecules act as accessory adhesion molecules by binding to class II or I, respectively.

Cytokines

- Although intimate cell contact is required for optimal T-cell responses, T cells and monocytes secrete cytokines, which can influence close or distant events.
- Cytokines are divided into several groups
  —Interferon (IFN; e.g., IFN-α, IFN-β, and IFN-γ)
  —Tumor necrosis factor (TNF; e.g., TNF-α, TNF-β, and TNF-γ)
  —Transforming growth factors
    ~ Hematopoietic colony-stimulating factors (CSFs)

- Cytokines act in concert, in tandem, or in conflict in a given immune response.
- A new family of cytokines, known as *chemokines*, were more recently identified.
  —These chemokines induce chemotaxis and migration of leukocyte subsets.
  —Four subsets of chemokines are known; they are defined by the number of intervening amino acids between the first two cysteine residues in the molecule.
    ~ Some of the receptors on chemokines may serve as the co-receptors for entry of human immunodeficiency virus (HIV) into monocytes/macrophages.
- T cells mature, acquire functional repertoires, and learn the concept of self in the thymus.
- T cells that express CD4 are referred to as T-helper (T_H) lymphocytes.
- Depending on the cytokine available, the precursors of TH_H cells develop into T_H1 or T_H2 cells; T_H1 cells favor the promotion of cellular immunity, whereas T_H2 cells favor the promotion of humoral immunity.
- Several types of killer cells exist, depending on MHC restriction, requirements for sensitization, specific targets, and response to cytokines.
  —MHC-restricted killers are
    ~ Cytotoxic T lymphocytes (CTLs)
    ~ Allogeneic CTLs
    ~ Antigen-specific CTLs (syngeneic CTLs)
  —MHC-nonrestricted killers: NK cells
    ~ Do not require sensitization to express their killer function
    ~ Make up 5% to 30% of normal peripheral blood lymphocytes
    ~ Express CD16, a receptor for immunoglobulin G (IgG)-Fc

Tests of Cellular Immunity

- Minimum quantitative evaluation tests
  —Lymphocyte count
  —T-cell subset numbers (CD3, CD4, CD8)
  —NK cell numbers by fluorescence analysis
- Qualitative evaluation tests
  —Delayed-type hypersensitivity (DTH) skin tests
  —In vitro tests
    ~ Proliferation in response to soluble antigen, to anti-CD3 antibody (Ab), and to alloantigen

~ The lytic activity of NK cells (spontaneously and after stimulation with interleukin [IL]-2 or IFN)

~ Ability to elaborate cytokines with emphasis on IFN-γ, TNF-α, IL-2, and IL-4

~ Ability to generate MHC-restricted CTL

B Cells and Humoral Immunity

• B cells seem to develop in a series of programmed steps, beginning in the bone marrow with the committed stem cell, then through the early and late pro-B cell stages and the pre-B cell stage, resulting in the immature B cell.

—B cells make up 5% to 15% of blood lymphocytes.

—B cells are morphologically indistinguishable from T cells.

• B cells in peripheral tissues are precommitted to respond to a limited number of antigens.

—The first antigen–B-cell interaction is the **primary immune response.**

—The **secondary (anamnestic or booster) immune response** takes place on subsequent encounters with the same antigen.

Antigens and Antibodies

• An antigen is a substance that can elicit specific immune responses.

• An Ab can combine with specific antigens, like jigsaw puzzle pieces.

—Substances are **immunogenic** (antigenic) if the immune system is able to recognize the antigenic determinants as foreign (nonself) and if the molecular weight of the substance is large enough.

—A **hapten** is a substance of lower molecular weight than an antigen and that is unable to induce Ab formation unless attached to another molecule, usually a protein (carrier protein) (e.g., penicillin is a hapten that can attach itself to albumin).

—**Antibody structure:** Ab molecules are Igs that have a particular amino acid sequence and tertiary structure to bind to a complementary structure on antigen; most Igs are probably Abs, but it is not always possible to know the antigen to which each Ig is directed.

—**Igs** are very heterogeneous and can combine with an almost limitless number of antigens.

~ Each class of antibodies serves different functions:

– IgM: the first Ab formed after immunization (new antigen); responsible for primary immune response

– IgG: the most prevalent type of Ab; the only Ig that crosses the placenta

– IgA: found in mucous secretions (saliva, tears, respiratory, genitourinary (GU), gastrointestinal (GI) tract, and colostrum); protects tissues from bacteria and viruses

– IgD: present in serum in very low concentrations; appears to be important in the growth and development of B cells

– IgE: (reaginic, skin-sensitizing, or anaphylactic Ab), found mostly in respiratory and GI mucous secretions

The Complement System

• **The complement system** is a system of more than 34 proteins interacting in a cascade (similar to the clotting system) that leads to a variety of biologic processes.

—Many complement proteins are enzymes in serum; others reside on cell surfaces.

—The three pathways of complement activation are:

~ Classical ⎫ All are directed at
~ Alternative ⎭ cleavage of C3.
~ Mannan binding lectin

—A common final pathway is the **terminal pathway** or the **membrane attack complex** (MAC).

Resolution of an Immune Response

• An immune response usually results in massive lymphocyte proliferation and differentiation (e.g., enlarged tonsils with strep throat).

• The immune response to invasion by bacteria or other pathogens is the secretion of several cytokines.

—When the infection is controlled and the antigens are removed, cytokine secretion stops.

~ When cytokine secretion stops, lymphocytes undergo apoptosis, which can occur either by necrosis of the cell or by apoptosis (programmed cell death).

IMMUNODEFICIENCY DISORDERS
Definition

Immunodeficiency disorders are a group of diverse conditions caused by one or more immune system defects and characterized clinically by increased susceptibility to infections with consequent severe, acute, recurrent, or chronic disease (Tables 15-1 and 15-2).

Etiology

- Immunodeficiency has no common cause.
  —A single gene defect is often present.
    ~ The defect can result in a missing enzyme (e.g., adenosine deaminase deficiency); a missing protein (e.g., complement component deficiencies); or developmental arrest at a specific stage (e.g., pre-B-cell arrest in X-linked agammaglobulinemia).
- Chromosome locations of defective genes have been identified for many of the primary immunodeficiencies.
- Intrauterine events may be implicated in some illnesses.
  —Maternal alcoholism in some cases of DiGeorge syndrome.
  —Drug ingestion (e.g., phenytoin in IgA deficiency)

Signs and Symptoms

- Most signs and symptoms of immunodeficiency are caused by recurrent infections (e.g., respiratory infections).
  —However, normal infants may have 6 to 8 respiratory infections/year, depending on exposure from older siblings.
- Most immunodeficient persons develop one or more severe bacterial infections that persist, recur, or lead to complications such as sinusitis, chronic otitis, and bronchitis, which follows repeated episodes of sore throat or upper respiratory infection (URI).
  —Bronchitis may lead to pneumonia, bronchiectasis, and respiratory failure, which is the most common cause of death.
  —Most patients with T-cell deficiencies develop opportunistic infections such as *Pneumocystis carinii* or cytomegaloviruses.
- Infections of skin and mucous membranes are also common.
  —Resistant thrush may be the first sign of T-cell immunodeficiency.
  —Oral ulcers and periodontitis are common in granulocytic deficiencies.
  —Conjunctivitis occurs in antibody-deficient adults.
  —Alopecia, eczema, severe warts, pyoderma, and telangiectasia are common.
- Other symptoms include the following:
  —Diarrhea
    ~ Often noninfectious but may be associated with *Giardia lamblia*, rotavirus, cytomegalovirus, or *Cryptosporidium* species
    ~ Some patients with diarrhea may have exudative loss of serum proteins and lymphocytes.
  —Malabsorption
  —Failure to thrive
- Less common signs and symptoms are
  —Hematologic abnormalities
    ~ Autoimmune hemolytic anemia
    ~ Leukopenia
    ~ Thrombocytopenia
  —Autoimmune phenomena
    ~ Vasculitis
    ~ Arthritis
    ~ Endocrinopathies
    ~ CNS problems (e.g., chronic encephalitis, slow development, seizures)

Diagnosis

- Family history is often helpful.
  —Early death
  —Similar signs and symptoms
  —Autoimmune illness
  —Early malignancy
- Type of infection may indicate nature of the immunodeficiency.
  —Infections with major gram-positive organisms (pneumonia, streptococcal infection)
    ~ These are common in Ab (B-cell) immunodeficiencies.
  —Severe infections with viruses, fungi, opportunistic organisms
    ~ Are associated with cellular (T-cell) immunodeficiencies
  —Recurrent staphylococcal and gram-negative infections are common in phagocytic deficiencies.
  —Recurrent *Neisseria* infections are seen in those with complement component deficiencies.

TABLE 15-1
Primary Immunodeficiency Disorders: Classification and Inheritance

Disorder	Associated Signs and Symptoms
B-CELL (ANTIBODY) DEFICIENCIES	
X-linked agammaglobulinemia	Pyogenic infection after age 6 mos
Ig deficiency with hyper-IgM (XL)	Neutropenia, lymphadenopathy
IgA deficiency	Autoimmunity; respiratory or food allergy; respiratory infection; usually asymptomatic
IgG subclass deficiencies	IgA deficiency
Antibody deficiency with normal or elevated Igs	
Immunodeficiency with thymoma	Aplastic anemia
Common variable immunodeficiency	Autoimmunity
Transient hypogammaglobulinemia of infancy	Prematurity
T-CELL (CELLULAR) DEFICIENCIES	
Predominant T-cell deficiency	
DiGeorge syndrome	Hypocalcemia, peculiar facies, aortic arch abnormalities, heart disease
Chronic mucocutaneous candidiasis	Endocrinopathies
Combined immunodeficiency with Igs (Nezelof syndrome)	Bronchiectasis
Nucleoside phosphorylase deficiency (AR)	
NK cell deficiency	Severe herpes viral infection
Idiopathic CD4 lymphocytopenia	Usually asymptomatic
Combined T- and B-cell deficiencies	
Severe combined immunodeficiency (AR or XL)	
Adenosine deaminase deficiency (AR)	Skeletal abnormalities
Reticular dysgenesis	Pancytopenia
Bare lymphocyte syndrome	Absence of HLA
Ataxia-telangiectasia (XL)	Dermatitis, neurologic deterioration
Wiskott-Aldrich syndrome (XL)	Eczema, thrombocytopenia
Short-limbed dwarfism	Cartilage-hair hypoplasia, severe varicella
XL lymphoproliferative syndrome	Severe EBV infection
PHAGOCYTIC DISORDERS	
Defects of cell movement	
Hyperimmunoglobulinemia E syndrome	Staphylococcal infections, eczema, dermatitis
Leukocyte adhesion defect type 1 (AR)	Prolonged attachment of umbilical cord, leukocytosis, periodontitis
Defects of microbicidal activity	
Chronic granulomatous disease (XL or AR)	Lymphadenopathy
Neutrophil G6PD deficiency	
Myeloperoxidase deficiency (AR)	
Chédiak-Higashi syndrome (AR)	Oculocutaneous albinism, giant granules of neutrophils
COMPLEMENT DISORDERS	
Defects of complement components	
C1q deficiency	Combined immunodeficiency; SLE-like syndrome
C1rs, C1s, C4, C2 (ACD)	SLE-like syndrome, glomerulonephritis
C3, C5 (ACD)	Pyogenic infections

From Beers MH, Berkow R, eds: Immunology, allergic disorders. *The Merck manual of diagnosis and therapy,* ed 17, Whitehouse Station, NJ, 1999, Merck & Co, Inc, pp 1024-1025.
XL, X-linked; *AR,* autosomal recessive; *EBV,* Epstein-Barr virus; *G6PD,* glucose-6-phosphate dehydrogenase; *SLE,* systemic lupus erythematosus; *ACD,* autosomal codominant. *Continued*

TABLE 15-1	
Primary Immunodeficiency Disorders: Classification and Inheritance—cont'd	
Disorder	**Associated Signs and Symptoms**
COMPLEMENT DISORDERS—cont'd	
C6 ⎫	⎫ Neisserial
C7 ⎬ (ACD)	⎬ infections
C8 ⎭	⎭
C9 } (ACD)	} None proven
Defects of control proteins	
C1 inhibitor deficiency (AD)	Agioedema, SLE
Factor I (C3b inactivator) deficiency (ACD)	Pyogenic infections
Factor H deficiency (ACD)	Hemolytic-uremic syndrome, glomerulonephritis
Factor D deficiency (ACD)	Pyogenic infections
Properdin deficiency (XL)	Neisserial infections

From Beers MH, Berkow R, eds: Immunology, allergic disorders. *The Merck manual of diagnosis and therapy*, ed 17, Whitehouse Station, NJ, 1999, Merck & Co, Inc, pp 1024-1025.
AD, Autosomal dominant.

- Age of onset
  - Infants less than 6 months usually have a T-cell defect.
- Physical examination
  - Appear chronically ill, with pallor, malaise, malnutrition, and distended abdomen
  - Macular rashes, vesicles, pyoderma, eczema, petechiae, alopecia, and telangiectasia are skin manifestations of immunodeficiency states.
  - Conjunctivitis is common in adults.
  - Cervical lymph nodes and adenoid and tonsillar tissue are often absent in B- or T-cell immunodeficiency.
    - ~ A lateral pharyngeal x-ray may show absent adenoidal tissue.
  - Lymph nodes may be enlarged and suppurative.
  - Tympanic membranes are often scarred or perforated.
  - Nostrils may be crusted and excoriated (indicating purulent nasal discharge).
  - Postnasal drip
  - Decreased gag reflex
  - Liver and spleen are often enlarged and palpable.
  - Muscle mass and fat deposits in the buttocks are often decreased.
  - Neurologic examination may show delayed development or ataxia.

Laboratory Tests

- Screening tests can be made in most offices or clinics.

- Specialized tests can be done only in laboratories or hospitals with sophisticated equipment.
- In cases of suspected immunodeficiency the following are performed:
  - Complete blood count (CBC) with differential and platelet count
  - Shows anemia, thrombocytopenia, neutropenia, leukocytosis
  - Lymphopenia $< 1500/\mu l$ suggests T-cell immunodeficiency
  - Peripheral smear
  - May show Howell-Jolly bodies, other unusual red blood cell (RBC) forms that may indicate asplenia or poor splenic fuction
  - Granulocytes may indicate morphologic abnormalities (Chédiak-Higashi syndrome).
  - Profound, prolonged lymphopenia indicates T-cell immunodeficiency.
  - IgG, IgM, and IgA levels
  - Assessment of antibody function
    - ~ B-cell (antibody) deficiency
  - Clinical and laboratory evaluation of the infection
  - Delayed hypersensitivity skin tests are valuable after age 2 years.
    - ~ Mumps, *Candida* infections, tetanus toxoid, *Trichophyton* infections
  - Total serum complement activity (CH_{50}), serum C3 and C4 levels
- Used to screen for complement abnormality

Prevention

- Prevention of primary immunodeficiency is limited to genetic counseling when identified genetic inheritance patterns are known.

TABLE 15-2
Secondary Immunodeficiency Disorders

Predisposing Factors	Specific Factors
Premature and newborn infants	Physiologic immunodeficiency due to immaturity of immune system
Hereditary and metabolic diseases	Chromosomal abnormalities (Down syndrome)
	Uremia
	Malnutrition
	Diabetes mellitus
	Vitamin and mineral deficiencies
	Protein-losing enteropathies
	Nephrotic syndrome
	Myotonic dystrophy
	Sickle cell disease
Immunosuppressive agents	Radiation
	Immunosuppressive drugs
	Corticosteroids
	Antilymphocyte or antithymocyte globulin
	Anti-T-cell monoclonal antibodies
Infectious diseases	Congenital rubella
	Viral exanthems (e.g., measles, varicella)
	HIV infection
	Cytomegalovirus infection
	Infectious mononucleosis
	Acute bacterial disease
	Severe mycobacterial or fungal disease
Infiltrative and hematologic diseases	Histiocytosis
	Sarcoidosis
	Hodgkin's disease and lymphoma
	Leukemia
	Myeloma
	Agranulocytosis and aplastic anemia
Surgery and trauma	Burns
	Splenectomy
	Anesthesia
Miscellaneous	SLE
	Chronic active hepatitis
	Alcoholic cirrhosis
	Aging
	Anticonvulsant drugs
	Graft-versus-host disease

From Beers MH, Berkow R, eds: Immunology, allergic disorders. *The Merck manual of diagnosis and therapy,* ed 17, Whitehouse Station, NJ, 1999, Merck & Co, Inc, p 1026.
SLE, Systemic lupus erythematosus.

- Prenatal testing of cultured amniotic cells or fetal blood may be done to detect X-linked agammaglobulinemia, Wiskott-Aldrich syndrome, most forms of severe combined immunodeficiency, adenosine deaminase deficiency, and chronic granulomatous disease.

Prognosis

- Prognosis for most primary immunodeficiencies is highly variable; many are genetic in origin and lifelong.

- Many patients with these conditions have a guarded prognosis throughout their lives.

Treatment

- Some immunodeficiencies are curable by stem cell transplantation.
- Most patients require an extraordinary amount of care to maintain optimal health and nutrition, manage infections, prevent psychologic problems as far as possible, and manage financial burden.

- Antibiotics are essential to treat infections.
  —Continuous prophylactic antibiotics are beneficial for many patients with recurrent infections.
- Antivirals (e.g., amantadine, rimantadine for influenza; acyclovir for herpes infections)
- Ig is effective replacement therapy in most forms of Ab deficiency.
- Stem cell transplantation (by bone marrow transplantation) often successfully corrects immunodeficiency.

SPECIFIC IMMUNODEFICIENCIES IN ADULTS

Most immunodeficiency diseases are diagnosed in infancy or early childhood, but must be treated for the life of the individual; the diseases listed become manifest in later childhood, teens, or young adulthood.
- Selective IgA deficiency
- Common variable immunodeficiency (acquired agammaglobulinemia)
- Hyperimmunoglobulinemia M immunodeficiency
- Chronic mucocutaneous candidiasis
- X-linked lymphoproliferative syndrome
  —Most patients appear to be normal until Epstein-Barr virus (EBV) infection occurs.
- Hyper-IgE syndrome
  —Recurrent staphylococcal infections of the skin are the most prominent feature.
- Chronic granulomatous disease
  —Onset occurs from early childhood to early teens, characterized by recurrent infections with various organisms (*Staphylococcus* organisms, *Serratia* organisms, *Escherichia coli*).

BIBLIOGRAPHY

Beers MH, Berkow R: Immunology; Allergic disorders. In Beers MH, Berkow R, eds: *The Merck manual of diagnosis and therapy*, ed 17, Whitehouse Station, NJ, 1999, Merck Research Laboratories.

Kishiyama JL, Adelman DC: Allergic & immunologic disorders. In Tierney LM, McPhee SJ, Papadakis MA, eds: *Current medical diagnosis & treatment 2000*, New York, 2000, Lange Medical Books/McGraw-Hill, pp 783-806.

Parkin JM, Morrow WJW, Pinching AJ: Immunology. In Kumar P, Clark M, eds: *Clinical medicine*, ed 4, Edinburgh, 1998, WB Saunders.

Valentine MD: Allergy and related conditions. In Barker LR, Burton JR, Zieve PD, eds: *Principles of ambulatory medicine*, ed 5, Baltimore, 1999, Williams & Wilkins.

REVIEW QUESTIONS

1. The immune system is best described as:
   a. A cellular complex
   b. A biochemical complex
   c. A reactive complex
   d. A protective complex
2. The immune system protects the body against invading organisms by creating:
   a. Local barriers and inflammation
   b. Tissue reaction
   c. Cellular destruction
   d. Activation of autoantibodies
3. The organs of the immune system include all of the following EXCEPT:
   a. Bone marrow
   b. Central nervous system
   c. Thymus
   d. Spleen
4. The humoral immune response:
   a. Is particularly effective against fungal infections
   b. Is particularly effective against bacterial and viral infections
   c. Uses T cells to produce antigens
   d. Always reacts immediately
5. Natural immunity:
   a. Is not present until early childhood
   b. Requires previous exposure to an allergen
   c. Develops memory
   d. Is the fast-reacting defense system
6. The cellular component of specific (adaptive) immunity is the:
   a. T cell
   b. B cell
   c. Lymphocyte
   d. Neutrophil
7. Lymphocytes originate from:
   a. Lymph nodes
   b. Bone marrow
   c. Thymus
   d. Spleen
8. Blood cells develop from:
   a. A pluripotent stem cell
   b. Lymphoid tissue
   c. The spleen
   d. The thymus
9. Lymphocytes that develop in the thymus are called:
   a. B cells
   b. T cells

c. CD4+ (helper) cells

d. CD8 (cytotoxic) cells

10. Tonsils function similarly to:
    a. Lymphocytes
    b. The spleen
    c. The thymus
    d. Lymph nodes

11. Human leukocyte antigens are derived from:
    a. Bone marrow
    b. The major histocompatibility complex
    c. The thymus
    d. The spleen

12. Cytokines are:
    a. Nonimmunoglobulin polypeptides
    b. Secreted by the lymph nodes
    c. Secreted by various cells
    d. High-molecular-weight proteins

13. The phagocytic process of killing and ingesting organisms is more effective if the particle is first coated with specific antibody and complement. The coating of organisms is called:
    a. Transduction
    b. Adhesion
    c. Binding
    d. Opsonization

14. Opportunistic infections occur because of:
    a. The virulence of the organism
    b. The specificity of the organism
    c. Impaired host defenses
    d. The number of invading organisms

15. Types of immunodeficiency include all of the following EXCEPT:
    a. Congenital
    b. Complement
    c. Whole-body
    d. Acquired

16. The primary cellular receptor for HIV is:
    a. Complement
    b. CD4+ T lymphocytes
    c. Immunoglobulin G
    d. B cells

17. The major and most characteristic feature in immunologic abnormalities is:
    a. Interleukin-2 depletion
    b. Complement depletion
    c. Depletion of cytotoxic T cells
    d. Depletion of CD4+ "helper" lymphocytes

18. Examples of autoimmune diseases include all of the following EXCEPT:
    a. Rheumatoid arthritis
    b. Amyotrophic lateral sclerosis
    c. Multiple sclerosis
    d. Type 1 diabetes mellitus

19. In clinical practice, immunodeficiency is:
    a. Very common
    b. Somewhat common
    c. Relatively rare
    d. Never encountered

20. The cause of immunodeficiency is usually:
    a. Defects in many of the major components of the immune system
    b. Certain drugs
    c. Unknown
    d. A single gene defect

16

Oncologic Disorders

OVERVIEW

The term *malignant disease* encompasses a wide range of illnesses, including common ones, such as lung, breast, and colon cancer, and rare ones, like acute leukemias.

Malignancies are widely prevalent and, in the West, almost a third of the population will develop cancer at some time during their life. It is second only to cardiovascular disease as the cause of death.

Whereas the mortality rate is still high in patients with cancer, many advances have been made in the last two decades, particularly with regard to treatment, and in knowledge about the etiology of the disease at the molecular level.

Treatment at the present time is given with curative or palliative intent, although the emphasis on curative intent may increase over time.

Definition

Cancer is defined as a proliferation of cells whose unique trait (loss of normal controls) results in unregulated growth, lack of differentiation, local tissue invasion, and metastasis.

Etiology

Molecular Abnormalities
- Mutations in genes are partly responsible for the growth or reproduction of malignant cells.
  —These mutations alter the quantity or behavior of the proteins encoded by growth: regulating genes and alter cell division.
- Two major categories of mutated genes are oncogenes and tumor suppressor genes.
  —The activation of oncogenes is not entirely understood, but many factors may con-

tribute (e.g., chemical carcinogens, such as tobacco smoke, or infectious agents, such as viruses).

—Oncogenes are abnormal forms of the genes that normally regulate cell growth (e.g., the *ras* gene is abnormal in about 25% of cancers).

—The Ras protein, which is encoded by the *ras* gene, regulates or signals cell division; in most circumstances, the gene is inactive, but in these malignant cells, the Ras protein is active and signals cells to divide, even though they should not.

—Another example of oncogene activity involves protein kinases, enzymes that help regulate many cellular activities, especially signaling from the cell membrane to the nucleus, thus initiating the cell's entrance into the cell cycle and controlling several other functions.

—Several human cancers (e.g., bladder cancer, breast cancer, chronic myelocytic leukemia [CML]) contain structurally altered protein kinase enzymes.

—When the kinase is overproduced or altered, it stimulates cell division continuously.

- Tumor suppressor genes normally suppress the development of malignancies by encoding for proteins that suppress tumor initiation and growth (e.g., the reticuloblastoma [RB] gene encodes for the protein pRB, which regulates the cell cycle by stopping deoxyribonucleic acid [DNA] replication).

—Mutations in the RB gene occur in 30% to 40% of all human cancers, allowing affected cells to divide continuously.

Chromosomal Abnormalities

- Although phenotypic heterogeneity occurs with any malignancy, genotypically a given cancer is believed to arise from a clone of transformed cells.
- The factors that ultimately cause genic or chromosomal changes are unknown; the deletion, translocation, or duplication of important genes gives a cancer cell a proliferative advantage over normal cells; and a tumor may develop.
- Chromosomal abnormalities are found in certain human cancers (e.g., about 80% of patients with CML have the Philadelphia t[9:22] chromosome).
  - Changes in cells indicate that a chromosomal change has occurred in the malignant cells.
  - For example, the loss of alleles on chromosome 17p and 18q appears important in the etiology of colorectal cancer.
  - The loss of alleles on chromosome 17p has also been implicated in breast cancer, gliomas, lung carcinoma, and osteosarcoma.
- The sites 17p and 18q have been suggested as the location of tumor suppressor genes.
- Patients with acute myelogenous leukemia who have normal chromosomes have a better prognosis than those with abnormal chromosomes.

Viruses

- Viruses linked with human malignancies include human papillomaviruses (cervical carcinoma), cytomegalovirus (Kaposi's sarcoma), Epstein-Barr virus (Burkitt's lymphoma, immunoblastic lymphoma, and nasopharyngeal carcinoma), and hepatitis B virus (hepatocellular carcinoma).
- Human retroviruses have been linked to T-cell lymphomas (human T-cell lymphotrophic virus [HTLV-1]), which have a predeliction for skin and bone involvement, hypercalcemia, and a leukemic phase.

Parasites

- Parasites such as *Schistosoma haematobium* have been linked to bladder cancer, which usually develops after chronic inflammation and fibrosis; *Opisthorchis sinensis* has been linked to carcinoma of the pancreas and bile ducts.

Chemical Carcinogenesis

- Chemical carcinogenesis is a multistep process:
  1. In initiation, a cell that experiences a carcinogenic event can potentially develop into a neoplastic clone.
  2. In promotion, which is reversible, continued existence of the neoplastic clonal proliferation depends on a chemical or agent with little carcinogenic activity.
  3. In progression, irreversible growth of altered (neoplastic) cells occurs.
- An agent that possesses little or no carcinogenic potency (a cocarcinogen) enhances the carcinogenic effect of another agent when exposure is simultaneous.
- Chemical carcinogenesis is influenced by age, endocrine status, diet, other exogenous agents (cocarcinogens or promoters) and immunologic status (Table 16-1).
- Ultraviolet light causes skin cancer (e.g., basal and squamous cell carcinoma, melanoma, and scleroderma pigmentosum in particular).
- Ionizing radiation is carcinogenic; survivors of the atomic bomb drop in Hiroshima and Nagasaki have a higher-than-expected incidence of leukemia and other cancers.
- Chronic irritation of the skin results in chronic dermatitis and, in some instances, squamous cell carcinoma.

Immunologic Disorders

- Patients with immunologic disorders are predisposed to lymphoreticular neoplasia, and they should be screened periodically.
  - Development of new or suspicious lymphadenopathy should be evaluated by biopsy.
  - In patients with ataxia-telangiectasia, the incidence of acute lymphoblastic leukemia (ALL), brain tumors, and gastric cancer is higher than that of the general population.
  - Patients with Wiskott-Aldrich syndrome and X-linked agammaglobulinemia are also at high risk for lymphoma and ALL.
  - Patients with immunodeficiency, as a result of either immunosuppressive drugs or

TABLE 16-1
Common Cancer-Causing Chemical Carcinogens

Carcinogen	Type of Cancer
OCCUPATIONAL CARCINOGENS	
Soot and mineral oil	Skin cancer
Arsenic	Lung and skin cancer
Asbestos	Lung cancer, mesothelioma
Hair dyes and aromatic amines	Bladder cancer
Benzene	Leukemia
Nickel	Lung cancer, nasal sinus cancer
Formaldehyde	Nasal cancer, nasopharyngeal cancer
Vinyl chloride	Hepatic angiosarcoma
Painting materials, nonarsenic pesticides, diesel exhaust, chromates, man-made mineral fibers	Lung cancer
LIFESTYLE CARCINOGENS	
Alcohol	Esophageal cancer, oropharyngeal cancer
Betel nuts	Oropharyngeal cancer
Tobacco	Head and neck cancer, lung cancer, esophageal cancer, bladder cancer
DRUG CARCINOGENS	
Alkylating agents	Leukemia
Diethylstilbestrol	Liver cell adenoma, vaginal cancer in exposed female fetuses
Oxymetholone	Liver cancer
Thorotrast	Angiosarcoma

From Beers MH, Berkow R, eds: Hematology and oncology. *The Merck manual of diagnosis and therapy,* ed 17, Whitehouse Station, NJ, 1999, Merck & Co, Inc, p 977.

human immunodeficiency virus (HIV) infection, are at risk for various neoplasms, especially large cell lymphoma and Kaposi's sarcoma.

—Patients with systemic lupus erythematosus (SLE), rheumatoid arthritis (RA), or Sjögren's syndrome are at risk for lymphoma, usually the B-cell type, presumably related to the altered immunologic status.

Diagnosis

- A complete history and physical examination are prerequisites to early diagnosis.
- Practitioners must be aware of predisposing factors and must specifically ask about familial cancer, environmental exposure, and prior illness (e.g., autoimmune diseases, previous immunosuppressive therapy, acquired immunodeficiency syndrome [AIDS]).
- In the review of symptoms, the focus should be on weight loss, fatigue, fevers or night sweats, cough, hemoptysis, hematemesis or hematochezia, change in bowel habits, and persistent pain.
- Physical examination should focus on the skin, lymph nodes, lungs, breasts, abdomen, and testes, and to the prostate, rectal, and vaginal examinations.

Staging

- Once a histologic diagnosis is made, staging (determination of the extent of disease) helps to formulate treatment decisions and prognosis (Box 16-1).
  —Staging relies on data from several sources: history, physical examination, serum chemistries and enzymes, endoscopy (depending on suspected location—mediastinoscopy is done in suspected small cell lung cancer, esophagoscopy in suspected esophageal or gastric cancer), axillary node removal and biopsy, laparotomy in colon carcinoma, laparotomy with splenectomy, lymph node removal, and liver biopsy is done in some patients with Hodgkin's disease, imaging

BOX 16-1
Tumor, Node, and Metastases* Classification for Cancer Staging

LUNG CANCER

Tx	Positive cytology only
T1	<3 cm
T2	>3 cm/extends to hilar region/invades visceral pleura/partial atelactasis
T3	Chest wall, diaphragm, pericardium, mediastinum, pleura, total atelactasis
T4	Heart, great vessels, trachea, esophagus, malignant effusion
N1	Peribronchial, ipsilateral hilar
N2	Ipsilateral mediastinal
N3	Contralateral mediastinal, scalene or supraclavicular
M0	No metastasis
M1	Metastases present

From Rohatiner AZS, Slevin ML, Tate T: Medical oncology. In Kumar P, Clark M, eds: *Clinical medicine,* ed 4, Edinburgh, 1998, WB Saunders, p 419.
*A T0/N0/M0 tumor has a much better prognosis than one that is staged as T4/N3/M1.

studies, ultrasonography, and liver-spleen scans may be necessary.

Complications

- Cancer may result in pain, wasting, neuropathy, nausea, anorexia, seizures, hypercalcemia, hyperuricemia, obstruction, and organ failure.
- Other complications include cardiac tamponade, pleural effusions, spinal cord compression, superior venus cava syndrome, and various syndromes: paraneoplastic syndromes, neurologic paraneoplastic, hematologic paraneoplastic, and renal paraneoplastic.

Treatment

- Tumor immunology
  - In the past decade, molecular biology has joined with classic tumor immunology to develop new approaches in cancer therapy.
  - Immune responses can be dramatically altered by single amino acid changes in either antigens or receptors.
  - A tumor-associated antigen (TAA) is an antigen that is relatively restricted to tumor cells.
  - Tumor-specific antigens (TSAs) are antigens unique to tumor cells.
  - Tumor antigens are present on tumor cells but are not present on normal cells.
  - Some TAAs and TSAs in human cancers have been identified (e.g., Burkitt's lymphoma, neuroblastoma, malignant melanoma, osteosarcoma, renal cell carcinoma, breast cancer, as well as in some gastrointestinal [GI] and lung carcinomas).

Cellular Immunity

- The T cell is the primary cell thought to be responsible for direct recognition and killing of tumor cells.
  - T cells carry out an immunologic surveillance, destroying newly transformed tumor cells after recognizing TAAs.
  - Some T cells require the presence of humoral antibodies directed against the tumor cells (antibody-dependent cellular cytotoxicity) to initiate the interactions that lead to the death of tumor cells.
- Natural killer (NK) cells, which can kill tumor cells, are found in persons without tumors.
  - NK cells appear to recognize certain common features of tumor cells, particularly low levels of class 1 major histocompatibility complex (MHC) molecules, whereas somewhat less effective than T-cell-mediated cytotoxic mechanisms, macrophages can kill specific tumor cells when activated in the presence of TAAs, lymphokines (soluble factors) produced by T cells, or interferon (IFN).
- Lymphokines produced by immune cells stimulate growth or induce activities of other immune cells; these lymphokines include interleukin-2 (IL-2), also known as T-cell growth factor, and the IFNs.
- More recently described growth factors, such as interleukin-12 (IL-12), specifically induce cytotoxic lymphocytes (CTLs) rather than suppress T-cell responses, and thus enhance antitumor immune responses.

Humoral Immunity

- Humoral antibodies that react with tumor cells in vitro are produced in response to various animal tumors induced by chemical carcinogens or viruses.
- Humoral antibodies directed against human tumor cells or their constituents have been shown in vitro in the sera of patients with Burkitt's lymphoma, malignant

melanoma, and lung, breast, and GI carcinomas.

- Cytotoxic antibodies are complement-fixing in general and are directed against surface antigens of relatively high density; immunoglobulin M (IgM) antibodies usually are more cytotoxic in transplantation systems than are IgG antibodies.

Immunotherapy

- Immunotherapy for cancer is considered part of a broader area—biologic therapy, or the application of biologic response modifiers (BRMs).
  —These agents can act through one or more mechanisms.
    ~ To stimulate the host's antitumor response by increasing the number of effector cells or by producing one or more soluble mediators (e.g., lymphokines)
    ~ To decrease host-suppressor mechanisms
    ~ To alter tumor cells to increase their immunogenicity or make them more susceptible to damage by immunologic processes
    ~ To improve the host's tolerance to cytotoxic drugs or radiotherapy (done by stimulating bone marrow function with granulocyte colony–stimulating factor (G-CSF) or other hematopoietic factors
- Active specific immunotherapy is designed to induce therapeutic cellular immunity in the tumor-bearing host by using autochthomous tumor cells (cells taken from the host), treating them with irradiation, neuraminidase, hapten conjugation, or hybridization with long-term cell lines in vitro and then replacing the cells.
- More recent work is the use of tumor cells that are genetically modified to produce immunostimulatory molecules, including cytokines (e.g., G-CSF factor or IL-2), costimulatory molecules such as B7-1, and allogeneic class 1 MHC molecules, which have been used successfully in animal studies and are being evaluated in human clinical trials.

Principles of Cancer Therapy

- Successful treatment of cancer requires elimination of all cancer cells, both at the primary and distant sites.

- The major methods of therapy are
  —Surgery and radiotherapy (for local or locoregional disease)
  —Chemotherapy (for systemic sites)
  —Endocrine therapy (for selected cancers such as prostate, breast, endometrium, liver)
  —Immunotherapy (BRMs to enhance endogenous immune cell kill and tumor vaccines)
  —Thermotherapy (cryotherapy and heat)
- Terms related to goals and progress of therapy include the following:
  —*Complete remission*, or *complete response*, indicates a potential cure.
    ~ These patients may appear to be cured but still have viable cancer cells that may in time cause recurrence.
  —*Partial response* is a greater than 50% reduction in the size of a tumor mass or masses and may result in significant palliation and prolongation of life, but tumor regrowth is inevitable.
  —*No response* indicates that the patient has no detectable change after therapy.
  —The time between disappearance of cancer and relapse is called the *disease-free interval*, or *disease-free survival*.
  —The *duration of response* is the time from partial response to the time of overt progression.
  —*Survival* is the time from diagnosis to death (Box 16-2).

Principles of Chemotherapy

- The ability to give anticancer treatment via the bloodstream was a major advance as it enabled therapy to potentially reach metastatic disease in any part of the body.
- However, the toxicity of the chemotherapy determined that drugs could be given only intermittently and that time had to be allowed for normal tissues to recover between each administration of new cytotoxic drugs.
- It was apparent that tumors rapidly developed resistance to single agents given on their own.
  —Based on these results, intermittent combination chemotherapy became the rule.
  —These drugs were given over a period of several days, followed by a few weeks of no treatment to allow normal tissues to regrow.
- It also became evident that normal tissues repaired more rapidly than cancer cells; it was therefore possible to deplete the tumor while

BOX 16-2
Karnowsky Performance Status (Response to Treatment)

100	Normal; no complaints
90	Able to carry on normal activity
	Minor symptoms of disease
80	Normal activity with effort
	Some symptoms of disease
70	Cares for self
	Unable to carry on normal activity or to work
60	Requires occasional assistance
	Able to care for most of own needs
50	Requires considerable assistance and frequent medical care
40	Disabled
	Requires special care and assistance
30	Severely disabled
	Hospitalization indicated although death not imminent
20	Very sick
	Hospitalization necessary, active supportive treatment necessary
10	Moribund
	Fatal processes progressing rapidly

From Rohatiner AZS, Slevin ML, Tate T: Medical oncology. In Kumar P, Clark M, eds: *Clinical medicine*, ed 4, Edinburgh, 1998, WB Saunders, p 420.

allowing the restoration of normal tissues between chemotherapy cycles.

Classification of Cytotoxic Drugs

- *Alkylating agents* act by covalently bonding alkyl groups, and their major effect is to cross-link DNA strands, interfering with DNA synthesis.
  - These were the earliest cytotoxic drugs developed, and they are still a mainstay of therapy.
  - Drugs include cyclophosphamide, chlorambucil, and busulfan.
- *Antimetabolites* are usually structural analogs of naturally occurring metabolites and interfere with normal synthesis of nucleic acids by falsely substituting purines and pyrimidines in metabolic pathways.
  - Antimetabolites are divided into folic acid antagonists, pyrimidine antagonists, and purine antagonists.
  - The classic folic acid antagonist, methotrexate, is structurally very similar to folic acid and binds preferentially to dihydrofolate reductase, the enzyme responsible for the conversion of folic acid to folinic acid; it is used widely in the treatment of solid tumors and hematologic malignancies, and plays a role in nonmalignant conditions such as rheumatoid arthritis.
  - The two major pyrimidine antagonists are 5-fluorouracil and cytosine arabinoside (cytarabine). 5-Fluorouracil consists of a uracil molecule with a substituted fluorine atom; it acts by blocking the enzyme thymidylate synthetase, which is essential for pyrimidine synthesis.
  - 5-Fluorouracil has a major role in treating solid tumors, particularly GI cancers.
  - Cytosine arabinoside is used almost exclusively in treating acute myeloid leukemia and remains the backbone of therapy.
  - 6-Mercaptopurine and 6-thioguanine are purine antagonists that are both used almost exclusively in treating acute leukemias.

Plant Alkaloids

- *Vinca alkaloids* are isolated from the periwinkle plant, and the major drugs in this class are vincristine and vinblastine.
  - These drugs act by binding to tubulin and inhibiting microtubule formation; they also have a role in treating hematologic and nonhematologic cancers.
  - They are likely best known for their potential for causing neurotoxicity.
- *Epipodophyllotoxins* are semisynthetic derivatives of podophyllotoxin, which is an extract from the mandrake plant.
  - Etoposide is used in a wide variety of cancers and works by producing DNA strand breaks by acting on the enzyme topoisomerase II.
  - Topoisomerase I inhibitors (e.g., irinotecan) are being tested; both of these enzymes unwind and uncoil the supercoiled DNA.
- *Taxanes*
  - Paclitaxel is isolated from the bark of the Western Yew.
  - Docetaxel is a semisynthetic taxane.
  - These drugs bind to tubulin dimers and prevent their assembly into microtubules.
  - These are active against ovarian and breast cancer.
  - Taxanes cause hypersensitivity reactions and patients should be premedicated with steroid H_1 and H_2 antagonists before treatment.

Cytotoxic Antibiotics

- Cytotoxic antibiotics act by intercalating adjoining nucleotide pairs on the same strand of DNA.
    —These include doxorubicin and daunorubicin, which have a wide spectrum of activity in hematologic cancers and solid tumors.
    —Doxorubicin is one of the most widely used of all cytotoxic drugs.

Platinum Analogs

- Cisplatin and carboplatin cause interstrand cross-links of DNA and are often regarded as nonclassical alkylating agents.
    —They have transformed the treatment of testicular cancer and have a major role against many other tumors, including ovarian cancer and head and neck cancers.

Side Effects of Chemotherapeutic Drugs

- Nausea and vomiting
- Hair loss
- Bone marrow suppression
- Cardiotoxicity
- Neurotoxicity
- Nephrotoxicity
- Sterility

Drug Resistance

- Drug resistance is one of the major obstacles to curing cancer with chemotherapy.
    —It is believed that most resistance occurs as a result of genetic mutation and becomes more likely as the number of tumor cells increases.
- The drugs themselves can also increase the rate of mutation to resistance.
- It has become clear that the death of cancer cells after damage by chemotherapy is not a passive event but an energy-dependent programmed event.
    —This process is called *apoptosis* or programmed cell death.
    —The process involves several oncogenes, particularly the tumor suppressor gene *p53*.
    —In tumors that have mutations of *p53* or other oncogenes involved in apoptosis, damage by chemotherapy may not lead to cell death.
    —It is increasingly apparent that failure to undergo apoptosis is a major mechanism of resistance to chemotherapeutic drugs.

Principles of Endocrine Therapy

- It has long been known that estrogen is capable of stimulating the growth of breast cancer, and androgens the growth of prostate cancer.
- Manipulation of the hormonal environment may result in regression of a number of tumors, particularly breast cancer, endometrial cancer, and prostate cancer.
- Hormonal therapy is generally not curative; however, it may provide control of a tumor for a period of time, often with few side effects.
- The presence of cell surface receptors for the hormone in question is a prerequisite for the therapy to be effective.
- The binding of hormone to receptors, and translocaton of the hormone-receptor complex into the nucleus, where it reacts with the DNA, is the action.
- Patients with breast cancer often have receptors for estrogen and progesterones.
    —Hormonal manipulation includes the use of tamoxifen, an antiestrogen drug, which blocks estrogen receptors.
    —This drug therapy and reduction of endogenous estrogen by oophorectomy or "medical oophorectomy" via pituitary down-regulation using a luteinizing hormone–releasing hormone (LH-RH) analog are effective in reducing the size of these tumors.
    —Goserelin and buserelin cause tumor regression in 30% of premenopausal women and in more than 50% of patients with estrogen-receptor–positive tumors.
    —Endometrial tumors also have receptors for both estrogen and progesterones, and frequently respond to the administration of progesterone and to the antiestrogen tamoxifen.

Principles of Biologic Therapy

- IFNs are naturally occurring cytokines normally produced in response to viral infection.
- The mechanism of action in malignant disease is uncertain.
    —IFNs have antiproliferative activity but can also increase NK cell activity and cause other immunologic changes that may result in an antitumor effect.
    —IFN-α is commercially available and has been used against several malignancies (e.g., melanoma, renal cell cancer, myeloma, and CML).

—In CML, IFN causes a reduction in the number of Philadelphia chromosome–positive cells in at least 50% of patients, and total elimination in 10%.

—Cytogenetic response has been shown to prolong survival, but IFN is not curative.

—Treatment with IFN has side effects: flu-like symptoms that tend to diminish with time and fatigue that generally does not.

—The major disadvantage is that the drug must be given as a subcutaneous injection.

- Colony-stimulating factors

  —G-CSF and granulocyte-macrophage colony–stimulating factor (GM-CSF) are used (1) to reduce the duration of neutropenia after chemotherapy, particularly in the United States, and (2) to stimulate the proliferation of hematopoietic progenitor cells in the marrow so that they enter the circulation and can be collected from the peripheral blood to support high-dose treatment.

- Monoclonal antibodies

  —Monoclonal antibodies directed against tumor cell surface antigens are used as treatment in several experimental settings.

  —They are used in vitro, in conjunction with complement, to deplete autologous bone marrow of tumor cells in patients with leukemia and lymphoma who are receiving high-dose treatment with autologous hematopoietic progenitor cell support.

  —They are also used in vitro in immunoadsorption columns, to select the CD34-positive (stem cell) fraction from peripheral blood progenitor cell, or in autologous bone marrow collections, to support high-dose treatment in hematologic and other malignancies.

  —They are used in vivo, as treatment for lymphoma (e.g., anti-CD20), which is a chimeric antibody (i.e., the molecule comprises a human constant region, with murine heavy and light chain regions); tumor cell lysis occurs by both complement and antibody-dependent cellular cytotoxicity.

    ~ The antibody is currently being evaluated as treatment for B-cell non-Hodgkin's lymphomas (NHLs), which express the antigen CD20 on their surface.

  —They are also used in vivo as a carrier molecule; antibody CD20 conjugated to radioactive iodine is being used as treatment for NHL; the antibody in these cases is being used to "carry" radiation to the CD20-bearing tumor cells.

ONCOLOGIC DISORDERS
Hematologic Malignancies (Leukemias)

See Chapter 12.

Myeloma

Definition

Myeloma is an osteolytic neoplasm consisting of a profusion of cells typical of the bone marrow that may develop in many sites and cause extensive destruction of the bone; bones most affected are the ribs, vertebrae, pelvic bones, and flat bones of the skull.

Risk Factors

- Older age

Etiology/Cause

- Myeloma is part of a spectrum of diseases characterized by the presence of a paraprotein in the serum that can be demonstrated as a monoclonal band on protein electrophoresis.
- The paraprotein is produced by abnormal, proliferating plasma cells that produce, most often, IgG or IgA and (rarely) IgD.
- The paraproteinemia may be associated with excretion of light chains in the urine that are either κ or λ; the excess light chains have for many years been known as Bence Jones protein.

Diagnosis

- Myeloma is a complex illness that reflects the interrelationships between the following:
  —*Bone destruction* causing vertebral collapse (which can cause spinal cord compression), fractures, and hypercalcemia
  —*Bone marrow infiltration* resulting in anemia, neutropenia, and thrombocytopenia, together with production of the paraprotein, which may (rarely) cause symptoms of hyperviscosity
  —*Renal impairment* due to a combination of factors: deposition of light chains, hypercalcemia, hyperuricemia, and (rarely) in patients who have had the disease for some time, deposition of amyloid

- These associated problems are complicated by a reduction in the normal Ig levels, contributing to the tendency for patients with myeloma to have recurrent infections.

Symptoms
- Bone pain—frequently, backache due to vertebral involvement
- Anemia and its associated symptoms (e.g., fatigue)
- Recurrent infections
- Renal failure
- Hypercalcemia
- Rarely, symptoms of hyperviscosity and bleeding due to thrombocytopenia

Laboratory Findings
- Complete blood count (CBC): hemoglobin (Hb) is normal or low; white blood cell count (WBC) is normal or low; platelet count is normal or low
- Erythrocyte sedimentation rate (ESR): almost always high
- Blood smear: may be rouleaux ("stacked coins") formation as a consequence of the paraprotein
- Urea and electrolytes: there may be evidence of renal failure
- Serum alkaline phosphatase: normal or increased
- Total protein: normal or increased
- Serum albumin: normal or low
- Protein electrophoresis: typically shows a monoclonal band
- Uric acid: normal or increased
- Skeletal survey: may show evidence of typical lytic lesions, most easily seen in the skull
- 24-Hour urine: to assess light chain excretion
- Bone marrow aspirate: shows characteristic infiltration by plasma cells

Treatment
- Anemia and infections are treated as in all other such cases.
- Bone pain is helped most rapidly by radiotherapy.
- Pathologic fractures may be prevented by prompt orthopedic surgery with pinning of lytic bone lesions.

- Renal impairment from hypercalcemia requires urgent attention, with the possibility of long-term dialysis.
  —Treatment of hypercalcemia is usually biphosphonates (disodium pamidronate); this therapy may also contribute to long-term control of bone disease.
  —Patients with spinal cord compression are given dexamethasone, followed by radiotherapy to the lesion delineated by a magnetic resonance imaging (MRI) scan.
- The use of alkylating agents (melphalan or cyclophosphamide) given in conjunction with prednisone has improved the median survival of patients from 7 months to 2.3 years.
- More intensive doxorubicin-containing regimens have been used recently and, in selected patients, high-dose melphalan supported by autologous bone marrow transplant (BMT) or peripheral stem cell transplantation (PSPC).
- Adjuvant interferon therapy after both standard chemotherapy and high-dose melphalan has been shown to prolong remission.

Patient/Family Education
- Instruct the patient and family regarding the nature of myeloma, its symptoms, course, treatment, and prognosis.
- Emphasize the fact that newer treatment modalities are continually being tried and perfected, the goal of which is to prolong life.
- Explain all medications and procedures as they are prescribed: reason for, what to expect, how long the treatment or procedure will last, the expected results, and the follow-up period.
- Although the outlook for most patients with myeloma is not favorable, it is important that an optimistic atmosphere be maintained.

Follow-up/Referral
- Patients can be followed closely by the primary care clinician most of the time, with continuing consultation of specialists as

needed: orthopedic surgeon, neurologist, psychiatrist, oncologist.

Bronchogenic and Lung Cancer

Definition
Bronchogenic carcinoma is a highly malignant primary lung cancer that accounts for most cases of lung cancer and has a very poor prognosis. Types of lung cancer are squamous cell, small cell, and adenocarcinoma.

Risk Factors
- History of smoking
- Second most common cancer in men (13%)
- Third most common cancer in women (13%)
- It is the leading cause of cancer death among men (32%) and women (25%).
- Most common in those 45 to 70 years

Etiology/Cause
- Cigarette smoking is the principal cause of bronchogenic cancer, accounting for 90% of cases in men and 80% in women.
- Of all lung cancers, 87% are attributed to tobacco exposure.
- A small proportion of lung cancers (15% in men, 5% in women) are related to occupational agents, often overlapping with smoking: asbestos, radiation, arsenic, chromates, nickel, chloromethyl ethers, mustard gas (poison war), and coke oven emissions.
- Radon gas in the home was thought to be a factor in some lung cancer, but a recent case-controlled study in Finland did not show an increased risk of lung cancer from indoor radon exposure.
- Damage to DNA, activation of cellular oncogenes, and stimulation by growth factors are now thought to be of primary importance in the pathophysiology of lung cancer.

Pathogenesis
- Four histologic types of bronchogenic carcinoma are distinguished.
  - Squamous cell, which usually arises in the larger bronchi, spreads by direct extension and lymph node metastasis.
  - Undifferentiated small cell, frequently associated with early hematogenous metas-

tases; spreads via the bloodstream and lymph system.
  - Undifferentiated large cell usually spreads through the bloodstream and lymph system.
  - Adenocarcinoma, usually peripheral, often spreads through the bloodstream and lymphatics.

Diagnosis
Signs and Symptoms
- Signs and symptoms depend on the tumor's location and type of spread.
- Most bronchogenic carcinomas are endobronchial, so that patients usually present with
  - Cough, with or without hemoptysis
- In patients with chronic bronchitis, increased intensity and intractability of preexisting cough suggest a neoplasm.
  - Sputum is usually not excessive but is often blood-streaked.
- Bronchial narrowing may cause air trapping with localized wheezing.
  - Atelectasis with ipsilateral mediastinal shift
  - Diminished expansion
  - Dull percussion sounds
  - Loss of breath sounds
- Infection of an obstructed lung causes the following:
  - Fever
  - Chest pain
  - Weight loss
- Persistent chest pain suggests tumor invasion of the chest wall.
- Late symptoms include the following:
  - Fatigue
  - Weakness
  - Decreased activity
  - Worsening cough
  - Pain
- Horner's syndrome, due to invasion of the cervical thoracic sympathetic nerves, is evident in
  - Enophthalmos
  - Miosis
  - Ptosis
  - Ipsilateral facial anhidrosis

- Pancoast syndrome (due to infiltration of the brachial plexus and neighboring ribs and vertebrae) causes
  —Pain
  —Numbness
  —Weakness of the affected arm
- A tumor may extend directly into the esophagus, causing
  —Obstruction
  —Formation of fistula(s)
- Phrenic nerve invasion may cause
  —Diaphragmatic paralysis
- Involvement of the heart causes
  —Dysrhythmias
  —Cardiomegaly
  —Pericardial effusion
- In case of superior vena cava syndrome, there is
  —Obstruction of venous drainage that results in dilation of collateral veins in the upper part of the chest and neck
  —Edema and plethora of the face, neck, and upper part of the body, including the breasts
  —Suffusion and edema of the conjunctiva
  —Breathlessness when supine
  —Central nervous system (CNS) symptoms: headache, visual distortion, disturbed states of consciousness

Diagnostic Data and Tests
- History
- Chest x-ray: locates the lesion; in symptomatic patients, cavitation or atelectasis may be visible
- Early detection of lung cancer does not appear to affect overall survival.
- Tissue samples for biopsy
- Computed tomography (CT) scan may be useful for staging.
- MRI of the chest is sometimes helpful in imaging the chest wall and vertebral body extension of apical Pancoast's tumors.
- Bronchoscopy is used to visualize and biopsy bronchial tumors.
- Exploratory thoracotomy is required in <10% of patients to establish the diagnosis and assess the resectability of the cancer.
  —Thoracotomy is not necessary if metastases have been demonstrated by other means.

- Staging is helpful with regard to prognosis and treatment.
  —The tumor, lymph nodes, metastasis (TNM) system is the standard staging classification for nonsmall carcinoma.
  —Small cell carcinoma has usually metastasized by the time it is diagnosed; it is staged as either limited (confined to one hemithorax with or without involvement of mediastinal and ipsilateral supraclavicular lymph nodes) or extensive (spread beyond these areas).

Differential Diagnosis
- Foreign bodies
- Nonsegmental pneumonia
- Endobronchial and focal pulmonary manifestations of tuberculosis (TB)
- Systemic mycoses
- Autoimmune disease
- Metastatic cancer caused by an extrathoracic primary cancer (e.g., breast)

Prognosis
- Bronchogenic carcinoma has a poor prognosis.
  —Untreated patients survive about 8 months.
  —About 10% to 35% of tumors are resectable, but the overall 5-year survival rate is about 13%.
  —In patients with well-circumscribed, slow-growing tumors, the 5-year survival rate after excision is from 15% in those with stage IIIA nonsmall cell carcinoma to 70% in those with stage I nonsmall cell carcinoma.
  —Best results are achieved in patients with peripheral nodular lesions treated by lobectomy.
  —Second primary lung cancers develop in 6% to 12% of survivors.
  —Because small cell carcinoma almost always has spread by the time of diagnosis, it is usually inoperable.
  —In rare cases, early small cell carcinoma can be surgically resected, but recurrence is common, so that adjuvant chemotherapy with cisplatin and etoposide usually follows surgery.
  —A second primary cancer develops after treatment of early-stage small cell carcinoma in 25% to 50% of patients.

Prevention
- Avoid tobacco and exposure to potentially carcinogenic substances in industry; second-hand smoke can also result in bronchogenic cancer.

Treatment
- Surgery is the treatment of choice for non-small cell carcinoma stages I and II.
- Patients with stage IV or IIIB carcinoma with a malignant pleural effusion are not candidates for surgery.
- Patients classified as T3N0M0 or T3N1M0 are considered for resection.
- CT scan of the chest and upper abdomen, including the liver and adrenal glands, is done before surgery.
- If patients have signs or symptoms of CNS involvement, an MRI of the brain is done before surgery.
- Older patients with lung cancer may also be candidates for surgery.
  - Untreated lung cancer patients usually survive less than 8 months, compared with an average normal life expectancy of 11.1 (men) and 14.8 (women) at age 70.
- Radiation therapy is of proven benefit for controlling bone pain, certain tumor types in the superior vena cava syndrome, spinal cord compression, brain metastasis, hemoptysis, and bronchial obstruction.
- Chemotherapy for patients in stages II, IIIA, and IIIB nonsmall cell carcinoma is promising.
  - Given before surgery in stage II or IIIA and before definitive radiation therapy in stage IIIA or IIIB, nonadjuvant chemotherapy can significantly reduce tumor burden and improve disease-free and overall survival.
- Chemotherapy with multiple drugs, particularly cisplatin and topoisomerase inhibitors (with or without radiation therapy), has yielded higher survival rates than surgery has in patients with small cell carcinoma.
  - However, cures are rare.
- Chemotherapy in unresectable stage IIIA, IIIB, or IV nonsmall carcinoma appears to improve median survival by 6 to 12 weeks on average, and can effectively ameliorate symptoms of the disease in those patients who respond to therapy.

Patient/Family Education
- Instruct the patient and family regarding the nature, cause, course, treatment, and expected outcomes of therapy.
- Patients with lung cancer survive for various periods of time, but much of that time may be spent in hospital or hospice because many of these patients die.
- Discussion with the family regarding end-stage care should be ongoing, and decisions should be made with the patient on managing the later stages of care.
- Because of severity of the patient's condition as death is near, home care may not be the best solution; this should be understood by family members.
- High-dose morphine via intravenous (IV) drip may be required to alleviate the distress of air hunger and pain experienced by many patients.

Follow-up/Referral
- Patients with lung carcinoma are followed closely from the time of presentation and diagnosis through end stage and death.
- The patient's wishes should be taken into account in decisions about care.
- Usually, many specialists are involved in the patient's care: pulmonologist, oncologist, thoracic surgeon, radiologist, and chemotherapist, who will together arrive at the best options for a particular patient.

Prostate Cancer
Definition
Prostate cancer (adenocarcinoma) occurs in the prostate gland, and is the most common malignancy in men over the age of 50.

Risk Factors
- Older age (>50)
- The incidence increases with each decade of life.
- About 209,000 new cases of prostatic cancer every year

Etiology/Cause
- Hormonal influences play a role in the development of adenocarcinoma of the prostate, but likely no role in sarcoma, undifferentiated cancer, squamous cell carci-

noma, or ductal transitional cell carcinoma.

Pathogenesis
- Prostate cancer is usually glandular, similar to the histologic configuration of normal prostate.
- Small cell proliferation and large nucleoli are characteristic.

Diagnosis
- Prostate cancer is slowly progressive and may cause no symptoms.
- A normal prostate on digital rectal examination (DRE) does not exclude carcinoma.
- In late disease, symptoms of bladder outlet obstruction, ureteral obstruction, and hematuria may appear.
- Metastases to the pelvis, ribs, and vertebral bodies may cause bone pain.
- Locally advanced cancer may show extension of induration to the seminal vesicles and fixation of the gland laterally.
- Cancer should be suspected on the basis of abnormal DRE, hypoechoic lesions on transrectal ultrasound (TRUS), or elevated levels of serum prostate-specific antigen (PSA).
- Often, cancer is diagnosed accidentally when malignant changes are found in the tissue removed during surgery for suspected benign prostatic hypertrophy (BPH).
- Whereas acid phosphatase and PSA levels decline after treatment and rise with recurrence, PSA is the most sensitive marker for monitoring cancer progression and response to therapy.
  —However, serum PSA is moderately elevated in 30% to 50% of patients with BPH, depending on the prostate size and degree of obstruction, and in 25% to 92% of those with prostate cancer, depending on tumor volume; its role in early detection and staging is still being evaluated.
  —Significantly elevated PSA levels suggest extracapsular extension of tumor or metastases.
  —Newer assays that determine the proportion of free versus bound PSA may decrease the need for biopsy in patients without cancer.

- Stony hard induration or a nodule of the prostate on DRE suggests malignancy and must be differentiated from granulomatous prostatitis, prostatic calculi, and other prostatic diseases.

Treatment
- Some older patients with localized prostate cancer, particularly if it is well-differentiated, may require no treatment but simply watchful waiting.
- Most patients elect to undergo definitive therapy with radical prostatectomy or radiotherapy.
- Radical prostatectomy is probably optimal for younger patients with long life expectancy.
  —These patients have the lowest risk of urinary incontinence (about 2%), and about 50% will be able to maintain erectile potency if at least one neurovascular bundle can be spared.
- Radiotherapy may offer comparable results, particularly in patients with low pretreatment PSA levels.
- An asymptomatic patient with a locally advanced tumor or metastases may benefit from hormonal therapy with or without adjuvant radiotherapy.
- Local radiotherapy is usually palliative in those with symptomatic bone metastases.

Prognosis
- Long-term local control, even cure, is possible in many patients.
- The potential for cure, even in patients with clinically localized cancer, depends on factors such as grade, stage, and pretreatment PSA level (Table 16-2).
- For patients with low-grade, organ-confined tumors, survival is almost identical to that for age-matched controls without prostate cancer.

Patient/Family Education
- Instruct the patient regarding the nature of the cancer, its status (level of staging), treatment options, and expected outcomes.
- Younger men are concerned about maintaining erectile potency, and this aspect

TABLE 16-2
Prostate Cancer Staging

Staging System		Characteristics of Tumor
Whitmore	AJCC/TNM	
A	T1	Clinically inapparent by palpation or imaging
	T1a	Is an incidental finding in ≤5% of resected tissue
	T1b	Is an incidental finding in ≥5% of resected tissue
	T1c	Is identified by needle biopsy performed for an elevated PSA level
B	T2	Is palpable or reliably visible on imaging, but is confined to prostate
	T2a	Involves one lobe
	T2b	Involves both lobes
C	T3	Extends through the prostate capsule
	T3a	Has extracapsular extension (unilateral or bilateral)
	T3b	Invades seminal vesicles
D	T4	Is fixed or invades adjacent structures

From Beers, MH, Berkow R, eds: Genitourinary disorders. *The Merck manual of diagnosis and therapy,* ed 17, Whitehouse Station, NJ, 1999, Merck & Co, Inc, p 1919.
AJCC, American Joint Committee on Cancer; *TNM,* tumor/node/metastasis.

should be discussed with the patient and his partner.

- Realistic treatment goals should be established as precisely as possible, depending on the factors that influence outcomes.

Follow-up/Referral

- The primary care clinician must carefully evaluate the routine DRE on all patients, and report immediately any suspicious finding, based on both symptoms and physical findings.
  —It is always better to err on the side of possibility of cancer when none exists, as opposed to not reporting minimal symptoms and findings when cancer is present.
- If cancer is strongly suspected, referral to a urologist is the next step for more comprehensive assessment and treatment.
- The primary care clinician can follow the patient through treatment and afterwards in evaluating the patient for possible recurrence.

Bladder Cancer

Definition

Bladder cancer is primary or secondary as metastasis from another source (e.g., prostate or uterine cancer).

Risk Factors

- Cigarette smoking accounts for ≥50% of new cases.
- Known urinary carcinogens are: phenacetin, cyclophosphamide, β-naphthylamine, ρ-aminodiphenyl (aniline dyes), certain chemical intermediates in the manufacture of rubber, and tryptophan metabolites.

Etiology/Cause

- As seen in risk factors, 50% or more of bladder cancers are caused by cigarette smoking.
- Chronic irritation (e.g., in schistosomiasis with bladder calculi) predisposes to bladder cancer.
- Metastasis from another site of a primary cancer

Pathogenesis

- Transitional cell carcinoma is the most common type of bladder cancer.
- At presentation, bladder cancer may range from a superficial, well-differentiated papillary tumor to a highly invasive, poorly differentiated tumor.
- Squamous cell carcinoma is less frequent and is usually associated with parasitic infestation or chronic irritation of the mucosa.

- Adenocarcinoma may occur as a primary tumor, and metastasis from a bowel carcinoma should be ruled out.

Diagnosis

Signs and Symptoms
- Microscopic hematuria may be the earliest sign.
- Pyuria, dysuria, burning, and frequency are also common early signs.
- Pelvic pain occurs with advanced disease.
- A mass may be palpable on bimanual examination.
- Filling defects of the bladder on cystography or in the cystographic phase of IVU suggest a bladder tumor.
- Urinary cytology is frequently positive for tumor cells.
- Diagnosis is by cystoscopy and transurethral biopsy or resection.
- Bimanual examination under anesthesia and pelvic CT, ultrasound (US), and MRI help in staging.

Treatment

- In patients with superficial malignancies, death from bladder cancer is very rare.
- In patients with deeply invasive lesions of the bladder musculature, survival is poor (about 50% at 5 years), but adjuvant therapy may improve these statistics.
- Squamous cell carcinoma of the bladder has a poor prognosis because it is usually highly infiltrative and presents at a more advanced stage.
- Early superficial malignancies, including superficial invasion of the bladder musculature, can be completely removed by transurethral resection and fulguration.
- Recurrence at the same or at another site in the bladder is relatively common, but may be reduced by repeated bladder instillations of chemotherapeutic drugs such as mitomycin C or doxorubicin.
- Bacille Calmette-Guérin (BCG) instillation controls superficial bladder cancer, particularly carcinoma in situ and other high-grade transitional cell carcinomas.
- Bladder instillation therapy is used to treat patients whose tumors cannot be completely resected.

- Photoradiation, now being used in investigational protocols, is available at a few institutions to treat highly selected cases of superficial bladder carcinoma.
  - A high-sensitive dye, hematoporphyrin derivative, is injected IV and taken up primarily by malignant cells.
  - Red laser light activates the dye, releasing highly reactive chemicals that kill the cancer cells.
  - Optimal case selection, dosing, and long-term results are still being evaluated.
- Tumors that deeply invade into or through the bladder wall usually require partial (about 5% of patients) or radical cystectomy.
  - For patients who cannot or will not undergo radical cystectomy, which requires concomitant urinary diversion, radiotherapy alone or in combination with chemotherapy may be curative.
- Urinary diversion usually involves routing urine to an abdominal stoma through an ileal conduit and collecting it in an external bag.
- Several other alternative methods, such as orthotopic neobladder and continent cutaneous diversion, are becoming increasingly common and are appropriate for some patients.
  - In both methods, an internal reservoir is constructed from the intestine.
  - For an orthotopic neobladder, the reservoir is connected to the urethra; the patient empties this reservoir by relaxing the pelvic floor muscles and increasing abdominal pressure so that urine passes through the urethra in an almost natural way; most patients maintain urinary control during the day, but some incontinence may occur at night.
  - For a continent cutaneous urinary diversion, the reservoir is connected to a continent abdominal stoma; the patient empties the reservoir by self-catheterization at regular intervals throughout the day.
- Metastatic malignancies require chemotherapy.
  - Several different combinations of drugs are active against this type of cancer, but relatively few patients are cured.

Patient/Family Education

- The patient and family should be instructed regarding the nature of the tumor, its size and location, course and method of treatment, and expected outcomes.
- Bladder cancer is problematic as to type, location, and staging assessment, all of which can be used to predict outcomes.
- Many menopausal women with a long history of smoking and who have some bleeding, mistakenly presumed to be from the uterus, may in fact have bladder cancer that goes undetected for months.
- The practitioner should keep in mind the possibility of bladder cancer in these patients, and question them closely on each visit regarding bleeding; the visit should include tests for hematuria and other signs of bladder cancer.
- All patients should be encouraged to stop smoking.

Follow-up/Referral

- Any patient who is suspected of having bladder cancer, or any other cancer, is referred immediately to the appropriate oncologic specialist (urologist, gynecologist, gastroenterologist) for additional evaluation and treatment.
- The primary care clinician usually follows the patient during or after treatment is concluded, paying particularly close attention to signs of recurrence.

Breast Cancer

Definition

Breast cancer is a neoplasm in any part of the breast or adjacent lymph nodes.

Risk Factors

- The cumulative risk of developing breast cancer in the United States is 12.64% (1 in 8) by age 95.
- The risk of dying is about 3.6%, with the greater proportion of the risk seen in those over age 75.
- Family history in a first-degree relative (parent, sibling, child) doubles or triples a woman's risk, but a history in more distant relatives increases the risk only slightly.
- In some studies, the risk was higher in women with relatives who had bilateral breast cancer or whose cancer was diagnosed before menopause.
- When two or more first-degree relatives have breast cancer, the risk may be five to six times higher.
- About 5% of women with breast cancer carry one of the two breast cancer genes, *BRCA1* or *BRCA2*.
  —However, women with either gene do not appear to have a greater risk of dying of breast cancer than women without the gene.
- Men who carry *BRCA2* also have an increased risk of developing breast cancer.
- The magnitude of risk is still uncertain, but may be as high as 50% to 85% by age 80.
- Women with early menarche, late menopause, or a late first pregnancy are at increased risk.
  —Women with a first pregnancy after age 30 are at higher risk than those who are nulliparous.
- Women who use oral contraceptives have a slightly higher risk than those who do not.
- Women who use postmenopausal estrogen replacement therapy have a slightly higher but less than twofold risk.

Etiology/Cause (see Risk Factors)
Diagnosis
Signs and Symptoms

- Over 80% of breast cancers are discovered as a lump by the patient.
- Less frequently, some women present with breast pain but no evidence of a mass, but some have breast enlargement or a nonspecific thickening of the breast.
- A typical cancer may be a slightly thicker area of tissue, which is not felt in the contralateral breast, may indicate cancer.
- More advanced cancers are characterized by fixation to the chest wall or to the overlying skin, by the presence of satellite nodules or ulcers of the skin, or by exaggerated skin markings (peau d'orange).
- If cancer is suspected during a physical examination, a biopsy should be scheduled soon after a mammogram that may delineate areas of the breast that should be biopsied; mammogram results should not alter the decision for biopsy.

- Increasingly, stereotactic biopsies are being done (needle biopsy performed during mammography) to improve diagnostic accuracy.
- Part of the biopsy specimen should be analyzed for estrogen and progesterone receptors.
- If metastasis is suspected, a thorough examination should be undertaken.
  —Lymphadenopathy
  —Hepatomegaly
  —Chest x-ray
  —Liver function studies
  —CBC
  —Carcinoembryonic antigen (CEA) and cancer antigen 15-3 are elevated in over 50% of patients with metastatic disease.
  —Bone scan in patients with lymphadenopathy
- Routine mammography reduces breast cancer mortality by 25% to 35% in asymptomatic women ≥ 50 years and by a smaller percentage in women ≤ 50 years.
- Ultrasonography helps distinguish a breast cyst from a solid mass.

Treatment

Invasive Cancer

- Survival rates for patients treated with modified radical mastectomy (simple mastectomy plus lymph node dissection) and for patients treated with breast-conserving surgery (lumpectomy, wide excision, partial mastectomy or quadrantectomy) plus radiation therapy appear to be identical, at least for the first 20 years.
  —The primary advantage of breast-conserving surgery with radiation therapy is cosmetic, with its resulting sense of body integrity, but it may not be possible in patients with a large mass.
  —The modified radical mastectomy removes all breast tissue but preserves the greater pectoral muscle and eliminates the need for skin graft; it has replaced the Halsted radical mastectomy.
  —Survival time after modified radical mastectomy and that after radical mastectomy are equivalent, and breast reconstruction is considerably easier after modified radical mastectomy.
- Patient preference plays a major role in the choice of treatment.

- Radiation therapy given as an adjuvant after mastectomy significantly reduces the incidence of local recurrence on the chest wall and in the regional lymph nodes, but does not improve overall survival time; as a consequence, radiation therapy after mastectomy is being used less often.

Adjuvant Systemic Therapy

- Chemotherapy or endocrine therapy begun soon after the completion of primary therapy and continued for months or years delays recurrence in almost all patients and prolongs survival in some.
  —Combination therapy may be given: cyclophosphamide, methotrexate, and 5-fluorouracil (CMF), or cyclophosphamide and doxorubicin (CA), and combination therapy is more effective than using a single drug.
  —Tamoxifen therapy is used alone and has some advantages over three-drug therapy, but it has both estrogenic effects on other parts of the body and antiestrogenic effects on breast tissue.
  —Tamoxifen carries a risk of producing endometrial cancer but significantly reduces cardiovascular mortality and osteoporosis.

Treatment of Metastatic Disease

- Breast cancer most commonly metastasizes to the lungs, liver, bone, lymph nodes, skin, and CNS.
- Treatment of metastatic disease increases median survival by 3 to 6 months.
- Even relatively toxic therapies (e.g., chemotherapy) palliate symptoms and improve quality of life.
  —Choice of treatment depends on the hormone receptor status of the primary tumor or metastatic lesion, the length of the disease-free interval from diagnosis to presentation of metastasis, and the number of metastatic sites and organs affected.
  —Tamoxifen is the endocrine therapy usually tried first.
- The most effective cytotoxic drugs for treating metastatic disease are cyclophosphamide, doxorubicin, paclitaxel, docetaxel, Navelbine, capecitabine, and mitomycin C.

Patient/Family Education

- Instruct the patient and family regarding the nature of the malignancy, its symptoms, course, response to treatments, and prognosis.
- Explain fully all procedures and medications as they are prescribed, to inform patient about the reason for the therapy, what to expect, how long it will take, and its expected effects.

Follow-up/Referral

- Patients with breast cancer are followed closely for months or years, depending on the course of the disease and the patient's response to treatment.
- Outcomes for breast cancer are much improved over those of the past, and a positive attitude on the part of health care professionals will help to bolster the patient's spirits.

Cervical Cancer

Definition

Cervical cancer is usually easily diagnosed at an early stage and treated.

Risk Factors

- In one sense, cervical cancer can be considered a sexually transmitted disease.
- Risk is inversely related to age at first intercourse and directly related to the lifetime number of sexual partners.
- Risk is increased for sexual partners of men whose previous partners had cervical cancer.
- Infection with human papillomavirus (HPV) is linked to all grades of cervical intraepithelial neoplasia (CIN) and invasive cervical cancer.
- Infection with HPV types 16, 18, 31, 33, 35, and 39 increases the risk of neoplasia.
- Cigarette smoking is associated with an increased risk of CIN and cervical cancer.

Etiology/Cause (see Risk Factors)
Pathogenesis

- Precursor cells (cervical dysplasia, CIN) develop into invasive cervical cancer over a number of years.
- CIN grades I, II, and III correspond to mild, moderate, and severe cervical dysplasia.

- CIN III, which includes severe dysplasia and carcinoma in situ, is unlikely to regress spontaneously and if untreated may eventually penetrate the basement membrane, becoming invasive carcinoma.
- Squamous cell carcinoma accounts for 80% to 85% of all cervical cancers, and adenocarcinoma accounts for most of the remainder.
- Invasive cervical cancer usually spreads by direct extension into surrounding tissues and the vagina, or via the lymphatics to the pelvic and paraaortic lymph nodes drained by the cervix.
- Hematologic spread is also possible.

Diagnosis
Signs and Symptoms

- CIN is usually asymptomatic and is discovered because of an abnormal Pap smear.
- Patients with early-stage cervical cancer usually present with irregular vaginal bleeding, most often postcoital; intermenstrual bleeding or menometrorrhagia may occur.
- Patients with larger cervical cancers or advanced-stage disease may present with foul-smelling vaginal discharge, abnormal vaginal bleeding, or pelvic pain.
- Obstructive uropathy, back pain, and leg swelling are symptoms of late-stage disease.
- More than 90% of early asymptomatic cases of CIN can be detected preclinically by cytologic examination of Pap smears obtained directly from the cervix.
  —However, the false-negative rate is 15% to 40%, depending on the patient population and the laboratory.
- About 50% of patients with cervical cancer have never had a Pap smear or have not had one for ≥10 years.
- Patients at higher risk for cervical neoplasia are the least likely to be tested regularly.
- A positive Pap smear requires further evaluation based on the descriptive diagnosis of the smear, and the patient's risk factors.
  —The cellular classification system (I to V) is no longer used.
- Suspicious cervical lesions should be biopsied directly.
- If there is no obvious lesion, colposcopy can be performed to identify areas that require biopsy and to localize the lesion; results of

the colposcopy can be correlated with the Pap smear as to color changes, vascular patterns, and margins of lesions.

- Colposcopy-directed biopsy usually provides sufficient clinical evidence to confirm a diagnosis.
- If the results of the colposcopy are inconclusive, a conization biopsy is required, performed by means of a loop-electric excision procedure (LEEP), laser, or cold knife.
- If cervical disease is invasive, staging is performed on the basis of the physical examination, with a metastatic survey that includes cystoscopy, sigmoidoscopy, IV pyelography, chest x-ray, and skeletal x-rays.
- For early-stage disease (IB or less), chest x-ray is usually the only other test needed.
- CT or MRI of the abdomen and pelvis is optional; these results cannot be used to determine clinical stage.

Treatment

- Distant metastases from invasive squamous cell carcinoma usually occur late, and this type of cancer often remains localized or regional for a considerable time.
- The 5-year survival rates are 80% to 90% for stage I, 50% to 65% for stage II, 25% to 35% for stage III, and 0% to 15% for stage IV.
- Nearly 80% of recurrences are detected within 2 years.
- Adverse prognostic factors are lymph node involvement, large tumor size, deep cervical stromal invasion, parametrial invasion, vascular space invasion, and neuroendocrine histology.
- For those with preinvasive cervical disease or microinvasive squamous cell carcinoma of the cervix, conization biopsy with LEEP, laser, or cold knife, or cryotherapy, is usually adequate treatment.
- Treatment must include the regional nodes.
- Radiation therapy or surgery may be selected; preserving surrounding tissues is a goal of treatment.
- Patients with stage IA2, IB, or IIA disease can be treated with radical hysterectomy, including bilateral pelvic lymph node dissection and removal of all adjacent ligaments (cardinal, uterosacral) and parametria.
  —Radiotherapy is also a choice; the 5-year cure rates for women with stage IB or IIA disease are 85% to 90% with either therapy.

—Advantages of surgery include a relatively short treatment time, provision of surgical staging data, preservation of ovaries in young women, and avoidance of vaginal stenosis and of late complications of radiation therapy.
—Advantages of radiotherapy are avoidance of the morbidity of major surgery, outpatient treatment, and preferred for poor surgical candidates.

- For patients with stage IIB, II, or IV disease, the treatment of choice is radiation therapy.
  —Advanced lesions require large doses.
  —The failure rate for bulky and advanced tumors within the pelvis is 40%.
  —The risk of pelvic and paraaortic lymph node metastasis and of distant metastases is significant.
  —The use of chemotherapy as a radiation sensitizer is often helpful.
- If tumors are restricted to the pelvis and involve the rectum or bladder, exenteration (excision of all pelvic organs) may be considered, but radiation therapy is tried initially.
  —Recent advances in exenteration include a continent urostomy, low anterior rectal anastomosis without colostomy, omental carpet to close the pelvic floor, vaginal reconstruction with gracilis or rectus abdominis myocutaneous flaps, and improved perioperative care.
- Systemic chemotherapy is not considered curative in this type of cancer.

Patient/Family Education

- Instruct the patient and family regarding the nature of the cancer, its location and size, treatment options, course of therapy, and expected outcomes.
- The earlier the diagnosis and treatment, the more positive the survival rates.
- Choice of therapy is usually based on the stage, location, and metastatic status of the cancer.

Follow-up/Referral

- As soon as cervical cancer is diagnosed, the patient is referred to a gynecologist/oncologist for further evaluation and treatment decisions.
- The primary care clinician can follow the patient throughout treatment and afterwards,

focusing on signs and symptoms of recurrence or of metastatic cancer.

Ovarian Cancer

Definition

Ovarian cancer is a malignant neoplasm of the ovaries rarely detected in the early stage and usually far advanced when diagnosed.

Risk Factors

- Perimenopausal and postmenopausal women ≥ 50 years of age
- Incidence is higher in industrialized countries in which dietary fat intake is high.
- History of nulliparity
- Late childbirth
- Delayed menopause
- Endometriosis
- Group A blood type
- Repeated spontaneous abortions
- Previous irradiation of pelvic organs
- Exposure to chemical carcinogens (e.g., asbestos, talc)
- Personal or family history of endometrial, breast, or colon cancer
- Over 5% of ovarian cancer cases are related to an inherited autosomal dominant gene, the *BRCA* gene
- Those with XY gonadal dysgenesis are predisposed to ovarian malignant germ cell tumors.
- The probability that an enlarged ovary represents ovarian cancer is directly proportional to the patient's age.

Etiology/Cause (see also Risk Factors)

- Any of the above factors, or a combination of factors, may cause ovarian cancer.
- Germ cell tumors, which arise from the primary germ cells of the ovary, occur in young women and are uncommon in women over age 30.

Pathogenesis

- Ovarian tumors are the most histologically diverse group of tumors.
- Over 80% of these tumors arise from the coelomic epithelium.
- The most common type is serous cystadenocarcinoma, which accounts for 75% of cases of epithelial ovarian cancer.

- Other types include mucinous, endometrioid, transitional cell, Brenner, clear cell, and unclassified carcinomas.
- The remaining cancers are germ cell and sex cord-stromal cell tumors, which are nonepithelial in origin, and metastatic tumors from the breast or GI tract.
- Ovarian tumors spread by direct extension, by intraperitoneal implantation via exfoliation of cells into the peritoneal cavity, by lymphatic dissemination in the pelvic and paraaortic region and, less commonly, hematogenously to the lungs or liver.

Diagnosis

Signs and Symptoms

- About 75% of women present with advanced-stage disease.
- Most women have vague, nonspecific symptoms such as dyspepsia, bloating, early-satiety anorexia, gas pains, and backache.
- The most common early finding is an adnexal mass that is usually solid, irregular, and fixed.
- Many are asymptomatic until an abdominal mass is palpated during a routine pelvic examination or until the disease is advanced.
- Some women present with severe abdominal pain due to torsion of the ovarian mass.
- Late symptoms include pelvic pain, anemia, cachexia, and abdominal swelling due to ovarian enlargement or accumulation of ascitic fluid.
- Nodular implants found on the rectovaginal examination point to pelvic malignancy.
- Functional effects of germ cell or stromal tumors include hyperthyroidism, feminization, and virilization.
- Benign functional cysts are common in young women and are distinguished from tumors by means of vaginal sonography or reexamination after 6 weeks.
- Tumor markers for germ cell malignancies, including the β-human chorionic gonadotropin (β-hCG), lactate dehydrogenase (LDH), α-fetoprotein, and cancer antigen 125 (CA-125), should be measured if a malignancy is strongly suspected.

Treatment

- Surgery is indicated when a mass is persistent or suspicious.

TABLE 16-3
Surgical Staging of Ovarian Carcinoma

Stage	Description
I	Limited to the ovaries
IA	Limited to one ovary; no tumor on the external surface, and capsule is intact
IB	Limited to both ovaries; no tumor on the external surface, and capsules are intact
IC*	Stage IA or IB but with tumor on the surface of one or both ovaries, with capsule ruptured, or with ascites or peritoneal washings containing malignant cells
II	Involving one or both ovaries, with pelvic extension
IIA	Extension or metastases to the uterus or tubes
IIB	Extension to other pelvic tissues
IIC*	Stage IIA or IIB but with tumor on the surface of one or both ovaries, with capsule ruptured, or with ascites of peritoneal washings containing malignant cells
III	Involving one or both ovaries with histologically confirmed peritoneal implants outside the pelvis or positive retroperitoneal or inguinal lymph nodes
IIIA	Grossly limited to the true pelvis with negative lymph nodes, but with histologically confirmed microscopic tumor outside the pelvis
IIIB	Involving one or both ovaries with histologically confirmed implants on abdominal peritoneal surfaces > 2 cm in diameter and with negative lymph nodes
IIIC	Abdominal implants > 2 cm in diameter and/or positive retroperitoneal or inguinal lymph nodes
IV	Involving one or both ovaries with distant metastases. If pleural effusion is present, cytologic test results must be positive to signify stage IV. Parenchymal liver metastasis equals stage IV.
Unconfirmed (Special category)	Unexplored cases thought to be ovarian carcinoma

From The International Federation of Gynecology and Obstetrics (FIGO), 1991.
*In stages IC and IIC, knowing whether capsule rupture was spontaneous or caused by the surgeon, and whether the source of malignant cells is ascites or peritoneal washings determines prognosis.

- A midline abdominal incision is made to allow access to all organs.
  - If the mass appears to be confined to the pelvis, the tumor is removed intact or unruptured.
  - All peritoneal surfaces, hemidiaphragms, and abdominal and pelvic viscera should be inspected and palpated.
- If a malignancy is confirmed, comprehensive surgical staging is required (Table 16-3).
- A large proportion of patients with apparently early-stage disease have extraovarian spread.

Postoperative Treatment
- Patients with stage IA or IB, grade I epithelial adenocarcinoma require no further treatment because their 5-year survival rate is not improved by adjuvant therapy.
- Those with stage IA or IB, grade 2 and 3 tumors, and those with stage II tumors require three to six courses of adjuvant chemotherapy.
  - Paclitaxel is combined with cisplatin or carboplatin.

- The 5-year survival rate is 70% to 100% for those with stage I disease, depending on tumor grade, and 50% to 70% for those with stage II disease.
- Patients with stage II or IV disease require six courses of paclitaxel and platinum-based chemotherapy: the median survival for those with microscopic residual disease at the beginning of chemotherapy is 30 to 40 months, versus 12 to 20 months for those with suboptimal cytoreductive surgery.
- Intraperitoneal chemotherapy and high-dose chemotherapy with bone marrow transplantation studies are now in clinical trials.
- Radiation therapy is rarely used.
- Advanced-stage ovarian cancer usually recurs; response to treatment is determined by measuring CA-125.
  - After chemotherapy, a second-look laparotomy is often done because about two thirds of those with stage III or IV disease have proven residual disease even after a

TABLE 16-4
Endometrial Carcinoma Risk Factors

Increased Risk	Diminished Risk
Unopposed menopausal estrogen	Ovulation
Replacement therapy	Progestin therapy
Menopause after 52 years	Combination oral contraceptives
Obesity	Menopause before 49 years
Diabetes	Multiparity
Feminizing ovarian tumors	
Polycystic ovarian syndrome	
Tamoxifen therapy for breast cancer	

From Smith JM, Huggins GR: Early detection of gynecologic malignancy. In Barker LR, Burton JR, Zieve PD, eds: *Principles of ambulatory medicine,* ed 5, Baltimore, 1999, Williams & Wilkins, p 1456.

complete clinical response to chemotherapy has occurred; the 5-year survival rate is 5% to 40%.

Patient/Family Education
- Instruct the patient and family as fully as possible (or feasible) regarding the nature of the cancer, its course, treatment, and expected outcomes.
- The family should be told the degree of severity of the cancer, and the usual prognosis in months or years.
- It is important to maintain hope in the patient, so the family and clinician need to confer about what and how much to communicate.
- Most patients prefer to know the truth so that they can prepare and make arrangements with regard to their possessions, finances, and funeral/burial arrangements.

Follow-up/Referral
- When the diagnosis of ovarian carcinoma is suspected or confirmed, the patient is referred to specialists: a gynecologist/oncologist, and others, as the need arises.

Endometrial Cancer
Definition
Endometrial cancer is an adenocarcinoma of the endometrium of the uterus.

Risk Factors (Table 16-4)
- Endometrial cancer is the most prevalent gynecologic malignancy, and occurs in those in their fifties or sixties.

- About 34,000 new cases of endometrial cancer were diagnosed in 1996.
- Medical history of infertility, anovulation, late menopause (>52 years), administration of exogenous estrogen, uterine polyps, and a combination of diabetes, hypertension, and obesity

Etiology/Cause
- The precise cause of endometrial cancer is not known for certain, but any of the risk factors may be involved.

Pathogenesis
- Adenocarcinomas make up about 90% of all endometrial tumors; the remaining 10% include mixed carcinomas, sarcomas, and benign adenoacanthomas.
- These carcinomas may spread to the cervix but rarely invade the vagina.

Diagnosis
Signs and Symptoms
- Staging is similar to that of ovarian cancer, ranging from stage IA to IVB.
- Abnormal vaginal bleeding, particularly in postmenopausal women, is usually the first sign of endometrial cancer.
- Lower abdominal and low back pain may also be present.
- A large, boggy uterus usually indicates advanced disease.
- Less than 50% of patients have a positive Pap smear because the cancer cells almost never exfoliate early in the disease.

- A Pap test of cells removed from the endometrium by means of jet washings of the uterine cavity provides the most accurate data.
- The preferred diagnostic test is dilation and curettage, in which each section of the uterus is curetted for biopsy.

Treatment
- These cancers metastasize to the broad ligaments, fallopian tubes, and ovaries so frequently that bilateral salpingo-oophorectomy with abdominal hysterectomy is the preferred treatment.
- Radiotherapy is usually given before and after surgery.
- High doses of a progestogen may be prescribed for palliation in advanced or inoperable cases.
- Chemotherapy may also be used in advanced cases.
  —Monthly regimens that combine doxorubicin 60 mg/m^2 and cisplatin 75 mg/m^2 IV may have overall response rates of ≥50%.

Prognosis
- Prognosis is based on the tumor's histologic appearance and grading, the patient's age (older women have a poorer prognosis), and metastatic spread.
- Overall, 63% of patients are cancer-free ≥ 5 years after treatment.
- For those with stage I disease, the 5-year survival rate is 70% to 95%.
- For those with stage III or IV disease, it is 10% to 60%.

Patient/Family Education
- As with all patients with cancer, communication is important, and information should be relayed as completely as possible, particularly to the family.
- Some patients want to know every last detail, whereas others do not want to hear anything; patients' questions should guide the clinician regarding how much to tell the patient after consulting with the surgeon/physician/oncologist and the family.

Follow-up/Referral
- Any patient with diagnosed cancer is followed closely by the clinician, the specialist of the particular body system involved, the surgeon, and the oncologist.
- Every known therapy is usually tried because there is wide variability in patients' response to any given treatment.
- The primary care provider is most often the one consistent health professional throughout the course of the patient's illness.

Colorectal Cancer
Definition
Colorectal cancer is a malignant neoplastic disease of the large intestine.

Risk Factors
- Age 50 or older
- The incidence is slightly higher in women than in men.
- The disease is prevalent in Western countries.
- Clustering in families is common.
- Personal history of ulcerative colitis, villous adenomas, and in particular familial adenomatous polyposis of the colon
- People who eat foods that are primarily low-fiber, high-fat, high-protein, and high in refined carbohydrates are more at risk of developing colon cancer.
- High alcohol consumption
- Those who do not regularly exercise relatively strenuously (e.g., brisk walk)
- Smoking
- Exposure to asbestos fibers
- Exposure to radiation

Etiology/Cause
- Any of the risk factors listed may be involved in development of colorectal cancer.
- It is often difficult to determine precise cause in any one individual, and cause may relate to a combination of factors.
- Familial polyposis and Lynch syndrome are two known types of familial colon cancer that occur across several generations, usually before age 40, and occur more often in the right colon.
  —At least four genes located on chromosomes 2, 3, and 7 have been shown to be mutated in some cases of the Lynch syndrome.

Pathogenesis
- Most lesions of the large bowel are moderately differentiated adenocarcinomas.

- These tumors have a long preinvasive stage and, when they invade, they tend to grow slowly.
- Typical napkin ring tumors in the sigmoid and descending colon grow circumferentially and constrict the intestinal lumen, causing partial obstruction and production of flat or pencil-shaped stools.
- Colorectal cancer spreads by direct extension through the bowel wall, hematogenous metastasis, regional lymph node metastasis, perineural spread, and intraluminal metastasis.

Diagnosis

Signs and Symptoms

- Because of the slow growth of adenocarcinoma of the colon and rectum, a long interval passes before the mass is large enough to produce symptoms.
- Symptoms depend on the lesion's location, type, extent, and complications.
- The right colon has a large caliber and a thin wall.
- The left colon has a smaller lumen, the feces are semisolid, and cancer tends to encircle the bowel, causing alternating constipation and increased stool frequency or diarrhea.
- Severe anemia that causes weakness and fatigue may be the only presenting symptoms.
- In cancer of the rectum, the most common symptom is bleeding with defecation.
- Tenesmus or a sensation of incomplete evacuation may be present.
- Pain is noticeably absent until perirectal tissue is involved.
- Whenever rectal bleeding occurs, even with known hemorrhoids or diverticular disease, coexisting cancer must be ruled out.
- Because the colon contents are liquid, obstruction is a late sign.
- Some large tumors may become palpable through the abdominal wall.
- Bleeding is usually occult.
- Testing for occult blood is advised for screening and high-risk surveillance.
  —Patients should eat a high-fiber, red meat–free diet for 3 days before stool sampling.
- About 60% of colorectal cancers are within reach of the flexible fiberoptic sigmoidoscope.

- If a cancerous lesion is detected on sigmoidoscopy, total colonoscopy and complete removal of all colonic lesions should be done.
- Endoscopic excision of synchronous polyps may reduce the amount of bowel that needs to be resected.
- Barium enema x-ray is often unreliable in detecting rectal cancer but may be important as a first step in diagnosing colon cancer.
- Elevated serum CEA is not specific to colorectal cancer, but levels are high in 70% of patients.
- CA-19-9 and CA-125 are other tumor markers that may be elevated.

Treatment

- Primary treatment is wide surgical resection of the colon cancer and regional lymphatic drainage after the bowel is prepared.
- The choice of procedure depends on the distance of the tumor from the anus, and on gross extent.
- Abdominoperineal resection of the rectum requires a permanent sigmoid colostomy.
- Staplers allow low anterior resection and anastomosis closer to the rectum with rectal sparing for more patients than in the past.
- Rectal cancer patients with one to four positive lymph nodes are treated with combined radiotherapy and chemotherapy; when there are more than four positive nodes in the resected colon, therapy of any kind is less effective.
- If a patient is an unacceptable surgical risk, some tumors can be controlled locally by electrocoagulation.
- Preliminary data from studies regarding adjuvant radiotherapy after curative surgery of rectal (but not colon) cancer indicate that local tumor growth can be controlled, recurrence delayed, and survival improved in patients with limited lymph node involvement.
- The only drug with proven efficacy for advanced colorectal cancer is 5-FU, but only 15% to 20% of 5-FU patients experience obvious tumor shrinkage and prolongation of life.
- A new drug, irinotecan (Camptosar) appears to have activity as a single agent in advanced colon cancer and is being evaluated as part of combination chemotherapy programs.

Prognosis
- Surgical cure is possible in 70% of patients.
- The best 5-year survival rate for cancer limited to the mucosa is nearly 90%, with penetration of the muscularis propria, 80%, and with positive lymph nodes, 30%.

Patient/Family Education
- Instruct the patient and family regarding the nature of the cancer, its location, treatment options, and expected outcomes.
- It is important to include both the patient and the family in decisions about treatment options, but recommendations can be made by the specialists.
- For whatever treatment regimen is selected, inform the patient and family about both the positive and negative potential outcomes.

Follow-up/Referral
- The frequency of follow-up after curative surgery for colorectal cancer is controversial.
  —Most authorities recommend two annual inspections of the remaining bowel with colonoscopy or x-rays; if negative, repeat evaluations at 2- and 3-year intervals.
- When surgery is not curative, limited palliative surgery may be indicated; median survival is 7 months.

BIBLIOGRAPHY

Anderson KN, Anderson LE, Glanze WD, eds: *Mosby's medical, nursing, & allied health dictionary,* ed 5, St. Louis, 1998, Mosby.

Baringa M: Cancer drugs found to work in new way. *Science* 288(5464)(April 14):245, 2000. Report of experimental results on laboratory mice at Harvard and University of Toronto.

Beers MH, Berkow R: Pulmonary disorders, gastrointestinal disorders, hematology and oncology. In Beers MH, Berkow R, eds: *The Merck manual of diagnosis and therapy,* ed 17, Whitehouse Station, NJ, 1999, Merck Research Laboratories, pp 328-330, 651-656, 1960-1962, 1962-1964.

Cookson MS, Smith JA: PSA testing: Update on diagnostic tools; to screen or not to screen. *Consultant: Consultations in Primary Care* 40(4):670-701, 2000.

Katz SJ, Zemencuk JK, Hofer TP: Breast cancer screening in the United States and Canada 1994: Socioeconomic gradients persist. *Am J Public Health* 90(5):799-803, 2000.

Prisco MK: Evaluating neck masses. *Nurse Pract* 25(4):30-51, 2000.

Rohatiner AZS, Slevin ML, Tate T: Medical oncology. In Kumar P, Clark M, eds: *Clinical medicine,* ed 4, Edinburgh, 1998, WB Saunders, p 415.

Rugo HS: Cancer. In Tierney LM, McPhee SJ, Papadakis MA, eds: *Current medical diagnosis & treatment 2000,* New York, 2000, Lange Medical Books/McGraw-Hill, pp 71-110.

Smith JM, Huggins GR: Early detection of gynecologic malignancy. In Barker LR, Burton JR, Zieve PD, eds: *Principles of ambulatory medicine,* ed 5, Baltimore, 1999, Williams and Wilkins, p 1452.

REVIEW QUESTIONS

1. In developed countries, the percentage of the population that will likely develop cancer at some time during their lives is:
   a. 10%
   b. 15%
   c. 25%
   d. 35%
2. Proliferation of cancer cells causes several characteristics of the disease. These characteristics include all but one of the following. The one characteristic that is NOT included is:
   a. Lack of differentiation
   b. Uncontrolled number of malignant cells
   c. Restriction to only one organ or tissue
   d. Local invasion of tissue
3. Molecular abnormalities in genes are partly responsible for the growth or reproduction of malignant cells. These abnormalities are known as:
   a. Cytolysis genes
   b. Extensor genes
   c. Mutations
   d. Prokaryotic genes
4. The gene that is abnormal in about 25% of cancers is:
   a. The α gene
   b. The β gene
   c. The ras gene
   d. The ρ gene
5. Another example of oncogene activity involves protein kinases—enzymes that help to regulate many cellular activities, particularly signaling from the cell membrane to the nucleus, thereby initiating the cell's entrance in the cell cycle and controlling several other cellular functions. Protein kinase enzymes that are structurally altered are found in several human cancers, including all but one of the following. The one cancer in which protein kinase enzymes are NOT found is:
   a. Bladder cancer
   b. Pancreatic cancer

c. Breast cancer

d. Myelocytic leukemia

6. Changes in cells indicate that:
   a. A change in deoxyribonucleic acid has occurred.
   b. A chromosomal change has occurred.
   c. A change on the cell's surface has occurred.
   d. A change in the cell's receptors has occurred.

7. The steps that occur in chemical carcinogenesis include all but one of the following. The one that does NOT belong is:
   a. Initiation
   b. Promotion
   c. Proliferation
   d. Progression

8. Patients who have a complete remission or a complete response to therapy indicate:
   a. A definitive cure
   b. A probable cure
   c. A potential cure
   d. A detectable cure

9. Methotrexate is a:
   a. Purine antagonist
   b. Folic acid antagonist
   c. Pyrimidine antagonist
   d. Vitamin B_{12} antagonist

10. The backbone of therapy for acute myeloid leukemia is:
    a. Cytosine arabinoside
    b. 5-Fluorouracil
    c. Vinca alkaloids
    d. Paclitaxel

11. Parts of the body most affected by myeloma include all but one of the following. The part that is NOT affected by myeloma is:
    a. Vertebrae
    b. Ribs
    c. Liver
    d. Pelvic bones

12. One of the first symptoms that patients with bronchogenic cancer have is:
    a. Hypoxia
    b. Anemia
    c. Breathlessness
    d. Cough

13. The number of new cases of prostate cancer that is diagnosed every year is more than:
    a. 50,000
    b. 100,000

c. 150,000

d. 200,000

14. In over 50% of bladder cancer, the primary cause is:
    a. Repeated infections of the urethra or bladder
    b. HIV/AIDS
    c. Cigarette smoking
    d. Exposure to chemicals that are carcinogenic

15. The risk of developing breast cancer in the United States by age 95 is:
    a. 1 in 3
    b. 1 in 5
    c. 1 in 6
    d. 1 in 8

16. The percentage of women who develop breast cancer and who carry one of the two breast cancer genes is:
    a. 5%
    b. 10%
    c. 20%
    d. 33%

17. Risk factors for cervical cancer are all but one of the following. The one that is NOT a risk factor for cervical cancer is:
    a. Older age
    b. Age at time of first intercourse
    c. Human papillomavirus
    d. Cigarette smoking

18. Ovarian cancer occurs primarily in women whose age is:
    a. Between 20 and 29
    b. Between 30 and 39
    c. Between 40 and 49
    d. 50 and older

19. The most prevalent gynecologic malignancy is:
    a. Cervical cancer
    b. Ovarian cancer
    c. Endometrial cancer
    d. Uterine cancer

20. The incidence and prevalence of colon cancer are increasing. All but one of the following is a risk factor. The one that is NOT a risk factor for colon cancer is:
    a. Young age
    b. Cigarette smoking
    c. Low-fiber, high-protein, and high-fat diet
    d. High alcohol consumption over time

21. Cancer may result in all but one of the following complications/symptoms. The one that is NOT a result of cancer is:
    a. Hypocalcemia
    b. Pain
    c. Neuropathy
    d. Seizures

22. Recent (May 2000) data for the 1990s indicate that both incidence and death rates of cancer are:
    a. Markedly increasing
    b. Gradually decreasing
    c. Markedly decreasing
    d. Staying about the same

23. The prognosis for bronchogenic carcinoma is:
    a. Poor
    b. Fair
    c. Good
    d. Excellent

24. A normal prostate on digital rectal examination:
    a. Definitely rules out prostate cancer
    b. Probably rules out prostate cancer
    c. Does not exclude the presence of prostate cancer
    d. Is of little diagnostic value

25. The early signs/symptoms of bladder cancer include all but one of the following. The one that is NOT an early indicator is:
    a. Pelvic pain
    b. Frequency
    c. Microscopic hematuria
    d. Dysuria

26. Family history of breast cancer in distant relatives increases the risk in a patient:
    a. Not at all
    b. Slightly
    c. Moderately
    d. Greatly

27. The percentage of women with breast cancer who carry one of the two breast cancer genes (i.e., *BRCA1, BRCA2*) is:
    a. 5%
    b. 10%
    c. 15%
    d. 20%

28. The risk of cervical cancer:
    a. Is directly related to age at first intercourse
    b. Is inversely related to the lifetime number of sexual partners
    c. Is directly related to the lifetime number of sexual partners
    d. Is not a factor in either age of first intercourse or lifetime number of sexual partners

29. At time of diagnosis, ovarian cancer is usually:
    a. At a very early stage
    b. At a localized stage
    c. At a stage that requires radiography
    d. At a far advanced stage

30. Ovarian carcinoma of grade I, stage IA or IB:
    a. Requires radical therapy
    b. Requires only chemotherapy
    c. Requires only radiation therapy
    d. Requires no treatment; 5-year survival is not changed

17

Musculoskeletal Disorders

These problems comprise 20% to 30% of the patient load of primary care providers. Many musculoskeletal problems are short-lived and self-limited, or resolve following rest and mild analgesics and physiotherapy. Early recognition and treatment of musculoskeletal problems, particularly inflammatory arthritis, by multidisciplinary teams, result in improved symptom control and prevention of chronic joint or muscle disability.

TAKING A MUSCULOSKELETAL HISTORY

As in other disorders, a carefully elicited history will often result in the diagnosis.

Questions to Ask

General Questions
- *Where is the pain? Is it localized or generalized?* Patterns of joint involvement are often important clues to the diagnosis (e.g., distal interphalangeal [DIP] joints in osteoarthritis).
- *Is the pain associated with the joint(s), the spine, muscles, or bones?* Soft tissue involvement and inflamed joints are point-tender.
- *Is the origin of the pain at another site, but referred?* Most joint pain is localized, but may radiate distally (e.g., shoulder to upper arm, hip to thigh and knee).
- *Is the pain constant, intermittent, or episodic? How severe is it—sharp, aching, or unbearable?* Pain from gout, or from septic arthritis, in a previously fit, nonimmunocompromised patient, is agonizing; joint pain that lasts a day or two may indicate palin-

dromic (recurrent) rheumatism, but pain that lasts longer indicates gout. Constant nagging pain, particularly if experienced at night, may indicate an underlying malignancy.
- *What are the precipitating and aggravating factors?* Mechanical disorders are usually worse with activity, and better with rest; pain in the spine or from inflammation usually improves with activity, and is made worse by inactivity. A common cause of musculoskeletal pain is trauma.
- *Are there any associated neurologic symptoms and signs?* Nerve pain is usually felt as numbness, pins and needles, or loss of strength (e.g., carpal tunnel syndrome, spinal problems such as disk prolapse or spondylosis, or neurologic disease). Nerve root pain, such as occurs because of a disk prolapse, generally reflects the anatomic distribution of the affected root.

Stiffness
- *Is it localized or generalized?* Joint or spine stiffness is common after injury.
- *Does it affect the limb girdles or periphery?* Joints that are stiff for more than 15 minutes every morning are usually inflamed (e.g., rheumatoid arthritis [RA] or other inflammatory arthritis). Spinal stiffness and pain that is much worse in the morning may be anklyosing spondylitis, particularly in those in their twenties or thirties. Shoulder and pelvic girdle stiffness and pain that are worse in the morning may be polymyalgia rheumatica, particularly in people over age 55.

Swelling

- *Is one joint affected, or several?* Always look for symmetry/asymmetry, a proximal or peripheral pattern, both of which are clues to the type of arthritis. RA is typically polyarticular, in symmetrical joints. Acute single-joint arthritis may be due to trauma, gout (in a middle-aged male), or sepsis (fever or immunosuppression).
- *Is it constant or episodic?*
- *Are episodes of swelling transient or of longer duration?*
- *Is there associated inflammation (redness, warmth)?*

Gender

- Reactive arthritis, gout, and ankylosing spondylitis are more common in men.
- Rheumatoid arthritis, polymyalgia rheumatica, and other autoimmune connective tissue diseases are more common in women.

Age

- *Is the patient young, middle-aged, or older?* Trauma is more common in young people, although it can occur at any age.
- *How old was the patient when the problem began?* Osteoarthritis and polymyalgia rheumatica rarely occur in those under 50. Rheumatoid arthritis is most common in women between 20 and 40.

General Health

- *Is there any other health problem, recent or long-standing, of concern (e.g., weight loss, intermittent fever, insomnia)?* **Fever may indicate joint sepsis due to infection, which is a medical emergency.**
- *Are there other medical conditions that may be relevant?* Anemia, psoriasis, and inflammatory bowel disease are associated with asymmetric arthritis; Charcot's joints are seen in patients with diabetes mellitus.

Medications/Drugs

- *What medications are you currently taking?* Diuretics may precipitate gout in older people; hormone replacement therapy (HRT) or oral contraceptives may precipitate systemic lupus erythematosus (SLE); steroids can cause avascular necrosis; some drugs (e.g., phenytoin) cause a lupus-like syndrome.

Transcultural Aspects

- Variations exist among diverse racial and ethnic groups and should be taken into consideration during assessment.
- *Are you of Mediterranean origin?* Some diseases occur almost exclusively in persons of a particular race/ethnicity: sickle cell anemia occurs in blacks; osteoporosis is uncommon in older blacks; thalassemia occurs more often in Mediterranean, Chinese, Asian, and Arabic people.

Other

- The long bones of blacks are significantly longer, narrower, and denser than those of whites. Black males have the densest bones, which likely accounts for the low incidence of osteoporosis in this population. Bone density in Chinese, Japanese, and Eskimos is below that of white Americans.
- Curvature of the long bones varies among culturally diverse groups. Native Americans have anteriorly convex femurs, blacks have markedly straight femurs, and in whites, the femoral curvature is intermediate. Thin blacks and whites have less curvature than the average. Obese blacks and whites have increased curvatures.

Past History

- *Have you had these symptoms before? When?* Gout is recurrent, and the episode resolves in about 10 days without treatment; acute episodes of palindromic rheumatism may precede the onset of RA.

Family History

- Does anyone in your family have a similar problem now? When they were younger? Osteoarthritis may be familial; seronegative spondyloarthritis is seen in families with a history of arthritis, psoriasis, ankylosing spondylitis, or inflammatory bowel disease; autoimmunity has a familial tendency.

Occupational History

- *What kind of work do you do now? In the past?* Heavy laborers and dancers often present with soft tissue problems and arthritis; work-related problems are becoming more common.

BOX 17-1
Examination of the Joints

THE UPPER LIMBS

Raise arms sideways to the ears (abduction). Reach behind the neck and back. If the patient has difficulty, could indicate a shoulder or rotator cuff problem.

Hold the arms forward, with elbows straight, fingers apart, palm up and palm down. With fixed flexion at the elbow, the problem is there. Examine hands for swelling, deformity, and wasting, which may indicate amyotrophic lateral sclerosis (ALS).

Place the hands in the "prayer" position with elbows apart. Flexion deformities of the fingers may be due to arthritis, flexor tenosynovitis, or skin disease. Painful restriction of wrists limits ability to move the elbows out with the hands held together.

THE LOWER LIMBS

Ask the patient to walk a short distance away from and toward you, and to stand still.

Move each ankle up and down. Examine the ankle, medial arch, and toes while the patient is standing.

THE SPINE

Stand behind the patient.

Ask the patient to (1) bend forward to touch the toes with straight knees, (2) bend backward, (3) flex, extend, and side-flex the neck. Observe abnormal spinal curves—scoliosis (lateral curve), kyphosis (forward curve), or lordosis (backward curve). Cervical or lumbar lordosis and thoracic kyphosis are normal. Muscle spasm is worse while standing and bending. Unequal leg length leads to scoliosis, which decreases on sitting or lying (lengths are measured while patient is lying).

Have the patient lie supine. Examine any restriction of straight-leg raising (disk dislocation).

Have the patient lie prone. Examine for anterior thigh pain during femoral stretch test (flexing knee while prone), which indicates a high lumbar disk problem.

Palpate the spine and buttocks for tender areas.

From Drury PL, Shipley M: Rheumatology and bone disease. In Kumar P, Clark M, eds: *Clinical medicine*, ed 4, Edinburgh, 1998, WB Saunders, p 450.

Psychosocial History

- *Has there been an injury in which a legal case for compensation is pending? Have there been any major stressors in your life, either with family or work?*
- Stress may precipitate an exacerbation of arthritis or decrease a person's ability to cope with pain or disability; the extent of a disability if present should be noted as baseline data.

EXAMINATION OF THE JOINTS
(BOX 17-1)

- As the patient walks into the room and sits down, look for signs of disability.
  - Are movements smooth and easy?
  - Is there a limp or other sign of weakness or pain?
  - Does sitting down cause the person to grimace, groan, or indicate in any way that pain in joints or spine is present?
- To examine a joint, the examiner must *look at*, *feel*, and *move* the joint.
  - Observe for swelling, redness, rash, muscle wasting, deformity, such as a distal bone displaced to the side as in knock knees (genu valgus) or bowed legs (genu varus), hyperextension or fixed flexion of an arm or leg, lack of smooth movements, decreased range of motion.
  - Feel the joint for inflammation, tenderness, warmth, redness, or swelling, which may be caused by fluid, tissue, or bone. Descriptors of swelling may be "fluctuant" (fluid), "firm" or "boggy" (synovial swelling), or "hard" (bone).
  - Move the joint to assess passive range of motion (e.g., flexion, extension, abduction, adduction, rotation), instability, pain on motion, or crepitus (grating sound when cartilage damage has occurred and the two bones of the joint rub together).

LABORATORY TESTS

- Complete blood count (CBC)—normochomic, normocytic anemia occurs in chronic inflammatory bowel disease; hypochromic, microcytic anemia indicates iron deficiency, which may be due to nonsteroidal antiinflammatory drugs (NSAIDs) that induce gastrointestinal (GI) bleeding.
  - White cell count: neutrophilia occurs in bacterial infection (e.g., septic arthritis) or with

BOX 17-2

Rheumatoid Factor in Serum Is Seen in These Conditions

DISEASES INVOLVING JOINTS
Sjögren's syndrome (90%)
RA (70%)
SLE (50%)
Systemic sclerosis (30%)
Polymyositis/dermatomyositis (≤50%)
Overlap syndromes (unknown)
Juvenile chronic arthritis (3%)

CHRONIC INFECTIONS (LOW TITERS)
Tuberculosis
Leprosy
Infective endocarditis
Kala-azar

NORMAL POPULATION
Elderly
Relatives of patients with RA

MISCELLANEOUS
Autoimmune hepatitis
Fibrosing alveolitis
Sarcoidosis
Waldenstrom's macroglobulinemia

From Drury PL, Shipley M: Rheumatology and bone disease. In Kumar P, Clark M, eds: *Clinical medicine*, ed 4, Edinburgh, 1998, WB Saunders, p 451.

BOX 17-3

Antinuclear Antibodies Are Seen in These Conditions

SLE (95%)
Systemic sclerosis (80%)
Sjögren's syndrome (60% to 70%)
Polymyositis and dermatomyositis (30%)
Juvenile chronic arthritis (variable)
Occasionally seen in
   Autoimmune hepatitis
   Primary biliary cirrhosis
   Infections (e.g., infective endocarditis)
   Normal elderly people

From Drury PL, Shipley M: Rheumatology and bone disease. In Kumar P, Clark M, eds: *Clinical medicine*, ed 4, Edinburgh, 1998, WB Saunders, p 451.

corticosteroid therapy; lymphopenia occurs with viral illnesses or active SLE; neutropenia may reflect drug-induced bone marrow suppression; eosinophilia is seen in polyarteritis nodosa and Churg-Strauss syndrome.
—Platelets: thrombocythemia occurs with chronic inflammation; thrombocytopenia is seen in drug-induced bone marrow suppression.
- Increases in erythrocyte sedimentation rate (ESR) and C-reactive protein (CRP) indicate inflammation.
- Bone and liver biochemistry—an elevated serum alkaline phosphatase may indicate liver or bone disease; elevation in liver enzymes is seen with drug-induced toxicity.

SERUM AUTOANTIBODY STUDIES

- Rheumatoid factors (RFs) (Box 17-2)
  —IgM rheumatoid factors are detected by agglutination tests using immunoglobulin G (IgG)-coated latex particles or sheep red

cells, the Rose-Waaler test, or the sheep cell agglutination test (SCAT).
  —These are antibodies (usually IgM, but sometimes IgG or IgA) against the *Fc* portion of immunoglobulin and are detected in 70% of patients with RA, but are not diagnostic; a high titer in early RA indicates a poor prognosis.
  —Positive titers occasionally predate the onset of RA (titers may fluctuate).
  —RFs are detected in many autoimmune rheumatic disorders (e.g., SLE), in chronic infections, and in asymptomatic older people.
- Antinuclear antibodies (ANAs) (Box 17-3)
  —ANAs are detected by indirect immunofluorescent staining of fresh-frozen sections of rat liver or kidney, or by Hep-2 cell lines.
  —Different patterns reflect a variety of antigenic specificities that occur with different clinical pictures (e.g., speckled, nucleolar, or anticentromere patterns).
  —ANAs are detected in many autoimmune diseases.
  —ANA is used as a screening test for SLE, but low titers occur in RA and chronic infection, as well as in normal persons, especially older people.

COMMON MUSCULOSKELETAL DISORDERS
Degenerative Joint Disease (Osteoarthritis)

Definition and Classification

Degenerative joint disease (DJD) (osteoarthritis) is an arthropathy (joint disease) with altered hyaline cartilage, characterized by loss of articu-

[handwritten top margin: OA — Osteophytes classified mono, oligo, poly. Prox: Bouchard's, Distal: Herberden's]

lar cartilage and hypertrophy of bone, producing osteophytes.

- The condition is usually divided into two types.
  - —**Primary,** which affects some or all of the DIP joints, causing Heberden's nodes, and less commonly the proximal interphalangeal (PIP) joints, causing Bouchard's nodes
  - —**Secondary,** which can occur in any joint after an articular injury: fracture, overuse, neurologic disorder, or metabolic disturbance (e.g., hyperparathyroidism)
- Osteoarthritis can also be classified according to the number of joints affected: monoarticular, oligoarticular, or polyarticular (generalized).

Incidence

- Osteoarthritis is the most common form of joint disease, and can occur at any age, in all races, and in all geographic areas of the world.
- At any one time, up to 70% of the U.S. population of adults over age 65 has some radiographic evidence of the condition, particularly in weight-bearing joints: ankles, kees, and hips.
- Signs and symptoms increase with age.
- DJD is second only to ischemic heart disease as a cause of work disability in men over age 50, and accounts for more annual hospitalizations than RA.

Etiology

- Age, inherited genetic makeup, and mechanical factors such as use of joints, obesity, and occupation are probably involved in the cause of disease.
- More recent evidence also points to certain enzymes and cytokines (e.g., interleukin-1 and tumor necrosis factor [TNF]) that cause cartilage degradation outweigh proteins that promote cartilage integrity (e.g., tissue inhibitor of metalloproteinases, kininogens, plasminogen activator inhibitor-1, transforming growth factor-β, insulin growth factor-I, interferon-γ).

Pathophysiology

- Focal destruction of articular cartilage occurs, along with subchondral bone changes, including microfractures, cyst formation, and osteophyte formation.
- X-rays show joint-space narrowing, osteophytosis, subchondral sclerosis, cyst formation, and abnormal bone contours.
- The joint cavity never becomes completely obliterated, however, and adhesions do not form.

Diagnosis

- DJD is diagnosed mainly on the basis of clinical and radiologic findings.

Signs and Symptoms

- Joint pain relieved by rest *[handwritten: ✳]*
  - —The joints most often affected include the DIP, PIP, first carpometacarpal, first metatarsophalangeal, hip, knee, and cervical and lower lumbar vertebrae. *[handwritten: sites]*
  - —Primary osteoarthritis rarely affects the metacarpophalangeal joint, wrist, elbow, or shoulder.
- Brief morning stiffness, seldom lasting >15 minutes *[handwritten: AM stiffness >15 min]*
- Later, pain on motion occurs in the affected joint(s), made worse by activity or weight bearing but relieved by rest. *[handwritten: Pain c̄ Activity]*
- Coarse crepitus may be felt in the joint.
- Joint effusion and other signs of articular inflammation are mild, if present.
- Joint enlargement, caused by soft-tissue changes, effusion, and osteophytosis.
- Later, gross deformity, subluxation, and decreased range of motion develop.

X-ray Findings

- Narrowed joint spaces, osteophytes (spurs), increased density of subchondral bone, and bony cysts may be seen. *[handwritten: ✳]*

Laboratory Findings

- Routine laboratory testing and synovial fluid analysis are not necessary in most cases.
- Blood cell counts, serum electrophoresis, serum calcium, phosphorus, and alkaline, phosphatase are usually within normal ranges.
- ANAs and RF are negative.
- ESR may be somewhat elevated.
- Synovial fluid analysis usually shows noninflammatory fluid with good viscosity and a

---

BOX 17-4

Suggested Steps to Manage Osteoarthritis in the Primary Care Setting

1. Confirm the diagnosis (history, physical, radiographic studies), and document extent of disease and disability.
2. A supervised walking program often results in clinical improvement, without aggravating joint pain.
3. Weight loss to decrease stress on all joints, particularly the weight-bearing joints—hips, knees, ankles.
4. A simple analgesic (acetaminophen, up to 4 g/day) along with nonpharmacologic methods (patient education, arthritis self-help class, physical therapy, assistive devices, hot or cool compresses or baths).
5. If pain is not relieved by acetaminophen, add a low-dose NSAID, such as ibuprofen 800 mg tid or qid, a nonacetylated salicylate, or topical capsaicin (Zostrix).
6. If required for pain relief: full-dose NSAID (ibuprofen 800 mg tid or qid); if risk factors for GI bleeding

are present, add misoprostol (Cytotec 200 μg bid), or a proton pump inhibitor.

7. Consider prescribing a selective cyclooxygenase-2 inhibitor (celecoxib [Celebrex] 200 mg/day; or rofecoxib [Vioxx] 12.5 to 25 mg/day).
8. Consider intraarticular glucocorticoid injections, particularly if effusion or inflammation is present.
9. Consider knee irrigation or joint arthroscopy with debridement in patients who are candidates for such therapy.
10. Consider referral to an orthopedic surgeon for total joint arthroplasty or osteotomy.
11. Newer surgical therapy includes experimental repair of focal cartilage loss by autologous chondrocyte transplantation, which has resulted in considerable improvement.

---

white blood cell (WBC) count of less than 2000/mm^3.
—Some fibrils and debris (wear particles), calcium pyrophosphate dihydrate, or basic calcium phosphate crystals may be present.

- Although DJD has not been considered an inflammatory disease, many patients have focal or scattered areas of inflammation caused by the release of cytokines in the synovial fluid.
  —These signs of inflammation are caused by crystals and wear particles produced by enzymatic and mechanical degradation of joint cartilage.

Differential Diagnosis

- Because of minimal systemic manifestations, the initial diagnosis is usually self-evident.
- The distribution of asymmetric joint involvement in hands distinguishes osteoarthritis from RA and other articular conditions.
- **One must be cautious of attributing all skeletal signs and symptoms to osteoarthritis, particularly in the spine, where metastatic neoplasia, osteoporosis, multiple myeloma, or other bone disease may be present.**

Treatment

- Goals: to preserve joint function, decrease pain, and educate about the disease and its management (Box 17-4)

Prognosis

- Significant disability in osteoarthritis is not nearly as common as it is in RA.
- However, symptoms can become quite severe, and activity may be limited.

Patient/Family Education

- Instruct about the condition, including its possible causes, usual course, treatment, and prognosis.
- Teach about how to preserve joints by programmed exercise, avoiding overuse as in running/jogging, and resting when pain develops.
- Instruct about medications: type, side effects, and wisdom of judicious use.
- Teach about other means of treating pain in joints: warm to hot shower or bath, massage, warm or cold compresses.
- Provide specific instructions regarding weight loss—low-calorie, low-fat diet.
- If patient smokes, encourage smoking cessation, which affects blood oxygen.

Follow-up/Referral

- Monthly telephone contact to answer questions and provide support.
- Have a list of recommended orthopedic surgeons who specialize in either hip or knee replacement surgery.
- Most patients are seen on a regular basis, usually every 3 to 4 months, or more often as needed, to monitor level of pain and activity, ability to carry out activities of daily living, medications: dosage and scheduling, weight loss, and range of motion of all joints.

Gout

Definition

Gout is a recurrent acute or chronic arthritis of peripheral joints resulting from deposition in and around joints and tendons of monosodium urate monohydrate crystals from supersaturated hyperuricemic body fluids.

Classification

- Primary gout occurs in men over age 30 and in postmenopausal women who take diuretics.
- Chronic polyarticular gout occurs over a period of years, which is the final, unremitting stage of the disease, known as tophaceous gout, and is characterized by persistent, painful polyarthritis; tophaceous gout occurs in fewer than 10% of patients with gout.

Incidence

- Gout is common among Pacific Islanders (e.g., Filipinos, Samoans).
- Males over age 30 make up 90% of patients with primary gout.
- Gout can occur in women during postmenopausal years, particularly if they take diuretics.

Etiology

- The specific cause of gout is not known.
- Sustained hyperuricemia (Box 17-5)
- The greater the degree and duration of hyperuricemia, the greater the chance of crystal deposition and of acute attacks of gout, although many hyperuricemic persons never develop gout.

> **BOX 17-5**
> ## Causes of Hyperuricemia in Patients with Gout
>
> **INCREASED URIC ACID PRODUCTION**
> **Genetic Causes**
> Enzymatic defects
> - Hypoxanthine-guanine phosphoribosyltransferase deficiency
> - Phosphoribosylpyrophosphate synthetase overactivity
> - Glucose-6-phosphatase deficiency
>
> **Acquired Causes**
> High purine diet/pancreatic extracts
> Obesity
> Hypertriglyceridemia
> Alcohol consumption
> Myeloproliferative disorders
> Lymphoproliferative disorders
> Chemotherapy
>
> **REDUCED URIC ACID CLEARANCE**
> **Genetic Causes**
> Polycystic kidney disease
> Down syndrome
> **Acquired Causes**
> Renal disease or hypertension
> Drugs (e.g., low-dose aspirin, diuretics)
> Endocrinopathies
> Metabolic abnormalities
> Postoperative dehydration or starvation

- Dietary purines contribute to serum uric acid, with marked rises in uric acid after ingestion of purine-rich foods, and particularly alcohol, but a strict low-purine diet lowers baseline serum urate by only about 1 mg/dl.

Diagnosis

- The "gold standard" for diagnosing gout is joint aspiration and identification of characteristics: needle-shaped, negatively birefringent monosodium urate crystals under compensated polarized light microscopy.

Signs and Symptoms

- Acute gouty arthritis begins without warning, but may be precipitated by minor trauma, overindulgence in purine-rich food or alcohol, surgery, fatigue, emotional stress, or medical stress (e.g., infection, vascular occlusion).

[handwritten: Gold Study Aspiration]

*[handwritten: *Urate 7 g/dL – supports DX]*

BOX 17-6

Drugs Used to Treat Gout

ACUTE ATTACK

NSAIDs: these have become first-line therapy for acute attacks because of many side effects from colchicine and its lack of efficacy beyond 24 hours after onset of attack.

Indomethicin (Indocin) 50 to 75 g PO initially, then 50 mg q6h, tapered over 7 days.

Ibuprofen 800 mg q8h, tapered over 7 days

Colchicine 0.6 mg PO q1-2h (maximum 4 mg/24 hours)—effective within first 24 hours of acute attack.

Corticosteroids: effective in patients who are unable to take NSAIDs and colchicine.

Prednisone 0.5 to 0.75 mg/day PO, tapered over 7 days

Triamcinolone acetonide 10 to 40 mg intraarticularly, depends on size of joint.

PREVENTION OF RECURRENCE

Colchicine 0.6 mg/day PO

NSAIDs

  Indomethacin 50 mg bid

  Ibuprofen 400 to 800 mg q8h

REDUCTION OF URIC ACID LEVELS

Uricosuric Drugs

Probenecid (Benemid, Benuryl) 250 mg bid × 7 days, increased to 500 to 1000 mg bid for maintenance dosage

Indications: Underexcretion of uric acid (<700 mg/24 hours), GFR >50 ml/minute, no acute gout, no history of kidney stones

Precautions: Avoid concomitant salicylate therapy and use in patients with sulfa allergy

Sulfinpyrazone (Anturane) 50 mg bid × 7 days, increase to 100 mg bid; maintenance dosage is 200 mg bid

Indications: Same as for probenecid

Precautions: Same as for probenecid

Xanthine Oxidase Inhibitors

Allopurinol (Purinol, Zyloprim) 300 to 600 mg/day, adjusted according to renal function (GFR)

Indications: Hyperuricemia associated with overproduction, urinary uric acid excretion >700 mg/24 hour, kidney stones, prophylaxis before chemotherapy, hyperuricemia associated with enzyme defects, intolerance to uricosuric agents, inability to lower uric acid to <7 mg/dl with uricosuric drugs, and patients with a history of kidney stones.

Precautions: Reduce dose by 75% if patient is also taking azathioprine (Imuran) or mercaptopurine (Purinethol).

GFR, Glomerular filtration rate.

- Acute monarticular pain, often nocturnal, is usually the first symptom.
- The pain becomes progressively more severe and is often excruciating.
- Signs are similar to those of infection: swelling, warmth, and redness, in addition to skin that is shiny and purplish.
- The metatarsophalangeal joint of the great toe is most often involved (podagra) but other areas may also be involved: instep, ankle, knee, wrist, and elbow.
- Fever, tachycardia, chills, malaise, and leukocytosis may occur.
- Initial attacks usually affect only one joint and last only a few days; later, attacks may affect several joints and persist for weeks if untreated.
- Asymptomatic periods vary but tend to be shorter as the disease progresses.
- Without treatment, the person may experience several attacks a year, with chronic joint symptoms with permanent erosive deformity developing.

Physical Findings

- History and physical examination are usually sufficient for a tentative diagnosis to be made.

Laboratory Findings

- Elevated serum urate 7 g/dl supports the diagnosis but is not specific.
  - About 30% of patients have a normal serum urate level at the time of the acute attack.
- Needle-shaped urate crystals seen in tissue or synovial fluid are pathognomonic.

Treatment

- Goals of treatment are to (1) terminate the acute attack with NSAIDs, (2) prevent recurrent frequent acute attacks with daily colchicine, (3) prevent further deposition of MSU crystals and resolution of existing tophi by lowering the urate concentration in extracellular fluid, and (4) treat obesity, hypertension, and hyperlipidemia if present (Box 17-6).

Avoid ASA, diuretics, Purines Alcohol

Conservative Measures

- Instruct patient regarding the nature, cause, treatment, course, and prognosis of the disease.
- Patient is advised to
  —Lose weight
  —Moderate use of alcohol, especially beer
  —Drink at least eight glasses of water a day
  —Avoid repetitive trauma
  —Control hyperlipidemia
  —Control hypertension
  —Reduce consumption of fat, cholesterol, and meat, especially organ meats, which contain high levels of purines
  —Drugs such as diuretics (loop and thiazides) should not be prescribed, as they may decrease the clearance of uric acid and reduce plasma volume.
  —Other drugs to be avoided (e.g., low-dose aspirin, ethambutol hydrochloride [Myambutol], pyrazinamide, niacin) decrease uric acid excretion by competing for secretion in renal tubules.

Patient/Family Education

- Instruct regarding the nature of the disease, its probable cause(s), treatment, course, and prognosis.
- Teach about all medications prescribed as to reason for taking, action, dosage and schedule, major side effects, and usual length of therapy.
- Provide a list of foods high in purine: anchovies, sardines, organ meats, (e.g., liver, kidneys), legumes, red meats, poultry. Foods lowest in purines include eggs, fruit, nuts, sugar, gelatin, and vegetables other than legumes.

Follow-up/Referral

- Patients are followed closely after initial attack and while medications are being adjusted.
- Most patients with gout require long-term treatment with either uricosuric agents or xanthine oxidase inhibitors.
- Monitor fluid intake, diet, weight loss, and response to drug therapy.
- Monitor weekly uric acid levels while drug dosages are being adjusted.
- CBC, hepatic function tests, uric acid level, and renal panel are done every 3 months.

Shoulder Pain (Bursitis) *Neer Impingement Test*

Definition

Pain in one or both shoulders from any one of various causes; presents diagnostic challenges for the practitioner because of the complexity of the structures involved. Shoulder function involves the thorax and three bones (humerus, glenoid, clavicle), and almost 30 muscles; four articulations must move normally for the shoulder to function correctly. Under the superficial layer is the *subacromial* or *subdeltoid bursa*, which aids free movement of underlying structures relative to the roof. Under the bursa lies the *rotator cuff*, a group of muscles and their tendons that consists of the supraspinatus superiorly, the infraspinatus and teres minor posteriorly, and the subscapularis anteriorly.

Etiology (Boxes 17-7 and 17-8)
Diagnosis

- History and physical examination are usually sufficient to establish a working diagnosis and to direct effective treatment.
- Physical examination consists of several parts including visual inspection, palpation, range-of-motion testing, strength testing, neurovascular assessment, and general physical evaluation.

Visual Inspection

- Examine the skin and contour of the entire shoulder girdle.
- Look for areas of swelling and muscle atrophy and compare one side with the other, allowing for dominant and nondominant sides.

Palpation

- Palpate from the neck to the fingers in all aspects of the upper extremities.
- Areas to be specifically palpated for tenderness: sternoclavicular joint, clavicle, acromioclavicular joint, anterior and posterior glenohumeral joint lines, biceps tendon, subacromial space, and scapula.
- Assess both active and passive motion of the shoulder.
- Patients with rotator cuff tear have full passive but reduced active range of motion; the rotator cuff muscles are tested for weakness (tear) or pain (tendinitis); always compare sides.

BOX 17-7
Causes of Shoulder Pain in Adults

MOST COMMON
Rotator cuff tendinitis (supraspinatus, infraspinatus-teres minor, subscapularis)

COMMON
Rotator cuff tears (partial more common than complete)
Subdeltoid/subacromial bursitis

INTERMEDIATE
Adhesive capsulitis/frozen shoulder

OCCASIONAL
Acromioclavicular arthritis/strain
Biceps (long head) tendinitis
Cardiac (referred pain)
Carpal tunnel syndrome (referred pain)
Cerebrovascular accident with hemiparesis
Cervical/neck disorders (referred pain)
Degenerative/osteoarthritis (may be posttraumatic)
Dislocation
Fracture (neck of humerus, greater tuberosity)
Glenohumeral instability/subluxation

Glenoid labral tears
Neoplasm (local or referred pain)
Rheumatoid arthritis

UNCOMMON
Arthritis, other causes (e.g., gout, pseudogout, psoriasis, neuropathic, ankylosing spondylitis)
Infection (intraarticular or extraarticular)
Nerve entrapment: axillary and suprascapular nerves (referred pain)
Osteonecrosis (avascular or aseptic necrosis)
Polymyalgia rheumatica
Reflex sympathetic dystrophy/shoulder-hand syndrome
Sickle cell crisis
Thoracic outlet syndrome (referred pain)
Visceral (referred from sources other than neck or heart, e.g., pleural irritation by lung cancer or other cause; irritation of phrenic nerve or diaphragm by pathologic process such as subdiaphragmatic abscess, ruptured viscus, or disease of the mediastinum, pericardium, spleen or gallbladder; dissecting aortic aneurysm)
Other traumatic or periarticular soft tissue disorders

From Kern DE: Shoulder pain. In Barker LR, Burton JR, Zieve PD, eds: *Principles of ambulatory medicine,* ed 5, Baltimore, 1999, Williams & Wilkins, p 893.

BOX 17-8
Periarticular and Glenohumeral Disorders of the Shoulder

PERIARTICULAR DISORDERS
Rotator cuff tendinitis
Subdeltoid (subacromial) bursitis
Rotator cuff tear
Bicipital tendinitis
Acromioclavicular disorders

GLENOHUMERAL DISORDERS
Adhesive capsulitis ("frozen shoulder")
Trauma
Arthritic and other conditions

From Kern DE: Shoulder pain. In Barker LR, Burton JR, Zieve PD, eds: *Principles of ambulatory medicine,* ed 5, Baltimore, 1999, Williams & Wilkins, pp 898-902.

- Severe impingement or capsulitis reduces both active and passive range of motion.

Diagnostic Tests
- The Neer impingement sign is the most reliable to identify nerve impingement: the patient's shoulder is rotated internally, and the

arm is brought passively into forward flexion; the sign is positive if pain is elicited in the midarc of motion.
- Impingement syndrome comprises a spectrum of conditions, including shoulder bursitis, rotator cuff tendinitis, and rotator cuff tears; each of these conditions has a similar cause and presentation; the end stage of impingement syndrome is a rotator cuff tear.
- The best signs for anterior shoulder instability are the apprehension sign and the relocation sign, which differentiate anterior instability from primary impingement.
  —With the patient supine and muscles relaxed, abduct the shoulder 90°, then gently rotate externally to the limit of motion; in this "apprehension" position, the patient may be afraid that the joint will dislocate, which is the positive apprehension sign.
  —In patients with more subtle instability, this maneuver produces posterosuperior glenohumeral joint pain as the tuberosity or the rotator cuff impinges against the

posterosuperior glenoid rim; when a gentle, anteriorly directed force is applied to the humeral head, the sign becomes more obvious.

- The relocation test is performed with the patient in the same position; a posteriorly directed force is applied to the humeral head; this force relocates the joint so that, in a patient with anterior instability, the apprehension and pain resolve.
- Routine use of imaging studies is not cost-effective for most patients with shoulder problems.
- Plain shoulder x-rays are done on patients with persistent pain, to detect calcification in the capsule or supraspinatus tendon, which suggests tendinitis.
- Other imaging studies (e.g., magnetic resonance imaging [MRI] computed tomography) reinforce the physical findings in difficult cases, and patients are usually referred to an orthopedist for these and other more sophisticated tests, if required.
- MRI is especially helpful in detecting subtle rotator cuff tears.
- Ultrasonography can show even partial rotator cuff tears.
- *Arthrography* is both sensitive (92%) and specific (about 98%) in detecting rotator cuff tears.
- *Arthrography and computed tomography (CT) (arthro-CT)* detects soft tissue lesions (e.g., partial tendon tears) and intraarticular pathology (e.g., labral tears, capsular tears, loose bodies, chondral defects), particularly in recurrent subluxation or dislocation.
- CT is noninvasive for evaluation of soft tissue lesions; MRI defines capsule anatomy, supraspinatus tendon integrity, site of impingement, and anatomy of bursae much better than CT.
- Use of CT is equal to arthrography and superior to ultrasound and is the technique of choice to diagnose early osteonecrosis.

Shoulder Bursitis   *Need Impingement Test*

Definition

- A bursa is a saclike cavity or potential cavity that contains synovial fluid located at tissue sites where friction occurs, such as where tendons or muscles pass over bony promi-

nences; bursae facilitate normal movement, minimize friction between moving parts, and may communicate with joints.
- Bursitis is simply an acute or chronic inflammation of a bursa, wherever it is located.
- The shoulder, or subacromial, bursa is located in the subacromial space, which is under the acromion and above the rotator cuff.
- Other shoulder problems besides bursitis are shoulder instability/dislocation, glenohumeral arthritis, and acromioclavicular joint problems (e.g., shoulder separation, osteoarthritis).

Incidence/Etiology

- The incidence of bursitis is extremely common.
- Causes include trauma, chronic overuse, inflammatory arthritis (e.g., gout, RA), or acute or chronic infection.

Diagnosis

Signs and Symptoms

- Shoulder bursitis typically is associated with an achy pain that becomes worse with activity; some patients report that the pain radiates into the biceps area in the front of the upper arm, and this pain can be worse than that in the actual bursa.
- Bursitis pain is usually mild-to-moderate but intensifies with overhead movement of the affected arm, although patients often do not volunteer this information unless asked specifically.
- Most patients are comfortable when the affected arm is at their side, and routine active and passive ranges of shoulder motion are usually normal.
- It is important to ask the patient to elevate the arm in forward flexion in the sagittal plane and in abduction in the coronal plane.
- The patient should be able to externally rotate the arm at the side with the elbow flexed to 90°.
- Finally, the patient is asked to reach as far up the midline of the back as he/she can reach, which helps to determine degree of internal rotation (normally, people can reach to about the tenth thoracic vertebra).
- For each of these tests, strength is normal, but pain occurs with resistance testing.

RICE, NSAIDS

- Eliciting pain with the Neer impingement sign usually confirms the diagnosis; injection of 10 ml of lidocaine into the subacromial space results in almost complete resolution of pain.

Treatment

Rest, ROM ex, Ice

- To relieve pain, 2 to 3 days of rest are usually necessary, with the arm in a sling.
- Many patients can begin range-of-motion exercises almost immediately to maintain mobility at maximum level.
- Strenuous exercise and overuse are discouraged.
- Long-term immobilization of the shoulder is avoided to prevent contracture.
- Patients with impingement disorders such as rotator cuff lesions or subdeltoid bursitis should avoid repetitive tasks that require that the arms be overhead, or elbows above the midtorso.
- Cooling of an injured part immediately after an injury is used to limit hemorrhage and relieve pain.
- Heat or ultrasound can be used to decrease pain and promote tissue extensibility in the subacute and chronic stages.
- Referral to a physical therapist is recommended.

Pharmacologic Therapy

- NSAIDs are generally more effective than placebo but less effective than steroid injections to decrease pain and restore function in periarticular disorders.
  —A 2-week course is usually prescribed.
  —Concerns exist about NSAIDs' effect on GI (peptic ulcer with bleeding, perforation) and renal toxicity (proteinuria, renal failure), particularly in older persons undergoing injection therapy.
  —Depocorticosteroid injections seem to reduce pain and speed functional recovery in patients with rotator cuff tendinitis/bursitis and are more effective than NSAIDs and analgesics.
  —The preferred therapy combines one to three depocorticosteroid injections with a planned program of exercise, which seem to be more effective than analgesic or no therapy in reducing pain and

speeding recovery of patients with adhesive capsulitis.
  —A 60% to 90% success rate is seen in steroid injections to treat bursitis and tendinitis of the shoulder.

Surgical Treatment

- Surgical intervention, such as manipulation under anesthesia or arthroscopic capsular release, often speeds recovery for some patients.

Patient/Family Education

- Teach the patient how to apply a sling or use other assistive devices, as appropriate.
- Reassure the patient regarding prognosis and likelihood of resuming previous activities within a reasonable length of time.
- Teach the patient how to protect his limbs, back, and joints in daily and occupational activities.
- Instruct about prescribed and over-the-counter medications as to side effects, interactions among drugs, and other information, including use of herbal remedies and their effect on prescription medications.

Follow-up/Referral

- In most cases, referral is not needed because a period of rest and analgesics will usually suffice for the patient's recovery.
- Regular monitoring regarding level of pain, range of motion, and ability to perform daily and occupational activities is necessary at gradually increasing intervals throughout convalescence, to rule out signs and symptoms of more serious conditions such as infection, cancer, or other.

Carpal Tunnel Syndrome

Median N compression

Definition

Carpal tunnel syndrome is a common painful disorder of the wrist and hand involving compression of the median nerve between the inelastic carpal ligament and other structures within the carpal tunnel.

Risk Factors

- Repeated trauma of hand/wrist
- Incidence is greater among women, aged 30 to 50 years.

Tinel, Phalen, + c dx of m. nerve

Etiology/Cause

- Often, no cause can be identified
- RA (may be the presenting manifestation)
- Cumulative trauma of the hand/wrist
- Activities or occupations that require repetitive flexion and extension of the wrist (e.g., keyboard use: computer, piano, organ)
- Often seen in association with
  —Hypothyroidism
  —Diabete mellitus
  —Pregnancy/obesity
  —Acromegaly

Pathogenesis

- Median nerve compression, resulting in nerve damage, thickened tendons, or synovitis in the carpal tunnel

Diagnosis

Signs and Symptoms

- Pain in the hand and wrist
- Tingling and numbness usually distributed along the median nerve (palmar side of the thumb, index, and middle fingers, and the radial half of the ring finger).
- Entire hand may be affected.
- Patient wakes at night with burning or aching pain, numbness, and tingling, and shakes the hand to obtain relief and restore sensation.
- Diagnosis is established by positive Tinel's sign, in which the tingling (paresthesia) is reproduced by tapping with a reflex hammer at the volar surface of the wrist over the site of the median nerve and the carpal tunnel.
- Other tests include wrist flexion maneuvers (e.g., Phalen's sign).
- Thenar atrophy and weakness on thumb elevation may develop late.
- Diagnosis is confirmed by electrodiagnostic testing of median nerve conduction velocity, which provides an accurate picture of motor and sensory nerve conduction.

Treatment

- Lightweight wrist splint, worn at night also
- Pyridoxine (vitamin B_6) 50 mg bid
- Mild analgesics (e.g., acetaminophen, NSAIDs)
- Adjusting position of computer keyboard, chair, seating at piano/organ

- If pain persists, injection of corticosteroid into the carpal tunnel at a site just ulnar to the palmaris longus tendon, and proximal to the distal crease at the wrist
- If symptoms persist or recur, or if hand weakness and thenar wasting progress, surgical decompression of the carpal tunnel is recommended.

Prognosis

- Carpal tunnel syndrome usually resolves with splinting, rest, and analgesics within 2 to 3 weeks.
- Surgical division of the volar carpal ligament to relieve nerve pressure is usually curative.

Patient/Family Education

- Patient and family require reassurance and support, as carpal tunnel syndrome is often a temporarily disabling condition.
- Teach the patient how to apply a splint, without making it too tight.
- Teach the patient how to perform gentle range-of-motion exercises, done at least twice a day.
- Emphasize the importance of splinting of the hand and forearm at night, and elevating the arm to relieve swelling of soft tissue and thus relieve some pain.
- Provide information and references about occupational counseling, if the patient needs to change jobs to prevent further carpal tunnel problems.
- Review the prescribed medication regimen; emphasize that drug therapy may require 2 to 4 weeks before maximum benefit is achieved.
- Some drugs (e.g., indomethacin, mefenamic acid, phenylbutazone, or piroxicam) should be taken with antacids to prevent gastric symptoms.

Follow-up/Referral

- The patient is followed weekly for several weeks to assess the need for injections of corticosteroids or surgery, if the condition does not abate.
- At any time, referral to an orthopedic surgeon may be necessary for further evaluation and treatment.

X SPLint, Rest, Analgesia X   RoM

BOX 17-9
Causes of Low Back Pain

TRAUMA
Falls
Accidents

MECHANICAL
Muscular pain
Postural back pain
Prolapsed disc
Lumbar spondylosis + spinal stenosis
Disseminated idiopathic skeletal hyperostosis (DISH)
Spondylolisthesis
Fibromyalgia

INFLAMMATORY
Infective lesions of the spine
Ankylosing spondylitis/sacroiliitis

METABOLIC
Osteoporosis + fracture
Osteomalacia
Paget's disease

NEOPLASTIC
Metastases
Multiple myeloma
Primary bone tumors

REFERRED PAIN

From Drury PL, Shipley M: Rheumatology and bone disease. In Kumar P, Clark M, eds: *Clinical medicine,* ed 4, Edinburgh, 1998, WB Saunders, p 457.

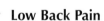 NSAIDs ↓ Neuro B/o Bowel Sx

Low Back Pain

Definition

Low back pain (LBP) is pain in the low lumbar, lumbosacral, or sacroiliac regions, possibly accompanied by pain radiating down one or both buttocks or legs in the distribution of the sciatic nerve (sciatica).

Risk Factors

- Chronic poor-quality or deficient sleep
- Fatigue
- Physical deconditioning
- Stress/psychosocial problems
- Overexertion
- Trauma

Etiology/Cause (Box 17-9) (see also Risk Factors)
- Often from work-related trauma (bending, lifting heavy objects, torsion movements)

- Between 70% and 80% of the population experience back pain sometime during their lives, ranging from 10% of adults in a 2-year period to a high of 20% of the population of a Western industrial society during a 2-week period.
- About 30% of those who develop low back problems do not seek medical help.

Pathogenesis
- Specific with each disorder

Diagnosis
- Taking the history of a patient with LBP (Tables 17-1 and 17-2)
- Past history of similar symptoms, course of treatment, and response to therapy
- Symptom onset or cause of current episode, location and character of pain
- Onset of current episode, mechanism of injury, and initial location of pain
- Compliance with current treatment and self-care
- Factors that exacerbate or alleviate pain
- Pain status: improving, deteriorating, or plateaued?
- Red flags: neurologic deficits, bowel or bladder dysfunction, systemic illness
- Physical and functional impairments due to pain

Laboratory Tests
- For most patients, routine testing is not necessary.
- Review results of any laboratory or radiologic studies done in the past or recently.
- "Red flags" warrant further investigation: cauda equina syndrome (saddle block anesthesia, recent onset of bladder or bowel dysfunction, especially urinary retention, severe or progressive lower extremity weakness); pain not relieved by rest, which could indicate cancer; systemic signs and symptoms: unexplained weight loss and risk of infection; risk factors for fracture (e.g., major trauma, minor trauma in a patient over 50 years old, prolonged corticosteroid use, osteoporosis, patients over age 70).

Treatment
- The majority of patients will improve within 1 to 4 weeks, with only the initial history

TABLE 17-1
Focused Physical Examination for Low Back Pain

Position	Test/Observation	Possible Findings
All positions	Observation	Behavioral factors, physical limitation
Standing	Posture and gait	Poor postural habits, change due to pain
	Heel and toe walking	L5 or S1 weakness
	Symmetry, asymmetry	Scoliosis, atrophy
	Range of motion	Pain response, physical limitation
Sitting	Straight-leg raise	Radicular pain
	Neurologic testing	Neurologic deficit
Supine	Leg length	Mechanical contribution
	Straight-leg raise	Radicular pain
	Patrick's test (fabere sign)	Hip involvement
Prone	Palpation	Muscle dysfunction
	Hip extension	Radicular pain (L2-4 nerve roots)
	"Prone prop"*	Facet joint dysfunction

*The "prone prop" patient is asked to extend the back by resting on bent elbows with the pelvis remaining on the examination table; results in passive extension of the lumbar spine and likely reduces compression on the intervertebral disk; ask about any pain associated with the position.

TABLE 17-2
Common Patterns of Acute Low Back Pain

Pain Source	Mechanism of Injury	Aggravating Actions
Musculoligamentous strain or sprain	Flexion	Flexion, twisting
Intervertebral disk	Flexion, compression	Flexion, sitting
Facet joint	Extension, rotation, compression	Extension, rotation
Sacroiliac joint	Fall onto buttocks	Walking, sitting
Nerve root irritation	Flexion, compression	Flexion, sitting

and physical examination needed to identify patients who require more extensive or urgent evaluation/treatment (e.g., infection, cancer, inflammatory disease such as ankylosing spondylitis, aortic aneurysm, or other) (Box 17-10).

- Other medications for LBP
  - Limited evidence supports the use of muscle relaxants such as diazepam, cyclobenzaprine, carisoprodol, and methocarbamol.
  - These drugs should be used only in those who have not responded to NSAIDs, and limited to 1 to 2 weeks of therapy.
  - Use of these drugs in older persons is not recommended, because of the risk of patients falling.

Patient/Family Education
- All patients should be taught how to protect their back in daily activities.
  - To not lift heavy objects
  - To use the legs rather than the back in lifting anything
  - To use only chairs with arms, to assist in rising
  - To get up from bed, roll to one side, then use the arms to push to an upright position
- Back manipulation for benign, mechanical LBP is shown to be as effective as therapies provided by other health care professionals.

Follow-up/Referral
- The patient who has presented with acute LBP should be followed at intervals of a few days to no more than 2 weeks.
- Monitor compliance with medication schedule, pain level, and activity level to emphasize self-care.
- Evaluate how much care the patient is using in protecting the back every day.
- Evaluate response to therapy.
- Perform a focused physical examination.
- Lack of improvement, uncertainty regarding diagnosis, or evidence of developing complex pain warrant referral to an orthopedist.

BOX 17-10

AHCPR* Guidelines for Management of Acute Low Back Pain

I. PATIENT EDUCATION

Patients with acute low back problems should be given accurate information about the following (strength of evidence = B):

A. Expectations for both rapid recovery and recurrences of symptoms based on natural history of low back symptoms.
B. Safe and effective methods of symptom control.
C. Safe and reasonable activity modifications.
D. Best means of limiting recurrent low back problems.
E. Lack of need for special investigations unless danger signs are present.
F. Effectiveness and risks of commonly available diagnostic and further treatment measures to be considered, should symptoms persist.

II. MEDICATIONS

Acetaminophen and NSAIDs

A. Acetaminophen is reasonably safe and is acceptable for treating patients with acute low back problems (strength of evidence = C).
B. NSAIDs, including aspirin, are acceptable for treating patients with acute low back problems (strength of evidence = B).
C. NSAIDs have a number of potential side effects. The most common complication is GI irritation. The decision to use these medications can be guided by comorbidity, side effects, cost, and patient and provider preference (strength of evidence = C).

III. PHYSICAL TREATMENTS

Spinal manipulation

A. Manipulation can be helpful for patients with acute low back problems without radiculopathy when used within the first month of symptoms (strength of evidence = B).
B. A trial of manipulation in patients without radiculopathy with symptoms longer than a month is probably safe, but efficacy is unproven (strength of evidence = C)

IV. ACTIVITY MODIFICATION

Activity recommendations for bed rest and exercise

A. A gradual return to normal activities is more effective than prolonged bed rest for treating acute low back problems (strength of evidence = B).
B. Prolonged bed rest for more than 4 days may lead to debilitation and is not recommended for treating acute low back problems (strength of evidence = B).
C. Low-stress aerobic exercise can prevent debilitation due to inactivity during the first month of symptoms and thereafter may help to return patients to the highest level of functioning appropriate to their circumstances (strength of evidence = C).

From Bigos SJ, Bowyer O, Braen G, et al: Acute low back problems in adults. Clinical Practice Guideline No. 14. AHCPR publication No. 95-0642. Rockville, MD, Agency for Health Care Policy and Research, Public Health Service, U.S. Department of Health and Human Services, December, 1994.
Ratings of strength of evidence: *A,* Strong research-based evidence (multiple relevant and high-quality studies); *B,* moderate research-based evidence (one relevant, high-quality or multiple adequate studies); *C,* limited research-based evidence (one adequate scientific study); *D,* studies did not meet inclusion criteria.
*As of January 1, 2000, this agency was renamed Agency for Health Care and Quality, but functions have not changed.

- Referral usually is not necessary unless pain becomes more acute or severe, or other signs and symptoms point to more severe problems.

Osteoporotic Crush Fracture of the Spine

Although osteoporosis is asymptomatic, it can result in an increased risk of fracture of peripheral bones, particularly the neck of the femur and wrist, and thoracic or lumbar vertebral crush fractures. Vertebral crush fractures occur without trauma, after minimal trauma, or as part of a major accident. They develop painlessly, or may cause agonizing localized pain that radiates around the ribs and abdomen. Multiple fractures result in an increased thoracic kyphosis ("widow's hump").

Diagnosis

- Diagnosis is confirmed by x-ray, which shows loss of anterior vertebral body height and wedging, with sparing of the vertebral end-plates and pedicles.

Treatment

- Bed rest and analgesics are given until the severe pain subsides over a few weeks, during which hospitalization may be required.
- Gradual mobilization begins.
- Management of established osteoporosis is unsatisfactory because the bone mass is already substantially reduced.
- Research shows that significant improvement can occur in bone density and rate of fractures.

Immobilize (handwritten note)

TABLE 17-3
Classification and Treatment of Ankle Sprain

Classification	Type of Sprain	Symptoms and Signs	Treatment
Grade 1	Mild or minimal, with no tear of ligament	Mild tenderness with some swelling	Strapping with elastic bandages or tape; Unna's paste boot immobilization; elevation; gradual gentle exercise and walking
Grade 2	Moderate sprain: incomplete or partial rutpure	Obvious swelling, ecchymosis, and difficulty walking	Below-knee walking cast; immobilization for 3 wks
Grade 3	Complete tear of ligament	Swelling, bleeding, ankle instability, unable to walk	Cast immobilization; possibly surgery

1 Grade, 2 Grade, 3 Grade (handwritten margin notes)

From Beers MH, Berkow R, eds: Musculoskeletal and connective tissue disorders: Common foot and ankle disorders. *The Merck manual of diagnosis and therapy*, ed 17, Whitehouse Station, NJ, 1999, Merck & Co, Inc, p 484.

- Ideally, future management will be largely prophylactic.
- Diet: adequate intake of calories, calcium, and vitamin D is required, with at least 1000 mg of calcium (1500 mg in postmenopausal women) and 400 to 800 IU of vitamin D daily.
- Weight gain in thin persons is necessary, as low body weight is itself a risk factor for fractures.
- Exercise: a minimum of 30 minutes of weight-bearing exercise three times a week has been shown to be beneficial.
- Smoking cessation: smoking appears to accelerate bone loss and may negate the beneficial effect of estrogen therapy, possibly by accelerating estrogen metabolism.
- Reduction in fall risk: physiotherapy and assessent of home safety may be required; hip protectors may be helpful

Ankle Sprain *Grade 1, 2, 3* (handwritten)

The ankle is supported laterally by the anterior talofibular ligament (ATL), the fibulocalcaneal ligament (FCL), and the posterior talofibular ligament (PTL). In ankle sprain, the ATL usually is ruptured first; only then can the FCL divide. About 64% of patients with ankle sprain injure only the ATL. About 17% of patients also injure the lateral FCL. The PTL rarely ruptures.

Risk Factors
- Weakness of the peroneal tendons
- Laxity of ligaments that support the ankle

- Persons whose gait involves forefoot valgus, in which the forefoot tends to evert during the gait cycle, causing the subtalar joint to compensate by inversion, may be more at risk for ankle sprain.

Diagnosis
Symptoms and Signs
- Palpation of the lateral ankle shows the site of injury of the ligament.

Treatment (Table 17-3)
- Adequate analgesic medication, particularly before exercise or walking
- Surgery is rarely necessary or possible because the extreme fragmentation of the ligament(s) makes surgical repair difficult.
  —Some surgeons use plaster casts for rupture of only one ligament (ATL) but recommend surgery if the FCL is torn.

Complications
- Meniscoid body: a small nodule is located at the ATL.
  —Impingement between the lateral capsular ligament, resulting from Grade 2 or 3 injury, causes persistent synovitis and over time fibrotic swelling and permanent induration.
  —Infiltration of soluble and insoluble corticosteroids with a local anesthetic between the talus and the lateral malleolus often results in dramatic and long-term improvement.

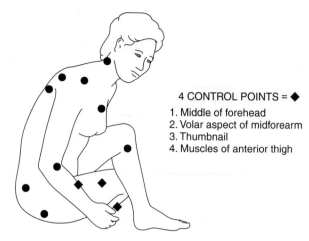

9 PAIRED TENDER POINTS = ●
1. Insertion of nuchal muscles into occiput
2. Upper trapezius (midpoint)
3. Pectoralis muscle—just lateral to second costo-chondral junction
4. 2 cm below lateral epicondyle
5. Upper gluteal region
6. 2 cm posterior to greater trochanter
7. Medial knee in area of anserine bursa
8. Paraspinous, 3 cm lateral to midline at the level of midscapula
9. Above the scapula spine near medial border

4 CONTROL POINTS = ◆
1. Middle of forehead
2. Volar aspect of midforearm
3. Thumbnail
4. Muscles of anterior thigh

Fig. 17-1 The tender point locations in fibromyalgia are remarkably consistent among patients. Multiple locations have been described. The nine paired (n = 18) tender points shown represent those that are seen most frequently in a wide distribution. Most patients have 11 or more tender points. Control points are not unusually tender and should be examined along with the nine pairs of most tender points. (From Kelley WN, Harris ED, Ruddy S, et al: *Textbook of rheumatology,* ed 5, Philadelphia, 1997, WB Saunders.)

- Other complications that may occur are
  —Neuralgia of the intermediate dorsal cutaneous nerve
  —Peroneal tenosynovitis
  —Reflex sympathetic dystrophy (Sudeck's posttraumatic reflex atrophy)
  —Sinus tarsi syndrome
- Most complications, if any occur, are treatable.
- Early mobility is the goal.

Prognosis
- Favorable in most cases, depending on the extent of injury.
- Symptomatic treatment—immobilization for a short time, strapping or casting, injection of corticosteroids and local anesthestic help to relieve inflammation and pain.

Patient/Family Education
- Reassurance from the time of injury is important.
- Relief of pain and urgent care are necessary.
- Keep the patient informed of procedures to be done: injection, manipulation, strapping, or casting as necessary.
- Explain in detail the program of gradual exercise and walking.
- Provide specific written instructions about analgesics and other medications.

Follow-up/Referral
- Treatment from the beginning should be under the supervision of an experienced orthopedist regarding initial evaluation, plan of treatment, strapping, or casting as needed.
- The nurse practitioner follows the patient after the initial evaluation and treatment plan are established, usually once a week × 2 to 3 weeks, then at longer intervals as healing occurs, monitoring pain level, compliance with medication and programmed exercise, and mobility.

Fibromyalgia (Fibrositis Syndrome)
Definition
Fibromyalgia (fibrositis syndrome) comprises a group of common nonarticular disorders characterized by achy pain, tenderness, and stiffness of muscles, areas of tendon insertions, and adjacent tissue structures (Fig. 17-1).
- Common terms used are myofascial pain syndrome, fibrotitis, and fibromyositis.
- The term *myalgia* indicates muscular pain.
- In contrast, myositis is caused by inflammation of muscle tissues and is an inappropriate term for fibromyalgia, in which inflammation is absent.
- Fibromyalgia indicates pain in fibrous tissues, muscles, tendons, ligaments, and other sites.

- Any fibromuscular tissues may be involved, but those of the occiput, neck (neck pain or spasm), shoulders, thorax (pleurodynia), low back (lumbago), and thighs (aches and charley horses) are particularly affected.
- **Primary fibromyalgia syndrome** (PFS) is a generalized, idiopathic form that is more commonly seen in healthy young or middle-aged women who tend to be stressed, tense, depressed, anxious, and striving, but may also occur in children or adolescents, particularly girls, or in older adults; it is often associated with a particular occupation or profession (e.g., myofascial pain syndrome).

Risk Factors
- May be unaccustomed to exercise
- Obesity
- Advancing age
- Women

Etiology/Causes
- Physical or mental stress
- Poor sleep
- Trauma
- Exposure to dampness or cold
- Systemic, usually rheumatic, disorder
- A viral or other systemic infection (e.g., Lyme disease) may precipitate the syndrome.
- Environmental factors
- The feet are subject to extreme pressures by weight-bearing and inappropriate shoes.
  —Broad, deep, thick-soled shoes are essential for sports activities, for prolonged walking or standing, and for persons with congenitally flat or arthritic feet.
- The feet are often painful.
- Two common foot deformities are
  —The feet stress the ankle and throw the hind foot into a valgus (everted) position—a flat foot is rigid and inflexible.
  —High-arched feet place pressure on the lateral border and ball of the foot.
- The foot is affected by a variety of *inflammatory arthritic conditions.*

Diagnosis
Signs and Symptoms
- Onset of pain and stiffness in PFS is gradual and diffuse, achy in nature.

- In localized disease, symptoms are more often sudden and acute, with typical "tender points" where pain is more evident.
- Some patients experience local tightness or muscle spasm but not to the point of contractions.
- Associated symptoms are also typically present.
  —Poor sleep
  —Anxiety
  —Fatigue
  —Irritable bowel
- Other similar conditions must be excluded.
  —Osteoarthritis
  —RA
  —Polymyalgia rheumatica
  —Other connective tissue diseases
  —Psychogenic muscle pain and spasm
  —Hypothyroidism should be excluded in older women (>45).

Treatment
- PFS may remit spontaneously with decreased stress but may recur frequently or become chronic.
- Stretching and aerobic exercises
- Improved sleep patterns
- Heat application
- Gentle massage
- Low-dose tricyclic antidepressant (e.g., cyclobenzaprine HCl 10 mg) at bedtime may improve sleep and relieve pain to some degree
- Aspirin and NSAIDs have not proven to be effective.
- Incapacitating tender areas may be injected with 1% lidocaine solution, 1 to 2 ml alone or combined with a 20- to 40-mg hydrocortisone acetate suspension.
- Despite thoughtful care, symptoms often persist, with intermittent remissions.

Prognosis
- Favorable with a comprehensive, supportive regimen, management of anxiety or depression with consultation of specialists as required
- The best management is a consistent, personalized approach, with maximum involvement of the patient.

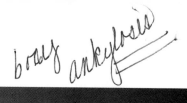

bony ankylosis

BOX 17-11
Stages of Rheumatoid Arthritis

CLINICAL STAGES

Stage I, Early
1. X-rays show no evidence of destructive changes.
2. X-rays may show evidence of osteoporosis.

Stage II, Moderate
1. X-rays show evidence of osteoporosis, possibly with slight destruction of cartilage or subchondral bone.
2. Joints are not deformed, but mobility may be limited.
3. Adjacent muscles are atrophied.
4. Extraarticular soft-tissue lesions (e.g., nodules, tenovaginitis) may be present.

Stage III, Severe
1. X-rays show cartilage and bone destruction, as well as osteoporosis.
2. Joint deformity (e.g., subluxation, ulnar deviation, hyperextension) exists but not fibrous or bony ankylosis.
3. Muscle atrophy is extensive.

4. Extraarticular soft-tissue lesions (e.g., nodules, tenovaginitis) are often present.

Stage IV, Terminal
1. Fibrous or bony ankylosis exists, in addition to all criteria listed in stage III.

FUNCTIONAL CLASSIFICATION

Class I
No loss of functional capacity

Class II
Functional capacity impaired, but sufficient normal activities despite joint pain or limited mobility

Class III
Functional capacity is adequate to perform only few, if any, occupational or self-care tasks

Class IV
Patient confined to bed or wheelchair and capable of minimal or no self-care

From Billings DM, Stokes LG: *Medical surgical nursing: common health problems of adults and children across the life span,* ed 2, St. Louis, 1987, Mosby.

Chronic Synovial Inflam.

Patient/Family Education
- Provide adequate reassurance about the benign nature of the condition.
- Enlist the patient's cooperation in managing symptoms, by analysis and evaluating effect of therapy and need for alternative medication or program.
- It is often helpful for the patient and the nurse practitioner if the patient keeps a daily record of how she is feeling, specific sites of pain, and whether there is improvement or worsening of symptoms each day, but if focusing on symptoms becomes obsessive, the journal should be discontinued.

Rheumatoid Arthritis *4 Stages*

Definition
RA is a chronic, inflammatory, destructive, sometimes deforming, collagen disease that has an autoimmune component.
- In the past 10 years, perspectives about the nature and treatment of RA have changed dramatically.
  - It is now apparent that RA is a serious systemic disorder, with 5-year survival similar to that of stage IV Hodgkin's disease or triple-vessel coronary artery disease.

- Investigators learned that in most patients, significant soft-tissue damage and bone erosions occur within 2 years of onset.
- Treatment has become increasingly aggressive and complex, particularly with regard to the new slow-acting antirheumatic drugs now available.
- RA is classified into four stages (Box 17-11).

Etiology/Cause
- Genetic factors—contribution to cause of RA is estimated at 15% to 30%.
- *Human leukocyte antigen (HLA) types*—a strong association exists between susceptibility to RA and certain HLA haplotypes.
  - HLA-DR4: occurs in 50% to 75% of patients correlates with a poor prognosis and the possession of a specific pentapeptide in the third allelic hypervariable region of HLA-Drβ-1 chain increases susceptibility.

Immunology
- The chronic synovial inflammation of RA may be caused by ongoing *T-cell activation*.
- Many factors are involved in the development and progression of RA that are too complex for inclusion here.

Pathology

infl of synovial lining

- RA is characterized by widespread persisting synovitis (inflammation of the synovial lining of joints, tendon sheaths, or bursae).
- The precise cause of these changes is unclear, but the production of RFs by plasma cells in the synovium and the local formation of immunocomplexes may play a part.
- The normal synovium becomes thickened, and becomes a palpable "boggy" swelling around the joints and tendons.
- Increased permeability of blood vessels and the synovial lining layer leads to joint effusions that contain lymphocytes and dying polymorphs.
- Activated lymphocytes and macrophages in the synovium produce a rich mixture of cytokines, including interleukins, prostaglandins, and TNF-α.
- The cartilage becomes thin and exposes the underlying bone.
- The size, site, and the joints affected lead to a variety of deformities and eventually to bony collapse.

Rheumatoid Factors

- These are circulating autoantibodies that have the *Fc* portion of immunoglobulin as their antigen.
  - The nature of the antigen causes them to self-aggregate into immunocomplexes and then activate complement and stimulate inflammation, which in turn causes chronic synovitis.
- Transient production of RFs is an essential part of the body's normal mechanism for removing immunocomplexes, but in RA their production is persistent and occurs into the joints; they may be of immunoglobulin class (IgM, IgG, or IgA), but the most common tests used clinically detect IgM RF.
- About 70% of patients with polyarticular RA have serum IgM RF in their serum.
- The term *seronegative RA* is used for patients in whom the standard tests for IgM RF are persistently negative; they tend to have a more limited pattern of synovitis.
- RFs are not found in synovitis associated with psoriasis, ankylosing spondylitis, inflammatory bowel disease, or reactive arthritis.

BOX 17-12
Diagnostic Approach to Polyarthritis

A. Define the host features
  1. Age, sex, ethnic background
  2. Family history
  3. Environmental factors
B. Describe the joint involvement
  1. Number
  2. Patterns
  3. Specific joints
  4. Symmetry/asymmetry
  5. Intensity of pain
  6. Course of signs/symptoms to date
C. Characteristics of extraarticular features
D. Supporting laboratory studies
E. Response to therapeutic trial

From Matsumoto AK, Wigley FM: Rheumatoid arthritis. In Barker LR, Burton JR, Zieve PD, eds: *Principles of ambulatory medicine*, ed 5, Baltimore, 1999, Williams & Wilkins, p 998.

- IgM RF is not diagnostic of RA, nor does its absence rule out RA, but it is useful in predicting prognosis.
  - A persistently high titer in early RA indicates more persistently active synovitis, more joint damage, and greater disability over time.

Diagnosis (Box 17-12)

Signs and Symptoms

- In about 70% of patients, RA begins as a *slowly progressive, symmetric, peripheral polyarthritis*, evolving over a period of a few weeks or months.
- Women are affected three times more often than men.
- The patient usually begins having symptoms during his or her thirties or forties, but RA can occur at any age.
- In about 15% of patients, the onset is rapid and can occur within a few days (or even overnight) with a severe symmetric polyarticular involvement.
  - These patients, surprisingly, often have a better prognosis.
- A worse than average prognosis (predictive accuracy of about 80%) is indicated if the patient is female, has a gradual onset over a few months, has a positive IgM RF, and develops anemia within 3 months of onset.

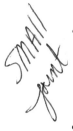

- Most patients complain of pain and stiffness of the small joints of the hands (metacarpophalangeal [MCP]), PIP and DIP, and feet (metatarsophalangeal [MTP]).
  —The typical joint deformity of the fingers is swan-neck deformity.
- The wrists, elbows, shoulders, knees, and ankles are all affected.
- Most patients present with involvement of many joints, but about 10% of patients present with monoarthritis of the knee or shoulder, or with carpal tunnel syndrome.
- Fatigue is common.
- Malaise ("I don't feel well")
- Joint pain and stiffness are significantly worse in the morning but usually improve gradually (within 1 to 2 hours) with gentle activity.
- Joints are warm and tender, with some swelling.
- Movement is limited.
- Evidence of muscle wasting
- Deformities develop as the disease progresses.

Other Signs
- Progression and signs and symptoms of RA vary considerably.
- Typically, RA has remissions and relapses, which occur either spontaneously or in response to drug therapy.
- Drugs may slow or halt the progression of RA.
- In some patients, RA remains active, continually producing joint damage, whereas in others, the inflammatory process stops ("burnt-out RA").
- A *seronegative limited synovitis* affects the wrists first, and has a less symmetric joint involvement.
  —This condition has a better long-term prognosis, but other cases progress to severe disability.
  —This form can be mistaken for psoriatic arthropathy, which has a similar distribution.
  —The patient may have a family history of psoriasis, or may develop psoriasis later.
- *Palindromic (recurrent) rheumatism* is unusual (5%) and is characterized by short-lived (24 to 48 hours) episodes of acute monoarthritis.
  —The joints become acutely painful, swollen, and red, which then resolves completely within a short time.

> **BOX 17-13**
> ## Nonarticular Manifestations of Rheumatoid Arthritis
>
> Scleritis
> Scleromalacia
> Sjögren's syndrome (dry eyes and mouth)
> Lymphadenopathy
> Pericarditis
> Bursitis/nodules
> Tendon sheath swelling
> Tenosynovitis
> Amyloidosis
> Sensorimotor polyneuropathy
> Atlanto-axial subluxation without cervical cord compression
> Pleural effusion ⎤
> Fibrosing alveolitis ⎥
> Caplan's syndrome ⎬ Lung
> Small airway disease ⎥
> Nodules ⎦
> Anemia
> Carpal tunnel syndrome
> Nailfold lesions of vasculitis
> Splenomegaly (Felty's syndrome)
> Leg ulcers
> Ankle edema

From Drury PL, Shipley H: Rheumatology and bone disease: Rheumatoid arthritis. In Kumar P, Clark M, eds: *Clinical medicine*, ed 4, Edinburgh, 1998, WB Saunders, p 475.

—Other attacks occur in the same or other joints.
—About 50% develop typical chronic rheumatoid synovitis, often after a delay of months or years.
—The remaining 50% remit or continue to have episodic arthritis.
—The appearance of IgM RF is a predictor of a change to chronic, destructive synovitis.

Nonarticular Manifestations of Rheumatoid Arthritis (Box 17-13)

Diagnostic Tests
CBC
- Anemia may be present.
- ESR and CRP are increased in proportion to the activity of the inflammatory process.

Serology
- RF is present in about 70% of cases.
- ANA at low titer in 30% of patients

X-rays
- May show cartilage or bone damage in affected joints

	Without any difficulty	Without some difficulty	Without much difficulty	Unable to do
A. Dress yourself, including tying shoelaces, doing buttons?	_____	_____	_____	_____
B. Get in and out of bed?	_____	_____	_____	_____
C. Lift a full cup or glass to your mouth?	_____	_____	_____	_____
D. Walk outdoors on flat ground?	_____	_____	_____	_____
E. Wash and dry your entire body?	_____	_____	_____	_____
F. Bend down to pick up clothing from the floor?	_____	_____	_____	_____
G. Turn regular faucets on and off?	_____	_____	_____	_____
H. Get in and out of car?	_____	_____	_____	_____

Fig. 17-2 Self-assessment of functional capacity. (From Matsumoto AK, Wigley FM: Rheumatoid arthritis. In Barker LR, Burton JR, Zieve PD, eds: *Principles of ambulatory medicine,* ed 5, Baltimore, 1999, Lippincott, Williams & Wilkins, p 1001.)

Aspiration

- Aspirate usually appears cloudy due to white cells.
- Specimen is sent for culture.
- In a suddenly painful joint, septic arthritis should be suspected.

Imaging

- In severe disease, extensive MRI or CT imaging is required to determine the extent of damage.

Treatment

- RA is a chronic disorder for which there is no known cure at present.
- Therapy requires a comprehensive plan that combines medical, social, and psychologic support.
- The goals of therapy are to reduce pain, prevent deformities and loss of joint function, and maintain the patient's productivity and activity.
- Knowing each patient's specific problems and needs forms the basis for long-term therapy.
- Chronic arthritis is a major stress that usually requires major changes in lifestyle.
- Realistic, attainable goals are possible and provide the patient with short-term goals to work toward.

- A self-assessment questionnaire provides an excellent periodic record of the patient's own perception of where they are (Fig. 17-2).

Pharmacologic Therapy

- NSAIDs, traditionally the first-line agents for treating RA, do not alter the course of the disease and have been shown to be as toxic as many of the slow-acting antirheumatic agents that may modify disease.
- Combinations of slow-acting agents are well tolerated and more effective than single-agent therapy; combination therapy early in the disease has become standard.
- Hydroxychloroquine sulfate (Plaquenil) and sulfasalazine (Azulfidine EN-tabs) are believed to be most effective as monotherapy in mild-to-moderate disease and are often used in combination with more potent drugs such as methotraxate (Rhematrex Dose pack) and cytotoxic agents.
  —These latter antiinflammatory and immunosuppressive drugs proved to be more predictably effective than older agents (e.g., parenteral gold compounds, penicillamine [Cuprimine, Depen]), and largely supplanted them.
- Methotrexate has become the "gold standard" of RA therapy; it is the slow-acting

agent against which all other agents of this type are measured.

—Methotrexate decreases deoxyribonucleic acid (DNA) synthesis, and inhibits synthesis of proteins.

—The result of these pharmacologic effects is impairment in function of inflammatory cells that mediate the rheumatoid process.

—Methotrexate is surprisingly well tolerated and is relatively inexpensive.

—On the negative side, the potential toxic effects of methotrexate include bone marrow suppression, hepatotoxicity, interstitial pneumonitis, pulmonary fibrosis, and increased susceptibility to infection; up to 15% of patients have some GI problem (e.g., adominal pain, anorexia, diarrhea, dyspepsia, gastritis); elevated liver enzyme levels may be seen in a significant number of patients, although moderate elevations tend to resolve without discontinuing therapy.

- Methotrexate and leflunomide are used in combination, or leflunomide is used alone in patients who cannot tolerate methotrexate.
- Infliximab (Remicade) is awaiting final approval by the U.S. Food and Drug Administration, but has been used in clinical trials in which patients with RA have shown definite clinical improvement after intravenous (IV) administration of the drug, which contains chimeric (mouse/human) monoclonal antibodies to TNF-α.

—The drug has resulted in significant improvement in joint swelling and tenderness, serum level of CRP, ESR, concentration of serum amyloid A, and scores on patient questionnaires regarding level of function.

—Side effects include headache, diarrhea, rash, infection (e.g., pharyngitis, rhinitis, upper respiratory infection [URI], urinary tract infection [UTI]) and infusion reactions (urticaria, pruritus, chills).

—In patients receiving infliximab alone, there was decreasing duration of therapeutic response with each cycle of drug administration; coadministration with methotrexate results in increased duration of clinical response, or even prolonged response.

- Etanercept (Enbrel) is the first truly effective biologic antirheumatic therapeutic agent to become available for clinical use; the drug has resulted in significant improvement in joint swelling and tenderness, morning stiffness, ESR, serum level of CRP, general pain level, and patient and physician assessments of disease activity, along with scores on patient questionnaires regarding function.

—Side effects are modest, and include self-limited reactions at the injection site and mild URI (cough, rhinitis, sinusitis, pharyngitis).

—Two major drawbacks of etanercept are that is must be given subcutaneously twice a week, and it is prohibitively expensive ($1100 to $1400/month).

Summary of Pharmacologic Management of Rheumatoid Arthritis

- No drug exists yet that results in a cure for RA; therefore the search for new, more effective drug therapy continues, such as minocycline hydrochloride (Minocin), which has inhibitory effects on matrix metalloproteinase that plays a major role in joint destruction.
- More effective inhibitors of this kind are being developed.

Gene Therapy

- Gene function controls every action of an immunocyte or inflammatory cell.
- Ongoing animal studies are using viral agents to introduce specific genes into target tissues, which could be engineered to control all functions, including up-regulation, cytokine production, cell division, and angiogenesis.
- Gene therapy may develop into a promising new treatment for RA in future.

Surgery

- Although surgery is not ordinarily performed for patients with RA, those with structural derangement of joints, excessive joint pain, or very limited mobility can be helped considerably with surgical intervention, a decision made with the patient, the primary clinician, the rheumatologist, and the orthopedic surgeon.

—Total joint arthroplasty, particularly of the knee, hip, wrist, and elbow, is highly successful.

—Arthroplasty of the MCP joints can reduce pain and improve function.

Patient/Family Education
- The nature, cause, treatment, and usual course of the disease should be explained to the patient.
- Reassurance and encouragement are essential throughout.
- All medications, including reason for giving, expected effects, potential side effects, dosage, and need for monitoring should be given in writing to the patient.
- Appropriate and effective physical and occupational therapy should be instituted as soon as possible and maintained specificly to the individual patient's needs as they change.
- Frequent consultations with the patient and family should take place, including the primary physician, nurse practitioner, rheumatologist, orthopedist, and physical and occupational therapists, to assess progress and current needs.

Prognosis
- RA is, over time, a progressive and debilitating disease.
- Care of the patient and family should be extremely supportive, consistent, sensitive, and compassionate.

Follow-up/Referral
- Patients with RA require continual follow-up and frequent referral to specialists (ophthalmologist, cardiologist, pain management) along with those listed previously, to provide long-term, consistent assessment and treatment (Box 17-14).

Reiter's Syndrome   *ChLAMydia*
Definition
Rieter's syndrome is a reactive arthritis seen in young adult males, resulting from *Chlamydia* myxovirus, *Mycoplasma* infection, or other genitourinary (GU) or GI infections.
- It primarily affects the ankles, feet, and sacroiliac joints.
- It is usually associated with conjunctivitis and urethritis.
- There exists a strong association with HLA-B27 (60% to 75% positive).

BOX 17-14

Indications for Referral of RA Patients to Specialist

TO A RHEUMATOLOGIST
If there is any question regarding the validity of the diagnosis
During the early phase of the disease to develop a comprehensive plan of care
If the therapeutic regimen requires the use of remitting agents
If severe manifestations of extraarticular disease are present
If arthrocentesis is indicated and the primary physician is not comfortable in undertaking to perform the procedure (rheumatologist or orthopedic surgeon)
If splinting is indicated, and specialist advice is needed
If corrective surgery is needed (rheumatologist or orthopedic surgeon)

TO AN ORTHOPEDIST
To advise about splinting
To advise regarding and to undertake corrective surgery

TO A PHYSICAL AND OCCUPATIONAL THERAPIST
Soon after diagnosis, to advise and institute physical therapy

From Matsumoto AK, Wigley FM: Rheumatoid arthritis. In Barker LR, Burton JR, Zieve PD, eds: *Principles of ambulatory medicine*, ed 5, Baltimore, 1999, Williams & Wilkins, p 1009.

Risk Factors
- Presence of HLA-B27 antigen
- Diarrhea caused by *Shigella* organism, *Yersinia* organism, or *Campylobacter pylori*

Etiology/Cause
- Infection with *Chlamydia trachomatis* is the most common causative agent.
- This disease often follows GU or GI infections (see Risk Factors).
- Both men and women are affected by the postenteric form.
- Men acquire the venereal form more often than women.

Pathogenesis (see also Risk Factors and Etiology/Cause)
Diagnosis
- The disease can begin abruptly and run a toxic course or begin insidiously and have an indolent course.

Signs and Symptoms

- Reiter's syndrome is characterized by a triad of symptoms: urethritis, conjunctivitis, and arthritis of the lower extremities and the sacroiliac joints.
- ① Urethritis, usually painless or with mild dysuria but with a mucopurulent discharge, is the first symptom.
- ② Conjunctivitis follows shortly after the urethritis—mild, with redness, weeping, and morning crusting, lasting only a few days.
- ③ Arthritis begins from several days to 1 month after the urethritis.
- Symptoms are pain, redness, and swelling in up to four joints: knees, ankles, and small joints of the feet.
- More than 50% of patients have nonarticular msuculoskeletal pain caused by inflammation of the insertion of tendons or fascia (enthesopathy).
- Heel pain resulting from inflammation of the plantar aponeurosis or of the Achilles tendon insertion is one of the most prominent symptoms and one of the most disabling; this may be the presenting symptom.
- Mucocutaneous features include the following:
  —Painless shallow oral ulcers on the tongue and palate
  —Circinate balanitis: moist, painless ulcers on the glans penis in uncircumcised men
  —Dry, scaling eruption on the glans in circumcised men
  —Papulosquamous skin eruption that begins on the palms and soles, resembling pustular psoriasis
  —These various lesions last from several days to several months.
- Fever (33% of patients)
- Weight loss
- Uveitis

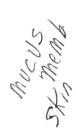

mucus memb, skin

Diagnostic Tests

- CBC
  —Normochromic, normocytic anemia characteristic of chronic disease
  —Hematocrit rarely falls below 30%.
  —Leukocytosis (10,000 to 15,000/mm³) is seen in 33% of patients.
  —Thrombocytosis with platelet counts between 400,000 and 600,000/mm³.
- Serology for RF and ANAs is negative.

- HLA typing shows the B27 antigen in 60% to 75% of patients.
- X-rays are normal early in the course of the disease, but later periostitis may be seen in the calcaneus or along the shafts of swollen digits.
- Sacroiliitis in seen in about 20% of cases and is usually unilateral.
- In severe disease, cartilage may be lost in joint spaces, and bony ankylosis may follow.
- Synovial fluid analysis shows characteristics of a moderate inflammatory process: poor mucin clot, elevated WBC count (5000 to 50,000/mm³), elevated protein, high complement (patients with RA have reduced complement), and normal glucose.
- Urethral stains and cultures are negative for gonococci, although concomitant gonococcal urethritis in Reiter's syndrome has been documented.
- *Chlamydia trachomatis* organisms are seen in urethral cultures in 30% to 50% of patients.
- Human immunodeficiency virus (HIV) infection should be tested for in all patients with sexually transmitted disease.

Treatment

- Rest
- Splinting of acutely inflamed joints
- Mild-to-moderate exercises are begun as soon as inflammation has subsided.
- Painful feet and heels may be helped by shoe inserts that shift weight to nonaffected areas.

Pharmacologic Therapy   *Chlamydia DOXYCYCLine, TCN*

- If *Chlamydia trachomatis* has been isolated in urethral cultures, a 3-month course of tetracycline or doxycycline 100 mg bid shortens the course of Reiter's syndrome.
- NSAIDs (e.g., indomethacin, tolmetin, sulindac) are effective in suppressing inflammation and relieving pain.
- Systemic corticosteroids may be required to treat severe uveitis or painful joints that have not responded to NSAIDs.
- If more intensive therapy is needed, consultation with a rheumatologist is required.

Patient/Family Education

- The nature, cause, treatment, course, and potential long-term effects (e.g., arthritis symptoms may last for months) should be explained to the patient.

- Information regarding safe sex practices should be provided in writing to the patient, and encourage patients to share the information with friends and sexual partners.
- If uveitis has occurred, close monitoring by an ophthalmologist is essential.

Prognosis

- Reiter's syndrome is generally self-limited and resolves within weeks to months with appropriate treatment.

Follow-up/Referral

- Patients with Reiter's syndrome require close monitoring during the course of the disease, particularly with respect to uveitis and infectious organisms.
- Posttreatment testing should be done to ensure eradication of *Chlamydia* organisms and other organisms.

Psoriatic Arthritis

Definition

Psoriatic arthritis is a form of arthritis associated with psoriasis primarily of the skin and nails, particularly at the DIP joints of the fingers and toes.

Risk Factors

- History of psoriasis
- Family history of psoriasis
- About 50% of these patients are HLA-B27 positive.

Pathogenesis

- The arthritis experienced in these patients is more limited in distribution and less severe than arthritis seen in osteoarthritis (OA) or RA.
- The most typical pattern of joint involvement is DIP arthritis, which is unsightly but rarely disabling.
- Nail dystrophy may occur close to the joints involved.
- Cutaneous lesions, interphalangeal joint synovitis, and tenosynovitis may cause "sausage" fingers or toes (dactylitis).
- A seronegative symmetric polyarthritis (a pattern similar to RA) occurs.

- In this type of arthritis, erosions occur but are central in the joint, not juxtaarticular, and produce a "pencil in cup" appearance.
- *Arthritis mutilans* occurs in about 5% of patients and causes marked periarticular osteolysis and bone shortening ("telescopic" fingers).
- Some patients may develop unilateral or bilateral *sacroiliitis* or *typical* ankylosing spondylitis (AS).

Etiology/Cause (see Risk Factors)
Treatment (see also Pathogenesis)

- NSAIDs and analgesics help relieve pain and inflammation.
- Some NSAIDs may worsen skin lesions.
- Local synovitis responds to intraarticular corticosteroid injections.
- In mild, polyarticular cases, sulfasalazine slows the development of joint damage.
- In severe disease, methotrexate or cyclosporine is given to control both the skin lesions and the arthritis.
- Oral corticosteroids may destabilize the disease and should be avoided.

Prognosis

- The outcome is favorable, with only minimal joint impairment in most cases.

Patient/Family Education

- With a history of psoriasis in either the patient or a family member, patients already understand the nature of the condition and the risk of arthritis occurring.
- Reviewing with the patient the nature, cause, course, and treatment of psoriatic arthritis will be helpful.
- Reassurance regarding outcome of the condition is also beneficial.
- Information about medications—reason for giving, dosage, and expected outcome—should be given.
- Effects should be provided in writing to the patient.
- Activity and exercises should be explained in detail to enable the patient to carry out the planned program.

Follow-up/Referral

- Patients with psoriatic arthritis are followed closely for the time that arthritis is present.

- The psoriasis itself may continue in its natural course, which is often lifelong.

Enteropathic Arthritis Associated with Inflammatory Bowel Disease

Definition
Enteropathic arthritis associated with inflammatory bowel disease occurs in conjunction with ulcerative colitis or Crohn's disease in some patients.

Risk Factors
- Ulcerative colitis
- Crohn's disease

Etiology/Cause
- The link between inflammatory bowel disease and arthritis is not known.

Pathogenesis
- Selective mucosal leaking may expose the patient to antigens that trigger synovitis.
- An HLA-B27–associated sacroiliitis or spondylitis is seen in 5% of patients with inflammatory bowel disease and is independent of disease activity.
- The joint symptoms may predate the development of bowel disease, or lead to its diagnosis.

Diagnosis
- Asymmetric arthritis that affects primarily the lower limb joints—knees, ankles

Treatment
- Treatment of the inflammatory bowel disease is necessary for the resolution of the associated arthritis.
- Remission of ulcerative colitis or total colectomy usually leads to remission of the joint disease, but arthritis may persist even in well-controlled Crohn's disease.
- The joint disease is managed symptomatically with NSAIDs.
  - Some NSAIDs make diarrhea worse, which may require trials of particular NSAIDs.
- A monoarthritis is often best treated with intraarticular corticosteroid injection.
- Sulfasalazine may benefit both the bowel disease and the arthritis.

Prognosis
- Each condition must be treated separately—ulcerative colitis, Crohn's disease, arthritis.
- Prognosis of arthritis is dependent on the outcome of the other condition.
  - Ulcerative colitis is chronic, with repeated exacerbations and remissions; surgery is usually required—total proctocolectomy is curative.
  - Established Crohn's disease is rarely cured but is characterized by intermittent exacerbations; with judicious care, most people with Crohn's disease function well.

Patient/Family Education
- The inflammatory bowel disease is usually the cause of the most anxiety and stress; the arthritis symptoms can be managed relatively well with the appropriate NSAID or other method.
- Patients with Crohn's disease or ulcerative colitis are already well versed in the disease, and have managed to live with the problems associated with the condition.
- Arthritis in persons with Crohn's disease usually persists despite therapy and perhaps because Crohn's disease is not permanently cured.

Follow-up/Referral
- The primary care provider is usually the professional who coordinates the care of those with multiple health problems.
- Consultation with specialists in each of the problem areas (gastroenterologist, rheumatologist) will likely be ongoing over time.
- Adequate support for the patient and family is essential.
- Social and psychologic interventions may be necessary to help with finances and psychologic problems developing during the course of the disease.

Autoimmune Diseases (Connective Tissue Disorders)

Systemic Lupus Erythematosus
Definition
SLE is a chronic inflammatory connective tissue disease of unknown cause that occurs predominantly in young women and can involve joints, kidneys, serous surfaces, and vessel walls.

Risk Factors
- Female sex
- Between 20 and 40 years of age

Etiology/Cause
- Although the precise cause is not known, several predisposing factors are known.
  - Heredity: there is a higher concordance rate in monozygotic twins (up to 85%) compared with dizygotic twins (37%).
  - First-degree relatives have a 3% chance of developing the disease, but about 20% have autoantibodies.
  - Genetics: there is an increased frequency of HLA-B8 and DR3 in whites.
  - There is a stronger association with HLA-DR2 in Japanese lupus patients.
  - Complement: there is an inherited deficiency of C2 and C4, which are in linkage disequilibrium with HLA-DR3 and DR2.
  - Sex hormone status: premenopausal women are affected; in addition, SLE has been seen in males with Klinefelter's syndrome (XXY); in New Zealand, a lupus-like disease is ameliorated by oophorectomy or treatment with male hormones.
- Immunologic factors
  - Loss of "self" tolerance has several consequences.
    - ~ *B-cell activation* results in increased autoantibody production to a variety of antigens (nuclear, cytoplasmic, and plasma membrane) and hypergammaglobulinemia.
    - ~ Development of and failure to remove *immunocomplexes* from the circulation leads to deposition of complexes in the tissue, causing vasculitis and disease (e.g., glomerulonephritis); immunocomplexes also form in situ (e.g., kidney glomerular basement membrane).
    - ~ *Impaired T-cell regulation* of the immune response
    - ~ *Abnormal cytokine production* (IL-1, IL-2), although its precise role in the pathogenesis is unknown; IL-6 and IL-10 levels are often raised
- Particular drugs can cause lupus-like symptoms (e.g., hydralazine, methyldopa, isoniazid, D-penicillamine).

- Flare-ups can be precipitated by oral contraceptives and hormone replacement therapy.
- Ultraviolet light can also trigger lupus-like symptoms.
- A viral agent causing SLE is a possible etiologic factor leading to the production of antibodies to nuclear material.

Pathology
- SLE is characterized by a widespread vasculitis affecting capillaries, arterioles, and venules.
- Fibrinoid (an eosinophilic amorphous material) is found along blood vessels and tissue fibers.
- The synovium of joints may be edematous and contain fibrinoid deposits, which contain immunocomplexes.
- Hematoxylin bodies (rounded blue homogeneous hematoxylin-stained deposits) are seen in inflammatory infiltrates and are believed to result from the interaction of ANAs and cell nuclei.

Diagnosis
Signs and Symptoms
- SLE is extremely variable in its manifestation.
- Most of the clinical characteristics are due to the consequences of vasculitis.
- Mild cases may present only with arthralgia, whereas severe cases may involve multiple systems.
- Fever is common in exacerbations, occurring in up to 50% of cases.
- Patients indicate marked malaise and fatigue.
- Joint involvement is the most common characteristic, occurring in over 90% of patients.
- Initially, symptoms are similar to RA with small joints affected in a symmetric manner.
- Joints are painful but typically appear normal on examination, although there may be slight soft-tissue swelling around the joint.
- Deformities due to joint capsule and tendon contraction and bony erosions are rarely seen.
- In a few cases, major joint deformity resembling RA, known as Jaccoud's arthropathy, is seen.

- Myalgia is present in up to 50% of patients, although a true myositis occurs in less than 5% of patients.
- The skin is affected in 75% of patients.
  —Erythema (redness) in a "butterfly" pattern on the cheeks and across the bridge of the nose is characteristic.
  —Vasculitic lesions on the fingertips and around the nail folds, purpura, and urticaria are evident.
  —In 33% of cases, there is photosensitivity; prolonged exposure to sunlight can lead to exacerbations of the disease.
  —Livedo reticularis, palmar and plantar rashes, pigmentation, and alopecia may be present.
  —Raynaud's phenomenon is common and may precede the development of arthralgia and other clinical symptoms by years.
  —Immunofluorescence of "normal" skin, obtained on biopsy, shows immunoglobulin and complement deposition at the dermoepidermal junction (called a positive band test).
- Lungs
  —Up to 50% of patients have lung involvement at some point in the course of the disease.
  —Recurrent pleurisy and pleural effusions (exudates) are the most common manifestations and are frequently bilateral.
  —Pneumonitis and atelectasis may occur.
  —Eventually, a restrictive lung defect develops with loss of lung volumes and raised hemidiaphragms.
  —Rarely, pulmonary fibrosis develops.
- Cardiovascular system
  —The heart is involved in about 25% of cases.
  —Pericarditis with small pericardial effusions detected by echocardiography is common.
  —A mild myocarditis may occur, which may cause dysrhythmias.
  —Aortic valve lesions and a cardiomyopathy involving the mitral valve (Libman-Sacks syndrome) are quite rare.
  —Raynaud's, vasculitis, and arterial and venous thromboses can occur kidneys.
  —The kidneys show histologic changes, although clinical renal involvement occurs in about 40% of patients.

—Most types of glomerulonephritis occur, including mesangial, focal, diffuse, and membranous.
—Proteinuria (1 g/24 hours) is common.
—Hypertension may develop because of the progression to either the nephrotic syndrome or renal failure.

- Central nervous system
  —Up to 60% of patients have involvement of the nervous system.
  —Symptoms often fluctuate.
  —Mild depression may occur and occasionally more severe psychiatric disturbances.
  —Epilepsy, cerebellar ataxia, aseptic meningitis, cranial nerve lesions, cerebrovascular accidents, or a polyneuropathy may occur.
  —Lesions may be due to vasculitis or to immunocomplex deposition.
- Eyes
  —Retinal vasculitis can cause infarcts (cytoid bodies), which appear as hard exudates, and hemorrhages.
  —There may be evidence of episcleritis, conjunctivitis, or optic neuritis.
  —Blindness is rare.
  —Secondary Sjögren's syndrome occurs in about 15% of patients.
- GI system
  —SLE causes GI symptoms, although these are usually not a major presenting feature.
  —Mesenteric vasculitis can cause inflammatory lesions involving the small bowel (infarction or perforation).
  —Liver involvement is uncommon, but lupoid antibodies are described in autoimmune hepatitis.
  —Pancreatitis is rare.

Lupus Variants

- *Chronic discoid lupus* is a benign type of the disease in which skin involvement is often the only sign, although systemic abnormalities may occur over time; the rash is typical and appears on the face as well-defined erythematous plaques that progress to scarring and pigmentation; subacute cutaneous lupus erythematosus, a rare variant, may develop.
- *Drug-induced SLE* is usually characterized by arthralgia and mild systemic symptoms, such as rashes and pericarditis, but rarely

Hydralazine Procainamide

renal or cerebral disease; these signs and symptoms usually disappear when the drug causing them is stopped; hydralazine and procainamide are the most likely causes, but other drugs have sometimes been implicated.

- *Overlap syndrome* occurs in patients who develop signs and symptoms of two or more autoimmune rheumatic diseases.
  —RA and SLE
  —RA, SLE, and Sjögren's syndrome
  —Polymyositis with scleroderma/systemic sclerosis or SLE

Diagnostic Tests

Autoimmune Disease

- CBC
  —Usually shows anemia (normochromic, normocytic), leukopenia, and thrombocytopenia.
  —An autoimmune hemolytic anemia may occur.
  —The ESR is elevated in proportion to disease activity.
  —The CRP is normal.
- Serum ANA
  —Are positive in almost all patients
  —Double-stranded DNA (dsDNA) binding is specific for SLE, but is present in only 50% of patients, particularly those with severe sytemic involvement (e.g., renal disease).
  —RF is positive in 30% to 50% of patients.
  —Serum complement levels are reduced during active disease.
  —Serologic tests for syphilis—33% of patients have a false-positive test for syphilis.
  —Immunoglobulins are elevated (usually IgG, IgM).
- Histology
  —Characteristic histologic and immunofluorescent abnormalities are seen in biopsies from the kidney and skin.
- Diagnostic imaging
  —CT of the brain sometimes shows infarcts or hemorrhage with evidence of cerebral atrophy.
  —MRI detects lesions in the white matter that are not seen on CT.

Treatment

- Patients need a caring and sympathetic approach.

- Reassure patients that the prognosis is good.
- Patients with photosensitivity should avoid direct sunlight.
- Drug therapy is used in active disease.
  —NSAIDs for arthralgia, arthritis, fever, and serositis
  —Antimalarial drugs (chloroquine, hydroxychloroquine) are beneficial for mild skin disease, fatigue, and arthralgias that are not responsive to NSAIDs.
  —Corticosteroids orally (PO) or as high-dose IV boluses or immunosuppressive drugs, such as azathioprine or cyclophosphamide, are essential in more severe disease (glomerulonephritis, vasculitis, cerebral disease, or blood dyscrasias) and when symptoms are not responsive to other therapy.

Prognosis

- The disease follows an episodic pattern, with exacerbations and remissions that may last for long periods.
  —Remissions may occur even in patients with renal disease.
- The 10-year survival rate is about 90%; if serious complications have not developed within this period, they likely will not occur.
- Arthritis is intermittent.
- Chronic progressive destruction of joints seen in RA and OA occurs in SLE rarely, although a few patients develop deformities such as ulnar deviation.

Patient/Family Education

- Because SLE is usually a long-term disease, the patient and family must be prepared for this situation, while assuring them that there are usually relatively long periods of wellness.
- All medications are listed and notes are made in writing regarding reason for taking, dosage, scheduling, and expected effects.
- The patient should be encouraged to actively participate in his or her own care regarding taking medications, protection from direct sunlight, skin care, and other aspects.

Follow-up/Referral

- Patients with long-term disorders are followed consistently by one team of providers.

- As indicated, SLE patients require compassionate, sympathetic attention.
- In disorders like SLE, a close relationship develops between patient and care providers, which is expected and is usually very helpful to the patient.
- Referral may be necessary to a rheumatologist, ophthalmologist, dermatologist, or other specialist.

Osteoporosis

Definition

Osteoporosis is a disorder characterized by low bone mass and microarchitectural deterioration of bone tissue, resulting in greater bone fragility and increased risk of fractures; unlike osteomalacia, the defect in osteoporosis is that *the existing bone is normally mineralized but is deficient in quantity, quality, and structural integrity.*

The World Health Organization (WHO) defines osteoporosis as a bone density more than 2.5 standard deviations (SDs) below the young adult mean value for individual matched for sex and race. Values between 1 and 2.5 SDs are termed *osteopenia.*

- Two types of osteoporosis are recognized, although the classification is a simplification.
  - Type I is the typical postmenopausal process
  - Type II is the more gradual senile osteoporosis that occurs in both men and women.

Risk Factors (Box 17-15)

- Female sex
- Older age (postmenopausal)—risk increases exponentially with age.
- White race

Pathogenesis

- Mismatch between the rates of bone resorption and bone formation during the remodeling process, which occurs over many years
- Postmenopausal state, hyperparathyroidism, and hyperthyroidism are associated with "high-turnover" osteoporosis.
- Anorexia nervosa and liver disease are associated with "low-turnover" osteoporosis.
- In the first 10 years after menopause, accelerated bone loss occurs.

BOX 17-15

Osteoporosis Risk Factors, Associated Disorders, and Drug Therapy

RISK FACTORS
Female sex
Increasing age
Early menopause (or ovariectomy)
White race
Slender habitus
Lack of exercise/mobility
Smoking
Family history
Excess alcohol
Nutrition (very low Ca^+, high protein intake over time)

DRUG THERAPY
Corticosteroids
Heparin
Cyclosporine
Cytotoxic therapy

ASSOCIATED DISORDERS
Endocrine
Cushing's syndrome
Hyperparathyroidism
Hypogonadism (or orchidectomy)
Acromegaly
Type I diabetes mellitus
Joint
Rheumatoid arthritis
Other
Chronic renal failure
Chronic liver disease
Mastocytosis
Anorexia nervosa

From Drury PL, Shipley H: Rheumatology and bone disease: Rheumatoid arthritis. In Kumar P, Clark M, eds: *Clinical medicine,* ed 4, Edinburgh, 1998, WB Saunders, p 508.

- The trabecular bones become thin and lose substance.

Diagnosis

Signs and Symptoms (Table 17-4)

- Osteoporosis per se does not cause symptoms.
- Fractures cause pain
  - Vertebral crush fractures and severe pain in the dorsal spine ensue, which resolve slowly over about 6 weeks.
  - These fractures result in diminished height of vertebrae, loss of height from the collapsed vertebrae, increased kyphosis, and abdominal protuberance.

TABLE 17-4

Factors and Conditions Associated with Osteoporosis

Factor	Type I	Type II
Age range for fractures	50-75	Over 70
	Mainly women	Both men and women
Major mechanism	Estrogen deficiency (androgens also)	Age-related changes, possible decreased calcium absorption
Pathology	Thinning, perforation, and disappearance of trabecular bone	Reduction in cortical thickness of trabecular bone
Common fracture types	Vertebral (Painful)	Hip
	Distal forearm (Colles)	Vertebral wedge (painless)
Main drug therapy	Estrogen replacement, bisphosphonates	Calcium and vitamin D; estrogen and bisphosphonates

From Drury PL, Shipley H: Rheumatology and bone disease: Rheumatoid arthritis. In Kumar P, Clark M, eds: *Clinical medicine,* ed 4, Edinburgh, 1998, WB Saunders, p 507.

—Lumbar vertebrae, the distal radius (Colles'), and the femoral neck are other usual sites of fractures.

- Osteoporosis is common in older people (senile osteoporosis), and fractures may not always be due to osteoporosis, but can occur with secondary deposits.

Diagnostic Studies

- X-rays: show a fracture and reveal earlier clinically unrecognized fractures and pedicle destruction of vertebrae suggestive of malignant destruction.
  - X-rays usually show generalized or localized rarefaction of the skeleton, if it is present.
  - X-rays are of limited value in assessing bone desnity because up to 30% to 40% of the bone mineral content has to be lost before any change in radiologic bone density is detectable.
- Bone scans are useful in showing fractures.
  - An osteoporotic fracture can be distinguished from a metastatic lesion.
- Bone density
  - Measurement of bone density is done by bone densitometry, usually dual-energy x-ray absorption scanning (DEXA).
  - CT can be used to assess bone density, but it requires a higher radiation dose.
  - Ultrasound of the calcaneum is used sometimes.
  - Iliac crest bone biopsy shows loss of trabecular bone but seldom needs to be done except in treatment trials and when the diagnosis is in doubt.
  - Serum calcium, phosphate, and alkaline are normal in osteoporosis alone, as no disorder of calcium *metabolism* is involved.
  - Biochemical markers of bone resorption can be used to evaluate treatment.

Treatment

- Management of established osteoporosis is unsatisfactory because bone mass is already substantially reduced.
- Therapy, particularly hormone replacement therapy, has been successful in improving bone density and reducing the fracture rate.
- Optimal therapy in the future will be prophylactic, not after fracture has occurred.
- Diet: an adequate intake of calories, calcium, and vitamin D is necessary, with at least 1000 mg of calcium daily (ideally, 1500 mg postmenopausally) and 400 to 800 IU of vitamin D.
- Exercise: a minimum of at least 30 minutes of weight-bearing exercise three times/week is encouraged.
- Smoking cessation: smoking appears to accelerate bone loss and may negate the beneficial effects of estrogen therapy, perhaps by accelerating estrogen metabolism.
- Reduction in fall risk: physiotherapy and assessment of home safety may be required; hip protectors may be of value.

Pharmacologic Therapy

- Estrogen therapy (HRT) is of proven value in preventing future fractures in post-menopausal women; it is the treatment of choice.
- Androgens are given to hypogonadal men.
- Bisphosphonates are increasingly used.
  —They are analogs of normal bone pyrophosphate.
  —They adhere to hydroxyapatite and inhibit osteoclastic bone resorption.
  —Alendronate 10 mg/day increases bone mass substantially.
- Agents used less fequently
  —Combination therapy: estrogens and bisphosphonates are being studied.
  —Calcitriol: the active metabolite of vitamin D produces some small improvement in bone density but not as much as HRT or bisphosphonates.
  —Calcitonin: nasal calcitonin, or the alternative subcutaneous salmon calcitonin, is recommended by some authorities, particularly where vertebral fracture pain is present.
  —Fluoride increases bone density, but there is concern about the quality of bone formed, and it is not currently recommended.

Prognosis

- At present, it is impossible to reconstruct bone that has been lost.
- As indicated, osteoporosis is often diagnosed only when a fracture occurs, at which time loss of bone mass is significant.
- Prevention is the key word for the future.

Patient/Family Education

- Teaching people about the effects of osteoporosis early in their lives is not too soon to prevent the development of osteoporosis.
- HRT should be initiated at the time of menopause to prevent the larger extent of bone mass loss in the first 10 years after menopause.
- Prevention of smoking in your patients is key to preventing many health problems, including osteoporosis.
- The benefits of exercise should be emphasized for all young people.

Follow-up/Referral

- Patients with osteoporosis are followed at frequent intervals to assess the status of bone mass, and to emphasize adherence to HRT and high-calcium intake.
- Fractures are treated as all fractures are treated, usually by open reduction and pinning by an orthopedic surgeon, or by total hip/knee replacement as needed.
- Treatment of fractures or joint replacement does not improve bone loss due to the disease, however.

BIBLIOGRAPHY

Arnett FC: Sacroiliitis, ankylosing spondylitis, and Reiter's syndrome. In Barker LR, Burton JR, Zieve PD, eds: *Principles of ambulatory medicine*, ed 5, Baltimore, 1999, Williams & Wilkins, pp 1010-1022.

Arthritis Foundation: http://www.arthritis.org

Beers MH, Berkow R: Musculoskeletal disorders. *The Merck manual of diagnosis and therapy*, ed 17, Whitehouse Station, NJ, 1999, Merck Research Laboratories, pp 407-508.

Biewen PC: A structured approach to low back pain. *Postgrad Med* 106(6):102-114, 1999.

Borenstein DG: Low back pain. In Barker LR, Burton JR, Zieve PD, eds: *Principles of ambulatory medicine*, ed 5, Baltimore, 1999, Williams & Wilkins, pp 913-927.

Davis JC: A practical approach to gout. *Postgrad Med* 196(4): 115-123, 1999.

Fye KH: New treatments for rheumatoid arthritis. *Postgrad Med* 106(4):82-92, 1999.

Hellmann DB, Stone JH: Arthritis and musculoskeletal disorders. In Tierney LM, McPhee SJ, Papadakis MA, eds: *Current medical diagnosis & treatment 2000*, New York, 2000, Lange Medical Books/McGraw-Hill, pp 807-859

Hellmann DG: Nonarticular rheumatic disorders. In Barker LR, Burton, JR, Zieve PD, eds: *Principles of ambulatory medicine*, ed 5, Baltimore, 1999, Williams & Wilkins, pp 928-938.

Kern DE: Shoulder pain. In Barker LR, Burton JR, Zieve PD, eds: *Principles of ambulatory medicine*, ed 5, Baltimore, 1999, Williams & Wilkins, pp 891-904.

Kessenich CR: Osteoporosis in primary care: The role of biochemical markers and diagnostic imaging. *Am Nurse Pract* 4(2):24-29, 2000.

Matsumoto AK, Wigley FM: Rheumatoid arthritis. In Barker LR, Burton JR, Zieve PD, eds: *Principles of ambulatory medicine*, ed 5, Baltimore, 2000, Williams & Wilkins, pp 988-1019.

McMahon PJ, Sallis RE: The painful shoulder. *Postgrad Med* 106(7):36-52, 2000.

Rehman Q, Lane NE: Getting control of osteoarthritis pain. *Postgrad Med* 106(4):127-134, 1999.

Skinner HB, Scherger JE: Identifying structural hip and knee problems. *Postgrad Med* 106(7):51-68, 1999.

Townes AS: Osteoarthritis. In Barker LR, Burton JR, Zieve PD, eds: *Principles of ambulatory medicine*, ed 5, Baltimore, 1999, Williams & Wilkins, pp 960-973.

Townes AS: Crystal-induced arthritis. In Barker LR, Burton JR, Zieve PD, eds: *Principles of ambulatory medicine*, ed 5, Baltimore, 1999, Williams & Wilkins, pp 974-987.

REVIEW QUESTIONS

1. The joints most commonly affected in osteoarthritis are the:
   a. Proximal interphalangeal joints (Bouchard's nodes)
   b. Distal interphalangeal joints (Heberden's nodes)
   c. Flexion of the distal interphalangeal joints, hyperextension of the proximal interphalangeal joints
   d. Ankle joint

2. Osteoarthritis:
   a. Causes chronic degeneration of the joints of the hip and knee
   b. Usually occurs in people in their twenties
   c. Is characterized by prolonged morning stiffness
   d. Is an inflammatory disease

3. Osteoporosis:
   a. Is commonly seen in blacks
   b. Is a metabolic disease
   c. Occurs in women of childbearing age
   d. Causes mainly loss of cortical bone *Trabecular*

4. Hypochromic, microcytic anemia may be caused by: *Fe def*
   a. Low-dose aspirin
   b. Septic arthritis
   c. Nonsteroidal antiinflammatory drugs
   d. Corticosteroids

5. Antinuclear antibodies are seen most often in patients with: *ANA*
   a. Systemic sclerosis
   b. Polymyositis
   c. Juvenile arthritis
   d. Systemic lupus erythematosus

6. Health care professionals must be careful not to attribute all skeletal signs and symptoms of the spine to osteoarthritis because:
   a. The spine has an unusually large number of nerves.
   b. The spine is subject to pain because of disk problems.
   c. Other diseases may be present (cancer, osteoporosis, or multiple myeloma).
   d. Aging often causes pain in the spine.

7. The major treatment goal of osteoarthritis is to:
   a. Preserve joint function
   b. Increase activity to maximal levels
   c. Have the patient run/jog every day
   d. Prevent destruction of cartilage

8. The initial medication to treat osteoarthritis pain is:
   a. Ibuprofen *2*
   b. Aspirin
   c. Acetaminophen *1*
   d. Vioxx (rofecoxib) *3*

9. Significant disability in osteoarthritis is not nearly as common or as severe as it is in:
   a. Systemic lupus erythematosus
   b. Rheumatoid arthritis
   c. Gout
   d. Bursitis

10. Gout, an acute or chronic type of arthritis, affects:
    a. The weight-bearing joints
    b. The peripheral joints
    c. Only the spine
    d. Only the great toe

11. Gout is caused by both acquired and *Genetic* _____ factors.
    a. Biologic
    b. Chemical
    c. Genetic *Enzymes, Down, Polycys Kid.*
    d. Environmental

12. Risk of crystal deposition and acute attacks of gout increases with: *overprod.*
    a. Degree of hyperuricemia *↓ excretion*
    b. Amount of high-purine foods ingested
    c. Level of obesity
    d. Amount of alcohol consumed

13. The "gold standard" for diagnosing gout is:
    a. Level of serum uric acid
    b. Joint aspirant that shows urate crystals
    c. Great toe inflammation and severe pain in the metatarsophalangeal joint
    d. Appearance of tophi soon after first attack

14. For an acute initial attack of gout, colchicine is given for:
    a. 12 hours
    b. 24 hours
    c. 3 days
    d. 7 to 10 days

15. The drug or category of drugs that has become the first-line therapy for gout is:
    a. Nonsteroidal antiinflammatory drugs
    b. Diuretics

c. Colchicine

d. Analgesics

16. Diuretics should not be prescribed for persons with gout because they may:
    a. Cause changes in plasma volume
    b. Decrease the clearance of uric acid from the kidneys
    c. Compete for secretion in renal tubules
    d. Reduce the glomerular filtration rate

17. The drug(s) used to prevent recurrence of gout is/are:
    a. Nonsteroidal antiinflammatory drugs
    b. Diuretics
    c. Colchicine
    d. Probenecid

18. Uricosuric drugs are prescribed for people who have:
    a. Underexcretion of uric acid
    b. Acute gout
    c. History of kidney stones
    d. Sulfa allergy

19. Xanthine oxidase inhibitors, such as allopurinol, are used in patients who have:
    a. Hyperuricemia because of overproduction
    b. No kidney stones
    c. Low urinary uric acid excretion
    d. No allergy or intolerance to uricosuric agents

20. Shoulder function involves the thorax, three bones, and almost _____ muscles.
    a. 9
    b. 15
    c. 24
    d. 30

21. The most common cause of shoulder pain in adults is:
    a. Adhesive capsulitis/frozen shoulder
    b. Biceps tendinitis
    c. Rotator cuff tendinitis
    d. Osteoarthritis

22. The primary basis for diagnosing shoulder problems is:
    a. X-rays of the affected shoulder
    b. Joint aspiration
    c. History and physical examination
    d. Cardiovascular evaluation

23. Carpal tunnel syndrome may be the presenting manifestation of:
    a. Osteoarthritis
    b. Rheumatoid arthritis

c. Acromegaly

d. Polymyalgia rheumatica

24. One of the major risk factors for low back pain is:
    a. Deficient or chronic poor-quality sleep
    b. Age
    c. Poor posture
    d. Type of work

25. The "tender points" seen in patients with fibromyalgia consist of _____ pairs.
    a. Three
    b. Five
    c. Seven
    d. Nine

26. Rheumatoid arthritis is currently seen as:
    a. Less serious than previously thought, with near-normal life span
    b. A serious systemic disorder with 5-year survival similar to stage IV Hodgkin's disease or triple-vessel coronary artery disease
    c. Having fewer classification stages than previously determined
    d. Being caused primarily by exposure to the Epstein-Barr virus

27. The drug(s) that is/are now the "gold standard" for treating rheumatoid arthritis is/are:
    a. Nonsteroidal antiinflammatory drugs
    b. Hydroxychloroquine sulfate (Plaquenil)
    c. Methotrexate
    d. Penicillamine (Cuprimine)

28. The most common cause of Reiter's syndrome is:
    a. *Chlamydia trachomatis* infection
    b. Epstein-Barr virus infection
    c. *Shigella* organism, *Yersinia* organism, or *Campylobacter pylori* infection
    d. *Neisseria gonorrhoeae* infection

29. Psoriatic arthritis is a form of arthritis associated primarily with psoriasis of:
    a. The trunk
    b. The hands and feet, particularly the distal interphalangeal joints of fingers and toes
    c. The scalp
    d. The extremities

30. The most common characteristic of systemic lupus erythematosus is:
    a. Mild arthralgias
    b. Mild-to-moderate fatigue and malaise
    c. Joint involvement
    d. Bony erosions

18

Dermatologic Disorders

EXAMINATION OF THE SKIN AND DERMATOLOGIC TERMS

The goals of the skin examination are to identify the lesion and assess the extent of the condition. Both the primary lesion and the entire skin should be examined, to discover any outlying lesions the same as the primary lesion or perhaps different from the primary lesion that may indicate the presence of more than one condition.

The Epidermis

- The epidermis is a stratified epithelium of ectodermal origin that arises from dividing basal keratinocytes.
- The lower cells (basal layer) produce a variety of keratin filaments and desmosomal connections, the so-called "cytoskeleton," which provides strength to the epidermis and prevents its shedding.
- Higher up in the granular layer, complex lipids are secreted by the keratinocytes; these form into intercellular lipid bilayers that act as a semipermeable skin barrier.
- The upper cells (stratum corneum) lose their nuclei and become surrounded by a tough impermeable "envelope" of various proteins (loricrin, involucrin, filaggrin, and keratin).
  —With changes in lipid metabolism, protein expression in the outer layers allows normal shedding of keratinocytes.
  —A relatively recent finding is that keratinocytes can secrete a variety of cytokines— interleukins, interferon, tumor necrosis factor-α—in response to tissue injury or in certain skin diseases, which play a role in immune

function, cutaneous inflammation, and tissue repair.

Other Cells in the Epidermis

- Melanocytes are found in the basal layer and secrete the pigment melanin; these cells protect against ultraviolet irradiation; racial differences are caused by variation in melanin production, not numbers of melanocytes.
- Merkel cells are also found in the basal layer and likely originate from the neural crest; they are numerous on fingertips and in the oral cavity, and play a role in sensation.
- Langerhans' cells are dendritic cells found in the suprabasal layer; they derive from the bone marrow and act as antigen-presenting cells.

Basement Membrane Zone

- The basement membrane zone is a complex proteinaceous structure consisting of type IV and VII collagen, hemidesmosomal proteins, integrins, and laminin; inherited or autoimmune-induced deficiencies of these proteins can cause skin fragility and a variety of blistering diseases.

The Dermis

- The dermis is of mesodermal origin and contains blood and lymphatic vessels, nerves, muscle, and appendages such as sweat glands, sebaceous glands, and hair follicles, as well as a variety of immune cells (e.g., mast cells, lymphocytes); the dermis is a matrix of collagen and elastin in a ground substance.

461

- The sweat glands, important with their vasculature in temperature control of the body, include the following two types:
  —Eccrine sweat glands are found throughout the skin, except the mucosal surfaces.
  —The apocrine sweat glands are found in the axillae, anogenital area, and scalp, and do not function until puberty.

Sebaceous Glands

- These glands too are inactive until puberty, and are responsible for secreting sebum or grease onto the skin surface by way of hair follicles; they are numerous on the face and scalp.

Nerves

- The skin is highly innervated; the nerve fibers allow sensation of touch, pain, itch, vibration, and change in temperature.

Hair

- Hairs arise from a downgrowth of epidermal keratinocytes into the dermis.
  —The hair shaft has an inner and outer root sheath, a cortex, and sometimes a medulla.
- The lower part of the hair follicle consists of an expanded bulb, which also contains melanocytes, surrounding a richly innervated and vascularized dermal papilla.
- The hair regrows from the bulb after shedding.
- The three types of hair are
  —Terminal: medullated coarse hair (scalp, beard, pubic)
  —Vellus: nonmedullated fine downy hair seen on women's faces and in prepubertal children
  —Lanugo: nonmedullated soft hair on newborns, particularly premature infants, and occasionally in people with anorexia nervosa

Nails

- Nails are tough plates of hardened keratin that arise from the nail matrix, just visible as the moon-shaped lunula, under the nailbed; it takes 6 months for a fingernail to grow out fully, and 1 year for a toenail.

The Subcutaneous Layer

- This layer consists mainly of adipose tissue, blood vessels, and nerves; this layer provides insulation and a lipid storage area.

The Patient's History

- Questions to pose to the patient
  —How long has the condition been present?
  —What is the distribution of the lesions?
  —What are the symptoms (rash, itch, pain)?
  —Family history, particularly regarding atopy and psoriasis
  —Past medical history
  —What makes the condition worse (sunlight, diet)?
  —What prior skin treatments have you had?

Dermatologic Terms

Atrophy: thinning of the epidermis or dermis resulting in fine wrinkling or depression of the skin such as seen in discoid lupus erythematosus, in steroid-induced atrophy, and in normal aging

Bulla: a blister, similar to a vesicle but larger than 5 mm in diameter, filled with serous or serosanguinous fluid, such as a friction blister or bullae seen in bullous pemphigoid

Burrow: a linear, threadlike elevation of the skin, usually several mm long, which is pathognomonic for scabies

Comedone: a plugged pilosebaceous or hair follicle, also known as whitehead, seen in acne

Crust: a yellowish-brown sticky debris made of dried serum, scales, and bacteria, such as seen in impetigo or eczema

Cyst: a spherical, firm, sometimes slightly compressible lesion, fixed in the dermis; an epidermal inclusion cyst

Erosion: loss of a portion of the epidermis such as candidiasis in the mammary crease with a moist surface, or in impetigo

Excoriation: similar to erosion but generally self-inflicted (witness or history) removal of some or all of the epidermis

Fissure: a vertical cut that extends into the dermis, such as cracks at the corners of the mouth, caused by *Candida* organisms, salivary enzymes, or vitamin deficiency

Hive: an erythematous or blanched edematous plaque with no surface changes, present for no longer than 24 hours

Hyperkeratotic: a lesion that is heaped up or stacked scale such as squamous cell carcinoma or wart

Macule: flat lesions that have changed color such as café-au-lait spots, brownish moles, or freckles

Morphology: the shape and appearance of the primary lesion, which can be described as linear, round, spherical, stellate, and so on

Nodule: a solid lesion up to 2 cm in diameter with a relatively deep component such as dermifibroma, nodular melanoma, and lipoma

Papule: an elevated, dome-shaped lump up to 10 mm in diameter such as an intradermal nevus or a lesion of molluscum contagiosum

Plaque: a flat-topped, elevated area of skin; the surface area is greater than the thickness such as lesions of psoriasis or cutaneous T-cell lymphoma

Pustule: a circumscribed area visibly filled with purulent material such as seen in folliculitis, acne pustule, pustular psoriasis

Scale: a change in the skin surface resembling flakes, caused by abnormal proliferation or desquamation of the outer epidermal layer (stratum corneum), as seen in psoriasis, tinea, or seborrheic dermatitis

Sclerosis: a scar-like induration such as seen in systemic sclerosis or localized scleroderma

Secondary changes: changes that occur as a result of the natural development or external manipulation of the primary lesion

Telangiectasia: dilated, superficial capillary or venule that may be linear, spiderlike, or star, as seen in basal cell carcinoma or in steroid- or lupus-induced atrophy

Tumor: a large mass, more than 2 cm in diameter with significant thickness (several mm), as seen in neglected squamous cell carcinoma or cutaneous lymphoma

Ulcer: loss of skin into the dermis that heals with scarring such as seen in venous stasis ulcer or pyoderma gangrenosum

Urticarial: localized area of edema and erythema such as seen in urticarial vasculitis or Sweet's syndrome

Vesicle: a blister up to 5 mm in diameter filled with serous or serosanguinous fluid, such as seen in herpes simplex infection

Wheal: same as hive (listed previously)

DERMATOLOGIC DISORDERS

Many dermatologists classify skin disorders according to the types of lesions they cause. To diagnose, the nurse practitioner should focus on the type of lesion the patient has, identify the morphologic category the lesions best fits, then use data from the patient's history, physical examination, and laboratory tests that can establish a working diagnosis.

The major morphologic types of skin lesions and disorders commonly associated with each type are seen in Box 18-1.

BACTERIAL INFECTIONS

- The skin's normal bacterial flora prevents colonization by pathogenic organisms.
- A break in epidermal integrity by trauma, leg ulcers, fungal infections such as athlete's foot, or abnormal scaling of the skin as in eczema can allow bacteria to enter.
  —If reinfection occurs after treatment, the cause may be asymptomatic nasal harboring of bacteria or the presence of other infected close contacts.

Cellulitis (Erysipelas)   *Staph*

Definition

Cellulitis is a diffuse, spreading, acute inflammation within solid tissues, characterized by hyperemia, white blood cell (WBC) infiltration, and edema without cellular necrosis or suppuration.

Risk Factors

- Exposure to causative organism
- A break in the skin anywhere on the body, particularly in the lower extremities

Etiology/Cause

- The causative organisms include the following, in descending order of incidence:
  —*Streptococcus pyogenes* (group A β-hemolytic streptococcus) is the most common cause of superficial cellulitis; diffuse infection occurs because the enzymes produced by the organism (streptokinase, DNase, and hyaluronidase) break down cellular components that otherwise would contain and localize the inflammation.
  —Group B, C, D, or G β-hemolytic streptococci are less common causes.

BOX 18-1

Morphologic Categories of Skin Lesions and Disorders

Pigmented	Freckle, seborrheic keratosis, nevus, blue nevus, halo nevus, melanoma, lentigo
Scaly	Psoriasis, dermatitis (atopic, stasis, seborrheic, contact), xerosis (dry skin), lichen simplex chronicus, tinea versicolor, secondary syphilis, pityriasis rosea, discoid lupus erythematosus, exfoliative dermatitis, Bowen's disease, intertrigo, Paget's disease
Vesicular	Herpes simplex, varicella, herpes zoster, vesicular dermatitis of palms and soles, vesicular tinea, dermatitis herpetiformis, miliaria, scabies, photosensitivity
Weepy, encrusted	Infections (impetigo), allergic contact dermatitis, vesicular dermatitis of all types
Pustular	Acne vulgaris, acne rosacea, folliculitis, candidiasis, any vesicular dermatitis
Figurate erythema	Urticaria, erythema multiforme, erythema migrans, cellulitis, erysipelas, arthropod bites
Bullous	Impetigo, blistering dactylitis, pemphigus, porphyria cutanea tarda, drug eruptions, erythema multiforme, toxic epidermal necrolysis
Papular	Hyperkeratotic: warts, corns, seborrheic keratoses
	Purple-violet: lichen planus, drug eruptions, KS
	Pearly: basal cell carcinoma, intradermal nevi
	Red, small, inflammatory: acne, miliaria, candidiasis, scabies
	Flesh-colored, umbilicated: molluscum contagiosum
Pruritus*	Xerosis, scabies, pediculosis, bites, systemic causes, anogenital
Cystic, nodular	Erythema nodosum, cystic acne, epidermal inclusion cyst
Morbilliform	Drug, viral infection, secondary syphilis
Erosive	Any vesicular dermatitis, infections, lichen planus, erythema multiforme
Ulcerated	Decubiti, herpes simplex, cancers, parasitic infections, chancre (syphilis), chancroid, vasculitis, stasis, arterial disease
Photodermatitis	(Characteristic distributions of rashes), drug eruptions, polymorphic light eruption, lupus erythematosus

*Not a category, but it is one of the most common symptoms of all skin disorders.

—*Staphylococcus aureus* occasionally produces a superficial cellulitis, usually less extensive than that of streptococcal origin and associated more often with an open wound or cutaneous abscess.

—Superficial cellulitis caused by other organisms (e.g., gram-negative bacilli) occurs rarely, usually under particular circumstances.

—In cases of granulocytopenia, diabetic foot ulcers, or severe tissue ischemia, aerobic gram-negative bacilli (e.g., *Escherichia coli, Pseudomonas aeruginosa*) may be the causative organisms.

—Cellulitis that develops after animal bites generally involves unusual organisms, especially *Pasteurella multocida* from dogs and cats.

—Immersion of injuries in fresh water may result in cellulitis caused by *Aeromonas hydrophila;* in warm salt water, *Vibrio vulnificus* is the causative organism, as a rule.

Pathogenesis

- A cutaneous abnormality, such as skin trauma, ulceration, tinea pedis, or dermatitis, may precede the infection.
- Areas of lymphedema or other edema are the most susceptible to cellulitis.
- Scars from saphenous vein removal for cardiac or vascular surgery are common sites for recurrent cellulitis, particularly if tinea pedis is present.

Diagnosis

Signs and Symptoms

- The major findings are local erythema and tenderness, frequently with lymphangitis and regional lymphadenopathy.
- The skin is hot, red, and edematous.
- Often, an infiltrated surface that looks like the skin of an orange (peau d'orange) is seen.
- The borders are usually indistinct, except in erysipelas.

- Petechiae are common.
- Vesicles and bullae may develop and rupture, sometimes with necrosis of the involved skin.
- Systemic manifestations including fever, chills, tachycardia, headache, hypotension, and delirium may precede the cutaneous findings by several hours, but many patients do not appear ill.
- Diagnosis is based on clinical findings because the causative organism is often difficult to locate and culture.

Laboratory Tests
- Blood cultures are sometimes positive.
- Serologic tests, particularly measurement of rising titers of anti-DNase B, confirm the diagnosis but are usually not necessary.
- Whereas cellulitis and deep vein thrombosis are usually easily differentiated, many physicians confuse these entities when edema occurs in the lower extremities.

Treatment *GRM(+)*
- For streptococcal cellulitis, penicillin is the drug of choice.
  —For outpatients with mild infection, penicillin V 250 to 500 mg orally (PO) qid or a single dose of benzathine penicillin 1.2 million U intramuscularly (IM)
  —For severe infections that require hospitalization, aqueous penicillin G 400,000 U intravenously (IV) q6h is indicated.
  —For patients allergic to penicillin, erythromycin 250 mg PO qid is effective for mild infections; for severe infections, IV clindamycin 150 to 300 mg IV q6h is effective.
- Although *S. aureus* is rarely the cause of cellulitis, many physicians prefer to treat for this with dicloxacillin 250 mg PO qid for mild infections and oxacillin or nafcillin 1 g IV q6h for severe infections.
  —For penicillin-allergic patients, vancomycin 1 g IV q12h is the preferred drug.
- When pus or an open wound is present, the Gram's stain will indicate antibiotic choice.
- In neutropenic patients, tobramycin 1.5 mg/kg IV q8h is effective against aerobic gram-negative bacilli.

- Elevation of the affected limb and cool compresses will help to reduce edema and relieve discomfort.

Prognosis
- Even without antibiotic therapy, most cases of superficial cellulitis resolve spontaneously, but recurrences in the same area are common, which sometimes causes serious damage to the lymphatics that results in chronic lymphatic obstruction, marked edema, and (rarely) elephantiasis.
  —Treating with antibiotics usually prevents any of these complications from occurring.
  —With antibiotics, signs and symptoms of superficial cellulitis usually disappear within a few days.

Patient/Family Education
- Treating ambulatory patients requires much more patient and family education than when the patient is hospitalized.
- Instruct about medications, use of topical or oral medications, application of compresses, the appropriate method for elevating one or both limbs, and signs and symptoms to look for if complications develop.
- Emphasize the importance of clearing the infection as quickly and effectively as possible.

Follow-up/Referral
- Patients should be followed closely until all signs of the infection are gone.
- If the infection persists despite therapy, referral to a dermatologist is recommended.

Furuncles (Boils) *macroides*
- Furuncles are rather deep-seated infections of the skin, usually caused by *Staphylococcus* organisms.
- They are usually painful swellings anywhere on the body but more commonly on the face, neck, and anogenital area.

Treatment
- Oral antibiotics such as erythromycin 500 mg qid for 10 to 14 days.
- Some boils require incision and drainage (I&D).

- Antiseptics such as povidone-iodine, chlorhexidine soap, and a bath oil such as Oilatum Plus, can act as prophylaxis to prevent recurrence.

DERMATITIS (ECZEMA)
Contact Dermatitis

Definition
Contact dermatitis is an acute or chronic inflammation, often asymmetric or oddly shaped, produced by substances contacting the skin and causing toxic (irritant) or allergic reactions.

Risk Factors
- Drugs, strong irritants (e.g., acids, alkalis, phenol)
- Weak irritants (e.g., soap, detergents, acetone)
- Anything known to cause dermatitis (e.g., wool, paint, cosmetics)

Etiology/Cause
- Contact with a chemical irritant or by an allergen (e.g., type IV delayed hypersensitivity reaction).
- Primary irritants may damage normal skin or irritate existing dermatitis.
- Allergic contact dermatitis may occur after years of exposure to a particular drug or detergent.
- Patients may become sensitized to various products, plants, or drugs after years of exposure.
  —On reexposure to the sensitizer, the patient may develop pruritus and dermatitis within 4 to 12 hours.

Pathogenesis
- The mechanisms by which irritants damage the skin are different for different agents.
  —Detergents activate keratinocytes, causing them to release inflammatory cytokines.
  —Allergens are captured by Langerhans' cells (a minor subpopulation of epidermal cells), which present them to T cells; cytokines released from keratinocytes and Langerhans' cells may contribute to sensitivity induction.
  —It takes between 6 and 10 days in the case of strong sensitizers, such as poison ivy, to

years (weaker sensitizers) for patients to become sensitized.

Diagnosis
Signs and Symptoms
- Signs and symptoms of contact dermatitis can range from transient redness to severe swelling with bullae.
- Pruritus and vesiculation are common.
- Any skin surface exposed to an irritant or sensitizing substance, including airborne ones, may be involved.
- Typically, the dermatitis is limited to the surface in contact with the irritant such as a leather sandal; the straps of the sandal cause redness, irritation, and skin changes in exactly the same pattern.
- If the causative agent is removed, erythema and blisters dry up and disappear.
- Vesicles and bullae may rupture, ooze, and crust.
- As inflammation subsides, scaling and temporary thickening of the skin occur.
- Continued exposure to the irritant will likely perpetuate the dermatitis and its symptoms.
- Skin changes in contact dermatitis may resemble other types of dermatitis.
- The pattern of skin changes and the history will facilitate an accurate diagnosis.
- Confirmation of the working diagnosis may require exhaustive questioning and extensive skin patch testing.

Treatment
- Treatment may be ineffective unless the causative agent is identified and removed.
- In acute dermatitis, gauze or thin cloths dipped in water and applied to the lesions (30 minutes 4 to 6 times/day) are soothing and cooling.
- An oral corticosteroid such as prednisone 60 mg/day for 7 to 14 days will help to alleviate symptoms.
  —The prednisone dose is decreased by 10 to 20 mg q 3 to 4 days.
- Blisters may be drained three times/day, but the tops should not be removed.
- Once the dermatitis has passed the acute phase, topical corticosteroid cream or ointment can be rubbed in gently tid.

- Antihistamines are ineffective in suppressing allergic contact dermatitis but may blunt the itching.

Patient/Family Education
- Instruct patient and family members about the nature of contact dermatitis, possible causes, course, usual treatment, and expected outcome.
- Patients are usually eager to be rid of bothersome signs and symptoms, and are cooperative in trying to pinpoint the cause of the dermatitis.
- Patients and families should receive written instructions regarding medications, application of compresses, and use of topical medicines.

Follow-up/Referral
- Patients are followed closely as long as the dermatitis is active.
- If therapy is not effective, or if the dermatitis persists despite therapy, the patient should be referred to a dermatologist for further evaluation and treatment.

Seborrheic Dermatitis

[handwritten: Pityrosporum Fungus, yeast]

Definition
Seborrheic dermatitis is an inflammatory scaling disease of the scalp, face, and sometimes other areas. The disorder affects areas with high densities of large oil glands.

Risk Factors
- None known.

Etiology/Cause
- Despite the name, the composition and flow of sebum are usually normal.
- Inflammation is caused by the body's reaction to *Pityrosporum* yeasts and to products that break down oil.

Pathogenesis
- Early dermatitis presents as dry or greasy diffuse scaling of the scalp (dandruff) with variable pruritus.
- In severe disease, yellow-red scaling papules appear along the hairline, behind the ears, in the external auditory canals, on the eyebrows, on the bridge of the nose, in the nasolabial folds, and over the sternum.

- Marginal blepharitis with dry yellow crusts and conjunctival irritation may be present.
- This disorder does not cause loss of hair.
- In newborns, seborrheic dermatitis presents as a thick, yellow, crusted area on the scalp (cradle cap), fissuring and yellow scaling behind the ears, red facial papules, and stubborn diaper rash.
- Older children may develop thick, tenacious, scaly plaques on the scalp up to 2 cm in diameter.

Diagnosis
- Diagnosis is made on the basis of clinical data and examination.

Signs and Symptoms (see Pathogenesis)

Treatment
- In adults, zinc pyrithione, selenium sulfide, sulfur and salicylic acid, or tar shampoo should be used daily or every other day until dandruff is controlled, then used twice a week.
- Corticosteroid lotion 0.01% fluocinolone acetonide solution; 0.025% triamcinolone acetonide lotion can be rubbed into the scalp or other hairy areas bid until scaling and redness are controlled.
- If shampoos alone are ineffective, 1% hydrocortisone cream rubbed in bid or tid will rapidly relieve seborrheic dermatitis of the postauricular areas, nasolabial folds, eyelid margins, and bridge of the nose.
  —The cream is then used qd.
  —Hydrocortisone cream is better than glucocorticosteroid cream because fluorinated corticosteroids may produce telangiectasia, atrophy, or perioral dermatitis.
- In some patients, 2% ketoconazole cream or other imidazoles bid for 1 to 2 weeks induce a remission that lasts for months.
- In infants, baby shampoo is used daily and 1% hydrocortisone cream is rubbed in bid.
- For thick lesions on the scalp of a young child, 2% salicylic acid in olive oil or a corticosteroid gel is applied at bedtime to affected areas and rubbed in with a toothbrush.
  —The scalp is shampooed daily until the thick scale is gone.

Prognosis

- The incidence and severity of the disorder seem to be affected by genetic factors, emotional or physical stress, and climate (it is usually worse in winter).
- This dermatitis may precede or be associated with the development of psoriasis.
- Patients with neurologic disease, especially Parkinson's disease, or human immunodeficiency virus (HIV) may have severe seborrheic dermatitis.
- Treating the disorder as indicated will relieve symptoms and lessen the thick yellow crust.

Patient/Family Education

- Instruct patient and family regarding application of cream or lotion, and how to gradually eliminate the thick yellow crust.
- Emphasize the importance of daily shampooing and application of the recommended medication.

Follow-up/Referral

- Patients are followed every 2 to 3 weeks for a time to assess response to therapy.
- If it seems necessary, referral to a dermatologist is made.

Stasis Dermatitis

Definition

Stasis dermatitis is a persistent inflammation of the skin of the lower legs, commonly associated with venous incompetency.

Risk Factors

- Venous stasis
- Obesity
- Poor hygiene

Etiology/Cause

- Venous insufficiency, particularly in older persons, is the underlying cause of the dermatitis.
- Because of the lack of symptoms, the condition is often neglected, resulting in increased edema, secondary bacterial infection, and eventual ulceration.
- Perivascular fibrin deposition and abnormal small-vessel vasoconstrictive reflexes may be the cause, not venous stasis per se.

Pathogenesis

- Pooling of blood in the lower extremities and deposition of fibrin acts over time on the tissues, causing erythema, edema, mild scaling, and brown discoloration to appear on the ankle; varicose veins may be present.

Diagnosis

- Often, patients neglect the early signs of the condition until the skin begins to break down, first as areas of weeping.
- Few patients have symptoms (e.g., pain, itching), which causes them to ignore the signs that appear gradually.

Treatment

- Elevating the feet above the level of the heart while sitting or lying helps to increase venous return to the heart, thus preventing edema of the ankles and feet.
- Properly fitted knee-high support stockings with the appropriate amount of pressure are essential and should be put on early each day, for life.
- Topical therapy may not be needed if support stockings are obtained and worn without fail every day.
  - Support stockings assist the venous blood to return to the heart, reduce edema, and reduce other factors that contribute to the developing condition.
- Walking for increasing distances each day is extremely helpful to also increase venous return and to prevent edema and the development of stasis ulcers.
- If stasis ulcers occur, they are treated with compresses either continuously or intermittently, using tap water, and dressings such as zinc oxide paste or DuoDerm.
- If the patient is ambulatory, Unna's paste (zinc gelatin) boot bandage or a newer colloid dressing is available commercially.
- More expensive absorptive, colloid-type dressings used under elastic support hose are more effective than the Unna's paste boot; the dressing is changed every 2 to 3 days, then once or twice a week as the ulcer heals.
- When the ulcer has healed, the patient should continue to wear support hose, put on before the patient rises in the morning.

Patient/Family Education

- The patient is instructed in the use of topical medications, compresses and how to apply them, putting on elastic support hose and their care, and other pertinent information and instructions.
- The patient must wear support hose every day for the rest of his/her life as a necessary preventive measure regarding ulcer development.
- Complex or multiple topical drugs or nonprescription remedies should not be used; the skin in stasis dermatitis is more vulnerable to direct irritants and to potentially sensitizing agents.

Follow-up/Referral

- The patient is followed closely during the time that the ulcer is healing, to make sure that the patient is following instructions absolutely correctly.
- Preventing stasis ulcers is much easier than healing them, and the preventive measures are simple, once the patient realizes that he or she must do those things that increase venous circulation in the lower legs.

FUNGAL SKIN INFECTIONS
Ringworm

zole

Definition

Ringworm infections are caused by dermatophytes—fungi that invade only dead tissues of the skin or its appendages (stratum corneum, nails, hair).

Risk Factors

- Exposure to the fungus

Etiology/Cause

- *Trichophyton, Epidermophyton,* and *Microsporum* organisms are the most common causes of fungal infections.
- Clinical differentiation of the dermatophytes is difficult.
- Transmission is usually from person to person or from animal to person.

Pathogenesis

- Some dermatophytes produce only mild or no inflammation or immunoreaction.

—In these cases, the organism may persist indefinitely, with intermittent remissions and exacerbations of a gradually extending lesion with a scaling, slightly raised border.
- Other dermatophytes produce an acute infection, typically causing a sudden vesicular and bullous disease of the feet or an inflamed, boggy lesion of the scalp (kerion) that results from a strong immunoreaction to the fungus.
  —In these cases, the infection is usually followed by remission or cure.

Diagnosis

- The diagnosis is made on clinical evidence according to the site of infection and is confirmed by direct microscopic examination of scales dissolved in a solution of potassium hydroxide or by culture that shows the pathogenic fungus in scrapings of lesions.

Treatment

- Topical preparations are usually effective in treating fungal infections of the skin.
  —Imidazoles (miconazole, clotrimazole, econazole, ketoconazole), ciclopirox, naftifine, or terbinafine
  —Resistant cases or those patients with widespread infection require systemic therapy.
- Newer systemic drugs include itraconazole and fluconazole, oral Triazole, and terbinafine, a second-generation allylamine.
  —These drugs appear to be safer and more effective than ketoconazole.

Tinea Corporis

Definition

Tinea corporis is ringworm of the body.

Risk Factors

- Exposure to the fungus

Etiology/Cause

- *Trichophyton* species are the usual cause of tinea corporis.

Diagnosis

Signs and Symptoms

- The characteristic pink-to-red papulosquamous annular plaques have raised borders, expand peripherally, and tend to clear centrally.

Differential Diagnosis
- Pityriasis rosea
- Drug eruptions
- Nummular dermatitis
- Erythema multiforme
- Tinea versicolor
- Erythrasma
- Psoriasis
- Secondary syphilis

Treatment
- For mild-to-moderate lesions
  —An imidazole, ciclopirox, naftifine, or terbinafine in cream, lotion, or gel form should be rubbed in twice daily for at least 7 to 10 days after lesions disappear.
- Extensive and resistant lesions occur in patients infected with *Trichophyton rubrum* and in those with debilitating systemic disease.
  —In these cases, oral itraconazole or terbinafine is best.

Tinea Pedis (Athlete's Foot)

Definition
Tinea pedis is ringworm of the feet.

Risk Factors
- Exposure to the fungus

Etiology/Cause
- *Trichophyton mentagrophytes* infections typically begin in the third and fourth interdigital spaces and later involve the plantar surface of the arch.

Pathogenesis (see Etiology/Cause)
Diagnosis
- Manifestations of the infection lead to the diagnosis, which is confirmed by microscopy of skin scrapings of the infected area.
- Toe web lesions are usually macerated and have scaling borders.
- Acute flare-ups with many vesicles and bullae are common during warm weather.
- Infected toenails become thickened and distorted.

- The fungus produces scaling and thickening of the soles, often extending just beyond the plantar surface in a "moccasin" distribution.
- Itching, pain, inflammation, or vesiculation may range from slight to severe.
- The initial infection may be complicated by bacterial infection, cellulitis, or lymphangitis.

Differential Diagnosis
- Maceration from hyperhidrosis and occlusive footwear
- Contact dermatitis
- Eczema
- Psoriasis

Treatment *Tinactin—*
- Itraconazole and terbinafine are the most effective treatments for mycologically proven tinea pedis.
- Topical agents can be used to treat interdigital areas.
- Systemic therapy is required for infection of nails (onychomycosis).
  —Treatment may need to continue for weeks or months, especially if toenails are infected.
- Good foot hygiene is essential.
  —Interdigital spaces must be dried thoroughly after bathing.
  —Macerated skin can be debrided gently
  —A bland, drying antifungal powder (e.g., miconazole) is applied.
  —Light, permeable footwear is recommended, especially during summer months.
- For acute vesicular flare-ups, bullae may be drained at the margin, but the blister roof should not be removed.
  —Drying agents include tap water or diluted Burow's solution soaks bid.

Prognosis
- Cure with topical treatment is difficult, but control may occur with long-term therapy.
- Recurrence is common after therapy is discontinued.

Patient/Family Education
- Instruct patient and family in proper foot hygiene—bathing, drying, application of powder or topical cream or lotion.

- Powder in the shoes may help to maintain foot hygiene.
- Open shoes or sandals allow for air-drying of the feet during summer.
- After therapy, maintaining a schedule of good foot hygiene and use of powder every day will help to prevent recurrences.

Follow-up/Referral

- The patient is followed every 2 to 3 weeks during the treatment phase.
- If bacterial infection or other complication occurs, referral to a dermatologist is recommended.
- Prophylaxis by maintaining good foot hygiene and daily powder after the infection clears is helpful.

YEAST INFECTIONS *Hyphae*
Candidiasis (Moniliasis)

Definition

Yeast infections are infections of the skin that is usually in moist, occluded, intertriginous areas, in skin appendages, or mucous membranes, caused by yeasts of the genus *Candida*. Candidiasis is usually limited to the skin and mucous membranes but occasionally may be systemic and cause life-threatening visceral lesions.

Risk Factors

- Exposure to yeast organisms (e.g., *Candida albicans*)
- Systemic antibacterial, corticosteroid, and immunosuppressive therapy
- Pregnancy
- Obesity
- Diabetes mellitus
- Other endocrine diseases
- Debilitating disease (e.g., HIV/acquired immunodeficiency syndrome [AIDS], cancer)
- Blood dyscrasias
- Immunologic defects

Etiology/Cause

- *Candida albicans* is a ubiquitous, usually saprophytic, yeast that can become pathogenic if a favorable environment or the host's weakened defenses allow the organism to proliferate (see Risk Factors).

Pathogenesis (see Risk Factors and Etiology)

Diagnosis

Signs and Symptoms

- Intertriginous infections are the most common type.
  —The lesions appear as well-demarcated, erythematous, sometimes itchy, exudative patches of varying size and shape.
  —The lesions are usually rimmed with small red-based papules and pustules that occur in the axillae, inframammary areas, umbilicus, groin, and gluteal folds (in infants, as diaper rash), between the toes, and on the finger webs.
  —Perianal candidiasis produces white macerated pruritus ani.
- Candidal paronychia
  —This condition begins around the nail as a painful red swelling that later develops pus.
  —It may develop as a result of improperly performed manicures.
  —The condition is common in kitchen workers and others whose hands are continually in water.
  —Subungual infections are characterized by distal separation of one or several fingernails (onycholysis) with white or yellow discoloration of the subungual area.
  —Defects in cell-mediated immune responses may lead to chronic mucocutaneous candidiasis, characterized by red, pustular, crusted, and thickened plaques resembling psoriasis, especially on the nose and forehead; this condition is almost invariably associated with oral moniliasis.
  —In immunodeficient patients, more typical candidal lesions or systemic candidiasis also occur.

Diagnostic Tests

- A Gram's stain of scrapings from the infected area, placed on a slide with a drop of potassium hydroxide, will show the typical yeast and pseudohyphae forms on microscopy.
- Because *Candida* species are a natural organism found in humans, specimens from the skin, mouth, vagina, urine, sputum, or stool should be interpreted cautiously.

—Confirmation of the diagnosis is made by finding the characteristic lesion, exclusion of other causes, and histologic evidence of tissue invasion if necessary.

- Oral candidiasis in a patient without a history of recent antibiotic therapy, chemotherapy, corticosteroid therapy, radiation therapy to the head and neck, or other immunosuppressive disorder may indicate the possibility of HIV infection.

Treatment

- Topical nystatin, the imidazoles, and ciclopirox are usually effective.
  —These agents suppress both the dermatophyte and candidal skin infections.
- Treatment is selected based on the location of the infection.
- Including an antifungal cream and a low-strength corticosteroid, such as hydrocortisone cream, both can be applied three to four times/day.
- Oral itraconazole is effective for many forms of acute and chronic mucocutaneous candidiasis, including vaginal.
  —Itraconazole 200 mg/day PO for 2 to 6 weeks is required.

Prognosis

- Yeast infections can be cleared within a few weeks with systemic itraconazole.
- Nystatin vaginal suppositories are effective, used bid for 5 to 7 days.

Patient/Family Education

- Emphasize that the organism that causes the yeast infection is normally present in humans.
- Instruct the patient about taking medications—oral, vaginal suppository, or mouth rinse.

Follow-up/Referral

- Patients are followed until the infection is resolved, usually within 6 weeks of oral therapy or less.
- If the infection persists, or recurs frequently, the patient should be referred to a urologist (male) or gynecologist (female).

PARASITIC SKIN INFECTIONS

Scabies

Definition

Scabies is a transmissible ectoparasite infection, characterized by superficial burrows, intense pruritus, and secondary infection.

Risk Factors

- Exposure to the causative parasite
- Insanitary, crowded living conditions
- Military personnel during battle conditions are susceptible to the parasite.

Etiology/Cause

- Scabies is caused by the mite *Sarcoptes scabiei.*
- Scabies is easily transmitted, with an entire household commonly infected by skin-to-skin contact.

Pathogenesis

- The impregnated female mite tunnels into the stratum corneum and deposits her eggs along the burrow; the larvae hatch within a few days.
- Although the patient may have hundreds of itching papules, often there are fewer than 10 burrows.
- The burrow is a fine, wavy, slightly scaly line a few mm to 1 cm long.
- A tiny mite (0.3 to 0.4 mm) is often visible at one end of the burrow.
- Burrows occur predominantly on the finger webs, in the flexor axillary folds, about the areolae of the breasts in females, on the flexor surface of the wrists, in the folds of the elbows, and on the genitals in males, along the belt line, and on the lower buttocks.
- The face usually remains free of infestation.

Diagnosis

- Definitive diagnosis requires demonstration of a burrow; observation of a burrow may be difficult because of being obscured by scratch marks, overlying dermatitis, or because of there being so few burrows.
  —It may be necessary to examine all of the skin area.
- The diagnosis is confirmed by microscopic examination of scrapings from the area of the burrow.

—The scrapings are placed on a slide, covered with mineral oil or immersion oil, and covered with a coverslip for viewing.

—Viewing the mite, ova, or fecal pellets provides a positive diagnosis.

Signs and Symptoms

- A delayed hypersensitivity reaction—an intensely itching papular eruption—is characteristic, beginning 30 to 40 days after infestation.
- Pruritus is most intense when the patient is in bed, although this nocturnal periodicity occurs in many pruritic dermatoses.

Treatment

- Topical medications (scabicide) are usually effective.
  - —The medication must be applied thoroughly to all skin from the neck down, particularly in the finger webs, genitalia, perianal areas, and toe webs.
  - —The medication remains on the skin for 12 to 24 hours (longer is better), then washed off.
- Improvement is slow, despite rapid eradication of mites.
  - —Prednisone 40 mg/day for 7 to 10 days provides prompt relief and prevents overtreatment dermatitis caused by repeated applications of the scabicide.
- The topical medication of choice is permethrin cream 5%, which is safe for all age groups.
- All members of a family, group, and others with known contact with infected persons should be treated at the same time.

Patient/Family Education

- Application of the medication is usually done by experienced health care personnel.
- Emphasize that all persons in the family/group and all contacts must receive treatment.
- Explain that extensive cleaning or fumigating of clothing and bedding is not required because the mite does not live long off the human body.

Follow-up/Referral

- Patients are followed and treated as needed for persistent pruritus or bacterial infection that may occur because of scratching.
- If complications develop, the patient may be referred to a dermatologist, urologist, or gynecologist.

Pediculosis

Permethrin

Definition

Pediculosis is an infestation by lice.

Risk Factors

- Crowded living conditions
- Exposure to someone who has lice
- Head lice is a common condition among schoolchildren, in college dormitories, and in military barracks.

Etiology/Cause

- *Pediculus humanus capitis* causes head lice.
- *Pediculus humanus corporis* causes body lice.
- *Phthirus pubis* causes pubic lice.
- Head and pubic (crab) lice live directly on the host.
- Body lice live in clothing.
  - —Body lice are important vectors of organisms that cause epidemic typhus, trench fever, and relapsing fever.

Pathogenesis (see Risk Factors and Etiology/Cause)

Diagnosis

Signs and Symptoms

- Head lice are transmitted by close personal contact and by such items as combs, hair ornaments, and hats.
- Although localized primarily on the scalp, head lice can infest the eyebrows, eyelashes, and beard.
- Severe itching occurs, sometimes resulting in secondary bacterial infection.
- In some children, there is mild posterior cervical adenopathy.
- The scalp is examined with the aid of a magnifying glass.
  - —Small, ovoid, grayish-white nits (ova) are seen fixed to the hair shafts, sometimes in great numbers.
  - —Unlike scales, nits cannot be dislodged.
  - —The ova mature into lice within 3 to 14 days.

—The mature lice are often found around the occiput and behind the ears.

- Body lice are uncommon with good hygiene.
  —Nits and body lice are easily seen in clothing worn next to the skin.
  —Lesions are especially common on the shoulders, buttocks, and abdomen.
  —Examination may show red puncta caused by bites, often seen with linear scratch marks.
  —Furunculosis is occasionally a complication.
- Pubic lice are usually transmitted venereally.
  —These lice infest the anogenital hairs but may involve other areas in hairy persons.
  —The anogenital area is examined carefully; lice may be few and be identified only by scratch marks.
  —Nits are usually attached to the skin at the base of the hairs.
  —One sign of infestation is a scattering of minute dark brown specks (louse excreta) on undergarments where they come in contact with the anogenital region.

Treatment

- Permethrin cream 5% is currently the treatment of choice.
  —It is left in place for 6 to 12 hours before being washed off.
  —Nits and lice can be removed with a comb in most cases.
- Resistance to permethrin is increasing.
- Keratolytic shampoos containing salicylic acid may be useful adjuncts in treating head lice.

Patient/Family Education

- Everyone, especially schoolchildren, must know that they are not to share clothing with others, especially combs, hats, scarves, or other garments.
- Family members, friends, and other personal contacts should be examined and treated if necessary.
- Instruct adults regarding personal hygiene and responsible sexual behavior that will prevent transmission of lice and sexually transmitted diseases.

Follow-up/Referral

- Those who are treated for lice are examined every few weeks after treatment to make sure that all nits and lice have been removed.
- If complications occur, antibiotic therapy for bacterial infections may be required, or referral to a dermatologist, urologist, or gynecologist may be necessary.

VIRAL SKIN INFECTIONS
Warts (Verrucae Vulgaris)

Definition

Warts are common, contagious, epithelial tumors caused by at least 60 types of human papillomavirus (HPV).

Risk Factors

- Exposure to persons with warts
- Patients with immunosuppression from organ transplants or other causes
- Autoinoculation

Etiology/Cause

- Viral infection caused by any one of the human papillomaviruses.

Pathogenesis

- The relative significance of humoral and cell-mediated immunity is not clear.
- Wart virus particles exist in the outer epithelium in the granular layer and beyond; these particles, however, are not likely to be deep enough to serve as effective antigens.
- Spontaneous disappearance of multiple warts in immunologically normal patients who later develop lifelong immunity requires further investigation.
- Warts may appear at any age but are most common in older children and uncommon in older persons.

Diagnosis

- Warts may occur either as a single or as multiple lesions.
- Size and appearance depend on the location, and on the degree of irritation and trauma.
- The course is variable among patients.
- Complete remission after many months is usual, but warts may persist for years and may recur at the same or at different sites.

- Some warts may become malignant.
- Common warts are sharply demarcated, rough-surfaced, round, or irregular in shape.
  —The lesions are firm, and may vary in color: light gray, yellow, brown, or gray-black nodules 2 to 10 mm in diameter.
- Warts appear most often on sites that are subject to trauma: fingers, elbows, knees, face.
  —The lesions may spread; periungual warts around the nail plate are common.
  —Plantar warts appear on the sole of the foot which are flattened by the pressure and surrounded by cornified epithelium; they are often exquisitely tender and are distinguished from corns and calluses by their tendency to bleed when the surface is pared away.
- Mosaic warts are plaques formed by the coalescence of myriad smaller, closely set plantar warts.
- Wart viruses contain circular, double-stranded deoxyribonucleic acid (DNA) with about 8000 base pairs.
  —Each type is indicated by a number and generally causes clinically distinct lesions.
  —To qualify as a separate type, DNA cross-hybridization must be less than 50%; for subtypes, greater than 50%.
- Although DNA is distinctive, most HPVs, including those of bovine origin, share a protein antigen that can be shown histologically on fixed tissue with a test that is positive for all types of HPV and is therefore useful for diagnosis.
  —DNA typing is available in only a few research laboratories but is important for prognosis of genital warts and their consequences.

Treatment

- Treatment depends on location, type, extent, and duration of the lesions and on the patient's age, immune status, and motivation to have the lesions treated.
- Most common warts disappear spontaneously within 2 years or with nonscarring therapy.
  —A flexible collodion solution containing 17% salicylic acid and 17% lactic acid applied daily, after gentle peeling

  —The clinician may freeze the wart with liquid nitrogen for 15 to 30 seconds; this treatment is curative but may need to be repeated in 2 to 3 weeks.
- Electrodesiccation with curettage of a few lesions is effective but may result in scarring.
- Laser surgery may also cause scarring.
- Plantar warts may require more aggressive maceration with 40% salicylic acid tape that is kept in place for several days.
  —The wart is debrided while damp and soft, and is then destroyed by freezing or caustics (e.g., 30% to 70% trichloroacetic acid).
- Flat warts can usually be treated with daily tretinoin (retinoic acid 0.05% cream).
  —Another irritant is 5% benzoyl peroxide or 5% salicylic acid cream that can be applied sequentially with tretinoin.
- Newer methods, whose effectiveness has not been established, include intralesional injection of small amounts of 0.1% solution of bleomycin in saline, which produces necrosis and cures stubborn plantar warts.
  —Reports of Raynaud's phenomenon and vascular damage to fingers where warts have been injected with bleomycin indicate that extreme caution should be used, despite the popularity and effectiveness of this technique among some experts.
- Extensive warts, even in formerly untreatable epidermodysplasia verruciformis, are improved or cleared with oral isotretinoin or etretinate, which are used only by dermatologists who are familiar with these drugs.
- Interferon, particularly interferon-α, given intralesionally or IM three times/week for 3 to 5 weeks, is also effective in clearing intractable skin and genital warts.

Patient/Family Education

- Instruct the patient/family regarding the nature, cause, course, treatment, and expected outcome of therapy.
- Explain all procedures and medications used, the reason for these, and their usefulness.
- Explain that newer medications and treatments are now used to effectively treat HPV infections that were once not responsive to therapy.

Follow-up/Referral

- Patients are followed throughout the course of treatment and until the lesions disappear, either spontaneously or with treatment.
- In patients who do not respond to usual treatment, or who develop extensive spread of lesions, referral to a dermatologist is recommended.

DISORDERS OF HAIR FOLLICLES AND SEBACEOUS GLANDS
Acne

Definition

Acne is a common inflammatory disease of the pilosebaceous glands characterized by comedones, papules, pustules, inflamed nodules, superficial pus-filled cysts, and (in severe cases) canalizing and deep, inflamed, sometimes purulent sacs.

Risk Factors

- Puberty: ages 9 to 13 years for girls, 12 to 14 years for boys

Etiology/Cause

- Acne usually begins at puberty, when an increase in androgens causes an increase in the size and activity of pilosebaceous glands.
  - An interaction among hormones, keratin, sebum, and bacteria determines the course and severity of acne.

Pathogenesis

- Inflammatory lesions include papules, pustules, and nodules or cysts.
- Noninflammatory lesions include open and closed comedones (whiteheads and blackheads).
- Intrafollicular hyperkeratosis results in blockage of the pilosebaceous follicles, which causes comedones to develop, which are composed of sebum, keratin, and microorganisms, particularly *Propionibacterium acnes*.
- Lipases from *P. acnes* break down triglycerides in the sebum to free fatty acids (FFA), which irritate the follicular wall.
  - Sebaceous secretions and dilation of the follicle often result in cyst formation.
  - Rupture of the follicle, with release of FFA, bacterial products, and keratin into the tissues, causes an inflammatory reaction that usually results in an abscess.
  - The abscesses heal, with scarring in severe cases.
- Acne often spontaneously remits, but the timing of remittance is not predictable.

Diagnosis
Signs and Symptoms

- Acne is often worse in winter and improves in the summer, perhaps because of the benefits of sunlight.
- Acne may cycle with the menses, and it may either improve or become worse during pregnancy.

Superficial Acne

- Blackheads (open comedones) or whiteheads (closed comedones), inflamed papules, pustules, and superficial cysts are characteristic.
- Large cysts sometimes occur after manipulation or trauma to an otherwise uninflamed blackhead.

Deep Acne

- Characterized by those signs and symptoms common to superficial acne, plus deep, inflamed nodules and pus-filled cysts that often rupture and become abscesses
  - Some of the abscesses open on the skin surface, then rupture and release their contents onto the skin surface.
- Lesions are most common on the face, but the neck, chest, upper back, and shoulders may also be affected, with frequent scarring.

Diagnostic Tests

- Usually, no diagnostic tests are required because clinical evidence clearly indicates the diagnosis.

Differential Diagnosis

- Rosacea (does not have comedones)
- Corticosteroid-induced acneiform lesions, which usually have follicular pustules in the same stage of development and no comedones

Treatment

- Despite the fact that acne is very common, its presence causes embarrassment to teenagers.

Superficial Acne

- Whereas frequent washing of the face has little effect, it does reduce skin oiliness, which improves appearance.
  —Any soap may be used; antibacterial soap has no benefit and irritation from abrasive soaps makes it difficult to use follicular drugs.

Superficial Pustular Acne

- Sunlight causes mild dryness
- Topical clindamycin or erythromycin alone or with one of the follicular drugs used to treat deep acne
- Azelaic acid cream 20% has antiproliferative and antibacterial effects, and may be effective in comedonal or inflammatory acne.
- Topical tretinoin (retinoic acid) 0.025% to 0.05% or a 0.1% cream, 0.05% liquid, or 0.01% to 0.025% gel is effective.
- A new topical retinoid, adapalene 0.1% gel, has been approved by the Food and Drug Administration (FDA) and may be slightly less irritating than topical tretinoin.
- With tretinoin or adapalene, acne may become worse initially, but improvement occurs within 3 to 4 weeks.
- Other topical drugs are 5% to 10% benzoyl peroxide, over-the-counter (OTC) drugs, and sulfur-resorcinol combinations.
  —Most of these are applied bid, or one preparation is applied in the morning and another one at bedtime.
- Oral antibiotics may also be useful in superficial pustular acne.

Deep Acne

- For severe, deep lesions, topical treatment is not effective.
- A broad-spectrum antibiotic effectively decreases bacterial organisms.
  —Tetracycline 250 mg qid or 500 mg bid, between meals and at bedtime for at least 4 weeks, then decreased to the lowest effective dose
  —In severe cases, the dosage may need to be increased to 500 mg qid.

- Because relapse occurs frequently after short-term therapy, treatment should be maintained for months to years.
  —Tetracycline 250 or 500 mg/day is usually sufficient.
- Many dermatologists recommend minocycline as the systemic antibiotic most effective, with no gastrointestinal (GI) side effects, more manageable dosage with regard to meals, and no photosensitization.
  —A dose of minocycline (100 mg bid) should be continued for at least 4 weeks before tapering.
  —Side effects with minocycline include dizziness and pigmentation of the skin and mucous membranes.
- The most common adverse effect of prolonged antibiotic therapy is candidal vaginitis.
- If topical and systemic antibiotics do not significantly improve the acne, they should be discontinued after a sufficiently long period of use because prolonged use of antibiotics may cause pustular folliculitis around the nose and in the center of the face.
  —This uncommon complication is sometimes difficult to treat.
  —The usual therapy is oral isotretinoin after stopping the oral antibiotic.
- Oral isotretinoin is the best treatment for patients who have not responded to oral antibiotics, or in patients with very severe deep acne.
  —Complete blood count (CBC), liver function tests, and triglyceride and cholesterol levels should be measured before initiating therapy and reassessed at 4 weeks, except for CBC, then again at the end of therapy unless abnormalities are noted before that time.
  —Isotretinoin is teratogenic, and women who are at risk of pregnancy must use two methods of contraception for 1 month before taking the drug, throughout the period of therapy, and for at least 1 month after discontinuing the drug.
  —The dose is usually 1 mg/kg/day for 20 weeks.
  —In patients who are slow to respond, the dosage may be increased to 2 mg/kg/day.
  —At the end of the treatment period, the acne may continue to improve; only rarely

is a second course required, which is instituted only after 4 months of not taking the drug.

—Side effects occur in about 15% of patients and include dryness of conjunctivae and mucosa of the genitalia, chapped lips, and pain or stiffness in large joints or lower back.

Cystic Acne

- Injection of 0.1 ml of triamcinolone acetonide (Azmacort, Triam-A) suspension 2.5 mg/ml into an inflamed cyst or abscess is helpful.
  - —Local atrophy resulting from the corticosteroid or destruction of tissue by the cyst is usually transient.
  - —For isolated, very boggy lesions, incision and drainage is usually the best method of treatment, although residual scarring may occur.
- Dermabrasion for small scars is sometimes useful, but its permanent effect is controversial.
- X-ray therapy is not justified.
- Topical corticosteroids, especially if fluorinated, may worsen acne.
- If the usual therapy fails and the acne seems to be associated with menses, an oral estrogen-progesterone contraceptive may be given, but therapy for at least 6 months is required to evaluate its effect.

Prognosis

- Acne vulgaris usually remits spontaneously, but no one can predict when this may occur.
- The condition may persist throughout adulthood, and may lead to severe scarring if untreated.
- Patients treated with antibiotics show improvement over the first 3 to 6 months of therapy.
- Relapse during treatment may indicate emergence of resistant *P. acnes*.
- The condition is chronic and usually flares intermittently despite treatment.
- Remissions in those treated with systemic isotretinoin may be lasting in up to 60% of patients.

- Relapses after isotretinoin occur within 3 years, and require a second course of treatment in up to 20% of patients.

Patient/Family Education

- If obvious acne is apparent to those around the affected individual, particularly adolescents, they may tend to withdraw to avoid difficult personal situations.
  - —Counseling for both patients and parents may be helpful.
- Misconceptions regarding alleged associations between acne and diet, athletics, and sex are common and should be discussed with health care professionals.
- Patients and families should be forewarned that treatment may need to be prolonged, but that gradual improvement does occur, given time and maturity of the individual.
- Because therapy takes at least several months, it can be relatively expensive.
  - —Patients and families should know this and be given an estimate of the cost for a definite period, perhaps 6 months.
- Treatment options should be explained in detail.
- Medications should be in writing, with the generic and trade names, dosage, side effects, expected outcomes, and relative cost.
- Counseling is usually very helpful, especially for adolescents.

Follow-up/Referral

- Patients are followed closely, preferably by the same nurse practitioner, over time so that a trusting relationship can be established and discussions about sensitive topics can take place more easily.
- Referral to a dermatologist may be necessary at some point, and the clinician should try to match the patient and the dermatologist as well as possible regarding empathetic attitude and sensitivity to patients' needs.

ROSACEA
Definition

Rosacea is a chronic inflammatory disorder, with affected persons usually developing initial signs of the disorder in their twenties or thirties. It is characterized by telangiectasis, erythema, papules, and pustules primarily in the central areas of the face.

Risk Factors

- Persons with fair complexions and blue eyes

Etiology/Cause

- Unknown

Pathogenesis

- Rosacea may resemble acne, but comedones are never present.

Diagnosis

Signs and Symptoms

- Central erythema, telangiectasias, and intermittent erythematous follicular papules and pustules occur.
- The disorder may also involve the eyes, causing a mild inflammation of the lid margins and manifested by mild erythema and a dry eye or foreign body sensation.
- Conjunctivitis, blepharitis, episcleritis, and recurrent chalazion and hordeolum may occur.
- Less than 5% of patients with rosacea develop a vision-threatening condition of the cornea, *rosacea keratitis*.

Treatment

- Treatment is the same as for acne.
  —Tetracycline 500 mg PO bid (or)
  —Erythromycin 333 mg PO tid
  —If the response is positive, the tetracycline dose is halved every 4 weeks twice, then stopped.
- Topical therapy is usually preferred, such as metronidazole gel or cream (MetroGel, Metro-Cream), and is applied to the central face bid after washing.
- One advantage of systemic over topical therapy is that oral antibiotics suppress ocular rosacea.

Patient/Family Education

- Because rosacea is so prominent, patients are often embarrassed and upset when the disorder occurs.

- Supportive counseling and reassurance that the condition is treatable and will become less noticeable will be helpful.
- Provide information in writing about medications, the reasons for giving them, side effects, dosage and scheduling, and expected outcomes of treatment.
- Instruct about treatment options that may be used.

Follow-up/Referral

- These patients are followed throughout treatment.
- Effectiveness of treatment is assessed every 2 to 4 weeks as necessary.
- If complications develop, referral to a dermatologist or ophthalmologist is recommended.

SCALING PAPULAR DISEASE

- Scaling papular diseases are either eczemas or papulosquamous disorders.
- Unlike eczemas, papulosquamous disorders typically have sharp margins and lack signs of epithelial disruption (e.g., wetness, crusts, fissures, and excoriations).

Psoriasis

Definition

Psoriasis is a common chronic, recurrent disease characterized by a dry, well-circumscribed, silvery, scaling papules and plaques of various sizes.

Risk Factors

- About 2% to 4% of whites are affected.
- Blacks have a much lower incidence.
- Onset is usually between ages 10 and 40, but the condition can occur at any age.
- A family history of psoriasis is common.

Etiology/Cause

- The cause of psoriasis is unknown, but the response to the immunosuppressive drug cyclosporine suggests that the primary pathogenic factor may be immunologic.

Pathogenesis (see also Etiology/Cause)

- The thick scaling is attributed to increased epidermal cell proliferation and concomitant dermal inflammation.

Diagnosis

Signs and Symptoms

- Onset is usually gradual.
- The course is usually chronic remissions and exacerbations that vary in frequency and duration.
- Factors that precipitate psoriatic flares include local trauma and irritation, such as severe sunburn, viremia, allergic drug reactions, topical and systemic drugs (e.g., chloroquine, antimalarial therapy, lithium, β-blockers, interferon-α), and withdrawal of systemic corticosteroids.
- Psoriasis usually involves the scalp, including the postauricular areas, the extensor surface of the extremities, particularly elbows and knees, the sacral area, buttocks, and penis; the nails, eyebrows, axillae, umbilicus, or anogenital region may also be affected.
- Rarely, the disorder is generalized.
- Typical lesions are sharply demarcated, variously pruritic, ovoid, or circinate.
- Erythematous papules or plaques covered with overlapping thick silvery micaceous or slightly opalescent shiny scales
- Papules sometimes extend and coalesce to produce large plaques in annular and gyrate patterns.
- The lesions heal without scarring, and hair growth is usually unchanged.
- Nail involvement occurs in 30% to 50% of patients and may clinically resemble a fungal infection, with stippling, pitting, fraying, discoloration, or separation of the distal and lateral margins of the nail plate and thickening, with hyperkeratotic debris under the nail plate.
- Psoriatic arthritis may occur and resembles rheumatoid arthritis (RA), but the rheumatoid factor is not present in the serum; however, crippling may be just as severe as in RA.
- Erythrodermic psoriasis (exfoliative psoriatic dermatitis) may be refractory to therapy.
  —The entire skin surface is red and covered with fine scales.
  —Typical psoriatic lesions may be obscured or absent.
  —This disorder may result in considerable debility and require hospitalization for the patient.

- Pustular psoriasis is characterized by sterile pustules that may be generalized or localized to the palms and soles.
  —Typical psoriatic lesions may be absent.

Differential Diagnosis

- Psoriasis may be confused with seborrheic dermatitis, squamous cell carcinoma in situ (Bowen's disease, especially when on the trunk), secondary syphilis, dermatophyte infections, cutaneous lupus erythematosus, eczema, lichen planus, pityriasis rosea, or localized dermatitis caused by scratching.
- Clinical diagnosis is rarely difficult because of the unique lesions.

Treatment

- Acute attacks of psoriasis generally resolve but permanent remission is rare.
- No therapy is curative, but most cases can be adequately controlled.
- Lubricants, keratolytics, topical corticosteroids, topical vitamin D derivatives, or anthralin should be tried first in patients with a small number of lesions.
- Exposure to sunlight is usually helpful, but occasionally sunburn may precipitate exacerbations.
- Hydrogenated vegetable (cooking) oils or white petrolatum is applied, either alone or with corticosteroids, salicylic acid, crude coal tar, or anthralin twice daily after bathing, while the skin is still damp.
- Crude coal tar ointment or cream may be applied at night and washed off in the morning, followed by exposure to natural or artificial ultraviolet B light (280 to 320 nm) in slowly increasing increments.
- Corticosteroids can be used twice daily, as adjunctive therapy to anthralin or coal tar treatment.
- Thick scalp plaques may be particularly difficult to treat.
  —A suspension of 10% salicylic acid in mineral oil may be rubbed into the scalp at bedtime, manually or with a toothbrush; the scalp is covered by a shower cap and shampooed in the morning with a tar or other type of shampoo.
- Recalcitrant or scalp patches may be treated with local intralesional injection of triam-

cinolone acetonide suspension diluted with saline to 2.5 or 5 mg/ml.

— Injections of lesions may cause local atrophy, which is usually reversible.

- Systemic corticosteroids are usually contraindicated.
- Psoralen plus ultraviolet A (PUVA) light therapy is usually effective in treating extensive psoriasis.

   — Oral methoxsalen is followed (after several hours) by exposure of the skin to longwave ultraviolet light (330 to 360 nm) in special phototherapy centers.

   — Although this treatment is less messy than topical therapy, repeated doses of ultraviolet light can induce skin cancer, especially in patients with a history of skin cancer.

- Oral methotrexate is the most effective treatment for severe disabling psoriasis, particularly severe psoriatic arthritis or widespread erythrodermic or pustular psoriasis.

   — Dosage varies, and should be administered only by physicians experienced in the use of this drug for patients with psoriasis.

- Etretinate and isotretinoin may be effective for severe and recalcitrant cases including pustular and hyperkeratotic palmo-plantar psoriasis.

   — Because etretinate and isotretinoin are teratogenic, women are warned against becoming pregnant while taking this oral retinoid, and for at last 2 years after discontinuation of therapy.

- Cyclosporine is extremely effective but is not yet approved in the United States for treatment of psoriasis and has potentially serious systemic side effects.

Patient/Family Education

- Because the skin plaques are a source of embarrassment to most patients, particularly women, they are often too eager to try new methods of treatment that may not yet be considered safe in this disorder.

   — Clinicians should be aware of and be sensitive to these feelings and encourage patients to remain with current established therapy.

- All medications, reason for giving, expected effect, side effects, and length of treatment should be provided in writing.
- Patients should understand that no treatment is curative, but that the clinician will work closely with the patient to control the disease as much as possible.

Follow-up/Referral

- Patients with psoriasis are followed closely throughout treatment, to assess for untoward drug effects, increasing severity of the extent or nature of the plaques, and general health, which is usually normal.
- If complications occur, or if the disorder does not respond to any of the usual therapies, referral to a specialist in treating psoriasis is recommended.

PITYRIASIS ROSEA
Definition

Pityriasis rosea is a mild inflammatory skin disease of unknown cause characterized by scaly lesions and a self-limited course.

Risk Factors

- None known.

Etiology/Cause

- None known.

Pathogenesis

- Pityriasis rosea can occur at any age but is most common in young adults.
- Attempts to isolate an infective agent have yielded mycoplasma, a picornavirus, and human herpesvirus 7.
- In temperate climates, incidence is highest during spring and autumn.

Diagnosis

Signs and Symptoms

- A herald path (primary plaque), usually on the trunk and having a diameter of 2 to 7 cm, precedes the generalized eruption by 5 to 10 days.
- The lesions are slightly erythematous, rose- or salmon-colored, circinate or oval in shape, with a slightly raised border (collarette).

- Many similar smaller plaques 0.5 to 2 cm in diameter follow the herald patch and sometimes continue to appear for weeks in a centripetal distribution, usually on the anterior trunk.
- On the back, they radiate from the spinal column in a Christmas tree–like pattern.
- In blacks, the eruption may be primarily papular, with little scaling.
- The distribution may sometimes be irregular, principally affecting the arms and occasionally the face.
- Systemic symptoms are usually absent, except for slight malaise and headache; however, itching may be troublesome.

Differential Diagnosis
- Tinea corporis
- Tinea versicolor
- Pityriasis lichenoides chronica
- Lichen planus
- Secondary syphilis—when palms and soles are affected, a serologic test for syphilis should be done
- Parapsoriasis en plaques should be ruled out if the eruption does not resolve within 10 weeks.
  —Two forms of parapsoriasis are
    ~ A small plaque type, which is benign
    ~ A large plaque type that is a precursor of cutaneous T-cell lymphoma

Treatment
- There is no specific treatment for pityriasis rosea; usually, none is needed.
- The patient should be reassured that the lesions will clear spontaneously.
- Natural or artificial sunlight may hasten involution.
- Weak to midstrength corticosteroid cream relieves redness and itching.
- Inflamed lesions and itching may be treated with 0.25% menthol in a vanishing cream base, topical preparations containing the local anesthetic pramoxine with or without a topical corticosteroid, and oral antihistamines.
- Prednisone 10 mg PO qid until the itching subsides, then tapered over 14 days, should be used only in severe cases, if at all.

Patient/Family Education
- This self-limiting disease usually resolves within a few weeks.
- Symptoms are mild, with only slight malaise and headache.
- Bathing in tepid water to which cornstarch has been added will often relieve itching and provide cooling of the skin.

Follow-up/Referral
- Most patients do not require follow-up, although they are encouraged to call the clinician if the plaques do not disappear within 2 months.
- Although the eruption may persist for as long as 2 months, remission within 4 to 5 weeks is usual and recurrence is rare.

Antihistamine,

LICHEN PLANUS *Steroid*
Definition
Lichen planus is a recurrent, pruritic, inflammatory eruption characterized by small discrete polygonal flat-topped violaceous papules that may coalesce into rough, scaly patches, often accompanied by oral lesions.

Risk Factors
- Exposure to arsenic, bismuth, or gold, and certain chemicals used to develop color photographs may produce an eruption that is indistinguishable from lichen planus.
- Long-term use of quinacrine or quinidine may produce hypertrophic lichen planus of the lower legs, and other systemic dermatologic disturbances.

Etiology/Cause (see also Risk Factors)
- Other causes include liver disease and graft-versus-host disease.

Pathogenesis
- The primary papules are 2 to 4 cm in diameter, with angular borders, a violaceous color, and a distinct sheen in cross-lighting.
- Rarely, bullae may develop.
- The lesions are usually distributed symmetrically, commonly on the flexor surfaces of the wrists, legs, trunk, glans penis, and oral and vaginal mucosa.

- Lesions may become large, scaly, and verrucous (hypertrophic lichen planus), particularly on the lower legs.
- During the acute phase, new papules may appear at sites of minor skin injury (e.g., scratch), known as Koebner's phenomenon.
- Hyperpigmentation and occasionally atrophy may develop if lesions persist.
- The oral mucosa is involved in about 50% of patients, usually before or in the absence of cutaneous lesions.
  - The buccal mucosa, tongue margins, and gingival mucosa in edentulous areas show asymptomatic ill-defined, bluish white linear lesions that may initially be reticulated or lacy or may coalesce and increase in size.
- Chronic remissions and exacerbations are common.
- The prevalence of chronic liver disease, including primary biliary cirrhosis, alcoholic cirrhosis, and hepatitis B and C, is increased.

Diagnosis (see also Pathogenesis)

- Histologically, lichen planus is distinctive.
- Persistent oral or vaginal lichen planus, with thickening and coalescence of the lesions, may sometimes be difficult to differentiate clinically from leukoplakia.
- Widespread oral lesions must be differentiated from candidiasis, carcinoma, aphthous ulcers, pemphigus, cicatricial pemphigoid, and chronic erythema multiforme.
- The periphery of the lesions should be examined for short dendritic extensions and characteristic delicate bluish white lacy patterns.
- Biopsy is often indicated but may not provide specific findings in old lesions.

Treatment

- Asymptomatic lichen planus does not require treatment.
- Any drug or chemical suspected of being the cause should be eliminated.
- An antihistamine, such as hydroxyzine 25 mg or chlorpheniramine 4 mg PO qid, may decrease the moderate itching.
- Local pruritic or hypertrophic areas may be treated with triamcinolone acetonide suspension diluted with saline to 2.5 to 5 mg/mL, and superficially injected into the lesion to elevate it slightly; this is not repeated more often than once every 3 weeks.
- Occlusive corticosteroid therapy, such as triamcinolone acetonide 0.1% cream, a more potent topical corticosteroid under polyethylene wrapping at bedtime, or flurandrenolide tape is effective.
- Tretinoin 0.1% solution combined with corticosteroid may be used to treat lichen planus on hairless skin.
  - This is applied with a cotton-tipped applicator at night, followed by three times daily application of a high-potency corticosteroid cream.
- For erosive oral lesions and widespread severely pruritic lesions, prednisone 40 to 60 mg every morning, tapering the dose by about one third every week
  - Itching may return after the drug is stopped.
  - Low-dose systemic corticosteroid every other morning may help to relieve itching; those patients with persistent itching may do better with PUVA therapy.
- Erosive oral lesions may respond to oral dapsone or cyclosporine rinses.

Prognosis

- Lichen planus tends to be self-limiting, but the course is variable.
- Recurrences are not uncommon, even after several years.

Patient/Family Education

- Instruction should be given regarding the nature, cause, treatment, and expected outcome of the disorder.
- Pruritus is often the most troublesome symptom, and the clinician must work closely with the patient to find the treatment that provides the most relief.

Follow-up/Referral

- Patients are followed closely throughout the course of the disorder, with special attention given to finding the therapy that provides the most relief.
- If itching persists, or if other complications occur, referral to a dermatologist is recommended.

MALIGNANT TUMORS OF THE SKIN

- Skin cancers are the most common type of cancer, and most are curable.

Basal Cell Carcinoma

Definition

Basal cell carcinoma is a superficial, eroding ulcer that derives from and resembles epidermal basal cells. Basal cell cancer is the most common type of skin cancer; more than 400,000 new cases are diagnosed each year in the United States.

Risk Factors

- Prolonged exposure to direct sunlight
  - The incidence is highest among outdoor workers, sportsmen, and sunbathers.
- The incidence is inversely related to the amount of melanin skin pigmentation.
  - Light-skinned persons are most susceptible.

Etiology/Cause (see Risk Factors)
Pathogenesis

- The biologic behavior of basal cell carcinomas is highly variable.

Diagnosis

Signs and Symptoms

- Basal cell carcinomas may appear as small, shiny, firm, almost transparent nodules (or)
- As ulcerated, crusted papules or nodules (or)
- As flat, scarlike indurated plaques (or)
- As red, marginated, thin papules or plaques difficult to differentiate from psoriasis or localized dermatitis
- Most frequently, the carcinoma begins as a shiny papule, enlarges slowly and, after a few months or years, shows a shiny, pearly border with prominent engorged vessels (telangiectasias) on the surface and a central dell or ulcer.
- Recurrent crusting or bleeding is common.
- The lesion continues to slowly enlarge.
- The lesion often crusts and heals, which may decrease the patient's and clinician's concern about its importance.

Diagnostic Tests

- Biopsy of lesion and surrounding normal-appearing skin
- Histologic evaluation of the biopsied specimen

Treatment

- The clinical and histologic findings determine therapy.
  - Curettage and electrodesiccation
  - Surgical excision
  - Cryosurgery
  - X-ray therapy occasionally
- Recurrent (5%) lesions, large lesions, and morphea-like cancers with indeterminate borders are treated by Mohs' surgery—microscopically controlled excision of the tissue.

Prognosis

- Basal cell carcinomas rarely metastasize, but may invade healthy tissues.
- In rare cases, death may be due to invasion of the cancer into vital structures (e.g., eyes, ears, mouth, bone, dura mater, other).

Patient/Family Education

- Once the lesion is diagnosed as basal cell cancer, the patient should be reassured regarding the fact that most skin cancers are curable and rarely metastasize.
- The nature of the carcinoma, course, treatment methods, and expected outcomes should be explained.
- The patient should be involved in decisions about type of treatment.
- The selected procedure should be explained in detail: preoperative, intraoperative (e.g., type of anesthesia), and postoperative care and expectations of the patient.

Follow-up/Referral

- The patient is referred to an oncology surgeon at the time of diagnosis; depending on the site of the lesion, an otolaryngologist may be the consultant of choice.
- After surgery, the patient is seen on a regular basis by the surgeon and the clinician to monitor the recovery process and to maintain the patient in a cancer-free state.

Squamous Cell Carcinoma

Definition

Squamous cell carcinomas arise from the malpighian cells of the epithelium and usually occur on sun-exposed areas.

Risk Factors
- Prolonged exposure to sunlight

Etiology/Cause
- Squamous cell carcinoma often develops in a preexisting actinic keratosis or patch of leukoplakia, or in burn scars.

Pathogenesis
- The clinical appearance of squamous cell carcinoma is highly variable.
- The neoplasm may begin as a red papule or plaque with a scaly or crusted surface that then may become nodular, sometimes with a warty surface.
- In some patients, the major part of the lesion may lie below the level of the surrounding skin.
- Eventually, it ulcerates and invades the underlying tissue.

Diagnosis (see also Pathogenesis)
- Biopsy of the lesion is the primary method for confirming the diagnosis.

Differential Diagnosis
- Many types of benign and malignant lesions, including basal cell carcinoma, keratoacanthoma, actinic keratosis, verruca vulgaris, and seborrheic keratosis

Treatment
- The treatment for squamous cell carcinoma is the same as for basal cell carcinoma.
- Surgical excision is the treatment of choice.

Prognosis
- The prognosis is excellent for small lesions that are removed early.
- However, about 33% of lingual or mucosal cancers have metastasized before diagnosis.
- In some cases, cure is difficult.
- The risk of metastasis in squamous cell cancers is greater than it is in basal cell carcinomas.

Patient/Family Education
- The patient should be instructed regarding the nature, cause, risks, treatment, and expected outcome of therapy.

- Because these cancers tend to metastasize, surgery may sometimes be disfiguring because the cancer occurs in sun-exposed skin such as on the face and neck.
  —Plastic surgery may be required after excision of the carcinoma.

Follow-up/Referral
- Treatment and follow-up must be monitored closely because of the greater risk of metastasis.
- Squamous cell carcinoma on the lip or other mucocutaneous junction is excised, but cure is sometimes difficult to achieve.
- Recurrences are treated with Mohs' microsurgery, the same as for basal cell carcinoma.

Malignant Melanoma
Definition
A malignant melanoma is a malignant melanocytic tumor that arises in a pigmented area: skin, mucous membranes, eyes, and central nervous system (CNS).

Risk Factors
- Sun exposure
- Family history
- Occurrence of lentigo maligna, large congenital melanocytic nevus, and the dysplastic nevus syndrome
- White race

Etiology/Cause
- About 40% to 50% of malignant melanomas develop from pigmented moles.
- The remainder arise from melanocytes in normal skin.

Pathogenesis
- Lentigo maligna melanoma arises from lentigo maligna (Hutchinson's freckle) or malignant melanoma in situ.
  —This nevus appears on the face or other sun-exposed area as an asymptomatic 2 to 6 cm, flat, tan or brown, irregularly shaped macule or patch with darker brown or black spots scattered irregularly on its surface.
  —In lentigo maligna, both normal and malignant melanocytes are confined to the epidermis.

—When the malignant melanocytes invade the dermis, the lesion is called lentigo maligna melanoma, and the cancer may metastasize.

- Superficial spreading melanoma accounts for two thirds of malignant melanomas.
  —Usually asymptomatic, it is usually diagnosed when smaller than lentigo maligna melanoma and occurs most commonly on women's legs and men's torsos.
  —The lesion is usually a plaque with irregular, raised, indurated white, black, and blue spots or small, sometimes protuberant, blue-black nodules.
  —Small notch-like indentations of the margins may be noted, along with enlargement or color changes.
  —Histologically, atypical melanocytes characteristically invade dermis and epidermis.
- Nodular melanoma makes up 10% to 15% of malignant melanomas.
  —It may occur anywhere on the body as a dark, protuberant papule or a plaque that varies from pearl to gray or black.
  —Sometimes a lesion contains little if any pigment or may look like a vascular neoplasm.
  —Unless it ulcerates, nodular melanoma is asymptomatic, but the patient usually seeks advice because the lesion enlarges rapidly.
- Acral-lentiginous melanoma, while uncommon, is the most common form of melanoma in blacks.
  —It arises on palmar, plantar, and subungual skin and has a characteristic histologic appearance similar to lentigo maligna melanoma.
- Malignant melanomas also occur on the mucosa of the oral and genital areas and the conjunctiva.
  —Mucosal melanomas, particularly anorectal melanomas that are more common in nonwhites, have an unfavorable prognosis.

Diagnosis

- Two classifications are used for evaluating stage I melanomas.
  —Melanoma thickness as measured from the granular layer of the epidermis to the greatest depth of tumor invasion (Breslow's index).
  —Anatomic level of invasion (Clark's index)
  ~ Level I is confined to epidermis.
  ~ Level II extends into papillary dermis.
  ~ Level III extends farther into papillary dermis with expansion of this layer.
  ~ Level IV extends into reticular dermis.
  ~ Level V extends into subcutaneous fat.
- Increased thickness (Breslow's criterion) and deeper invasion (Clark's levels) correlate with poorer prognosis.
  —Melanomas arising in the CNS and subungual areas are not classifiable by these systems.

Diagnostic Test

- Biopsy should include the full depth of the dermis and extend slightly beyond the edges of the lesion; biopsy should be excisional for small lesions and incisional for larger lesions.
  —By doing step sections, the pathologist can determine the maximal thickness of the melanoma.
- Radical surgery should not precede definitive histologic diagnosis.

Differential Diagnosis

- Basal cell carcinomata
- Seborrheic keratoses
- Dysplastic nevi
- Blue nevi
- Dermatofibromas
- Moles
- Hematomas (particularly on the hands or feet)
- Pyogenic granulomas
- Warts
- Venous lakes

Treatment

- The clinical type of tumor is less important in the survival rate than the thickness of the tumor at the time of diagnosis.
  —If the thickness is less than 0.76 mm, the 5-year survival rate is 98% to 100%.
  —If the thickness is more than 3.0 mm, the 5-year survival rate is 46%.
- Metastasis of melanoma occurs by way of the lymphatic system and blood vessels.

—Sometimes, enlarged lymph nodes are discovered before the primary lesion is identified.

- Melanomas arising from mucous membranes have a poor prognosis, even though their extent appears quite limited when discovered.
- Treatment is by surgical excision.
  —Most experts agree that a 1-cm lateral tumor-free margin is adequate for lesions less than 1 mm thick.
  —Larger lesions usually require more radical surgery and sentinel node biopsy.
- Lentigo maligna melanoma and lentigo maligna are usually treated with wide local excision and, if necessary, skin grafting.
  —Only controlled cryosurgery is able to reach deep enough into involved follicles, which must be removed.
- Spreading or nodular melanomas are usually treated by wide local excision extending down to the fascia.
  —When there is node involvement, node dissection is usually recommended.
- Thick malignant melanomas and regional or distant metastasis may be treated with chemotherapy (dacarbazine or the nitrosoureas carmustine and lomustine).
  —However, in these cases, the prognosis is poor.
  —Cisplatin and other drugs are under investigation as potential effective chemotherapeutic agents.
  —New forms of immunotherapy such as interleukin-2 and lymphokine-activated killer cells appear to hold some promise.

Patient/Family Education

- The public's knowledge of melanomas is little; explaining the nature, cause, course, treatment, and expected outcome of therapy is the first step.
- When the patient's definitive diagnosis has been established, the patient and the family should be informed.
- In most cases, surgical excision is the only choice available currently.
  —Drawing a picture of the area to be excised, with its dimensions, may be helpful for family members.

—An indication of whether or not a skin graft will be necessary may also help the patient and family know what to expect.

- Reassurance is essential for both the patient and the family, but it is important not to raise expectations that are unrealistic.
- The patient, and perhaps other family members, should be advised to avoid prolonged exposure to direct sunlight.

Follow-up/Referral

- All patients who have had excisional surgery for melanoma are followed for at least 10 years, when possible.
- The oncologic surgeon is the specialist who evaluates the patient's status every 2 to 3 months initially, then every 6 months to 1-year intervals thereafter.

Kaposi's Sarcoma

Definition

Kaposi's sarcoma (KS) is a multicentric vascular neoplasm caused by herpesvirus type 8 that has three forms: indolent, lymphadenopathic, and AIDS-related.

Risk Factors

- Unprotected sex
- Sexual contact with a partner known to have AIDS

Etiology/Cause

- The cell of origin is the endothelial cell, seen in specific staining for factor VIII.
- KS used to occur most often in Eastern Europe, Italy, and the United States, primarily in the indolent form in men of Italian or Jewish ancestry greater than 60 years old.
- Because of AIDS, KS is endemic in equatorial Africa, where it is a more aggressive form, occurs commonly in children and young men, and accounts for nearly 10% of all malignancies in Zaire and Uganda.
- Since 1981, aggressive KS has occurred in at least one third of patients with AIDS, and has assumed epidemic proportions in the United States and many other countries.

Pathogenesis

- KS originates from multifocal sites in the middermis and extends to the epidermis.

- Histopathology shows spindle cells and vascular spaces admixed to various degrees.
- The cells of origin are the endothelial cells; tumor cells resemble smooth muscle cells, fibroblasts, and myofibroblasts.
- The indolent form manifests nodular or plaquelike dermal lesions.
- The lymphadenopathic form is disseminated and aggressive, involving lymph nodes, viscera, and occasionally the GI tract.
- In AIDS-related KS, there may be a few lesions, or lesions may be widely disseminated in skin, mucous membrane, lymph nodes, and viscera.

Diagnosis

Signs and Symptoms

- In older men without AIDS, KS usually appears on the toes or legs as purple or dark brown plaques or nodules that may fungate or penetrate soft tissue and invade bone.
  - —Disseminated lymph node and visceral involvement occurs in 5% to 10% of those affected.
- In patients with AIDS, KS may be the first notable manifestation of AIDS.
  - —Slightly elevated purple, pink, or red papules or round or oval brown or purple plaques appear first mainly on the upper body or mucosa.
  - —The lesions may become widely disseminated on the skin and are associated with visceral lesions and disseminated lymph node involvement.
  - —Bleeding, including from internal organs, may be extensive.

Treatment

- For indolent superficial lesions, cryotherapy, electrocoagulation, or electron beam radiotherapy flattens and fades most lesions.
  - —Unresponsive dermal or lymph node disease with lymphedema is treated locally with 10 to 20 Gy of x-ray therapy.
- AIDS-related KS has been treated with single agent or combination chemotherapy (e.g., etoposide, vincristine, vinblastine, bleomycin, and doxorubicin).
  - —Interferon-α effectively slows progression of early lesions and cures others.
  - —Intralesional vinblastine is also very helpful.

—The course of KS in HIV infection is dictated by the level of immunosuppression, which determines the likelihood of opportunistic infections occurring simultaneously.
- Treatment of KS does not prolong life in most patients because infections dominate the clinical course.

Patient/Family Education

- The patient and family members are instructed regarding the nature, cause, course, treatment, and expected outcome of therapy for KS.
- The type of therapy preferred in particular persons should be outlined fully.
- The patient should be adequately prepared for procedures that are recommended in the individual case.
- Signs and symptoms that may present should be explained as soon as necessary.

Follow-up/Referral

- Consultation with appropriate specialists (e.g., oncologist, radiologist, chemotherapist) should occur in a timely manner.
- Patients are followed closely during hospitalization periods, and after discharge on home care.
- Patients may be asked to keep a daily log about signs and symptoms, and response to therapy.
- As indicated, patients with KS usually do not survive, but individual life spans vary.

BIBLIOGRAPHY

Beers MH, Berkow R: Dermatologic disorders. In Beers MH, Berkow R, eds: *The Merck manual of diagnosis and therapy*, ed 17, Whitehouse Station, NJ, 1999, Merck Research Laboratories, pp 777-846.

Berger TG: Skin & appendages. In Tierney LM, McPhee SJ, Papadakis MA, eds: *Current medical diagnosis & treatment 2000*, New York, 2000, Lange Medical Books/McGraw-Hill, pp 124-188.

Elston DM: Dermatology clinic: A smattering of spots. *The Clinical Advisor* 2(9):48-50, 1999.

Fenn WH: Derma diagnosis. *Clin Rev* 9(6):65-66, 1999.

Fenn WH: Derma diagnosis. *Clin Rev* 9(10):33-34, 1999.

Paige D, Leigh IM: Dermatology. In Kumar P, Clark M, eds: *Clinical medicine*, ed 4, Edinburgh, 1998, WB Saunders, pp 1149-1210

Whitmore SE: Common problems of the skin. In Barker LR, Burton JR, Zieve PD, eds: *Principles of ambulatory medicine*, ed 5, Baltimore, 1999, Williams & Wilkins, pp 1499-1539.

REVIEW QUESTIONS

1. The goal of the skin examination is to:
   a. Diagnose the disorder
   b. Identify the lesion
   c. Determine the depth of the lesion
   d. Estimate the number of lesions
2. The basement membrane zone consists of:
   a. Collagen
   b. Fascia
   c. Blood vessels *dermis*
   d. Nerves
3. A bulla is a blister, similar to a vesicle, but is:
   a. Smaller than a vesicle
   b. Larger than a vesicle
   c. Lacking in any fluid
   d. Bluish in color
4. Another name for cellulitis is:
   a. Ulcers of the skin
   b. Cellular necrosis
   c. Erysipelas
   d. Tissue ischemia
5. The typical appearance of impetigo is:
   a. Blistering
   b. Dark brownish exudate
   c. Honey-colored crusts
   d. Irregular, rough surface similar to warts
6. The usual cause of a furuncle is:
   a. *Candida albicans*
   b. Group A *Streptococcus* organisms
   c. Human papillomavirus
   d. *Staphylococcus aureus*
7. One of the most common forms of dermatitis is:
   a. Seborrheic dermatitis
   b. Contact dermatitis
   c. Stasis dermatitis
   d. Drug reaction dermatitis
8. Ringworm of the skin is a condition caused by:
   a. Dermatophytes
   b. Dermacentor
   c. Dermatophagoides
   d. Dermatomyocites
9. Yeast infections are most commonly found on areas that:
   a. Are dry and open to the air such as the arms and legs
   b. Are along the neckline

c. Are moist and covered or occluded such as under the breasts and in the axillae
   d. Are the mucous membranes of the nose and mouth
10. Scabies is a skin infection often found in:
    a. Places that are crowded, unhygienic, and unsanitary
    b. Tropical climates where rain is frequent
    c. Military camps
    d. Neighborhoods where there is a large rodent population
11. The cause of warts is:
    a. Several different viruses
    b. The human papillomavirus
    c. The same virus that causes herpes simplex
    d. Contact with frogs
12. Acne is an inflammatory disorder of the:
    a. Pilosebaceous glands
    b. Eccrine sweat glands
    c. Hair follicles
    d. Keratin components of the skin
13. Rosacea is a chronic inflammatory disorder primarily involving:
    a. The extremities
    b. The scalp
    c. The interdigital areas of the fingers and toes
    d. The central areas of the face
14. Pityriasis rosea is a mild inflammatory skin disease whose lesions are found primarily on the:
    a. Face and neck
    b. Hands and feet
    c. Arms and legs
    d. Trunk
15. Exposure to arsenic, bismuth, or gold may cause:
    a. Acne
    b. Rosacea
    c. Lichen planus
    d. Psoriasis
16. Skin cancers are becoming increasingly common, largely because of people's tendency to spend long hours in the sun, either working or sunbathing. The most common form of skin cancer is:
    a. Basal cell carcinoma
    b. Squamous cell carcinoma
    c. Malignant melanoma
    d. Blue nevi

17. Squamous cell carcinoma, too, is often seen in people who are exposed to the sun for long periods. The difference between basal cell and squamous cell cancers is:
    a. That squamous cell cancer of the tongue or oral mucosa frequently metastasizes before it is diagnosed
    b. That they are treated differently
    c. That squamous cell cancer occurs primarily in older men and women
    d. That squamous cell cancer is more easily cured than basal cell cancer

18. Malignant melanoma may also be affected by exposure to sun by light-skinned people. About 40% to 50% of malignant melanomas arise from:
    a. Melanocytes in normal skin
    b. Sun exposure—face, neck, arms
    c. A genetic basis
    d. Pigmented moles

19. Sebaceous glands are responsible for secreting _____ onto the skin surface via hair follicles.
    a. Fatty acids
    b. Grease
    c. Sodium chloride
    d. Waste products

20. Lentigo maligna melanoma arises from:
    a. Hutchinson's freckle
    b. Melanocytes
    c. Malignant melanoma of the dermis
    d. Sun exposure

21. Two classifications are used to evaluate stage I melanomas. The index used to measure the thickness of the melanoma from the granular layer of the epidermis to its greatest depth is:
    a. Clark's index
    b. Hutchinson's index
    c. Breslow's index
    d. Depth index

22. Survival rates in patients with malignant melanoma are determined by:
    a. Origin of the melanoma
    b. Duration of sun exposure over 10 years
    c. Thickness of the tumor when diagnosed
    d. Color of the melanoma

23. Kaposi's sarcoma is caused by:
    a. Human papillomavirus
    b. Herpesvirus type 8
    c. Human herpesvirus ty
    d. AIDS virus

24. Since 1981, aggressive Kaposi's sarcoma has occurred in at least _____% of patients with AIDS.
    a. 5
    b. 10
    c. 20
    d. 33

25. Warts occur most often on sites that are subject to:
    a. Trauma
    b. Exposure to organisms
    c. Exposure to extremes in temperatures
    d. Pressure

26. Candidiasis is usually limited to the:
    a. Skin
    b. Mucous membranes
    c. Both skin and mucous membranes
    d. Viscera

27. The most common type of *Candida* infections are:
    a. Seen on the surface of the skin
    b. Seen on dry mucous membranes
    c. Seen in intertriginous areas
    d. Seen in areas usually not covered by clothing

28. Stasis dermatitis is associated with:
    a. Intertriginous areas of the skin
    b. Areas around joints
    c. Skin in the groin area
    d. Venous incompetency

29. Signs and symptoms of contact dermatitis can range from transient redness to:
    a. Severe swelling with bullae
    b. Deep redness and pruritus
    c. Redness and papules
    d. Redness and pustules

30. A significant risk factor for cellulitis (erysipelas) is:
    a. Bruising of the skin
    b. History of repeated sunburn
    c. A break in the skin, particularly in the lower extremities
    d. History of joint pain

19

Eye Disorders

When a patient presents with eye complaints, and a specific cause for the complaints cannot be identified, a complete history and examination of all parts of the eye are required to discover the cause of the problem (Fig. 19-1 and Box 19-1).

Conditions of the eye that can usually be managed by the nurse practitioner are acute and chronic bacterial conjunctivitis, viral conjunctivitis, inclusion conjunctivitis, allergic conjunctivitis, chemical conjunctivitis, foreign body, and subconjunctival hemorrhage (Boxes 19-2 and 19-3).

Symptoms of eye disorders include the following:

- Redness, due to hyperemia of the conjunctival, episcleral, or ciliary vessels
- Erythema of the eyelids
- Subconjunctival hemorrhage
- Ocular discomfort
- Ocular pain
- Foreign body sensation
- Photophobia
- Itching
- Scratching, burning
- Tearing
- Eyestrain
- Headache

THE EYE EXAMINATION

Box 19-4 lists elements of the basic eye examination.

Visual Acuity

- One eye at a time is tested, beginning with the right eye, using a standardized chart (e.g., Snellen's), and with the patient wearing his/her glasses or contact lenses.
- If refractive correction equipment is not available, a pinhole will overcome most refractive errors, and will also allow the clinician to ascertain whether refractive error is the cause of the patient's decreased vision.
- Visual acuity is expressed as the following fraction:

$$\frac{\text{Distance (usually 20 feet)}}{\text{Lowest line patient can see}}$$

- Visual acuity of less than 20/30 is considered abnormal.
- Visual acuity can also be tested by counting fingers (CF), hand movements (HM), and perception of light (PL) versus no light perception (NLP).

Pupils

- The pupils are examined for absolute and relative size and reactions to light and accommodation.
- A large, weakly reacting pupil may be caused by third nerve palsy, injury to the iris from acute glaucoma, or pharmacologic mydriasis.
- A small, weakly reacting pupil is seen in Horner's syndrome (oculo-sympathetic paralysis), inflammatory adhesions between iris and lens, or neurosyphilis (Argyll Robertson pupils).
- Unequal pupils that react normally may be due to anisocoria (an inequality of the diameter of the two pupils).
- Optic nerve disease may be seen when the pupillary light reaction in one eye is of less intensity

491

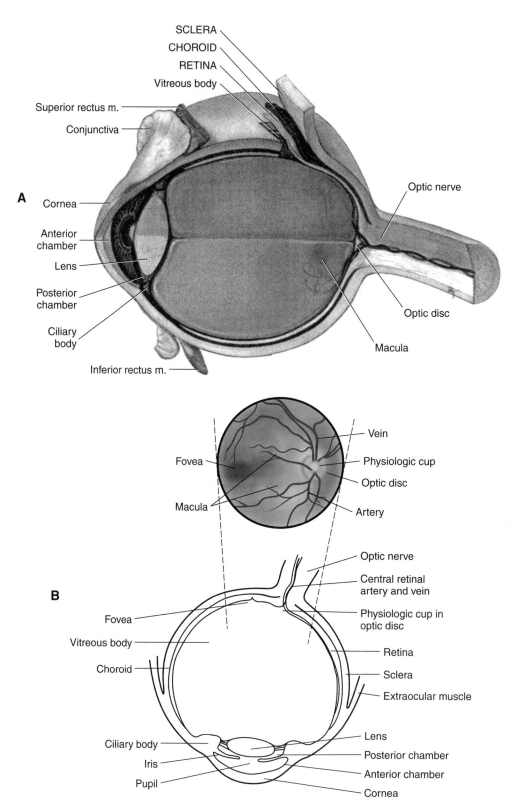

Fig. 19-1 Cross-sections of the eye. (**A,** From Bickley LS, Hoekelman RA: *Physical examination and history taking,* ed 7, Philadelphia, 1999, Lippincott Williams & Wilkins, p 166; **B,** From Jarvis C: *Physical examination and health assessment,* Philadelphia, 1992, WB Saunders, p 313.)

BOX 19-1
Internal Structures of the Eye

Cornea
Anterior chamber—The space between the cornea and the iris
Angle—In the area of the limbus, where the cornea and the iris form an "angle," is the area that houses the drainage system for the aqueous
Trabecular meshwork—The drainage system of the aqueous
Schlemm's canal—The trabecular meshwork drains into Schlemm's canal, which in turn drains into the venous system of the eye.
Ciliary body—A continuation of the iris that creates the liquid aqueous
Zonules—Fibrils that hold the lens in place
Lens—A cellular structure just behind the iris containing crystalline matter; it is biconvex and transparent, allowing images to be focused on the retina.
Pars plana—The continuation of the retina as it approaches anteriorly
Retina—The sensory network; it transforms light impulses to electric impulses that are transmitted through the optic nerve to the brain
Choroid—Vascular tissue of the globe
Optic nerve—The second cranial nerve that connects the eye with the brain for accurate vision and correctly interpreted images

BOX 19-2
Eye Disorders that Require Referral

Eye trauma
Loss of vision (sudden or gradual)
Severe eye pain

From Wu G: *Ophthalmology for primary care*, Philadelphia, 1997, Saunders, p 173.

BOX 19-3
Major Causes of Blurred Vision

Refractive error
Macular degeneration
Cataract
Diabetic retinopathy
Open-angle glaucoma, end stage
Corneal dystrophy
Migraine, usually transient binocular peripheral vision loss
Binocular optic nerve disease

From Bezan DJ, LaRussa FP, Nishimoto JH, et al: *Differential diagnosis in primary eye care*, Boston, 1999, Butterworth-Heinemann, p 10.

BOX 19-4
Elements of the Basic Eye Examination

Visual acuity testing using Snellen's chart for both distance and near vision
Pupillary examination: reaction to light and near/far accommodation
Evaluation of the optic nerve by visualization with the ophthalmoscope

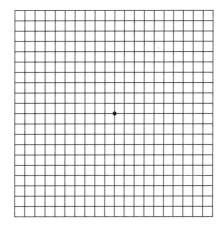

Fig. 19-2 The Amsler grid. Minimal changes within the central visual field can be assessed with an Amsler grid. Macular alterations are symptomatic as scotomas or distortion of lines. (From Krieglstein GK, Jonescu-Cuypers CP, Severin M, et al: *Atlas of ophthalmology*, New York, 2000, Springer-Verlag New York, Inc, p 237.)

compared with the normal eye; moving the light between the two eyes will usually enable the examiner to see this difference.

OTHER COMPONTENTS OF THE EYE EXAMINATION
Visual Fields

- Amsler grids are the easiest method of detecting central field abnormalities due to central vision disorder (Fig. 19-2).

Extraocular Movements

- Assess whether the two eyes are correctly aligned.

- Misalignment of the visual axes is called a manifest deviation **(tropia)**.
- A deviation that is apparent only when binocular function is disrupted is called latent deviation **(phoria)**.
- Testing for axial deviation can be done by observing the corneal light reflex in both eyes, or using the **cover test**.

Examination Using the Ophthalmoscope

- Examination of the interior of the eye with the ophthalmoscope can detect the following important ocular disorders:
  —Glaucoma
  —Diabetic retinopathy
  —Hypertension
  —Optic disk edema
  —Papilledema
  —Cataract

COMMON EYE DISORDERS
Nearsightedness (Myopia) and Farsightedness (Hyperopia)

Definition

Myopia is the inability of the patient to see clearly because the point of focus is in front of the retina. Hyperopia is the inability of the patient to see clearly because the point of focus is beyond the retina (hyperopia). Presbyopia, or the ability to focus far and near alternately, involves the process of accommodation, in which the lens changes shape slightly to provide clear vision by changing the focus of incoming light rays.

Risk Factors
- Heredity (parents who have refractive errors)

Etiology/Cause
- Familial
- All refractive errors represent mismatch between axial length of the eye and the power of refractive surfaces (cornea and/or lens).
- Astigmatism, in which patients focus a point of light on the horizon into a complex form that can be in front of, behind, or straddling the retina
- More rarely, patients with normal axial length and refractive surface power have a refractive error due to movement of the lens-iris diaphragm: myopia occurs if the lens moves forward, hyperopia occurs if the lens moves backward.

Pathogenesis
- The optic disk in myopia is oblique; the temporal edge is flattened and the nasal edge is elevated.
- The retinal pigment epithelium and Bruch's membrane do not extend to the temporal disk edge; the choroid extends farther.
- The exposed sclera is viewed through transparent retina as a white crescent.
- Patients with very high myopia are at risk for retinal breaks and detachments, breaks in Bruch's membrane with macular hemorrhage, and vitreous degeneration.

Diagnosis
Signs and Symptoms
- Decreased visual acuity of distance and/or near vision
- Visual discomfort (asthenopia)
- Squinting
- Holding objects either close to or far away from the eyes

Diagnostic Tests
- Refraction
- Visual acuity examination

Differential Diagnosis
- Decreased vision from any pathologic ocular condition
- High hyperopia: seen in nanophthalmos, in which the eye is small but there are no other gross abnormalities
- Macular hypoplasia and thickened sclera: thickened sclera predisposes the patient to choroidal effusion and retinal or choroidal detachment

Treatment
- Corrective glasses or contact lenses are the traditional method of treating refractive errors.
- Radial keratotomy or photorefractive keratotomy surgery performed by laser is the newer method for correcting refractive errors. Patients need to be carefully screened to establish eligibility for the procedure.

- Surgery carries the risk of corneal infection or perforation.
- Patients with unequal refractive errors (anisometropia) may need special lenses to provide equal image sizes in both eyes; aniseikonia (unequal image sizes) may prevent comfortable single binocular vision).

Prognosis
- Use of corrective glasses or contact lenses provides near-normal visual acuity.

Patient/Family Education
- Parents of children with refractive errors should attend to the amount of close work that the child does (homework, computer time, reading) because it is speculated that prolonged close work for young children may cause increased axial length and accommodation tone.

Follow-up/Referral
- Patients should be evaluated annually at first, then every 2 years.

Lid Inflammation (Blepharitis)

Definition
Blepharitis is red, sometimes painful, edematous eyelids; multiple conditions are associated with swollen eyelids, so that a careful history is required to differentiate among possible causes.

Risk Factors
- Ocular trauma
- Systemic disease
- Allergic reactions
- Reaction to medications
- Insect bite

Etiology/Cause
- Staphylococcal blepharitis
- Seborrheic blepharitis
- Meibomian gland dysfunction
- Allergic blepharitis
- Viral blepharitis
- Hordeolum
- Chalazion
- Preseptal cellulitis
- Canaliculitis
- Orbital cellulitis
- Allergies (see Diagnosis)

Diagnosis
- Lid inflammation can be caused by multiple problems; each will be addressed separately.
- Allergies usually produce marked crinkly lid edema with scaling of one or both eyes.
- The acute type, seasonal allergic lid edema is caused by hypersensitivity to airborne pollens or direct hand-to-eyelid application of pollens (e.g., after working in the garden).
- Chronic allergic reactions occur from contact sensitivity due to topical drugs (e.g., atropine, neomycin) or cosmetics or metals (nickel) and perennial allergic lid edema, which is believed to be due to a hypersensitivity to molds or to animal or dust mite dander.
- Hereditary angioedema due to C1 esterase inhibitor deficiency can also cause acute lid edema.

Treatment
- In allergic lid edema, removal of the offending cause is often the only treatment needed.
- Cold compresses over the closed lids may speed resolution.
- Topical corticosteroid ointment (e.g., fluorometholone 0.1% tid for not longer than 7 days) may be used if swelling persists for longer than 24 hours.

Prognosis
- The inflammation should begin to clear rapidly (1 to 2 days), with appropriate treatment.

Patient/Family Education
- Instruct regarding the nature of the condition and possible causes.
- Encourage the patient to find out the specific allergen that may be the cause of the lid edema.
- Teach how to give cold compresses or to instill eye drops or eye ointment.
- Teach regarding eye hygiene and the importance of washing hands frequently to avoid autoinoculation with debris or organisms.

Follow-up/Referral
- Usually, no follow-up is necessary; however, if the condition seems to be getting worse

despite therapy, an ophthalmologist should be consulted.

Angular Blepharitis

Definition
Angular blepharitis is commonly caused by *Staphylococcus* and *Moraxella* organisms.

Risk Factors
- Exposure to organisms by transmission from contaminated hands, unclean towels, or from infected individuals

Etiology/Cause
- Organisms (bacterial or viral)

Pathogenesis
- Organisms invade the areas of the eyelids through eyelash follicles, in which colonization of organisms/viruses occurs to cause local infection and the signs and symptoms of inflammation: redness, swelling, itching, pain.

Diagnosis
Signs and Symptoms
- Hyperemia
- Maceration
- Excoriation } near the lateral canthus
- Ulceration (rarely)
- Tenderness

Treatment
- Culture and sensitivity of exudate or scrapings of the eyelid.
- Bacitracin or erythromycin eye ointment is effective against staphylococcal infection.
- Polymyxin B sulfate-trimethoprim eye drops are effective for staphylococcal infections.
- Zinc sulfate eye ointment is used for *Moraxella* infections.

Patient/Family Education
- Warm compresses } essential in treating
- Lid scrubs } marginal blepharitis, regardless of cause

Follow-up/Referral
- Return appointment within 1 week, gradually increasing time between check-ups as the condition improves.

- If complications (e.g., ulceration, increased swelling) occur, the patient should be seen by an ophthalmologist as soon as possible.

Seborrheic Blepharitis

Definition
Seborrheic blepharitis is seen more commonly in older persons, in whom it may be chronic, or it may occur in association with staphylococcal blepharitis.

Risk Factors
- Older age
- Dandruff of the brows or scalp
- Poor hygiene, particularly around the eyes

Etiology/Cause
- Infection resulting from seborrheic dermatitis or dandruff

Pathogenesis
- Seborrhea invades the eyelash follicles, resulting in inflammation and associated with the signs and symptoms of dandruff.

Diagnosis
Signs and Symptoms
- May be asymptomatic
- Greasy scales or scurf on the lids and lashes are characteristic of this condition.
- Less redness and less inflammation than are seen in bacterial or viral blepharitis

Treatment
- Warm compresses for 10 to 15 minutes four times/day
- Lid scrubs once or twice a day (washcloth wrung out of very warm water; several drops of baby shampoo may be added to the water)
- Selenium sulfide–based dandruff shampoo to manage seborrheic scalp condition
- If there appears to be an associated staphylococcal infection, prescribe an antibiotic eye ointment (bacitracin or erythromycin).

Patient/Family Education
- Provide careful instructions regarding need to treat all areas where seborrhea is evident: scalp, eyebrows, eyelids.
- Instruct thoroughly in care of eyelids by means of warm compresses, application of

eye ointment or eye drops, lid scrubs on a regular basis, even after current condition is under control.

Follow-up/Referral
- Patient should be seen within a week to verify that the condition is clearing without complications.
- If condition is resolving and hygiene seems to be effective, increase interval between appointments by 1 to 2 weeks each time, until the condition has cleared.

Meibomian Gland Dysfunction

Definition
In meibomian gland dysfunction, inflammation and swelling of the upper eyelid occur, usually on only one side. The condition may occur alone (meibomianitis) or secondary to rosacea or seborrheic blepharitis.

Risk Factors
- History of chronic eyelid inflammation
- Poor eye/eyelid hygiene

Etiology/Cause
- Infectious condition of the eyelids or meibomian glands
  —Bacterial: *Staphylococcus aureus, S. epidermidis, Streptococcus pneumoniae, Haemophilus influenzae, Moraxella lacunata*
  —Viral: herpes simplex, herpes zoster, molluscum contagiosum
- Noninfectious condition
  —Acne rosacea
  —Eczema
  —Seborrhea
  —Meibomian gland dysfunction

Pathogenesis
- Inflammation of the upper eyelid, from either infectious or noninfectious cause (see Etiology/Cause)

Diagnosis

Signs and Symptoms
- Itching, burning, tearing
- Mild pain
- Sensation of foreign body in the eye
- Crusting on the eyelids on awaking
- Crusty, red, thickened eyelid margins with prominent blood vessels
- Hardened oil gland at the eyelid margin (meibomianitis)
- Superficial punctate keratitis (SPK), marginal infiltrates
- Elevated milky white nodules on the conjunctiva (rarely, cornea)

Diagnostic Tests
- History
- Complete external examination: periorbital area, facial skin, scaling, vesicles
- Visual acuity test
- Intraocular pressure (IOP) measurement
- Examination of fundus (with dilated pupil)
- If persistent, swab culture of eyelids and conjunctiva

Differential Diagnosis
- Preseptal cellulitis
- Sebaceous gland carcinoma
- Discoid lupus

Treatment
- Lid hygiene
- Eyelid scrubs twice a day using baby shampoo in water on cotton-tipped applicator
- Warm compresses 10 to 15 minutes, four times/day
- For bacterial and seborrheic blepharitis
  —Instill artificial tears four to eight times/day.
  —Topical antibiotic eye ointment (erythromycin, bacitracin, gentamicin, or sulfacetamide) to eyelids two to three times/day.
  —Apply topical corticosteroids (fluorimethalone or prednisolone acetate) three to four times/day, but taper quickly and stop drug as soon as resolution of the blepharitis occurs.
- For herpetic blepharitis and conjunctivitis
  —Trifluridine 1% solution eight times/day for 10 days
    ~ Chronic trifluridine therapy may cause a toxic superficial keratitis and conjunctivitis; apply topical ointment on the skin lesions to prevent bacterial superinfection.
- For recurrent meibomianitis
  —Tetracycline 250 mg orally (PO) 4 times/day
    ~ If tetracycline is taken by pregnant women, it can be deposited in the de-

veloping teeth of the fetus, causing discoloration.
~ Patients taking tetracycline may develop photosensitivity and should avoid sun exposure.

Prognosis
- Patients respond well to appropriate treatment.
- Encourage ongoing eyelid hygiene and lid scrubs.

Follow-up/Referral
- If patient is taking steroids, need to monitor IOP every 2 weeks until drug is discontinued.
- Schedule patient return visits every 3 to 4 weeks as appropriate.

Orbital Cellulitis

Definition
Orbital cellulitis is an inflammatory response associated with infections of the sinus, orbit, teeth, or with orbital trauma, including surgery.

Risk Factors
- Dental abscess
- Sinusitis
- Trauma to the head, particularly in the area of the eyes

Etiology/Cause
- Most cases (>60%) develop from infection of contiguous sinuses, especially ethmoid sinuses.
- Staphylococcal or streptococcal infections
- Secondary to trauma, upper respiratory infection, dental abscess, or other infections of the head

Pathogenesis
- An acute inflammatory reaction characterized by neutrophils and necrosis; special stains may show bacterial cause, usually *S. aureus* or *Streptococcus* organism.

Diagnosis
Signs and Symptoms
- Decreased vision, usually resulting from abnormalities in the tear film, not spread of the infection to the optic nerve
- Pain and redness in the area of inflammation
- Swelling, pressure
- Tearing
- Blurred vision
- Diplopia
- Redness of eyelids
- Chemosis of conjunctiva
- Lid swelling, causing almost complete closure of the eyes
- Exophthalmus (ocular proptosis) due to inflammation posterior to the septum orbitale (e.g., postseptal extension)
- Patient appears acutely ill, generally

Diagnostic Tests
- Ocular examination
- Dilated pupil, marked ophthalmoplegia, loss of vision, and afferent pupillary defect are warning signs of serious orbital cellulitis.
- Laboratory: complete blood count (CBC) (white count and differential), culture of ocular material
- Special computed tomography (CT), magnetic resonance imaging (MRI), or orbital ultrasound, especially if swelling precludes an adequate ocular examination

Differential Diagnosis
- Graves' diseases
- Allergic reaction (angioneurotic edema)
- Parinaud's oculogranular syndrome (granulomatous conjunctivitis and ipsilateral enlargement of the preauricular lymph nodes)
- Wegener's granulomatosis
- Orbital mucocele
- Carotid cavernous fistula
- Orbital neoplasms

Treatment
- Bed rest, warm compresses, parenteral antibiotics
- Culture of purulent material
- Antibiotic therapy based on sensitivity tests
- Sinus or abscess incision and drainage (needed in about 90% of adult patients)
- Blood cultures as indicated

Prognosis
- With prompt antibiotic therapy and drainage of any sites of infection, the prognosis for visual and ocular outcomes is excellent.

Follow-up/Referral
- Close follow-up initially is imperative to prevent complications and provide early administration of antibiotics PO or intravenously (IV), with surgical drainage of infected sites as needed.
- Close supervision should be discontinued only when all danger of further development of infectious sites is eliminated and the patient is recovering without complications.

Hordeolum *sty*

Definition
Hordeola are acute infections involving the glands of the eyelids. Internal hordeola involve the glands of Zeis and Moll, and external hordeola involve the meibomian glands.

Etiology/Cause
- Bacterial infections of the glands of the eyelid, usually staphylococcal, streptococcal, or viral organisms

Diagnosis
Signs and Symptoms
- Focal areas of redness and swelling on the lid(s)
- These areas may develop a yellow point, and drain spontaneously within a few days of onset.
- Reddened areas tend to be quite painful until rupture and drainage occur.

Treatment
- Warm compresses for 15 to 20 minutes three to four times/day
- Antibiotic eye ointment is often prescribed to prevent spread of infection.
- Stab incision and drainage will likely help to reduce pain from pressure and speed resolution.
- For resistant cases, oral antibiotics (e.g., doxycycline, minocycline, erythromycin, or dicloxacillin) may be prescribed to eradicate the infection.

Prognosis
- With appropriate treatment, the infection usually resolves within a week.
- However, patients often develop a history of recurrent infections unless adequate

teaching about eyelid hygiene is provided and followed.

Patient/Family Education
- Instruct in proper eyelid hygiene, warm compresses, and instillation of eye drops or eye ointment.
- Emphasize the importance of prompt treatment for any recurrences.

Chalazion *under lid*

Definition
A chalazion is a focal granuloma of a meibomian gland.

Etiology/Cause
- May be a sequela of chronic blepharitis or hordeolum
- Compared with hordeolum, the chalazion is relatively asymptomatic.

Diagnosis
Signs and Symptoms
- Appears on the lid as a firm, nontender, flesh-colored lump of variable size

Treatment
- Small chalazia may be treated conservatively with warm compresses.
- Resistant small lesions (<6 mm in diameter) may respond to intralesional injections of triamcinolone.
- Larger lesions may require surgical incision and curettage.

Prognosis
- Chalazia have a tendency to recur; therefore appropriate follow-up is necessary for prompt treatment.

Acute Conjunctivitis ("Red Eye")

Definition
Acute conjunctivitis is an inflammation of the conjunctiva caused by viral, herpetic, or bacterial infection.

Risk Factors
- Herpes simplex virus infection on the face
- Contact with person with the condition, regardless of cause

Etiology/Cause
- **Infectious** (bacterial): *S. aureus, S. pneumoniae, H. influenzae, Neisseria gonorrhoeae;* viral: herpes simplex
- **Noninfectious:** allergy, seasonal/atopic

Diagnosis
Signs and Symptoms
- Discharge
- Eyelid sticking
- Red eye
- Foreign-body sensation of less than 4 weeks' duration
- Marked chemosis
- Preauricular adenopathy (particularly associated with gonococcal conjunctivitis)
- Purulent moderate discharge with conjunctival papillae (bacterial conjunctivitis other than gonococcal)
- Mucus discharge, conjunctival follicles, preauricular adenopathy, subconjunctival hemorrhage, subepithelial infiltrates (viral conjunctivitis)
- Thick, ropy discharge, large conjunctival papillae under the upper lid or along the limbus, superior corneal-shield ulcer, limbal or palpebral raised white dots (Horner-Trantas dots) (vernal/atopic conjunctivitis)

Diagnostic Tests
- History: severe purulent discharge within 12 hours (gonococcal); recent upper respiratory infection or contact with someone with red eye (adenoviral); seasonal recurrence (vernal, history of allergies)
- Visual acuity test
- Slit-lamp examination by ophthalmologist
- Conjunctival swab for culture and sensitivity (blood agar, chocolate agar, Thayer-Martin plate, and immediate Gram's stain if severe)

Differential Diagnosis
- Episcleritis
- Scleritis
- Uveitis
- Acute angle-closure glaucoma
- Corneal ulcer
- Dural-cavernous fistulae
- Kawasaki syndrome

Treatment
- For adenoviral conjunctivitis
  - Instill artificial tears four to eight times/day.
  - Vasoconstrictor/antihistamine to alleviate itching
  - Fluorometholone or prednisolone acetate 0.125%, four times/day
  - Used for pseudomembranes or corneal subepithelial infiltrate, or if vision is reduced; taper steroid slowly after resolution; gently peel off membrane if present.
- For herpes simplex conjunctivitis
  - Cool compresses several times/day
  - Trifluorothymidine 1% (Viroptic), four times/day
- For bacterial conjunctivitis
  - Ciprofloxacin drops, four times/day (or)
  - Erythromycin ointment, four times/day for 7 days
- For *H. influenzae* conjunctivitis
  - Amoxicillin/clavulanate 20 to 40 mg/kg/day PO in three divided doses
  - Oral dose due to nonocular involvement (e.g., otitis media, pneumonia, meningitis)
- For gonococcal conjunctivitis*
  - Treatment is initiated if Gram's stain shows gram-negative intracellular diplococci or if there is a high suspicion of gonococcal conjunctivitis clinically.
  - Ceftriaxone 1 g IM in single dose (or)
  - Ceftriaxone 1 g IV q 12-24h if severe with lid swelling and corneal involvement (patient should be hospitalized until there is a satisfactory response to therapy)
  - Topical bacitracin or erythromycin ointment four times/day for 2 to 3 weeks
  - Tetracycline or erythromycin 250 to 500 mg PO four times/day for 2 to 3 weeks
  - Irrigate the eye with saline four times/day until the discharge is eliminated.
- For vernal or allergic conjunctivitis
  - Instill artifical tears as needed (mild infection).
  - Livostin or alopatadine HCl 0.1% (antihistamine) four times/day } moderate infection
  - Ketorolac four times/day

*Patients with this eye infection should be referred immediately to an ophthalmologist for evaluation and therapy.

—Fluorometholone four times/day for 1 to 2 weeks (severe infection)
  ~ Add topical cromolyn sodium 4% or alomide for vernal/atopic disease.
  ~ If shield ulcer is present, add topical steroid and topical antibiotic (e.g., erythromycin ointment or Polytrim drops four times/day).

Prognosis
- Acute conjunctivitis usually lasts ≤4 weeks, and is usually self-limited except in gonococcal conjunctivitis; recurrence of vernal/atopic conjunctivitis is common.

Patient/Family Education
- Provide information about the nature and cause of the condition and usual course of treatment.
- Instruct about application of compresses and instillation of eye drops or eye ointment as appropriate.
- Explain likelihood (or not) of recurrence and preventive measures.

Follow-up/Referral
- Adenovirus: every 1 to 3 weeks
- Herpes simplex: every 2 to 3 days initially to monitor corneal involvement, then every 1 to 3 weeks
- Bacterial: every 1 to 2 days initially, then every 2 to 5 days until resolved; gonococcal conjunctivitis needs to be followed daily until improvement is obvious, then every 2 to 3 days until complete resolution

Chlamydial Keratoconjunctivitis

Trachoma (*Chlamydia trachomatis* Serotypes A to C)

Definition
Trachoma is a chronic infectious disease of the eye caused by the bacterium *C. trachomatis,* characterized by symptoms of inflammation initially, which if untreated progresses to follicle formation on the upper eyelids that grow larger until granulations invade the cornea, eventually causing blindness.

Risk Factors
- History of exposure to sexually transmitted diseases: vaginitis, cervicitis, or urethritis may be present in chlamydial inclusion conjunctivitis, which could point toward a possible diagnosis.
- History of exposure to areas with a high incidence of trachoma: North Africa, Middle East, India, Southeast Asia.
- History of eye drop use, especially for glaucoma.

Etiology/Cause
- *C. trachomatis* organism

Diagnosis
Signs and symptoms
- Trachoma stage 1
  —Superior tarsal follicles
  —Mild superficial punctate keratitis
  —Pannus (often preceded by purulent discharge and tender [PAN])
    ~ Pannus is an abnormal condition of the cornea, which has become vascularized and infiltrated with granular tissue just beneath the surface; may develop in the inflammatory stage of trachoma or after detached retina, glaucoma, iridocyclitis, or other degenerative eye disorder.
- Trachoma stage 2
  —Significant superior tarsal follicular reaction and papillary hypertrophy associated with pannus, subepithelial infiltrates (SEI), and limbal follicles
- Trachoma stage 3
  —Follicles and scarring of superior tarsal conjunctiva
- Trachoma stage 4
  —Extensive conjunctival scarring

Diagnostic tests
- Visual acuity test
- Slit-lamp examination by ophthalmologist
- Dilated fundus examination
- Conjunctival scraping for Giemsa stain (basophilic and intracytoplasmic inclusion bodies in epithelial cells): chlamydial inclusion conjunctivitis and trachoma

Treatment
- Tetracycline 250 to 500 mg PO four times/day (or)
- Doxycycline 100 mg PO four times/day (or)
- Erythromycin 250 to 500 mg PO four times/day

  } for 3 to 4 weeks

- Both patient and sexual partners should be treated.

Prognosis
- Trachoma must be treated in early stages to prevent significant corneal scarring.

Patient/Family Education
- Fully explain the nature of the condition, potential problems if untreated, and usual course of treatment.
- Make certain that the patient understands autoinoculation.
- Emphasize the importance of treating the patient and all sexual partners.
- Emphasize the possibility/probability of blindness if not treated.
- Outline preventive measures that can be taken against reinfection.

Follow-up/Referral
- Patient and treated others should be seen every 1 to 3 weeks, depending on severity of the infection.

Inclusion Conjunctivitis (*C. trachomatis* Serotypes D to K)

Definition
Inclusion conjunctivitis is similar to trachoma and is more common in sexually active adults.

Etiology/Cause
- *C. trachomatis* serotypes D to K

Diagnosis
- Acute redness, discharge, and irritation of eyes
- Follicular conjunctivitis with mild keratitis
- Nontender preauricular lymph nodes can often be palpated.
- Cytologic examination of conjunctival scrapings shows a picture similar to that of trachoma.
- Inferior tarsal conjunctival follicles
- Superior corneal pannus
- Palpable PAN
- Gray-white SEI
- Stringy mucous discharge

Treatment
- Same as for trachoma, but with duration of therapy only for 2 to 3 weeks

Prognosis
- Treatment is usually curative.

Patient/Family Education
- Instruct regarding transmission of genital organisms to other areas of the body, including the eyes.
- Instruct about the potential threat to vision by causative organism.
- Emphasize the benefits of frequent, thorough handwashing.
- Emphasize the need for prompt treatment of sexually transmitted diseases.

Follow-up/Referral
- Every 1 to 3 weeks, depending on severity and response to treatment

Keratoconjunctivitis Sicca (Dry Eyes)

Definition
- Keratoconjunctivitis sicca is a common disorder, particularly in older women.

Risk Factors
- Older age
- Hypofunction of lacrimal glands
  —Due to aging, hereditary disorder, systemic disease (e.g., Sjögren's syndrome), systemic or topical drugs, climate (dry, hot, windy), or abnormalities of the lipid component of the tear film

Etiology/Cause
- Occurs when the quantity or quality of the tear film is insufficient to maintain the integrity of the epithelial surface
  —The cause is a deficiency in the aqueous, mucin, or lipid layers of the tears.
  —Can also develop because of lid-surfacing disorders, neurologic disorders, epitheliopathies, and environmental factors (see Risk Factors)

Diagnosis
- Patient's history
- History of sensitivity to drafts or wind (e.g., air conditioning, driving with windows open)
- Reading may exacerbate the condition because the blink frequency decreases during tasks requiring concentration and close work.

- A history of pemphigoid, Stevens-Johnson syndrome, rosacea, or rheumatoid arthritis may lead to dry-eye problems.
- Medications: prescribed and over-the-counter (e.g., chlorpheniramine, isotretinoin, hydrochlorthiazide, and propranolol hydrochloride)

Signs and Symptoms
- Photophobia
- Scratchy feeling
- Difficulty in moving the eyelids
- Irritation
- Redness
- Ocular discomfort
- Excessive secretion in the eyes (due to reflex lacrimation triggered by ocular irritation)
- In severe cases: marked conjunctival injection, loss of the normal conjunctival and corneal luster, epithelial keratitis that may progress to ulceration of the cornea, and mucous strands.

Diagnostic Tests
- Formation of corneal mucoid filaments (seen with sodium fluorescein dye)
- Tear breakup time
- Rose bengal stains devitalize epithelial cells, mucin, and filaments.
- Schirmer's, Sno-strip, and phenol red thread tests to determine whether the filamentary keratitis is associated with very low tear production

Treatment
- Replacement of the aqueous component of tears with artificial tears (0.9% physiologic saline or hypoosmotic [0.45%] saline 3 to 4 times/day)

Patient/Family Education
- Explain the nature of the problem.
- Emphasize the importance of adhering to the schedule for instilling artificial tears.

Follow-up/Referral
- Initially, the patient should be seen every week until it is apparent that the solution used to correct the condition is effective.
- When the patient is comfortable, return visits can be scheduled as indicated, 2 to 4 weeks to begin and then at longer intervals.

Corneal Ulcer

Definition
Corneal ulcers involve epithelial and stromal defects, corneal infiltration and edema, neovascularization, corneal thinning, and scarring.

Risk Factors
- Infection from any source
- Diabetes mellitus (DM)
- Topical corticosteroids (cause immunosuppression and contribute to the development or exacerbation of corneal infections)

Etiology/Cause
- Infections
- Noninfectious causes
  —Neurotropic keratitis (resulting from loss of corneal sensation)
  —Incomplete eyelid closure, causing exposure keratitis
  —Severe dry eyes
  —Severe allergic eye disease
  —Various inflammatory conditions that may be purely ocular or partly a systemic vasculitis

Pathogenesis
- Infection or environmental or physical conditions that place the cornea at risk for ulcer formation

Diagnosis
Signs and Symptoms
- Pain
- Photophobia
- Tearing
- Reduced vision
- Redness
- Circumcorneal injection
- Purulent or watery discharge
- Appearance of the cornea varies, depending on the organism(s) involved

Treatment
- Essential to begin treatment as early as possible
  —Delayed therapy may result in intraocular infection or corneal scarring.
- Choice of antibiotic ointment or eye drops depends on culture and sensitivity.
- Artificial tears may alleviate some of the symptoms.

Prognosis

- Usually favorable, depending on the duration of the infection and length of time between onset of infection and beginning of treatment

Patient/Family Education

- Fully explain the condition and its probable cause.
- Describe the usual treatment.
- Instruct regarding application of eye ointment or eye drops.

Follow-up/Referral

- Frequent follow-up for the first several weeks of therapy is necessary.
- If complications develop (no response to treatment, signs of more severe or spreading infection), refer immediately to ophthalmologist.

Bacterial Keratitis

Definition

Bacterial keratitis is an infection of the cornea caused by bacterial organisms.

Risk Factors

- Wearing of contact lenses, particularly soft lenses worn overnight
- Exposure to bacteria from any source
- History of eye infections

Etiology/Cause

- *Pseudomonas aeruginosa*
- Pneumococci
- *Moraxella* organisms
- Staphylococci

Pathogenesis

- Organisms invade the cornea, causing ulceration and destruction of tissue.
- Severe ulceration may require corneal transplantation.

Diagnosis

Signs and Symptoms

- Pain
- Redness
- Irritation
- Cornea appears hazy
- Central ulcer
- Stromal abscess

Diagnostic Tests

- Scraping of ulcer to obtain material for Gram's stain and culture before beginning therapy with fortified topical antibiotics

Treatment

- Choice of antibiotics depends on results of culture and sensitivity.
  - —For gram-positive organisms
    - ~ Cephalosporin (cefazolin 100 mg/ml)
  - —For gram-negative organisms
    - ~ Aminoglycoside (tobramycin) 15 mg/ml (or)
    - ~ A fluoroquinolone (ciprofloxacin) 3 mg/ml (or) exfloxacin 3 mg/ml may be given instead of the aminoglycoside.
  - —If no organisms are isolated, these drugs are used together.
    - ~ Topical antibiotics should be given at least every hour night and day for the first 24 hours.
    - ~ Patient must be checked frequently regarding appearance and condition of the cornea.

Prognosis

- Usually favorable, with intensive antibiotic therapy and careful observation

Patient/Family Education

- Explain the nature of the problem, its probable cause, and usual course of treatment.
- Instruct regarding instillation of eye ointment or eye drops.
- Ensure that the patient understands the length of treatment.
- Define preventive measures that will obviate recurrences of infection.

Follow-up/Referral

- If no response to treatment is observed within 8 to 12 hours, immediate referral to an ophthalmologist is mandatory.
- Patient requires frequent examination for several weeks after resolution of the keratitis.

Herpes Simplex Keratitis

Definition

Herpes simplex keratitis is an infection of the cornea with the herpes simplex virus.

Risk Factors
- Presence of a herpes simplex infection elsewhere on the body (face, lip)
- Frequent recurrence of infection

Etiology/Cause
- Herpes simplex viral infection of one or both corneas

Pathogenesis
- This infection is a major cause of ocular morbidity in adults.
- The virus has the ability to colonize the trigeminal ganglion, which results in recurrent infections that may be precipitated by fever from any cause, exposure to sunlight, or immunodeficiency (e.g., human immunodeficiency virus [HIV] infection).
- The corneal ulcer characteristically is a dendritic (branching) ulcer.
- More extensive ("geographic") ulcers may develop.
- Each recurrence causes increasingly severe corneal opacity and scarring.

Diagnosis
- Examination of ulcers with a blue light after instilling sterile fluorescein
- Identification of the herpes simplex virus

Treatment
- **Topical corticosteroids must not be used.**
  - Corticosteroids may enhance viral replications, resulting in severe epithelial disease.
  - If used at all in patients infected with herpes virus, an ophthalmologist must provide strict supervision.
  - Steroid dependence is common
- Trifluridine eye drops (or) idoxuridine drops or ointment q2h during the day
- Acyclovir ophthalmic ointment may reduce the rates of recurrence and complications, but this agent is not commercially available in the United States.
- Oral acyclovir 200 to 400 mg five times/day may be helpful in atopic or HIV-infected persons.
- Corneal grafting may be necessary due to extensive scarring.

Prognosis
- Even with aggressive therapy with fortified antibiotics and corneal grafting, the overall outcome for these patients is relatively poor.

Patient/Family Education
- Inform the patient about the nature of the condition, its likely cause, and the course of treatment.
- Emphasize the potential severity of the problem and the need to adhere closely to pharmacologic therapy.
- Stress the need for frequent follow-up visits.

Follow-up/Referral
- Most of these patients should be followed regularly and frequently by an ophthalmologist.
- Recurrences should be prevented through patient/family education, with clear instructions regarding preventive measures.

Fungal Keratitis

Definition
Fungal keratitis is an infection of the cornea with a fungus.

Risk Factors
- Contact lens wearer, especially soft contact lenses
- Corneal abrasion or trauma involving some kind of vegetable matter
- HIV or acquired immunodeficiency syndrome (AIDS) infection
- Immunocompromised patients, due to use of immunosuppressive agents such as corticosteroids

Etiology/Cause
- Fungal infection from any source, usually from plant material or in an agricultural setting
- Fungi most frequently found are *Candida* and *Aspergillus* organisms
- Corneal abrasion, which permits fungus to enter the cornea

Pathogenesis
- Fungal ulcers often have a greenish-white area of infiltration with an elevated, rough, textured surface.

- The margins of the ulcer are irregular and feathery, and extend into adjacent stroma.
- Satellite lesions, or remote foci of infiltrations, can be seen several millimeters from the main area of involvement.
- The course may be indolent.
- The cornea develops multiple stromal abscesses with relatively little epithelial loss.
- Intraocular infection is common.

Diagnosis
Signs and Symptoms
- Decreased vision
- Pain
- Photophobia
- History of corneal abrasion
- History of contact lens wear
- Conjunctival infection
- Purulent discharge may be present, even with apparently mild infection.

Diagnostic Tests
- Material from a suspected fungal ulcer should be cultured on Sabouraud agar.
- Microscopic evaluation of a scraping prepared with potassium hydroxide adds important information regarding the kind of fungus.

Treatment
- Treatment of fungal keratitis is often difficult.
- Initially, the lesion is treated as bacterial until proven otherwise.
- Available fungal agents tend only to inhibit growth, and the host must eradicate the infection.
- Amphotericin B, natamycin, scopolamine, or 5% homatropine help to minimize secondary anterior chamber reaction.

Prognosis
- Variable, depending on the ability of the person to fight the infection

Patient/Family Education
- Explain the nature of the infection and its probable cause.
- Inform about the course of treatment.
- Emphasize the importance of frequent follow-up and adherence to medication.

- Instruct regarding preventive measures to obviate recurrences.

Follow-up/Referral
- Patients with fungal infection of the cornea should be followed regularly by an ophthalmologist.
- A major goal of follow-up is to prevent reinfection with fungus.

Acanthamoeba Keratitis
Definition
Acanthamoeba keratitis is an infection of the cornea with the *Acanthamoeba* organism, a condition that is being more frequently seen in primary care practice.

Risk Factors
- Contact lens wearer
- Use of tap water to make a saline solution for cleaning contact lenses
- Wearing contact lenses in hot tubs

Etiology/Cause (see also Risk Factors)
- Exposure of the eye to *Acanthamoeba* organism
- Repeated wearing of contaminated contact lenses

Pathogenesis
- The ameba is introduced into the eye, causing suppurative keratitis.
- Early signs such as changes in the corneal epithelium are identifiable.
- Over time, the organism is able to encyst within the corneal stroma.

Diagnosis
Signs and Symptoms
- Pain
- Photophobia
- Reduced vision
- Early corneal signs include infiltrates in the central or paracentral area and pseudodendrites
- Signs in the later stages of the condition include radial neuritis, a complete or partial ring of infiltrates in the stroma, and recurrent epithelial defects

Diagnostic Tests

- Gram's or Giemsa stains are used to rule out other organisms, and to identify dormant amebic cysts.
- Slit-lamp biomicroscopy shows lid edema, conjunctival injection, keratitis, and a mild anterior chamber reaction.
- Calcofluor white and immunofluorescent antibody staining of corneal tissue from scrapings or biopsies add other diagnostic information.
- Laboratory analysis of the patient's contact lenses and solutions may prove helpful.

Treatment

- *Acanthamoeba* keratitis is difficult to treat.
- Prompt, aggressive therapy is essential.
- Combination antibacterial, antifungal, and antiamebic agents are used initially, from among the following:
  —Propamidine isethionate
  —Neomycin
  —Paromomycin sulfate
  —Miconazole
  —Clotrimazole
  —Ketoconazole
  —Itraconazole
- Topical corticosteroids are sometimes added to control inflammation.
- Penetrating keratoplasty may be necessary if a corneal scar develops that causes loss of vision.
- Corneal grafting may be performed in the acute stage to arrest the progression of infection, or to restore vision after resolution of the infection.

Prognosis

- Variable, depending on degree of infection and other factors

Patient/Family Education

- Comprehensive instruction regarding the dangers of improper contact lens care and cleaning and of wearing contact lenses while swimming or soaking in hot tubs may help to prevent reinfection in patients, or to prevent initial infection in others (if they are educated in a timely manner).

Acute (Angle-Closure) Glaucoma

Definition

Glaucoma is an abnormal condition of elevated pressure within an eye caused by obstruction of the outflow of aqueous humor. Acute (angle-closure, closed angle, or narrow-angle) glaucoma occurs if the pupil in an eye with a narrow angle between the iris and cornea dilates markedly, causing the folded iris to block the exit of aqueous humor from the anterior chamber.

Risk Factors

- Older age
- Hyperopes
- Asian race
- Pupillary dilation (sitting in a darkened movie theater)
- Stress
  —Stress from primary pupillary block, which pushes the iris forward, resulting in closure of the angle
  —Mydriasis for ophthalmoscopic examination
  —Medications such as anticholinergics (e.g., atropine)
- Shallow anterior chamber (determined by oblique illumination of the anterior segment of the eye)

Etiology/Cause

- Primary acute angle-closure glaucoma can occur only with closure of a preexisting narrow anterior chamber angle, often found in elderly persons because of physiologic enlargement of the lens.
- May occur secondary to long-standing anterior uveitis or dislocation of the lens

Pathogenesis

- Patients who develop acute glaucoma usually experience extreme pain and blurred vision due to sudden elevation of IOP caused by backup of aqueous humor.

Diagnosis

- Severe pain in the eye or brow pain on the affected side
- Haloes around lights

- Abdominal discomfort
- Nausea

} in older persons, these symptoms may be due to acute glaucoma, rather than problems in the GI tract

- Slit-lamp biomicroscopy usually shows a steamy, edematous cornea, a slightly injected conjunctiva, and a pupil fixed in a mid-dilated position.
- IOP is usually above 40 mm Hg.
- Gonioscopy reveals a closed angle.

Treatment
- In primary acute angle-closure glaucoma, laser peripheral iridotomy usually results in a permanent cure.
- IOP must be lowered before the iridotomy is performed, by means of a single 500 mg IV dose of acetazolamide, followed by 250 mg PO four times/day.
- An antiemetic may be needed before beginning acetazolamide, if the patient is nauseated.
- Once the IOP is below 50 mm Hg, 2% pilocarpine eye drops are effective in continuing to lower the pressure.
- Pilocarpine is not given if the patient is aphakic or pseudophakic (has no lens in the eye as a result of congenital or surgical cause).

Prognosis
- Untreated acute glaucoma results in severe and permanent loss of vision within 2 to 5 days after onset of symptoms.
- With appropriate treatment, including iridotomy, the outcome is favorable.

Patient/Family Education
- Older persons should know about glaucoma because they are the age group in whom the condition is most frequent.
- Literature about glaucoma should be available in all clinics and clinicians' offices.

Open-Angle Glaucoma

Definition
Open-angle glaucoma occurs because of consistently elevated IOP from abnormal drainage of aqueous humor through the trabecular meshwork.

Risk Factors
- Older age, but younger than those persons who develop acute glaucoma
- Black race
- First-degree relatives with open-angle glaucoma
- Steroid therapy can cause elevated IOP
- History of uveitis or eye trauma

Etiology/Cause
- The cause of decreased rate of aqueous outflow is not clearly understood.
- Recently, a mutation on chromosome 1 has been found to cause abnormal production of a trabecular meshwork protein (trabecular meshwork inducible glucocorticoid response [TIGR]) because of its association with glaucoma secondary to steroid therapy.
- This mutation has been found in only a small percentage of patients.

Pathogenesis
- Open-angle glaucoma produces a characteristic optic neuropathy in which there is loss of the neuroretinal rim of the optic disk, with associated enlargement of the optic cup, an increase in the area of pallor of the disk, excavation of the neuroretinal rim, and exposure and backward bowing of the lamina cribrosa.
- This is accompanied by loss of the retinal nerve fiber layer.
- Two patterns of damage to the optic nerve and nerve-fiber layer are recognized: **diffuse** (concentric loss of neuroretinal rim, cup enlargement, thinning of retinal nerve fiber layer) and **focal** (preferential loss of neuroretinal rim and cup enlargement in one area, marked defect in one area of nerve fiber layer).
- There is degeneration of the collagen of the trabecular beams, degeneration and loss of trabecular endothelial cells, and collapse of the intertrabecular spaces.
- There is a reduction in the pore density and number of giant vacuoles in the endothelium of Schlemm's canal.
- Optic nerve shows loss of nerve fibers, capillaries, and glial cells.

- Thinning and backward bowing of the lamina cribrosa, and undermining of the disk margin, which results in the characteristic "bean pot" appearance.

Diagnosis

Signs and Symptoms

- Most patients are asymptomatic and not aware of any vision problem.
- Patients with very advanced disease at diagnosis may complain of decreased vision; some may be aware of defects in their field of vision at some time in the past.
- Patients may indicate problems with night driving, fluctuating vision with close work or reading, and going from brightly lit to dim environments.
- Visual field loss
  —Most common form is the nerve fiber bundle defect, characterized by the tendency to respect the horizontal midline, especially in the nasal portion of the visual field.
  —This defect is not specific to open-angle glaucoma, and can be seen in other optic nerve disorders.
- Afferent pupil defect
  —Asymmetric damage to the optic nerve, as occurs in open-angle glaucoma, causes an afferent pupil defect in the eye with the greater degree of cupping.
- Elevated IOP
  —Most patients with open-angle glaucoma have an IOP of 21 mm Hg at least some of the time.
  —Research shows that between 10% and 40% of these patients do not have elevated IOP (these patients are said to have normal-tension glaucoma).
  —In some patients, IOP is quite variable, and shows diurnal fluctuation.

Diagnostic Tests

- Imaging of the optic disk and nerve-fiber layer
  —Stereo photography of the optic disk and red-free photography of the nerve-fiber layer are done to detect glaucomatous damage and to provide a baseline record of the appearance of the optic disk at the time of diagnosis.
- Automated static perimetry is done to detect and monitor visual field defects.
- Serial tonometry or diurnal tension curves to define the role of IOP and the effects of treatment
- Neuroimaging: carotid flow studies
- Systemic, vascular, and neurologic evaluation are done in some patients with atypical features such as low levels of IOP, in younger patients or patients with rapidly progressive visual loss, in markedly asymmetric disease, or in atypical patterns of visual field loss or changes in the optic disk.

Treatment

- Initially, medications are given.
- Some drugs lower IOP by enhancing the outflow of aqueous.
- Other drugs act by reducing the production of aqueous by the ciliary body.
- Most clinicians try two medications, one from each group.
- If the combination of two drugs does not achieve the target IOP (a theoretic IOP for any given patient that is usually 30% to 50% below the pretreatment level), either a third drug is added, or a recommendation is made for laser or surgical procedure.
- The miotics and prostaglandin analogs enhance aqueous outflow.
- Epinephrine and dipivefrin seem to have dual action on both outflow and production.
- Other drugs inhibit the formation of aqueous humor.
- Surgical and laser therapy
  —Argon laser trabeculoplasty
  —Filtering surgery

Prognosis

- Untreated chronic glaucoma that begins at age 40 to 45 will likely cause complete blindness by age 60 to 65.
- Early diagnosis and treatment will preserve useful vision throughout life, in most cases.

Patient/Family Education

- It is imperative to fully inform the patient about the nature of the condition and the best course of treatment.
- The patient should assume responsibility for taking medications as directed.

- The patient should know about the potential for blindness, but reassure him or her that early diagnosis and treatment can preserve eyesight for the life span.

Follow-up/Referral
- Regular follow-up with optic disk evaluation and visual-field testing is required, under the supervision of an ophthalmologist.
- Treatment for open-angle glaucoma has a high failure rate over time and often produces adverse effects.
- Once the target pressure has been achieved and the disease appears stabilized, the patient should be seen every 3 to 6 months, with detailed optic disk evaluation and perimetry every 6 to 12 months.
- Those with more advanced disease require more frequent follow-up.

Uveitis

Definition
Uveitis is inflammation of the uveal tract, which is formed by the iris (iritis), ciliary body (cyclitis), and choroid (choroiditis).
- Classifications of uveitis
  —Anterior uveitis ⎫ depending on the
  —Posterior uveitis ⎬ location of the
  —Panuveitis ⎭ most prominent inflammation
- Categories of uveitis
  —Acute
  —Chronic
  —Granulomatous
  —Nongranulomatous

Risk Factors
- HIV/AIDS
- Immunodeficiency states

Etiology/Cause
- Systemic disorders associated with acute nongranulomatous anterior uveitis are the human leukocyte antigen (HLA)-B27–related conditions.
  —Sacroiliitis
  —Ankylosing spondylitis
  —Reiter's syndrome
  —Psoriasis
  —Ulcerative colitis
  —Crohn's disease

- Behcet's syndrome produces both anterior uveitis with recurrent hypopyon (an accumulation of pus in the anterior chamber of the eye, which appears as a gray fluid between the cornea and the iris), and posterior uveitis with marked retinal vascular changes.
- Both herpes simplex and herpes zoster infections may cause nongranulomatous anterior uveitis.
- Disorders that cause granulomatous anterior uveitis and often posterior uveitis are
  —Sarcoidosis
  —Tuberculosis
  —Syphilis
  —Toxoplasmosis
  —Vogt-Koyanagi-Harada syndrome (bilateral uveitis associated with alopecia, poliosis [depigmented eyelashes, eyebrows, or hair], vitiligo, and hearing loss)
- The principal organisms that cause ocular inflammation in AIDS and other immunodeficiency states are
  —Cytomegalovirus
  —Herpes simplex and herpes zoster viruses
  —Mycobacteria
  —*Cryptococcus* organism
  —*Toxoplasma* organism
  —*Candida* organism
- Autoimmune retinal vasculitis and pars planitis (intermediate uveitis) are idiopathic disorders that cause posterior uveitis.
- Retinal detachment, intraocular tumors, and central nervous system lymphoma may masquerade as uveitis.

Pathogenesis
- Inflammation of the uveal tract is caused by specific disorders listed previously for each type of uveitis, with varying signs and symptoms.

Diagnosis
Signs and Symptoms
- Anterior uveitis
  —Inflammatory cells and flare within the aqueous
  —Cells are also seen on the corneal epithelium as keratotic precipitates (KPs).
  —In severe anterior uveitis, hypopyon (layered collection of white cells) and fibrin may be in the anterior chamber.

—Small pupils, which may become irregular if posterior synechiae develop (adhesions between the iris and anterior lens capsule)
- Granulomatous uveitis
  —KPs that are large and "mutton-fat"–like
  —Iris nodules may be present.
  —Granulomatous anterior uveitis begins less acutely, with blurred vision and a mildly inflamed eye.
- Nongranulomatous anterior uveitis
  —Acute onset with pain, redness, photophobia, and visual loss
- Posterior uveitis
  —Usually presents with history of gradual visual loss, and a relatively quiet eye
  —Bilateral involvement is common.
  —Vision loss may be due to vitreous haze and opacities and inflammatory lesions of the macula with resulting macular edema, retinal vein occlusion, and rarely, optic neuropathy.
  —Inflammatory cells present in the vitreous.
  —New lesions are yellow, with indistinct margins, and are often pigmented.
  —Retinal vessel sheathing may occur near new lesions, or diffusely.
  —In severe cases, vitreous opacity precludes visualization of the retina.

Treatment
- Anterior uveitis usually responds to topical corticosteroids.
- In some cases, periocular steroid injections or systemic steroids may be required to bring the inflammation under control.
- Posterior uveitis usually requires systemic corticosteroid therapy and less commonly immunosuppressive therapy with azathioprine or cyclosporine.
- Dilation of pupils is usually not necessary.
- If an infectious agent is identified, specific chemotherapy is indicated.

Prognosis
- The outcome for anterior uveitis, particularly the nongranulomatous type, is more favorable than for posterior uveitis.

Patient/Family Education
- Provide information about the specific disorder relevant to the patient, the possible cause, and the course of treatment.
- Keep the patient and family informed about symptoms, response to therapy, and care at home.

Follow-up/Referral
- Patients with uveitis are usually followed closely by an ophthalmologist.
- Primary care clinicians are closely involved in patients care also, in discovering causes of the disorder and assisting in giving antimicrobials, high-dose systemic corticosteroids, and systemic immunosuppressants if they are needed.

Cataract

Patients with diagnosed cataracts are managed by the ophthalmologist; however, the primary care practitioner often diagnoses the disorder, refers the patient, and follows the postsurgical patient in consultation with the physician.

Definition
A cataract is an abnormal progressive condition of the lens of the eye, characterized by loss of transparency of the lens and reduced vision.

Risk Factors
- Older age
- Heredity
- DM
- Oral or inhaled corticosteroid therapy
- Exposure to ultraviolet B (UVB) radiation
- Poor nutrition
- Smoking

Etiology/Cause (see also Risk Factors)
Pathogenesis
- The pathology depends on the type of cataract.
- Generally, degenerative changes are found in the nucleus, cortex, or anterior or posterior subcapsular areas.
- Early changes in the cortex appear as tiny areas of liquefaction called morgagnian degeneration, seen clinically as cortical spoke.
- The liquefaction can progress to involve the entire cortex, at which point the lens appears milky-white.

Diagnosis
- The patient complains of very gradual loss of visual acuity.

- The insidious loss of vision may go largely unnoticed by the patient until he or she happens to close or cover one eye, and immediately recognizes the difference in visual acuity between the eyes.
- Many patients say that at night they see haloes around lights, often while driving.
- On examination of the eye by ophthalmoscope, lens opacity may be evident.

Diagnostic Tests

- **As soon as cataract is known or suspected, the patient is referred to an ophthalmologist for confirmation of diagnosis and treatment, usually surgery.**
- Visual acuity tests
- Refraction
- IOP determination
- Undilated and dilated slit-lamp examination
- Dilated fundus examination

Differential Diagnosis

- Cystoid macular edema
- Age-related macular degeneration
- Diabetic retinopathy
- Retinal detachment
- Vitreous hemorrhage
- Corneal edema

Treatment

- Surgical lens replacement by means of small-incision, no-stitch, outpatient intracapsular cataract extraction (ICCE) surgery
- The patient can usually resume normal activities the day after surgery.
- Glasses, if needed, are prescribed in 2 to 4 weeks.
- In operative surgery, in which a larger incision is necessary, the recovery time is longer, and glasses, if needed, are prescribed in 6 to 8 weeks after surgery.

Prognosis

- Cataract surgery results in about 95% improvement to a visual acuity of 20/40 or better.

Patient/Family Education

- Explain the disorder to the patient in simple terms.

- Explain the options for surgery—laser or operative surgery, and conditions under which each is selected.
- Before surgery, outline the procedure that will be done and what to expect afterward.

Follow-up/Referral

- Long-term follow-up is needed to ensure proper visual rehabilitation and to check for postoperative complications (corneal edema, opacification of the posterior lens capsule, glaucoma, intraocular inflammation, and retinal detachment.

Diabetic Retinopathy

Definition

Retinopathy is a noninflammatory eye disorder resulting from changes in the retinal blood vessels; in this case, the cause is DM. Types of diabetic retinopathy include background retinopathy, preproliferative retinopathy, and proliferative retinopathy.

Risk Factors

- Older age
- History of DM
- Type I DM

Etiology/Cause

- The major effect of DM on the retina is a microangiopathic process that results in microvascular damage and occlusion of retinal capillaries.

Pathogenesis

- Progressive thickening of the retinal capillary basement membrane
- Vascular occlusion
- Breakdown of the blood retinal barrier
- Intraretinal lipid exudates
- Background retinopathy results in damage to the microvasculature of the retina.
  —Capillaries become damaged and cause microaneurysms, which are identified as tiny red dots by ophthalmoscopy.
  —Capillary fluid leaks out of the microaneurysms, causing intraretinal hemorrhage and eventually hard exudates.
  —Vision is affected if the macula becomes edematous.

- Preproliferative retinopathy results in a stage of progression from background retinopathy, with further destruction of retinal capillaries and development of capillary dropout.
- Proliferative retinopathy results in abnormal blood vessels (neovascularization), which grow on the surface of the retina.
  —Vessels can grow into the surface of the vitreous chamber and hemorrhage, filling the chamber with blood, thus preventing light from reaching the retina.
  —Untreated, more than 50% of patients with proliferative retinopathy will become blind.
  —Diabetes accounts for 10% of new cases of legal blindness every year in the United States.
- Incidence of diabetic retinopathy depends on the age of patients, duration of the disease, Type I (insulin-dependent) DM.
- Between 25% and 50% of Type I DM patients who have had DM for 10 to 15 years will have signs of retinopathy; those with Type II DM for 11 to 13 years will develop signs of retinopathy.

Diagnosis

Signs and Symptoms
- Gradual decreased vision
- Floaters
- Acute loss of vision
- Intraretinal hemorrhages
- Retinal edema
- Intraretinal microvascular abnormalities
- Cotton-wool spots
- Microaneurysms
- Neovascularization of the disk and other areas of the retina
- Venous beading
- Venous omega loops
- Vitreous hemorrhage
- Tractional retinal detachment
- Iris neovascularization

Diagnostic Tests
- Careful slit-lamp examination to rule out neovascularization of the iris
- Gonioscopy if there is suspicion of neovascular glaucoma
- Dilated fundus examination
- Fluorescein angiography

Differential Diagnosis
- Ocular ischemic syndrome
- Hypertension
- Vasculitis
- Central, hemiretinal, or branch retinal vein occlusion

Complications
- Cataracts
- Neovascular glaucoma secondary to ischemia with iris or angle neovascularization
- Tractional retinal detachment
- Vitreous hemorrhage
- Preretinal hemorrhage
- Macular edema
- Optic nerve damage

Treatment
- The goals of treatment are to
  —Stabilize vision or decrease the rate of visual loss
  —Decrease macular edema
  —Achieve regression of proliferative retinopathy
  —Release of traction if macula is threatened
  —Clear vitreous hemorrhage if present for longer than 3 to 4 months

Pharmacologic Therapy
- Maintain a normal blood glucose level.
- Increase or maintain exercise patterns.
- For neovascular glaucoma
  —Nonselective β-blockers, one drop twice/day
  —Selective β-blockers, one drop twice/day
  —Topical carbonic anhydrase inhibitor 250 mg four times/day (or) one 500 mg Sequel twice/day
  —Oral carbonic anhydrase inhibitor 250 mg four times/day (or) one 500 mg Sequel twice/day
- For iris neovascularization
  —Atropine sulfate 1%, one drop twice/day to maintain long-term pupil dilation
- Nonpharmacologic therapy
  —Focal laser therapy: for macular edema if it is within 500 μm of the fovea with or without intraretinal lipid or if there is an area of macular edema that is equal or greater in size within one disk diameter of the fovea.

—Panretinal photocoagulation for prolifative diabetic retinopathy if there is neovascularization of the disk or moderate-to-severe neovascularization elsewhere with associated vitreous hemorrhage.

—Pars plana vitrectomy for nonclearing vitreous hemorrhage or tractional retinal detachment that threatens the fovea.

Prognosis
- Variable, depending on the severity of the disease

Patient/Family Education
- It is hoped that patients will have received sufficient education about DM, particularly those with Type I DM, from the time of diagnosis that they will be aware of the natural history of the condition and the long-term risk of total loss of vision due to retinal damage.
- Provide support in every way possible for these patients as they undergo therapy.
- Explain procedures, why they are being done, what the objectives of the procedure are, how they are relevant to the patient, and the expected results of therapy.
- Provide vision aids as visual loss occurs over time, to help patients cope with loss of vision.

Follow-up/Referral
- Annual screening dilated fundus examinations should be performed on all patients with diabetes.
- Consultation with a retinal specialist is mandatory throughout.
- If diabetic retinopathy begins to develop, examinations should take place every 2 to 3 months to observe the rate of progression and to plan therapy accordingly.

Hypertensive Retinal Changes

Definition
Hypertensive retinal changes are vascular changes in the retina that occur as a result of high blood pressure and resulting stress on the microvasculature of the retina (where the changes can be seen) and in other organs of the body.

- Classification
  —Essential hypertension is characterized by lower systolic and diastolic pressures.
  —Malignant hypertension includes the findings related to essential hypertension, plus exudative retinal detachment and optic nerve edema.
- The high prevalence of hypertension among the U.S. population results in 10% to 15% of the total population having hypertensive retinal changes.

Risk Factors
- Older age
- Black race
- History of hypertension

Etiology/Cause
- Acute or chronic systemic hypertension

Pathogenesis
- The retinal arterioles develop thickening of their walls as a result of intimal hyalinization, medial hypertrophy, and endothelial hypertrophy.

Diagnosis
- Many patients are asymptomatic.

Signs of Essential Hypertension
- Focal narrowing and straightening of retinal arterioles
- Nicking of the retinal veins, seen in arteriovenous-crossing changes
- Increased light reflex and loss of transparency of blood column
- Arteriolar and venous tortuosity
- Cotton-wool spots
- Dot and blot hemorrhages
- Flame hemorrhages
- Retinal edema
- Optic nerve edema
- Venous-venous collaterals

Diagnostic Tests
- Blood pressure measurement
- Visual acuity testing
- Slit-lamp and dilated fundus examinations

- Fluorescein angiography to look for evidence of impedance to blood flow, microaneurysms, focal areas of nonperfusion, and leakage from dilated capillaries

Differential Diagnosis
- Congenital venous tortuosity
- Involutional sclerosis (atherosclerosis associated with aging)

Complications
- Vascular occlusive disease (venous and arteriolar)
- Macroaneurysm formation
- Optic neuropathy
- Optic nerve edema
- Blindness

Treatment
- Goal of therapy: to normalize systemic blood pressure
- Lose weight and exercise
- Watch sodium intake
- Control blood pressure with antihypertensive medication, with consultation of the primary care physician

Prognosis
- Good, if patient adheres to weight-loss diet and medication regimens

Patient/Family Education
- Patient should clearly understand the consequences of high blood pressure, and the need to maintain the blood pressure within normal limits.
- Particular antihypertensive medications have adverse effects; these should be listed for patients taking a specific medication so that they can monitor themselves and report to the nurse practitioner.
- Teach patients to take their own blood pressure, if they have access to the equipment, and record readings.

Follow-up/Referral
- Return visits every 3 to 4 months to monitor weight, exercise, and blood pressure
- Annual dilated-eye examination to monitor blood vessel changes

BIBLIOGRAPHY

Beers MH, Berkow R: Ophthalmologic disorders. In Beers MH, Berkow R, eds: *The Merck manual of diagnosis and therapy,* ed 17, Whitehouse Station, NJ, 1999, Merck Research Laboratories, p 700.

Bezan DJ, LaRussa FP, Nishimoto JH, et al: *Differential diagnosis in primary eye care,* Boston, 1999, Butterworth-Heinemann.

Bohn RL, Gurwitz JH, Yeomans SM, et al: Which patients are treated for glaucoma? An observational analysis. *J Glaucoma* 9(1):38-44, 2000.

Brilliant RL: *Essentials of low vision practice,* Boston, 1999, Butterworth-Heinemann.

Fechtner RD: Initial medical management of open-angle glaucoma. *J Glaucoma* 9(1):83-86, 2000.

Lee BL, Wilson MR: Health-related quality of life in patients with cataract and glaucoma. *J Glaucoma* 9(1):87-94, 2000.

Riordan-Eva P, Vaughan DG: Eye. In Tierney LM, McPhee SJ, Papadakis MA, eds: *Current medical diagnosis & treatment 2000,* ed 39, New York, 2000, Lange Medical Books/McGraw-Hill, pp 189-222.

Smith SC, Wilbur ME: Nursing assessment of the visual and auditory systems. In Lewis SM, Heitkemper MM, Dirksen SR, eds: *Medical-surgical nursing: assessment and management of clinical problems,* ed 5, St. Louis, 2000, Mosby, p 417.

Valentine V: Nursing management of the patient with diabetes mellitus. In Lewis SM, Heitkemper MM, Dirksen SR, eds: *Medical-surgical nursing: assessment and management of clinical problems,* ed 5, St. Louis, 2000, Mosby, p 1367.

Wu G: *Ophthalmology for primary care,* Philadelphia, 1997, Saunders.

Yanoff M, ed: *Ophthalmic diagnosis and treatment,* Boston, 1998, Butterworth-Heinemann.

REVIEW QUESTIONS

1. Which of the following is an ophthalmic emergency?
   a. Cataract
   b. "Red eye"
   c. Gonococcal conjunctivitis
   d. Viral conjunctivitis
2. The cause of inclusion conjunctivitis is:
   a. A species of *Chlamydia*
   b. Trauma to the conjunctiva (e.g., exposure to toxic fumes)
   c. Overexposure to sunlight and ultraviolet light
   d. Allergy to grasses, pollens, and molds
3. The appearance of a purulent, creamy yellow discharge from the eyes in a patient with conjunctival hyperemia is a sign of:
   a. Bacterial conjunctivitis
   b. Allergic conjunctivitis
   c. Viral conjunctivitis
   d. Giant papillary conjunctivitis

4. The eye infection that results in symptoms such as mucopurulent discharge, tearing, local irritation, and eyelids sticking together during sleep is:
   a. Chronic bacterial conjunctivitis
   b. Acute bacterial conjunctivitis ("red eye")
   c. Hyperacute bacterial infection
   d. Viral conjunctivitis (acute follicular)

5. The reason that corticosteroid pharmaceutical preparations are NOT recommended for the treatment of eye infections or other conditions, is that these drugs cause:
   a. Damage to the eighth cranial nerve
   b. Partial loss of vision
   c. Retinal detachment
   d. Corneal ulceration

6. Blepharitis is:
   a. Inflammation of the optic nerve
   b. Inflammation of the cornea
   c. Inflammation of the eyelids
   d. Inflammation of the conjunctiva

7. Corneal ulcers occur as a result of:
   a. A corneal abrasion
   b. Local necrosis
   c. Infection of the cornea
   d. Trauma to the cornea from exposure to toxic fumes

8. An external hordeolum is:
   a. Caused by trauma to the eyelid
   b. An area of blockage of a gland
   c. A localized infection of a sebaceous gland in the eyelid
   d. A swelling caused by overgrowth of tissue

9. Uveitis is inflammation of part or all of the eye's:
   a. Choroid layer
   b. Ciliary body
   c. Iris
   d. All of the above

10. In 40% of patients with uveitis, an underlying systemic disease may be present such as:
    a. Osteoarthritis
    b. Cancer of the gastrointestinal tract
    c. Syphilis
    d. Chronic obstructive pulmonary disease

11. A key diagnostic test used by the ophthalmologist when there is a suspicion of corneal trauma is:
    a. Examination with the ophthalmoscope with pupils dilated
    b. Magnetic resonance imaging of the eye
    c. X-rays of the eye
    d. Fluorescein staining and slit-lamp examination

12. The immediate treatment for chemical burns of the eye is:
    a. Instillation of erythromycin drops in both eyes
    b. Instillation of oxymetazoline hydrochloride drops in the eyes
    c. Irrigation of both eyes with polyvinyl alcohol ophthalmic solution
    d. Irrigation of both eyes with copious amounts of normal saline or lactated Ringer's solution, if available, or plain tap water.

13. The most serious emergency situation involving the eye(s) is:
    a. Sudden partial or complete loss of vision
    b. Infection with *Neisseria gonorrhoeae*
    c. Conjunctival hemorrhage
    d. Swelling and hyperemia of both eyelids

14. Among persons over 65 years of age, the following percentage have some degree of opacity of the lens of the eye:
    a. 20%
    b. 50%
    c. 70%
    d. 95%

15. Glaucoma is characterized by:
    a. Decreased intraocular pressure
    b. Retinal detachment
    c. Increased intraocular pressure
    d. Retinal hemorrhages

16. One of the major risk factors for retinal detachment is:
    a. Hypertension
    b. Pulmonary disease
    c. Rheumatoid arthritis
    d. Peripheral vascular disease

17. The treatment for detached retina is:
    a. Administration of antihypertensive drugs
    b. Scleral buckling
    c. Complete bed rest for 2 weeks
    d. Ice packs to the eyes for 10 minutes every hour

18. The area of decreased vision in people with macular degeneration is:
    a. Peripheral vision
    b. Near vision
    c. Far vision
    d. Central vision

19. The procedure that most likely will result in a permanent cure of patients with primary acute angle-closure glaucoma is:
    a. Laser peripheral iridotomy
    b. Panretinal photocoagulation
    c. Laser photocoagulation
    d. Laser trabeculectomy
20. Refractive surgery is being performed on more persons, allowing them to have:
    a. Near-normal vision with glasses or contact lenses
    b. Near-normal vision without glasses or contact lenses
    c. Clearer night vision
    d. Clearer peripheral vision
21. Which of the following is NOT a risk factor for primary open-angle glaucoma?
    a. Normal intraocular pressure
    b. Older age
    c. Family history
    d. Black race
22. Angular blepharitis is diagnosed by all but one of the following signs/symptoms. The one that is NOT an indication of this condition is:
    a. Hyperemia
    b. Scarring
    c. Excoriation
    d. Maceration
23. The risk factors for seborrheic blepharitis include all but one of the following signs/symptoms. The one that is NOT a risk factor is:
    a. Younger age
    b. Dandruff of the eyebrows or scalp
    c. Poor hygiene, especially around the eyes
    d. Presence of staphylococcal blepharitis
24. In meibomian gland dysfunction, inflammation and swelling occur in which one of the following?
    a. Both lower lids
    b. Both upper lids
    c. Only one upper lid
    d. Only one lower lid
25. The most frequent cause of orbital cellulitis is:
    a. Infection of nearby sinuses, usually the ethmoid sinus
    b. Trauma
    c. Bacterial infections of the eye
    d. Dental abscess
26. Internal hordeola involve which of the glands listed?
    a. Meibomian
    b. Sebaceous
    c. Eyelid glands
    d. Zeis and Moll
27. The most predominant symptom of detached retina is:
    a. Blurred vision
    b. Irritation of the eyelids and tearing
    c. Sudden partial or complete loss of vision in one eye
    d. Pain in the affected orbit
28. Trachoma must be treated in the early stages to prevent:
    a. Uveitis
    b. Significant retinal hemorrhage
    c. Blindness
    d. Orbital infection
29. Inclusion conjunctivitis caused by *Chlamydia trachomatis* D to K is seen most often in:
    a. Young children living in unhygienic environments
    b. Sexually active adults
    c. Adolescents with severe acne
    d. Older people with history of eye infections
30. The cause of many corneal ulcers is:
    a. Habitual rubbing of eyes
    b. Hypertension
    c. Incomplete eyelid closure
    d. Use of contact lenses

Ear, Nose, and Throat Disorders

The evaluation and treatment of problems of the ears, nose, throat, head, and neck are reasons for frequent visits of patients to the nurse practitioner in the primary care setting. Because the structures of the head and neck are relatively small and so intertwined, it is important to have a good grasp of the anatomy (Fig. 20-1).

MAJOR SYMPTOMS OF EAR PROBLEMS

Hearing loss, tinnitus, vertigo, earache, and otorrhea are the main symptoms of ear problems. The examination of the ear is limited to the external and a small portion of the middle ear. Abnormal conditions of the middle and inner ear are made primarily by inference based on the patient's history and screening tests (Fig. 20-2).

The external ear includes the auricle and the external ear canal. The canal's outer portion is cartilage covered with skin that contains glands that produce cerumen. The inner portion of the canal is bone covered with skin. The canal curves inward about 24 mm. The mastoid process, the lowest portion of the temporal bone, sits below the canal and is palpable behind the ear lobes. The tragus is the anterior border of the external canal.

The middle ear begins at the tympanic membrane (TM), a translucent membrane that is stretched over the three bones of the middle ear—the ossicles, which include the incus, malleus, and stapes (Fig. 20-3). The malleus provides several clear landmarks seen in the otoscopic examination of the TM. The tip of the malleus (the umbo) is the point at which the cone of light starts, and stretches to the perimeter of the TM.

When a patient presents with symptoms of ear problems, the physical examination should focus on the ears, nose, nasopharynx, and paranasal sinuses. The teeth, tongue, tonsils, hypopharynx, larynx, salivary glands, and temporomandibular joint should also be examined, to rule out referred pain from these areas to the ears.

THE PHYSIOLOGY OF HEARING

Hearing is initiated by the transmission of vibrations through the air of the external canal, through the TM and the bones of the middle ear, to the cochlea. There, the cochlear nerve (a portion of the eighth cranial nerve) is stimulated and nerve impulses are sent to the brain (air conduction). Sound can also be transmitted by bone conduction, during which vibrations of the bones of the skull are transmitted directly to the cochlea, bypassing the external and middle ear. Air is normally more sensitive.

HEARING LOSS

The severity and probable cause for hearing impairment are often determined by means of the history, testing the patient's ability to hear the spoken voice, and testing with a tuning fork.
- In taking the history, pertinent questions to ask the patient are the following:
  —Is one ear involved, or both?
  —Was the onset of hearing loss sudden or gradual?
  —Has the hearing loss progressed rapidly?
  —Has hearing acuity fluctuated?

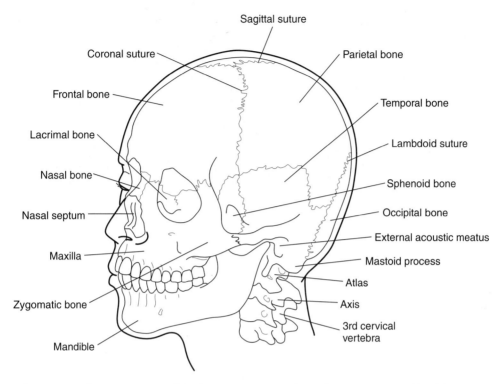

Fig. 20-1 Schematic aspect of skull. (From Jarvis C: *Physical examination and health assessment,* Philadelphia, 1992, WB Saunders, p 276.)

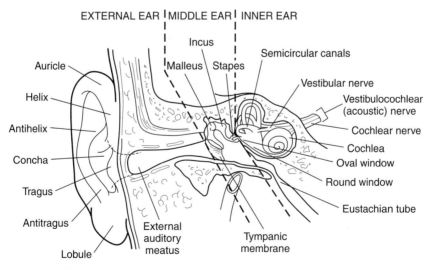

Fig. 20-2 Schematic structures of the ear. (From Lewis SM, Heitkemper MM, Dirksen SR: *Medical surgical assessment and management of clinical problems,* ed 5, St. Louis, 2000, Mosby, p 432.)

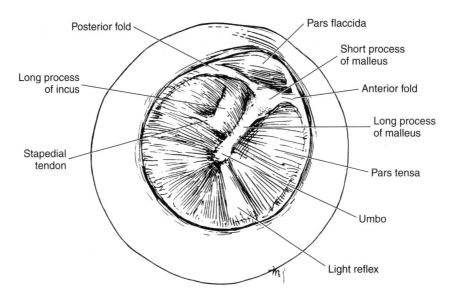

Fig. 20-3 Right tympanic membrane showing important landmarks. (From Lewis SM, Heitkemper MM, Dirksen SR: *Medical surgical assessment and management of clinical problems,* ed 5, St. Louis, 2000, Mosby, p 436.)

—Is tinnitus, vertigo, pain, discharge, or facial weakness associated?
—Is there a family history of hearing loss?
—Is there a history of noise exposure?
—Are there potential causes of hearing loss?
  ~ Diabetes mellitus
  ~ Syphilis
  ~ Hypothyroidism
  ~ Head trauma
  ~ Autoimmune disease
—Has the patient been exposed to ototoxic agents?
  ~ Aspirin
  ~ Aminoglycosides
  ~ Diuretics
  ~ Chemotherapeutic agents
• Evaluation
—Severity of hearing loss
  ~ Historical estimate of speech recognition impairment in noisy settings
  ~ Response to voice testing in the office
  ~ Audiogram findings
  ~ *Slight* impairment is difficulty in hearing distant speech in noise (e.g., group meetings, social gathering).
  ~ *Moderate* impairment is some difficulty with short-distance speech and conversation.

  ~ *Severe* impairment is no understanding of the conversational voice, but understanding of the amplified voice.
  ~ *Profound* (total) impairment is the inability to hear and understand the spoken voice despite maximal amplification.
• Level of sound
—A soft whisper is about 25 decibels (dB).
—A moderate whisper is about 40 dB.
—Conversational speech is about 60 dB.
• Classification of hearing loss (Table 20-1)
—Conductive hearing loss
  ~ Results from external or middle ear disease
—Sensorineural hearing loss
  ~ Results from inner ear or auditory neuronal problem
• Tuning fork tests
—The mechanism of hearing loss can be classified as conductive or sensorineural by means of a 512-Hz tuning fork.
—Weber's test: the vibrating tuning fork is held against a spot in the midline of the forehead; the patient is asked in which ear he hears the sound louder (Table 20-2).
  ~ A unilateral conductive hearing loss with normal bilateral ear function produces a louder sound in the affected ear.

TABLE 20-1
Estimating Severity of Hearing Loss in the Office

Severity of Loss	Social Setting	Office Voice Test	Audiogram
Normal hearing	None	≥18 ft—normal voice	No loss over 10 dB
Slight hearing loss	Long-distance speech	≤12 ft—normal voice	10-30 dB loss
Moderate loss	Short-distance speech	≤3 ft—normal voice	p to 60 dB loss
Severe hearing loss	Unamplified voices	Raised voice at ear	>80 dB loss
Profound loss	Voices never heard	Unable to hear	>90 dB loss

Barker LR, Burton JR, Zieve PD, eds: *Principles of ambulatory medicine,* ed 5, Baltimore, 1999, Williams & Wilkins, p 1462.

TABLE 20-2
Classification of Hearing Loss Using Tuning Fork Tests

Classification	Rinne's Test	Weber's Test
NORMAL HEARING		
Both ears	AC > BC	Midline
CONDUCTIVE LOSS		
Right ear	Right ear: BC > AC	Lateralized to right ear
	Left ear: AC > BC	
Left ear	Right ear: AC > BC	Lateralized to left ear
	Left ear: BC > AC	
Both ears	Right ear: BC > AC	Lateralized to poorer ear
	Left ear: BC > AC	
SENSORINEURAL LOSS		
Right ear	AC > BC bilaterally	Lateralized to left ear
Left ear	AC > BC bilaterally	Lateralized to right ear
Both ears	AC > BC bilaterally	Lateralized to better ear

Barker LR, Burton JR, Zieve PD, eds: *Principles of ambulatory medicine,* ed 5, Baltimore, 1999, Williams & Wilkins, p 1464.

~ A unilateral sensorineural hearing loss produces a louder sound in the normal ear.

—Rinne's test: the vibrating tuning fork stem is placed against the mastoid bone and held in place until it can no longer be heard, then it is held about an inch away from the external meatus of the ear.

~ Air conduction is perceived longer than bone conduction with normal hearing.

~ With sensorineural hearing loss, the reverse is true for conductive losses.

• Sound transmission by air is much more efficient than by bone. Air conduction may remain greater than bone conduction in early or minimal conductive hearing loss (Table 20-3).

AUDIOMETRY

Audiometric evaluation establishes the precise level of hearing loss. Pure tone air conduction and bone conduction measurements are made for sounds of varying intensity (dB) and frequency.

DISORDERS OF THE EXTERNAL EAR
Cerumen Impaction

Definition
Cerumen impaction is a collection of cerumen ("ear wax") in the ear canal.

Risk Factors
• Self-cleaning of the ear canal with hairpins, cotton-tipped applicators, or other means

TABLE 20-3
Causes of Hearing Loss in Adults

Causes	Mechanism	Onset*	Unilateral/Bilateral
EXTERNAL AUDITORY CANAL			
Cerumen impaction	C	Either	Usually unilateral
Foreign body	C	Rapid	Unilateral
Otitis externa	C	Rapid	Unilateral
New growth	C	Gradual	Unilateral
MIDDLE EAR			
Serous otitis media	C	Either	Either
Acute otitis media	C	Rapid	Unilateral
Barotrauma	C or SN	Rapid	Unilateral
Traumatic perforation of TM	C	Rapid	Unilateral
Chronic otitis media	C	Gradual	Unilateral
Cholesteatoma	C	Gradual	Either
Ossicular chain problem	C or SN	Gradual	Unilateral
Adhesive otitis media	C	Gradual	Either
Tympanosclerosis	C	Rapid	Unilateral
Traumatic injury	C or SN	Gradual	Bilateral
Otosclerosis	C and/or SN	Gradual	Unilateral
New growths	C or SN		
INNER EAR			
Presbycusis	SN	Gradual	Bilateral
Acoustic trauma	SN	Gradual	Bilateral
Drug-induced	SN	Either	Bilateral
Meniere's syndrome	SN	Rapid	Usually unilateral
CNS infection			
Meningitis	SN	Rapid	Either
Syphilis	SN	Either	Either
Tuberculosis	SN	Either	Either
Acoustic neuroma	SN	Gradual	Unilateral
Mumps	SN	Rapid	Unilateral
ATRAUMATIC SUDDEN SENSORINEURAL HEARING LOSS			
	SN	Rapid	Unilateral

Barker LR, Burton JR, Zieve PD, eds: *Principles of ambulatory medicine*, ed 5, Baltimore, 1999, Williams & Wilkins, p 1465.
C, Conductive; *SN*, sensorineural.
*Rapid = hours to days; Gradual = months to years.

Etiology/Cause
- Manipulation of the ear canal by self-cleaning

Pathogenesis
- Self-cleaning of the ear canal pushes the cerumen back toward the TM, opposite to its normal forward movement, resulting in impaction of the canal with cerumen.

Diagnosis
- Itching, pain, feeling of fullness in the canal, diminished hearing

- The examiner can see the cerumen in the canal with the otoscope, partially or completely blocking visualization of the TM.

Differential Diagnosis
- External otitis
- Bony overgrowths in the canal
- Foreign body in the canal

Treatment
- Hydrogen peroxide 3% ear drops, or carbamide peroxide 6.5% ear drops

- Irrigation with normal saline if the TM is intact, suction, or mechanical removal may be used.
- After removal of the cerumen, the canal should be thoroughly dried, either by instilling isopropyl alcohol or by using a hair dryer on low-power setting, to prevent the development of external otitis.
- Referral to an otolaryngologist may be necessary if the impaction cannot be removed by the measures described.

Prognosis
- Simple measures to remove impacted cerumen are usually successful.

Patient/Family Education
- Emphasize to the patient that self-cleaning of the ears is not necessary. The only appropriate method is to cover the index finger with a washcloth to cleanse the auricle, pinna, and external opening of the ear.
- Caution against the use of hairpins, cotton-tipped applicators, and electric jet irrigators such as the WaterPik, which should be used only for cleaning the teeth.

Foreign Bodies
Definition
A foreign body is any object that enters or is placed in the ear canal that does not belong there.

Risk Factors
- Toddler-aged children
- Play things such as beads, buttons
- Objects that fall on the floor unheeded: beans, peas, other small objects

Etiology/Cause
- Small children frequently put small objects into their ears, mouths, and noses, not recognizing the potential danger of their presence.
- Insects may get into the ears, such as flies, mosquitoes, ants, roaches, or other small insects.

Pathogenesis
- Any object put into a body opening has the potential for causing infection from organisms that are normally present on the skin and mucous membranes.

Diagnosis
Signs and Symptoms
- Often, the parents are not aware that a foreign object has been put into the child's ear until the child complains of itching or pain.
- A foul odor may develop caused by developing infection around the foreign object.
- Redness or drainage may develop in the ear canal.

Differential Diagnosis
- The signs and symptoms may resemble infection from other causes (e.g., external otitis, otitis media).

Treatment
- As soon as the parents recognize that something is wrong, they should take the child to the clinic or hospital emergency room.
- Firm objects (bead, button) may be removed with a hook or loop.
- Irrigation should not be done if the object is thought to be organic (bean, pea) because the water may cause the object to swell.
- Living insects should be immobilized by filling the ear canal with lidocaine before attempting removal.

Prognosis
- Removal of the object results in the disappearance of all signs and symptoms.
- The child should be observed closely for several days to ascertain that no complications are developing (e.g., infection, incomplete removal).

Patient/Family Education
- The parents or family should be cautioned to pick up dropped objects immediately, and not to buy toys that have small parts attached (e.g., small bead-like eyes on stuffed animals).
- The child should be discouraged from putting objects in the mouth, nose, or ears.

Follow-up/Referral
- Usually not required

External Otitis ("Swimmer's Ear")
Definition
External otitis is an infection of the ear canal. Types include localized (furuncle) and diffuse (entire canal is affected).

Risk Factors

- Exposure to water, irritants such as hair spray, shampoo, dye, or other substance in the canal
- Persons with allergies, psoriasis, eczema, or seborrheic dermatitis
- Cleaning the canal with fingernails, hairpins, or other objects that may transmit organisms and cause a break in the skin

Etiology/Cause

- Gram-negative rods, e.g., *Escherichia coli, Pseudomonas aeruginosa,* or *Proteus vulgaris*
- *Staphylococcus aureus*—causes furuncles
- Fungus (rare)

Pathogenesis

- Ordinarily, the ear canal cleans itself by the movement of foreign material to the opening of the canal. If there are skin breaks from scratches or attempts to clean the canal with sharp objects, pathogens that may enter cause infection to develop.

Diagnosis

Signs and Symptoms

- Itching
- Pain
- Foul-smelling discharge
- Hearing loss if canal becomes edematous or filled with debris
- If the pinna is pulled slightly, or even touched, by the examiner, exquisite pain results.
- The examiner can usually see that the skin of the ear canal is red and swollen, and the canal is filled with debris, obscuring the TM.
- Sensation of fullness in the outer ear
- Fever, usually low-grade, but can go as high as 40° C (104° F)
- Lymphadenopathy anterior to the tragus, upper neck, or in mastoid area

Diagnostic Tests

- Culture of exudate from the ear
- Organisms that may be present include *Pseudomonas, Proteus, Streptococcus, Staphylococcus, Aspergillus,* and *Candida* species.

Differential Diagnosis

- Acute diffuse otitis media
- Otomycosis (fungal infection caused by *Aspergillus niger* or *C. albicans*)
- Chronic external otitis/dermatitis (psoriasis, seborrheic dermatitis)
- Impacted cerumen
- Perforated TM from chronic suppurative otitis
- Persistent external otitis in patients with diabetes or who are immunocompromised may evolve into osteomyelitis of the skull base (called malignant external otitis), which is usually caused by *P. aeruginosa,* begins in the floor of the ear canal, and may extend into the middle fossa floor, the clivus, and even the contralateral skull base.

Complications

- Symptoms of chronic external otitis include persistent foul aural discharge, granulations in the ear canal, deep otalgia, and progressive cranial nerve palsies involving CN VI, VII, IX, X, XI, or XII. In these cases, the diagnosis is confirmed by computed tomography (CT) and radionuclide scanning, which show osseous erosion.

Prevention and Treatment

- External otitis can often be prevented by irrigating the ears gently with a 1:1 mixture of rubbing alcohol and vinegar immediately after swimming.
- In the presence of external otitis, the canal is gently and thoroughly cleaned of debris and exudate, by suction or dry cotton wipes.
- Topical antibiotics and corticosteroids are the usual treatment.
  - A solution or suspension containing neomycin sulfate 0.5% and polymyxin B sulfate 10,000 U/ml is effective against gram-negative rods.
  - Hydrocortisone 1% helps to reduce swelling and relieve discomfort, 5 drops tid for 7 days.
- Altering the pH of the canal by means of
  - Topical acetic acid 2%, 5 drops tid for 7 days is effective for milder cases.
- For pain, codeine 30 mg orally (PO) q4h may be necessary for 24 to 48 hours.

- If cellulitis develops, penicillin V 500 mg PO q6h for 7 days or erythromycin at the same dosage and schedule is given if the patient is allergic to penicillin.
- Furuncles should be allowed to open and drain spontaneously because incision may spread the infection.
  - Topical antibiotics are not effective.
  - Dry heat and codeine 30 mg PO q4h will relieve pain.

Prognosis
- Good, after treatment

Patient/Family Teaching
- Explain the nature, cause, course, treatment, and expected outcome of the condition.
- Write out information about medications: brand and trade names, reason for giving, action, major side effects if any, dosage and scheduling.
- Stress preventive measures, particularly immediately after swimming in any location: pool, ocean, lake, river.
- Because cerumen is a natural barrier to invasion of bacteria, stress the importance of never using the fingers, hairpins, applicators, or other means to self-clean the ear canal.
- Emphasize the importance of seeking professional help for the earliest symptoms of external otitis, to clear the infection quickly and to prevent complications.
- These instructions should be doubly emphasized for patients with diabetes or who are immunocompromised.

Follow-up/Referral
- The patient should be seen by the nurse practitioner once after treatment is completed, to make certain that the treatment has been successful and no complications are present.
- Patients who develop malignant external otitis or complications from external otitis should be referred to an otolaryngologist at once.

Tumors of the External Ear
Definition
Tumors may be referred to as neoplasia, which means "new growth."

- Types
  - Benign growths: sebaceous cysts, osteomas, keloids
  - Ceruminomas
  - Basal cell and squamous cell carcinomas

Risk Factors
- Persistent inflammation as in chronic otitis media may predispose the patient to the development of squamous cell carcinoma.

Etiology/Cause
- Unknown

Pathogenesis
- Any neoplasm within a confined space, whether benign or malignant, will result in partial or complete obstruction of the canal, with subsequent decrease or complete loss of hearing.

Diagnosis
Signs and Symptoms
- Itching or irritation
- Pain
- Feeling of fullness
- Neoplasm may be seen or felt.
- Any lesion suspected of being malignant must be biopsied and examined microscopically.

Differential Diagnosis
- All lesions must be differentiated between being benign or malignant.

Treatment
- Sebaceous cysts, osteomas, and keloids may develop and occlude the ear canal, resulting in retention of cerumen and a conductive hearing loss.
- These benign growths are excised as completely as possible, which is the treatment of choice.
- Ceruminomas develop in the outer third of the ear canal and are thus seen early and treated early; although these neoplasms are benign, histologically, they behave in a malignant way, and must be excised widely.
- Basal cell and squamous cell carcinomas often begin in the pinna, after regular exposure to the sun.

—Either of these malignancies may arise in the ear canal, with squamous cell carcinoma being somewhat more common than basal cell tumors.

—Early lesions are treated successfully with cautery and curettage or radiation therapy.

—More advanced lesions that affect the cartilage must be surgically excised in V-shaped wedges or larger portions of the pinna.

~ When malignant cells invade cartilage, radiation therapy is less effective, and surgical excision becomes the preferred treatment; generally, extensive resection is required, followed by radiation therapy.

—En bloc resection of the ear canal, sparing the facial nerve, is performed when lesions are localized to the ear canal and have not invaded the middle ear.

Prognosis
- The outcome is favorable in all cases of benign growths, but variable in cases of malignancy, depending on the extent of the neoplasm.

Patient/Family Teaching
- Emphasize the importance of seeking professional care for any growth anywhere in the body because, regardless of past history, a new growth may be malignant.

Follow-up/Referral
- All new growths should be referred to an otolaryngologist for biopsy and diagnosis.
- Follow-up is usually necessary for patients with excision and radiation of malignant growths for variable lengths of time.

DISORDERS OF THE TYMPANIC MEMBRANE AND MIDDLE EAR
Trauma

Definition
Trauma to the TM (eardrum) is relatively common, particularly puncture of the TM, which may result in dislocation of the ossicles, fracture of the stapes footplate, injury to the facial nerve, or a perilymph fistula from the oval or round window.

Risk Factors
- Accidents, explosions, diving, being hit or beaten, other
- The TM may be punctured by objects placed in the ear canal (e.g., applicator, hairpin) or those that enter the ear canal accidentally (e.g., twigs, pencils), or by sudden pressure; changes occur with explosions, hitting or slapping, or diving, or sudden negative pressure that may occur when strong suction is applied to the ear canal.

Etiology/Cause
- Most trauma to the eardrum is caused by accidents or sudden changes in pressure from blows to the ear, diving, explosions, or gunshots close to the person's ear.

Pathogenesis
- It depends on the cause of the trauma, but infection may develop if organisms are introduced into the ear canal, or the trauma may cause damage to structures in the inner ear.

Diagnosis
Signs and Symptoms
- Sudden severe pain followed by bleeding from the ear (puncture of the TM)
- Loss of hearing, partial or complete
- Tinnitus
- Vertigo (if there is injury to the inner ear)
- Purulent discharge may develop within 24 to 48 hours if water enters the middle ear.

Diagnostic Tests
- Examination of the ear by otoscope
- Hearing test using tuning forks and voice

Differential Diagnosis
- History of trauma usually makes it unnecessary to make a differential diagnosis until evaluation of the damage from the trauma is conducted.

Treatment
- Referral to an otolaryngologist is mandatory.
- Many TM perforations can be managed without the need for invasive therapy.
- If infection is present or likely to occur, oral penicillin V 250 mg q6h for 7 days is given.

- Aseptic technique should be maintained while examining the ear.
- The ear, nose, and throat (ENT) specialist may try to place the flaps of the TM in place, using local anesthesia and microscopic control, which will facilitate healing.
- The ear is kept as dry as possible.
- If infection develops, acetic acid 2% ear drops, 5 drops tid, may be started.
- No ear drops should be used to prevent infection.
- Spontaneous closure of the eardrum usually occurs within 1 to 2 months.
- If closure and healing of the TM have not occurred within 2 months, surgical repair is performed.
- If conductive hearing loss persists, which may indicate disruption in the ossicular chain, the middle ear should be explored surgically and repaired.
- If a sensorineural hearing loss or vertigo persists for hours to 1 or 2 days after the injury, the inner ear should be surgically explored and repaired as soon as possible.

Patient/Family Education
- Throughout the treatment period, the patient and the family should be kept informed of the findings, recommended therapy, and progress.
- Patient or family consent must be obtained for surgical or other procedures, with full explanations of the rationale for the procedure, the attendant risks and benefits, and likely outcome.

Follow-up/Referral
- For any patient who has had injury to the ears, an otolaryngologist should be the primary diagnostician and provider of care from the outset.
- This specialist should also see the patient after hospitalization for several weeks or months, to make sure that no complications or untoward sequelae result from the injury.

Acute Otitis Media

Definition
Acute otitis media is a bacterial or viral infection in the middle ear and in the mucosally lined air-containing spaces of the temporal bone, usually secondary to an upper respiratory infection (URI).

Risk Factors
- Young age (3 months to 3 years)
- Secondhand smoke
- URI

Etiology/Cause
- In newborns, gram-negative bacilli (e.g., *Escherichia coli* and *Staphylococcus aureus* are the organisms that usually cause acute otitis media.
- After the neonatal period, *E. coli* is rarely the cause of acute otitis media.
- In older children (under 14 years) *Streptococcus pneumoniae, Haemophilus influenzae,* group A β-hemolytic streptococci, *Moraxella (Branhamella) catarrhalis,* and *S. aureus* are the organisms that cause acute otitis media.
- Viral otitis media is often complicated by secondary invasion by one of the bacteria mentioned previously.
- In patients over 14 years, *S. pneumoniae,* group A β-hemolytic streptococci, and *S. aureus* are the primary causative organisms.
- The causative organism in a community at any given time depends on which microorganisms are epidemic.
- The frequency of otitis media caused by multi-drug-resistant *S. pneumoniae* has increased.

Diagnosis
Signs and Symptoms
- Persistent, severe earache
- Diminished hearing
- Fever (up to 40.5° C [105° F])
- Nausea, vomiting
- Diarrhea (young children)
- Erythematous, bulging eardrum
- TM landmarks become indistinct or unseen
- TM light reflex is displaced
- Bloody, then serosanguinous, then purulent otorrhea usually follows spontaneous or surgical perforation of the TM.

Symptoms of Impending Complication
- Headache, increasing in severity
- Sudden profound hearing loss
- Vertigo
- Chills
- Fever

Complications
- Acute mastoiditis
- Petrositis
- Labyrinthitis
- Facial paralysis
- Conductive and sensorineural hearing loss
- Epidural abscess
- Meningitis (most common intracranial complication)
- Brain abscess
- Lateral sinus thrombosis
- Otitic hydrocephalus

Diagnosis
Signs and Symptoms
- Clinical picture
- History of current ear disorder
- Visualization of the TM by otoscope
- Culture of exudate from the middle ear

Treatment
- Pharmacologic therapy
  —Penicillin V 250 mg PO q6h for 12 days (>14 years)
  —Amoxicillin 20 to 40 mg/kg/day PO q8h (equal doses) for 7 to 12 days (<14 years) because of *H. influenzae* infections
    ~ This regimen is often continued for up to 14 days to ensure resolution and prevent sequelae.
  —Follow-up therapy depends on clinical course and on culture and sensitivity results.
- For patients allergic to penicillin
  —Erythromycin 50 mg/kg/day PO q6h (or)
  —Combined erythromycin 30 to 50 mg/kg/day PO and sulfisoxazole 150 mg/kg/day PO both q6h in equal doses for 12 to 14 days (<14 years) (or)
  —TMP-SMX 160/800 mg q12h for 12 days (adults)
- For pain relief
  —Tylenol at recommended dosage, depending on age
- Nonpharmacologic therapy
  —Heat to affected ear/side helps to relieve pain and promote suppuration
  —Plenty of fluids, especially when fever is present
  —Patient's hearing, visualization of TM, and movement of TM should be monitored until resolution is complete.

Patient/Family Education
- Instruct regarding the nature, cause, treatment, usual course, and expected outcome.
- Write out information about medications: generic and trade name, dosage, administration, and scheduling.
- Stress importance of taking antibiotics at scheduled times for maximum benefit.
- Discuss preventive measures to take against potential episodes of acute otitis media.

Follow-up/Referral
- The patient is followed closely in first 2 weeks, to make certain that patient is compliant and that no medication side effects occur, to monitor resolution of infection, and to ensure that no complications develop.

Serous Otitis Media
Definition
Serous otitis media is an effusion in the middle ear resulting from incomplete resolution of acute otitis media or obstruction of the eustachian tube. The effusion may be sterile, but pathogenic bacteria are often present. Obstruction in the eustachian tube may result from inflammatory processes in the nasopharynx, allergic manifestations, hypertrophic adenoids, or benign or malignant neoplasms.

Incidence
- It occurs primarily in children but can occur at any age.

Risk Factors
- Incomplete resolution of previous acute otitis media
- Impaired patency of eustachian tube
- History of allergies

Etiology/Cause
- Recent acute otitis media
- Obstruction in the eustachian tube
- Enlarged adenoids
- Inflammation of the TM, middle ear, or eustachian tube

Pathogenesis
- The middle ear normally is ventilated three to four times/minute as the eustachian tube opens during swallowing, and oxygen is ab-

sorbed by the blood in the vessels of the middle ear mucous membrane.

- If obstruction occurs in the eustachian tube, oxygen absorption and gas exchange are restricted, resulting in relative negative pressure in the middle ear, causing retraction of the TM, displacement of the light reflex, and immobility of the TM.
- A fluid level or air bubbles may be seen behind the TM.

Diagnosis
Signs and Symptoms
- TM: immobile, retracted
- Fluid level or air bubbles visible behind the TM
- TM landmarks become pronounced and the light reflex displaced.
- Transudate develops in the middle ear, which gives a gray or amber appearance of the TM.
- Conductive hearing loss develops.

Treatment
- Trial of antibiotic therapy based on possible presence of pathogens in the middle ear, same drugs and dosages as for acute otitis media.
  —Purpose: effective against pathogens, relief of obstruction in eustachian tube, and sterilization the middle ear
- Systemic sympathomimetic amines such as ephedrine sulfate, pseudoephedrine, or phenylpropanolamine 30 mg PO tid (adults)
  —Purpose: vasoconstrictive effect may open obstructed eustachian tube
- Myringotomy may be necessary to relieve obstruction of the eustachian tube by aspiration of fluid.
- Valsalva's maneuver to ventilate the middle ear temporarily
- Treat underlying nasopharyngeal disorders (e.g., adenoidectomy).
- Treat allergies, and eliminate allergens from patient's environment.

Patient/Family Education
- Explain the condition, symptoms, usual treatment, and expected outcomes.
- Describe the Valsalva's maneuver and its effects on the eustachian tube.

- List all medications, dosages, schedule, and reason for giving.
- Emphasize the importance of taking antibiotics on time, without skipping doses.
- Arrange a series of follow-up appointments to determine the status of the TM, amount of drainage if any, and degree of resolution of the disorder.
- Inform regarding dates and times of follow-up appointments and the need to keep all appointments.

Chronic Otitis Media and Cholesteatoma
Definition
Chronic otitis media (COM) is a condition that develops when there is a permanent perforation of the TM, with or without permanent changes in the middle ear. Depending on the type of perforation, COM can be divided into two major categories: (1) COM caused by central perforations of the pars tensa and (2) COM caused by the more dangerous attic perforations of the pars flaccida or marginal perforations of the pars tensa.

Cholesteatomas tend to develop during healing of acute necrotizing otitis media, when the remaining epithelium of the mucous membrane and the stratified squamous epithelium of the ear canal migrate to cover the denuded areas. After the squamous epithelium is established in the middle ear, it begins to desquamate and accumulate, thus creating cholesteatoma.

Risk Factors
- Recent acute otitis media
- Unresolved acute otitis media
- Mechanical trauma
- Perforations of the TM (central, marginal, or attic, which lead into the epitympanum and may result in more complications than central perforations)

Etiology/Cause
- Acute otitis media
- Eustachian tube obstruction
- Mechanical trauma
- Thermal or chemical burns
- Blast injuries

Pathogenesis
- Any of the causes listed can result in permanent perforations of the TM and possible

permanent damage to the middle ear, resulting in cholesteatomas or conductive hearing loss. Cholesteatomas are seen during otoscopic examination, and appear like white debris in the middle ear, with destruction of the ear canal bone nearest to the perforation. Aural polyps frequently accompany cholesteatomas. Cholesteatomas, particularly associated with attic perforation, increase the likelihood of serious complications such as purulent labyrinthitis, facial paralysis, intracranial suppuration, mastoiditis, osteomyelitis of the skull base, sigmoid sinus thrombosis, and central nervous system infection.

Diagnosis

Signs and Symptoms
- Typical major sign: purulent aural discharge
- Ear drainage may be intermittent or continuous, increasing with upper respiratory infections and after exposure to water (e.g., swimming).
- Perforation of the TM
- Mucosal changes: polypoid degeneration, granulation tissue, and osseous changes such as osteitis and sclerosis
- Little if any pain
- Conductive hearing loss due to perforation of the TM and destruction of the ossicular chain

Diagnostic Tests
- Culture of aural discharge
  —Often shows mixed flora: (aerobes): *E. coli, S. aureus, P. mirabilis, P. aeruginosa,* diphtheroid bacilli, or (anaerobes): *Bacteroides fragilis, B. melaninogenicus,* or *Peptococcus magnus*
- If cholesteatomas are present—CT scan

Treatment
- The definitive treatment is surgery.
  —Repair of the TM by means of temporalis muscle fascia or homograft of middle ear structures
  —Reconstruction of the TM is achieved in about 90% of patients, resulting in elimination of infections, improved hearing, and decreased chance of complications.

  —Mastoidectomy is performed when the mastoid air cells are involved.
  —When cholesteatomas are present, surgical marsupialization of the sac or removal of the sac is performed.
- Nonsurgical treatment
  —Regular removal of infected debris
  —Use of earplugs to protect against water exposure
  —Topical antibiotic drops for exacerbations
  —Ciprofloxacin 500 mg PO bid for 1 to 6 weeks helps to dry out a chronically discharging ear and protect against *Pseudomonas* organisms.

Patient/Family Education
- Explain the nature of the disorder, its cause(s), and its treatment.
- Emphasize the importance of protecting the ear from exposure to water or other potential dangers (blasting, loud noises).
- Explain treatment modalities and the need for patient cooperation.
- If surgery becomes necessary, explain the procedure(s) to be done, the reason for them, and expected outcomes.

Follow-up/Referral
- Patients with COM often require regular visits to the otolaryngologist.
- Write out a list of dates and times of appointments to enable the patient to make long-term arrangement at work, school, or other.

Mastoiditis

Definition
Acute mastoiditis occurs when there is a bacterial infection in the mastoid process, which results in coalescence of the mastoid air cells.

Risk Factors
- Recent acute purulent otitis media

Etiology/Cause
- A chronic infection of the middle ear, with extension to the mastoid process

Pathophysiology
- Chronic infectious process in the mastoid can result in necrosis of the bone of the mas-

toid process and breakdown of the bony structure.

- If untreated, the infection can cause formation of subperiosteal abscesses and extension into the coverings of the brain as meningitis, or facial paralysis, brain abscesses, or sigmoid sinus thrombosis, which are all serious complications.

Diagnosis
Signs and Symptoms
- In most cases, large accumulation of thick, purulent material fills the external auditory canal, indicating perforation of the TM.
- The soft tissue near the eardrum may rupture and sag.

Diagnostic Tests
- X-rays or CT scan may show clouding of the air cells, decalcification of the bony walls, and complete coalescence of the air cells.
- Audiometry, to determine extent of hearing loss and degree of middle ear obstruction

Treatment
- Intensive antibiotic therapy is initiated.
- Myringotomy may be required to debride the area.
- Mastoidectomy is preformed to completely eradicate the affected tissues.

Patient/Family Education
- Provide clear explanation of the problem and the usual course of treatment.
- Discuss potential for hearing loss.
- Reassure patient and family that many support services are available if needed.
- Explain that noises (e.g., crackling, popping) usually follow mastoid surgery for variable lengths of time.
- Instruct about usual degree of pain, and that any sudden increase in pain level should be reported to the clinician at once.
- Emphasize that water must be kept out of both ears by use of earplugs or by placing cottonballs coated with petroleum jelly into the external ear before bathing.
- Instruct the patient to request permission of the otolaryngologist for air flight, should travel be necessary.

Otosclerosis
Definition
Otosclerosis is a progressive disease with a marked familial tendency that affects bone surrounding the inner ear. This disorder is often the cause of progressive conductive hearing loss in adults with a normal TM.

Risk Factors
- Autosomal dominant inheritance
- White race
- Age: late teens, early twenties

Etiology/Cause
- Inherited autosomal dominant genes
- About 10% of white adults have foci of otosclerosis.

Pathogenesis
- Otosclerotic lesions involving the footplate of the stapes result in decreased sound transmission through the ossicular chain, resulting in conductive hearing loss.
- When otosclerotic lesions impinge on the cochlea, permanent sensory hearing loss occurs.

Diagnosis
Signs and Symptoms
- Otosclerosis becomes clinically apparent in the late teens or early twenties with slowly progressive, asymmetric hearing loss.
- Fixation of the stapes may occur rapidly during pregnancy.

Treatment
- Initial trial with a hearing aid or microsurgical techniques to improve hearing
- One microsurgical technique is removal of the stapes and replacement with a prosthesis (stapedectomy), which corrects the hearing loss.
- Oral sodium fluoride—Florical 8.3 mg—and calcium carbonate 364 mg (2 tabs PO every morning) may stabilize hearing loss.

Patient/Family Education
- Explain the disorder, its likely cause(s), and treatment.
- Treating hearing loss requires patients to have a great deal of patience.

- Describe the treatment and expected outcomes.
- If the patient is prescribed medications, describe the medication, reasons for giving them, and action.
- If surgery is to be done, explain the procedure(s) and how they will affect the patient's hearing.

Prognosis
- Prognosis is favorable, as long as hearing loss can be minimized or stabilized.

Follow-up/Referral
- Regular check-ups and hearing tests will evaluate patient's progress over time. Always provide new information as it becomes available.

DISORDERS OF THE INNER EAR

The inner ear consists of the auditory portion (cochlea, saccule, acoustic nerve) and the vestibular portion (semicircular canals, utricle, superior and inferior vestibular nerves).

Meniere's Disease
Definition
Meniere's disease (or syndrome) is characterized by recurrent, severe vertigo, sensory hearing loss, tinnitus, and a sensation of fullness or pressure in the ear. It is associated with generalized dilation of the membranous labyrinth (endolymphatic hydrops).

Risk Factors
- Head trauma
- Syphilis

Etiology/Cause
- No precise cause for the syndrome is known.
- The two risk factors are also causes, but the syndrome can develop in the absence of either syphilis or head trauma.

Pathogenesis
- Pathophysiology of the syndrome is not fully understood.
- The primary lesion seems to be in the endolymphatic sac, which is thought to be re-

sponsible for endolymph filtration and excretion.

Diagnosis
Signs and Symptoms
- Episodic vertigo, lasting from 1 to 8 hours
- Low-frequency sensorineural hearing loss, often fluctuating
- Tinnitus, usually low-pitched and "blowing" in quality
- Sensation of aural fullness or pressure
- These manifestations come and go as the endolymphatic pressure rises and falls.

Diagnostic Tests
- Caloric testing may show loss or impairment of thermally induced nystagmus on the affected side (test involves instillation of cold water into the ear canal, which normally causes nystagmus).

Treatment
- Therapy is aimed at lowering endolymphatic pressure.
- Low-sodium diet (<2 g sodium daily)
- Diuretic (usually hydrochlorothiazide 50 to 100 mg qd) as required to supplement the low-sodium diet by decreasing body fluid, thus decreasing the endolymphatic pressure in the inner ear.
- If medical treatment fails to relieve symptoms, surgical decompression of the endolymphatic sac may eliminate symptoms.

Prognosis
- Vertigo and tinnitus can be extremely disruptive for the patient, particularly if the symptoms persist; the prognosis is good with appropriate and timely therapy.

Patient/Family Education
- Explain the nature and cause of the condition.
- Describe the usual treatment, and that surgery is not done unless medical management fails to relieve symptoms.
- Reassure the patient that the symptoms can be relieved.
- Emphasize the importance of physical activity in preventing attacks of vertigo.

DISORDERS OF THE CENTRAL AUDITORY AND VESTIBULAR SYSTEMS

Lesions of the eighth cranial nerve and central audiovestibular pathways produce neural hearing loss and vertigo. Neural hearing loss is characterized by deterioration of speech discrimination out of proportion to the decrease in pure tone thresholds. Another characteristic is auditory adaptation, in which a steady tone seems to the listener to diminish and then disappear.

Vertigo resulting from central lesions tends to be more chronic and debilitating than that seen in labyrinthine disorders. The associated nystagmus is often nonfatigable, vertical rather than horizontal, and is not suppressed by visual fixation.

Evaluation of central audiovestibular dysfunction usually requires imaging of the brain with CT scans or magnetic resonance imaging (MRI), along with the paramagnetic contrast agent gadolinium-gadopentetate dieglumine (DTPA) (with MRI), which significantly improves the diagnostic sensitivity in detecting central audiovestibular lesions.

Vestibular Schwannoma (Acoustic Neuroma)

Definition
Vestibular schwannomas are eighth nerve tumors that arise from Schwann cells and are among the most common of intracranial benign tumors, accounting for about 7% of these tumors.

Risk Factors
- None known.

Etiology/Cause
- Whereas Schwann cells are implicated in the development of these tumors, other etiologic factors are not known.

Pathogenesis
- Acoustic neuromas develop within the auditory canal and gradually grow to involve the cerebropontine angle, eventually compressing the pons and resulting in hydrocephalus.

Diagnosis
- Auditory symptoms include unilateral hearing loss, with deterioration of speech discrimination greater than that associated with the degree of pure tone loss.
- Sudden unilateral hearing loss is an atypical presentation but occurs fairly frequently.
- Any person with unilateral or asymmetric sensorineural hearing loss should be evaluated for an intracranial mass lesion.
- Vestibular dysfunction usually occurs in the form of continuous dysequilibrium rather than episodic vertigo.
- Definitive diagnosis is made by enhanced MRI.

Treatment
- Excision by microsurgery is indicated.
- Small tumors in older patients may be managed with stereotactic radiotherapy, or they may be followed with just serial imaging studies.

Patient/Family Education
- Provide an explanation of the condition, and what is known about cause and incidence.
- Emphasize the fact that acoustic neuromas are benign tumors, which, if small enough, do not require immediate surgery.
- Instruct the patient to report symptoms on a regular basis, and to come for serial imaging studies regularly, to determine whether the tumor is growing, and at what rate, so that plans can be formulated for surgical excision.

Prognosis
- Favorable

OTOLOGIC MANIFESTATIONS OF AIDS

Manifestations of acquired immunodeficiency syndrome (AIDS) with respect to the ear include Kaposi's sarcoma of the pinna and external canal and persistent invasive fungal infections, usually caused by *Aspergillus fumigatus*.

The most common middle ear manifestation of AIDS is serous otitis media due to auditory tube dysfunction resulting from adenoidal hypertrophy (human immunodeficiency disease [HIV] lymphadenopathy), recurrent mucosal viral infections, or an obstructing nasopharyngeal tumor (e.g., lymphoma). Insertion of ventilating tubes in AIDS patients when middle ear effusions are present is not helpful and may trigger profuse watery otorrhea.

Acute otitis media is usually caused by the typical bacterial organisms that occur in immunocompromised patients.

Inner ear manifestations in AIDS patients include sensorineural hearing loss, which is common and likely caused by viral central nervous system infection. In cases of progressive hearing loss, the patient should be evaluated for cryptococcal meningitis and syphilis.

Facial paralysis due to herpes zoster infection (Ramsay Hunt syndrome) is common and follows a clinical course similar to that in nonimmunocompromised patients. Treatment is with high-dose acyclovir, and corticosteroids may be helpful.

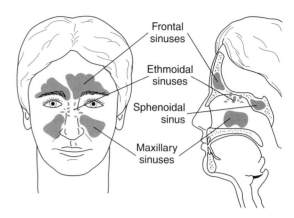

Fig. 20-4 Location of sinuses (sphenoid sinuses are directly behind ethmoid sinuses). (From Lewis SM, Heitkemper MM, Dirksen SR: *Medical surgical assessment and management of clinical problems,* ed 5, St. Louis, 2000, Mosby, p. 587.)

DISORDERS OF THE NOSE AND SINUSES

The primary functions of the nose are to cleanse, humidify, and warm inspired air. The upper portion of the nose is supported by bone; the lower portion by cartilage. Inside, the nose is covered by well-vascularized mucosa. The most anterior portion—the vestibule—is, unlike the rest of the nose, covered by hair-bearing skin rather than mucous membrane, for further protection against inhaled foreign substances.

The inferior, middle, and superior turbinates are bony structures within the nose that are covered with mucosa. The inferior meatus or groove is situated below the inferior turbinate and drains the nasolacrimal duct. The middle meatus drains the paranasal sinuses.

The paranasal sinuses (maxillary, frontal, ethmoid, and sphenoid) are cavities in the bones of the skull that normally are filled with air, and are lined with mucous membrane (Fig. 20-4). These sinuses open into the nasal cavity. Their purpose is not clear. Only the frontal and maxillary sinuses can be directly examined.

Viral Rhinitis (Common Cold)
Definition
Rhinitis is an inflammation of the nasal mucous membrane, causing edema and vasodilation, nasal discharge, and obstruction due to swelling and mucous drainage.

- Types include the following:
  —Acute rhinitis: the usual manifestation of the common cold
  —Chronic rhinitis: a prolongation of subacute inflammatory or infectious rhinitis
  ~ May occur in patients with syphilis, tuberculosis (TB), rhinoscleroma, rhinosporidiosis, blastomycosis, and histoplasmosis.
  ~ Any of these conditions are characterized by granuloma formation and destruction of soft tissue, cartilage, and bone.
  ~ These conditions result in nasal obstruction, purulent rhinorrhea, and frequent bleeding.
  ~ Rhinosporidiosis is characterized by bleeding polyps.

Risk Factors
- Exposure to others with a URI
- Poorly nourished or immunocompromised persons

Etiology/Cause
- Rhinitis is most frequently caused by viral infection, but may also be caused by streptococcal, pneumococcal, or staphylococcal organisms.

Diagnosis
Signs and Symptoms
- Headache
- Nasal congestion
- Watery rhinorrhea
- Sneezing
- Scratchy sore throat
- General malaise
- Low-grade fever may be present, and subnormal temperature is common.
- Examination of the nose usually shows reddened, inflamed, edematous mucosa and a watery discharge.
- If a purulent nasal discharge is present, it indicates bacterial infection.

Treatment
- Supportive measures help to relieve discomfort and symptoms.
- A decongestant (e.g., pseudoephedrine 30 mg q4h, or 120 mg bid) may relieve nasal congestion and rhinorrhea.
- Nasal sprays (e.g., oxymetazolone, phenylephrine) are effective but should not be used for more than 2 to 3 days, because chronic use results in rebound congestion.
- Tylenol at dosages recommended on the label, depending on the age of the patient, are helpful in relieving headache and general malaise.
- Provide plenty of fluids and light meals as desired.

Patient/Family Education
- As far as possible, the patient should be segregated from other family members to avoid spread of the virus.
- Patients should use paper tissues, which should be collected in a paper bag for disposal by burning.
- Paper tissues should be used to cover the mouth and nose when coughing or sneezing.
- Encourage the patient to drink a lot of fluids of various kinds: orange juice, water, hot or cold tea.
- Encourage the patient to be as active as possible without causing undue fatigue.

Allergic Rhinitis
Definition
Immunoglobulin E (IgE)–mediated rhinitis is characterized by seasonal or perennial sneezing, rhinorrhea, nasal congestion, pruritus, and conjunctivitis and pharyngitis. Hay fever (pollinosis) is the acute seasonal form of allergic rhinitis

Risk Factors
- Exposure to known allergens (tree, grass, or weed pollens), airborne fungal spores
- Family history of allergies

Etiology/Cause
- Specific allergy to plants, trees, or other allergens
- Reaction to allergens, specific to individuals

Pathogenesis
- The precise interaction of allergens in persons with known allergies to specific substances is not clearly understood.
- Allergy develops only after one exposure has occurred.
- In antigen-antibody interactions, mast cell degranulation and chemical mediator release occur, causing slower ciliary action, stimulation of mucosal glands, and leukocyte (eosinophil) infiltration.
- Histamine is the primary mediator of the inflammation, with other factors.
- Hyperplasia and thickening of the mucosal epithelium occur.
- Proliferation of connective tissue is evident.

Diagnosis
Signs and Symptoms
- Redness and edema of local tissues
- Intermittent nasal obstruction
- Clear nasal discharge
- Postnasal drainage
- Sneezing
- Tearing and itchiness of eyes
- Irritation of nose, palate
- Mucosa covering the turbinates is pale

Diagnostic Tests
- Positive skin tests—responses correspond to history and symptoms
- Serology—radioallergosorbent test (RAST) shows increased IgE levels.
- Sinus x-rays
- Microscopic scrapings of nasal mucosa show eosinophils.
- CT scan of sinuses

Treatment
- The goal of therapy is to alleviate symptoms.
- Increase fluid intake.
- Oral decongestant, antihistamine medication
- Intranasal steroid spray—beclomethasone, flunisolide
- Antibiotic agents for secondary bacterial infection, if present
- Analgesic therapy for patient comfort

Patient/Family Education
- Provide information about allergies: if condition is first-time occurrence, give comprehensive instructions about self-care.
- Explain about the length of time needed to detect causative allergen(s).
- Instruct about medication and use of nasal spray for limited time.
- Instruct about use of warm salt-water solution mouthwash and nasal spray.

Acute Sinusitis

Definition
Acute sinusitis is the inflammation of the paranasal sinuses due to viral, bacterial, or fungal infections or allergic reactions.
- Types
  —Acute (see Etiology/Cause)
  —Chronic sinusitis may be exacerbated by a gram-negative rod or anaerobic microorganisms; in some cases, chronic maxillary sinusitis may be secondary to dental infection.

Risk Factors
- Recent acute viral respiratory tract infection

Etiology/Cause
- Acute sinusitis is usually caused by streptococci, pneumococci, *H. influenzae,* or staphylococci

Pathogenesis
- When an upper respiratory tract infection is present, the swollen nasal mucous membrane obstructs the ostium of a paranasal sinus and the oxygen in the sinus is absorbed into the blood vessels of the mucous membrane, which creates a relative negative pressure in the sinus (vacuum sinusitis), causing pain.

- If the vacuum is not relieved, a transudate from the mucous membrane develops and fills the sinus, with the transudate serving as a medium for bacteria that enter the sinus through the ostium or by way of a spreading cellulitis or thrombophlebitis in the mucous membrane.
- This stimulates an outpouring of serum and leukocytes to combat the infection, which causes painful positive pressure in the obstructed sinus, causing the mucous membrane to become hyperemic and edematous.

Diagnosis
Signs and Symptoms
- The area over the affected sinus becomes tender and swollen.
- Pain can be felt in the maxillary or frontal areas, depending on which sinus(es) are affected.
- Ethmoid sinusitis causes pain behind and between the eyes and a "splitting" frontal headache.
- Sphenoid sinusitis results in more diffuse pain, often referred to the frontal or occipital areas.
- Malaise, fever, and chills suggest an extension of the infection beyond the sinuses.
- Dizziness may occur due to congested mucous membranes in the nose and throat.
- The mucous membrane of the nose is red and inflamed, and a yellow or green purulent discharge may be present.

Diagnostic Tests
- The infected sinuses may appear opaque on x-ray because of the exudate filling the cavities; CT provides better definition of the extent of the infection.

Treatment
- Steam inhalation effectively produces nasal vasoconstriction and promotes drainage.
- Saline nasal washes may promote drainage.
- Topical vasoconstrictors (e.g., phenylephrine 0.25% spray q3h) are effective but limited to a maximum of 7 doses.
- Systemic vasoconstrictors (e.g., pseudoephedrine 30 mg PO q4-6h [adult dose]) are less effective.

- If antibiotics seem necessary, they should be given for at least 10 to 12 days.
- For acute sinusitis, penicillin V 250 mg PO q6h is the drug of choice.
- Erythromycin 250 mg PO q6h is the second choice.
- In exacerbations of chronic sinusitis, broad-spectrum antibiotics, such as ampicillin 250 to 500 mg or tetracycline 250 mg PO q6h, are indicated, given for 4 to 6 weeks to ensure complete resolution.
- Sinusitis that does not respond to medical therapy may require surgery.

Patient/Family Education

- Explain the nature of sinusitis, both acute and chronic, and the symptoms.
- Explain the need for treatment, beginning with steam inhalation and proceeding to antibiotic therapy if indicated.
- If the patient is given antibiotics, emphasize the need to take every dose as prescribed and on schedule for the full 4 to 6 weeks to ensure complete resolution of the infection.
- Stress good nutrition, dental hygiene, and plenty of fluid intake, both during treatment and afterward.

Follow-up/Referral

- Any patient who does not respond to a reasonable course of therapy should be referred to an otolaryngologist for further evaluation and perhaps surgery.
- Patients with poorly controlled diabetes who develop sinusitis should be referred to an otolaryngologist from the outset because they sometimes develop mucomycosis due to fungi of the order Mucorales, which is characterized by devitalized, black tissue in the nasal cavity and neurologic signs secondary to retrograde thromboarteritis in the carotid arterial system.
- Aspergillosis and candidiasis of the paransal sinuses may occur in patients who are immunocompromised due to cytotoxic drugs or underlying disease processes of leukemia, lymphoma, multiple myeloma, AIDS, or other immunosuppressive diseases.
- These patients may require extensive paranasal sinus surgery and intravenous (IV) amphotericin B.

Neoplasms

Definition

Neoplasms are tumors of the nose and paranasal sinuses that are frequently malignant.

Risk Factors

- Smoking or other tobacco use
- Wood dust (causes cancer of the nasal cavity)
- Chronic irritation from any source (chemicals, cleaning compounds)
- Long-term use of alcohol
- Epstein-Barr virus (EBV)
- Poor oral hygiene

Etiology/Cause

- Cancerous growths can appear in the nose and paranasal sinuses.
- Exophytic papillomas are squamoous cell papillomas that have a branching, vascular connective tissue stalk with fingerlike projections on the surface; these growths are seen in the nasal cavity and require repeated excision but tend to run a benign course.
- Inverted papillomaas are squamous cell papillomas in which the epithelium is invaginated into the vascular connective tissue stroma.
  —**These neoplasms are invasive and are malignant.**
  —Excision requires a large margin of normal tissue, including bone of the lateral wall of the nasal cavity—a procedure called lateral rhinotomy.
- Fibromas, hemangiomas, and neurofibromas are benign tumors that occur in the nasal cavity and require excision only if they create obstruction.
- Squamous cell carcinoma is the most common malignant tumor in the nose and paranasal sinuses; radical resection and radiation therapy provide the best survival rates for patients with cancerous tumors.

Diagnosis

Signs and Symptoms

- Early symptoms are vague, nonspecific (e.g., sinusitis, rhinitis)
- Unilateral nasal obstruction
- Discharge
- Pain, localized
- Recurrent bleeding (significant sign)

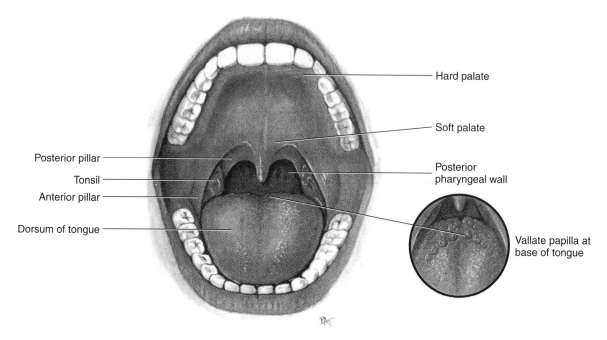

Fig. 20-5 Parts of the mouth (From Jarvis C: *Physical examination and health assessment,* Philadelphia, 1992, WB Saunders, p 402.)

- Unilateral unresolved serous otitis media
- Hearing loss
- Neck mass
- Diplopia
- Cranial neuropathy (especially CN VI)
- Loose teeth
- Proptosis
- Swelling around sinuses, cheeks, eyes
- Lymphadenopathy—neck, jaw, face

Diagnostic Tests
- CT scan
- MRI
- Biopsy of lymph nodes

Treatment
- If you suspect cancer in any patient, refer immediately to a specialist: oncologist, otolaryngologist, and others.
- Management depends on the extent of the tumor, type of tumor, and current therapy: surgical resection, radiation therapy, or chemotherapy.

Patient/Family Education
- Explain the nature of the neoplasm, its location, and usual treatment.
- If referral to a specialist is required, let the patient know.
- Provide a list of specialists and recommend several from which the patient can choose.
- Reassure the patient, but do not give details about therapy; say that the specialist will decide about treatment, after consultation with the patient and family.

DISORDERS OF THE PHARYNX (FIG. 20-5)

Thirty-two teeth are present in the adult's mouth, based in and surrounded by the gums (gingivae). The gingivae are thick, fibrous tissue covered by pale pink mucous membrane. The anterior part of the palate is the soft portion, and posterior to the soft palate is the hard palate, which becomes lighter in color toward the back. The uvula hangs from the roof of the mouth at the back. The dorsal aspect of the tongue is covered with papillae, the largest of which are at the back of the tongue. These papillae help to move food along so that it can be swallowed easily. The tonsils, which atrophy with age if they are not removed surgically before then, lie between the anterior and posterior pillars at the back of the throat.

Acute Pharyngitis

Definition
Pharyngitis is acute inflammation of the pharynx.

Risk Factors
- Recent upper respiratory infection
- Exposure to someone infected with viral or bacterial URI

Etiology/Cause
- Although pharyngitis is usually a viral infection, it may also be caused by other organisms: group A β-hemolytic streptococci, *Mycoplasma pneumoniae*, *Chlamydia pneumoniae*, or other bacteria.

Pathogenesis
- Differentiating viral from bacterial pharyngitis on the basis of physical examination alone is difficult. In both, the pharyngeal mucous membrane may be mildly injected or severely inflamed and may be covered by a membrane and a purulent exudate.

Diagnosis
- Examination of the mouth and throat shows a reddened, inflamed mucous membrane, sometimes with drainage at the back of the throat.
- The throat is quite painful, making swallowing difficult.
- Fever may be present, whether the inflammation is viral or bacterial, and may reach 39° C (102° F); bacterial infection usually exhibits a higher fever.
- Cervical adenopathy and lymphadenopathy may be present, sometimes with painful nodes.
- Leukocytosis is present in both viral and bacterial infections but may be more marked in bacterial infection.

Diagnostic Tests
- Complete blood count with differential culture of exudate at back of throat

Treatment
- Acetaminophen to relieve discomfort
- Antibiotic therapy is usually begun at the first visit, without waiting for the results of the throat culture.
  - Penicillin V 250 mg PO q6h for 10 days (for group A streptococcal pharyngitis)
  - Alternatively, parenteral penicillin G benzathine, oral erythromycin, or a first-generation cephalosporin may be prescribed.

Patient/Family Education
- Instruct the patient to increase the normal intake of fluids.
- Warm saline gargles may help relieve the pain and decrease the amount of drainage at the back of the throat.
- Rest and a light diet of soft foods will prevent added injury to the throat.
- Emphasize that the antibiotic and acetaminophen should be taken as prescribed, on schedule.
- Instruct the patient to call or come to the clinic if the infection seems to be getting worse (e.g., greater lymphadenopathy, increased pain, difficulty swallowing, which may indicate peritonsillar abscess).

Peritonsillar Cellulitis and Abscess

Definition
A peritonsillar abscess (quinsy) is an acute infection between the tonsil and the superior pharyngeal constrictor muscle. This condition is rare in children and more common in young adults.

Risk Factors
- Exposure to organisms that may cause peritonsillar abscess
- Poor nutritional state

Etiology/Cause
- Although group A β-hemolytic streptococcus is the primary organism, others may be the cause as well, including anaerobic microorganisms such as bacteroides.

Diagnosis

Signs and Symptoms
- Swallowing causes severe pain.
- The patient is usually febrile and toxic.
- The patient tilts his/her head toward the side of the abscess.
- The patient shows marked trismus.
- The tonsil is displaced medially by the peritonsillar cellulitis and abscess.
- The uvula is edematous and displaced to the opposite side.

Treatment
- Cellulitis without pus formation responds to penicillin in 24 to 48 hours.
- Penicillin G 1 MU IV q4h is given initially.
- If pus is present and does not drain spontaneously, aspiration or incision and drainage is required, performed by an otolaryngologist.
- Penicillin V 250 mg PO q6h is then given for 12 days unless cultures and sensitivity indicate that another antibiotic is preferable.
- Throat irrigations with warm saline provide some pain relief and aid in drainage.
- Acetaminophen or codeine is given for pain as needed.
- If the patient has a history of recurrent peritonsillar abscesses, tonsillectomy may be considered, performed either 6 weeks after the acute infection has subsided, or during the acute episode, if antibiotic therapy is given concomitantly.

Patient/Family Education
- Explain the problem and the usual course of therapy to the patient.
- Describe the medications and the reasons they are being prescribed.
- If throat irrigations are initiated, demonstrate the equipment set-up and how to direct the flow of solution.
- Instruct the patient to request pain medication when needed.
- If tonsillectomy is planned, explain the procedure to the patient.
- Instruct the patient to call the otolaryngologist at once if excessive bleeding occurs after surgery.

DISORDERS OF THE LARYNX
Vocal Cord Polyps

Definition
Vocal cord polyps are chronic edema in the lamina propria of the true vocal cords.

Risk Factors
- Smoking
- Long-term inhalation of irritants such as cleaning compounds

Etiology/Cause
- Voice abuse (e.g., singing)
- Allergic reactions that affect the larynx
- Cigarette smoking
- Industrial fumes

Pathogenesis
- If the larynx is exposed to irritants over time, it becomes inflamed, causing hoarseness and a breathy voice.

Diagnosis
- If a patient exhibits symptoms suggesting vocal cord polyps, referral to an otolaryngologist is mandatory.
- Biopsy of a few lesions, performed by microlaryngoscopy, to rule out carcinoma

Treatment
- Surgical removal of polyps to restore the voice
- Elimination of underlying cause (e.g., smoking, voice abuse)

Patient/Family Education
- Explain the nature of the problem, possible cause(s), and usual treatment.
- Reassure the patient that treatment will correct the problem.
- After surgery, elimination of causative factors is required (e.g., stop smoking, distance from industrial fumes, stop voice abuse).

Cancer, Leukoplakia, and Erythroplakia

Definition
Leukoplakia and other similar plaques are precancerous lesions that can be found on mucous membranes in many areas of the body, including the oral cavity.

Risk Factors
- Male sex
- Between 40 and 60 years of age
- Cigarette smoking
- Alcohol abuse
- Use of betel nut, snuff, or oral tobacco

Pathogenesis
- Most common sites of these lesions are the inner cheeks, lips, and lower gingivae.
- Exposure to cigarette smoke, oral tobacco, and other tobacco products causes epithelial tissue to break down, predisposing the area to development of precancerous and cancerous lesions.
- Leukoplakia are white patches that develop and adhere tightly to mucous membranes, and cannot be removed by simple rubbing.
- Of these leukoplakia lesions, between 2% and 8% become malignant.
- Erythroplakia are lesions similar to leukoplakia, except that they are red, and 90% are or become cancerous.
- Ninety percent of oral cancers are squamous cell carcinoma.

Diagnosis
- Most lesions are painless and remain undetected until the lesions are ≥2 cm or more in diameter.
- Any oral sore or lesion that bleeds easily or does not heal is suspected of being cancerous.
- Any lump or thickening in the mouth is also suspect.
- Difficulty in chewing or moving food around in the mouth is an indication of advanced disease.
- Biopsy of any suspicious area/lesion
- X-ray or bone scan of mandible
- CT scans of all areas of the mouth, throat, and neck
- Endoscopy with examination under anesthesia to determine extent of lesions

Treatment
- Referral of patients with suspicious lesions, lumps, or plaques to an otolaryngologist is mandatory.
- If areas prove to be precancerous or cancerous, surgery with reconstruction is indicated.
- Surgery may be total laryngectomy, modified radical neck dissection, or mandibular resection and reconstruction.
- Surgery is followed by radiation therapy or chemotherapy as appropriate.

Patient/Family Education
- Instruct all patients about oral hygiene and how to self-examine their mouth—floor, inside of cheeks, and palate—using palpation and visualization with a mirror.
- Explain the nature of any lesions found and usual treatment.
- Strongly encourage all patients to stop smoking, use of oral tobacco, and drinking alcohol.
- Emphasize the importance of keeping all appointments, and following the instructions of the otolaryngologist as to surgery and follow-up therapy.

Candidiasis
Definition
Candidiasis is a yeast infection of the mouth (visible) or esophagus (invisible except by endoscopy).

Risk Factors
- HIV/AIDS
- Chronic disease
- Recent treatment with antibiotics
- Pregnancy
- Diabetes mellitus
- Poorly nourished
- Radiation therapy to the mouth
- Persons who wear dentures

Pathogenesis
- The mouth, throat, or esophagus may be affected after exposure to the organism *Candida albicans*.
- Fungal spores lodge between cells, gradually increasing in number, resulting in separation of epithelial layers, which predisposes to the spread of yeast within the mouth.

Diagnosis
Signs and Symptoms
- Pain, irritation, or discomfort in the mouth and throat
- Difficulty swallowing

- Soft, creamy white patches that look like milk curd, which are easily wiped away with gauze or cotton-tipped applicator, leaving areas of erythema
- Generalized erythema of mucosa
- It is necessary to distinguish candidiasis from leukoplakia or erythroplakia.
- Cells can be stained with Schiff purple stain.
- Culture and sensitivity of lesions
- Complete blood count (CBC), serum B_{12} and folic acid levels
- X-ray with dental film floor of the mouth from below the jaw
- Barium swallow or esophagoscopy if extension to the esophagus is suspected

Treatment
- Topical oral antifungal
  —Nystatin 500,000 units as a gargle five times/day
  —Clotrimazole troches 10 mg five times/day
- Systemic antifungal
  —Fluconazole 100 mg PO once
- Thorough cleaning of the mouth, teeth, or dentures one to two times/day
- Refer if patient does not respond to therapy previously described.

Patient/Family Education
- Preventive measures regarding treatment of underlying problems that predispose to yeast infections
  —Control of diabetes
  —Oral hygiene and thorough cleaning of dentures twice a day
  —Regular examination/self-examination of mouth, teeth, and gingivae
  —Dental checkups every 6 months

DISORDERS OF THE NECK

The side of the neck can be divided into two triangles bordered by the sternocleidomastoid muscles. The posterior triangle is bordered by the trapezius muscle posteriorly, the clavicle inferiorly, and the sternocleidomastoid muscle anteriorly. The anterior triangle is bordered by the sternocleidomastoid muscle posteriorly, the edge of the mandible superiorly, and the midline of the neck anteriorly. These landmarks help to place the locations of the vital structures of the neck.

The lymph nodes of the head and neck are located in front of and behind the ear; above, beneath, and along the edges of the sternocleidomastoid muscles; and inferior to the edge of the mandible and chin. These nodes play an extremely important role in diagnosis and follow-up of problems of the head and neck. Normally, lymph nodes are round or oval, smooth, soft, small (1 cm), and nontender.

Neck Masses
Definition
Head and neck masses include any neoplasm anywhere in these areas.

Risk Factors
- The average age of persons with head and neck cancers is 59 years.
- Persons who develop sarcomas or carcinomas of the salivary glands, thyroid gland, or paranasal sinuses are usually less than 59 years of age.
- Those who develop squamous cell carcinoma of the oral cavity, pharynx, or larynx are usually older than 59 years.

Etiology/Cause
- The most common cancer of the upper respiratory and alimentary tracts is squamous cell carcinoma of the larynx; next is squamous cell carcinoma of the palatine tonsil and hypopharynx.
- About 85% of patients with cancer of the head and neck have a history of ethanol or tobacco abuse.
- The EBV is associated with the pathogenesis of nasopharyngeal cancer.
- Patients treated with small doses of radiation ≥25 years ago are predisposed to develop thyroid and salivary gland cancer.
- Patients with HIV/AIDS or who are otherwise immunocompromised tend to develop hematogenous metastases from large or persistent tumors.

Pathogenesis
- A primary lesion develops at some point in the neck or head, and gradually increases in size until it becomes apparent to the patient or the examiner; many tumors of the head and neck, however, remain undetected for

years, until their growth becomes noticeable, which may also be at an advanced stage.

Diagnosis

- Head and neck cancers are classified according to size and site of the primary lesion (T), number and size of metastases to the cervical lymph nodes (N), and evidence of distant metastases (M).
- Stages are also used to classify these cancers.
  - —Stage I: The primary neoplasm is ≤2 cm at greatest dimension, or localized to one anatomic site without regional or distant metastases (T1N0M0).
  - —Stage II: The primary neoplasm is 2 to 4 cm at greatest dimension, or affects two areas in a specific site (e.g., larynx), with no regional or distant metastasis (T2N0M0).
  - —Stage III: The primary neoplasm is >4 cm at greatest dimension, or affects three adjacent areas in a specific head and neck site, and/or has an isolated neck metastasis of ≤3 cm at greatest dimension (T3N0M0 or T1-3N1M0).
  - —Stage IV: The cancer is massive, invades bone and cartilage, and/or extends outside of its site of origin into another site (e.g., oral cavity into oropharynx). The neck metastasis measures >3 cm and affects multiple ipsilateral, contralateral, or bilateral lymph nodes, or is fixed to surrounding tissue, and/or there is evidence of distant metastases (T1-4N1-3M0-1).
- Clinical staging is usually supplemented or confirmed by CT or MRI.

Treatment

- Stage I: most primary neoplasms, whether in the respiratory or alimentary tract, respond the same to surgery and to radiation therapy; other factors usually determine choice of therapy.
  - —In radiation therapy, it is delivered to the primary site and, if the likelihood of regional, nonpalpable metastasis is >20%, then also to the bilateral cervical lymph nodes. In these cases, there is a 5-year cure rate in 90% of patients.
  - —Lesions >2 cm or with bone or cartilage invasion (with or without regional neck

metastasis) require surgical resection of the primary site and possible resection of regional lymph nodes

  - ~ If lymph node metastases are found or considered very likely to occur, postoperative radiation therapy to the primary site and bilaterally to any remaining cervical lymph nodes
  - ~ An alternative to surgery, radiation therapy—with or without chemotherapy—is given; if the cancer recurs, the patient may choose surgery.
- —In advanced squamous cell cancer (most of Stage II and all of Stages III and IV), combined surgery and radiation therapy offers a better chance of cure than with either one alone.
  - ~ Surgery is more effective than radiation therapy or chemotherapy in controlling large primary tumors.
  - ~ Radiation is more effective in controlling the periphery of primary lesions, and of microscopic or nonpalpable metastases; radiation therapy may be given preoperatively or postoperatively but is usually given after surgery.

Prognosis

- With appropriate treatment, survival rates are
  - —Stage I: 90%
  - —Stage II: 75%
  - —Stage III: 45% to 75%
  - —Stage IV: <35%
- Patients over age 70 often have longer disease-free periods and better success rates than do younger patients.

SYSTEMIC DISORDERS WITH ENT SYMPTOMS AND MANIFESTATIONS
Infectious Mononucleosis

Definition

Infectious mononucleosis is an acute infection due to EBV, characterized by fever, pharyngitis, and lymphadenopathy.

Risk Factors

- Exposure to the EBV
- Adolescent age

Etiology/Cause

- The EBV enters through the upper respiratory or digestive tracts.
- Transmission may occur by transfusion of blood products but more often occurs by oropharyngeal contact (kissing).
- Transmission in early childhood occurs more often among lower socioeconomic groups and in crowded conditions.

Pathogenesis

- After initial replication in the nasopharynx, the virus infects beta lymphocytes, which are induced to secrete immunoglobulins, including antibodies called heterophil antibodies, which are useful in diagnosis.
- The EBV-transformed lymphocytes are the target of a multifaceted immune response, both humoral and cellular.
- After primary infection, the EBV remains within the host for life and is intermittently shed from the oropharynx.
  - The virus is detectable in oropharyngeal secretions of 15% to 25% of healthy EBV-seropositive adults.
  - Shedding is greater and more frequent in immunocompromised patients (e.g., organ allograft recipients and HIV-infected persons).
- Reactivation of EBV is usually subclinical, unlike the herpes simplex or varicella-zoster virus.
- The EBV is relatively labile, has not been found in environmental sources, and is not very contagious.
- The incubation period is probably 30 to 50 days.

Diagnosis

Signs and Symptoms

- Fever, fatigue, pharyngitis, and lymphadenopathy are common.
  - Fatigue is maximal in the first 2 to 3 weeks.
  - Fever peaks in the late afternoon or early evening, at about 39.5° C (103° F), although it can reach 40.5° C (105° F).
- When fever and fatigue predominate (typhoidal form), onset and resolution may be much slower.

- The pharyngitis may be severe, painful, and exudative, resembling streptococcal pharyngitis.
- Lymphadenopathy may involve any nodes, but is usually symmetric.
- Splenomegaly is present in about 50% of cases and is most pronounced during the second or third week.
- Mild hepatomegaly and tenderness on hepatic percussion may occur.

Diagnostic Tests

- CBC with differential—mild leukocytosis, atypical lymphocytes may be absent or may account for up to 80% of the white blood cell (WBC) differential count.
- Heterophil titer—heterophil antibodies
- EBV-viral capsid antigen (VCA) antibodies are seen during the incubation period.
- IgM antibodies to viral copied antigen (VCA) are present in all patients with primary EBV infection and disappear 2 to 3 months after recovery, showing that these antibodies are diagnostic of primary EBV infection.

Differential Diagnosis

- Group A β-hemolytic streptococcal infection
  - Presence of these organisms does not rule out infectious mononucleosis.
  - When heterophil antibody is absent, the mononucleosis may be due to cytomegalovirus (CMV).
- Primary HIV infection

Treatment

- Infectious mononucleosis is usually self-limited, with the acute phase lasting about 2 weeks.
- Therapy is largely supportive.
  - Rest is encouraged during the acute phase, with return to normal activity as soon as the fever, pharyngitis, and malaise subside.
- Acetaminophen is the first choice for fever and discomfort.
- Corticosteroids usually hasten defervescence and relieve pharyngitis, but are prescribed only to treat specific complications such as impending airway obstruction.

- Oral or IV acyclovir decreases oropharyngeal shedding of EBV but is generally not used in uncomplicated cases.

Patient/Family Education
- Encourage fluids by mouth.
- Monitor fever and urinary output.
- Instruct about infectious nature of the disorder and complications (e.g., streptococcal pharyngitis).
- Instruct about possible long-term effects (e.g., shedding of EBV).
- Causing fever, coryza, cough, headache, malaise, and inflamed respiratory mucous membranes

BIBLIOGRAPHY

Beers MH, Berkow R, eds: *The Merck manual of diagnosis and therapy,* ed 17, Whitehouse Station, NJ, 1999, Merck Research Laboratories, pp 661-683.

Dykewicz MS, Spector SL: Sinusitis: making the diagnosis, *Consultant* 40(3):603-606, 2000.

Jackler RK, Kaplan MJ: Ear, nose, and throat. In Tierney LM, McPhee SJ, Papadakis MA, eds: *Current medical diagnosis & treatment 2000,* ed 39, New York, 2000, Lange Medical Books/McGraw-Hill, pp 223-263.

Niparko JK: Hearing loss and associated problems. In Barker LR, Burton JR, Zieve PD, eds: *Principles of ambulatory medicine,* ed 5, Baltimore, 1999, Williams & Wilkins, pp 1461-1473.

Slavin RG: What you should know about sinusitis, *Consultant* 40(3):607-617, 2000.

REVIEW QUESTIONS

1. Diagnosis of middle and inner ear disorders is made primarily by:
   a. Examination with the otoscope
   b. X-ray, computed tomography scan, or magnetic resonance imaging
   c. The clinical picture (symptoms)
   d. Audiometry
2. The ear canal consists of the following:
   a. Bone covered with cartilage
   b. Cartilage covered with skin
   c. Skin covered with mucous membrane
   d. Cartilage covered with mucous membrane
3. The middle ear begins at the:
   a. Tragus
   b. Back portion of the ear canal
   c. Tympanic membrane
   d. Auricle

4. The cone of light that is reflected from the tympanic membrane begins at the:
   a. Malleus
   b. Incus
   c. Stapes
   d. Umbo
5. Hearing is possible because of:
   a. Vibrations of air
   b. Vibrations of the tragus
   c. Vibrations of the external canal
   d. Vibrations of the cochlea
6. The cochlear nerve is a part of the:
   a. Fifth cranial nerve
   b. Sixth cranial nerve
   c. Seventh cranial nerve
   d. Eighth cranial nerve
7. Pain in acute sinusitis is due to:
   a. Congestion of mucous membranes
   b. Relative negative pressure in the sinus (vacuum sinusitis)
   c. The transudate from the infection
   d. Immunoglobulin E–mediated reaction
8. The major purpose of the labyrinth of the middle ear is to:
   a. Protect the cochlea
   b. Ensure the appropriate transmission of sound through the middle ear
   c. Connect with the ossicles to transmit sound
   d. Maintain the person's balance by sensing position and movements of the head
9. In the primary care setting, hearing impairment can be adequately determined by means of:
   a. Examination of the tympanic membrane with the otoscope
   b. Palpation of the mastoid process
   c. The patient's history, repeating words of the examiner, and testing with a tuning fork
   d. Indicating whether he or she hears the ticking of a watch
10. Treatment of acute sinusitis includes all but one of the following. Which one is NOT included as part of therapy?
    a. Long-term use of vasoconstrictors
    b. Steam inhalation
    c. Saline nasal irrigations
    d. Surgery if patient does not respond to other treatment

11. Two classifications of hearing loss are used. They are:
    a. Conductive and sensorineural hearing loss
    b. Traumatic and displaced ossicles hearing loss
    c. Nerve damage and perforated eardrum hearing loss
    d. Labyrinthine and cochlear hearing loss

12. Conductive hearing loss usually results from a/an:
    a. Inner ear or auditory nerve problem
    b. Labyrinthine problem
    c. Cochlear nerve problem
    d. External or middle ear disease

13. The basis for using Weber's test is that:
    a. A unilateral conductive hearing loss with normal bilateral ear function produces a softer sound in the unaffected ear
    b. A unilateral conductive hearing loss with normal bilateral ear function produces a louder sound in the affected ear
    c. A unilateral sensorineural hearing loss produces a softer sound in the affected ear
    d. A unilateral sensorineural hearing loss produces a louder sound in the affected ear

14. Evaluation of hearing by means of audiometric testing results in determination of the precise level of hearing loss by using sounds that:
    a. Vary in pitch
    b. Vary in quality
    c. Vary in intensity (dB)
    d. Vary in timing

15. A major cause of acute suppurative otitis media is:
    a. *Streptococcus pneumoniae*
    b. External ear infection
    c. Labyrinthitis
    d. Dysfunction of the tympanic membrane

16. Antibiotic therapy for acute otitis media must be given for at least:
    a. 5 days
    b. 7 days
    c. 10 days
    d. 12 days

17. In chronic otitis media, there is:
    a. Conductive hearing loss
    b. Severe pain
    c. Spiking fever
    d. Isolation of one specific causative organism

18. Meniere's disease is associated with conditions that affect:
    a. The middle ear
    b. The ossicles
    c. The vestibular apparatus
    d. Trauma to the ear

19. Treatment of acute pharyngitis is:
    a. Routine among all clinicians
    b. Routine as to whether to culture or length of antibiotic therapy
    c. Uncertain because of the difficulty of differentiating between viral and bacterial infection
    d. Assumed to be bacterial until proven otherwise

20. Several systemic illnesses are associated with ear, nose, and throat symptoms. Included among these is:
    a. Infectious mononucleosis
    b. Tuberculosis
    c. Pneumonia
    d. Amyotrophic lateral sclerosis

21. All but one of the following can be included in the differential diagnosis of cerumen impaction. The one that is NOT among these is:
    a. External otitis
    b. Otitis media
    c. Bony overgrowths in the canal
    d. Foreign body in the canal

22. External otitis is seen frequently in:
    a. Runners
    b. Skiers
    c. Swimmers
    d. Soccer players

23. A sign of gout is often seen on the external ear as:
    a. Redness and swelling
    b. Infection
    c. Discharge
    d. Tophi

24. Sudden severe pain followed by bleeding, partial or complete loss of hearing, tinnitus, and purulent discharge that develops within 24 to 48 hours are signs and symptoms of:
    a. Ruptured tympanic membrane
    b. Acute viral infection of the middle ear
    c. Mononucleosis
    d. Acute mastoiditis

25. Relative negative pressure, retraction of the tympanic membrane, displacement of the light reflex, and immovable tympanic membrane are signs and symptoms of:
    a. Acute otitis media
    b. Serous otitis media
    c. Meniere's syndrome
    d. Acute infection in the inner ear
26. Treatment for serous otitis media includes all but one of the following. Which one is NOT considered appropriate therapy in this condition?
    a. Valsalva's maneuver by the patient
    b. Trial of antibiotic therapy
    c. Instillation of antibiotic drops tid
    d. Myringotomy
27. The condition that produces progressive conductive hearing loss in young adults with normal tympanic membranes is:
    a. Chronic otitis media
    b. Cholesteatoma
    c. Neoplasm of the middle ear
    d. Otosclerosis
28. Recurrent, severe vertigo; sensory hearing loss; tinnitus; and a sensation of fullness or pressure in the ear are signs and symptoms of:
    a. Trauma to the ear, often seen in boxers
    b. HIV/AIDS infection
    c. Meniere's disease
    d. Tertiary syphilis
29. Lesions of the eighth cranial nerve and central audiovestibular pathways produce:
    a. Conductive hearing loss
    b. Neural hearing loss and vertigo
    c. Facial palsy
    d. Horizontal nystagmus
30. Acoustic neuroma:
    a. Arises from Schwann cells
    b. Is a highly malignant neoplasm of the inner ear
    c. Accounts for almost 75% of benign tumors of the ear
    d. Causes minimal compression in the auditory canal

21

Infectious Diseases

- Infectious diseases are the most common afflictions of humans, and a major source of morbidity and mortality in all countries.
- Prevalence of infectious diseases varies widely, depending on geography, climatic conditions, sanitation, the quality and abundance of water and food supplies and, to some degree, the resistance of indigenous populations to specific diseases.
- Continuation of infectious diseases in human populations requires
  —Reservoirs of infection
  —Effective modes of transmission

RESERVOIRS
Reservoirs of Infection

- Human reservoirs are necessary for those organisms/agents of diseases that afflict only humans (e.g., hepatitis A and B, cholera, shigellosis), and include the following:
  —Skin (e.g., *Staphylococcus epidermis*)
  —Nasopharynx (e.g., meningococci)
  —Intestinal tract (e.g., *Giardia* species, *Entamoeba histolytica:* both can continue to colonize after recovery from an acute episode)
- Viruses remain in the body for months or years (e.g., hepatitis B, herpes viruses).
- Helminths may stay in the circulation for many years (e.g., schistosomes in the portal vein), constantly producing millions of ova, a high proportion of which are deposited back into the environment or in the lymphatic system (e.g., filarial worms).

Animal Reservoirs

- Animal reservoirs that harbor organisms/agents that afflict humans are a significant source of infections throughout the world; infections that can be transmitted from animals (except via arthropods, which include crabs, lobsters, ticks, spiders, and insects; they are distinguished by a joined exoskeleton [shell] and paired, jointed legs, which can act as vectors of diseases) to man are called zoonoses, and include the following:
  —*Salmonella* or *Campylobacter jejuni* infections from battery-farmed chickens
  —*Toxoplasma gondii* infection from domestic cats
  —*Giardia* infection from domestic and wild animals
  —*Cryptosporidium parvum*, enterohemorrhagic *Escherichia coli* O157:H7, and prions such as Creutzfeldt-Jakob disease from cattle
- Diseases that rely on arthropods for their transmission include malaria, many viruses (e.g., yellow fever, dengue fever), and rickettsial infections.

Environmental Reservoirs

- These sources act as a temporary lodging place for some bacteria, viruses, and parasites.
  —Water: enteropathogens, hepatitis A virus, cysts and oocysts of some protozoa *(Giardia, Cryptosporidium parvum)* may remain viable despite effective water purification procedures.
  —Soil: spore-forming bacteria (e.g., *Clostridium* spp, *Bacillus anthracis*), whose spores can re-

main viable under suitable climatic conditions for months.

TRANSMISSION

Airborne spread: bacteria, viruses, bacterial spores can be carried by the wind; some are carried in droplets in the air (e.g., influenza viruses), and other organisms (e.g., *Legionella*), which are spread by aerosol, typically from air conditioning units

Direct Contact

- Person-to-person: skin contact (impetigo, ringworm, scabies) and sexually transmitted diseases; entry through the skin of larval forms of some helminths that can survive in soil or water—*Schistosoma, Strongyloides,* and hookworm
- Fecal-oral spread, particularly among children in residential institutions (e.g., shigellosis, giardiasis, hepatitis A)
- Inoculation of infection (transfusions of blood or blood products that contain hepatitis B, C, or human immunodeficiency virus [HIV]); by contaminated needles (drug abusers, medical and paramedical personnel)
- Insect bites (mosquitoes—malaria; sandfly—leishmaniasis; Tsetse fly—African trypanosomiasis; ticks—babesiosis, Lyme disease; bugs—Chagas' disease)

Spread by Food and Water

- Enteropathogens are generally transmitted through food and water:
  - *Shigella*
  - *Vibrio cholerae*
  - "Food poisoning" can be caused by preformed bacterial toxins such as staphylococcal enterotoxin.
  - Cysts of parasites, such as *Giardia* organisms and *E. histolytica*, that can survive in water, and water-treatment procedures, for months; these are often found in swimming pools.

Spread by Fomites

Transmission of disease between persons via an inanimate object such as books, paper money, and bed linen.

HOST DEFENSES

- Skin: the skin is an effective barrier against all microorganisms as long as it is intact and is not physically disrupted by cuts, lesions, trauma, intravenous (IV) catheter, surgical incision, or insect bite.
  - The only exceptions are human papillomavirus, which causes warts and can invade normal skin, and some parasites that can penetrate intact skin: *Schistosoma mansoni, Strongyloides stercoralis;* no bacteria are known to be capable of penetrating intact skin.
- Mucous membranes that are bathed with secretions that have antimicrobial properties (e.g., cervical mucus, prostatic fluid, and tears, all of which contain lysozyme that can split bacterial cell walls).
- Respiratory tract filtering system of the upper airway and tracheobronchial tree and the mechanisms of sneezing and coughing.
- GI tract: the acid pH of the stomach and the antibacterial activity of pancreatic enzymes, bile, and intestinal secretions are natural barriers.
- Genitourinary (GU) tract: protection is provided by the length of the urethra (20 cm in an adult); bacteria seldom gain entrance unless they are introduced by instrumentation; women are protected by the acid pH of the vagina; the hypertonic state of the kidney medulla is an unfavorable environment for most microorganisms; Tamm-Horsfall protein is a glycoprotein produced by the kidney and excreted in large amounts in the urine, and particular bacteria avidly bind to it, which prevents them from gaining entrance into the urinary tract.
- Immune responses also protect the body from infection (see Chapter 15).

PRINCIPLES AND BASIC MECHANISMS

Steps that occur during the pathogenesis of infections are seen in Fig. 21-1.

INFECTIOUS DISEASES
Fever of Unknown Origin

Definition

Fever of unknown origin (FUO) is a body temperature >38.3° C (≥101° F) rectally for 3 weeks or longer without discovering the cause, despite extensive investigation for at least 1 week. Pa-

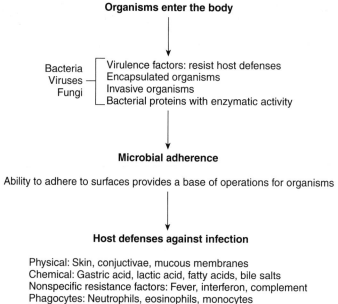

Fig. 21-1 Pathogenesis of infection.

tients with FUO are often difficult to diagnose. The fever, intermittent or continuous, may be an unusual presentation of a common disease or some other more exotic condition.

Risk Factors
- Foreign travel
- Ingestion of contaminated food or water
- Bites or stings of insects or ticks
- Meat handlers

Etiology/Cause (Box 21-1)
- Common causes include infections, connective tissue diseases, and occult neoplasms (leukemia, lymphoma).
- Most cases of FUO are found to be caused by systemic diseases (e.g., Still's disease, sarcoidosis, temporal arteritis).

Diagnosis

Signs and Symptoms
- Fever that occurs every third day—48 hours (tertian) or every fourth day—72 hours (quartan) may indicate malaria.
- In cyclic neutropenia, the peripheral neutrophil count falls to very low levels every

21 days, often resulting in infection and fever.
—Patients may present with periodic fever, which raises suspicion of Hodgkin's disease.

Diagnostic Tests
- Include all routine and relevant tests based on signs and symptoms, history, and other factors: computed tomography (CT), magnetic resonance imaging (MRI), biopsy of particular site (liver, bone marrow, lymph nodes, intestine, muscle).

Treatment
- Specific therapy depends on the diagnosis, either probable or definitive.
- May include pharmacologic therapy (antibiotics, corticosteroids, vitamins, other).
- Surgery may be required for incision and drainage of abscesses, resection of cancerous tissue, or other.
- Patient should be encouraged to exercise in accordance with status: minimal would be passive range of motion every 3 to 4 hours, and maximal would be working out on exercise equipment to tolerance.

BOX 21-1
Some Causes of Fever of Unknown Origin

INFECTION (40%)
Pyogenic abscesses (e.g., liver)
TB
UTI
Biliary infection
Subacute infective endocarditis
EBV infection
CMV virus
Q fever
Toxoplasmosis
Brucellosis
Septic arthritis in prosthetic joint

CANCER (30%)
Lymphomas
Leukemia
Solid tumors
   Renal carcinoma
   Hepatocellular carcinoma
   Pancreatic carcinoma

IMMUNOGENIC (20%)
Drugs
Connective tissue and autoimmune diseases
RA
Systemic lupus erythematosus
Polyarteritis nodosa
Polymyalgia/cranial arteritis
Sarcoidosis

MISCELLANEOUS
Thyrotoxicosis
Chronic liver disease
Inflammatory bowel disease
   Familial Mediterranean fever
   Kawasaki syndrome

FACTITIOUS (1%-5%)
Switching thermometers
Injection of pyrogenic material

REMAIN UNKNOWN (5%-9%)

From Farthing MJG, Jeffries DJ, Anderson J: Infectious diseases, tropical medicine and sexually transmitted diseases. In Kumar P, Clark M, eds: *Clinical medicine,* ed 4, Edinburgh, 1998, WB Saunders, p 7.
EBV, Epstein-Barr virus; *CMV,* cytomegalovirus.

- Nourishing diet and adequate fluid intake are essential.
- Sufficient rest to repair body tissues, replenish body stores of essential components.

Patient/Family Education
- FUO poses specific problems for the patient because knowing what is wrong usually allays most of the fears and anxiety that patients have before knowing the specific cause, and therefore specific treatment, for the condition.
- The patient may have to undergo repeated diagnostic testing, sometimes of an invasive nature such as sigmoidoscopy or bronchoscopy; each should be explained in detail as to what will happen, the reason for doing the test, and the expected gain to be achieved from the test.
- Encouraging activity and continued interest in previous involvements (e.g., sports, news, politics) can help to allay anxiety by inferring that the cause will be discovered in time, and that patience and courage in the face of the unknown are called for during the period of diagnostic testing.

Follow-up/Referral
- Specialist consultants may be called in during the diagnostic testing phase, if specific test results point to a specific condition.
- In almost all cases, a definitive diagnosis is derived at some point, and treatment instituted that is specific for the condition.
- Even after recovery, however, these patients are followed fairly closely for several weeks or months, to determine that treatment was successful and that no recurrence seems evident.

Septicemia
Definition
- **Bacteremia** and **septic shock** are related conditions.
- Bacteremia denotes bacteria in the bloodstream.
- Septic shock is sepsis with hypoperfusion and hypotension refractory to fluid therapy.

- **Sepsis** refers to a serious infection, localized or bacteremic, that is accompanied by systemic manifestations of inflammation.
- **Septicemia** is a term used to indicate sepsis due to bacteremia, but the term is rarely used now because of its nonspecificity.
- **Systemic inflammatory response syndrome** is the more general term, and one that is used most commonly now to indicate the possibility of any one of several severe conditions: infection, pancreatitis, burns, or trauma, all of which can trigger an acute inflammatory reaction, associated with release into the circulation of a large number of endogenous mediators of inflammation.

Risk Factors
- Surgical manipulation of infected oral tissues
- Catheterization of an infected lower urinary tract
- Incision and drainage of an abscess
- Colonization of indwelling devices (e.g., IV and intracardiac catheters, urethral catheters, ostomy devices and tubes)

Etiology/Cause
- Gram-negative organisms are often implicated.
  —Although these organisms may not affect healthy persons, they are a serious threat to patients who are immunocompromised, have debilitating diseases after chemotherapy, or are malnourished.
  —The primary site of infection is often the lungs, the GU or gastrointestinal (GI) tracts, or soft tissues (e.g., skin in patients with pressure ulcers).
  —Chronically ill or immunocompromised patients are also susceptible to bloodstream infections caused by aerobic bacilli, anaerobes, and fungi.
- Enterococcus, staphylococcus, and fungus may be the cause of endocarditis.
- Staphylococcal bacteremia is common among IV drug users.
- Staphylococcus is a major cause of gram-positive bacterial endocarditis of the tricuspid valve.

Diagnosis
Signs and Symptoms
- Mild bacteremia is often asymptomatic.
- The typical presentation includes signs and symptoms of systemic infection: tachypnea, shaking chills, temperature spikes, GI symptoms (abdominal pain, nausea, vomiting, diarrhea), diminished mental alertness, and hypotension.
- Infections above the diaphragm are more likely to be caused by gram-positive organisms.
- Abdominal, biliary, and urinary tract infections are more often due to gram-negative bacteria.
- Between 25% and 40% of patients with persistent bacteremia develop hemodynamic instability, which indicates septic shock.

Diagnostic Tests
- Gram's stain and culture should be done on all fluids taken from potentially infected sites: body cavities, joint spaces, skin lesions, sputum, catheter insertion sites, and wounds.
  —Two blood cultures, 1 hour apart, taken from two different sites, are usually sufficient to diagnose bacteremia.
- Negative Gram's stain or culture results do not exclude bacteremia, particularly in patients who have had prior antibiotic therapy.
- The systemic inflammatory response syndrome (formerly called the sepsis syndrome) is diagnosed on the basis of two or more of the following:
  —Temperature $> 38°$ C ($>100.4°$ F) or $< 36°$ C ($<96.8°$ F)
  —Heart rate > 20 beats/minute or $Paco_2 < 32$ mm Hg
  —White blood cell (WBC) count of $>12,000$ or <4000 cells/μl, or $>10\%$ immature forms
  —Typically, the WBC count is at first decreased to $<4000/\mu$l, then rises to $15,000/\mu$l, with a marked increase in immature forms over a period of 2 to 6 hours.

Treatment
- Mild, transient bacteremia due to surgical procedures with indwelling IV or urinary

catheters is often not detected and requires no therapy except in patients with valvular heart disease, intravascular prostheses, or immunosuppression.

—For these patients, a prophylactic regimen of antibiotic therapy is usually ordered, primarily to prevent endocarditis.

- The outcome of more serious bacteremia depends on two primary factors.

—How rapidly and effectively the source of infection can be discovered and eliminated

—The nature, extent, and severity of the underlying condition; some cases (e.g., internal abscesses, gangrene of the bowel or gallbladder) require surgery with its attendant risks

- Antibiotic therapy in all cases is required, and usually is effective in eliminating the bacterial source.
- When many different types of organisms are evident on culture (polymicrobial bacteremia), the prognosis is poor.

Patient/Family Education
- Instruct the patient and family regarding the nature, cause, treatment, and expected outcome.
- The patient is encouraged to increase fluid intake above normal, as tolerated.
- The patient is encouraged to walk and do mild exercise up to capability.
- All medications are explained, listed in writing, along with dosages and scheduling.
- If surgery is required, the procedure should be explained in some detail, the reason for the surgery, and preoperative, intraoperative, and postoperative events.

Follow-up/Referral
- While being treated, either in the ambulatory or hospital setting, specialist consultants may be called to examine, assess, and treat particular problems (e.g., gastroenterologist, neurologist, neurosurgeon, infectious disease specialist, or other), and may follow the patient for some time after recovery to ensure against recurrence of infection and to assess wound healing and recovery.

Septic Shock
Definition
- Septic shock is caused by systemic bacteremia that produces changes in circulation such that tissue perfusion is critically reduced.
- Shock caused by staphylococcal toxins is called **toxic shock,** a condition that occurs more frequently in young women.

Risk Factors
- Hospital-acquired gram-negative bacilli
- Patients who are immunocompromised or who have chronic disease
- Diabetes mellitus
- Cirrhosis
- Leukopenia
- Patients with carcinoma who have received treatment with cytotoxic drugs
- Prior infection, especially in the urinary, biliary, or GI tracts
- Invasive devices: catheters, drainage tubes
- Recent antibiotic or corticosteroid therapy, or use of ventilatory devices

Etiology/Cause
- Pathogens that produce bacterial toxins in systemic infection

Pathogenesis
- The pathogenesis of septic shock is not entirely understood.

—Bacterial toxins produced by the infecting organism(s) trigger complex immunologic reactions.

—Many mediators (e.g., tumor necrosis factor, leukotrienes, lipoxygenase, histamine, bradykinin, serotonin, and interleukin-2, have been implicated, along with endotoxin.

- Initially, vasodilation of arteries and arterioles occurs, with decreased peripheral arterial resistance with normal or increased cardiac output, even though the ejection fraction may be decreased as the heart rate increases.
- Later, cardiac output may decrease and peripheral resistance may increase.
- Despite increased cardiac output, blood flow to the capillary exchange vessels is impaired, resulting in decreased exchange of essential

substrates, particularly oxygen, and decreased removal of CO_2 and waste products.

—The decreased perfusion significantly affects the kidneys and brain, and usually causes failure of one or more of the visceral organs.

- Finally, cardiac output is decreased markedly, and the typical signs of septic shock appear.

Diagnosis

Signs and Symptoms

- Signs and symptoms of bacteremia are present initially.
- When septic shock develops, the initial sign may be decreased mental alertness.
- Blood pressure falls, although the skin and extremities feel warm.
- Tachycardia, tachypnea, and oliguria develop.
- Pale, cool extremities with peripheral cyanosis and skin mottling appear later.
- As decreased perfusion continues, multiple organ failure develops in kidneys, lungs, and liver.
- Disseminated intravascular coagulopathy (DIC) and heart failure may develop.

Diagnostic Tests

- Septic shock should be distinguished from hypovolemic, cardiogenic, and obstructive shock.
- Urine specific gravity and osmolality are helpful measurements.
- Volume depletion responds rapidly to fluid replacement.
- Cardiogenic shock is associated with myocardial infarction.
- Obstructive shock results from pulmonary artery or other major bloodstream artery obstruction by pulmonary emboli or dissecting aortic aneurysm.
- A distributive defect is identified in septic shock.
  —At first, a hyperdynamic state occurs that is unique to sepsis: normal or increased cardiac output with decreased peripheral arterial resistance and warm, dry skin.
  —The hypodynamic state is represented by decreased cardiac output and increased peripheral resistance and is a late stage of septic shock.

—Neither central venous pressure (CVP) nor pulmonary artery occlusive pressure is likely to be decreased.

—ECG may show nonspecific sinus tachycardia (ST)-T wave abnormalities and supraventricular and ventricular dysrhythmias, partly related to hypotension.

- At the beginning of septic shock, the leukocyte count is usually significantly reduced, the polymorphonuclear leukocytes (PMNs) may be as low as 20%, and there is a sharp decrease in platelets to $\leq 50,000/\mu l$.
  —However, within 1 to 4 hours, a turnaround occurs, in which there is a significant increase in both the total WBC count and PMNs to 80% with a predominance of immature forms.
- Urinalysis may indicate that the GU tract is the source of the infection, noted frequently in those with indwelling catheters.
- Respiratory alkalosis with a low P_{CO_2} and increased arterial pH is present early in the process, and compensates for lactic acidemia.
- Serum bicarbonate is usually low; serum and blood lactate are increased.
- As shock progresses, metabolic acidosis becomes paramount.
- Early respiratory failure results in hypoxemia, with $P_{O_2} < 70$ mm Hg.
- An electrocardiogram (ECG) may show depressed ST segments with T-wave inversions and occasionally atrial and ventricular dysrhythmias.
- Blood urea nitrogen (BUN) and creatinine concentrations usually increase progressively as renal failure develops, with decreased creatinine clearance.

Treatment

- Mortality from septic shock ranges from 25% to 90%.
- Poor outcome often results from failure to begin therapy early.
- Once severe lactic acidosis with decompensated metabolic acidosis becomes established, particularly with simultaneous multiorgan failure, septic shock is likely to be irreversible, regardless of therapy.
- Therapy should occur in an intensive care unit (ICU), with continuous monitoring of all body systems, and frequent measure-

ments of blood gas levels, blood lactate levels, electrolyte levels, renal function, and perhaps tissue P_{CO_2}.

- CVP and pulmonary artery pressure should also be monitored.
- Tracheal intubation is usually necessary; oxygen support is provided by nasal cannula or mask.
- Antibiotic therapy should be instituted immediately, without waiting for sensitivity results to be known; **antibiotic therapy may be lifesaving.**
  - —Gentamicin or tobramycin plus a third-generation cephalosporin (cefotaxime or ceftriaxone or, if *Pseudomonas* is suspected, ceftazidime)
  - —If line sepsis (gram-positive organisms) is the source of infection, vancomycin is given, and is mandated when resistant staphylococci or enterococci are suspected.
  - —Dosages are set at maximum levels and continued for several days after shock resolves and the primary source of infection is eradicated.
- Other therapy is given according to patient symptoms (e.g., diuretics for oliguria, dopamine for hypotension).

Patient/Family Education

- Often, the patient is too ill to take in information, so the family becomes the major focus of instruction.
- Frequent reports to the family about the patient's status, progress, and responses, if any, are necessary.
- Explain in as much detail as seems necessary the nature, cause, treatment, and expected outcome of therapy.
- Maintain an optimistic demeanor without raising false hopes, depending on the patient's condition over several hours or days.

Follow-up/Referral

- While in the ICU, specialists are often called in to assess the patient and order drugs or other therapy as required.
- These specialists, along with the patient's primary care clinician, follow the patient after discharge to ensure that complete recovery has occurred, and that no relapse is evident on the basis of appropriate monitoring.

- Oral antibiotics may be continued after discharge, and the patient's compliance must be assessed at each visit.

Bacterial Skin Infections

Most skin infections are mild and can be treated at home without medical supervision. However, every year, about 5% of the population develop skin infections that require medical intervention. As in other infections, severity depends on the virulence of the invading organism and the defenses of the host. Organisms most often implicated include *S. aureus* and *Streptococcus pyogenes*.

Superficial Skin Infections

- Impetigo, ecthyma, and erysipelas are the most common skin infections caused by group A hemolytic streptococci *(S. pyogenes)* and *S. aureus.*
- *Impetigo* begins as a pruritic, focal, superficial eruption of small (1 to 2 mm) vesicles, often on the face near the nose, on the chin, or on the lower extremities.
- In several days, the vesicles change to pustules that break, become crusted, and have an erythematous base.
- Regional lymphadenopathy is often associated.
- The infection often spreads because of scratching.
- Healing occurs without scarring.
- *Ecthyma* is characterized by 3- to 10-mm discrete, ulcerating lesions with an adherent necrotic crust and surrounding erythema.
  - —A small amount of pus often is present beneath the crusts.
  - —The lesions are deep enough to cause permanent scarring.
  - —Lesions are most commonly seen on the anterior tibial surface at sites of minor trauma or insect bites.
  - —Untreated, the lesions spread widely, and lymphadenopathy may be present.
  - —Culture may show both *S. aureus* and *S. pyogenes.*
- *Erysipelas* is usually caused by *S. pyogenes,* and is characterized by a rapidly spreading area of marked erythema with warmth, local pain, an elevated sharp margin between involved and uninvolved skin, and firm edema that gives the skin a typical "orange peel" appearance.

TABLE 21-1
Antibiotic Drugs for Superficial and Pustular Skin Infections

Infection	Antibiotic*	Route
SUPERFICIAL INFECTIONS		
Impetigo	Mupirocin	Topical
	Dicloxacillin†	Oral
	Cephalexin†	Oral
	Erythromycin	Oral
Ecthyma	Same as for impetigo	
Erysipelas		
Mild	Penicillin V	Oral
	Erythromycin	Oral
Severe	Penicillin G	IV
PUSTULAR INFECTIONS		
Folliculitis	None	
Furunculosis, boils	Dicloxacillin†	Oral
	Cephalexin†	Oral
	Erythromycin	Oral
Bullous impetigo	Same as for furunculosis	
Carbuncle	Same as for furunculosis	
	Nafcillin	IV
	Vancomycin	IV
Cellulitis	Same as for carbuncle	

From Pierce NF: Bacterial infections of the skin. In Barker LR, Burton JR, Zieve PD, eds: *Principles of ambulatory medicine*, ed 5, Baltimore, 1999, Williams & Wilkins, p 313.
*Give a single antibiotic. Choices are in order of preference and include alternatives for patients allergic to penicillin; if patient cannot tolerate one, continue down the list. Dosages are seen in Table 17-4.
†Other penicillinase-resistant oral β-lactams may also be given.

—Facial lesions are especially dangerous because of potential intracranial spread by way of draining lymphatics or veins.
—Extensive involvement of the trunk also has an increased risk of death.
—Erythema often extends centrally along superficial draining lymphatics.
—Regional lymphadenopathy is usually present.
—Systemic toxicity, chills, and fever are common.
—If untreated, metastatic infection may occur, with significant mortality.

Treatment (Tables 21-1 and 21-2)
• Cultures of the lesions of impetigo, bullous impetigo, and ecthyma are not helpful.
• Blood cultures should be obtained when erysipelas is extensive or associated with marked systemic toxicity (e.g., temperature >102° F [39° C], shaking chills, severe malaise).
• Minor episodes of erysipelas are treated with penicillin V or erythromycin.

• Application of moist heat to the affected area hastens healing.
• Patients at risk (e.g., severe erysipelas infection involving systemic toxicity, extensive lesions, facial lesions, particularly in those with diabetes) require hospitalization and parenteral penicillin G.
• Patients who have preexisting damage to the veins or lymphatics of an extremity often have repeated episodes of erysipelas that cause further damage.
—These patients should receive prophylactic therapy (penicillin V 250 mg bid, benzathine penicillin 600,000 units intramuscularly [IM]) every month, or erythromycin 250 mg bid.
—Elastic support stockings and diuretics to reduce edema reduce susceptibility to erysipelas.

Prognosis
• Superficial infections usually respond rapidly to appropriate therapy.

TABLE 21-2
Antibiotic Dosage and Schedule for Skin Infections Caused by *S. pyogenes* and *S. aureus* in Adults

Antibiotic	Dosage
AMBULATORY TREATMENT	
Mild infection	
Mupirocin	2% ointment bid
Dicloxacillin	250 mg PO tid
Cephalexin	500 mg PO qid
Erythromycin	250-500 mg PO tid
Penicillin V	500 mg PO tid
PARENTERAL TREATMENT	
Severe infection	
Penicillin G	600,000-2,000,000 units IV q6h
Nafcillin	1.0-1.5 g IV q4h
Vancomycin	0.25-0.5 g IV q6h

From Pierce NF: Bacterial infections of the skin. In Barker LR, Burton JR, Zieve PD, eds: *Principles of ambulatory medicine,* ed 5, Baltimore, 1999, Williams & Wilkins, p 313.

—Systemic toxicity and erythema associated with erysipelas usually disappear within 3 to 4 days, and skin lesions heal almost completely within 10 days.

Complications
- Streptococcal infections may cause *acute glomerulonephritis* if the strain is nephritogenic; symptoms of nephritis appear about 2 weeks after the onset of the streptococcal infection.
  —Most patients who develop nephritis are asymptomatic.
  —Some patients have symptoms that indicate the need for evaluation related to glomerulonephritis; symptoms include the following:
  ~ Hematuria
  ~ Acute hypertension
  ~ Signs of salt and water retention (e.g., dependent edema, congenital heart failure [CHF])
  —Nephritis is not prevented by antibiotic therapy.
  —Initial and follow-up evaluation should include urinalysis.
  —Metastatic infection may include meningitis, endocarditis, septic arthritis, infec-

tion of preexisting pleural effusion or ascites, and solid organ abscesses (liver or spleen).

Patient/Family Education
- The nature, cause, treatment, and expected outcome are outlined for the patient and family.
- All medications, including dosage and scheduling, are written out for the patient and family before discharge.
- Emphasize the importance of compliance in taking antibiotics, wearing support hose, and any other instructions specific to the individual.

Follow-up/Referral
- These patients are evaluated every 1 to 2 weeks after discharge, with respect to symptoms or signs of recurrent infection.
- The lower legs, if there had been prior damage to the veins or tissues, are examined carefully at each visit and, if necessary, a dermatologist should also follow the patient.

Pustular Infections Caused by *Staphylococcus aureus*
- These infections include folliculitis, furunculosis, hidradenitis suppurativa, and carbuncles, and usually indicate increasingly severe effects of infections of hair follicles, sebaceous glands, or sweat glands by *S. aureus*, resulting in inflammation and abscess formation (Box 21-2)

Folliculitis
- Folliculitis involves minor inflammation of individual hair follicles, often with formation of small superficial pustules.
  —Little or no pain is experienced.
  —In some patients, lesions may recur for months or years.
  —A commonly affected area is the bearded part of the face, where minor trauma from shaving may be a contributing factor.

Furunculosis
- Deeper infection of follicles or cutaneous glands results in formation of pustular furuncles (boils are large furuncles).
  —They may range in diameter between 15 mm and 2 to 3 cm.

BOX 21-2

Clinical Conditions Caused by *Staphylococcus aureus*

DUE TO INVASION	Miscellaneous
Skin	Parotitis
Furuncles	Pyomyositis
Cellulitis	Septicemia
Impetigo	Enterocolitis
Carbuncles	
Lungs	**DUE TO TOXIN**
Pneumonia	Staphylococcal food
Lung abscesses	poisoning
Heart	Scalded-skin syndrome
Endocarditis	Bullous impetigo
Pericarditis	Staphylococcal scarlet
CNS	fever
Meningitis	Toxic shock syndrome
Brain abscess	
Bones and Joints	
Osteomyelitis, arthritis	

From Farthing MJG, Jeffries DJ, Anderson J: Infectious diseases, tropical medicine and sexually transmitted diseases. In Kumar P, Clark M, eds: *Clinical medicine*, ed 4, Edinburgh, 1998, WB Saunders, p 21.

—They occur most often in hairy areas that are exposed to trauma, friction, or maceration (e.g., buttocks, neck, axillae, groin, forearms, thighs, upper back).

—Furunculosis may be a complication of adolescent acne.

—The infections begin with pruritus, local tenderness, and erythema, followed by swelling and marked local pain as the infection entrenches.

—Pus forms in the center portion, and the overlying skin becomes thin, the lesion becomes raised, pain increases, and spontaneous drainage of pus then occurs, usually with prompt relief of pain and rapid healing.

—Furunculosis may be recurrent in some persons, especially diabetic patients and those who are chronic nasal carriers of *S. aureus*.

Hidradenitis Suppurativa

- Hidradenitis suppurativa is caused by obstruction of apocrine sweat glands, usually in the axilla, perineum, or groin.
  - —The process is chronic, partly because of scars, abscesses, and sinus tracts that develop in the affected skin.

Carbuncle

- A carbuncle is a coalescent mass of deeply infected follicles or sebaceous glands with multiple interconnecting sinus tracts and cutaneous openings that drain pus ineffectively.
  - —These lesions usually appear in the thick skin on the back of the neck or the upper back.
  - —Once formed, the lesions steadily worsen, with increasing pain, erythema, swelling, purulent drainage, and lateral enlargement.
  - —They range in diameter from 3 to 10 cm or larger.
  - —Fever and systemic toxicity are common.
  - —These lesions occur often in diabetic patients and in those with damaged areas of skin.

Treatment

- Cultures of pustular lesions are usually not necessary because almost all are caused by *S. aureus*, and most are resistant to penicillin G.
- Minimal lesions (e.g., folliculitis) require little treatment other than careful, twice-daily cleansing with a mild soap, preferably one that contains hexachlorophene, and avoidance of minor trauma and irritants such as cosmetics or abrasive soaps.
- Furuncles are treated initially by application of warm moist heat (compresses or baths) for 30 minutes four times a day, and by immobilizing the affected area (e.g., splinting of digits, instructing the patient to avoid pressing on the furuncle); lesions less than 1 cm in diameter often drain spontaneously after 1 to 2 days.
  - —Larger lesions that do not drain spontaneously should be surgically incised while avoiding downward pressure, then packing with iodoform gauze for 1 to 2 days to control oozing.
- Antibiotic therapy is needed only for extensive lesions of any kind, those with marked surrounding inflammation, or in diabetic patients.
- Antibiotic therapy often resolves indurated furuncles before they become fluctuant.
- Carbuncles may require extensive surgical drainage that can be performed in an out-

patient setting; those (especially diabetic patients) with extensive lesions and severe systemic toxicity require hospitalization and parenteral penicillinase-resistant penicillin; vancomycin is an effective alternative for patients allergic to penicillin.

- Recurrent furunculosis may prove to be frustrating.
  - —Patients with nasal infections should be cultured and treated with mupirocin ointment to the anterior nares bid for 5 days.
  - —Alternatively, bacitracin ointment may be applied three to four times daily for 14 days.
- Recurrent furunculosis is often persistent in patients who have conditions that impair their defenses (e.g., diabetes).
  - —In some patients, defects in polymorphonuclear leukocyte function are a rare cause; if such a defect is suspected, the patient should be referred to a medical center with the capability to investigate these disorders.
- Hidradenitis suppurativa is a difficult problem that may require prolonged, perhaps lifelong, treatment, using multiple methods, and cared for by a dermatologist knowledgeable about these particular disorders.
  - —Selective surgical drainage of abscesses
  - —Elimination of irritants such as tight clothing, antiperspirants, and shaving the axillae.
  - —Long-term systemic antibiotic therapy
  - —In some cases, irradiation or excisional surgery

Complications
- Spread to other sites, particularly in those patients at increased risk (e.g., ventricular septal defect, artificial heart, artificial heart valve, arthritis of a joint).
- Any patient whose symptoms persist despite treatment with antibiotics should be considered to have metastatic infection and be referred to a specialist for further evaluation and treatment.

Patient/Family Education
- Patients and families should be instructed about the nature, cause, course, treatment, and expected outcomes of therapy.

BOX 21-3

Diseases Caused by Streptococci

SUPPURATIVE	Peritonitis
Skin	Necrotizing fasciitis and
Impetigo	myositis
Pyoderma	Lymphangitis
Erysipelas	Bacteremia
Cellulitis	
Pharyngeal	**INFECTIONS**
Pharyngitis	**CONFINED TO**
Tonsillitis	**WOMEN**
Peritonsillar abscess	Puerperal sepsis
Pulmonary	Endometritis
Pneumonia	Toxic shock syndrome
Empyema	
Others	**NONSUPPURATIVE**
Osteomyelitis	Rheumatic fever
Infective endocarditis	Glomerulonephritis
Meningitis	Scarlet fever

From Farthing MJG, Jeffries DJ, Anderson J: Infectious diseases, tropical medicine and sexually transmitted diseases. In Kumar P, Clark M, eds: *Clinical medicine,* ed 4, Edinburgh, 1998, WB Saunders, p 22.

- Medications should be written, with dosages and scheduling.
- Emphasize the importance of adhering to the schedule, particularly with antibiotics.
- Emphasize the need to return or call if infection seems to be recurring.
- If prolonged prophylactic drug therapy is needed, explain the rationale and the importance of compliance and keeping appointments for return visits.

Follow-up/Referral
- Patients are followed on a regular basis for several months after hospitalization or after a course of antibiotic therapy to determine whether additional medication should be given.
- If necessary, a specialist in skin diseases (dermatologist) may be consulted to further evaluate and suggest therapy.

Streptococcal Infections
- Streptococci are round or ovoid gram-positive bacteria (Box 21-3).
- Virulence is attributed to the cell-wall M protein and the production by some streptococci of hyaluronidase, the deoxyribonuclease (DNases), or streptokinase.

- The spread of streptococci is mediated by direct contact, fomites, or airborne droplet infection.
- Group A β-hemolytic streptococci *(S. pyogenes)* are responsible for over 95% of human infections; the most common are pharyngitis and tonsillitis.
- Necrotizing fasciitis and myositis are aggressive infections of subcutaneous tissue and skin that require surgical debridement of infected tissue, along with antibiotics.
  —Progressive destruction of the tissues may occur, which can be life-threatening.
- Group B streptococci frequently cause neonatal sepsis and meningitis.
- Groups C, F, and G organisms can cause pharyngitis.
- Group D causes endocarditis and septicemia.
  —An estimated 75% of all streptococcal endocarditis infections are caused either by α-hemolytic streptococci, commonly found in the mouth (known collectively as *S. viridans*), or by *S. mutans,* a nonhemolytic streptococcus.
- *S. pneumoniae* is the most common cause of pneumonia.

Streptococcal Pyoderma (Impetigo)
- Impetigo can also be caused by *S. aureus.*

Signs and symptoms
- Streptococcal infections can be divided into three groups.
  —The carrier state in which the patient harbors streptococci without apparent infection
  —Acute infection, often suppurative, caused by streptococcal invasion of tissues
  —Delayed, nonsuppurative complications that occur usually 2 weeks after a clinically overt infection, but the infection may be asymptomatic and the interval between infection and evidence of complications may be longer than 2 weeks.
- Primary and secondary infections spread through the affected tissues and along lymphatic channels to regional lymph nodes, and the organisms can cause bacteremia.
- The development of suppurative infection depends on the virulence of the organism, the severity of the infection, and the susceptibility of the host.

Streptococcal Pharyngitis
- This is the most common streptococcal infection caused by group A β-hemolytic streptococci.
- Signs and symptoms include the following (may be mild to severe):
  —Fever
  —Sore throat
  —Beefy red pharynx
  —Purulent tonsillar exudate
  —Cough, laryngitis, and stuffy nose are uncharacteristic of streptococcal pharyngeal infection; these symptoms are more typical of viral infection or allergy.

Scarlet Fever (Scarlatina)
- This infection is rarely seen today, probably because antibiotics prevent the disease from developing and spreading.
- The streptococci (group A or other strains) produce an erythrogenic toxin that causes a diffuse pink-red cutaneous flush that blanches on pressure, seen on the abdomen and lateral chest as dark red lines in skinfolds (Pastia's lines), a strawberry tongue resulting from inflamed papillae that protrude through a dark red coating (must be distinguished from toxic shock and Kawasaki syndromes).

Streptococcal Toxic Shock Syndrome
- Similar to that caused by *S. aureus*
- Attributed to group A β-hemolytic streptococci strains capable of producing pyrogenic exotoxins

Signs and symptoms
- Erythrocyte sedimentation rate (ESR) is usually >50 mm/hour in the acute phase.
- WBC count can range from 12,000 to 20,000/μl, with 75% to 90% neutrophils with many immature cells.
- The specific organism can be established by overnight incubation on a sheep blood agar plate or, for group A organisms, by immediate staining with fluorescent antibodies.

Treatment
- Antibiotics have little effect on streptococcal infections (pharyngeal, scarlet fever) but can shorten the course in young children.
  —Antibiotics can prevent complications (peritonsillar abscess, otitis media, sinusi-

tis, mastoiditis), as well as rheumatic fever that may follow untreated infections and that may have long-term effects.

- Penicillin is the drug of choice for most group A β-hemolytic streptococcal infection.
  —A single injection of benzathine penicillin G, 600,000 U IM for small children, or 1.2 MU IM for adolescents and adults
  —Oral penicillin V 125 to 250 mg tid or qid for patients who can be relied on to maintain the regimen
- If penicillin is contraindicated, erythromycin 250 mg qid or clindamycin 300 mg may be given orally for 10 days.
- For headache and fever, analgesics can be taken.
- Bed rest and isolation are not necessary.
- Enterococci that are resistant to many antibiotics (e.g., vancomycin, gentamicin, streptomycin) are prevalent in many hospitals, and are now a cause of serious, refractory infections from vancomycin-resistant enterococci (VRE).

Patient/Family Education

- The nature, cause, course, treatment, and expected outcome of the infection can be explained to the patient and family.
- Physicians and nurses can emphasize the importance of seeking treatment for infections that may appear mild at first, but that can have serious complications if untreated.
- Provide written information about all medications: reason for giving, dosage, scheduling; **emphasize the importance of taking all of the pills, even though the infection seems to have abated.**

Follow-up/Referral

- Patients are seen in the office/clinic in 1 week to make certain that signs and symptoms are resolving, to assess for development of complications, and to stress compliance in completing the prescription.
- Rarely is a specialist (e.g., ear, nose, and throat [ENT]) required for consultation or treatment of complications.
- A final visit can confirm that the infection has cleared completely, and the patient should be instructed to call if any other symptoms develop.

Pneumococcal Infections (Formerly *Diplococcus pneumoniae*)

- *S. pneumoniae* is a gram-positive, encapsulated diplococcus, with a lancetlike shape; it sometimes is seen as short chains.
  —Old cultures or purulent exudates may stain gram-negative.
  —The capsule, visible in smears stained with methylene blue, consists of a complex polysaccharide that determines the serologic type and contributes to virulence and pathogenicity.
  —Over 85 types of *S. pneumoniae* exist.
- Pneumococci can be found in about 50% of the population in winter and early spring; they inhabit the respiratory tract.
  —The organisms are spread in droplets.

Risk Factors

- Patients with lymphoma, Hodgkin's disease, multiple myeloma, splenectomy, chronic debilitating disease, immunologic deficiencies, or sickle cell disease
- Damage to the respiratory epithelium from chronic bronchitis or viruses, especially influenza virus, may predispose to pneumococcal invasion.

Diseases Caused by Pneumococcus

- *Pneumonia:* the most frequent serious infection, usually lobar but often presents as bronchopneumonia or tracheobronchitis.
- *Empyema:* complicates more than 3% of pneumococcal pneumonia; the exudate may resolve spontaneously or during treatment for the pneumonia, or the exudate may become thick and fibrinopurulent and may require surgical drainage.
- *Acute otitis media:* primarily in infants and children; formerly serious complications of otitis media (e.g., mastoiditis, meningitis, lateral sinus thrombosis) are now rare because of antibiotic therapy.
- *Infection of the paranasal sinuses:* infection of the ethmoid or sphenoid sinus may extend into the meninges, causing bacterial meningitis; sinusitis may become chronic and polymicrobic.
- *Acute purulent meningitis:* can occur at any age; cause may be infection of any of the structures of the head or from bacteremia.

- *Bacteremia:* may accompany the acute phase of pneumococcal pneumonia, meningitis, endocarditis, or paranasal sinus infection; internal ear infection; or mastoiditis.
- *Pneumococcal endocarditis:* may result from bacteremia even in patients without previous valvular heart disease; signs and symptoms may include a new murmur or other changes.
- *Pneumococcal arthritis:* a rare extension of pneumococcal infection that can result in septic arthritis; bacteremia usually precedes the development of the purulent arthritis.
- *Pneumococcal peritonitis:* a rare occurrence, primarily in young women, probably as an ascending infection from the vagina through the fallopian tubes, or in women with nephrotic syndrome.

Treatment
- Therapy of choice is penicillin G or one of its analogs.
  —Penicillin G IV 6 to 10 MU/day
  —Penicillin V 250 to 500 mg orally (PO) for 5 to 7 days for acute pneumococcal otitis media or sinusitis
  —Parenteral administration is preferred for arthritis.
  —For pneumococcal meningitis or endocarditis, aqueous penicillin G 20,000 to 40,000 U/day IV for 10 days to 2 weeks after the patient is afebrile and cultures of blood and cerebrospinal fluid (CSF) have become sterile
- Penicillin-resistant organisms may be treated with vancomycin, ceftriaxone, or cefotaxime alone or in combination with rifampin.

Patient/Family Education
- Instruct the patient and family regarding the nature, cause, course, treatment, and expected outcome of the infection.
- Write out all medications: reasons for giving, action, dosage and schedule, and expected outcome.

Follow-up/Referral
- If the patient is seriously ill and hospitalized, specialist consultants in relevant areas may be called: neurologist, neurosurgeon, pulmonologist, ENT, or other; the specialist(s) may follow the patient for a time after discharge or resolution of the infection/complications.
- Return visits are scheduled every 2 to 3 weeks after discharge, more often for older persons who may be more debilitated from the infection and who may therefore be more susceptible to complications or recurrence of infection.

Diseases Caused by Gram-negative, Aerobic Cocci

Neisseria Infection
(See section on sexually transmitted diseases.) Organisms of the genus *Neisseria* include *N. meningitidis,* the causative organism in meningitis, bacteremia, and other serious infection in both children and adults, including *N. gonorrhoeae,* a major cause of sexually transmitted diseases (e.g., urethritis, cervicitis, proctitis, pharyngitis, salpingitis, epididymitis, and bacteremia/arthritis).

Diagnosis
- The infection is confirmed by identification of the organism by Gram's stain (small gram-negative cocci, often in pairs or chains).

Diseases Caused by Gram-positive Bacilli

Erysipelothricosis
Definition
Erysipelothricosis is an infection caused by *Erysipelothrix rhusiopathiae* that most often takes the form of *erysipeloid,* an acute but slowly evolving skin affliction.

Etiology/Epidemiology
- *E. rhusiopathiae* (formerly called *E. insidiosa*) is a gram-positive, capsulated, nonsporulating, nonmotile, microaerophilic bacillus with worldwide distribution; it is primarily a saprophyte (an organism that lives on dead organic matter).
- The organism infects a variety of living animals (insects, shellfish, fish, birds, mammals [especially swine]).
- In humans, the infection is mainly occupational and typically follows a penetrating wound in persons who handle animal matter, either edible or nonedible (infected car-

casses, rendered products such as fat, grease, fertilizer), bones, and shells.

Diagnosis
- Culture of a full-thickness biopsy of the skin is better than needle biopsy.
- Aspiration of the advancing edge of a lesion to isolate *E. rhusiopathiae*

Signs and symptoms
- Infection becomes apparent about 1 week after a skin wound.
- Purplish red, nonvesiculated, indurated, maculopapular rash appears first, with itching and burning.
- Local swelling, although sharply demarcated, may inhibit use of the hand, which is the most common site of infection.
- The lesion's border usually slowly extends outward and may cause pain and disability lasting about 3 weeks.
- The infection is usually self-limited; complications, such as endocarditis or arthritis, are rare.

Treatment
- Benzathine penicillin G 1.2 million U IM (a single 600,000-U dose in each buttock), or erythromycin 0.5 g qid PO for 7 days is curative.
- If arthritis is a complication, the same drug may be given, but repeated needle aspiration drainage of the infected joint is necessary.

Patient/Family Education
- Explain the nature, cause, course, treatment, and expected outcome to the patient and family.
- Emphasize the importance of protecting hands from injury at work, and suggest the possibility of wearing gloves, if permissible.
- Write out all medications, dosage, schedule, and any other information required by the individual in self-treating the infection.

Follow-up/Referral
- Return visits every week for 3 to 4 weeks are necessary to monitor the progress of the infection and patient compliance, and to re-emphasize protection of hands at work, frequent hand-washing without causing surface abrasion, and wearing protective gloves.

- At the time the infection seems to have completely cleared, and the patient is asymptomatic and ready to return to work, return visits are no longer necessary, but instruct the patient to call immediately if any signs of infection recur, so that early treatment will curtail the course.

Listeriosis
- This gram-positive anaerobic organism is found worldwide in the environment and in the gut of nonhuman mammals, birds, arachnids, and crustaceans.
- Because it is so rare ($\leq$7 cases/1,000,000 cases/year), it will not be discussed here, other than to list it among the gram-positive bacilli.

Anthrax

Definition
Anthrax is a highly infectious disease of animals, particularly ruminants, transmitted to humans by contact with the animals or their products.

Etiology/Epidemiology
- The organism is *B. anthracis*, a large, gram-positive, facultatively anaerobic, encapsulated rod; the spores resist destruction and remain viable in soil and animal products for decades.
- Transmission to humans is usually through the skin but can occur as the result of ingesting contaminated meat; inhaling spores when a respiratory infection is present in the person may cause pulmonary anthrax (woolsorters' disease), which is often fatal.
- Although this infection is an important disease of animals, it is extremely rare in humans, and therefore discussion will not be presented here.

Nocardiosis
This is another uncommon disease, caused by the gram-positive bacillus *Nocardia asteroides*, a soil saprophyte.

Diseases Caused by Gram-negative Bacilli

Enterobacteriaceae Infections
Enterobacteriaceae infections include *Salmonella, Shigella, Escherichia, Klebsiella, Enterobacter, Serratia, Proteus, Morganella, Providencia, Yersinia,*

and other less common genera. These organisms are oxidase-negative, gram-negative, catalase-positive bacilli that are readily cultured on ordinary media, ferment glucose, and reduce nitrates to nitrites.

Escherichia coli
- Normally inhabits the GI tract
- When the organisms have colonizing, enterotoxic, cytotoxic, or invasive virulence traits, they become major causes of watery, inflammatory, or bloody diarrhea, sometimes with the hemolytic-uremic syndrome.
  —If normal anatomic structures are disturbed, the organism may spread to adjacent structures or invade the bloodstream.
  —*E. coli* often infects the GU tract; hepatobiliary, peritoneal, cutaneous, and pulmonary infections also occur.
- This organism is an important cause of bacteremia and is an opportunistic pathogen causing disease in patients who have defects in resistance because of other existing diseases (e.g., cancer, diabetes, cirrhosis) or who received corticosteroid therapy, radiation, antineoplastic drugs, or antibiotics.

Diagnosis
- The organism must be observed in culture and appropriate biochemical or virulence tests because Gram's stain does not differentiate *E. coli* from other gram-negative bacteria.

Treatment
- Antibiotic therapy is begun immediately, then modified according to antibiotic sensitivity results.
- Although many strains are still sensitive to ampicillin and tetracyclines, therapy is increasingly turning to other antibiotics: ticarcillin, piperacillin, the cephalosporins, aminoglycosides, trimethoprim-sulfamethoxazole (TMP-SMX), and quinolones (adults).
- Surgery may be needed to drain pus, excise necrotic lesions, or remove foreign bodies.

Klebsiella, Enterobacter, and Serratia Infections
Klebsiella, Enterobacter, and *Serratia* infections are usually acquired in the hospital, primarily in those patients with diminished resistance. These organisms cause disease in the same sites as *E. coli* and are also important causes of bacteremia.

Treatment
- These organisms are sensitive to broad-spectrum antibiotics (e.g., ticarcillin, piperacillin) and the aminoglycosides; sensitivity is required, however, because many isolates are resistant to multiple antibiotics.
- *Klebsiella* pneumonia is a rare pulmonary infection usually seen in diabetics and alcoholics, characterized by severe pneumonia, sometimes with expectoration of dark brown or red ("currant-jelly") sputum, lung abscess formation, and empyema; it responds to cephalosporins and aminoglycosides.

The Protei
- Protei are gram-negative organisms that do not ferment lactose, and rapidly deaminate phenylalanine.
- They make up at least three groups.
  —*Proteus* (*P. mirabilis, P. vulgaris,* and *P. myxofaciens*)
  —*Morganella* (*P. morganii*)
  —*Providencia* (*P. rettgeri, P. alcalifaciens,* and *P. stuartii*)
- *P. mirabilis* causes most human infections and is distinguished from the others by its failure to form indole.
- These organisms are normally found in soil, water, and the flora of normal feces; they are often present in superficial wounds, draining ears, and sputum, particularly in patients whose normal flora has been eradicated by antibiotic therapy.
- They may cause deep-seated infection, especially in the ears and mastoid sinuses, peritoneal cavities, and urinary tracts of patients with chronic urinary tract infections (UTIs) or with renal or bladder stones; they also cause bacteremia.

Treatment
- *P. mirabilis* is often, but not always, sensitive to ampicillin, carbenicillin, ticarcillin, piperacillin, the cephalosporins, and aminoglycosides.
  —The other species are generally more resistant but are sensitive to most of the previously listed antibiotics, except for ampicillin, and to gentamicin, tobramycin, and amikacin.

Salmonella Infections

- The known serotypes of *Salmonella* (n = 2200) can be classified into the following groups:
  —Highly adapted to human hosts: *S. typhi, S. paratyphi A, B (S. schottmülleri),* and *C (S. hirschfeldii),* which are pathogenic only in humans and commonly cause enteric fever.
  —Adapted to nonhuman hosts: these cause disease almost exclusively in animals, but two of the strains also infect humans.
  —Unadapted to specific hosts: designated *S. enteritidis,* includes 2000 serotypes that cause gastroenteritis and account for 85% of all *Salmonella* infections in the United States.

Typhoid Fever

Definition

Typhoid fever is a systemic disease caused by *S. typhi* and characterized by fever, prostration, abdominal pain, and a rose-colored rash.

Epidemiology/Pathogenesis

- About 400 to 500 cases of typhoid fever are reported each year in the United States.
- Typhoid *bacilli* are shed in the feces of asymptomatic carriers or in the stool or urine of those with active disease.
- About 3% of untreated patients shed organisms in their stool for over a year, and are referred to as **chronic enteric carriers.**
  —Some carriers have no history of clinical illness, and apparently were asymptomatically infected.
  —Obstructive uropathy related to schistosomiasis may predispose some typhoid patients to develop a urinary carrier state.
- Most of the carriers in the United States are older women with chronic biliary disease.
- Studies show that typhoid carriers are more likely than the general population to acquire hepatobiliary cancer.
- Inadequate hygiene after defecation may spread the organism to communal food or water supplies.
- In geographic areas where sanitary measures are inadequate, the organism is transmitted by water more often than by food.

- In developed countries, transmission is usually by food that has been contaminated by healthy carriers during preparation.
- Flies may be the vector that transmits the organism from feces to food.
- Transmission may occur by means of fecal-oral route among children playing together or by adults during sexual practices.
- The disease is rarely seen in hospital personnel who have not taken proper precautions after changing bed linen or assisting a person to toilet.
- The organism enters the body via the GI tract and gains access to the bloodstream by way of the lymphatic channels.
- Monocytic inflammation occurs in the ileum and colon, within the lamina propria and Peyer's patches, where local tissue necrosis is common.
- In severe cases, ulceration, hemorrhage, and intestinal perforation may occur.

Diagnosis

Signs and Symptoms

- The incubation period—usually 8 to 14 days—is inversely related to the number of organisms ingested.
- Onset is gradual, with fever, headache, arthralgias, pharyngitis, constipation, anorexia, and abdominal pain; less common symptoms are dysuria, nonproductive cough, and epistaxis.
- If no treatment is begun, the temperature increases in steps over 2 to 3 days, remains elevated (usually 39.4° C to 40° C [103° F to 104° F]) for another 10 to 14 days, then begins to fall at the end of the third week, and reaches normal levels during the fourth week.
  —Prolonged fever is usually accompanied by bradycardia and prostration, and by central nervous system (CNS) symptoms such as delirium, stupor, or coma in severe cases.
- In about 10% of patients, discrete pink, blanching lesions (rose spots) appear in crops on the chest and abdomen during the second week and resolve in 2 to 5 days.
- Intestinal perforation, usually involving the distal ileum, occurs in 1% to 2% of patients,

which may be indicated by an acute abdomen and leukocytosis during the third week of illness.

- Splenomegaly, leukopenia, anemia, liver function abnormalities, proteinuria, and a mild consumption coagulopathy are common.
- Acute cholecystitis and hepatitis may develop.
- Late in the disease, florid diarrhea may begin, with blood (20% occult, 10% gross).
  —In about 2% of patients, severe bleeding occurs during the third week, with a mortality rate of about 25%.
- Pneumonia may develop from a pneumococcal infection, although *S. typhi* can also cause infiltrates.
- Convalescence may last several months.
- In 8% to 10% of untreated patients, signs and symptoms similar to the initial clinical syndrome may recur about 2 weeks after defervescence.
- For unknown reasons, antibiotic therapy during the initial illness increases the incidence of febrile relapse to 15% to 20%.
- If antibiotic therapy is reinstituted at the time of relapse, the fever abates rapidly unlike the slow defervescence seen during the primary illness.
- In some patients, a second relapse occurs.

Diagnostic Tests

- The diagnosis is confirmed by isolating the typhoid bacilli in cultures, although the clinical setting and hematologic abnormalities may suggest typhoid fever; the organisms can be isolated from cultures of blood or bone marrow only during the first 2 weeks of the illness, although stool cultures remain positive during the third to fifth weeks.
- Urine cultures are often positive.
- Cultures of liver biopsies or rose spots may also yield the organism.

Differential Diagnosis

- Other *Salmonella* infections that cause enteric fever, the major ricksettsioses, leptospirosis, disseminated tuberculosis (TB), malaria, brucellosis, tularemia, infectious hepatitis, psittacosis, *Yersinia enterocolitica* infection, and lymphoma; early in the infection, typhoid may resemble viral upper respiratory infection (URI) or UTI

Prognosis

- Without antibiotics, the mortality rate is about 12%; with timely therapy, the mortality rate is less than 1%.
  —Most deaths occur in patients who are malnourished, infants, and the elderly.
  —Stupor, coma, or shock indicates severe disease and a poor prognosis.
  —Complications occur in patients who are untreated, or in whom treatment is delayed.

Treatment

- Antibiotics have markedly decreased the severity and duration of illness, and also decrease complications and mortality.
  —Ceftriaxone 30 mg/kg/day IM or IV in two divided doses, for 2 weeks, and cefoperazone 60 mg/kg/day IV in two divided doses for 2 weeks are first-choice drugs.
  —Chloramphenicol is still widely used throughout the world but resistance is increasing.
  —Quinolones may be helpful but are not recommended for use with prepubertal children.
  —Glucocorticoids are used, in addition to antibiotics, to treat severe toxicity.
  —Patients are usually kept on bed rest while febrile.
- Salicylates, laxatives, and enemas should be avoided.
  —Diarrhea may be minimized with a clear liquid diet and if necessary parenteral nutrition.
  —Intestinal perforation and associated peritonitis require broader gram-negative and anaerobic antibiotic drugs; surgery to repair perforation is preferred, with antibiotics after the repair.
- Carriers must be reported to the local health department and prohibited from handling food.
- Typhoid bacilli may be isolated for up to 6 months after the acute illness in those who do not become carriers.
  —After that, three negative stool cultures at weekly intervals are required to exclude a carrier state.

- In carriers with normal biliary tracts, the cure rate is about 60% with antibiotics such as ampicillin or amoxicillin.
  —In those with gallbladder disease, eradication of the bacilli has been achieved with TMP-SMX and rifampin.
  —In other cases, cholecystectomy with antibiotics for 2 days preoperatively and 2 to 3 weeks postoperatively has been successful.

Patient/Family Education

- Explain the nature, cause, course, treatment, and expected outcome of therapy.
- Provide rationale for postrecovery testing to define potential carrier state.
- Give written information about all medications, dosages, and schedules.
- Instruct about how typhoid is transmitted, and precautions to take to avoid contamination of food and water.

Follow-up/Referral

- Many recovered typhoid patients are followed for weeks to months, sometimes years, depending on the patient's status.
- All known contacts are screened for possible infection.
- Carriers are prohibited from handling food or beverages (e.g., restaurants, grocery stores, food warehouses).
- Three negative stool cultures, one week apart, are required to verify full recovery and noncarrier status.

Haemophilus Infections

Haemophilus is a gram-negative, pleomorphic, coccobacillus. *Haemophilus* pathogens that affect humans include *H. influenzae, H. ducreyi,* and *H. parainfluenzae.* Noncapsulated forms produce luminal infections (e.g., bronchitis), and encapsulated organisms produce invasive disease (e.g., meningitis).

- *Haemophilus* is a normal commensal of the upper respiratory tract and is found in about 80% of healthy individuals.
- Of the six antigenic types of *H. influenzae* identified, type b is the most significant in humans, and demonstrates the greatest pathogenicity, particularly in children under 5 years of age.
- An effective vaccine is now available; all children in developed countries are vaccinated.

- Many less developed countries (i.e., Gambia) have instituted mass immunization programs.
- Patients undergoing splenectomy or those with hyposplenism (e.g., sickle cell disease) and patients who are HIV-positive should receive the vaccine.
- *H. influenzae* can cause disease in several organs: URI, respiratory (sinusitis, bronchitis, pneumonitis, pneumonia); CNS (meningitis, brain abscess); heart (endocarditis, pericarditis); joints (septic arthritis); skin, soft tissues (cellulitis); ENT (epiglottitis, otitis media).
- Many formerly very serious diseases caused by *H. influenzae* have now been almost or entirely eliminated by the use of antibiotics (e.g., meningitis, epiglottitis).

Diagnosis

- The diagnosis of an *H. influenzae*–caused infection is by isolation and culture of the organism.
  —Counterimmunoelectrophoresis can detect type b capsular antigen in 75% of patients.

Treatment

- Therapy is urgent because delay may result in a high mortality.
- In cases of meningitis and epiglottitis, the drug of choice is chloramphenicol 50 to 100 mg/kg/day for children, and 4 g/day for 7 to 10 days for adults.
- Cefuroxime can be given orally or, for meningitis, 3 g q8h.
- Ampicillin can be used for less severe cases, but resistance to this drug is increasing.
- Those in close contact with an infected individual are at increased risk of developing the disease.
- Rifampin 20 mg/kg/day for 4 days is helpful in preventing development of the disease or diminishing its effects.
- Conjugate vaccines have been developed in which a purified capsular polysaccharide is linked to a protein to improve immunogenicity.
- These are highly effective; 99% of children have protective levels after 3 days.

Patient/Family Education

- Instruct patients and families about the infectious nature of *H. influenzae,* and the need for urgent treatment once the disease is diagnosed.

- Inform patients and families about the availability of vaccines and new advances in the area of prevention.

Follow-up/Referral

- Patients are seen once a week until complete recovery is evident.
- Specialists may be called in consultation at any time during the course of illness: neurologists, ENT specialists, cardiologists, or others according to the system involved.
- After full recovery, the patient returns to his or her preinfection schedule of regular appointments.
- The patient is asked to call in case of recurrence, new symptoms, or suspicion of reinfection.

Shigella Infections

Shigellosis (Bacillary Dysentery)

Definition

Shigellosis is an acute, self-limiting intestinal infection caused by one of four species of gram-negative nonspore-forming bacilli: *Shigella dysenteriae, S. flexneri, S. boydii,* and *S. sonnei.*

- All of these are enteroinvasive, but *S. dysenteriae* type 1 and some strains of *S. flexneri* and *S. sonnei* are known to elaborate a toxin that is enterotoxic, neurotoxic, and cytotoxic.
  —Like salmonellosis, shigellosis is found worldwide and is more prevalent in areas with poor hygiene and overcrowding.
- Transmission is via the fecal-oral route; a very low dose is sufficient to produce the disease.

Diagnosis

- The diagnosis is confirmed by positive stool culture.

Signs and symptoms

- Children under 5 years are those most commonly affected, but people of all ages are at risk.
- The incubation period is quite short—2 days.
- Onset is acute, with fever, malaise, abdominal pain, and watery diarrhea.

- As the disease progresses in severity, bloody diarrhea with mucus, tenesmus, fecal urgency, and severe cramping abdominal pain become prominent.
- Nausea, vomiting, headache, and convulsions in small children are likely due to the neurotoxin.
- When the infection is caused by *S. dysenteriae,* which is responsible for the more fulminant forms of shigellosis, cholera-like symptoms may occur.

Diagnostic tests

- Sigmoidoscopy shows the presence of a markedly hyperemic and inflamed mucosa with transversely distributed ulcers with ragged undermined edges; these signs are often indistinguishable from other dysenteric infections, and from nonspecific inflammatory bowel disease.
- Complications may be mild (e.g., arthritis, conjunctivitis, and morbilliform rash); or life-threatening (e.g., colonic perforation, septicemia, and the hemolytic anemia syndrome).

Treatment

- Treatment is symptomatic: oral fluid replacement as necessary.
  —In severe cases, trimethoprim 200 mg bid or ciprofloxacin 500 mg bid may be used.
- Public health measures, particularly the disposal of excreta and availability of potable water, prevent spread of the infection.

Patient/Family Education

- Patients and family members should be instructed about the nature, cause, course, treatment, prophylaxis, and expected outcome of therapy.
- Diseases, such as shigellosis, provide an excellent opportunity to convey the importance of handwashing, particularly after toileting, general hygiene, and noncontaminated food and water.

Follow-up/Referral

- Patients are followed for several weeks after recovery to assess for recurrence or new symptoms.

- Repeat instructions regarding hygiene, hand-washing, and uncontaminated food and water.

Campylobacter Infections

C. jejuni is a gram-negative, motile, curved spiral rod that is microaerophilic and therefore fails to multiply under aerobic or strict anaerobic conditions.

- It invades the mucosa of both the small and large bowel, causing inflammation and sometimes ulceration.
- It causes acute gastroenteritis and, in many parts of the world, is the most common cause of dysentery-like disease.
- In developing countries, asymptomatic carriers are found among young children.

Diagnosis

Signs and Symptoms

- Symptoms begin 2 to 5 days after consuming infected material (usually chicken or milk).
  —Fever, headache, and malaise are the initial symptoms.
  —These are rapidly followed by diarrhea, often with blood, and severe cramping abdominal pain.
  —The patient appears ill.

Diagnostic Tests

- Sigmoidoscopy may show the changes of acute colitis, which are usually indistinguishable from those of ulcerative colitis.
- Complications include cholecystitis, pancreatitis, a reactive arthritis, the Guillain-Barré syndrome, and the hemolytic uremic syndrome.
- Diagnosis is confirmed by direct phase microscopy of a wet mount of stool, which may show the motile curved rods resembling "flying birds."
- The organism may be cultured on special media within 48 hours.
- In severe cases, the organism may be cultured from blood.

Treatment

- In most cases, *Campylobacter* enteritis is self-limiting, resolving in 5 to 7 days.

- Although the organism is sensitive to erythromycin, there is no supportive evidence to show that treatment alters the natural history of the infection.
- If symptoms persist, and if bacteremia develops, antibiotics are initiated.

Patient/Family Education

- Instruct the patient and family about the nature, cause, course, treatment, and expected outcome of the disease.
- It is extremely important that fluids be replaced if they are being lost through vomiting or diarrhea, either orally or parenterally.
- Care is largely supportive: maintaining the comfort of the patient as much as possible, making sure that fluids are readily available 24 hours a day and that discomfort is relieved by analgesics.

Follow-up/Referral

- After recovery, the patient is seen in the office every 1 to 2 weeks to assess for any signs of recurrence of symptoms, complications, or reinfection.
- Vital signs are taken and recorded, and the state of hydration/nutrition is noted.

Helicobacter Infections

Definition

Helicobacter pylori is now considered to be the cause of peptic ulcer disease.

- It is a gram-negative organism that colonizes the gastric epithelium beneath the mucus layer and in areas of gastric metaplasia that occur in the duodenum.
  —*H. pylori* and nonsteroidal antiinflammatory drugs (NSAIDs) may disrupt the normal mucosal defense and repair, making the mucosa more susceptible to the attack of acid.
- *H. pylori* is noted for its ability to produce urease, which is thought to be involved in the pathogenesis of disease.
- *H. pylori* is found in 10% of healthy people under age 30, and in 60% of healthy people over age 60; it is seen in over 90% of people with a duodenal ulcer.
- Eradication of the organism appears to result in accelerated duodenal ulcer healing,

and significantly decreases ulcer recurrence 1 and 2 years after treatment.

Risk Factors
- Cigarette smoking: increases the risk and delays the healing of duodenal ulcer.
  —Nonsmokers who do have *H. pylori* eradicated and who are not placed on maintenance drug therapy have an annual recurrence rate of about 20%, which is equal to that of smokers treated with maintenance therapy.
  —Nontreated smokers in whom *H. pylori* is not eradicated have a recurrence rate of 70%.
  —Smoking may also predispose patients to bleeding and perforation.
- Aspirin and NSAIDs are risk factors for gastric erosion and ulcers.

Diagnosis
Signs and Symptoms
- Signs and symptoms are the same as for peptic ulcer disease.
  —Epigastric distress—vague discomfort or a feeling of gnawing hunger, usually in the midline
  —If pain occurs, it is typically aching or burning.
  —The symptoms occur 1 to 3 hours after a meal, and may awaken the patient from sleep, usually between 1 and 2 AM.
  —Symptoms are relieved within minutes by food, antacids, or vomiting.
  —Pain is minimal before breakfast.
  —Weight loss occurs in up to 50% of patients with benign gastric ulcer and is not a helpful feature in distinguishing benign from malignant disease.

Diagnostic Tests
- The gold standard for diagnosing *H. pylori* infection is histologic testing, with tissue samples obtained by endoscopy from different parts of the antrum; this method has a sensitivity and specificity of 85% to 100%.
  —This procedure is expensive and time-consuming.
  —*H. pylori* is identified by using hematoxylin and eosin, Warthin-Starry, or Giemsa stains; sensitivity ranges from 50% to 95%, specificity is nearly 100%.
- For patients having endoscopy, the least expensive and quickest test is the urease (CLO) test, which is commercially available, with a sensitivity and specificity of 95%.
- Another test to confirm the diagnosis of *H. pylori* infection is by fingerstick; the antibody (immunoglobulin G [IgG]) is shown in the blood, which is >90% specific and sensitive.
- The diagnosis of peptic ulcer disease is also made by barium studies or endoscopy.
- A test used for both diagnosis and to monitor the eradication of *H. pylori* is the urea breath test; sensitivity is 96% and specificity is 98%; however, results of this test are read by a mass spectrometer, and must therefore be sent out of the office for reading.

Treatment
- Pharmacologic therapy to eradicate *H. pylori* and thus heal gastric or peptic ulcers requires a combination of drugs (Table 21-3).
  —Dual therapy with omeprazole 20 mg bid and clarithromycin 500 mg tid given for 14 days is a well-tolerated regimen with eradication rates between 75% and 85%; omeprazole 20 mg/day should be continued for 2 additional weeks.
  —Triple therapy with bismuth subsalicylate 2 tablets qid, metronidazole 250 mg qid, and tetracycline with bismuth
- **Surgery:** except in cases of emergency (e.g., hemorrhage, perforation) surgery now is almost never necessary.

Patient/Family Education
- Instruct the patient and family about the nature, cause, course, treatment, and expected outcome of therapy.
- As with other drug regimens, strict adherence to dose and schedule is essential for optimal outcome.
- Advise the patient to avoid foods or beverages that cause discomfort; otherwise, no dietary restrictions are necessary.

Follow-up/Referral
- Periodic evaluations are necessary to determine whether eradication of *H. pylori* has occurred after therapy.

TABLE 21-3
Therapeutic Options for Eradication of *H. pylori*

Regimen	Drugs	Dosage	Duration
Dual therapy	Omeprazole	40 mg qd	2 wks
	Clarithromycin (or)	500 mg tid	
	RBC	400 mg bid	4 wks
	Clarithromycin	500 mg tid	2 wks
Bismuth-based triple therapy	Bismuth subsalicylate	2 tablets qid	2 wks
	Metronidazole	250 mg qid	
	Tetracycline (or)	500 mg qid	
	amoxicillin	500 mg qid	
PPI-based triple therapy	Metronidazole (or)	500 mg bid	10-14 days
	amoxicillin	1000 mg bid	
	Omeprazole	20 mg bid	
PPI + 2 antibiotics	Clarithromycin	500 mg bid	
Quadruple therapy	Bismuth-based triple therapy + omeprazole	Triple therapy + omeprazole 20 mg qd	14 days

From Katz PO: Peptic ulcer disease. In Barker LR, Burton JR, Zieve PD, eds: *Principles of ambulatory medicine,* ed 5, Baltimore, 1999, Williams & Wilkins, p 486.
RBC, Ranitidine and bismuth citrate; *PPI,* proton pump inhibitors.

- Consultation with specialists (e.g., gastroenterologist) may be necessary if complications occur.

Lyme Disease

Definition
Lyme disease is a tick-transmitted, spirochetal, inflammatory disorder characterized by a rash that may be followed weeks to months later by neurologic, cardiac, or joint abnormalities. Lyme disease was recognized in 1975 based on clustering of cases in Lyme, CT; it has since been reported in 49 states, but over 90% of cases occur from Massachusetts to Maryland, in Wisconsin and Minnesota, and in California and Oregon; it also occurs in Europe, Russia, China, and Japan.

Risk Factors
- Walking or camping in thickly wooded areas where the deer population is known to be high.

Etiology/Cause
- Lyme disease is caused by a spirochete, *Borrelia burgdorferi,* which is transmitted primarily by tiny ticks of the *Ixodes ricinus* complex.
  —In the United States, the white-footed mouse is the primary animal reservoir for *B. burgdorferi* and the preferred host for nymphal and larval forms of *I. scapularis (dammini),* the deer tick.
  —Deer are the preferred host for the adult ticks in the United States; sheep are the preferred host in Europe.
  —Other animals (e.g., dogs) can be incidental hosts and can develop the disease.

Pathogenesis
- Deer ticks in the nymphal stage, which attack humans, are very small and difficult to see.
  —Once attached to the skin, they continue to gorge on blood for days.
  —Transmission of *B. burgdorferi* does not usually occur until the infected tick has been in place for at least 36 to 48 hours; therefore screening for ticks after potential exposure, and removing them, can help prevent infection.
  —*B. burgdorferi* enters the skin at the site of the tick bite; it may spread to lymph, producing regional adenopathy, or disseminate in blood to organs or other skin sites.
  —The relatively small number of organisms in the affected tissue suggests that most manifestations of infection are due to host immune response rather than to the destructive properties of the organism.

Diagnosis

Signs and Symptoms

- **Erythema migrans** is the hallmark and best clinical indicator of Lyme disease, and develops in at least 75% of patients, beginning as a red macule or papule, generally on the proximal portion of an extremity or on the trunk, particularly the thigh, buttock, or axilla, between 3 and 32 days after a tick bite.
  —The area of erythema expands, sometimes with central clearing, up to a diameter of 50 cm.
  —Soon after onset, nearly 50% of untreated patients develop multiple smaller lesions without indurated centers.
  —Cultures of these lesions are positive, indicating dissemination of infection.
  —Erythema migrans usually lasts for several weeks; evanescent lesions sometimes appear during resolution; resolved lesions may reappear faintly, occasionally before recurrent attacks of arthritis.
- A musculoskeletal, flu-like illness with malaise, fatigue, fever, chills, and arthralgias often accompanies erythema migrans, or precedes it by a few days.
  —Less frequently, backache, nausea and vomiting, adenopathy, sore throat, and splenomegaly may occur.
  —Some patients may develop fibromyalgia.
- Neurologic abnormalities develop in about 15% of patients within weeks to months or erythema nigrans, usually before arthritis appears, often lasts for months, and then resolves completely.
  —These abnormalities include lymphocytic meningitis, meningoencephalitis, cranial neuritis (similar to Bell's palsy), which may be bilateral, and sensory or motor radiculoneuropathies; these symptoms may occur singly or in combination.
- Myocardial abnormalities occur in about 8% of patients within weeks of erythema migrans, including fluctuating degrees of atrioventricular block (first-degree, Wenckebach, or third-degree) and, rarely, myopericarditis with reduced ejection fractions and cardiomegaly.
- Arthritis develops in about 60% of patients within weeks to months (up to 2 years) of disease onset (erythema migrans).

—Intermittent swelling and pain in the large joints, particularly the knee, recur for several years, although the affected knees are usually more swollen than painful, and may be warm but not red.
—Baker's cysts may form and rupture.
—Malaise, fatigue, and low-grade fever may precede or accompany attacks of arthritis.
—About 10% of patients develop chronic (unremittent for ≥6 months) knee involvement.
—Later symptoms that may occur years after onset include antibiotic-sensitive skin lesions (acrodermatitis chronica atrophicans) and chronic CNS abnormalities.

Diagnostic Tests

- Laboratory tests are usually reserved for patients in whom probability of the disease is high, based on history and symptoms.
  —Skin biopsy that is positive for erythema migrans, which resembles an insect bite: epidermal and dermal involvement at the center that is often indurated; all layers of the dermis are heavily infiltrated with mononuclear cells around blood vessels and skin appendages
  —At the center, the papillary dermis is edematous and the epidermis has a thickened keratin layer and intracellular and extracellular edema.
  —Titers of antispirochetal antibodies (e.g., IgM, then IgG) are determined by enzyme-linked immunosorbent assay (ELISA) or by indirect immunofluorescence, but these are not useful until the patient has made antibodies.
  —Confirmation of positive titers is best made by Western blot initially.
  —ESR may be elevated.
  —WBC are differential, and Hct are usually normal.
  —Serum complement components are either normal or elevated during active disease.
  —Aspartate transaminase (AST) and lactate dehydrogenase (LDH) levels are often slightly elevated when erythema migrans is present.
  —Patients who develop arthritis have an increased frequency of the B-cell alloantigen

BOX 21-4

Current Antibiotic Therapy for Adult Lyme Disease

EARLY LYME DISEASE
Amoxicillin 500 mg PO tid × 10-21 days
Doxycycline 100 mg PO bid × 10-21 days
Cefuroxime axetil 500 mg PO bid × 10-21 days
Azithromycin 500 mg qd × 7 days (less effective than
   other regimens)

NEUROLOGIC MANIFESTATIONS
(Bell's-like palsy, no other neurologic
   abnormalities)
Doxycycline or amoxicillin (as for early disease)
Meningitis (with/without radiculoneuropathy or
   encephalitis)
Ceftriaxone 2 g IV qd × 14-28 days
Doxycycline 100 mg PO bid × 14-28 days
Chloramphenicol 1 g PO qid × 14-28 days

CARDIAC MANIFESTATIONS
Ceftriaxone 2 g IV qd × 14 days
Penicillin G 20 MU IV × 14 days
Doxycycline 100 mg PO bid × 21 days*
Amoxicillin 500 mg PO tid × 21 days

ARTHRITIS
Amoxicillin and probenecid 500 mg PO each, qid ×
   30 days
Doxycycline 100 mg PO bid × 30 days
Ceftriaxone 2 g IV qd × 14-28 days
Penicillin G 20 MU IV qd × 14-28 days

ACRODERMATITIS CHRONICA ATROPHICANS
Penicillin V 1 g PO tid × 30 days or 3 g/day
Penicillin G 20 MU IV qd × 14-28 days for 30 days
Doxycycline 100 mg PO bid × 30 days

Modified from Rahn DW, Malawisa SE: Treatment of Lyme disease. Special article. In Mandell GL, Bone RC, Cline MJ, et al, eds: *1994 Year book of medicine,* St. Louis, 1994, Mosby-Year Book, pp xxi-xxxvi.
*These are guidelines, to be modified by new findings and applied always with primary focus on the clinical context of individual patients.

human leukocyte antigen (HLA)-DR4, but not HLA-B27, which is common in patients with spondyloarthropathies.
—Synovial fluid analysis shows a WBC count increase of about 25,000/μl (normal range is <2000/μl).
—Synovial membrane from affected joints may be indistinguishable from that of rheumatoid arthritis (RA) patients.
—X-ray findings usually show only soft tissue swelling, but some patients have erosion of cartilage and bone.

Differential Diagnosis
• Lyme disease should be distinguished from juvenile RA in younger persons and from Reiter's syndrome and atypical RA in adults, and from other tick-transmitted diseases; other conditions that should be excluded are peripheral neuropathies, chronic fatigue, and CNS syndromes.

Treatment
• Most cases of Lyme disease respond well to antibiotics (Box 21-4).

Patient/Family Education
• Many patients are not yet aware of tick-transmitted diseases, so instruction regard-

ing preventive measures, what to look for, and treatment is helpful.
• History of allergic reactions to any antibiotics to be used should be documented.
• Explain in detail the treatment to be carried out, its duration, and expected outcomes, including potential long-term complications and their signs, symptoms, and therapy.
• Instructions about when to call the clinician in case of recurring symptoms or evidence of new symptoms should be in writing.

Follow-up/Referral
• Patients are monitored every 1 to 2 weeks after completion of antibiotic therapy to make certain that the condition has resolved completely.
• Consultation with or referral to a specialist in infectious diseases may be required at any time during therapy or after resolution.

Mycobacterial Infections
Tuberculosis
Definition
TB is a chronic, recurrent infection, usually in the lungs.

Risk Factors
• HIV infection
• Black race

- IV drug users
- Urban-dwelling men between ages 25 and 44
- Incidence is lower in white, middle-class homosexual men with acquired immunodeficiency syndrome (AIDS).
- Alcoholism
- Poor nutrition

Incidence

- About 27,337 cases were reported in 1996 in the United States (8/100,000), but two thirds of patients were people born in other countries (e.g., Haiti, Mexico, India, China, Vietnam, or the Philippines).
- Prevalent in people over 70 years, all races, in whom the incidence may be as high as 200/100,000.
- Signs of a potentially dangerous epidemic of TB have appeared.
  —HIV-infected persons (up to 30% in New York state in 1992 to 1993)
  —Drug-resistant organisms are increasing.

Etiology

- TB is caused by *Mycobacterium tuberculosis*, *M. bovis*, or *M. africanum*.
- Other mycobacteria cause diseases similar to TB; these respond poorly to the drugs used to treat TB.
  —*M. kansasii*
  —*M. avium-intracellulare*
- Fungi that cause diseases similar to TB
  —*Cryptococcus neoformans*
  —*Histoplasma capsulatum*

Pathogenesis

- Human TB occurs almost exclusively from inhalation of organisms dispersed as droplet nuclei from a person with pulmonary TB whose sputum smear is positive.
- *M. tuberculosis* may float in the air for several hours.
- Spread can occur in hospitals, mycobacteriology laboratories, and autopsy rooms.

Stages of Tuberculosis

- Primary (initial) infection: 90% to 95% of new infections are not diagnosed; they result in a positive tuberculin test and a latent or dormant infection.
  —Primary TB may become active at any age, producing clinical TB in any organ, most commonly in the apical area of the lung, but also in the kidney, long bones, vertebrae, lymph nodes, and other sites.
  —Activation may occur within 1 to 2 years of infection, but in other people, activation may not occur for many years, becoming active only after the patient has developed diabetes mellitus, during periods of high stress, or after treatment with corticosteroids or other immunosuppressive drugs.
  —The initial infection leaves nodular scars in the apices of one or both lungs, called **Simon foci,** which are the most common seeds for later active TB.
  —Frequency of activation is apparently unaffected by calcified scars of primary infection **(Ghon foci)** or by residual calcified hilar lymph nodes.
  —Subtotal gastrectomy and silicosis also predispose patients to development of active TB.
  —A healthy adult newly infected with TB has about a 5% chance of developing clinical TB in the first 5 years after infection, and a total lifetime risk of about 10%.
  —The other 90% of normal people infected with TB have a positive skin test but never develop clinical disease.
  —People who are tuberculin-positive due to long-standing infection and who then acquire HIV infection have an annual incidence of 8% to 10% and nearly a 100% lifetime incidence.
- Even more devastating are people with HIV infection who contract TB, in whom the annual incidence of severe clinical TB is much higher, perhaps as much as 50% to 100%.
- Latent or dormant infection
  —Most sporadic, symptomatic cases of TB develop in those who were infected many years ago and who were never treated or were inadequately treated.
- Adult-type (recrudescent) is the type of TB that occurs in people many years after the initial infection (e.g., activation of latent or dormant infection).

TABLE 21-4
Drugs Used to Treat Mycobacterial Diseases in Adults

Drug*	Once Daily Dose	Twice Weekly Dose
Isoniazid (INH)	5-10 mg/kg up to 300 mg PO or IM	15 mg/kg PO up to 900 mg
Rifampin	10 mg/kg up to 600 mg PO	10 mg/kg up to 600 mg PO
Streptomycin	15-20 mg/kg up to 1 g IM	25-30 mg/kg up to 1 g IM
Pyrazinamide	15-30 mg/kg up to 2 g PO	50-70 mg/kg up to 4 g
Ethambutol	15-25 mg/kg PO	50 mg/kg PO up to 2.5 g

From American Thoracic Society: Treatment of tuberculosis and tuberculosis infection in adults and children. *Am Rev Respir Dis* 134:355, 1986.
*Duration of therapy is variable according to drug or combination of drugs; consult most current literature.

Prophylaxis
- Prophylaxis is indicated primarily in those whose tuberculin skin test converted from negative to positive within the previous 2 years, for any HIV-infected person whose tuberculin reaction is ≥10 mm because the protective effect of T-cell immunity is lost, and for any child <4 years of age who is in a household with a person whose sputum is positive for acid-fast bacilli.
- Prophylaxis is usually isoniazid unless resistance is suspected.
  - 300 mg/day × 6 to 9 months for adults
  - 10 mg/kg/day up to 300 mg, as a single morning dose
  - In infected children and elderly tuberculin converters, isoniazid therapy is 98.5% effective in preventing development of clinical TB.
- Isolation of TB patients is no longer necessary because any risk of transmission will already have occurred by the time of diagnosis and treatment.
- Patients usually become noninfectious within 10 to 14 days after beginning treatment.

Treatment
- Antituberculous drugs include five that are *bactericidal* in the usual doses, and three that are *bacteriostatic* in usual doses (Table 21-4).
- Patients who are given a drug may improve at first, then worsen as the resistant mutants multiply.
- To prevent development of resistance to drugs, all patients with TB are treated with at least two drugs that act through different mechanisms.

Patient/Family Education
- Instruct the patient about the nature, cause, transmission, treatment, and expected outcome of therapy.
- Health departments now supervise therapy, test contacts, provide prophylactic isoniazid (INH) if necessary, provide free drugs, and perform sputum cultures and radiographs to determine cure.
- In ambulatory care settings, patients with active TB are placed in a separate waiting area apart from other patients, and not in open waiting areas.

Follow-up/Referral
- Appointments in health department clinics should be scheduled so that HIV-infected patients and others who are immunocompromised are not there at the same time.
- After treatment has begun, patients are seen or contacted at least once a month to ensure compliance with the drug regimen and to monitor drug side effects.
  - Sputum samples are cultured every month for 3 months; *sputum cultures should be negative after 3 months of therapy.*
  - A test-of-cure sputum culture should be done on all patients at 5 or 6 months.
  - Chest x-rays are done at 3 months, and between 6 and 12 months.

Viral Diseases

Several hundred different viruses infect humans primarily. Many of these have only recently been recognized and their clinical effects are not fully understood.
- Most viruses are spread mainly via respiratory and enteric excretions.

—Many viruses infect hosts without producing symptoms; however, their widespread prevalence causes important medical and public health problems.

—Spread of many viruses is limited because of inborn resistance of the host, prior immunization or vaccination, sanitary and other public health measures to improve health status of individuals and communities, and use of prophylactic antiviral drugs.

• Viruses are the smallest of parasites and are completely dependent on cells (bacterial, plant, or animal) to reproduce.

—They range in size from 0.02 to 0.3 micron, too small for light microscopy, but are visible under the electron microscope.

• Viruses are made up of an outer cover of protein, and sometimes lipid, and a nucleic acid core of ribonucleic acid (RNA) or deoxyribonucleic acid (DNA).

—In many cases, this core penetrates susceptible cells and initiates the infection.

—Like most other parasites, viruses stimulate host antibody production.

• Some viruses have oncogenic properties: human T-cell lymphotropic virus type 1 (a retrovirus) is associated with human leukemia and lymphoma; Epstein-Barr virus has been associated with malignancies such as nasopharyngeal carcinoma, Burkitt's lymphoma, Hodgkin's disease, lymphomas in immunosuppressed organ transplant recipients, Kaposi's sarcoma, primary effusion lymphomas, and Castleman's disease, a lymphoproliferative disorder.

• Slow viral diseases are characterized by prolonged incubations and cause some chronic degenerative diseases, including subacute sclerosing panencephalitis (measles virus), progressive rubella panencephalitis, progressive multifocal leukoencephalopathy (JC virus), and Creutzfeldt-Jakob disease (a prion disease).

• Latency, a quiescent infection by a virus, permits recurrent infection despite immune responses and facilitates person-to-person spread; hyperviruses exhibit latency.

Diagnosis

• Only a few viral diseases can be diagnosed clinically or epidemiologically (e.g., by well-known viral syndromes).

• Diagnosis usually requires testing using culture, polymerase chain reaction, or viral antigen tests; histopathology can sometimes aid in diagnosis.

Prophylaxis and Treatment

• Effective vaccines used for active immunity are available: influenza, measles, mumps, poliomyelitis, rabies, rubella, yellow fever, hepatitis A, hepatitis B, and varicella.

—An effective adenovirus vaccine is available but is used only in high-risk groups (e.g., military recruits).

• Immunoglobulins are available for passive immune prophylaxis.

• Therapeutic or prophylactic drugs against some viruses are available: amantadine or rimantadine for influenza A; acyclovir, valacyclovir, and famciclovir for herpes simplex or varicella-zoster infections; ganciclovir, foscarnet, and cidofovir for cytomegaloviruses; and reverse transcriptase inhibitors, protease inhibitors, and others for HIV; currently, interferon use is limited to hepatitis B and C and human papillomavirus.

Respiratory Viral Diseases

• Respiratory viral infections cause acute local and systemic illnesses, and include the following:

—Common cold
—Influenza
—Pharyngitis
—Laryngitis
—Tracheobronchitis
—Pneumonia

• The most serious and damaging viral respiratory diseases are influenza and respiratory syncytial viruses.

• Immunity to reinfection by viruses is usually brief because of the short life of immunologic responses and the antigenic diversity of most viruses.

Influenza
Definition

Influenza is an acute viral respiratory infection, a virus that causes fever, coryza, cough, headache, malaise, and inflamed respiratory mucous membranes.

Risk factors

- Young or old age
- Exposure to the influenza virus
- Poor nutrition
- Chronic pulmonary disease (e.g., chronic obstructive pulmonary disease [COPD], pulmonary edema)
- Persons with valvular heart disease
- Immunocompromised persons (e.g., HIV-infected, immunosuppressive drugs)

Etiology/cause

- Many people mistakenly label as "flu" all respiratory infections, even those not caused by the influenza virus.
- Spread of viral influenza is by airborne droplets, person-to-person contact, or contact with contaminated items.

Pathogenesis

- Influenza viruses are orthomyxoviruses, and are classified as types A, B, or C by complement-fixing antibodies to the nucleoprotein and matrix proteins.
- Influenza C virus infection does not cause classic influenza.
- Influenza types A and B have two principal surface glycoproteins, hemagglutinin (HA) and neuraminidase (NA).
  - These permit the virus to attach to and infect susceptible hosts and are targets of significant host immunologic responses.
  - HA allows the virus to bind to cellular sialic acid and to fuse with the host membrane.
  - NA functions as an enzyme to remove sialic acid, preventing self-aggregation and promoting dispersion during binding of new virions from the infected cell.
- Currently, only a single serologic type of influenza B virus is recognized, although strain variability is shown by the antigenicity of HA and NA.
- On the other hand, influenza A viruses have been categorized into subtypes based on direct antigenic divergence of HAs and NAs.
  - Mutations of HA and NA within a type of influenza virus are known as antigenic drift, a continuous process for both influenza A and B viruses.
  - Antigenic drift can be substantial, leading to severe epidemics with severe disease.
- Exchange of entire gene segments between viruses of human and animal (usually avian) origin produces new reassortant viruses in a process known as antigenic shift.
  - Antigenic shift has occurred only in influenza A viruses, resulting in pandemics.
- An avian strain of influenza A (H5N1) emerged as a cause of human influenza in 18 documented cases in Hong Kong in 1997, but pandemic spread did not occur.

Diagnosis

Signs and symptoms

- In uncomplicated influenza, the leukocyte count is normal.
- Fever and severe constitutional symptoms differentiate influenza from the common cold.
- Although rarely needed, a specific diagnosis can be made definitively by isolating the virus, demonstrating infected cells in secretions using immunologic or molecular methods to detect viral constituents or showing a rise in antibodies specific for HA or NA in serologic tests.
- The virus is most easily recovered from respiratory secretions by replication in tissue cultures.

Serologic tests

- To establish infection, complement fixation (CF) and hemagglutination inhibiting (HI) tests are done, although enzyme-linked immunosorbent assay techniques are being increasingly used.
- Leukocytosis with a shift toward immature granulocytes in the blood smear is a valuable sign of complicating bacterial or mixed viral-bacterial pneumonia.
- Purulent sputum specimens should be collected for smear, Gram's stain, and examination for leukocytes and bacteria.
- During the 48-hour incubation period after infection, virus replicates in the respiratory tract and transient asymptomatic viremia may occur.
- In mild cases (e.g., resistant or partially immune hosts), the symptoms are like those of a common cold.
  - Chills and fever up to 39° C to 39.5° C (102° F to 103° F) begin suddenly.

—Prostration and systemic aches and pains, most often in the back and legs, occur early.

—Headache is prominent, often with photophobia and retrobulbar aching.

—Respiratory symptoms may be mild at first, with scratchy sore throat, substernal burning, nonproductive cough, and sometimes coryza.

—Later, the respiratory symptoms become dominant, in which cough can be persistent and productive.

—In severe cases, sputum may be bloody.

—The skin is warm and flushed.

—The soft palate, posterior hard palate, tonsillar pillars, and posterior pharyngeal wall may be red, without exudate.

—Conjunctivitis may be present, and the eyes water easily.

—After 2 to 3 days, acute symptoms rapidly subside and fever ends, although fever may last up to 5 days without complications.

—Abnormal lung clearance and altered bronchiolar air flow can be observed.

—Weakness, sweating, and fatigue may persist for several days, up to several weeks.

—Hemorrhagic bronchitis and pneumonia may occur and progress rapidly.

—Fulminant, fatal pneumonia may be viral, bacterial, or mixed viral-bacterial.

—When this occurs, dyspnea and bloody sputum associated with pulmonary congestion and edema may end with death in as little as 48 hours after onset.

—When pneumonia develops, cough worsens and purulent or bloody sputum is produced.

—Crepitant or subcrepitant rales can be detected over the involved pulmonary segments.

- Severe disease usually occurs during a pandemic caused by a new influenza serotype, and in persons with cardiac or pulmonary risk factors.

Complications

- Encephalitis, myocarditis, and myoglobinuria occur infrequently as complications of influenza infection, occurring usually during the convalescent period.

Differential diagnosis

- Includes other viral causes of respiratory illness that resemble influenza, parainfluenza viruses, respiratory syncytial virus, and rhinoviruses and echoviruses.

Treatment

- For most patients with influenza, treatment is symptomatic rest, increased fluid intake, and antipyretics and analgesics to reduce symptoms during the acute phase.
- Cool water vapor inhalation may help to relieve mucous membrane dryness and promote drainage of nasal passages.
- Complicating bacterial infections require appropriate antibiotic therapy.

Patient/family education

- Provide information about immunization against influenza viruses.
- Most patients know about "flu" and its uncomfortable symptoms.
- Give a list of potential drugs to decrease fever, relieve headache and musculoskeletal pain, and alleviate mucous membrane dryness.

Follow-up/referral

- Patients are followed closely during the acute phase, usually by phone.
- Return visits to the office or clinic should be scheduled for 7 to 10 days from onset of illness to monitor progress, detect complications if they occur, and order new medications if warranted (e.g., antibiotics).

Herpesvirus Infections

Herpes Simplex

Definition

Herpes simplex is an infection with herpes simplex virus (HSV) characterized by one or more clusters of small vesicles filled with clear fluid on slightly raised inflammatory bases.

Risk Factors

- Direct contact (usually sexual) with HSV
- Multiple sexual partners
- Unprotected or oral sex

Etiology/Cause

- The two types of HSV are HSV-1 and HSV-2.
- HSV-1 usually causes herpes labialis, herpetic stomatitis, and keratitis.

- HSV-2 causes genital herpes and is transmitted by direct contact with lesions.
- The time of initial HSV infection is often not known.
  —After initial eruption, HSV remains dormant in the nerve ganglia; recurrent herpetic eruptions can occur, precipitated by overexposure to sunlight, febrile illnesses, physical or emotional stress, or immunosuppression.
  —Recurrent disease is usually less severe than the primary infection.

Diagnosis
- The diagnosis is confirmed by cultures for the virus, seroconversion and a progressive increase in serum antibodies to the appropriate serotype (in primary infections), and biopsy findings.
- A Tzanck preparation of the base of a lesion usually shows multinucleate giant cells in HSV or varicella-zoster virus infection.
- Newer techniques, such as the polymerase chain reaction of CSF, may allow early noninvasive diagnosis of herpes simplex encephalitis.

Differential diagnosis
- HSV should be distinguished from herpes zoster ("shingles"), which rarely recurs and usually causes more severe pain and larger groups of lesions distributed along a dermatome.
- Other differential diagnoses include varicella, genital ulcers, or gingivostomatitis due to other causes, and vesicular dermatoses, particularly dermatitis herpetiformis, and drug eruptions.

Signs and symptoms
- The lesions of HSV may appear anywhere on the skin or mucosa but are most often seen around the mouth, on the lips, on the conjunctiva and cornea, and on the genitalia.
- After a prodromal period (usually <6 hours in recurrent HSV-1) of tingling discomfort or itching, small tense vesicles appear on an erythematous base.
  —Single clusters vary in size from 0.5 to 1.5 cm, but clusters may coalesce.
  —Skin lesions on the nose, ears, or fingers may be particularly painful.

—The vesicles persist for a few days, then begin to dry, forming a thin yellowish crust.
—Healing occurs within 8 to 12 days from onset.

Primary Infection of HSV-1
- Generally causes a gingivostomatitis and is most often seen in infants and young children.
  —Symptoms include irritability, anorexia, fever, gingival inflammation, and painful ulcers of the mouth.

Primary Infection of HSV-2
- Lesions usually appear on the vulva and vagina, or on the penis in young adults.
- The illness is accompanied by fever, malaise, and tender inguinal adenopathy.
  —If the disease occurs in newborns, it causes severe disseminated disease.
  —The infection can cause severe encephalitis.
  —The infection may also cause self-limited aseptic meningitis and lumbosacral myeloradiculitis syndromes, which may include urinary retention or obstipation.
- In patients with AIDS, herpetic infections can be particularly severe.
  —Persistent and progressive esophagitis, colitis, perianal ulcers, pneumonia, and neurologic syndromes with eczema are common.
- HSV outbreaks may be followed by typical erythema multiforme.
- Herpetic whitlow is a swollen, painful, and erythematous lesion of the distal phalanx, caused by inoculation of HSV through a cutaneous break or abrasion, and is most common in health care workers.

Treatment
- In serious herpes infections, acyclovir is the treatment of choice for herpes simplex encephalitis, disseminated neonatal disease, and immunocompromised patients.
- Acyclovir, valacyclovir, and famciclovir can be used for suppression of recurrent eruptions.
- Under supervision of an ophthalmologist, topical trifluridine is used to treat herpes simplex keratitis.

- Topical penciclovir is used to treat recurrent orolabial HSV, and topical acyclovir is used for initial herpes genitalis.
  - —IV foscarnet is used to treat HSV that is mucocutaneous, and those with immunosuppression.
  - —Secondary infections are treated with topical antibiotics (e.g., neomycin-bacitracin ointment) or if severe with systemic antibiotics.

Patient/Family Education
- Emphasize that this infection can be transmitted by direct/sexual contact and by contact with fluid from a ruptured vesicle.
- Instruct regarding the nature, cause, transmission, course, treatment, and expected outcome of therapy.
- Write out all prescription drugs, including dosage and schedule.

Follow-up/Referral
- Herpes simplex infections tend to recur frequently, so that follow-up of patients with regard to complete recovery from the primary infection is necessary.
- Explain in detail how best to avoid direct contact with the virus (lesions anywhere on the body of the infected individual).
- Emphasize the importance of consistently using safe sexual practices.
- Write out signs and symptoms that indicate need for an appointment with the clinician.

Herpes Zoster
Definition
Herpes zoster is an infection with varicella-zoster virus primarily involving the dorsal root ganglia and characterized by vesicular eruption and neurologic pain in the dermatome of the affected root ganglia.

Risk Factors
- Previous infection with chickenpox (varicella-zoster virus)
- Older patients can develop postherpetic neuralgia.

Etiology/Cause
- The varicella-zoster virus causes the infection, but this infection is a result of the re-activation of the virus from its latent or dormant state in the posterior root ganglia.
  - —Inflammation occurs in the sensory root ganglia and in the skin of the associated dermatome.
  - —Vesicles that develop are distributed along the pathway of the dermatome, and can involve the ganglion in the eye, causing ophthalmic herpes zoster involving the gasserian ganglion of the fifth nerve.

Diagnosis
- Diagnosis of herpes zoster is difficult in the preeruption phase but is easily made as soon as the vesicles appear.
- The Tzanck preparation shows multinucleate giant cells for both varicella-zoster virus and HSV.

Differential diagnosis
- Pleurisy
- Trigeminal neuralgia
- Bell's palsy
- Chickenpox

Signs and symptoms
- Pain along the path of the impending eruption precedes the rash by 2 to 3 days.
- Characteristic crops of vesicles on an erythematous base appear, and follow the cutaneous distribution of one or more adjacent dermatomes.
- Vesicles occur most often in the thoracic and lumbar areas and are unilateral.
  - —The vesicles continue to form over 3 to 5 days.
- Herpes zoster can disseminate to other regions of the skin and to visceral organs, particularly in immunosuppressed patients.
- The pain of herpes zoster is often severe and continuous.

Treatment
- Application of wet compresses to the vesicles is usually soothing, along with analgesics to relieve the persistent burning/aching quality of pain.
- In immunosuppressed patients who develop herpes zoster, acyclovir IV is recommended at a dosage of 10 mg/kg q8h for 7 days for adults, and 500 mg/m^2 q8h for 7 days for children.

—Famciclovir and valacyclovir have better bioavailability with oral dosing than does acyclovir.

- Management of postherpetic neuralgia is difficult and may include tricyclic antidepressants.

Patient/Family Education

- Herpes zoster is relatively uncommon, and many patients know little or nothing about its cause and treatment.
- Instruct the patient and family regarding the nature, cause, course, signs and symptoms, treatment, and expected outcome of therapy.
- Prescribe adequate analgesics to relieve the pain that is usually severe.
- Suggest additional measures (e.g., wet cool compresses), which will also help to relieve pain.

Follow-up/Referral

- Patients are followed for several weeks after recovery from the acute phase of the disease to determine that complete recovery has occurred and to monitor for complications, particularly after ophthalmic herpes zoster infection.

HIV Infection

Definition

HIV is an infection caused by one of two related retroviruses (HIV-1 and HIV-2), resulting in a wide range of clinical manifestations varying from asymptomatic carrier states to severely debilitating and fatal disorders related to defective cell-mediated immunity. Since AIDS was first recognized in 1981 when cases of *Pneumocystis carinii* pneumonia and Kaposi's sarcoma were reported in homosexual men in California and New York, over 581,000 cases and 357,000 deaths have been reported through December 1996 in the United States. Worldwide, over 30 million HIV infections and 10 million AIDS cases are estimated. In the United States, women now make up about 20% of AIDS cases.

Risk Factors

- Exposure to body fluids containing infected cells: blood, semen, vaginal secretions, breast milk, saliva, wound exudates.

Etiology/Cause

- HIV-1 was identified in 1984 as the cause of a widespread epidemic of severe immunosuppression called **AIDS.**
- HIV transmission requires contact with body fluids that contain infected cells: blood, semen, vaginal secretions, breast milk, saliva, wound exudates, and plasma.
- HIV is NOT transmitted by casual contact or even by close nonsexual contact that occurs at work, school, or home.
- The most common cause of HIV is direct transfer of bodily fluids either through sharing contaminated needles or sexual relations.

Pathogenesis

- The two closely related retroviruses HIV-1 and HIV-2 have been identified as causing AIDS in different geographic regions.
    - HIV-1 causes most of the cases of AIDS in the Western Hemisphere, Europe, Asia, and Central, South, and East Africa.
    - HIV-2 is the principal agent of AIDS in West Africa, and seems to be less virulent than HIV-1.
    - In particular areas of West Africa, both organisms are prevalent.
- All retroviruses contain an enzyme called reverse transcriptase that converts viral RNA into a proviral DNA copy that becomes integrated into the host cell DNA; these integrated proviruses are duplicated by normal cellular genes each time the cell divides.
    - Therefore all progeny of the originally infected cell will contain the retroviral DNA.
    - The proviral HIV DNA is both transcribed to RNA and translated to proteins to produce hundreds of copies of the infectious virus.
- Critical to the final step in the life cycle of HIV is another enzyme—HIV protease, which converts immature, noninfectious HIV to its infectious form by splitting crucial proteins so that they can rearrange within the virus after it has budded from an infected human cell.
- HIV infects a major subset of T lymphocytes defined phenotypically by the T4 or CD4 transmembrane glycoprotein and functionally as helper/inducer cells.

- HIV also infects nonlymphoid cells such as macrophages, microglial cells, and various endothelial and epithelial cells.

Predictors of Onset
- The best predictors of onset of the serious opportunistic infections that define AIDS are the total number of circulating CD4$^+$ lymphocytes (CD4 count) and the level of HIV RNA in plasma (viral load), also known as the number of HIV-1 RNA copies in 1 ml of plasma.
  - The risk of progression to AIDS or death appears to increase about 50% for every threefold increase in plasma viral RNA.

Laboratory Diagnosis
- Detection of antibodies to HIV is sensitive and specific at most stages of infection, is inexpensive, and is widely available.
  - Rapid (10 min) serum tests, home collection systems, and tests for HIV antibody in oral secretions and urine are useful in some situations, but they require confirmation by standard serum testing.
  - Detection of HIV RNA in blood provides a sensitive and specific diagnosis of HIV infection in the very early stages of infection when antibodies may not yet have developed.
- Tests for detecting antibody to HIV include ELISA, which can detect antibodies to HIV proteins.
- The Western blot test is more specific, using an immunoelectrophoresis procedure to identify antibodies to specific viral proteins separated by their molecular weight.

Signs and Symptoms
- Primary HIV infection
  - Fever
  - Malaise
  - Rash
  - Arthralgias
  - Generalized lymphadenopathy that lasts 3 to 14 days
  - This early stage is then followed within days to 3 months by seroconversion for antibody to HIV.
- The acute symptoms disappear, except for lymphadenopathy, which usually persists,

and patients then become antibody-positive, asymptomatic carriers.
  - Some of these patients develop mild, remittent symptoms and signs that do not meet the definition of AIDS (e.g., thrush, diarrhea, fatigue, fever); leukopenia is common and anemia and immune-mediated thrombocytopenia may also occur.
- *Neurologic symptoms:* These may be the first manifestation of AIDS: acute aseptic meningitis; encephalopathy with seizures; peripheral neuropathies; focal motor, sensory, or gait deficits; and cognitive dysfunction progressing to dementia
- *Hematologic symptoms:* Anemia, immune-mediated thrombocytopenia
- *GI symptoms:* Abdominal pain, nausea and vomiting, diarrhea; opportunistic infections frequently invade the GI tract: *Candida,* Kaposi's sarcoma, lymphoma, and various organisms (e.g., *Salmonella, C. difficile*) and other internal organs
- *Dermatologic manifestations:* Herpes zoster, rash, genital ulcers, Kaposi's sarcoma
- *Oral symptoms:* thrush (oral candidiasis), oral hairy leukoplakia probably caused by Epstein-Barr virus and treatable with acyclovir, periodontal disease
- *Pulmonary symptoms:* TB, fungal infections of the lung: *P. carinii, H. neoformans, Coccidioides immitis,* and others
- *AIDS in women:* Most frequent early signs are refractory vaginal candidiasis and increased risk of cervical intraepithelial neoplasia
- *Cardiovascular complications:* Thrombotic or bacterial endocarditis, particularly among IV drug users, or cardiomyopathy with CHF

Treatment
- Combination of drugs usually targeting two enzymes (HIV reverse transcriptase and protease); therapy using two to four drugs can promptly halt viral reproduction, preserve immune function, and decrease the likelihood of emergence of drug-resistant viral mutants (Table 21-5)

Prognosis
- Opportunistic infections have continued to be the immediate cause of death for almost all AIDS patients.

TABLE 21-5
Antiretroviral Drugs*

Generic Drug Name	Abbreviation	Usual Adult Dose
NUCLEOSIDE REVERSE TRANSCRIPTASE INHIBITORS		
Zidovudine	ZDV, AZT	300 mg bid
Didanosine	ddI	200 mg bid (>60 kg)
		125 mg bid (<60 kg
Zalcitabine	ddC	0.75 mg tid
Stavudine	d4T	40 mg bid (>60 kg)
		30 mg bid (<60 kg)
Lamivudine	3TC	150 mg bid
Abacavir	—	300 mg bid
PROTEASE INHIBITORS		
Saquinavir	SAQ	600 mg tid
Indinavir	IND	800 mg tid
Ritonavir	RIT	600 mg bid
Nelfinavir	NEL	750 mg tid
NONNUCLEOSIDE REVERSE TRANSCRIPTASE INHIBITORS		
Nevirapine	NVP	200 mg qd × 2 wks, then
		200 mg bid
Delavirdine	DLV	400 mg q8h
Loviride	LVD	Investigational
Efavirenz	—	Investigational (600 mg qd)
NUCLEOTIDE REVERSE TRANSCRIPTASE INHIBITOR		
Adefovir	bis-POM PMEA	Investigational (125 mg qd)

From Beers MH, Berkow R, eds: Infectious diseases. *The Merck manual of diagnosis and therapy,* ed 17, Whitehouse Station, NJ, 1999, Merck & Co, Inc, p 1322.
*All of these drugs have side effects, more or less, from rashes to CNS symptoms, kidney stones, leukopenia; refer to Physicians' Drug Reference (PDR) for most current information. Antiretroviral drugs listed here have been FDA approved, as of 1998, except those under investigation.

- Combination antiretroviral drug therapy has dramatically prolonged the survival of patients with AIDS over periods of 2 to 3 years, but length of benefit is variable and to date is incompletely defined.

Patient/Family Education
- A great deal of misinformation has been published and communicated by word of mouth that needs to be clarified for many people who are not familiar with HIV and AIDS.
- Instruct the patient and family regarding the nature, cause, signs and symptoms, complications, course, treatment, and expected outcome for the individual.
- Drug therapy has been able to prolong survival of HIV-infected patients and those with AIDS to a remarkable extent, compared with what was known and what was available in the mid-1980s.

- Care for patients with AIDS remains complex and comprehensive.

Follow-up/Referral
- HIV patients are followed closely throughout, from diagnosis until the patient develops AIDS and beyond.
- AIDS patients, depending on symptoms and severity of the illness, require frequent hospitalizations.
- Specialists may be consulted at any time during the illness: neurologists, dermatologists, infectious disease specialists, and others as needed, who will follow the patient with the clinician.

Sexually Transmitted Diseases
Overview
- The incidence of sexually transmitted diseases (STDs), which are among the most common communicable infections in the

world, increased steadily from the 1950s until the 1970s, but then stabilized in the 1980s.

- The incidence of some STDs (e.g., syphilis, gonorrhea) decreased between the mid-1980s and the mid-1990s in the United States and in other countries.
- Nonspecific urethritis, trichomoniasis, chlamydial infections, genital and anorectal herpes and warts, pediculosis pubis, and molluscum contagiosum are probably more prevalent than the five historically defined venereal diseases: syphilis, gonorrhea, chancroid, lymphogranuloma venereum, and granuloma inguinale, which are reported more consistently than the others, for which incidence rates are not reliable.
- In 1995, the worldwide incidence of gonorrhea was estimated at more than 250 million cases (United States about 400,000); syphilis—50 million cases (United States about 70,000), including about 16,000 primary and secondary cases and 1500 congenital cases).
- Chlamydial infections now affect about 500,000 annually in the United States, but only between 10% and 20% of cases are reported.
- Infections such as giardiasis, salmonellosis, amebiasis, shigellosis, campylobacteriosis, hepatitis A and B, and cytomegalovirus are sexually transmitted, but can also be spread by other means.
- Research shows a strong association between cervical cancer and papillomaviruses, which are sexually transmitted.
- Since 1978, HIV has spread rapidly among many populations.
- Incidence of all STDs remains high in most of the world, despite diagnostic and therapeutic advances that can identify specific STDs and rapidly render affected persons either noninfectious or cured.
- Availability of various contraceptives and changing sexual practices have eliminated sexual limitations, particularly among women, which has affected the incidence and prevalence of STDs.
- Many organisms that cause STDs have become drug-resistant, which hinders treatment.

- Effective vaccines for STDs have still not been perfected but continue to be investigated and evaluated by means of clinical trials.

Prevention
- Prevention of STDs requires a multifaceted approach.
  —Clinics and laboratories for diagnosis and treatment
  —Identifying and treating patients' sexual partners
  —Follow-up of treated patients to ensure that they have indeed been cured
  —Educating health care workers and the public about STDs
  —Teaching and disseminating materials about safe sexual practices
  —Funding programs to develop effective vaccines for STDs

Gonorrhea

Definition
Gonorrhea is an infection of the epithelium of the urethra, cervix, rectum, pharynx, or eyes by *N. gonorrhoeae*, which may result in bacteremia and metastatic complications.

Risk Factors
- Contact with the organism, usually through sexual activity
- Asymptomatic carrier status, often among women
- Asymptomatic infection is often found in the oropharynx and rectum in homosexual men, and occasionally found in the urethra of homosexual men.

Etiology/Cause
- Gonorrhea is caused by the specific organism *N. gonorrhoeae*.

Diagnosis/Signs and Symptoms
- Gram's-stained smear of urethral discharge is a rapid method to identify the gonococcus in over 90% of men.
- The Gram's-stained cervical smear is only about 60% sensitive.
- Symptoms of rectal or pharyngeal infection require cultures or genetic methods for diagnosis, since Gram's stains are neither sufficiently sensitive nor specific.

—Cultures of exudates from the urethra, cervix, rectum, and other infected areas are inoculated onto a medium, such as Thayer-Martin, and incubated in a controlled environment for 24 to 48 hours.

Gonorrhea in men

- At the time of examination, the patient should also have a serologic test for syphilis (STS) and be tested for other STDs.
- The incubation period is from 2 to 14 days.
- Onset is marked by mild discomfort in the urethra and then, a few hours later, dysuria and a purulent discharge occur.
- Frequency and urgency become prominent as the infection spreads to the posterior urethra.
- Examination shows a purulent, yellowish-green urethral discharge and the lips of the meatus may be red and swollen.
- Severe rectal infection is more common in homosexual men than in heterosexual men or in women.

Gonorrhea in women

- Symptoms begin between 7 and 21 days after infection.
- The onset can be mild or severe; many women are asymptomatic.
- Usually, they experience perianal discomfort and a rectal discharge.
- Women may report seeing a coating of mucopus on stools and report pain on defecation and rectal intercourse.
- Patients with oropharyngeal gonorrhea are often asymptomatic, but some may complain of sore throat and discomfort on swallowing.
  - On examination, the pharynx and tonsillar area may be red, exudative, and sometimes edematous.

Complications

Men

- Postgonococcal urethritis
- Epididymitis (uncommon, unilateral)

Women

- Salpingitis is significant
- Disseminated gonococcal infection (DGI) with bacteremia is more common in women than in men.
  - Signs and symptoms include low-grade fever, malaise, migratory polyarthralgias or polyarthritis, or a few pustular skin lesions, usually on the periphery of the limbs.
  - Each of these signs and symptoms is present in two thirds of patients.
- Gonococcal arthritis is a more focal form of DGI, often occurring after symptomatic bacteremia.
  - Onset is often acute, with fever, severe pain, and limitation of movement in one or a few joints; joints are swollen and tender, and the overlying skin is warm and red.

Treatment

- The emergence of drug-resistant gonococci has limited the utility of previous antibiotic therapy.
  - Coexisting chlamydial infection is often present.
  - Simultaneous presumptive treatment is often required to treat both gonorrhea and chlamydia.
  - Ceftriaxone 125 mg IM as a single dose for gonococci, plus either doxycycline 100 mg PO for 7 days, or azithromycin 1 g PO once for chlamydia are recommended as the initial therapy for urethral, endocervical, pharyngeal, and rectal infections.
  - For DGI, ceftriaxone 1 g IM or IV daily, ceftizoxime 1 g IV q8h, or cefotaxime 1 g IV q8h are the choices, and are equivalent in effectiveness.
  - Duration of treatment is usually defined as 3 days of parenteral therapy, followed by 4 to 7 days of oral therapy with antibiotics.
- To treat gonococcal arthritis, an NSAID may be effective in controlling pain and joint effusion.
  - Repeated aspirations are not necessary; the limb is usually kept immobilized in a functional position, with passive range-of-motion exercises begun as soon as possible and, if the knees are involved, quadriceps strengthening exercises.
  - Once the pain abates, more strenuous exercises may be encouraged, including stretching and active range-of-motion exercises done twice daily.

TABLE 21-6
Classification and Stages of Syphilis

Acquired	Congenital
Primary stage: chancre, regional lymphadenopathy Secondary stage: (immediately follows primary stage): varied skin lesions that mimic other disorders (e.g., rashes, erosion of mucous membranes, alopecia, many other manifestations) Latent stage: asymptomatic; may persist for years, or be followed by late stage; early latent: infection < 2 yrs duration; infectious lesions may recur; late latent: infection > 2 yrs duration Late or tertiary stage: not contagious, symptomatic: benign tertiary syphilis; cardiovascular syphilis; neurosyphilis (general paresis)	Early congenital syphilis; seen in infants up to 2 yrs (overt infection) Late congenital syphilis: later in life (e.g., Hutchinson's teeth, scars of interstitial keratitis, bony abnormalities)

From Beers MH, Berkow R, eds: Infectious diseases. *The Merck manual of diagnosis and therapy,* ed 17, Whitehouse Station, NJ, 1999, Merck & Co, Inc, p 1328.

—Over 95% of patients treated for gonococcal arthritis regain complete joint function.

Patient/Family Education
- The nature, cause, transmission, course, treatment, and expected outcome should be explained to the patient and the family as soon as the diagnosis is made.
- The patient should abstain from sexual activity throughout the treatment period.
- The patient's sexual contacts should be located and treated.
- Testing to confirm that the patient is no longer infectious after therapy is not necessary, as long as symptomatic response is adequate.

Follow-up/Referral
- Rescreening for reinfection with gonococcus or chlamydia is done at 4 to 8 weeks, including a STS, although if any coexisting syphilis was present, the drug regimen for the other STDs would also cure syphilis.
  - Once full recovery and noninfectious state is confirmed, the patient is not followed.
- Before discharge, the patient should be questioned regarding knowledge of how transmission of gonorrhea and chlamydia occur and how to prevent reinfection.

Chlamydial, Mycoplasmal, and Ureaplasmal Infections
- These patients usually present with the same symptoms as those of gonorrhea, and treatment is the same.
  - In cases of complications or relapse, antibiotic therapy may be prolonged until full recovery and noninfectious status are confirmed.
  - Sexual partners are also located and treated.

Syphilis
Definition
- Syphilis is a contagious systemic infection caused by the spirochete *Treponema pallidum* and characterized by sequential infectious stages and long-term latency (Table 21-6).

Risk Factors
- Exposure to the causative organism
  - Congenital: the risk of transplacental infection of the fetus (about 60% to 80%) depends on the mother's stage of infection and pregnancy; untreated primary or secondary infection is usually transmitted, but latent or tertiary syphilis is not.
  - Acquired: *T. pallidum* enters through the mucous membranes or skin, reaches the regional lymph nodes within hours, and rapidly disseminates throughout the body.

- In the 1980s and 1990s, rates of primary and secondary syphilis doubled in the black population, in association with cocaine abuse and prostitution.
- However, rates in all populations declined in the mid-1990s, probably because of aggressive contact tracing and mandatory treatment.

Etiology/Cause (see Definition and Risk Factors)

Pathogenesis

- Infection is almost always transmitted by sexual contact, including orogenital and anorectal contact, but it sometimes is transmitted by kissing or close bodily contact.
  —Skin lesions of primary, secondary, or early latent syphilis account for all acquired infections.
- Treated infection does not confer immunity against subsequent reinfection.
- Once established, and in all stages of infection, perivascular infiltration of lymphocytes, plasma, cells, and later fibroblasts causes swelling and proliferation of the endothelium of the smaller blood vessels, resulting in **endarteritis obliterans.**
- In late syphilis, *T. pallidum* elicits a granulomatous-like (gummatous) reaction that causes masses, ulcerations, and necrosis of tissue.
  —Inflammation may abate, despite progressive damage, particularly in the cardiovascular system and CNS.
- The CNS is affected early in the infection.
  —In the secondary stage, 30% of patients have abnormal CSF and many have symptoms of meningitis.
  —In the first 5 to 10 years of infection, the meninges and blood vessels are primarily involved, leading to meningovascular neurosyphilis.
  —Later, the parenchyma of the brain and spinal cord are damaged, resulting in parenchymatous neurosyphilis.
  —Involvement of the cerebral cortex and overlying meninges results in general paresis.
  —Destruction of the posterior columns and root ganglia of the spinal cord causes tabes dorsalis.

Diagnosis

- Diagnostic studies for syphilis include a targeted history and physical examination, serologic tests and darkfield examination of fluids from lesions, CSF tests, and radiologic examination.
- Diagnosis is confirmed by viewing *T. pallidum,* a delicate spiral organism about 0.25 μm wide and from 5 to 20 μm long, with characteristic morphology and motility, by darkfield microscopy or fluorescent techniques.
- STS include the Venereal Disease Research Laboratory (VDRL) and the rapid plasma reagin (RPR) tests.
- Specific treponemal tests detect antitreponemal antibodies and include the fluorescent treponemal antibody absorption (FTA-ABS) test, microhemagglutination assay for antibodies to *T. pallidum* (MHA-TP), and *T. pallidum* hemagglutination assay (TPHA).

Signs and symptoms

- The incubation period can range from 1 to 13 weeks, but is usually 3 to 4 weeks.
- Signs and symptoms can appear at any stage, and long after the initial infection because of the many manifestations of syphilis; it is not found often among populations in developed countries; the clinician may not recognize the presenting signs and symptoms as being caused by syphilis.

Primary stage

- The primary lesion **(chancre)** evolves and heals usually within 4 to 8 weeks in untreated patients.
- After infection, a red papule rapidly erodes to form a painless ulcer with an indurated base, which when abraded exudes a clear serum containing many spirochetes; chancres can occur on the penis, anus, rectum in men, and on the vulva, cervix, and perineum in women; they may also occur on the lips or the oropharyngeal or anogenital mucous membranes, but rarely on the hands or other parts of the body; they produce minimal symptoms and are often ignored by the patient as trivial.
- Regional lymph nodes enlarge, becoming firm, discrete, and nontender.

Secondary stage
- Skin rashes appear within 6 to 12 weeks of infection and become florid after 3 to 4 months.
    - The lesions may be transitory or may persist for months.
    - Untreated, they usually heal, but new lesions appear within weeks or months; about 25% of patients have a residual chancre in this stage.
- Often, generalized, nontender, firm, discrete lymphadenopathy and hepatosplenomegaly are palpable.
- Over 80% of patients have mucocutaneous lesions; 50% have generalized lymphadenopathy; 10% have lesions of the eye (uveitis), bones, joints, meninges, and kidneys.

Latent stage
- This stage may resolve spontaneously within a few years or may last for the remainder of the patient's life.
- In the early latent phase the patient may continue to have infectious mucocutaneous lesions.
- After 2 years, contagious lesions rarely occur, and the patient appears normal.
- About one third of patients develop late syphilis but usually not for many years after the initial infection.
    - If patients are treated with antibiotics for other diseases, syphilis may be serendipitously cured.

Late (tertiary) stage
- *Benign tertiary syphilis* is rarely seen now, but the characteristic lesion is a **gumma,** an inflammatory mass that evolves to necrosis and may diffusely infiltrate an organ or tissue.
- *Cardiovascular syphilis* results in a dilated aneurysm of the ascending or transverse aorta, narrowing of the coronary ostia, or aortic valvular insufficiency, which appears 10 to 25 years after initial infection.
- *Neurosyphilis* is asymptomatic at first and is seen in about 15% of patients originally diagnosed as having latent syphilis, and in 5% of those with benign tertiary syphilis.
    - Meningovascular neurosyphilis begins with headache, dizziness, poor concentration, lassitude, insomnia, neck stiffness and blurred vision; mental confusion,

epileptiform attacks, papilledema, aphasia, and monoplegia or hemiplegia may develop; the **Argyll Robertson pupil** occurs almost exclusively in neurosyphilis, and is a small, irregular pupil that accommodates normally with convergence but does not react to light.
    - *Parenchymatous neurosyphilis* generally affects patients in their forties or fifties, and is manifested by general paresis or dementia paralytica, resulting in progressive behavioral deterioration that may mimic a psychiatric illness or Alzheimer's disease; the more common symptoms include headache, irritability, difficulty in concentrating, insomnia, fatigue, and lethargy; the posterior column lesions of **tabes dorsalis (locomotor ataxia)** cause insidious pain, sensory changes, and loss of tendon reflexes, but often the first symptom is an intense, stabbing (lightning) pain in the back of the legs that recurs irregularly.

Treatment
- Penicillin is used in all stages of syphilis.
    - Benzathine penicillin G 2.4 MU IM (1.2 MU in each buttock) once produces a satisfactory blood level for 2 weeks.
    - Two additional injections of 2.4 MU q 7 days are given for secondary and latent syphilis.
    - In penicillin-allergic patients, ceftriaxone 1 g IM q 3 days diluted in 3.6 ml of 1% lidocaine for four doses, or erythromycin or tetracycline 500 mg PO q6h for 15 days, or doxycycline 100 mg PO bid for 14 days, although the effectiveness of the alternative drugs has not been well defined

Patient/Family Education
- The nature, cause, course, treatment, and expected outcome should be explained to the patient and appropriate family members.
- Emphasize the absolute necessity of therapy and the need to take all drugs exactly as ordered.
- Signs and symptoms can be outlined in brief form for the patient so that he or she knows what to expect.
- The importance of repeated tests to confirm cure is emphasized; these are done at 1, 3,

6, and 12 months or until no reaction is found; however, the treponemal tests (FTA-ABS and MHA-TP) usually remain positive for years or for life.

- After successful treatment, lesions heal rapidly.
- Patients with neurosyphilis have the CSF examined q 6 months until it has been normal for 2 years; abnormal CSF should be examined q 3 months until it is normal, then annually for another 2 years.

Follow-up/Referral

- Patients who have had syphilis should be encouraged to be tested for HIV.
- Testing for cure is done at 1, 3, 6, 12, 18, and 24 months for those patients with persistently positive STS, and these patients are usually seen once a year indefinitely.
- Patients with cardiovascular syphilis are usually followed for the rest of their lives.
- Specialists in conditions caused by syphilis (e.g., uveitis) may be called in consultation at any time, along with others (e.g., gastroenterologists, nephrologists).
- All sexual contacts are located and treated.

Trichomoniasis

Definition

Trichomoniasis is an infection of the vagina or male genital tract with *Trichomonas vaginalis*.

- *T. vaginalis* is a flagellated protozoan found in the GU tract of both men and women.
  —The organism is pear-shaped, averaging 7 to 10 μm but sometimes reaching 25 μm.
  —It has four anterior flagella, and a fifth flagellum embedded in an undulating membrane.

Risk Factors

- The infection is more common in women, and affects about 20% of those in the reproductive years.
  —The infection may account for 5% to 10% of all cases of male urethritis in some areas.

Etiology/Cause (see Definition)
Diagnosis

- In women, an immediate diagnosis can be made with an unstained saline suspension of vaginal secretions from the posterior fornix examined by ordinary light microscopy; the lashing movements of the flagella and motility of the oval-shaped organisms are readily seen.
- Examination should be done early in the morning before voiding, when a slight mucoid discharge may be present and some fine mucous threads may be seen in the 2-glass urine test.
- A wet film of the urethral secretions may be examined the same as in women.

Signs and symptoms

- In women, onset is characterized by a copious greenish-yellow, frothy vaginal discharge, with irritation and tenderness of the vulva, perineum, and thighs.
  —The patient usually reports dyspareunia and dysuria.
  —Some women have only slight symptoms, and others may be asymptomatic carriers for long periods, with symptoms developing at any time.
  —In severe cases, the vulva and perineum are inflamed, with edema of the labia.
- Men are usually asymptomatic but may have transient frothy or purulent urethral discharge with dysuria and frequency, usually early in the morning, discomfort in the perineum or deeper in the pelvis, and subpreputial discharge.

Treatment

- Metronidazole 2 g PO in a single dose cures up to 85% of women, if sexual partners are treated at the same time.
- Single-dose therapy for men is less clear; treatment may be metronidazole 500 mg bid for 7 days.
- No alternative treatment is available.
- Metronidazole may cause leukopenia, disulfiram-like reaction to alcohol, or candidal superinfection.
- All sexual contacts should be examined and treated.

Patient/Family Education

- Instruct the patient regarding the nature, cause, course, treatment, and expected outcomes of therapy.
- Written instructions about metronidazole, its dose and schedule, should be given if the

patient is to receive more than single-dose treatment.

- Emphasize the need to examine and treat all sexual partners.

Follow-up/Referral

- Patients are followed for 1 to 2 weeks after therapy to ensure that cure has taken place.
- Provide the patient with information about available office hours and telephone number(s) to call in case reinfection occurs.
- All known sexual partners are contacted and asked to come in for examination and treatment, if necessary.

Genital Candidiasis

Definition

Genital candidiasis is a symptomatic overgrowth of commensal yeasts on the mucosa of the vagina or penis.

Risk Factors

- Treatment with broad-spectrum antibiotics
- Use of oral contraceptives
- Pregnancy
- Menstruation
- Diabetes mellitus
- Constrictive undergarments
- Suppression of cell-mediated immunity by drugs or HIV infection

Etiology/Cause

- Infection by *C. albicans* is not considered a sexually transmitted disease, although it usually involves the external sexual organs of both sexes.
- Infection is usually caused by the patient's normal skin or intestinal flora, which overgrows because of predisposing (risk) factors (see Risk Factors).

Pathogenesis

- Normal flora proliferate under certain conditions, causing, in women, symptoms such as vulval irritation, or in men, a slight urethral discharge.

Diagnosis

- Immediate diagnosis is made by taking smears from the vagina, glans penis, or pre-

puce, and staining with Gram's stain or potassium hydroxide, then examining them under ordinary light microscope.

- The organisms are gram-positive, oval, budding yeast with typical elongated, filamentous pseudohyphae.
- Because candidiasis is not transmitted sexually, testing for coexisting STDs should be done only if clinically indicated.

Signs and symptoms

- Women usually have vulval irritation and vaginal discharge.
  —Often, the irritation is severe and the discharge is slight.
  —The vulva usually appears inflamed, with excoriation and fissures in the tissues.
  —The vaginal wall is usually covered with white, cheesy, adherent patches of yeast.
- Men are usually asymptomatic carriers, but may occasionally have slight urethral discharge, and may complain of irritation and soreness of the glans penis and prepuce, particularly after intercourse.
  —The glans penis and prepuce may be inflamed, and white, cheesy material, vesicles, or erosions may be present.
  —In severe cases, the prepuce may be edematous, causing phimosis (constriction of the foreskin).

Treatment

- Vaginal candidiasis is treated locally with the following:
  —Clotrimazole, one 100-mg tablet/day intravaginally for 6 days, or 200 mg/day for 3 days.
  —Miconazole 200 mg/day intravaginally for 3 days
  —Butoconazole 2% cream 5 g/day intravaginally for 3 days
  —Terconazole one 80-mg suppository/day for 3 days or 0.4% cream 5 g/day for 7 days
  —Econazole 1% vaginal cream or 100-mg suppository for 3 days
  —Fluconazole 150 mg PO once is also effective but may be more expensive.
- All of these agents are used once daily at bedtime.

Patient/Family Education

- Adolescent girls may also develop genital candidiasis, and instructions to the mothers may be necessary.
- Emphasize the relatively benign nature of the infection and that it is easily treated.
- Explain the nature, cause, course, treatment, and expected outcome of therapy.
- Instruct regarding the use of vaginal suppositories or creams, whichever is selected as the most appropriate for the individual patient.
- If the patient is male, instructions about application of cream on areas of the glans penis or prepuce should be given and demonstrated.
- Encourage patients to seek treatment immediately should reinfection occur.

Follow-up/Referral

- Patients are usually seen once after treatment to ensure that the infection has been eradicated and that healing is occurring satisfactorily.

Genital Herpes

Definition

Genital herpes is an infection of the genital or anorectal skin or mucous membranes by either of two closely related HSVs (HSV-1 or HSV-2).

Risk Factors

- Exposure to the herpes simplex virus of an infected sexual partner, or self-inoculation of the virus from another part of the body (e.g., lip) to the genital area

Etiology/Cause

- The usual virus that results in genital herpes is HSV-2, although 10% to 30% of patients are infected with HSV-1.
- This infection is the most common ulcerative STD in developed countries.

Pathogenesis

- The skin or mucous membranes of the genital and anorectal areas are infected.
- Recurrences are common because the virus chronically infects the sacral sensory nerve ganglia, from which it reactivates and reinfects the skin.

Diagnosis

- Immediate presumptive diagnosis is made by identifying the characteristic multinuclear giant cells in Wright's-Giemsa–stained smears of cells from lesions (Tzanck test).
- The diagnosis can be confirmed by culture, direct immunofluorescent assay, or serology.

Signs and symptoms

- Primary lesions develop 4 to 7 days after contact.
  - A small cluster of variably painful vesicles develops, erodes, and forms superficial, circular ulcers with a red areola, which may coalesce.
  - The ulcers become crusted after a few days and generally heal in about 10 days, sometimes with scarring.
- Lesions may be seen on the glans penis, prepuce, and penile shaft in men, and on the labia, clitoris, perineum, vagina, and cervix in women.
  - During the initial outbreak, the lesions are more painful, prolonged, and widespread than those of recurrent outbreaks.
  - Fever, malaise, and regional adenopathy usually are present in the initial outbreak.
- Patients may have difficulty urinating, dysuria, or difficulty walking due to bladder paresis.
- In recurrent episodes, paresthesia with itching, tingling, or burning usually precedes the localized erythema of the skin or mucous membranes.
- Neuropathic symptoms of pain in the hips or legs may be severely troubling.
- Patients with depressed cell-mediated immunity from HIV infection or other causes
- Many experience prolonged symptoms or progressive lesions that may persist for weeks to months; failure to heal or frequent recurrences indicate the need to test for HIV.

Treatment

- Antiviral therapy for HSV reduces viral shedding and symptoms in severe primary infections; marginally reduces shedding and symptoms in recurrent infection; heals chronic infections in immunocompromised patients; and reduces rates of recurrence when used prophylactically.

—Acyclovir 200 mg PO 5 times/day or 400 mg PO q8h for 5 to 10 days

—Valacyclovir 500 mg PO q12h for 5 to 10 days

- Both medications are effective in treating primary herpetic infections of the mouth, genitalia, and rectum.

  —Even early treatment does not prevent latent infections or recurrences.

- For frequent recurrent (>once/month) infections, prophylaxis with either of the two antiviral agents is appropriate.

Patient/Family Education

- Explain the nature, cause, course, treatment, and expected outcome of therapy.
- Emphasize that recurrences may occur.
- Write signs and symptoms of recurrent infection, so that the patient may recognize these early, and seek treatment immediately.

Follow-up/Referral

- Referral to a gynecologist or dermatologist may be required at any time.
- Patients are seen once a week, then once every 2 weeks after completion of therapy to ensure that the infection is eradicated.

BIBLIOGRAPHY

Anderson KN, Anderson LE, Glanze WD: *Mosby's medical, nursing, & allied health dictionary,* ed 5, St. Louis, 1998, Mosby Year-Book, Inc.

Beers MH, Berkow R: Infectious diseases. In Beers MH, Berkow R, eds: *The Merck manual of diagnosis and therapy,* ed 17, Whitehouse Station, NJ, 1999, Merck Research Laboratories, pp 1085-1340.

Bennett RC: Acute gastroenteritis and associated conditions. In Barker LR, Burton JR, Zieve PD, eds: *Principles of ambulatory medicine,* ed 5, Baltimore, 1999, Williams & Wilkins, pp 319-330.

Bockhold KM: Who's afraid of hepatitis C? *Am J Nurs* 100(5):26-32, 2000.

Bouckenooghe A, Shandera WX: Infectious diseases: viral and rickettsial. In Tierney LM, McPhee SJ, Papadakis MA, eds: *Current medical diganosis & treatment 2000,* New York, 2000, Lange Medical Books/McGraw-Hill, pp 1295-1333.

Carlini ME, Shandera WX: Infectious diseases: viral & rickettsial. In Tierney LM, McPhee SJ, Papadakis MA, eds: *Current medical diagnosis & treatment 1999,* Stamford, Conn, 1999, Appleton & Lange, pp 1255-1290.

Chambers HF: Infectious diseases: bacterial & chlamydial. In Tierney LM, McPhee SJ, Papadakis MA, eds: *Current medical diagnosis & treatment 2000,* New York, 2000, Lange Medical Books/McGraw-Hill, pp 1334-1375.

Farthing MJG, Jeffries DJ, Anderson J: Infectious diseases, tropical medicine, and sexually transmitted diseases. In Kumar P, Clark M, eds: *Clinical medicine,* ed 4, Edinburgh, 1998, WB Saunders, pp 1-124.

Flynn JA, Rompalo AM: Selected spirochetal infections: syphilis and Lyme disease. In Barker LR, Burton JR, Zieve PD, eds: *Principles of ambulatory medicine,* ed 5, Baltimore, 1999, Williams & Wilkins, pp 372-385.

Hamil RJ: Infectious diseases: Mycotic. In Tierney LM, McPhee SJ, Papadakis MA, eds: *Current diagnosis & treatment 1999,* Stamford, Conn, 1999, Appleton & Lange, pp 1418-1430.

Hollander H, Katz MH: Infectious diseases: HIV infection. In Tierney LM, McPhee SJ, Papadakis MA, eds: *Current medical diagnosis & treatment 1999,* Stamford, Conn, 1999, Appleton & Lange, pp 1228-1254.

Horn J, Fantry L: Ambulatory care for the HIV-infected patient. In Barker LR, Burton JR, Zieve PD, eds: *Principles of ambulatory medicine,* ed 5, Baltimore, 1999, Williams & Wilkins, pp 425-456.

Jacobs RA: General problems in infectious diseases. In Tierney LM, McPhee SJ, Papadakis MA, eds: *Current diagnosis & treatment 2000,* New York, 1999, Lange Medical Books/McGraw-Hill, pp 1241-1265.

Jacobs RA: Infectious diseases: Spirochetal. In Tierney LM, McPhee SJ, Papadakis MA, eds: *Current diagnosis & treatment 2000,* New York, 2000, Lange Medical Books/McGraw-Hill, pp 1376-1395.

Koster FT, Barker LR: Respiratory tract infections. In Barker LR, Burton JR, Zieve PD, eds: *Principles of ambulatory medicine,* ed 5, Baltimore, 1999, Williams & Wilkins, pp 342-362.

Murphy PA: Genitourinary infections. In Barker LR, Burton JR, Zieve PD, eds: *Principles of ambulatory medicine,* ed 5, Baltimore, 1999, Williams & Wilkins, pp 331-341.

Murphy PA: Tuberculosis in the ambulatory patient. In Barker LR, Burton JR, Zieve PD, eds: *Principles of ambulatory medicine,* ed 5, Baltimore, 1999, Williams & Wilkins, pp 362-372.

Pierce NF: Bacterial infections of the skin. In Barker LR, Burton JR, Zieve PD, eds: *Principles of ambulatory medicine,* ed 5, Baltimore, 1999, Williams & Wilkins, pp 312-318.

Shovein JT, Damazo RJ, Hyams I: Hepatitis A—How benign is it? *Am J Nurs* 100(3):43-48, 2000.

Stokstad E: Drug-resistant TB on the rise. *Science* 287(5462): 2391, 2000.

REVIEW QUESTIONS

1. Viruses remain in the body for:
   - a. Days
   - b. Weeks
   - c. Months
   - d. Years

2. The transmitter of disease can be ticks, spiders, insects, and other forms of life; however, the transmitter does not become infected with the organism that it transmits. This transmitter is known as a:
   a. Mechanical vector
   b. Biologic vector
   c. Transport
   d. Messenger

3. Infections that can be transmitted from animals to man are called:
   a. Arthrophones
   b. Zoonoses
   c. Zooparasites
   d. Zoopaths

4. Probably the best host defense against invasion of organisms is:
   a. The immune system
   b. Sunlight
   c. Mucous membranes
   d. The skin

5. Resistance to antimicrobial therapy can occur in all but one of the following ways. The one that does NOT affect resistance is:
   a. Failure to reach the target site
   b. Enzyme inactivation
   c. Conjugation
   d. Transformation

6. Fever of unknown origin is diagnosed when a fever of 38.3° C (≥ 101° F) or higher is present for at least:
   a. 1 week
   b. 2 weeks
   c. 3 weeks
   d. 4 weeks

7. A fever that occurs every third day or 48 hours (tertian) or every fourth day or 72 hours (quartan) may indicate:
   a. Tuberculosis
   b. Pneumonia
   c. Influenza
   d. Malaria

8. A systemic infection caused by bacteria is called:
   a. The inflammatory response syndrome
   b. Bacteremia
   c. Infection of the lymphatic system
   d. Hemodynamic instability

9. All but one of the following are among the most common skin infections. The one that is NOT as common is:
   a. Impetigo
   b. Erysipelas
   c. Cellulitis
   d. Ecthyma

10. Before the advent of antibiotics, erysipelas was a greatly feared infection because it is highly infectious and can involve systemic toxicity, extensive lesions, and the need for hospitalization. Most patients who had the infection:
    a. Were treated at home
    b. Were isolated
    c. Were quarantined
    d. Died

11. All but one of the following is the name of a group of streptococcal infections. The one that is NOT among the streptococcal groups is:
    a. Carrier state
    b. Acute infection
    c. Chronic infection
    d. Delayed symptoms

12. In the winter and early spring months, pneumococci can be found in _____% of healthy individuals.
    a. 10
    b. 20
    c. 40
    d. 50

13. Gastrointestinal infections are most often caused by:
    a. Staphylococcal organisms
    b. Streptococcal organisms
    c. Gram-negative organisms
    d. *Proteus mirabilis* organisms

14. The major cause of peptic ulcer disease is now considered to be:
    a. *Haemophilus influenzae*
    b. *Shigella flexneri*
    c. *Helicobacter pylori*
    d. *Campylobacter jejuni*

15. Lyme disease was first recognized in 1975 as an infection transmitted by all of the following except one. The one that is NOT implicated in transmission of the infection is:
    a. The white-footed mouse
    b. The deer tick
    c. The sheep tick
    d. The groundhog tick

16. The largest population group that develop tuberculosis is:
    a. Adolescents between ages 13 and 19
    b. White, middle-class homosexual men with AIDS
    c. City-dwelling men between ages 25 and 44
    d. Alcoholics

17. Viruses are the smallest parasites, and their ability to reproduce depends entirely on:
    a. Cells of other living things
    b. Size
    c. Number of viruses in the immediate area
    d. Other organisms (spirochete)

18. HIV is caused by a particular type of virus, known as:
    a. Retrovirus
    b. Adenovirus
    c. Arenavirus
    d. Rhinovirus

19. Of venereal diseases, five are considered historically significant. Among these are all but one of the following. The one that does NOT belong to the group of five is:
    a. Syphilis
    b. Molluscum contagiosum
    c. Granuloma inguinale
    d. Gonorrhea

20. Complications of chlamydia infections (*Chlamydia trachomatis*) include all but one of the following. The one condition that is NOT a complication of chlamydia is:
    a. Reiter's syndrome
    b. Cholelithiasis
    c. Infertility
    d. Ectopic pregnancy

21. *Escherichia coli* is a member of the following group:
    a. Gram-positive bacilli
    b. Gram-negative bacilli
    c. Gram-positive bacteria
    d. Gram-positive diplococcus

22. *Proteus mirabilis* causes:
    a. Very few human infections
    b. Some human infections
    c. Many human infections
    d. Most human infections

23. About _____ new cases of typhoid fever are reported each year in the United States.
    a. 50
    b. 100
    c. 300
    d. 500

24. Asymptomatic typhoid fever carriers shed the bacilli in:
    a. Sputum
    b. Feces
    c. Urine
    d. Tears

25. Typhoid patients have prolonged fever, along with:
    a. Pneumonia
    b. Tachycardia
    c. Bradycardia
    d. Extreme diuresis

26. *Campylobacter jejuni* is transmitted by ingestion of infected:
    a. Water
    b. Chicken
    c. Vegetables
    d. Fruits

27. *Helicobacter pylori* is found in _____ % of healthy people over age 60.
    a. 10
    b. 40
    c. 60
    d. 90

28. The gold standard for diagnosing *H. pylori* is:
    a. Blood smear
    b. Tissue sample
    c. Urine culture
    d. Stool culture

29. Lyme disease, weeks to months after initial symptoms, may cause:
    a. Cardiac symptoms
    b. Musculoskeletal symptoms
    c. Respiratory symptoms
    d. Urologic symptoms

30. The characteristic lesion seen in patients with primary syphilis is called a/an:
    a. Gumma
    b. Erosion
    c. Chancre
    d. Eruption

22

Psychosocial Disorders

In primary care settings in the United States, one in three patients has a significant psychosocial problem. The rates of both occupational and physical disability were higher in patients with mental illness than in those without. These data emphasize the importance of evaluating patients for mental illness.

DIAGNOSIS OF PSYCHOSOCIAL PROBLEMS

Accurate diagnosis of a psychosocial problem is essential for prognosis and management. The *Diagnostic and Statistical Manual of Mental Disorders*, fourth edition (DSM-IV), published by the American Psychiatric Association, is a useful reference because it provides diagnostic criteria, epidemiologic information, and prognostic profiles for most of the psychosocial syndromes encountered in ambulatory practice.

GATHERING INFORMATION: HISTORY AND CURRENT STATUS

When the patient expresses somatic complaints (physical symptoms), the clinician must always consider physical illness, even though the patient's demeanor indicates a psychosocial problem. Psychosocial symptoms often do not relate to a specific syndrome. Information to establish a diagnosis of a psychosocial problem is different from that needed to evaluate physical symptoms and must be obtained by asking about or observing the patient's feelings, behaviors, events, relationships, and thoughts. After initial questioning,

which may take some time, it is usually possible to decide in which area the problem lies: anxiety, depression, somatization, cognitive impairment, or maladaptive behavior. A general diagnosis (e.g., depression) can be formulated more specifically under the following likely areas:

- Major depression
- Dysthymic disorder (depressive neurosis)
- Depression related to a recently prescribed drug
- Adjustment disorder with depressed mood
- Alcoholism presenting as depression

From the patient's statements at the beginning, the clinician can focus on and assess general aspects of the patient's life and history.

- Family history of psychosocial problems
- Patient's mental status
- Patient's personality
- Patients' coping styles
- Patient's social history
- Patient's occupation and work history
- The chronologic development of the current symptoms
- Patient's current medication, both prescribed and over the counter
- Patient's current life situation: marital status, household members, family structure, educational level, recreational activities and interests, use of tobacco, alcohol, and drugs by patient and family members
- Review of the patient's life patterns, events, and people that have influenced the patient from childhood to the present: relationships with parents and siblings, school experiences, friends, teachers, religious affiliations, level of perceived

success in school and work, losses (e.g., death of parent or other close family member)

- As the patient as a person with a problem becomes clearer, more specific questions can be directed toward the link between symptoms and when they occur: during conflicts with spouse or children, in groups of people, in particular locations where environment may play a role (e.g., heights, subway [underground], in crowds).

Many psychosocial problems are related to stressors and maladjustments that the patient may unknowingly reveal during questioning: loneliness, fear of spouse, anxiety about children, and worries about money.

Common social factors that frequently are linked to psychosocial illness include the following:

- Loss (personal by death, loss of material things: home, job, children)
- Conflict (in family, with neighbors, or with co-workers; internal conflicts that working mothers often have)
- Change (time of life, menopause, move to a new city/town)
- Maladjustment (conflicts without open anger with spouse or children, failure to adjust to new location, living at a higher level than one can afford)
- Stress (unexpected, acute—sudden death or major illness of parent, spouse, or child; long-term stress of unhappy marriage or feeling of being stuck in one place with no recourse)
- Isolation (in general: friends have died, new location, older age makes getting out more difficult, fear of neighborhood)
- Failure or frustrated expectations (dreams of youth are shattered by realities of life: advancement in work never happens, feels that he or she has failed as a spouse/parent)

Any of these underlying problems can, over time, be a cause of psychosocial illness.

Other specific questions to ask regarding the patient's mental status are

- Orientation to time, place, person
- Speech: use of correct syntax and words to express thoughts, speech problems (slurring, inability to find right words, flight of ideas, inability to express self)
- Memory: knowledge of recent events; ability to remember physicians' names who are currently treating; ability to remember past history and illness in proper chronologic sequence
- Concentration, attention span: ability to understand and follow instructions
- Mood: an obvious, persistent emotion as described by the patient: angry, depressed, anxious, little emotion
- Affect: an emotion that is immediately obvious and one that is freely expressed—anger, fear, sadness, humorous—that is consistent with the spoken message, behavior, and expressed thought
- Perceptions: presence of hallucinations, whether visual, auditory, or of another kind; paranoia, phobias; delusions (fixed beliefs that are false)
- Suicidal thoughts: words or actions that indicate a wish to harm self
- Homicidal or violent thoughts: spoken intent to harm or kill others
- Judgment: ability to understand one's current situation or to show an appropriate level of compliance with this current situation
- The Mini-Mental Status Examination (MMSE) is the most commonly used test to determine whether a person has a cognitive disorder (Box 22-1).
  —For those patients who describe cardinal symptoms of anxiety, affective, or psychotic disorders, focused interviewing is necessary (identified under each of the types of disorder).

PERSONALITY

- Personality is the enduring attitudes and patterns of behavior that typify an individual.
  —The clinician becomes acquainted with a patient's personality through caring for the person over months or years, particularly observing the patient's behavior during illnesses.
  —In those patients who show maladaptive behaviors, recognizing the problem will be helpful in planning the person's care.

COPING RESPONSES

- Coping responses are behaviors that people use to adapt to life stresses.
- Several commonly used coping behaviors should be recognized in patients who may use

BOX 22-1
Mini-Mental State Examination*: Instructions for Administration and Scoring

ORIENTATION
1. Ask for year, season, date, day, month. Then ask specifically for parts omitted. One point for each correct response. (0-5)
2. Ask in turn for name of state, county, town, hospital or place, floor or street. One point for each correct. (0-5)

REGISTRATION
Ask the patient whether you may test his or her memory. Then say the names of three unrelated objects, clearly and slowly, about 1 sec for each. After you have said all three, ask the patient to repeat them. This first repetition determines his or her score (0-3) but keep saying them until he or she can repeat all three up to six trials. If the patient does not eventually learn all three, recall cannot be meaningfully tested.

ATTENTION AND CALCULATION
Ask the patient to begin with 100 and count backward by 7. Stop after five subtractions (93, 86, 79, 72, 65). Score total number of correct answers, one point for each. (0-5) If the patient cannot or will not perform this task, ask him or her to spell the word *world* backward. The score is the number of letters in correct order, e.g., dlrow − 5, dlrwo = 3. (0-5)

RECALL
Ask the patient whether he or she can recall the three words you previously asked him or her to remember. (0-3)

LANGUAGE
Naming: Show the patient a wrist watch and ask him or her what it is. Repeat for pencil. (0-2)

Repetition: Ask the patient to repeat this phrase after you: "No ifs, ands, or buts." Allow only one trial. (0 or 1)

Three-stage command: "Take a piece of paper in your right hand, fold it in half, and put it on the floor." Give the patient a piece of blank paper and repeat the command. Score 1 point for each part correctly executed. (0-3)

Reading: On a blank piece of paper print the sentence, "Close your eyes," in letters large enough for the patient to see clearly. Ask him or her to read it and do what it says. Score 1 point only if the patient actually closes his or her eyes. (0-1)

Writing: Give the patient a blank piece of paper and ask him or her to write a sentence for you. Do not dictate a sentence; it is to be written spontaneously. It must contain a subject and verb and be sensible. Correct grammar and punctuation are not necessary. (0-1)

Copying: On a clean piece of paper, draw intersecting pentagons, each side about 1 inch, and ask him or her to copy it exactly as it is. All 10 angles must be present and 2 must intersect to score 1 point. Tremor and rotation are ignored. (0-1)

Estimate the patient's level of sensorium along a continuum, from alert on the left to coma on the right.

*Total possible score is 30 points. Patients with a total of 23 points or less are highly likely to have a cognitive disorder.

them to avoid confronting a problem for which they need help.

- When maladaptive coping is seen, the clinician can help the patient to disclose the major problem and to help him or her to achieve a healthier attitude to resolve it.
  - —*Denial:* a response that enables the patient to avoid considering a distressing problem; the denial response may be **silent** about a suspected problem (e.g., blood in stools that is not acknowledged because of fear of cancer); or **openly expressed** (e.g., a person who, after surviving a life-threatening heart attack and is fearful of dying, denies having any signs or symptoms of heart disease)
  - —*Rationalization:* a process in which a person gives plausible explanations for behavior

that is obviously designed to avoid unpleasant realities (e.g., an alcoholic explains that his work demands have increased so much that it has made it impossible for him to attend Alcoholics Anonymous [AA] meetings)
  - —*Regression:* is reversion to dependent behavior that is typical of childhood, and is a common response to major illness or other circumstances that threaten a person's autonomy (e.g., a woman who is recovering slowly from a hip fracture gets upset easily about small problems, such as when her daughter misses a visiting time one evening, or expects her daughter to feed her dinner every evening during her visit)
  - —*Projection:* a process in which an unpleasant aspect of one's self is ascribed to another per-

BOX 22-2

Axis IV: Categories for Psychosocial and Environmental Problems

Problems with primary support group
Problems related to the social environment
Education problem
Occupation problem
Housing problem
Economic problem
Problems with access to health care services
Problems related to interaction with the legal system/ crime
Other psychosocial problem

Reprinted with permission from the *Diagnostic and statistical manual of mental disorders,* ed 4, text revision, Copyright 2000, American Psychiatric Association.

son (e.g., a wife who is unfaithful to her husband accuses him of being unfaithful to her)
—*Displacement:* a process in which feelings toward one person are directed toward someone else (e.g., a man who is furious at his boss for keeping him late at work several evenings becomes angry with his wife for no apparent reason)

FORMULATION OF THE PROBLEM

- When all of the important information about the patient's psychosocial history has been gathered, a useful way to formulate the problems is the five-axis approach recommended by the American Psychiatric Association.
  —*Axis I:* Psychosocial syndromes, plus conditions not attributable to a formal mental disorder that are a focus of attention (e.g., psychologic factors affecting medical condition, malingering, uncomplicated bereavement, noncompliance with medical treatment, or academic or occupation problems)
  —*Axis II:* Personality disorders or styles and specific developmental disorders
  —*Axis III:* General medical conditions
  —*Axis IV:* Psychologic and environmental problems (Box 22-2)
  —*Axis V:* Global Assessment of Functioning (GAF): current level and highest level for at least a few months during the past year (Box 22-3)

- Box 22-4 presents a sample case study that utilizes this five-axis approach.

COMORBIDITY IN THE PATIENT'S FAMILY

- Psychosocial problems often create significant stress for the spouse, children, and other people with close ties to the affected patient, particularly in cases of chronic problems such as alcoholism, affective disorders, anxiety disorders, and the somatoform disorders. The impact on the patient's family should always be considered in evaluating psychosocial problems because the comorbidity of the family can be alleviated as part of the overall approach to these difficult problems.

LEVEL OF COMPETENCE, DECISION-MAKING CAPACITY, AND NEED FOR COMMITMENT

- Level of competence, decision-making capacity, and need for commitment are problem areas that usually require input from one or more specialists who know the patient, and who have examined him or her.
- *Competence* and *incompetence* are legal terms, and their use should be limited to only those situations in which a formal determination has been made about them.
  —Under the law, people are presumed to be competent to manage their own affairs until a judicial determination has been made, in which a clinician may be required to provide testimony in a particular case.
  —Common civil issues that require determination of mental competence include competence to accept or refuse medical care, commitment to hospitals, contesting of wills, and guardianship decisions.
  —In the primary care setting, the most common problem among marginally competent persons is their ability to provide self-care, in which information provided by a family member or a visiting nurse is necessary, in addition to the measures needed to obtain a legal decision about competence.
  —Decision-making capacity, also called *clinical competence,* is a clinical term that refers to

BOX 22-3

Global Assessment of Functioning Scale

Consider psychologic, social, and occupational functioning on a hypothetical continuum of mental health-illness. Do not include impairment in functioning caused by physical or environmental limitations.

CODE

100
91   Superior functioning in a wide range of activities, life's problems never seem to get out of hand, is sought out by others because of his or her many positive qualities. No symptoms.

90
81   Absent or minimal symptoms (e.g., mild anxiety before an exam), good functioning in all areas, interested and involved in a wide range of activities, socially effective, generally satisfied with life, no more than everyday problems or concerns (e.g., an occasional argument with family members)

80
71   If symptoms are present, they are transient and expected reactions to psychosocial stressors (e.g., difficulty concentrating after family argument); no more than slight impairment in social, occupational, or school functioning (e.g., temporarily falling behind in schoolwork)

70
61   Some mild symptoms (e.g., depressed mood and mild insomnia) OR Some difficulty in social, occupational, or school functioning (e.g., occasional truancy, or theft within the household), but generally functioning pretty well, has some meaningful relationships

60
51   Moderate symptoms (e.g., flat affect and circumstantial speech, occasional panic attacks) OR moderate difficulty in social, occupational, or school functioning (e.g., no friends, unable to keep a job)

50
41   Serious symptoms (e.g., suicidal ideation, severe obsessional rituals, frequent shoplifting) OR any serious impairment in social, occupational, or school functioning (e.g., no friends, unable to keep a job)

40
31   Some impairment in reality testing or communication (e.g., speech is at times illogical, obscure, or irrelevant) OR major impairment in several areas such as work or school, family relations, judgment, thinking, or mood (e.g., depressed man avoids friends, neglects family, and is unable to work; child frequently beats up younger children, is defiant at home, and is failing at school)

30
21   Behavior is considerably influenced by delusions or hallucinations OR serious impairment in communication or judgment (e.g., sometimes incoherent, acts grossly inappropriately, suicidal preoccupation) OR inability to function in almost all areas (e.g., stays in bed all day; no job, home, or friends)

20
11   Some danger of hurting self or others (e.g., suicide attempts without clear expectation of death, frequently violent, manic excitement) OR occasionally fails to maintain minimal personal hygiene (e.g., smears feces) OR gross impairment in communication (e.g., largely incoherent or mute)

10
1   Persistent danger of severely hurting self or others (e.g., recurrent violence) OR persistent inability to maintain minimal personal hygiene OR serious suicidal act with clear expectation of death

0   Inadequate information

Reprinted with permission from the *Diagnostic and statistical manual of mental disorders,* ed 4, text revision, Copyright 2000, American Psychiatric Association.

BOX 22-4
Case Study

Mr. D, a 67-year-old married newspaper reporter, underwent coronary artery bypass graft (CABG) surgery in December 1996. His postoperative hospital course was uneventful except for mild reaction to one drug, which was immediately discontinued. Soon after discharge, he came twice in the same day to the emergency department complaining of severe chest pain and cold lower extremities. Evaluation revealed mild tenderness at the incision site. The next day he returned, this time describing inability to sleep, and still complaining of severe chest pain and cold lower extremities. A comprehensive evaluation, including an exercise stress test, did not disclose any physical basis for his symptoms.

The patient's wife described instances of regressive behavior since the patient's discharge: he wanted her to bring his meals on a tray to his bed, asked her to pick out his clothes each day, had occasional urinary incontinence, and had her dispensing all of his medications. He was not sleeping well and always awakened his wife when he awoke. Additional questions revealed a somewhat diminished sense of self-worth and some doubts about whether he would be able to return to work as he had expected before surgery. He knew that his income would be significantly lower if he applied for social security benefits.

The patient also said that he thought that he had been on the pump too long and he was afraid that his incision would break down (which had happened to a friend after CABG).

Previously, Mr. D had always been a self-reliant person, had worked at his newspaper job for almost 30 years, and had been fully compliant with his medical regimen for several years before surgery. The CABG was recommended when his angina worsened in October 1996, and he was unable to cover his assignments in all parts of the city. He had never before shown regressive tendencies, although he depended on his wife to help in making decisions about large purchases they made, and they had never been separated except when they both worked during their 40-year marriage. There was history of psychiatric illness in his family.

Based on this information and additional data from questions, the formulation of Mr. D's illness was:

Axis I: Adjustment disorder, with depressed mood and somatic complaints.

Axis II: No personality disorder; history of dependency that made him vulnerable to the behavior he exhibited after CABG

Axis III: (a) Coronary artery disease; (b) status post-CABG with good results

Axis IV: Financial problems

Axis V: Global Assessment of Functioning (GAF): Current GAF—moderate symptoms and functional impairment (Code 60 in Box 22-3); past year GAF = slight symptoms and functional impairment (Code 80 in Box 22-3).

---

the capacity of the patient to make a particular decision; decision-making capacity is considered to be present when the patient is able (1) to understand information that is relevant to the decision, (2) to deliberate about the options in accordance with personal values and goals, and (3) to communicate (verbally or nonverbally) with caregivers.

— Many patients are able to make some decisions but not all, depending on the complexity and circumstances; each situation that requires a decision by the patient is considered separately.

— Commitment laws in most states require examination by a physician, and do not specify that the examination must be conducted by a psychiatrist; the test for commitment is to evaluate whether the patient is potentially a danger to themselves or to others.

PSYCHOTHERAPY IN THE PRIMARY CARE SETTING

- Psychotherapy consists of verbal and behavioral processes that are used for the purpose of relieving symptoms and resolving intrapersonal and interpersonal conflicts.
  — Many different techniques are presented in the literature, but fundamental principles are basic in all psychotherapeutic techniques.
- Most patients who require psychotherapy in the outpatient setting are those who suffer from demoralization, a painful sense of disappointment and personal inadequacy in the face of life circumstances.
- The state of demoralization is usually defined as the product of interactions between environmental stressors and personal vulnerabilities.
  — Environmental stressors may be temporary (e.g., unemployment) or unchangeable (e.g., conjugal bereavement).

—Personal vulnerabilities may be constitutional (e.g., mental retardation) or learned (e.g., excessive dependency, perfectionism).

—When these patients seek help, their usual problem-solving methods have failed and their usual support systems have been exhausted.

• Psychotherapy, then, can be seen as an interactive process in which the goal is to restore morale; the process involves both cognitive and relational tasks.

—The major cognitive tasks are

~ To develop a working formulation of patients' difficulties as a product of environmental stressors and personal vulnerabilities.

~ To assess and appreciate the personal strengths and resources available to patients for problem solving.

~ To ameliorate emotional distress and to help the patient apply these strengths and resources to regain a sense of mastery over life's problems.

—The relational task is to promote in patients what Jerome Frank calls "expectant trust," which is an attitude on the part of patients that their clinician cares about them, is competent to help, is confident of their recovery, and is committed to remain available until relief is achieved.

• Expectant trust is an essential element in the success of psychotherapy, and is enhanced by several specific techniques used with patients; its effective mobilization requires an understanding of the concepts of transference and countertransference.

TRANSFERENCE

• Patients' expectations of their physicians relates partly to the patients' experiences with their parents in circumstances of fear, pain, and other forms of distress; patients may therefore consciously or unconsciously expect that new people in their lives will treat them as their parents did.

—These expectations are known as transference phenomena: patients transfer expectations onto the physician.

—When the transfer expectations are positive (positive transference), therapists have at their disposal a powerful resource to help their patients feel better; positive transference may explain placebo effects and must be taken into consideration when the responses to a new intervention are being evaluated.

—Not all transference phenomena are positive; everyone experiences frustration, anger, disappointment, and other painful emotions that occur throughout growth from child to adult.

—These negative experiences may leave psychologic scars that may influence the relationship of the patient with authority figures or others (e.g., physicians, therapists); a patient who was abandoned by parents may cling to the therapist with pathologic dependency.

—Other experiences of early life may lead to passivity, hostility, compulsiveness, and other maladaptive behaviors.

• In psychotherapy, therefore transference is viewed as both a tool and a potential obstacle.

—In short-term counseling, intense therapeutic relationships usually do not develop, and the transference is primarily positive.

COUNTERTRANSFERENCE

• Like their patients, physicians and therapists must experience the trials and tribulations of childhood and adolescence and may therefore develop positive and negative expectations that are transferred to other people, including their patients.

—This countertransference may limit the ability of the therapist to care for particular patients (e.g., if the therapist had an abusing alcoholic parent, he may become enraged and ineffective in dealing with a patient who is alcoholic and who relapses).

TREATMENT TECHNIQUES

• The first goal of the therapist is to establish an effective therapeutic relationship, which requires several components.

—The patient must trust the therapist, which is engendered when the therapist shows consistent interest, accepts sensitive information without being judgmental, takes the patient's concerns seriously, and controls inappropriate reactions to patients who are difficult.

—Another element is for the therapist to be sure that the patient understands how to gain access to them, and to recognize limits regarding access during ongoing treatment; the therapist needs to know that these trust-promoting, limit-setting actions are accomplished before counseling can begin.

Eliciting Information

- Patients' misinformation or lack of information may cause much emotional distress (e.g., fear of serious illness, conviction that one's symptoms must be caused by physical illness).
  —Among therapists' powerful aids during the counseling process is to help patients identify and clarify their information needs and to provide information that is specific to the patient's needs.
  —Clear, unequivocal explanations of normal physiology, diseases, treatment regimens, and the close relationship of mind and body are tools that the therapist can use to the patient's advantage.

Responding to Feelings

- The therapist can be extremely helpful when they use empathetic listening with patients; attending closely to what the patient is saying, allowing the patient time to reflect, remembering details of the patient's story, and responding readily and appropriately to the patient's feelings tell the patient that the therapist is concerned, which diminishes the patient's sense of isolation that is associated with unexpressed feelings and enhances the patient's self-esteem.

Legitimizing Feelings

- Patients often feel embarrassed or off-base by their reactions to a situation.
  —The therapist can point out that anyone in a similar situation would likely have the very same reactions, which is helpful to the patient.

Ventilating Feelings

- Encouraging the patient to express feelings openly usually helps to loosen the patient's defenses, so that he or she is able to ventilate their deeper feelings.

Showing Respect and Facilitating Choice

- The therapist should avoid acting as a powerful, all-knowing figure.
- Most patients have tried to resolve their problems before seeking professional help.
  —Asking about and acknowledging prior efforts, even when those efforts have been unsuccessful, and supporting the patient as a problem solver can assist the patient to consider and think through a current problem by pointing out personal strengths, supportive people, and enjoyable activities, and allows the patient to identify options and make choices that will likely be effective in resolving current problems.

Contingency Planning

- Once the particular problem is dissected as to its causes, effects, and possible changes that can make it more manageable, the therapist and the patient can together devise a plan of operations for dealing with a particular problem and other related problems that may occur over the next several days or weeks.

Giving Advice and Persuading

- The patient considers the therapist to be an expert, and the therapist can and should use this expertise in providing concrete advice when the patient is unable to use their own judgment and coping skills.
  —The therapist can offer specific suggestions that the patient can accept and use until his or her own coping mechanisms become functional once again.

Managing Abnormal Illness Behavior

- Abnormal illness behavior occurs when the patient's symptoms or impairments or actions are disproportionate to detectable disease.
  —These patients have somatoform disorders and express their emotional distress in terms of somatic complaints and dreaded conditions.
- The therapist, in these cases, does not reinforce abnormal illness behavior by
  —Avoiding unnecessary tests
  —Avoiding unnecessary prescriptions
  —Avoiding unnecessary referral to specialists

—Scheduling regular visits (not making visit contingent on new symptoms)

—Allowing the patient to have some symptoms rather than eliminating all symptoms as a treatment goal

—Encouraging the patient to talk about his or her life situation rather than about somatic symptoms

Using Family, Friends, and Community Resources

• The therapist takes every opportunity to address the informational needs of the patient's family.

• The therapist enlists the family's help in assisting the patient to make positive choices and decisions.

• The therapist encourages the patient to try new and unexplored experiences or activities that are of interest (e.g., painting, writing, taking a job that enables the patient to meet new people every day and see other people's problems).

• The therapist can point out various community resources of which the patient may not be aware, and that will be helpful in meeting needs.

Forms of Counseling

• Supportive therapy helps the patient cope with ongoing medical problems and stressful life circumstances; this type of counseling is usually open-ended and is often part of routine management of a chronic disease.

• Short-term counseling is particularly useful for a patient who accepts a psychologic basis for symptoms and who wants help in resolving a crisis related to the symptoms.

—The goal here is to strengthen the patient's defenses and to relieve symptoms without uncovering long-standing intrapsychic conflicts underlying the current problem.

—Generally, a therapeutic contract is established in which the purpose, length, frequency, and cost of the sessions are clearly set at the beginning; patients often react to the boundaries as part of the transference phenomenon by objecting to them or by trying to change or violate them; however, the terms of the contract should not be altered, but should remain the same throughout the course of therapy.

—The therapist's schedule usually requires that sessions be brief (15 to 20 minutes) and limited in number (5 to 10 patients).

—Patients are usually seen individually, but couples or family members may be involved in therapy at the same time, as well.

—Therapy focuses on problems that are specific, conscious, readily accessible, unrepressed, and current.

—The interactive style is conversational and natural, not remote and analytical.

—The therapist's role is to facilitate problem solving, not to prescribe solutions.

—The process includes the following:

~ Help patients to identify their strengths and resources

~ Praise their adaptiveness

~ Help them to explore how they can build on their strengths

~ Encourage them to try options discussed in the sessions through homework assignments carried out between sessions

—Throughout short-term therapy, it is essential to continually screen for evidence of a major psychiatric disorder (e.g., panic disorder, major depression, substance abuse that may require pharmacotherapy or other intervention).

Family Counseling

• The goals of family counseling are to

—Facilitate communication among family members

—Enable them to be aware of maladaptive patterns of behavior that may be destructive to one or more family members

—Help the family to change maladaptive behaviors to constructive behaviors

—The techniques used are similar to those used in short-term counseling.

PSYCHOSOCIAL DISORDERS
Somatization

• Patients who seek medical help are supposed to have a physical cause for their symptoms.

—Their complaints and the associated physical disability should be proportional to the disease diagnosed.

—With appropriate treatment, they are supposed to follow and cooperate with the cli-

nician's prescriptions and suggestions and to resume their normal functioning as soon as possible.
- These events are called *normal illness behavior.*
- Many patients, however, exhibit abnormal illness behavior by manifesting somatization, a phenomenon in which unexplained or amplified physical symptoms are linked to psychologic factors or conflicts.
- The causes of somatization are not fully understood.
- Four distinctive perspectives help to explain somatization; it may be viewed
  —As a symptom of a disease
  —As a manifestation of personality
  —As a modeled or reinforced behavior
  —As an understandable consequence of a patient's life history
- Patients with a major affective disorder often exhibit abnormal illness behavior.
  —However, up to 30% of somatizing patients were ultimately diagnosed as having a specific medical or neurologic disease.
- Personality is considered to consist of enduring attitudes and habitual patterns of response and as an approximation of ideal prototypes, such as histrionic or obsessive-compulsive, or clusters of individual traits.
  —Patients with these types of personality may be predisposed to develop somatization or hypochondriasis.
  —People who are introspective, who focus their attention on their own thoughts and feelings, and those who are considered to be neurotic (emotionally unstable), vulnerable to stress, and self-conscious often experience unexplained physical symptoms.
  —For some patients, their somatization is reinforced by those in their surroundings, such as might occur if a particularly doting father expressed much sympathy whenever his daughter was ill, which encouraged the daughter to somatize to gain her father's attention.
  —Patients whose early years were marked by parental neglect and abuse may likely carry into adulthood their feelings of both hostility and dependency, which may be activated in their relationships with physicians or other authority figures.
  —Patients with this history and current symptoms are usually hostile and demanding; physicians and therapists, knowing and understanding the impact of early childhood deprivation, can more realistically assess the patient and be objective in meeting the patient's needs without reinforcing the abnormal illness behavior.

Adjustment Disorders

- These disorders are reactive emotional states that result from the patient's difficulty in meeting the demands of the environment (Box 22-5).
  —It is understandable that in today's rush-rush atmosphere, both at home and at work, patients do react by exhibiting somatic complaints.
- In many patients, the diagnosis of adjustment disorder may be difficult if the somatic symp-

---

BOX 22-5

Diagnostic Criteria for Adjustment Disorder

A. The development of emotional or behavioral symptoms in response to an identifiable stressor(s) occurring within 3 months of the onset of the stressor(s)
B. These symptoms or behaviors are clinically significant as evidenced by either of the following:
  1. Marked distress that is in excess of what would be expected from exposure to the stressor
  2. Significant impairment in social or occupational (academic) functioning
C. The stress-related disturbance does not meet the criteria for any specific Axis I disorder and is not merely an exacerbation of a preexisting Axis I or Axis II disorder
D. Does not represent bereavement
E. The symptoms do not persist for more than 6 months after the termination of the stressor (or its consequences).
Acute: If the symptoms have persisted for less than 6 months
Chronic: If the symptoms have persisted for 6 months or longer

toms resemble those of an established disease process; the nurse practitioner must first address three areas.

—Elicit a comprehensive history.

—Rule out major depression.

—A routine physical examination and laboratory tests are done, but no extensive work-up is conducted because it may place the patient in a definitive sick role and prolong the symptoms.

Treatment

- Many patients get better after just one office visit that is conducted as a short-term counseling session with empathetic listening, a partial physical examination, and reassurance that there is no serious physical problem.
- Short-term prescription of drugs for anxiety or insomnia has no effect on patients' improvement; about two thirds of patients show significant improvement within 1 month even without medications.
- Evaluate within a week the benefit of one visit should occur before considering prescribing a psychotropic drug for an adjustment disorder.
- If a patient does not respond to conservative therapy, further evaluation to rule out other syndromes should be conducted, especially for panic disorder, major depression, alcoholism, chemical dependency, or domestic violence that affects the patient or another member of the family.

Conversion Disorders

Definition

Conversion disorders are disorders in which physical symptoms are caused by psychologic conflict, unconsciously converted to resemble those of a neurologic disorder.

Risk Factors

- Female sex
- Young age: adolescence to early adulthood

Etiology/Cause

- A socially or psychologically stressful event
- An unexplained loss or change of body functioning develops in the presence of evidence that the symptoms *solve or express a psychologic conflict or need.*

- Patients may have histrionic or dependent personalities, and may show remarkable serenity *(la belle indifference)* in the face of their impairments.

Pathogenesis

- The patient has had an extraordinarily stressful event occur that causes him or her to assume a physical problem that resembles a neurologic disorder.
- The stress apparently causes an internal conflict or need that is overwhelming in its significance to the patient.

Diagnosis

Signs and Symptoms

- Symptoms develop unconsciously and are limited to those that suggest a neurologic deficit—usually impaired coordination or balance, weakness, paralysis of an arm or a leg, or loss of sensation in part of the body.
- The most common conversion disorder symptoms observed are amnesia, aphonia, blindness, paralysis, numbness, and seizures.
- Secondary gain is the object when unexplained symptoms allow the patient to avoid onerous tasks or undesirable duties.
- Primary gain is the goal when conversion symptoms appear to resolve an internal conflict by a feeling, impulse, or wish that the individual finds frightening or morally unacceptable (e.g., violent behavior against someone close to the patient).

Treatment

- A trusting physician-patient relationship is essential.
- Rule out any undiagnosed medical disorder.
- Review those relevant factors that may be promoting conversion symptoms: psychiatric illness, major depression, personality disorder, environmental reinforcers, and aspects of the patient's life story.
- Emphasize to the patient the absence of serious disease and express optimism that full recovery is expected.
- Avoid confronting the patient with the psychologic basis of the behaviors, but emphasize that emotional factors may have played a role in exacerbation of symptoms.

- Behavior modification therapy, including relaxation training, is effective in some patients.

Prognosis

- Hospitalized patients usually improve within 2 weeks, but 20% to 25% of patients have recurrences within a year and symptoms become chronic in some.

Patient/Family Education

- It is important to emphasize that no serious illness is present.
- The psychologic basis for symptoms is not mentioned directly to the patient, and perhaps not to family members either, who may use it against the patient in terms of anger, threats, abusive behavior, or other untoward actions.
- The general nature of the condition is explained, primarily that the patient has had an experience or faced a severe threat that has caused symptoms to occur.
- Hypnotherapy or narcoanalysis may be helpful for some patients.

Follow-up/Referral

- Patients with conversion disorders often require continuing follow-up for months to years.
- Referral to a psychiatrist may be necessary for both the patient and the family if symptoms become chronic and cause disruptions among family members.

Hypochondriasis

Definition

Hypochondriasis is a chronic disorder in which the patient unrealistically interprets physical symptoms as a serious, life-threatening disease, despite repeated reassurances that no serious disease exists.

Risk Factors

- Onset is usually in the thirties
- Both sexes are equally affected
- Obsessive-compulsive personality traits
- Alcohol or drug dependence

Etiology/Cause

- The cause is unknown.

Pathogenesis

- A stressful event (e.g., death of a parent) may cause the susceptible patient to believe that he or she may have the same disease that caused the death of the parent, and begin to focus on symptoms that are inconsequential or that occur normally, but that the patient believes are due to a serious, life-threatening illness.

Diagnosis

Signs and Symptoms (Box 22-6)

Treatment

- Patients with hypochondriasis firmly believe that they are physically ill, and so do not accept psychiatric therapy.

BOX 22-6
Diagnostic Criteria for Hypochondriasis

A. Preoccupation with fears of having, or the idea that one has, a serious disease based on the person's misinterpretation of bodily symptoms

B. The preoccupation persists despite appropriate medical evaluation and reassurance

C. The belief in A is not of delusional intensity (as in delusional disorder, somatic type) and is not restricted to a circumscribed concern about appearance (as in body dysmorphic disorder)

D. The preoccupation causes clinically significant distress or impairment in social, occupational, or other important areas of functioning

E. The duration of the disturbance is at least 6 months

F. The preoccupation does not occur exclusively during the course of generalized anxiety disorder, OCD, panic disorder, a major depressive episode, separation anxiety, or another somatoform disorder

Specify with poor insight if, for most of the time during the current episode, the person does not recognize that the concern about having a serious illness is excessive or unreasonable

- Treatment is the same as for other chronic somatoform disorders.
  - —Do a careful history and physical examination to convince the patient that the diagnosis and treatment are based on data collected as usual.
  - —Review the four explanatory perspectives for factors that might be promoting hypochondriasis.
    - ~ Psychiatric illness
    - ~ Personality disorder
    - ~ Environmental reinforcers of the hypochondriasis
    - ~ Aspects of the patient's life history as a basis for physical illness
- Do not indicate that the patient will be cured.
- Assure the patient of your continuous availability; schedule brief visits that do not hinge on the development of new symptoms.
- Do not indicate to the patient that the symptoms are entirely psychologic, but point out that emotional factors worsen physical distress, and encourage the patient to discuss stressors, past and present.
- Some patients may accept short-term counseling; the development of a relationship characterized by expectant trust is critical if patients are to be persuaded that their worries are excessive and that they should participate more actively in outside activities.

Patient/Family Education
- Reassure family members that despite the persistence of symptoms, there is no serious illness present and encourage them to support a strategy de-emphasizing expensive and elaborate diagnostic tests and stressing the maintenance of function despite symptoms.

Follow-up/Referral
- Patients with hypochondriasis do not accept the fact that they do not have a serious illness, and continue in their belief despite repeated reassurance.
- Psychiatric referral is usually unnecessary and incurs added cost for the patient and family.
- The nurse practitioner continues to look for evidence of an underlying physical disorder but invariably finds none.

- Continuous encouragement of the patient regarding the need to remain active and to participate in social activities and family events is essential.
- Support for the family may be provided by community support groups, as well as by the clinician and health professional staff.
- Visits are scheduled on a regular basis, rather than on the appearance of new symptoms.

Dysmorphic Disorder
Definition
Dysmorphic disorder is a condition in which the person has an excessive or completely unfounded preoccupation with a defect in personal appearance.

Risk Factors
- Onset is usually between adolescence and age 30.
- Women are more often affected than men, but both sexes may have the disorder.
- Dependent personality
- Extreme self-consciousness
- Obsessive-compulsive personality
- Early experiences with overly critical parents who caused the patient to feel inferior.

Etiology/Cause (see also Risk Factors)
- The specific cause is unknown.

Pathogenesis (see also Risk Factors)
- Predisposed patients develop misconceptions about their body image, perhaps influenced by comments from parents, siblings, or classmates.
- The patient begins to focus on one or a few body parts: the face, head, or jaw is often the center of their concern.

Diagnosis (Box 22-7)
Signs and Symptoms
- Symptoms may develop gradually or abruptly.
- Although the intensity of symptoms may vary, the course is one of few symptom-free intervals.
- The patient's focus is often the face or head, but any part of the body may be involved, and may change from one part to another.

- Specific areas of concern may be thinning hair, wrinkles, acne, scars, vascular markings, complexion color, excessive facial hair, or shape and size of a particular body part (e.g., abdomen, buttocks, breasts).
- Some patients have difficulty controlling their preoccupation and often spend hours thinking about their perceived defect.
- Some patients may persistently check their appearance in mirrors, others avoid mirrors.
- Camouflage efforts may be made (e.g., wearing the hair in a style that covers part of the face, growing a beard to cover scars).
- Some patients undergo cosmetic, dental, or other types of therapy, which may intensify their preoccupation with their appearance.
- Patients' self-consciousness often prevents them from socializing, appearing in public, and even going to work, which leads to social isolation and greater inwardness.
- Dysmorphic disorder is different from normal concern about one's appearance because it is time consuming, causes significant distress, and impairs functioning.
- If body size and shape are a major concern, anorexia nervosa is likely to develop.
- The diagnosis is made only when the preoccupation is not explained more definitively by another psychiatric disorder.

Treatment
- Patients are reluctant to talk about their obsessive thinking, so the condition can persist for years.
- The data about treatment and prognosis are very limited.
- Some preliminary evidence indicates that selective serotonin reuptake inhibitors (SSRIs), such as clomipramine and fluoxetine, may be helpful.

Prognosis
- Because of the duration of symptoms before diagnosis and treatment, outcome of therapy is largely unknown.
- It is likely that the patient, regardless of treatment, will continue to have persistent preoccupation with only brief periods that are symptom-free.

Patient/Family Education
- The patient is difficult to reach in terms of elucidating behavior, its causes, and possible ways in which to eliminate the obsessive thinking.
- In many, if not most, patients, the preoccupation began in childhood or early adolescence and has become part of the patient's behavioral pattern.

Follow-up/Referral
- Patients may seek medical help, perhaps hoping for surgical intervention that will solve the problem of the physical fault.
- After taking a history, the primary care provider may conclude that the problem is primarily psychologic, and refer the patient to a psychiatrist well versed in treating dysmorphic disorders.

Anxiety Disorders
Definition
Anxiety includes a wide range of feelings and fears, from a mild sense of impending disaster to a state of intense anxiety and panic, with physical signs and symptoms that reflect inner feelings: palpitations, shortness of breath, dizziness, faintness, profuse sweating, and restlessness. In many cases, the patient cannot relate the intense anxiousness to any specific cause for fear. Generalized anxiety disorder (GAD) occurs in 3% to 5% of ambulatory patients, often seen as a medical disorder initially, both by the patient and the nurse practitioner.

BOX 22-8
Diagnostic Criteria for Generalized Anxiety Disorder

A. Excessive anxiety and worry (apprehensive expectation), occurring more days than not for at least 6 months, about a number of events or activities (e.g., work or school performance)
B. The person finds it difficult to control the worry.
C. The anxiety and worry are associated with at least three of the following six symptoms (with at least some symptoms present for more days than not for the past 6 months)
   1. Restlessness or feeling keyed up or on edge
   2. Being easily fatigued
   3. Difficulty concentrating or mind being blank
   4. Irritability
   5. Muscle tension
   6. Sleep disturbance (difficulty falling or staying asleep, or restless unsatisfying sleep)

D. The focus of the anxiety and worry is not confined to features of an Axis I disorder, e.g., the anxiety or worry is not about having a panic attack (as in panic disorder), being embarrassed in public (as in social phobia), being contaminated (as in OCD), being away from home or close relatives (as in separation anxiety disorder), gaining weight (as in anorexia nervosa), or having a serious illness (as in hypochondriasis), and is not part of PTSD.
E. The anxiety, worry, or physical symptoms cause clinically significant distress or impairment in social, occupational, or other important areas of functioning.
F. Not due to the direct effects of a substance (e.g., drugs of abuse, medication) or a general medical condition (e.g., hyperthyroidism), and does not occur exclusively during a mood disorder, psychotic disorder, or pervasive developmental disorder.

Reprinted with permission from the *Diagnostic and statistical manual of mental disorders,* ed 4, text revision, Copyright 2000, American Psychiatric Association.

Risk Factors
- A specific, recent stressor (e.g., death of a parent)
- Attention deficit/hyperactivity disorder
- Somatoform disorder
- Affective disorder
- Cognitive impairment
- Substance abuse

Etiology/Cause
- Symptoms usually begin in the teens or twenties, during times of high stress.
- The precise cause of anxiety disorder is not clear, although anxiety may develop in persons as a reaction to acute stress.
- Patients with another psychosocial problem may develop anxiety disorder in addition to the prior disorder.
- Hyperthyroidism
- Use of corticosteroids or cocaine may produce symptoms and signs identical to those of primary anxiety disorders.

Pathogenesis (see also Risk Factors and Etiology/Cause)
- Psychiatrists and other physicians believe that anxiety disorder stems from both physiologic and psychologic factors.
- The underlying cause may be some frightening event that occurred in the patient's childhood that was perhaps misinterpreted as a personal threat.

Diagnosis (Box 22-8)
Signs and Symptoms (see also Definition)
- In addition to the signs and symptoms of the disorder previously listed, the patient may experience gastrointestinal (GI) or genitourinary (GU) symptoms (e.g., diarrhea, constipation, urinary incontinence), blood pressure (BP) spikes with flushed face and dizziness, dyspnea, and an overwhelming feeling of doom or death.
- The initial anxiety episode is usually followed by continuing anxiety, with the severity of symptoms varying widely as life stresses come and go.
- Symptoms may develop suddenly, as in a panic attack, or gradually over hours or days.
- Longer duration of anxiety is usually associated with anxiety disorder.
- Feelings of anxiety may be so distressing and disruptive that the patient develops depression; these two disorders often coexist.
- Diagnosis of a specific anxiety disorder is based primarily on its characteristic symptoms and signs.

- If a state of anxiety is very distressing, interferes with functioning, and does not terminate spontaneously, anxiety disorder is present and warrants therapy.
- On the initial visit, the nurse practitioner takes a history that includes inquiries about consumption of alcohol, caffeine, and other drugs, and performs a focused physical examination to look for signs of hyperthyroidism, pheochromocytoma, or hypoglycemia that may present with symptoms of anxiety.

Treatment
- Some experts believe that anxiety should be regarded as a symptom rather than as a distinct entity.
- An understanding practitioner can do much to allay the anxious patient's fears and provide hope for recovery, or at least greatly diminish anticipatory anxiety and the number and intensity of episodes of acute anxiety.
- Pharmacotherapy is useful for these patients.
  - A trial of buspirone is well tolerated and effective in treating generalized anxiety disorder but may not be effective in patients who have taken benzodiazepines for long periods; buspirone is given for 6 to 12 months.
  - If the patient is hypervigilant, with autonomic hyperactivity and muscle tension, a 1- to 2-month course of benzodiazepines may prove beneficial, prescribed on an as-needed rather than a continuous dosage.
  - If symptoms do not change with the previously listed therapy, an antidepressant, such as trazodone or a tricyclic agent, may be beneficial.
  - In a recent study, imipramine, trazodone, and diazepam were prescribed together; results showed that 70% of patients on this regiment improved markedly, compared with 47% of placebo-treated patients.
- Anxious patients are usually demoralized and benefit from short-term counseling aimed at solving problems and restoring self-esteem.
- If the patient shows no response to treatment, or if relapse occurs, the clinician should re-

assess the diagnosis, examine the patient for medical and psychologic comorbidity, and consider possible psychiatric referral.

Patient/Family Education
- The patient and the family should be told that anxiety disorder results from both biologic and psychologic dysfunction.
- Reassurance that, with appropriate treatment (medication and behavior therapy), improvement is likely, and even full recovery
- Instruct the patient in techniques such as progressive muscle relaxation, and encourage regular use of these and other similar techniques.
- Patients may be encouraged to keep a diary of symptoms that will help to guide therapy.

Follow-up/Referral
- Patients with anxiety disorder are followed closely for 6 to 12 months.
- Referral to a psychiatrist for more intensive therapy may be required.

Obsessive-Compulsive Disorder
Definition
Obsessive-compulsive disorder (OCD) is characterized by recurrent, unwanted, intrusive ideas, thoughts, images, or impulses that seem silly, weird, nasty, or horrible **(obsessions)**, and by repetitive, purposeful, but senseless actions (e.g., washing hands 100 times a day) **(compulsions)** due to the obsessions. The presence of these obsessions and compulsions distinguishes OCD from obsessive-compulsive personality disorder, which is characterized by meticulousness, perfectionism, and rigidity.

Risk Factors
- Slightly more women than men are affected.
- About 1% to 2% of the population and in the general medical clinic meet the criteria for OCD.
- Onset occurs between adolescence and early adulthood.

Etiology/Cause and Pathogenesis
- Explanations for OCD have been presented in the psychiatric literature.
  - Many psychoanalytic professionals view obsessive-compulsive symptoms as prod-

ucts of reaction formation against unacceptable wishes and impulses, often related to aggression and sexuality.

—Behavioral theorists and practitioners stress the anxiety-reducing effects of compulsive rituals and propose that compulsions are maintained precisely because of their positively reinforcing ameliorating effects on conditioned anxiety.

—The importance of personality traits is suggested by research showing that preexisting obsessive traits (e.g., meticulousness, perfectionism, indecisiveness) are very common in clinical samples of patients who go on to develop OCD.

—More recent research indicates that OCD has biologic origins.

~ Studies show high concordance for OCD among monozygotic twins and increased risk for OCD among first-degree relatives of probands with Gilles de la Tourette's syndrome.

—Brain imaging studies show abnormalities of the left orbital frontal gyri and the caudate nuclei in patients with OCD.

—Clinical studies link OCD with head trauma and other neurologic disorders, which adds to the evidence that OCD may be a manifestation of brain disease.

—Further evidence is shown in the finding that certain antidepressant medications, especially the tricyclic agent clomipramine and agents that inhibit the reuptake of serotonin (e.g., fluoxetine) may dramatically diminish obsessive-compulsive symptoms.

~ The effectiveness of fluoxetine suggests a role for central serotonergic neuronal systems in the pathophysiology of OCD.

Diagnosis (Box 22-9)
Treatment

• In the history and physical examination, look for evidence of medical conditions, medications, or dietary practices that may

---

BOX 22-9

Diagnostic Criteria for Obsessive-Compulsive Disorder

A. Either obsessions or compulsions:
Obsessions as defined by 1, 2, 3, and 4:
1. Recurrent and persistent thoughts, impulses, or images that are experienced at some time during the disturbance as intrusive and inappropriate and cause marked anxiety or distress.
2. The thoughts, impulses, or images are not simply excessive worries about real-life problems.
3. The person attempts to ignore or suppress such thoughts or impulses or to neutralize them with some other thought or action.
4. The person recognizes that the obsessional thoughts, impulses, or images are a product of his or her own mind (not imposed from without as in thought insertion).

Compulsions are defined by 1 and 2:
1. Repetitive behaviors (e.g., handwashing, ordering, checking) or mental acts (e.g., praying, counting, repeating words silently) that the person feels driven to perform in response to an obsession, or according to rules that must be applied rigidly
2. The behaviors or mental acts are aimed at preventing or reducing distress or preventing some dreaded event or situation; however, these behav-

iors or mental acts either are not connected in a realistic way with what they are designed to neutralize or prevent, or are clearly excessive.
B. At some point during the course of the disorder, the person has recognized that the obsessions or compulsions are excessive or unreasonable. Note: This does not apply to children.
C. The obsessions or compulsions cause marked distress, are time-consuming (take more than an hour a day), or significantly interfere with the person's normal routine, occupational functioning, or usual social activities or relationships with others.
D. If another Axis I disorder is present, the content of the obsessions or compulsions is not restricted to it (e.g., preoccupation with food in the presence of an eating disorder, hair pulling in the presence of trichotillomania, concern with appearance in the presence of body dysmorphic disorder, preoccupation with drugs in the presence of a substance use disorder, preoccupation with having a serious illness in the presence of hypochondriasis, or guilty ruminations in the presence of major depressive disorder).
E. Not due to the direct effects of a substance (e.g., drugs of abuse, medication) or a general medical condition.

simulate or exacerbate symptoms of anxiety.

- Consider use of psychosocial therapy.
  —Cognitive-behavioral therapy may be effective as a first-line therapy for every patient willing to participate; this therapy is considered helpful on the fact that compulsions are maintained by their temporary amelioration of conditioned anxiety.
    ~ Patients are taught to control their obsessive ruminations by commanding themselves to stop ruminating when obsessive ideas arise (thought stopping).
    ~ They are strongly encouraged to resist carrying out their compulsive acts to learn that no dire consequences occur with nonexecution of the rituals (response prevention).
  —Consider use of antidepressant medications known to be effective in patients with OCD.
    ~ The tricyclic clomipramine
    ~ The SSRIs fluvoxamine, fluoxetine, and sertraline
    ~ Patients improve while on medication, but symptoms recur when medications are stopped.
  —Consider short-term problem-solving counseling; although this may not achieve total relief, we know that symptomatic exacerbations of OCD occur during times of stress and change; short-term counseling may help to reduce the impact of these influences.
    ~ However, insight-oriented, introspective psychotherapy has generally not been effective in the treatment of OCD.

Prognosis
- By using all therapies that have been proven effective in treating patients with OCD, at least a decrease in the obsessive-compulsive thoughts and behaviors may be achieved.
- Long-term intervals of freedom from obsessive-compulsive thoughts and behaviors are variable among individuals.

Patient/Family Education
- Explain in as much detail as possible the nature, potential causes, course, and treatment available.

- Provide the patient with information relevant to each suggested type of therapy, and obtain their permission for each one in turn that is implemented.
- Ask the patient/family members to keep a log of the patient's symptoms in as much detail as possible, which will help to evaluate the effectiveness of therapy and guide future treatment.

Follow-up/Referral
- Patients with OCD are followed closely for months to years.
- New signs and symptoms are treated as they arise.
- If all therapies have been tried with little change in the patient's OCD symptoms, referral to a psychiatrist who is expert is treating OCD is recommended.

Posttraumatic Stress Disorder

Definition
Posttraumatic stress disorder (PTSD) is a disorder in which an overwhelming traumatic event is experienced, causing intense fear, helplessness, horror, and avoidance of stimuli associated with the trauma. The disorder is characterized by intrusive recollections or dreams of the event and a heightened level of arousal. When these symptoms are present for less than 3 months, a diagnosis of acute PTSD is appropriate. If the symptoms have been present for at least 3 months, the diagnosis of chronic PTSD is made (Box 22-10).

Risk Factors
- Severe physical or emotional trauma in the recent past
- The prevalence in the community is about 1%.
- In American men, the full syndrome is found among Vietnam veterans who were in combat.
- In women, the most common precipitant is physical assault.
- In individuals, symptoms of PTSD occur in about 15% of the population: nightmares, feelings of jitteriness, and sleep disturbance.
- Combat, physical assault, seeing someone seriously hurt or die, or experiencing a serious threat or close call are the most common traumata seen in PTSD.

BOX 22-10

Diagnostic Criteria for Posttraumatic Stress Disorder

A. The person has been exposed to a traumatic event in which both of the following have been present:
   1. The person has experienced, witnessed, or been confronted with an event or events that involve actual or threatened death or serious injury, or a threat to the physical integrity of oneself or others.
   2. The person's response involved intense fear, helplessness, or horror. Note: In children, it may be expressed instead by disorganized or agitated behavior.

B. The traumatic event is persistently reexperienced in at least one of the following ways:
   1. Recurrent and intrusive distressing recollections of the event, including images, thoughts, or perceptions. Note: In young children, repetitive play may occur in which themes or aspects of the trauma are expressed.
   2. Recurrent distressing dreams of the event. Note: In children, there may be frightening dreams without recognized content.
   3. Acting or feeling as if the traumatic event were recurring (includes a sense of reliving the experience, illusions, hallucinations, and dissociative flashback episodes, including those that occur upon awakening or when intoxicated). Note: In young children, trauma-specific reenactment may occur.
   4. Intense psychologic distress at exposure to internal or external cues that symbolize or resemble an aspect of the traumatic event.
   5. Physiologic reactivity on exposure to internal or external cues that symbolize or resemble an aspect of the traumatic event.

C. Persistent avoidance of stimuli associated with the trauma and numbing of general responsiveness (not present before the trauma), as indicated by at least three of the following:
   1. Efforts to avoid thoughts, places, or conversations associated with the trauma.
   2. Efforts to avoid activities, places, or people that arouse recollections of the trauma.
   3. Inability to recall an important aspect of the trauma.
   4. Markedly diminished interest in participation in significant activities.
   5. Feeling of detachment or estrangement from others
   6. Restricted range of affect (e.g., unable to have loving feelings)
   7. Sense of a foreshortened future (e.g., does not expect to have a career, marriage, children, or a normal life span)

D. Persistent symptoms of increased arousal (not present before the trauma), as indicated by at least two of the following:
   1. Difficulty falling or staying asleep
   2. Irritability or outbursts of anger
   3. Difficulty concentrating
   4. Hypervigilance
   5. Exaggerated startle response

E. Duration of the disturbance (symptoms in B, C, and D) is more than 1 month

F. The disturbance causes clinically significant distress or impairment in social, occupational, or other important areas of functioning.

Acute: If duration of symptoms is less than 3 months
Chronic: If duration of symptoms is 3 months or more
With delayed onset: Onset of symptoms at least 6 months after the stressor

Reprinted with permission from the *Diagnostic and statistical manual of mental disorders,* ed 4, text revision, Copyright 2000, American Psychiatric Association.

- Coexistence of another psychiatric disorder (see Etiology/Cause)
- Risk of PTSD is increased in those with a history of childhood behavioral problems (e.g., lying, stealing, truancy, vandalism, school expulsion).

Etiology/Cause

- PTSD usually develops soon after the traumatic event.
- Onset may be delayed in combat veterans and survivors of burn injury.
- Whereas symptoms may persist for years in some patients, about 50% of patients report resolution of symptoms within 6 months of onset.

- Those who develop PTSD are twice as likely as those without PTSD to have another psychiatric disorder (e.g., OCD, dysthymia, substance abuse, bipolar affective disorder, or antisocial personality).
- Explanations of PTSD have been proposed from several perspectives.
  —Behavioral theorists and practitioners state that the posttraumatic symptoms (e.g., hyperarousal, intrusive recollections) are products of classically conditioned linkages between innocuous stimuli (e.g., a news report about a fire) and the original traumatic event (e.g., painful injury in a fire).

—Avoidance symptoms are explained in terms of operant conditioning: avoidance of stimuli reminiscent of the traumatic event is reinforced by its protection of the patient from the symptoms of phobic anxiety (hyperarousal).

—Biologic theorists propose that PTSD is caused by changes in central adrenergic autonomic arousal, and in cerebral mechanisms regulating sleep cycles.

—Personality theorists say that early life experience and personality traits are important, as seen in burn patients and other trauma victims who demonstrate relationships between maladaptive personality traits, early life behavioral problems, and poor posttraumatic adjustment.

Pathogenesis (see Etiology/Cause)
Diagnosis (see Box 22-10)
Treatment
Behavioral Treatment
- Techniques such as desensitization are required to help patients overcome the conditioned avoidance of stimuli that are reminiscent of the traumatic event.

Psychotherapy
- Psychotherapy is virtually always needed to assist patients to deal with anger about the injury, guilt about survival, and similar themes common among those with PTSD.

Pharmacotherapy
- Antidepressant and anxiolytic medications have been used with variable efficacy; tricyclic antidepressants and monoamine oxidase (MAO) inhibitors may be effective in ameliorating hyperarousal, intrusion, and avoidance symptoms, and in relieving concurrent major depression.
- SSRIs, such as fluoxetine, may be effective in ameliorating "numbing," particularly in noncombat trauma victims.
- Benzodiazepines have been used, but there is no empiric evidence for their effectiveness in persons with PTSD, and they are contraindicated for persons who are at high risk for chemical dependency.
- Neuroleptic drugs are essentially never used for persons with PTSD.

Prognosis
- Most people with PTSD resolve the symptoms associated with the disorder within 6 months.
  —Behavioral therapy, psychotherapy, and pharmacotherapy are usually effective in shortening the recovery period, in alleviating symptoms, and in providing long-term relief from the effects of PTSD.
- Time for complete recovery is variable, depending on the severity of the trauma and the individual affected.
- Partial recovery may be a realistic goal for some patients, in whom symptoms are diminished and occur far less frequently than without therapy.

Patient/Family Education
- Instruct the patient (as fully as possible depending on status) and the family regarding the nature of the problem, its cause, course, treatment, and expected outcome.
- Enlist the cooperation of the patient in complying fully with treatment regimen(s) selected by both the patient and the clinician.
- Reassure the patient and family regarding the expected favorable outcome of therapy, within broad time limits.
- Instruct regarding what is meant by complete recovery and partial recovery, and why both are desirable, although perhaps only partial recovery is possible.

Follow-up/Referral
- Patients with PTSD are followed for as long as it takes for either partial or full recovery to be accomplished.
- Referral to a specialist in PTSD may be recommended at any time during treatment, as needed or requested by the patient/family.

Maladaptive Personalities

Concept of Personality
- The enduring attitudes, behaviors, and capacities that distinguish individuals from one another are collectively called personality.
- Two concepts of personality are currently used.
  —Specification and classification of categories of personality in Greek topology was: phlegmatic, melancholic, sanguine,

and choleric; the *DSM-IV* also classifies personality disorders.

—Another concept is to consider personality as a *mosaic of dimensional traits,* each of which is possessed by individuals in differing degrees.

~ Intelligence quotient (IQ)

—Setting rigid guidelines that separate, for example, those who are mentally retarded from those who are not, by specific numbers on a scale, may be misleading and obscure areas of vulnerability that a dimensional approach may bring to light.

~ We use dimensional thinking when we recognize that some people are more meticulous, more argumentative, more gregarious than others.

~ It is useful to recognize that certain persons are more meticulous or introverted than others even when they are not categorically obsessional or schizoid.

- Personality evolves from interactions between constitutional (inborn) factors and the molding influences of the environment.

—Constitutional factors include capacities, such as intelligence, and aspects of temperament, such as sociability and emotionality, all of which may have neurobiologic correlates and genetic determinants.

—The most important environmental influences are interpersonal relationships, usually with parents.

- Many theories of personality have been developed, but none has proved to be fully adequate.

Personality Disorders

- Personality disorders are among the most controversial conditions in psychiatry.
- Most experts accept the fact that some people have enduring patterns of maladaptive attitudes and behaviors that interfere with their ability to work effectively and to develop and sustain gratifying interpersonal relationships.

—Many of these persons are at increased risk for long-term social impairment and for many major psychiatric illnesses.

- The controversy refers to how best to conceptualize and subdivide these disorders; several possible conceptualizations and subdivisions exist.

—The dominant approach in the United States is that adopted by the American Psychiatric Association in their *DSM-IV,* the most current (as of this writing); this approach is prototypical and categorical.

~ The diagnostic criteria for the personality disorders are lists of attitudes and behaviors (e.g., self-dramatizing, attention seeking) which in combination evoke an ideal prototype (e.g., the histrionic personality).

~ Only a person exhibiting the requisite number of such attitudes and behaviors (at least four, in the case of histrionic personality) is said to have the condition; personality disorder is rare when defined in this way.

~ The *DSM-IV* classifies personality disorders into 10 types, and groups them under three clusters: the dramatic (histrionic, borderline, narcissistic, and antisocial types); the anxious or fearful (obsessive-compulsive, dependent, and avoidant types); and the odd or eccentric (schizoid, schizotypal, and paranoid types).

—Maladaptive personalities can also be conceptualized in terms of quantitative deviations from normal along specific personality dimensions.

~ Many important personality traits may be viewed dimensionally: people may be high or low in obsessionality, dependency, or self-importance.

~ Excesses likely lead to special vulnerabilities (e.g., excessive obsessionality may lead to great distress in circumstances that require flexibility and emotional spontaneity; poor self-esteem may predispose one to demoralization in response to criticism from a superior)

—A third conceptualization of personality disorders is one in which disorders are viewed as incomplete or atypical expressions of schizophrenia, mood disorders, or other major psychiatric illnesses.

- It is clear, from descriptions of the categorical disorders that follow, that many of the personality disorders may be viewed as manifestations of extreme positions on dimensions of personality such as emotionality, narcissism, trust, social ability, self-esteem, and assertiveness.

—It can also be seen that the types within each cluster tend to share traits and vulnerabilities and also share implications for treatment.

—A few disorders are linked to major psychiatric illnesses; it is important to emphasize that a patient with clinically obvious disturbances involving dimensions of personality may meet criteria for several *DSM-IV* personality disorders or may meet criteria for none.

Treatment of Personality Disorders

- Several points are useful to keep in mind when treating personality-disordered patients of any subtype.

  —Many maladaptive trait(s) are of long standing and deeply ingrained, so that it is doubtful that they will change in response to the clinician's efforts.

    ~ The approach is to recognize these sources of vulnerability, take them into account when interacting with the patient, and minimize their adverse impact on medical care.

  —Patients often become angry or depressed when their maladaptive traits are pointed out, and either of these responses defeats the practitioner's purposes; it is often important to call patients' attention to ways in which they are undermining their medical care.

    ~ When such action is necessary, it is most helpful to refer to specific behaviors rather than to general aspects of personality, and to present one's observations plainly but compassionately, and without criticism (e.g., "It is difficult for us to provide you with care that you need when you curse at us and criticize every effort we make. I need to ask you to stop behaving in this way.").

  —Counseling by the general practitioner, if undertaken at all, is best symptom-focused and short-term.

  —For long-term treatment, patients with seriously disturbed personalities are referred to a mental health professional.

Descriptions of Personality Types within Clusters

Dramatic Cluster

- Most patients in this group with disturbances usually are on extreme ends of emotionality and narcissism.

  —Symptoms are impulsiveness, self-absorption, and aggressive or self-destructive behaviors. They lack empathy for others and have either unrealistically high or low self-concepts. They are demanding and their relationships are unstable, tempestuous, and exploitive.

Histrionic personality

- Patients with histrionic personalities demonstrate excessive emotionality, self-dramatization, and attention-seeking behaviors.

  —Diagnostic criteria for this category of disorders include self-centered, unusually eager for approval and praise, overly concerned with physical beauty, often inappropriately sexually seductive or flattering (e.g., "Of all the nurses I've had, you are the first to really listen to me").

  —They speak as though on stage, are impressionistic, and factually imprecise; their expression of emotions is usually exaggerated, shifts rapidly, and is openly shallow. They may be frequently seductive with the male clinician and present with complaints that are dramatically expressed but vague in relevance to any medical problem. These patients often develop somatic disorders.

Narcissistic personality

- Patients with narcissistic personality are characterized by an exaggerated sense of self-importance, intolerance of criticism, and insensitivity to the needs of others. They often exploit others for their own needs, require constant admiration and attention, believe themselves entitled to special treatment, and envy those who are more successful, attractive, intelligent, or otherwise esteemed.

  —Most of these patients are difficult to care for because they believe that their problems are unique and solvable only by the very best clinicians. They frequently challenge the clinician's knowledge, skills, and judgment. They fully expect that scheduling of tests and appointments will be made at their convenience.

Borderline personality

- Patients with borderline personalities are characterized by extreme instability—their mood, interpersonal relationships, and self-regard
  - —Recent data indicate a link between borderline personalities and depressive disorders.
  - —Substance abuse, sexual impulsiveness, poor self-esteem, self-mutilation, recurrent suicidal threats that are usually manipulative attempts, with brief periods of deep depression and rage superimposed on chronic feelings of emptiness or boredom are typically seen in these patients.
  - —They tend to view others as all good or all bad and to react to them with extremes of idealization and devaluation, which creates difficulty in all interpersonal relationships, including those with clinicians and therapists, whom they see as either good or bad and thus pit them against one another (staff splitting).

Antisocial personality

- Patients with antisocial personalities are characterized by a chronic and pervasive pattern of irresponsible and socially unacceptable behavior: truancy, vandalism, fire setting, lying, and theft during childhood precede the move toward impulsiveness, recklessness, aggressiveness, sexual promiscuity, financial irresponsibility, and outright criminal acts in adulthood. Although continually complaining of being mistreated, they openly exploit others. In medical settings, they may be malingerers, feigning disease for personal gain. In dealings with medical professionals, they are either demanding and abusive or flattering and ingratiating, whichever they believe is most expedient at the moment.

Treatment of dramatic subtypes

- In treating these patients, the clinician should expect extremes of emotions and pressure to provide emotional and material favors along with excellent medical care.
- The health care professional must maintain dignity and equanimity in facing these extremes, to avoid being defensive when challenged, and to provide special attention within professional limits.
- Socializing or becoming familiar with histrionic or borderline patients is especially high-risk for being exploited.
- It is often necessary to point out, firmly but nonpunitively, the limits of acceptable behavior with professional staff.
- Limits are particularly needed by narcissistic and antisocial patients.

Anxious or Fearful Cluster

- Patients with personality disturbances in this group are usually self-doubting, timid, and tense, lack self-confidence, and have a tendency to avoid making decisions, preferring to have others decide and do things for them, but they tend to be dissatisfied and critical of others. They are socially unassertive, and submit to the wishes of others and even avoid friendships for fear of ultimate rejection. Anxiety levels are persistently high.

Avoidant personality

- Patients with avoidant personalities crave social contact but avoid it because of intense social discomfort related to expectations of criticism and rejection; they frequently complain of being lonely but are too shy to make the social contacts needed to overcome the problem unless they are certain to be accepted; major depression and social phobia are commonly associated with these personality types.
- Knowing that physicians are usually accepting of their patients, the avoidant person usually feels quite comfortable in the presence of their clinicians, and often develops symptoms that will justify regular visits to alleviate their loneliness.

Dependent personality

- Patients with dependent personalities lack self-confidence and go to great lengths to ensure the availability of others on whom they can depend for advice and reassurance.
- Because they feel uneasy and helpless when alone, they may put up with abuse, or perform unpleasant or demeaning tasks to preserve the dependent relationship.
- They are exceedingly sensitive to criticism and abandonment.

- This type of person may become very dependent on their physicians, especially when other relationships are unsatisfactory, and may use vague, chronic complaints as a means of staying in close touch, particularly during periods of unusual stress.
- Some dependent persons will become ill just before the physician is scheduled to be away from the office for a time.

Obsessive-compulsive personality

- Patients with obsessive-compulsive personalities are rigid, parsimonious, morally scrupulous, and emotionally restricted.
- They are exceedingly committed to work, are reluctant to delegate duties, convinced that no one else can do things correctly, but they are often indecisive and sometimes become ineffective because of their perfectionism and preoccupation with trivial details.
- They describe upsetting emotional experiences in a cool, detached manner (isolation of affect).
- When ill, they often present the physician with very detailed descriptions of symptoms, request lengthy descriptions of their condition, and require precise instructions about medications and their potential side effects.
- They are aware of hospital routines and rules, and are intolerant of lateness and inefficiency.
- Those with obsessive-compulsive personalities are prone to develop hypochondriasis and OCD.

Passive-aggressive personality

- Passive-aggressive personality type is not listed in *DSM-IV*, but requires description because of its potential impact on providing medical care.
- This type of person does not want to meet the expectations of others, nor to be held responsible for this decision.
- Therefore they do not say no directly but express hostile inefficiency and pretend forgetfulness.
- Usually dependent and lacking in self-confidence, they seek advice from others, but often resist following the advice given.
- In seeking medical care, they earnestly promise to follow treatment recommendations, but then forget to keep a symptom log

that was requested by the clinician, to assess the effectiveness of a new drug, or to go to the laboratory for an essential blood test.

Treatment of anxious subtypes

- Managing dependency is a major component because these patients tend to develop attachments to their physicians.
- The practitioner may have to allow patients to be excessively dependent within set limits, particularly during times of increased stress for the patient.
- Make short, regular appointments so that new symptoms cannot be the reason for seeing the physician, and advise them to call on a weekly basis, for an update on their status may be helpful to them and prevent emergency calls at inconvenient times.
- These patients require advanced notice of vacations and will benefit from meeting the covering physician ahead of time.
- In some cases, treatment of general anxiety disorder, phobias, and major depression may be indicated.

Odd or Eccentric Cluster

- Patients under this category take extreme positions on the dimensions of sociability and trust; they are usually highly suspicious and tend to isolate themselves from other people because of anxious mistrust, awkwardness, or indifference.

Paranoid personality

- Patients with paranoid personalities are prone to perceive threats and insults at every turn.
- In expecting to be exploited or harmed by others, they hear veiled threats in the most innocuous remarks and readily question the loyalty of friends and the fidelity of spouses.
- They are guarded, easily slighted, defensive, and unforgiving; although their suspiciousness does not carry the intensity or conviction of a true delusion, schizophrenia and delusional disorders are common in their family histories.
- When receiving care, they are reluctant to give a complete history, especially a social history. "What does this have to do with my medical problem?" is a frequently heard reaction, and they may not agree to undergo laboratory tests ("You doctors are all trying to make money off me").

Schizotypal personality

- Patients with schizotypal personalities exhibit odd behavior, have peculiar beliefs, and suffer social isolation as a result of their own social anxiety and the impact of their beliefs and behavior on others.
- Their affect is often constricted, their talk vague and digressive, and their appearance unkempt.
- They are suspicious and superstitious; those with this disorder are usually severely impaired, often meeting criteria for other personality disorders simultaneously.
- There are family links with schizophrenia and some experts contend that this disorder should be classified as a variant of schizophrenia rather than a personality disorder.
- In giving a history, these patients may present unusual symptoms (e.g., feelings of electricity in their scalp), and odd theories of illness cause (e.g., "Could my neighbors be doing this to me?").

Schizoid personality

- The central features of patients with schizoid personalities are indifference to the company of others and constricted emotionality.
- They are loners who seldom marry, prefer solitary activities, and appear cold and aloof.
- Despite its name, this disorder does not seem to be linked with schizophrenia; schizoid people tend to shun contact with physicians and may appear very uncomfortable when hospitalization places them in close and constant contact with others.

Treatment of eccentric subtypes

- The most important principle of treating these patients is to work gradually toward establishing rapport by meticulous honesty, composure in the face of patients' suspiciousness and reserve, and a consistent demonstration of sincere concern for their well-being and respect for their privacy.

Adjustment (Mood) Disorders

Definition

Affective (mood) disorders (now known as adjustment disorders) are a group of heterogeneous, typically recurrent illnesses, including unipolar (depressive) and bipolar (manic-depressive) disorders that are characterized by pervasive mood disturbances, psychomotor dysfunction, and vegetative symptoms.

Impact of Adjustment Disorders on Public Health

- Depressive conditions are major public health problems.
  - In a medical outcome study of community-dwelling people, the *poor functioning uniquely associated with depressive symptoms* was comparable to or worse than that uniquely associated with **nine** major chronic medical conditions: arthritis, advanced coronary artery disease, recent myocardial infarction, angina, back problems, severe lung problems, inflammatory bowel disease, diabetes, and hypertension.
  - High death rate in depressive disorders is usually related to suicide (15% of this population); suicide is the ninth leading cause of death in the United States; among persons age 19 to 24, suicide is the third leading cause of death; 50% to 75% of suicides (30,000/year) occur in people with depressive disorders.
  - Substance abuse is considered to be a major factor in the recent increase in adolescent suicide rates, which doubled between 1960 and 1980 in white males.
  - Other recent research data show that the incidence and outcome of other medical disorders are adversely affected by depression.
    - ~ The incidence of myocardial infarction is increased fourfold in those with a prior episode of major depression.
    - ~ The risk of dying within 18 months of having a myocardial infarction is three times greater in patients with concurrent depression than in those with no depression.
  - In terms of economics, a recent, systematic study estimated that the annual cost of depressive disorders in the U.S. economy was $44 billion, in contrast to the annual cost of stroke ($18 billion).

Dying, Death, and Bereavement

Sociopsychologic Issues

- Humans are the only creatures known who bury their dead, and have done so from the beginning of time on earth for humans.

- Before the 11th century CE, death was calmly accepted, without fear.
- Then the concept of the last judgment began to be taken seriously.
  - Awe and fear of death became manifest in art and culture.
  - Images of hell, purgatory, and heaven preoccupied the minds of medieval people, and continue to exert its influence on a significant segment of society now.
- Even though we know that death is inevitable for all of us, many people cannot face the thought of their own death.
- Fear of dying should not be confused with fear of death.
  - Fear of dying is really a combination of fear of death and fear of living in dread of death.
- Whether at home, surrounded by loved ones, or in a hospital with myriad machines, lights, and noise, the thought of dying is not welcome to anyone.
- A dying person often continues to hope for a miraculous recovery, but after periods of failed treatments, an overwhelming sense of helplessness falls over the patient.
  - Often, there is self-blame for not having taken better care of oneself, and guilt about one's conduct may cause the patient to see terminal illness as punishment.
  - Fears of drastic treatment, chemotherapy, or surgery, combined with fears of a crippled existence and being left alone to die in isolation away from family, friends, and children, are in the mind of many people who are nearing death.

Emotional Reactions in the Face of Death

- The stages of grief that are felt by dying patients in facing the reality of their impending death consist of the following:
  - Shock and denial
  - Anger
  - Bargaining
  - Depression
  - Acceptance
- If the death of a loved one has been unexpected, grief usually begins with an initial stage of shock and disbelief accompanied by a general numbing of all affect.

- If death has been anticipated, this stage is less prominent.
  - There is often a feeling of relief that the dead person's suffering has ended.
- Within hours to days, there is a more demonstrative phase characterized by protest and anguish, often accompanied by tears.
  - These feelings come in waves and may be precipitated by even an indirect reference to the lost person; these feelings rarely last longer than 1 to 2 months.
- Other symptoms of mourning normally occur throughout the first year after the death.
- During this period, survivors are continuing to grieve while they reorient their lives.
- As time passes, there is often a preoccupation with memories of the lost person.
- Guilt feelings for not having done enough for the deceased are very common.
- About 80% of bereaved people are depressed and have disturbed sleep.
- *New research being conducted at the National Institutes of Health (NIH) regarding surviving spouses may show data that refute this percentage of depression in this population.*
- About 40% have a poor appetite, weight loss, difficulty in concentrating, and general loss of interest in daily life.
- Depression is particularly common in spouses in the middle or later years of their lives; about 33% have symptoms that meet the criteria for major depression.
  - Although depression may last for many months, about 80% of persons show improvement within 10 weeks.
  - Two thirds of bereaved spouses at the end of the first year of bereavement continue to have some symptoms of apathy, aimlessness, and a disinclination to look to the future.

Management of Normal Grief During the First Year

- Management is individualized, depending on the patient's personal, family, and social background.
- All bereaved people need to be reminded that their grief and its psychophysiologic concomitants are normal.

- This reassurance must be given with care by acknowledging the irreparable loss while encouraging them to lead a full life without feeling guilty.
- Some patients may experience physical symptoms or exaggeration of preexisting symptoms.
- In time, with the completion of their grieving reaction, these patients stop having physical symptoms and again become active participants in a new life.
- The clinician can support the bereaved patient by writing a note of sympathy, visiting the funeral parlor or gravesite, and responding to questions about the person's death posed by the survivor(s).
- Special attention is usually needed at holidays of special significance, anniversaries, and the birthday of the dead person.
- The nurse practitioner is often the one to recognize signs of pathologic mourning such as social isolation, immoderate feelings of guilt or anger, panic attacks, and other symptoms that indicate the need for help.
- Providing consistent, thoughtful support is often the best kind of therapy needed by bereaved persons.

Diagnosis (Box 22-11)

Signs and Symptoms
- Most patients who seek medical attention do not complain of depressed mood as a primary symptom.
- If patients acknowledge depressed feelings, it is in relation to other complaints, which they see as primary.
- Three complaints are most common.
  - Many somatic symptoms: vegetative symptoms of depression: loss of energy, inability to concentrate, poor sleep, poor appetite, weight loss, and decreased motivation or interests.
    - ~ Includes autonomic anxiety symptoms: tachycardia, chest discomfort, and lightheadedness.
  - Aches and pains that may have musculoskeletal basis but are out of proportion to what the patient usually experiences (e.g., worsening of migraine, irritable bowel, and back pains).

BOX 22-11
Diagnostic Criteria for Adjustment Disorder

A. The development of emotional or behavioral symptoms in response to an identifiable stressor occurring within 3 months of the onset of the disorder
B. These symptoms or behaviors are clinically significant as evidenced by either of the following:
   1. Marked distress that is in excess of what would be expected from exposure to the stressor
   2. Significant impairment in social or occupational (academic) functioning
C. The stress-related disturbance does not meet the criteria for any specific Axis I disorders and is not merely an exacerbation of a preexisting Axis I or Axis II disorder
D. Does not represent bereavement
E. The symptoms do not persist for more than 6 months after the termination of the stressor (or its consequences).
Acute: If the symptoms have persisted for less than 6 months
Chronic: If the symptoms have persisted for 6 months or longer

Reprinted with permission from the *Diagnostic and statistical manual of mental disorders*, ed 4, text revision, Copyright 2000, American Psychiatric Association.

  - Nervous complaints (e.g., increased tension and feelings of anxiety).
- Coexistence of psychiatric and medical disorders is the rule rather than the exception, so complaints of any nature must be evaluated carefully.
- *Atypical depression* refers to major depression or dysthymic states in which hypersomnia, overeating, and psychomotor agitation occur.
  - These patients seem to be predisposed to panic-type anxiety symptoms.
  - Patients with atypical depression have the characteristic depressive changes in self-attitude and vital sense but describe their mood more as a fatigued feeling than as sadness.
- In evaluating patients with adjustment disorder, the clinician should ask family members to corroborate and augment the information given by the patient.
- With the patient's consent, the clinician should share with the family the diagnostic assessment, plans for treatment, and the prognosis because the depressed patient usually does not remember what he or she

and the clinician have discussed, and may interpret everything too negatively.

Patient/Family Education

- The clinician should instruct the patient and family regarding the nature, usual course, treatment, and expected outcome in as much detail as feasible and within the capacity of each family member.
- In treating patients with depression of any degree, it is of benefit to encourage the cooperation and participation of the family in assisting the patient to full recovery.

Follow-up/Referral

- Most patients, with short-term counseling and the full support of their family, recover from depression within 6 months.
- If, with counseling and perhaps antidepressant medication as a trial, the patient does not respond, referral to a psychiatrist whose specialty is adjustment disorders is recommended.

Dysthymic Disorder

Definition

Dysthymia is a chronic (lasting 2 years or more) depressive state in which the number of depressive symptoms experienced is fewer than what is required for the diagnosis of major depressive disorder (see Boxes 22-9 and 22-11).

Risk Factors

- Previous history of depression
- Identifiable related stressor before the onset of symptoms

Etiology/Cause (see also Risk Factors)

- The cause of dysthymia is unknown.
- The depressive symptoms typically begin insidiously in childhood or adolescence and follow an intermittent, low-grade course over many years or even decades.

Pathogenesis

- No physiologic basis for dysthymia has been identified.
- Personality disorder may be at the root of dysthymia, although this link has not been established other than the chronicity of the disorder and its persistence.

Diagnosis (Box 22-12)
Signs and symptoms

- Patients with dysthymia usually have the characteristic sustained changes in self-attitude and vital sense seen with major depression.

BOX 22-12

Diagnostic Criteria for Dysthymic Disorder

A. Depressed mood for most of the day, for more days than not, as indicated either by subjective account or observation made by others, for at least 2 years

B. Presence, while depressed, of at least three of the following:
1. Low self-esteem or self-confidence, or feelings of inadequacy
2. Feelings of pessimism, despair, or hopelessness
3. Generalized loss of interest or pleasure
4. Social withdrawal
5. Chronic fatigue or tiredness
6. Feelings of guilt, brooding about the past
7. Subjective feelings of irritability or excessive anger
8. Decreased activity, effectiveness, or productivity
9. Difficulty in thinking reflected by poor concentration, poor memory, or indecisiveness

C. During the 2-year period of the disturbance, the person has never been without the symptoms in A and B for more than 2 months at a time

D. No major depressive episode during the first 2 years of the disturbance, that is, not better accounted for by chronic major depressive disorder or major depressive disorder in partial remission.

E. Has never had a manic episode, or an unequivocal hypomanic episode

F. Does not occur exclusively during the course of a chronic psychiatric disorder such as schizophrenia or delusional disorder

G. Not due to the direct effects of a substance (e.g., drugs of abuse, medication), or a general medical condition (e.g., hypothyroidism)

Reprinted with permission from the *Diagnostic and statistical manual of mental disorders*, ed 4, text revision, Copyright 2000, American Psychiatric Association.

- In pure dysthymia, depressive manifestations occur at a subthreshold level and overlap considerably with those of a depressive temperament.
  —Habitually gloomy
  —Pessimistic
  —Humorless
  —Incapable of fun
  —Skeptical
  —Passive, lethargic
  —Introverted
  —Self-critical, self-reproaching, self-derogatory
  —Preoccupied with inadequacy, failure, and negative events

Treatment

- Recent studies show greater similarities between patients with dysthymia and those with major depression, and treatment for both is the same.
- Several SSRIs and tricyclic antidepressants are effective in reducing depressive symptoms.
- Brief psychotherapies are also beneficial for most patients.
- The primary difference in treatment for the two types of depression is the increased rate of comorbid problems in behavior, personality, and life problems associated with the more chronic form of depression (dysthymia).
  —Recognizing that depression plays an important part in their life problems can be helpful for dysthymic patients.

Prognosis

- Although patients with chronic forms of depression (dysthymia) may never fully recover to the point of not having symptoms, the frequency and severity of symptoms can be controlled and enable them to live a more normal life, with more appropriate self-attitudes.

Patient/Family Education

- Patients should be instructed regarding the impact of their depressive mood on all aspects of their life: work, personal image, and relationships with others.
- Psychotherapy and counseling may help, over time, to help dysthymic patients to adopt a more positive attitude about themselves, about those around them, and about life in general.
- Group therapy may prove beneficial after a relatively long period of individual counseling, which allows them time to accommodate new behaviors and attitudes into their repertoire of thinking and acting.
  —Hearing other patients' stories about the impact that negative thinking has had on their ability to function at an optimal level may help individuals to focus on more positive habits, and increase their self-worth.

Follow-up/Referral

- The chronicity of dysthymia is a challenge to the most adept counselor/therapist; to overcome years of negativity and provide the incentive and motivation for people to change their lifelong attitudes requires time and patience, which may be completely lost.
- However, the effort is usually of value in many respects, both in teaching the therapist more about managing dysthymic patients and in helping the patients to better cope with their condition and to be more satisfied with their efforts.

Major Adjustment Disorders

Manic Depressive Disorder

Definition

Mania and major depression are the two syndromes that give the traditional name *manic depressive disorder* to this group of disorders. These disorders are characteristically episodic, with complete remissions between episodes. Most patients suffer only recurrent depressive episodes (the *unipolar group*). Few suffer only manic episodes (they are grouped with patients with bipolar disorder). The remainder suffer from both manic and depressive episodes (the *bipolar group*).

Risk Factors

- Family history of bipolar disorders
- Females are affected by depression about twice as often as men.
- Bipolar disorder occurs in only about 0.6% to 1.2% of adults and is equally common

---

BOX 22-13

Possible Etiologic Factors in Adjustment Disorders

BIOLOGIC
Genetic
10% to 15% of first-degree relatives have an affective disorder (risk in community: 1% to 2%).
Monozygotic twins reared together or apart are concordant for manic-depressive disorder.
23% of dizygotic twins are concordant for manic-depressive disorder; possible links with genetic markers.
Biochemical
Imbalance in neurotransmitters (e.g., monoamine neurotransmitters are depleted in depression, but increased in mania).
Loss of diurnal rhythm of plasma cortisol in depression
Hormonal factors (e.g., depression is common after childbirth, in premenstrual phase, use of oral contraceptives, menopause, and posthysterectomy)
Electrolytes: intracellular sodium is high in affective disorders

PSYCHOLOGIC
Maternal Deprivation
Psychoanalysis suggests that the loss of maternal affection in early life or early childhood predisposes persons to affective disorder later in life (68%).

Learned Helplessness
Experimental animals put in a position where they cannot escape or control punishing stimuli develop a behavioral syndrome that resembles depression in humans; it is suggested that a similar mechanism is at work in humans.

SOCIAL
Stressful Events
An excess of life events is found in the months before the onset of depression.
Includes bereavement, loss of job, moving, marriage, going on vacation
Vulnerability Factors
In women, it has been claimed that certain factors render them vulnerable to becoming depressed. Include lack of a job outside the home, presence of three or more young children in the family, and lack of a confiding, intimate relationship.

From Clare AW: Psychological medicine: mood (affective) disorders. In Kumar P, Clark M, eds: *Clinical medicine,* ed 4, Edinburgh, 1998, WB Saunders, p 1123.

---

in men and women, with the first manic episode occurring before age 30.

Etiology/Cause (Box 22-13)

Major Depressive Disorder
Definition
Major depressive disorder is a disorder of mood characterized by a persistent dysphoric mood, anxiety, irritability, fear, brooding, appetite and sleep disturbances, weight loss, psychomotor agitation or retardation, decreased energy, feelings of worthlessness or guilt, difficulty in concentrating or thinking, possible delusions and hallucinations, and thoughts of death or suicide. The most common form of clinical depression is major depressive disorder. Most depressed people visit a health care facility during the depressive episode but only about 30% are diagnosed and given treatment for depression.

Risk Factors
- Family history of depressive disorder (or bipolar disorder)
- Previous history of depression
- Recent (within 2 months) stressful life event
- History of alcohol or drug abuse

Etiology/Cause (Box 22-14, see Box 22-11)
- The precise cause of most types of depressive disorders is unknown.
- Experts tend to agree that the disorder is caused by multiple factors: genetic, biologic, psychologic, social, cultural, and interpersonal.

Pathogenesis (see Definition)
Diagnosis (Box 22-15)
Differential diagnosis
- The differential diagnosis of symptoms that indicate major depression varies, depending on age, patient's presenting manifestation, and other associated factors.
- In older patients with complaints of memory deficits, the diagnosis is complex because memory complaints without substantial memory performance problems are common.

BOX 22-14

Drugs and Substances that May Cause or Precipitate Mood Disorder

DEPRESSED STATES
Alcohol
Amphetamine or cocaine withdrawal
Antihypertensive drugs (clonidine, methyldopa, reserpine, (β-blockers)
Benzodiazepines
Cyclosporine
Dapsone
Glucocorticoids
Interferon
Oral contraceptives

HYPOMANIC OR MANIC STATES
Antidepressants (all classes)
Bromocriptine
Cyclobenzaprine
Cyclosporine
L-Dopa
Glucocorticoids
Interferon
Metoclopramide
Quinacrine hydrochloride
Stimulant drugs (amphetamine, cocaine, phencyclidine)
Thyroid hormones
Zidovudine

From Drugs that cause psychiatric symptoms, *Medical Letter: Drugs and Therapy* 35:65, 1993.

- A mild, reversible dementia can result from the depression alone (so-called pseudo-dementia).
- Also, depression and dementia syndromes can be related to underlying neuropathologic disorders (e.g., Parkinson's disease, stroke).
- In younger patients, it is important to distinguish major depression from schizophrenia, especially when hallucinations or delusions are part of the presenting picture.
  - —In younger patients, when there are no symptoms of schizophrenia, the differentiation is between adjustment disorder and major depression in those with recent onset of symptoms, and between adjustment disorder and dysthymia in those with a longer history of symptoms.
- Stressful life events are common triggers of major depressions, but their presence is not useful for making or excluding the diagnosis.

BOX 22-15

Diagnostic Criteria for Major Depressive Episodes

A. At least five of the following symptoms have been present during the same 2-week period and represent a change from previous functioning; at least one of the symptoms is either (1) depressed mood or (2) loss of interest or pleasure.
  1. Depressed mood most of the day, nearly every day, as indicated by either subjective report (e.g., feels sad or empty) or observation made by others (e.g., appears tearful)
  2. Marked diminished interest or pleasure in all, or almost all, activities most of the day, nearly every day (as indicated either by subjective account or observation made by others)
  3. Significant weight loss or weight gain when not dieting (e.g., more than 5% of body weight in a month), or decrease or increase in appetite nearly every day
  4. Insomnia or hypersomnia nearly every day
  5. Psychomotor agitation or retardation nearly every day (observable by others, not merely subjective feelings of restlessness or being slowed down)
  6. Fatigue or loss of energy nearly every day
  7. Feelings of worthlessness or excessive or inappropriate guilt (which may be delusional) nearly every day (not merely self-reproach or guilt about being sick)
  8. Diminished ability to think or concentrate, or indecisiveness, nearly every day (either by subjective account or as observed by others)
  9. Recurrent thoughts of death (not just fear of dying), recurrent suicidal ideation without a specific plan, or a suicide attempt or a specific plan for committing suicide
B. The symptoms cause clinically significant distress or impairment in social, occupational, or other important areas of functioning.
C. Not due to the direct effects of a substance (e.g., drugs of abuse, medication) or a general medical condition (e.g., hypothyroidism)
D. Not occurring within 2 months of the loss of a loved one (except if associated with marked functional impairment, psychotic symptoms, or psychomotor retardation).

Reprinted with permission from the *Diagnostic and statistical manual of mental disorders*, ed 4, text revision, Copyright 2000, American Psychiatric Association.

- In patients with panic attacks or obsessive-compulsive symptoms, it is important to remember that both of these may occur in the context of a major depressive syndrome.
- All depressed patients should be screened for alcoholism and checked for use of other

substances or medications that can cause or exacerbate symptoms of depression.

Treatment

- Antidepressants
  - The mechanism of therapeutic action of antidepressants is unknown.
  - Indirect evidence indicates that they exert their therapeutic effects by enhancing catecholaminergic and serotonergic neurotransmission, but this is not known for certain.
  - Antidepressant medication is the appropriate initial treatment for patients who are in good physical condition, who are not overwhelmed with depressive delusions, and who are not suicidal.
- Any of these drugs is effective in 70% of cases.
  - Patients who do not respond to an antidepressant from one class often respond to one from a different class.
  - Patients with depression with associated delusions, hallucinations, and profound psychomotor retardation are generally less responsive to drugs than those without these manifestations.
- No antidepressant medication has been shown to be more effective than others.
- Depressed patients tolerate side effects (or perceived side effects) poorly and often stop medication without completing the full 8-week trial.
  - The choice of antidepressant therefore is related more to convenience of scheduling and side effects than to the likelihood of a favorable response.
- In patients with expressed suicidal intent, antidepressants, particularly tricyclics, should be prescribed with extreme caution, in small amounts, to prevent a lethal overdose.

Characteristics of antidepressants

- Tricyclic antidepressants (TCAs) are the oldest class and are listed in two subgroups: secondary and tertiary amines.
- The MAO inhibitors are not listed and are rarely used today, even by psychiatrists specializing in the treatment of depression.
- There are five SSRIs.
  - Fluoxetine (Prozac)
  - Fluvoxamine (Luvox) ⎫ these two are more
  - Paroxetine (Paxil) ⎬ sedating than the other two
  - Sertraline (Zoloft)
  - Citalopram (Celexa)
  - A newer antidepressant, *nefazodone* (Serzone), is less sedating than its older relative, *trazodone* (Desyrel).
- *Bupropion* (Wellbutrin) is an antidepressant of the aminoketone class, unrelated to the tricyclic and SSRI antidepressants but related to the phenylethylamines.
  - It inhibits serotonin, norepinephrine, and dopamine reuptake.
  - A serious side effect is seizures, which occur in 0.4% of patients taking 450 mg/day, the total recommended dosage, with 150 mg as the largest single dose, and single doses separated by at least 4 hours.
  - This is only slightly more than the rate of seizures associated with tricyclics.
- *Venlafaxine* (Effexor) is a newer antidepressant of the phenylethylamine class, given in dosages of 150 to 300 mg/day.
  - Diastolic hypertension may occur in a small number of patients, so monitoring of BP for 2 weeks after any increase in dosage is recommended.
- *Mirtazapine* (Remeron) is a new antidepressant with limited use in the United States.
  - It is associated with significant sedation and has a half-life long enough to allow bedtime dosing.
  - A less common but serious side effect is granulocytopenia.
- Nutritional supplements and herbs are commercially available, which patients ask about and many prefer these to the pharmaceutical drugs.
  - St. John's wort is frequently advertised as being a "natural antidepressant."
  - Several studies indicate that it has antidepressant properties, but further investigation is needed to make comparisons of its effectiveness against that of antidepressant drugs.
- The SSRIs have become the drugs of first choice for depressed patients, because of few side effects and ease of use.

—Their cost is a prohibitive factor: they cost between $1.50 and $2.00/day, whereas the oldest tricyclic antidepressant, imipramine, costs about $0.05/day.

- In otherwise healthy patients who have depression, treatment can reasonably begin with either *fluoxetine* or *paroxetine,* which can be administered at a daily dose of 20 mg and requires no titration.
- Most antidepressant drugs are started at a low dose, then increased to the next highest dose (e.g., from 25 to 50 mg) every week or every 2 weeks until the patient is responding well.
  —Most older patients are started at half the usual starting dose of antidepressants.

Side effects of antidepressants

- Most antidepressants have common side effects.
  —SSRIs cause transient mild nausea, transient insomnia, and transient nervousness and muscular irritability.
  —All SSRIs cause *sexual dysfunction* in about 20% of patients: delayed orgasm, decreased interest, and erectile dysfunction may occur.
- Side effects of tricyclics are anticholinergic: dry mouth, constipation, delayed micturition, blurred vision, and an anticholinergic delirium.
  —The effects on sexual function in this class of drugs are just as prominent as in the SSRIs, usually related to erectile dysfunction.
  —Tricyclics also have *cardiac side effects* and should be prescribed with caution in patients with preexisting conduction abnormalities or any unstable cardiac condition (e.g., recent myocardial infarction [MI]).
  —Nortriptyline has been studied in cardiac patients and can be given to patients with preexisting stable heart disease.
- Bupropion is contraindicated in patients with seizure disorders.
- The most concern regarding the use of MAO inhibitors is acute hypertension caused by foods containing the sympathomimetic agent tyramine: cheeses, wines, beers, broad bean pods, and some drugs.
  —More common adverse reactions are headaches, hypotension, and nausea.

Duration of drug therapy

- For most patients with depression, the minimum length of treatment is a 2-month trial period.
- If the drug is effective and well tolerated, treatment should continue for at least a year, the time when relapse most frequently occurs.
  —It is not recommended that patients be told that the duration of treatment is "for the rest of your life," or "for an indefinite period," which conveys a sense of pessimism.
  —Most patients who have a history of episodes and relapses should continue therapy for several years.
  —The use of a lower dosage of the effective medication as prophylaxis is not recommended; patients on half the usual dose have no better outcome than patients on placebo, according to published data.
- When an antidepressant drug is stopped, regardless of the reason, the patient should be warned that withdrawal symptoms may occur: nausea, dizziness, headache, and increased perspiration and salivation.

Patient/Family Education

- The nurse practitioner and consulting psychiatrist should lay out the plan of treatment at the outset, when the diagnosis of major depressive disorder is made.
  —The length of treatment, use of trial periods to find the most effective drug, counseling, scheduling of appointments, probable length of treatment, and expected outcome
- The patient is usually so eager to be free of depressive symptoms that he is willing to try anything.
- The development of a trusting relationship must be established as soon as possible in the course of therapy.

Follow-up/Referral

- At the beginning, patients are seen every other week for 6 to 8 weeks, for monitoring medication and for short-term counseling.
- Consistent answers to three common questions that depressed patients ask are necessary.
  —"What is wrong with me?"
  —"Is the treatment going to work?"
  —"What will happen if it doesn't work?"

- The answer to all three questions is: "You have clinical depression, We don't understand how it is caused but it is not your fault. It is a medical disease. You will get better. We are going to continue to care for you and fight the depression with you until you are better."
    —This response is important for both the patient and the family, particularly the assurance that the patient will get better.
- Patients are followed for at least 8 weeks by the primary care provider.
- Referral to a psychiatrist should be made if the diagnosis is not definite enough to allow for confident treatment, for those who after 8 weeks of treatment show no improvement, and for those who cannot or who will not take the prescribed medications.
    —These patients require the expertise of a psychiatrist and may require more intensive treatment in or out of the hospital or perhaps electroconvulsive therapy (ECT).

Mania

Definition
Mania is a sustained change in mood, self-attitude, and vital sense. The patient's mood may be euphoric or irritable or may alternate between the two.

Risk Factors
- Same as for other adjustment disorders

Etiology/Cause
- The cause of bipolar disorder, manic phase, is not well understood.
- The basis for the disorder is generally accepted as multifaceted, a combination of genetic, physiologic, psychologic, personality, social, and cultural factors.
- There is growing evidence of a strong genetic cause for bipolar disorder.
    —A sibling or offspring of a patient with a major affective disorder has a 10% chance of developing the disorder.
    —In some families, the risk may be 50%.
- No genes have been isolated so far, although linked loci on two chromosomes have been identified that are likely to harbor genes related to bipolar disorder.

Pathogenesis (see Etiology/Cause)
Diagnosis (Box 22-16)
Signs and symptoms
- The patient has a dramatically increased energy level and a decreased need for sleep.
- An overconfident ease in making decisions is evident.
- The patient has a sense of heightened perception of almost everything in the envi-

---

BOX 22-16
Diagnostic Criteria for a Manic Episode

A. A distinct period of abnormally and persistently elevated, expansive, or irritable mood, lasting at least 1 week (or any duration if hospitalization is necessary)
B. During the period of mood disturbance, at least three of the following symptoms have persisted (four if the mood is only irritable) and have been present to a significant degree:
   1. Inflated self-esteem or grandiosity
   2. Decreased need for sleep (e.g., feels rested after only 3 hours of sleep)
   3. More talkative than usual or pressured to keep talking
   4. Flight of ideas or subjective experience that thoughts are racing
   5. Distractibility (i.e., attention too easily drawn to unimportant or irrelevant external stimuli)

6. Increase in goal-directed activity (either social, at work, or school, or sexually) or psychomotor agitation
7. Excessive involvement in pleasurable activities that have a high potential for painful consequences (e.g., the person engages in unrestrained buying sprees, sexual indiscretions, or foolish business investments)
C. The mood disturbance is sufficiently severe to cause marked impairment in occupational functioning or in usual social activities or relationships with others, or to necessitate hospitalization to prevent harm to self or others.
D. Not due to the direct effects of a substance (e.g., drugs of abuse, medication) or a general medical condition (e.g., hyperthyroidism)

ronment: colors are brighter, tastes are enhanced, and sounds are distinctive and pleasant.

- In this heightened state, the patient sees only continued supreme well-being in the future.
- The family members observe that the patient is very distractible in speech, jumping from topic to topic, and in the same way, jumping from project to project without completing any.
- Judgment ranges from poor to catastrophic as spending sprees increase, and the patient gives away money to friends and strangers alike.
- Self-attitude is usually one of overconfidence; when more severe, it is reflected in an inflated sense of power, position, and importance.
- Delusions and hallucinations, when present, are either grandiose or persecutory.

Treatment

- Patients with mania are more difficult to manage because of the disruptive and disinhibited behavior.
- The patient's acceptance of the need for help is the exception rather than the rule.
- The family's and patient's physician may be the one to diagnose and treat the mania at an early stage.
- Knowledge about the use of neuroleptic drugs and mood stabilizing drugs, such as lithium and sodium valproate, is essential for primary care practitioners.
- Severe acute mania requires treatment initially with neuroleptics and later with both mood stabilizers, such as lithium, and neuroleptics.
- It is often the case that the patient must be hospitalized for 1 to 2 weeks, where treatment begins.
- For acute manic agitation, the use of parenteral fluphenazine (Prolixin) or another high-potency neuroleptic is usually effective.
  - Small dosages of 5 to 10 mg intramuscularly (IM) calm most patients with little or no depression of BP and little sedation.
  - The calming effect of drugs of this type usually last for several hours.

- However, patients may develop extrapyramidal side effects from the drug such as dystonic reactions.
- This condition is relieved by 50 mg of IM diphenhydramine (Benadryl) or 1 to 2 mg of trihexyphenidate (Cogentin).
- Newer neuroleptics recently available, or that will soon be available (e.g., olanzapine, quetiapine, seroquel), may prove useful in treating patients in the manic state.

Maintenance Therapy for Bipolar Disorder

- To date, lithium is the only medication for which efficacy has been unequivocally established for preventing relapses in patients with bipolar disorder or mania after acute episodes have remitted.
  - Lithium is prescribed in divided doses, beginning with 300 to 600 mg on the first day and increasing the dosage in small increments every 3 to 4 days until the therapeutic blood level is achieved.
  - The usual maintenance dosage is 600 to 1800 mg given in divided doses (two to three times/day with standard preparations, and one to two times daily with slow release preparations).
  - Blood levels, measured 12 hours after a dose (trough levels) should be monitored one to two times/week at first.
  - Blood levels in a completely stabilized, compliant patient should be measured six times/year.
  - Because of the possibility of long-term renal effects, maintenance dosage is aimed at the lowest therapeutic level (0.6 to 0.9 mEq/L).
- Controlled comparisons of carbamazepine and lithium show that they are about equivalent in prophylactic efficacy.
- Side effects of lithium may occur at three levels.
  - Early side effects, associated with rapidly rising blood levels: nausea, vomiting, diarrhea, mild lassitude, and drowsiness.
  - Side effects from maintenance dose: may be a large number of side effects (e.g., hand tremor, thyroid disturbances, and renal toxicity).
  - Renal concentrating defect (partial nephrogenic diabetes insipidus due to vaso-

pressin resistance: polyuria and polydipsia occurs in about 10% of patients).
- Toxic side effects are exaggerated side effects in other stages of dosage: nausea, vomiting, diarrhea, tremor, confusion, delirium, stupor, and coma may occur.

Prognosis
- Before modern treatment developed, patients with unipolar and bipolar disorders usually recovered spontaneously within 6 to 18 months.
- With antidepressants, mood stabilizers, such as lithium, and ECT, remissions can be achieved more quickly.
- However, even with modern therapy, about 20% of patients with severe major depression may not recover fully in a 2-year period after entering treatment.
- Manic episodes are briefer and less likely to become chronic.
- Predictors of poor outcome are severity sufficient to require hospitalization and long duration of symptoms (1 year) before treatment.
- Some patients who do not recover have not been treated aggressively enough after failure to respond to a trial of antidepressant medication.
- Clinical experience shows that patients who do not respond to an initial therapy will eventually respond to a second, third, or fourth treatment effort.
- *Relapse* is a hallmark of the course of unipolar and bipolar disorders.
    —The frequency of relapse is variable.
    —Fewer than 20% of major affective syndromes resolve without relapse at some point.
    —Relapses become more frequent later in life, or later in the course of the illness.
- Maintenance medication is usually continued indefinitely, particularly in patients who have relapsing disorder.

Patient/Family Education
- The patient and family should be instructed regarding the nature of the disorder, its usual course, treatment, effects of treatment, outcome, and prognosis.
- In particular, the relapsing and remitting course of the disorder should be explained and is expected in many cases.
- The clinician should develop a plan for treatment of relapses if and when they occur, so that the family is prepared to do whatever is necessary to have the patient treated as early as possible.
- The patient and family should be reassured that the frequency and severity of relapses will be fewer and milder with drug therapy than without.
- Family members of patients with affective disorders often feel confused, hopeless, helpless, and guilty, and may take out these feelings as recriminations against the patient.
    —Health care professionals and psychotherapists need to meet regularly with both the patient and the family, together and separately, to discuss aspects of the illness and how best to manage the patient at home, so that they understand that these disorders are actual diseases, such as physical disease, that can occur without cause but that are also treatable.
- Both patient and family members benefit from regular, close contact with the health care professionals and should feel free to contact them at any time for advice and help.

Schizophrenia
Definition
Schizophrenia is a common, serious mental disorder characterized by loss of contact with reality (psychosis), hallucinations (false perceptions), delusions (false beliefs), abnormal thinking, flattened affect (restricted range of emotions), diminished motivation, and disturbed work and social functioning. Familiarity with schizophrenia is important to the generalist for two reasons: (1) in the prodromal stage, the patient often presents first to a general practitioner, and (2) the interested generalist can provide much of the care for a patient with this lifelong disorder.

Risk Factors
- Both sexes are equally affected.
- In men, the peak age of onset is 18 to 25 years.

- In women, the peak age of onset is 26 to 45 years.
- Lower socioeconomic groups, likely because of a downward social drift resulting from deterioration of social and vocational functioning
- Single people seem to be affected more often than married persons.
- Maternal exposure to famine, influenza in the second trimester of pregnancy, and Rh incompatibility in a second or subsequent pregnancy are associated with an increased risk of schizophrenia in offspring.

Etiology/Cause
- The precise cause of schizophrenia is unknown, but many experts believe that the disorder has a biologic basis.
- A vulnerability-stress model, in which schizophrenia is viewed as occurring in persons with neurologically based vulnerabilities, is the most widely accepted explanation.
  —Onset, remission, and recurrence of symptoms are seen as products of interaction between these vulnerabilities and environmental stressors.
- Vulnerability to the disorder may include genetic predisposition.
- Vulnerability to the disorder may also include viral infections of the central nervous system (CNS).
  —Deficits in information processing, attention, and sensory inhibition may be markers for vulnerability.
- Vulnerability may be reflected by impaired social competence, cognitive disorganization or perceptual distortion, diminished capacity to experience pleasure, and other general coping deficiencies.
  —The presence of these deficits, when severe, may impair social, academic, and vocational functioning in vulnerable persons before onset of the disorder.
  —These premorbid disabilities often limit functional recovery once the disorder is established.
- Although most persons with schizophrenia do not have a family history of it, genetic factors have been implicated.
  —Those with a first-degree relative with the disorder have about a 15% risk of developing the disorder, compared with 1% risk among the general population.
  —A monozygotic twin whose co-twin has the disorder has a >50% probability of developing schizophrenia.
  —In children of one schizophrenic parent, the risk for offspring developing the disorder ranges between 7% and 15%.
  —In children of two schizophrenic parents, the risk for developing the disorder increases to 40%.
- Excessive activity of the dopamine systems may be part of a biochemical defect in schizophrenic patients, based on data from studies related to the effects of antipsychotic drugs.

Natural History of Schizophrenia
- Although the first episode of acute psychosis usually occurs in late adolescence or early adulthood, prodromal manifestations of the disease are often present for years before the acute episode.
  —Gradual withdrawal from social relationships into their own inner psychologic world
    ~ Withdrawal often results in gradual deterioration of scholastic and vocational abilities.
  —Persons, usually older patients, who have already achieved substantial social, educational, and vocational skills show little deterioration of their baseline function.
    ~ Younger patients have not yet acquired social, educational, or vocational skills, and deterioration in this younger group seems more insidious.
  —Indifference to grooming
  —Growing suspicious attitudes about others
  —Increasingly ignore social graces and social rituals
  —Seem to others to be different, peculiar, and sometimes bizarre
- In a study of the prodromal stage of schizophrenia, some patients had dysphoria (anxiety or depression) along with the social deterioration, and over 50% presented to the primary care practitioner with vague somatic complaints.

Diagnosis (Box 22-17)

Signs and symptoms

- No pathognomonic symptoms, signs, or laboratory findings point to the diagnosis.
- The family history provides only partial information regarding the diagnosis.
- Diagnosis therefore is based on findings of the symptoms of psychosis elicited by a mental status examination and a history that documents the prodromal phase.

Differential diagnosis

- Any kind of psychotic state may resemble acute schizophrenia.
- Differences in symptoms allow for differentiation and diagnosis.
- The psychotic symptoms of major affective disorders (both mania and depression) can also be similar to those seen during acute episodes in the course of schizophrenia.
- The primary difference between affective disorders and schizophrenia is that, in affective disorders, delusions and hallucinations appear after the development of the disturbance (either mania or depression), whereas in schizophrenia, marked depression or mania may appear, but the affective disturbance occurs *after* the onset of the psychotic symptoms.
- However, the principles of differential diagnosis are not laid down in stone, and it can happen that a person with an affective disorder can be diagnosed as schizophrenic, and vice versa; but because of the poor prognosis associated with schizophrenia, mislabeling has serious consequences (e.g., attitudes toward the patient by others, and the actual treatment provided.
- *Schizophrenic personality* is a personality type that is not accompanied by the psychotic features seen in schizophrenia, the disorder.

Treatment

- The primary treatment of the acute and chronic psychotic manifestations of schizo-

---

BOX 22-17

Diagnostic Criteria for Schizophrenia

A. Characteristic symptoms: Two or more of the following, each present for a significant portion of time during a 1-month period (or less if successfully treated):
 1. Delusions
 2. Hallucinations
 3. Disorganized speech (e.g., frequent derailment or incoherence)
 4. Grossly disorganized or catatonic behavior
 5. Negative symptoms, i.e., affective flattening, alogia, or avolition
  (Note: Only one criterion A symptom is required if delusions are bizarre or hallucinations consist of a voice keeping up a running commentary on the person's behavior or thoughts, or two or more voices conversing with each other)
B. Social/occupational dysfunction: For a significant portion of the time since the onset of the disturbance, one or more major areas of functioning, such as work, interpersonal relations, or self-care, is markedly below the level achieved before the onset (or when the onset is in childhood or adolescence, failure to achieve expected level of interpersonal, academic, or occupational achievement).
C. Duration: Continuous signs of the disturbance persist for at least 6 months. This 6-month period must in-clude at least 1 criterion A (i.e., active-phase symptoms), and may include periods of prodromal or residual symptoms. During these prodromal or residual periods, the signs of the disturbance may be manifested by only negative symptoms or two or more symptoms listed in criterion A present in an attenuated form (e.g., odd beliefs, unusual perceptual experiences).
D. Schizo-affective and mood disorder exclusion: Schizo-affective disorder and mood disorder with psychotic features have been ruled out because either (1) no major depressive, manic, or mixed symptoms have occured or (2) if mood episodes have occurred during active-phase symptoms, their total duration has been brief relative to the duration of the active and residual periods.
E. Substance/general medical condition exclusion: The disturbance is not due to the direct psychologic effects of a substance (e.g., a drug of abuse, a medication) or a general medical condition.
F. Relationship to a pervasive developmental disorder: If there is a history of autistic disorder or another pervasive developmental disorder, the additional diagnosis of schizophrenia is made only if prominent delusions or hallucinations are also present for at least a month (or less if successfully treated).

phrenia in ambulatory or hospitalized patients is with the neuroleptic antipsychotic agents (these agents may produce unwanted symptoms that resemble neurologic disease).

- There are several classes of neuroleptics, with numerous drugs in each class; some of the most common drugs are (not by class): Thorazine, Vesprin, Serentil, Quide, Stelazine, Taractan, Navane, Maxolon, Haldol, Clozaril, Risperdal, and Syrex.
- The drugs produce effects within 1 hour of oral administration, and within 10 to 15 minutes after IM injection; they are lipid soluble and are distributed throughout the CNS with no local or regional accumulation; metabolites are partially excreted every day, with significant portions retained in lipid-rich tissues and connective tissues; as these tissues become saturated, the drugs undergo slow turnover.
  —The drugs are detoxified and inactivated mainly through oxidation by hepatic microsomal enzymes, and they are excreted through the bile and the kidneys.

Treatment of acute psychotic episodes

- Any of the neuroleptic antipsychotic drugs is effective in controlling psychotic symptoms in schizophrenia.
- Any differences stem from individual reactions and side effects peculiar to each individual.
  —Initially, one drug is selected (e.g., Thorazine), and the dose is 300 to 1000 mg/day, given in three divided doses IM, usually, if the patient cannot take the drugs by mouth.
  —This dosage controls combativeness, hyperactivity, and agitation within 24 to 48 hours.
  —If symptoms are not controlled within this time period, the dosage should be increased 100 to 200 mg/day, up to the equivalent of 800 to 1000 mg.
- Delusions, hallucinations, associational deficits, negativism, and withdrawal begin to subside within 1 to 2 weeks from when treatment begins, with continual improvement over the next 4 to 8 weeks.
- High dosage should be reduced to the equivalent of 400 to 600 mg as soon as possible, and the adjustment can usually be made 1 to 2 weeks after reaching the peak dosage of Thorazine.
- Side effects may include: sedation, anticholinergic symptoms (dry mouth, stuffy nose, blurred vision, sometimes urinary retention in older patients). Parkinson's syndrome symptoms, occasionally, dystonia may occur, orthostatic hypotension, or cholestatic jaundice (reversible), which may occur as an allergic reaction.
- Dosage for older patients, who are more susceptible to side effects, should be 100 to 200 mg less than the dose for younger patients.

Long-term treatment of schizophrenia

- The primary care practitioner can assume the long-term care of schizophrenic patients, which is primarily drug therapy.
  —Many studies indicate that these patients usually relapse within 1 year if they are not receiving medication.
  —Most patients should be treated for at least 2 years after an acute episode.
  —The goal of long-term therapy is to minimize psychotic symptoms with the lowest possible dose of antipsychotic drugs.
  —Moderate maintenance dosages seem to be as effective as, and safer than, the larger dosages that had been ordinarily given in the past.
  —Most patients can be maintained on the equivalent of 100 to 200 mg of Thorazine daily.
  —Some patients may continue to have psychotic symptoms while on this dosage but do not seem to be disturbed by them (e.g., "I still hear the voices, but they don't bother me").
- Side effects from long-term use of neuroleptic drugs sometimes occur after months to years of therapy.
  —Tardive dyskinesia is an extrapyramidal syndrome, occurring in about 27% of women and 22% of men.
  —This condition is characterized by voluntary or semivoluntary movements of choreiform, ticlike nature, sometimes associated with a dystonic component that classically involves the tongue, facial, and neck muscles.

—Early signs include fine wormlike movements of the tongue, facial tics, and jaw movements.

—Later signs include bucco-lingual-masticatory movements, chewing motions, lip smacking, blinking of eyes, and choreoathetoid movements of the extremities.

—The prognosis for remission of tardive dyskinesia is poor, regardless of treatment, and symptoms last for years, if not for the life of the patient.

—Use of neuroleptics should therefore emphasize the prevention of tardive dyskinesia.

—In younger patients who begin to develop signs and symptoms of tardive dyskinesia, gradual tapering and discontinuation of the drug, if possible; symptoms usually gradually diminish and disappear over several months in about 33% of patients who can be taken off drugs early.

Overall treatment of patients with schizophrenia

- These patients are sensitive to change or instability in any aspect of their lives.
- When possible, one practitioner should provide continuous care so that person becomes a predictable resource for helping the patient to maintain their role in the community.
  —Although a few (<20%) of these patients work full time, most should be referred for vocational rehabilitation or sheltered workshops.
  —Most patients determine their own levels of social activity, and it is useless to push them into unwanted situations.
- The practitioner should always be available to the family for periodic review of the patient's progress and status.
- Regular office visits should be scheduled; the frequency is determined by many factors: patient's status, degree of compliance, reliability of the patient in reporting symptoms, and patient's ability to recognize early signs of onset of acute episodes.
  —These office visits are often in the nature of supportive care, to check the patient's general status, to allow time for questions

and discussions, and to provide encouragement to the patient in dealing with day-to-day activities.

- For patients who are having difficulty within their families, a *family management approach* may be useful.
  —Sessions devoted to educating the patient and family about the nature, course, and treatment of the disorder.
  —Family sessions aimed at reducing existing family tensions and improving problem-solving skills of the family in coping with causes of stress.
- Management of patients is enhanced if there is easy access to social services, psychiatric day-care, and inpatient services.
  —Social services are often needed to facilitate welfare, food stamps, and disability payments, to prevent acute episodes caused by threatened or actual withdrawal of financial support from these sources.

Patient/Family Education

- Schizophrenia is a lifelong disease that requires an open-ended commitment by the clinician.
- The patient's and the family's lives are disrupted periodically by psychotic episodes, sometimes requiring hospitalization, and usually accompanied by arrest or deterioration of the patient's social functioning.
- Many patients lead lonely, withdrawn, socially marginal existences.
- Suppression of psychosis may allow the patients to use their intellectual and social talents more effectively in developing and maintaining some role in the community.
  —The newer antipsychotic drugs are reported to have a positive effect on the deterioration of social function that is so characteristic of schizophrenia.

Follow-up/Referral

- As indicated, this is usually a lifelong disorder with periodic episodes of acutely psychotic behaviors and deterioration of the patient's status from earlier.
- Caring for these patients requires commitment, skill, a caring and supportive environment, and maintaining the patients to a

TABLE 22-1
Medical Conditions that May Affect Sexual Responses in Men

Organic Factor	Sexual Disorders
Dyspareunia (genital pain during intercourse)	Hypoactive desire, hypoactive arousal, hypoactive orgasm
Disturbed penile anatomy (chordee, Peyronie's disease, traumatic fracture, traumatic amputation)	
Penile skin infections	
Prostatic infections	
Testicular diseases (orchitis, epididymitis, tumor, trauma)	
Urethral infections (gonorrhea, nonspecific urethral infections)	
Hypogonadal androgen-deficiency states	Hypoactive desire, hypoactive arousal, hypoactive orgasm
Klinefelter's syndrome, testicular agenesis, testicular tumors, orchitis, hyperprolactinemia, castration	
Mechanical problems (inguinal hernia, hydrocele)	Hypoactive arousal
Surgical procedures:	
Abdominoperineal bowel resection	Hypoactive arousal
Lumbar sympathectomy	Hypoactive orgasm
Radical perineal prostatectomy	Hypoactive arousal

From Schmidt CW: Sexual disorders. In Barker LR, Burton JR, Zieve PD, eds: *Principles of ambulatory medicine,* ed 5, Baltimore, 1999, Lippincott, Williams & Wilkins, p 201.

degree that allows them to assume some role in the family and in the community.

- Family support and education are just as important as that provided to patients.

Sexual Disorders

Definition

Psychosexual disorders include sexual dysfunction (the most common form of psychosexual disorder seen in the primary setting), gender disorders, and paraphilias. Sexual dysfunction is defined as disturbances in the sexual response cycle or pain associated with sexual arousal or intercourse.

- About 4% to 5% of the population are preferentially homosexual their entire lives.
  —Since 1973 the American Psychiatric Association has not considered homosexuality a disorder.
  —For most, homosexuality is not a matter of choice.

Risk Factors
- Genetic factors
- Environmental factors
- Biologic factors

Etiology/Cause (see also Risk Factors) (Table 22-1 and Box 22-18)
- Psychologic factors: anger directed toward the partner; fear of the partner's genitals, of

BOX 22-18
Medical Conditions that May Affect Sexual Response*: Women

COMPLICATIONS OF SURGERY
Ovarian approximation to vagina
Posthysterectomy scarring
Shortened vagina

DYSPAREUNIA (PAINFUL INTERCOURSE)
Agenesis of the vagina
Clitoral phimosis
Imperforate hymen, rigid hymen, tender hymenal tags
Infections of external genitalia: herpes genitalis, labial cysts, furuncles, Bartholin cyst infections
Infections of the vagina: herpes genitalia, *Candida albicans, Trichomonas* species
Injuries due to birth trauma: episiotomy scars, tears, uterine prolapse
Irritations of the vagina: chemical dermatitis (douches), atrophic vaginitis, intercourse with insufficient lubrication

MISCELLANEOUS PELVIC PROBLEMS
Cystitis, urethritis, urethral prolapse
Endometriosis, ectopic pregnancy, pelvic inflammatory disease, ovarian cysts and tumors, pelvic tumors
Intrauterine device complications

From Schmidt CW: Sexual disorders. In Barker LR, Burton JR, Zieve PD, eds: *Principles of ambulatory medicine,* ed 5, Baltimore, 1999, Lippincott, Williams & Wilkins, p 201.
*The sexual disorders that may be caused by the problems listed above are: hypoactive desire, hypoactive arousal, hypoactive orgasm, and vaginismus.

intimacy, of losing control, of dependency, or of pregnancy; guilt after a pleasurable experience; depression; anxiety due to marital discord, stressful life situations, aging, ignorance of sexual norms (e.g., frequency and duration of intercourse, oral-genital sex, or sexual practices); belief in sexual myths (e.g., deleterious effects of masturbation, hysterectomy, or menopause).

- Immediate causes of anxiety include: fear of failure, demand for performance, spectating (observing one's physical responses), an exaggerated wish to please the partner, and avoidance of sex or of talking about sexual concerns.

- These factors further impair performance and satisfaction, and continued avoidance of sexual activity with impaired communication creates a vicious cycle.

- Many medical conditions and drugs can impair normal function, because sexual functioning involves neural, vascular, and endocrine physiologic mechanisms, along with cellular activity.

Pathogenesis

- Proper sexual functioning in men and women depends on the sexual response cycle, which consists of an anticipatory mental set (sexual motive state or state of desire), effective vasocongestive arousal (erection in men; swelling and lubrication in women), orgasm, and resolution.

- In men, the sensation of orgasm includes emission followed by ejaculation.
  - Emission, mediated by contractions of the prostate, seminal vesicles, and urethra, produces a sensation of ejaculatory inevitability.
  - In women, orgasm is accompanied by contractions (not always subjectively experienced as such) of the muscles of the outer third of the vagina.
  - In both men and women, generalized muscular tension, perineal contractions, and involuntary pelvic thrusting (every 0.8 second) usually occur.
  - Orgasm is followed by resolution—a sense of general pleasure, well-being, and muscular relaxation.
    - ~ During this period of resolution, men are physiologically refractory to erec-

tion and orgasm for a variable period of time, but women may be able to respond to additional stimulation almost immediately.

- The sexual response cycle is mediated by a delicate, balanced interplay between the sympathetic and parasympathetic nervous systems.
  - Vasocongestion is mediated primarily by parasympathetic (cholinergic) outflow; orgasm is predominantly sympathetic (adrenergic).
  - Orgasm is almost entirely sympathetic; emission involves sympathetic and parasympathetic stimulation.

- These responses are easily inhibited by cortical influences or by impaired hormonal, neural, or vascular mechanisms α- and β-adrenergic blockers may desynchronize emission, ejaculation, and perineal muscle contraction during orgasm, and serotonin agonists frequently interfere with desire and orgasm.

- Disorders of the sexual response cycle may involve one or more of the cycle's phases.
  - Usually, both the subjective components of desire, arousal, and pleasure and the objective components of performance, vasocongestion, and orgasm are disturbed, but any one of the components may be affected independently.

- Sexual dysfunctions may be lifelong (no effective performance ever, usually due to intrapsychic conflicts) or acquired (after a period of normal function); generalized or limited to particular situations or particular partners; and total or partial.
  - Most patients complain of anxiety, guilt, shame, and frustration, and may develop physical symptoms.

Diagnosis

- Patients often have difficulty initiating questions or discussion about sexual concerns; it is therefore essential for the clinician to inquire about sexual orientation and function as a part of the history for each patient (Box 22-19).
  - In one study in a general medicine practice, 90% of patients appreciated being asked about sexual function.

- If the patient's problem involves a partner, it is important to have the partner's view.

BOX 22-19

Questions for the Clinician to Ask About Sexual Problems and Practices

OPENING (LEGITIMIZING STATEMENT)
"Something that I ask each of my patients about is sexual activity. Is that all right with you?"

INITIAL QUESTIONS
"Can you tell me about your present sexual activity (practices)?" (or)
"Have you noticed any problem in your ability to have and enjoy sexual relations?" (or)
"Do you have any problems or questions related to your current sexual activities?"

SCREENING QUESTIONS FOR SEXUAL DYSFUNCTION (ASK FOR CLARIFICATION OF ANY POSITIVE RESPONSE)
"Have you noticed any loss of interest in having sex?" (both sexes)
"Any problems having an erection?" (men)
"Any problems with lubrication or swelling of the vagina when you are sexually aroused?" (women)

"Any problems having an orgasm?"
"Any pain during intercourse?"

SCREENING QUESTIONS REGARDING SEXUAL ORIENTATION
"Have you ever had sex with men, women, or both?" (or)
"Do you ever have sex with another man?" (men)
"Do you ever have sex with another woman?" (women)

SCREENING QUESTIONS FOR RISK OF OR HISTORY OF SEXUALLY TRANSMITTED DISEASE
"In the past few years about how many partners have you had for sexual relations?"
"Have you ever had any kind of infection that you got from having sex?"

QUESTION TO ELICIT FURTHER INFORMATION
"Is there any other information or any other questions about your sexual activities that you would like to discuss with me?"

From Schmidt CW: Sexual disorders. In Barker LR, Burton JR, Zieve PD, eds: *Principles of ambulatory medicine*, ed 5, Baltimore, 1999, Lippincott, Williams & Wilkins, p 203.

Sexual Desire Disorders

Sexual desire disorders are predominantly psychogenic in origin and are classified in the *DMS-IV* as follows:

- Hypoactive sexual desire (loss of libido)
  —Persistently or recurrently deficient (or absent) sexual fantasies and desires for sexual activity; the judgment of deficiency or absence is made by the clinician, taking into account factors that affect sexual functioning (e.g., age, sex, context of the person's life).
  —The disturbance causes marked distress or interpersonal difficulty.
  —Does not occur exclusively during the course of another Axis I disorder (except another sexual dysfunction) and is not caused exclusively by the direct physiologic effects of a substance (e.g., drugs of abuse, medication) or a general medical condition
- Sexual aversion disorder
  —Persistent or recurrent extreme aversion to and avoidance of all or almost all genital sexual contact with a sexual partner
  —The disturbance causes marked distress or interpersonal difficulty.

  —The sexual dysfunction is not caused by another Axis I disorder (except another sexual dysfunction).
- In men, congenital or acquired *hypogonadism* may be associated with decreased sexual interest.
  —The testosterone level needed for full stimulation of the prostate and seminal vesicles, the patient should also complain about a decrease or absence of emission when loss of sexual desire is due to hypogonadism.
- In both sexes, *prolactin-secreting microadenomas* of the pituitary gland may cause loss of sexual interest.
- Hyperprolactinemia causes amenorrhea and galactorrhea in females, but galactorrhea is rare in affected men.
- In both sexes, alcohol or other substance abuse can cause decreased sexual desire.
  —Patients who abuse drugs are usually guarded or untruthful about their habits; persistence and use of collateral interviews may be necessary to diagnose the primary problem.
- Depression is a common cause of loss of sexual desire.

- Marital strife is often the cause of decreased sexual desire among married couples.
- Repeated sexual failure may result in decreased loss of sexual desire.

Treatment

- Hypogonadism in men can be treated by surgery, radiotherapy, hormone replacement, or hormone suppression (in the case of hyperprolactinemia).
- If drug abuse is suspected of interfering with sexual desire, it should be discontinued when possible as a diagnostic-therapeutic test.
- If drugs of abuse appear to be the cause of decreased sexual desire, treatment is aimed at controlling addiction and use.
- Transient hypoactive sexual desire disorders secondary to psychologic factors (e.g., stress, anger, other interpersonal problems) are managed effectively with short-term counseling.
  —An agreement among the clinician and patient or couple is made to meet for a specific number of sessions (usually 2 to 5) for about 30 minutes per session.
- Sexual aversion disorders usually require psychotherapy and treatment of associated panic attacks with low-dose antidepressant medication.
- There is no scientific basis for prescribing drugs for sexual desire disorders other than testosterone for treating confirmed hypogonadism and bromocriptine to treat hyperprolactinemia.

Sexual Arousal Disorders

- Psychogenic disorders are classified by the *DSM-IV* as follows:

Female Arousal Disorders

- Persistent or recurrent inability to attain or to maintain until completion of the sexual activity an adequate lubrication-swelling response of sexual excitement
- Disturbance causes marked distress or interpersonal difficulty
- Sexual dysfunction is not better accounted for by another Axis I disorder (except another sexual dysfunction) and is not caused by the direct physiologic effects of a substance (e.g., drugs of abuse, medication) or a general medical condition.

Male Erectile Dysfunction (Impotence)

- Persistent or recurrent inability to attain or maintain an adequate erection until completion of the sexual activity
- Disturbance causes marked distress or interpersonal difficulty
- Dysfunction is not better accounted for by another Axis I disorder (other than a sexual dysfunction) and is not caused exclusively by the direct physiologic effects of a substance (e.g., a drug of abuse, medication).

Treatment

- The initial history, including psychosocial evaluation, usually leads to a formulation that the problem is either organic or predominantly psychogenic.

Symptoms of Organic Cause of Arousal Disorders

- Usually insidious decline from previous competency (90% to 95% of cases)
- Usually persistent, with progressive deterioration
- Unable to obtain erection with masturbation, erotic stimuli, other partner
- Nocturnal or morning erection is generally absent or reduced in frequency and intensity

Symptoms of Psychogenic Cause of Arousal Disorders

- Usually abrupt, with temporal relationship to specific stress (e.g., marital difficulties, loss of job, bereavement, fatigue)
- Selective, intermittent, episodic, transient
- Evidence of potential to respond to erotic stimuli and fantasies, with masturbation, other partner
  —Nocturnal or morning erection is usually present
- If the sexual disorder is likely to have an organic basis, treatment of the underlying condition (e.g., diabetes, hypertension, other) is the primary aim.
- If a drug is suspected of causing the disorder, stopping the drug or treating the substance abuse problem is of paramount concern.
- If the disorder seems to have a psychogenic basis, possible causes should be identified (e.g., life stresses, environmental factors, interpersonal difficulties) and treated.

- Many psychogenic sexual arousal disorders can be treated with removal of the cause and short-term counseling, with short-term antidepressant drugs if necessary.
- If a disease process has caused permanent impairment of neural, vascular, or anatomic function in males, prosthetic devices that cause erection or pharmacologic measures can be considered, in consultation with a urologist.

Disorders of Orgasm

Female Orgasmic Disorder

- Persistent or recurrent delay in or absence of orgasm after a normal sexual arousal phase
- Women exhibit wide variability in the type and intensity of stimulation that triggers orgasm.
- Diagnosis of female orgasmic disorder should be based on the clinician's judgment that the woman's orgasmic capacity is less than would be reasonable for her age, sexual experience, and the adequacy of sexual stimulation she receives.
- Disturbance causes marked distress or interpersonal difficulty
- Orgasmic disorder is not better accounted for by another Axis I disorder (except another sexual dysfunction) and is not caused exclusively by the direct physiologic effects of a substance (e.g., a drug of abuse, medication) or a general medical condition.

Male Orgasmic Disorder

- Persistent or recurrent delay in or absence of orgasm after a normal sexual excitement phase during sexual activity that the clinician, taking into account the person's age, judges to be adequate in focus, intensity, and duration.
- The disturbance causes marked distress or interpersonal difficulty.
- The orgasmic disorder is not better accounted for by another Axis I disorder (except another sexual dysfunction) and is not caused exclusively by the direct physiologic effects of a substance (e.g., a drug of abuse, medication) or a general medical condition.

Premature Ejaculation

- Persistent or recurrent ejaculation with minimal sexual stimulation before, on, or shortly after penetration and before the persons wishes it; the clinician must take into account factors that affect duration of the arousal phase, such as age, novelty of the sexual partner or situation, and recent frequency of sexual activity
- The disturbance causes marked distress or interpersonal difficulty.
- The premature ejaculation is not caused exclusively by the first effects of a substance (e.g., withdrawal from opioids).

Treatment

- Premature ejaculation is the most common male orgasmic disorder.
  —There are no known organic causes for this condition.
  —Treatment should therefore focus on psychologic therapy.
  —The personality structure of the premature ejaculator is often passive-aggressive.
  —Evaluation of the relationship usually indicates an ongoing struggle between the partners.
- Psychologically caused orgasmic disorder is a common problem in women.
  —Many studies show that about 10% of women are anorgasmic to any stimuli.
  —About 30% to 50% of all married women are occasionally anorgasmic with intercourse.
  —Although some women present with a complaint of anorgasmia, evaluation reveals that the patient actually has a sexual arousal disorder.
- Treatment of premature ejaculation focuses on techniques to increase awareness of the sexual response cycle and to practice techniques to control timing of ejaculation.
- Treatment of orgasmic disorder in women is limited to discontinuing possible causal drugs.
  —The goal of therapy is to help the patient adjust to the permanent loss of sexual responsiveness.
  —Short-term counseling is of some help for some women.
  —Referral to a psychiatrist who is expert at treating anorgasmic patients is recommended.

Sexual Pain Disorders

- Diagnostic classification of psychogenic dyspareunia can be made only when all possible causes have been ruled out.
- The *DSM-IV* diagnostic criteria for sexual pain disorder are the following:
  - I. Dyspareunia
    - A. Recurrent or persistent genital pain associated with sexual intercourse in either a male or a female
    - B. The disturbance causes marked distress or interpersonal difficulty.
    - C. The disturbance is not caused exclusively by vaginismus or lack of lubrication, is not better accounted for by another Axis I disorder (except another sexual dysfunction), and is not caused exclusively by the direct physiologic effects of a substance (e.g., drug of abuse, medication) or a general medical condition.
  - II. Vaginismus
    - A. Recurrent or persistent involuntary spasm of the musculature of the outer third of the vagina that interferes with sexual intercourse
    - B. The disturbance causes marked distress or interpersonal difficulty.
    - C. The disturbance is not better accounted for by another Axis I disorder (e.g., somatization disorder) and is not caused exclusively by the direct effects of a general medical condition.
- The common causes of genital pain during intercourse (dyspareunia) are identified in Box 22-16.
- Complaint of discomfort or pain during intercourse requires a careful history, physical examination, and laboratory testing.
- The most common causes are infections or atrophic vaginitis in women, and urethral or prostatic infections in men.
- There are few causes of organic vaginismus, and these are usually secondary to dyspareunia.
  - —The diagnosis may be made at the time the clinician attempts to perform a pelvic examination and finds it impossible to pass a finger or speculum into the vagina because of contraction of the musculature around the vaginal outlet; the history may show that the patient is unable to be penetrated during coitus because of tightness of the vaginal outlet caused by muscular spasm.

Treatment

- The focus of therapy is on the organic cause of painful intercourse: infection or atrophic vaginitis in women, and infections in men.
- Few patients have psychogenic dyspareunia over a sustained period.
  - —Most such patients have severe underlying psychiatric conditions and require referral for expert evaluation and therapy.
- For functional vaginismus, the couple is counseled and given a series of exercises to do in their own home that involves gradual desensitization of the woman by progressive touching and introduction of dilators until coitus is possible.

Homosexuality

- The American Psychiatric Association removed homosexuality from its list of mental disorders in 1973.
- The term *Sexual Disorder, Not Otherwise Specified* may be used for patients who experience persistent and marked distress about their sexual orientation.
  - —In a recent study of homosexual men, Cochran and Mays (2000) reported greater prevalence of suicidal symptoms than was found in men reporting only female partners.
  - —Results also showed a small, increased risk of recurrent depression among gay men, with symptom onset occurring, on average, during early adolescence.
- Although Kinsey and others estimated that 10% of white men and 5% of white women were homosexual, Cochran and Mays (2000) reported 2.2% same-sex partners in men.
- Recent reports from several European and American studies indicate that only 1% to 2% of the population of adult men and women is exclusively homosexual.

Risk Factors

- No studies have demonstrated psychosocial precipitants of homosexuality.
- Evidence of a genetic basis is sparse.

- A relationship between hormonal abnormalities (pituitary and sex hormone functioning) and homosexuality has not been shown.
- There is no evidence that homosexuals are subject to or manifest greater levels of major psychopathology than do heterosexuals.

Complications
- Social stigma attached to homosexuality, perhaps becoming less so now
- Many local legislative bodies have enacted or are considering legislation that explicitly protects homosexuals from job, housing, and other types of discrimination.

Treatment
- For patients who express concerns about homosexual fantasies or experiences, the focus is on the frequency of the experiences, the patient's decisions to continue the homosexual experiences, and whether they feel comfortable with their decisions.
- Patients who are anxious or depressed about their homosexual inclinations may need therapy.
- Sexually transmitted diseases are of concern to the clinician who is seeing homosexual patients.
  —Lesbians may present with three forms of vaginitis: candidiasis, trichomonas, and nonspecific vaginitis.
  —Cancer screening for lesbian patients is the same as for heterosexual women.

Patient/Family Education
- Both sexes should be instructed about safe sex practices and avoidance of sexually transmitted diseases.
  —Known contacts of infected patients should be treated also.
- It is possible that lesbians have a greater risk of breast cancer than do heterosexual women because breast-feeding seems to lower the risk of breast cancer.
- Regular gynecologic or urologic check-ups should be scheduled for homosexual patients.

Gender Identity Disorders
Definition
Gender identity disorders are characterized by a strong, persistent cross-gender identification and by continuous discomfort about one's anatomic (assigned) sex or by a sense of inappropriateness in the gender role of that sex.

- **Core gender identity** is a subjective sense of knowing to which gender one belongs (e.g., "I am a male").
- **Gender identity** is the inner sense of masculinity or femininity.
- **Gender role** is the objective, public expression of being male, female, or androgynous (blended).
  —Everything that one does or says indicates to others and to oneself the degree to which one is male or female.
  —Those with gender identity disorders experience a severe incongruity between their anatomic sex and their gender identity.
- Childhood gender identity disorders are usually present by 2 years of age.

Diagnosis
- Requires the presence of both cross-gender identification (the desire to be or insistence that one is the other sex) and a sense of discomfort about one's sex or of inappropriateness in one's gender role.
  —Cross-gender identification must not be merely a desire for perceived cultural advantages of being the other sex.
- Requires the presence of significant distress or obvious impairment in social occupational or other important areas of functioning.

Transsexualism
Definition
Transsexualism is a gender identity disorder in which the person believes he or she is the victim of a biologic accident, cruelly imprisoned in a body incompatible with his or her subjective gender identity.

Risk Factors
- The incidence of transsexualism is estimated to be about 1 in 30,000 male births, and 1 in 100,000 female births.
- Genital ambiguity is rare.
- Most transsexuals are males who claim a feminine gender identity and regard their genitalia and masculine features with repugnance.

Etiology/Cause
- The manifestations of this disorder usually become apparent in early adulthood, although most adults state that they have been aware of gender discomfort since childhood or adolescence.

Diagnosis
- Diagnosis is confirmed by the patient and by the insistent, persistent desire to change all aspects of his or her sex to conform to his or her inner conviction regarding the true sexual identity.
- Evaluation of these disorders in adults is fairly simple.
- Most patients identify themselves as being unhappy with their anatomic sex and interested in a surgical reassignment.
- No endocrinologic studies are indicated, and physical findings show that the people seeking surgical reassignment are genetically normal men or women.

Treatment
- Patients with gender identity disorders are referred to psychiatrists or to special programs that have the expertise to treat these problems.
- Patients who are in a cross-gender program and who need continuous administration of cross-gender hormones (e.g., estrogen) may be transferred to the generalist.
- Some clinicians are not comfortable working with these patients, who should be referred to experts who are familiar with the disorder and know how best to treat it.

Patient/Family Education
- The parents of those with gender identity disorder are probably the ones most affected by the decision to seek help and surgical reassignment.
  - The mother or father of a child whom they considered to be a male but who now states that he really is female in every aspect of his thinking can be a difficult issue to assimilate.
  - In most cases, counseling for the parents is recommended, so that they become knowledgeable about the disorder and can learn to accept that they have not lost a child, but have lost a son and gained a daughter.
- Patients are treated conservatively and gradually, with counseling to assure the therapist that the gender identity disorder is valid and requires therapy: hormonal, counseling, group therapy, and finally surgical reassignment to match the person's anatomy with his or her psychologic self.
- There may be legal ramifications for the transsexual person, also, and legal counsel is usually sought.

The Paraphilias
Definition
The paraphilias are disorders that are characterized by long-standing, intense, sexually arousing fantasies, urges, or behaviors that involve inanimate objects, actual or imagined suffering or humiliation of oneself or one's partner or nonconsenting partners, and that are associated with clinically important distress or disability.

Risk Factors
- Far more males than females have paraphilia disorders.
- The need for males to transfer their infantile identification with their mothers to their fathers during the preschool or oedipal period (e.g., age 3 to 6 years) may make males more vulnerable to developing paraphilias.

Etiology/Cause
- No biologic basis for the disorders is known, although some deviant behavior has been reported in association with temporal lobe epilepsy.
- A history of physical or sexual abuse during childhood appears in a small number of cases.
- Psychiatric disorders, mainly depression secondary to loss, may precipitate bursts of deviant behavior in these patients.
- Many of the paraphilias are rare; the most common are pedophilia, voyeurism, and exhibitionism.

Pathogenesis
- The arousal patterns that these patients develop are considered deviant because they are

often obligatory for sexual functioning (i.e., erection or orgasm cannot occur without the stimulus), may involve inappropriate partners (children), and cause significant distress or impairment in social, occupational, or other important areas of functioning.

- Patients with paraphilia are those whose sexual drive is absorbed almost entirely in performing or submitting to flagellation or similar practices, is directed toward articles of clothing, or is largely expressed in exhibitionism or voyeurism.
- The capacity for affectionate, reciprocal emotional and sexual intimacy with a partner is usually impaired or nonexistent, and other aspects of personal and emotional adjustment are impaired.
- Objects of sexual attraction may be articles of clothing (e.g., female underclothes), exhibitionism, fetishism (e.g., an object or a body part other than those usually associated with genital sexuality); zoophilia (e.g., the person prefers achieving sexual excitement through animals); frotteurism; pedophilia; voyeurism; and sadism/masochism in which sexual arousal and gratification depend on either inflicting pain (sadism) or experiencing it (masochism), with a wide range of behaviors, from the dim awareness of cruelty or suffering as part of the sexual experience to overt behavior, including extreme physical injury and murder; aspects of sadism and masochism are usually found in the same person, although one or the other behavior is dominant.

Diagnosis

- The formal diagnosis of each of these conditions includes as criteria that the person has acted on the specific urges or is markedly distressed by them, and that the problem has been present for at least 6 months.
- Unless the paraphilia causes the patient intolerable distress, or involves criminal activity (e.g., pedophilia), the person may not be diagnosed.

Treatment

- Psychotherapy or other psychologic treatment aimed at controlling or eliminating

paraphiliac behavior is best provided through a skilled psychiatrist.

- The clinician's role is to manage any concurrent medical problems.
- Diagnosis and treatment of sexually transmitted disease in patients whose sexual behavior is promiscuous is of major concern.
- Evidence of child abuse should be sought if families have a paraphiliac member.

Patient/Family Education

- Paraphiliac behaviors may be the result of childhood punishment or sexual abuse, and the adult behaviors may perpetuate those behaviors inflicted on the child generation after generation.
- Explain the nature, possible causes, course, treatment, and expected outcome of therapy.
- The course of these disorders is usually chronic, with peaks of deviant activity occurring with life stress or in association with psychiatric symptoms, primarily depressive episodes.
- Fear of discovery, arrest, and incarceration may cause the patient to be very circumspect regarding the deviant behavior; if these fears are allayed for any reason, there is little motivation for treatment or behavior changes.

Follow-up/Referral

- As soon as the paraphilia is diagnosed, the patient is referred to a competent psychiatrist for follow-up evaluation and treatment.

BIBLIOGRAPHY

Barker LR, Schmidt CW: Evaluation of psychosocial problems. In Barker LR, Burton JR, Zieve PD, eds: *Principles of ambulatory medicine*, ed 5, Baltimore, 1999, Williams & Wilkins, p 125.

Beers MH, Berkow R: Psychiatric disorders. In Beers MH, Berkow R, eds: *The Merck manual of diagnosis and therapy*, ed 17, Whitehouse Station, NJ, 1999, Merck Research Laboratories, pp 1503-1598.

Cochran SD, Mays M: Lifetime prevalence of suicide symptoms and affective disorders among men reporting same-sex sexual partners: Results from NHANES III. *American Journal of Public Health* 90(4):573-578, 2000.

DePaulo JR: Affective disorders. In Barker LR, Burton JR, Zieve PD, eds: *Principles of ambulatory medicine*, ed 5, Baltimore, 1999, Williams & Wilkins, p 167.

Kinsey AC, Pomeroy WB, Martin CE: *Sexual behavior in the human male*, Philadelphia, 1948, Saunders.

Roca RP: Somatization. In Barker LR, Burton JR, Zieve PD, eds: *Principles of ambulatory medicine*, ed 5, Baltimore, 1999, Williams & Wilkins, p 137.

Roca RP: Anxiety. In Barker LR, Burton JR, Zieve PD, eds: *Principles of ambulatory medicine*, ed 5, Baltimore, 1999, Williams & Wilkins, p 148.

Roca RP: Maladaptive personalities. In Barker LR, Burton JR, Zieve PD, eds: *Principles of ambulatory medicine*, ed 5, Baltimore, 1999, Williams & Wilkins, p 163.

Roca RP, Barker LR: Psychotherapy in ambulatory practice. In Barker LR, Burton JR, Zieve PD, eds: *Principles of ambulatory medicine*, ed 5, Baltimore, 1999, Williams & Wilkins, p 131.

Schmidt CW: Schizophrenia. In Barker LR, Burton JR, Zieve PD, eds: *Principles of ambulatory medicine*, ed 5, Baltimore, 1999, Williams & Wilkins. p 183.

Schmidt CW: Sexual disorders. In Barker LR, Burton JR, Zieve PD, eds: *Principles of ambulatory medicine*, ed 5, Baltimore, 1999, Williams & Wilkins, p 199.

Waterbury L, Purtell M.J: Dying, death, and bereavement. In Barker LR, Burton JR, Zieve PD, eds: *Principles of ambulatory medicine*, ed 5, 1999, Baltimore, 1999, Williams & Wilkins, p 215.

REVIEW QUESTIONS

1. Of patients in primary care settings in the United States, the percentage who have a psychosocial disorder is:
   a. 10%
   b. 20%
   c. 30%
   d. 40%

2. Social factors that are often linked to psychosocial illness include all but one of the following. The one area that is NOT linked to possible psychosocial illness is:
   a. Personal loss (death of a loved one, loss of job, loss of home)
   b. Major recent change (move to a new area, change in job)
   c. Stress (unexpected, acute: damage to home, accident)
   d. Educational level (less than eighth grade, less than high school)

3. Personality is defined as:
   a. Physical appearance and mannerisms
   b. Long-established attitudes and patterns of behavior
   c. A combination of cultural and social factors
   d. Typical values and responses

4. Coping mechanisms are used by people to:
   a. Adapt to life stresses
   b. Deal with difficult people
   c. Preserve one's self-esteem
   d. Overcome problems at work

5. The American Psychiatric Association has developed a particular approach to formulate psychosocial problems, called:
   a. The two-axis system
   b. The three-axis system
   c. The four-axis system
   d. The five-axis system

6. Psychotherapy consists of:
   a. Helping the patient to resolve conflicts
   b. Helping the patient through a period of demoralization
   c. Verbal and behavioral processes used to relieve patients' symptoms and resolve patients' intrapersonal and interpersonal conflicts
   d. Helping the patient to cope with personality defects

7. Transference is:
   a. A process in which a patient may transfer his or her feelings of anger, frustration, and inadequacy onto the therapist
   b. When patients transfer expectations to the therapist regarding how they consider that the therapist should respond to them as their parents did during their growing-up years
   c. When patients exploit the therapist for their own ends by rationalizing behaviors that they know are or were unacceptable
   d. When patients assume knowledge and expertise regarding their own psychologic status, when in reality they are ignorant of these problems

8. Countertransference is:
   a. When the physician or therapist develops positive or negative expectations regarding the patient
   b. When the physician or therapist expects the patient to respond in a certain way
   c. When the physician or therapist expects the patient always to respond positively to their care
   d. When the physician or therapist and the patient have antagonistic or different expectations of one another

9. Patients with somatoform disorders:
   a. Often have severe psychosocial problems
   b. Express their emotional distress in crying jags and self-pity

c. Express their emotional distress in somatic complaints, thinking that they have an incurable physical disease

d. Express their emotional distress in symptoms that are not attributable to any specific disease process

10. Supportive counseling serves two purposes, which are:
   a. To help the patient cope with personal and family problems
   b. To help the patient cope with stressful life circumstances and his or her responses to them
   c. To help the patient with both medical problems that are present, and to cope with the stresses of life (family, occupational, or other)
   d. To help the patient with medical problems and to help the patient recognize that they have underlying emotional problems

11. Dysmorphic disorders are conditions in which the person:
   a. Places undue emphasis on a particular personality trait
   b. Places undue emphasis on a particular physical characteristic
   c. Places undue emphasis on interpersonal relations
   d. Places undue emphasis on physical symptoms

12. Anxiety encompasses a wide range of feelings and fears, including:
   a. A mild sense of impending disaster
   b. Mental anguish
   c. A relationship between the anxiety and a specific cause
   d. Physical symptoms: palpitations, profuse sweating, restlessness

13. Obsessive-compulsive disorder is characterized by:
   a. Occasional thoughts or mental images that are weird or horrible, but transient
   b. Meticulousness, perfectionism, and rigidity
   c. Repetitive, purposeful, but senseless actions such as washing hands 100 times a day
   d. A combination of frequent intrusive thoughts, images, or ideas that appear silly, weird, nasty, or horrible, and of repetitive, senseless actions that result from the thoughts and images; the thoughts (obsessions) and the actions (compulsions) are linked.

14. Most psychosocial disorders must be present for a specific period of time before a definitive diagnosis can be made. The period of time is usually:
   a. 1 month
   b. 2 months
   c. 6 months
   d. 12 months

15. Personality evolves from:
   a. Genetic inheritance
   b. Environmental influences throughout infancy and childhood
   c. Interactions between inborn factors and environmental influences
   d. A combination of inborn factors: intelligence, temperament, sociability, emotionality, and relationships with parents and others

16. The impact of affective disorders on public health is:
   a. Minimal
   b. Moderate
   c. Severe
   d. Extremely severe

17. The risk for first-degree relatives to develop a major affective disorder is:
   a. 2% to 3%
   b. 5% to 7%
   c. 10% to 15%
   d. 20%

18. The only drug that has been unequivocally established as effective in preventing relapses in patients with bipolar disorder is:
   a. Benadryl
   b. Cogentin
   c. Selective serotonin reuptake inhibitor
   d. Lithium

19. Even with modern therapy, the percentage of patients with severe major depression may not fully recover for:
   a. 6 months
   b. 1 year
   c. 2 years
   d. 3 years

20. The cause of schizophrenia is:
   a. Unknown
   b. Believed to have a genetic basis

c. Viewed as occurring in persons with neurologically based vulnerabilities

d. The result of interaction between the patient and the environment

21. Disorders formerly called "affective" are now termed:
    a. Transient disorders
    b. Depressive disorders
    c. Adjustment disorders
    d. Unipolar disorders

22. Persons with depressive symptoms function more poorly than those with _____ major chronic medical conditions (e.g., arthritis, coronary artery disease, myocardial infarction):
    a. 3
    b. 6
    c. 9
    d. 12

23. Patients who have terminal illnesses and who may fear death are overwhelmed with:
    a. Helplessness
    b. Terror
    c. Regret
    d. Hopelessness

24. Bereaved persons usually show at least partial recovery from grief by:
    a. 3 weeks
    b. 5 weeks
    c. 10 weeks
    d. 5 months

25. Most patients with depression who seek professional help do not complain of:
    a. Physical symptoms
    b. Emotional (depressive) symptoms
    c. Sleeplessness
    d. Anorexia

26. One of the plants used as alternative medicine is said to be a "natural antidepressant." That plant is:
    a. St. John's wort
    b. Peppermint
    c. Licorice
    d. Ginseng

27. The only medication to date that prevents relapses in patients with bipolar disorder is:
    a. Prozac
    b. Zoloft
    c. Prolixin
    d. Lithium

28. All but one of the following are signs and symptoms of schizophrenia. The one that is NOT applicable to these patients is:
    a. Loss of contact with reality
    b. Hallucinations
    c. Wide range of emotions
    d. Delusions

29. In _____, the American Psychiatric Association (APA) stated that homosexuality is not a psychiatric disorder, since for most it is not a matter of choice:
    a. 1965
    b. 1973
    c. 1989
    d. 1997

30. "Core gender identity" is:
    a. The objective expression of one's gender
    b. The inner sense of masculinity or femininity
    c. The genetic determination of gender
    d. The subjective sense of knowing to which gender one belongs

23

Care of the Aging Adult

AGING

Definition

- Biologic aging: refers to changes in structure and functions of the body that occur over the life span.
- Functional aging: refers to the capacities of individuals for functioning in society, as compared with those of others of the same age.
- Psychologic aging: refers to behavioral changes, alterations in self-perception, and reactions to the biologic changes that occur over time.
- Sociologic aging: has to do with the roles and social habits of individuals in society.

Incidence

- Persons over age 65 are generally placed in the category of older persons.
- About 33.2 million Americans are over age 65, which is 13% of the total population.
  —19.7 million: 65 to 74 years of age
  —12 million: 75 to 84 years of age
  —5 million: 85+ years of age
- In the year 2000, one in every five Americans is 65 or over.
- The most rapidly growing segment of elderly are those 85 and older.
  —In year 2000, the number is over 5 million.

The Process of Aging

- One does not suddenly become "old" at age 65.
- Aging, as with all other developmental stages, is a linear process.
  —The rate at which the elderly lose functions does not increase with age.

—A 35-year-old is aging as fast as an 85-year-old.
- Illness is common among the elderly, but symptoms cannot be ascribed simply to "aging."
- Hypochondria is far less common among the elderly than among younger people.
- When an elderly person calls for an ambulance, it is usually with good reason, although the reason may not be what the patient says it is.
- Dementia occurs in no more than 10% of the elderly and is not a normal part of the aging process.

THEORIES OF AGING

- Different disciplines have developed theories of aging, which include the following:
  —Biologic theories of aging
  —Sociologic theories of aging
  —Psychologic theories of aging

Biologic Theories

- **Biologic theories of aging** are divided into three major categories (Table 23-1).
—Genetic mutation theories
  ~ Age is the result of accumulated mutations in the deoxyribonucleic acid (DNA) in the body cells → progressive impairment of function.
  ~ Research has focused on the role of telomerase, an enzyme expressed in germ cells, not in body cells.
  ~ Telomeres, the ends of chromosomes, appear to shorten with each cell cycle in body cells → decrease in cell reproductive capacity and, ultimately, cell death.

TABLE 23-1
Biologic Theories of Aging: Alternative Concepts

Theory	Components
Cellular senescence	Other than stem cells, human cells have a finite capacity to replicate; limited replication is an expression of programmed genetic events.
Programmed loss of genetic material (codon restriction)	Loss of redundant DNA sequences with repeated cell divisions results in decreased functional capacity. At afixed point in life, cells begin to manufacture a substance that inhibits protein synthesis.
Accumulation of random errors (disposable soma)	Random mutations progressively accumulate during transcription or translation. Random errors in protein synthesis ultimately impair synthesis or function.
Error catastrophe (obligate aging)	Cells develop serious defects in genes normally repair errors in DNA synthesis or in transcription, resulting in faulty protein synthesis or function.
Free radical oxidative damage (waste product accumulation)	Oxygen-free radicals produced during oxidative metabolism or resulting from radiation exposure may result in damage to DNA, particularly mitochondrial DNA.
Telomere shortening	Duplication of DNA during cell division is incomplete in somatic cells, leading to shortening of chromosome ends (telomeres). Length of telomeres is proportionate to remaining replicative capacity. Telomerase protects against shortening in germ and stem cells.
Decreased heat shock response	Heat shock proteins, which mediate cellular response to various stressors, exhibit reduced expression with aging.
Glycosylation of proteins and nucleic acids (cross-linkage)	Advanced glycosylation end (AGE) products increase with age, cross-linking proteins (e.g., collagen) and nucleic acids, and altering their function.
Age-of-onset modifier	Modifier genes, which normally suppress degenerative effects, are inactivated because reproductive potential has been exhausted.
Rate of living	Life span is inversely related to the metabolic rate of the organism.
Endocrine deficiency	The endocrine system acts as a pacemaker for aging.
Neural pacemaker	The central nervous system determines the time of onset of aging and the rate at which it proceeds.
Immune system decline	Decline of immune function results in decreased defense and increased autoantibody formation.

From Hansen, M: *Pathophysiology: foundations of disease and clinical intervention,* Philadelphia, 1998, WB Saunders, p 127

~ Telomerase protects germ cells from this process by making a DNA copy of its own ribonucleic acid (RNA), then fusing this strand to the chromosomal end, which prevents shortening.
~ Manipulation of telomerase to inhibit cancer growth or to slow the aging process is currently under intensive investigation.
—Oxidative stress theories
~ Derived from current knowledge that reactive oxygen species (oxygen-free radicals) are generated randomly in any cell with oxidative metabolism.
  – These are believed to be potentially damaging to cells because of their ability to combine chemically with enzymes and structural proteins and to induce breaks in DNA.
  – Mitochondrial DNA is probably particularly vulnerable to this type of damage because of its proximity to the oxidative metabolism machinery.
  – Antioxidant enzymes (e.g., superoxide dismutase) usually clear most of the radicals before cell damage occurs.
  – Activity of these enzyme systems decreases with age.
  – Lipofuscin, the purported biomarker of aging, may be an auto-oxidation product of lipids, proteins, and perhaps DNA.
—Genetic program theories
~ Specific genes program senescence and cell death.
~ Those who support this theory say that because maximal life span is genetically determined, the aging process is, too.

~ According to this theory, regulatory processes turn off expression of some genes, and turn on others.

~ Evidence that supports this theory is the degree of variability of life span in mammals, from 2 to 100 years, which indicates a developmental basis for longevity.

~ Additional evidence is attributed to patients with progeria, a condition that produces accelerated aging due to a known genetic defect, who display pronounced shortening of chromosomal telomeres.

Sociologic Theories

- These theories focus on the roles and relationships in which individuals participate in their later years and an adaptation to accepted societal values.
- *Disengagement theory*—this theory proposes that aging is a developmental task in and of itself, associated with particular patterns of behavior that result from simply growing older.
  —This theory assumes that the aging person ceases to focus on society and the community, and gradually withdraws by virtue of becoming "old" (Cumming and Henry, 1961).
  —As might have been expected, people (particularly older people) dismiss this theory as not being valid; older people do not tend to withdraw but continue to be active in their churches and communities for as long as they are able (Havighurst, Neugarten, and Tobin, 1963).
- *Activity theory*—proposes the opposite of the disengagement theory, in that older people remain active, which in itself is a sign of "healthy aging."
- *Continuity theory*—proposes that how a person has been throughout life is how the person will continue through the remainder of life; individuals change very little over time. If they were active and outgoing when they were younger, they most likely would behave in exactly the same way as they aged.
- *Age-stratification theory*—in the 1970s, aging theories began to focus more on societal and structural factors: how the aging person is viewed by others. The major premise of this theory is the interdependence of the older adult with society, and how each influences the other in many ways (Riley, Johnson, and Foner, 1972).

- *Person-environment fit theory*—presented by Lawton (1982), this theory relates the individual's personal competence within the environment in which he or she interacts; it examines the concept of interrelationships between the competence of a group of people, older adults, and their society or environment.
  —As the person ages, changes may occur in some of his or her individual competencies.
  —As a person ages, the environment may become more threatening and make one feel incompetent to deal with it.
  —With rapid advances in technology in all areas, this theory may explain why older persons might feel intimidated by the chaos and noise around them and tend to become more isolated.

Psychologic Theories

- There is no one theory or definition of aging.
- Using an eclectic approach by incorporating concepts from all areas (biology, sociology, psychology) will provide a comprehensive perspective of aging.
- Psychologic theories of aging are intertwined with both biologic and sociologic theories of aging and thus cannot be separated from either (Birren and Cunningham, 1985).
- As a person ages psychologically, adaptive changes take place that assist the person to cope with or accept some of the biologic changes.
  —These adaptive mechanisms include memory, learning capacity, feelings, intellectual functioning, and motivation to engage or not engage in particular activities.
- Psychologic aging incorporates both behavioral changes and also developmental aspects related to the older adult.

Maslow's Hierarchy of Human Needs Theory

- Maslow (1954) proposed that all persons have specific needs that motivate behavior.
- The needs are prioritized automatically, without thinking; like a step ladder, as the lowest order of needs are satisfactorily met, and only then, the person moves to the next level.
  —Basic biologic and physiologic needs (e.g., food, shelter, clothing)

—Next in priority are safety and security needs (e.g., a lock on the door)
—Belonging: being loved, cherished, accepted
—Self-esteem comes when the lower order needs are satisfied
—At the highest level is self-actualization: the individual at this level is able to perceive reality; accepts himself or herself, others, and all of nature; exhibits spontaneity; is able to problem solve; becomes self-directive; develops a need for privacy and time alone; finds freshness and joy in new experiences; identifies with other human beings; develops satisfying and changing relationships; has a democratic character structure; has a sense of values; and is able to be creative.
• Some analysts of this theory estimate that complete self-actualization is achieved by only 1% of the population, including older persons; age alone does not guarantee self-actualization.

Jung's Theory of Individualism
• In 1960 Swiss-born Carl Jung proposed this theory of personality development as continuing throughout life stages: childhood, adolescence, young adulthood, middle age, and old age.
—The personality, he said, is composed of the ego, the personal unconsciousness, and the collective unconsciousness.
—Individual personality is oriented either toward the external world (extroverted) or toward the subjective, inner experiences (introverted).
~ These two characteristics are present in everyone; a balance between them is essential for good mental health.
—Jung's theory states that it is during middle age that individuals question their values and beliefs, as well as past accomplishments and those things that, although considered very important, are still not accomplished, thus constituting the so-called "midlife crisis," which may last variable lengths of time.
~ Part of this process is determining whether one's "true self" has emerged and has reached certain goals.

—Successful aging, says Jung, is when a person can look deeply inside himself or herself and is able to evaluate and value past accomplishments and accept one's limitations.

Course of Human Life Theory
• Buhler (1968) proposed this theory that describes human development based on an extensive study of biographic materials and personal interviews.
—The author identifies five phases that individuals pass through in attaining personal life goals.
~ Childhood: the future is vague, and no formal goals are set.
~ Adolescence and young adulthood: by age 25, most persona have a sense of their own potential, and begin to set definite life goals (but keep in mind Maslow's hierarchy of needs).
~ Middle years: the individual begins the process of "life review," evaluates what has or has not been accomplished, and revises his or her life goals in a more realistic context.
~ Old age (65 to 70), says Buhler, is a time to no longer aspire to accomplish major life goals.

Erikson's Stages of Life Theory
• In 1950 Eric Erikson proposed a theory regarding psychologic development that reflects cultural and societal influences, involving the individual's ego structure (sense of self).
• In each stage, a "crisis" occurs that influences the development of the person's ego, having to do with the degree of success, or lack of success, in mastering the stage of development.
• The stages of development for people 40 to 65 years of age and for those over 65 years of age, their characteristics, and consequences are outlined in Table 23-2.
• Peck (1968) revised Erikson's eighth stage of life because of increased longevity of people. He developed a stage for "old-old," expanding the stage of ego integrity versus despair into three stages:
—Ego differentiation versus work role preoccupation

TABLE 23-2
Erikson's Theory: Middle and Late Adulthood

Stages and Ages	Characteristics of Stage	Consequences
Generativity versus *Self-Absorption* or *Stagnation* ages 40-65 yrs Mode: Nurturing Virtue: Care	Middle-aged adult becomes concerned about guiding and supporting next generation; looks beyond self, expresses concern for future of world in general.	Self-absorbed adult will be preoccupied with personal well-being and material gains. Preoccupation with self leads to stagnation in life.
Ego integrity versus *despair* (age 65 yrs to death) Mode: Acceptance Virtue: Wisdom	Older adult can look back with sense of satisfaction and acceptance of life and death.	Unsuccessful resolution of this crisis may result in sense of despair in which individual views life as a series of misfortunes, disappointments, and failures.

Modified from Potter PA, Perry AG: *Fundamentals of nursing*, ed 3, St. Louis, 1993, Mosby.

~ The task for the older adult is to achieve identity and feelings of worth from sources other than the work role.

~ The person with a well-differentiated ego, who is defined by many dimensions, can replace the work role as the major defining factor regarding self-esteem.

~ The task can be accomplished by focusing on satisfactions derived from interacting with family and friends.

—Body transcendence versus body perception

~ The task is to adjust to or transcend the declines that may occur to maintain feelings of well-being.

~ The task can be unsuccessfully resolved by focusing on the satisfaction obtained from interpersonal interactions and psychosocial-related activities.

—Ego transcendence versus ego preoccupation

~ The task is for the individual to reach acceptance of impending death without morbidly dwelling on it.

~ Acceptance can be achieved by remaining actively involved with the future that extends beyond one's mortality.

PREVENTION OF DISEASE IN THE ELDERLY

• Measures to prevent disease, or to limit its effects, are important for all age groups and particularly for the elderly.

—Current immunizations for influenza, pneumococcal pneumonia, and tetanus

—Mammogram every 2 years until age 75

—Risk/benefits are the basis for prescribing daily low-dose aspirin and hormone replacement therapy (HRT).

~ Data to date do not support these as routine practice, but if the patient is taking one or both without side effects (e.g., bleeding from aspirin), the person can continue.

• Osteoporosis

—Calcium intake: about 1500 mg with 400 to 800 IU of vitamin D daily.

—Consider prescribing drug that diminishes bone loss.

• Regardless of age, individuals should be encouraged to stop using tobacco, and to limit intake of alcohol to two drinks/day, preferably wine over hard liquors.

• Treat hypertension to reduce both systolic and diastolic pressure.

—Older patients apparently derive greater benefit from hypertensive therapy than younger individuals.

~ Begin with low dose of thiazide diuretic, add low-dose reserpine, atenolol, or angiotensin-converting enzyme (ACE) daily; these drugs have minimal side effects.

• Annual dental care should be provided as needed.

• Annual visual examination by an ophthalmologist is needed to diagnose and treat eye problems (e.g., glaucoma, retinal signs of disease).

• Both hypothyroidism and hyperthyroidism are difficult to detect clinically in older persons.

—Require serum thyroid-stimulating hormone (TSH) test annually
- Test for cholesterol levels if indicated and if the patient has heart disease, or, in the absence of heart disease, the patient is amenable to treatment to lower cholesterol.
- The Papanicolaou test should be done every 2 years but need not be done after two negative test results have been obtained.
- Tuberculosis (TB) test (purified protein derivative [PPD]) should be done on everyone at risk of having or contracting TB: residents of nursing homes, those living in group homes, those with a family history.
- Exercise to tolerance should be encouraged, regardless of age, particularly walking and resistance training.

- Achievement of ideal weight for height and age
  —Increase or decrease intake to achieve weight gain or loss
    ~ Assessment/screening of older people (Box 23-1)
- High-risk elderly
  —Over age 75
  —Living alone
  —Depressed/bereaved
  —Cognitively impaired
  —Frail: history of falls, bruising, trauma
  —Bowel or bladder dysfunction
  —Weight problem: obese or anorectic
- Unique problems among older people
  —Dysfunction should be related to disease rather than to age in years; most older people are relatively well.

BOX 23-1

Annual Screening Assessment* for People 70 Years of Age and Older

HISTORY
Medications currently taking
Physical activity—activities of daily living
Falls in past 12 months
Appetite—increase or decrease in weight
Tobacco/alcohol use
Bowel and bladder function: incontinence, constipation, diarrhea, flatus, bleeding
Problems with driving
Activity, exercise
Socialization—groups, meetings, concerts
Ability to manage money, shopping, make telephone calls (instrumental activities of daily living

LABORATORY TESTS
CBC*
Vitamin B_{12}, folate
Electrolytes, liver function tests
Cholesterol, lipids
Glucose
TSH
TB—2-step Mantoux
Urinalysis
ECG*
Chest x-ray

REFERRAL AS INDICATED
Gynecologist
Ophthalmologist
Dentist
Ear, nose, and throat
Gastroenterologist
Home care organization/provide

PHYSICAL EXAMINATION
Skin
Gait
BP*—both arms, standing, sitting
Weight, height
Vision
Hearing
Heart, lungs
Breasts
Rectal—men and women
Pelvic
Reflexes
Legs and feet—ulcers, varicosities, toenails
Mini-Mental State Examination (MMSE)
Geriatric Depression Scale (GDS)

IMMUNIZATIONS
Influenza
Pneumovax
Tetanus
Other as indicated

CANCER SCREENS
Mammogram
Papanicolaou
Fecal occult blood
Sigmoidoscopy/colonoscopy
PSA*—men

CBC, Complete blood count; *ECG,* electrocardiogram; *BP,* blood pressure; *PSA,* prostate-specific antigen.
*Annual assessment: monitors all of the areas listed, with specific action (specific test, referral) decided on every year to maintain optimal health.

—Respond differently to illness, injury, and medications than younger people do

—More likely to develop toxic reactions to drugs

—Do not tolerate fluid loads well, particularly intravenously (IV)

—Many physiologic capacities are diminished.

—The "normal" signs and symptoms of disease may be markedly altered in the elderly.

~ Myocardial infarction may occur without chest pain.

~ Pneumonia may be present with minimal fever.

~ Diabetes that is out of control may present more as hyperosmolar coma than as ketoacidosis.

~ Some serious diseases (e.g., congestive heart failure, acute abdomen) may present as an acute confusional state (delirium).

• The older the patient, the more likely it is that he or she has multiple problems.

—One study showed that people over 65 years of age had an average of 3.5 disabilities.

—Among older people admitted to a hospital, the average number of problems is six.

—The most common problems are hypertension, heart disease, diabetes, depression, chronic renal failure, venous insufficiency in the lower legs, and arthritis.

—When several organ systems are borderline in function, the effects of only one disease may have repercussions throughout the body, leading to the failure of one system after another—the "domino effect" (Table 23-3).

TABLE 23-3
Effects of Aging on Organ Systems

Organ System	Physiologic Effects	Related Diseases
Immune	Thymic involution, decreased immune response, increased circulating autoantibodies, increased circulating immunocomplexes	Infections, neoplasia, autoimmune disorders
Hematopoietic	Inconclusive evidence of decreased bone marrow function	Anemia, leukemia, gammopathy, multiple myeloma, polycythemia
Endocrine	Increased thyroid nodules, decreased glucose tolerance, decreased immune function of Langerhans' cells	Hypothyroidism and hyperthyroidism, type II diabetes mellitus
Cardiovascular	Some cardiac enlargement, decreased aortic compliance, decreased cardiac output, decreased cardiac reserve, arteriosclerosis	Atherosclerosis, aortic stenosis, coronary heart disease, peripheral vascular disease, hypertension, congestive heart failure, dysrhythmias
Respiratory	Weaker intercostal muscles, thoracic rigidity, decreased pulmonary defenses	Pneumonia, influenza, tuberculosis, chronic obstructive pulmonary disease, lung cancer
Musculoskeletal	Decreased bone mass, decreased joint mobility, postural changes	Osteoarthritis, rheumatoid arthritis, gout, osteoporosis, fractures, Paget's disease
Gastrointestinal	Atrophy of secretory cells, decreased motility, decreased salivation, decreased absorptive surface area, decreased gallbladder emptying, decreased liver function	Dental caries, periodontal disease, dysphagia, hiatal hernia, esophageal cancer, gastritis, gastric cancer, bowel obstruction, malabsorption, cholecystitis, cholelithiasis, constipation, incontinence, colorectal cancer, polyps, diverticulitis, hemorrhoids
Reproductive	Decreased sexual function, menopause, breast changes: fibrosis, vulvar and vaginal atrophy	Benign prostatic hyperplasia, prostatic cancer, uterine prolapse, cystocele, rectocele, erectile dysfunction, ovarian cancer, breast cancer
Integumentary	Uneven pigmentation, dryness, wrinkling, flattened epidermal junction, hair loss, hair graying, increased epidermal turnover, increased or decreased dermal vasculature, decreased subcutaneous fat, decreased sweating	Hypothermia, hyperthermia, xerosis, pruritus, skin tumors, pressure ulcers, herpes zoster, photoaging

From Hansen M: *Pathophysiology: foundations of disease and clinical intervention,* Philadelphia, 1998, WB Saunders, p 129.

—Drug therapy for a major condition may be contraindicated for problems in one or more other body systems (e.g., renal failure).
- Older persons are more likely to have adverse reactions to drugs.
  —Changes in drug metabolism because of diminished hepatic function
  —Changes in body composition and distribution of drugs through the different body compartments
  —Changes in elimination of drugs because of diminished renal function
  —Changes in the responsiveness to drugs by the central nervous system
- Older people experience greater influence on physical disease from psychosocial factors.
  —Although the body and the mind operate simultaneously throughout life, particular stresses are associated with aging that can make people more susceptible to illnesses.
    ~ Retirement
    ~ Bereavement
    ~ Loneliness
    ~ Isolation

PROBLEMS ENCOUNTERED IN OLDER PERSONS
Signs and Symptoms

- Clinical manifestations of aging include those related to decreased cellular proliferation: poor wound healing, cataracts, osteoporosis, decreased glucose tolerance; and those related to increased cellular proliferation: cancer, prostatic hypertrophy, osteoarthritis, and skin lesions/masses.
- Older persons become more dissimilar as they age, contrary to prevailing stereotypes, which indicate that people become more alike.
- As people age, they are more likely to have multiple health problems, disability, and side effects from drugs.
- Because of impaired compensatory mechanisms, older persons often present with disease at earlier stages.
- Disease presentation is frequently atypical in the elderly.

SPECIFIC DISORDERS OF OLDER PEOPLE

- Sleep disorders
  —Sleep disorders are classified into four groups according to signs and symptoms.
    ~ Disorders of initiating sleep (insomnia)
    ~ Disorders of excessive somnolence
      - Excessive DAYTIME sleep (pickwickian syndrome)
      - Hypersomnia sleep apnea (hypersomnia sleep apnea [HAS] syndrome—lack of breathing during sleep)
    ~ Disorders of the sleep-wake cycle
    ~ Dysfunctions of sleep, the sleep stages, or partial arousals
- Dehydration
  —Dry mucous membranes in tongue
  —Longitudinal furrows in tongue
  —Weak upper body muscles
  —Confusion
  —Difficulty in speaking
  —Sunken eyes, cheeks
- Trauma
  —About 9500 elderly die every year as a result of falls.
  —About 40% of older people fall at least once a year.
  —The risk of falling increases markedly after age 65.
  —Most falls do not result in serious injury.
    ~ Risk of fractures or death from falls increases with age.
  —Because many older women have osteoporosis, falls can result from fractures, rather than fractures occurring as the result of falls.
  —The cause of falls in the elderly is divided between extrinsic or accidental causes (tripping over a doorway), and intrinsic, as a result of dizziness or palpitations that result in faintness.
  —Motor vehicle accidents are the second leading cause, after falls, of accidental death among older persons.
    ~ There are 13 million licensed drivers over age 65 in the United States.
    ~ The risk of fatal injury in a traffic accident is five times higher than for younger people.
    ~ Causes of motor vehicle accidents include impaired vision and/or hearing, errors in judgment, underlying medical conditions, impaired reflexes/rapid responses.
    ~ About 2000 pedestrian fatalities occur among older people every year.

- Specific injuries
  —Head trauma: from falls (can result in intracranial bleeding)
  —Enlarged subarachnoid space
  —Decrease in supportive tissue of the meninges
  —Subdural hematoma
    ~ Often develops slowly, over days or weeks.
    ~ Initial trauma may be trivial.
    ~ Headache, worse at night
    ~ Change in level of consciousness → drowsy
- Cervical spinal cord injury/cord compression
  —Degenerative changes in the cervical spine—cervical spondylosis → pressure on the nerve roots
- Rib fractures, flail chest from brittle bones, stiffening of chest wall
- Abdominal trauma → liver injury: tear, bruise
- Hip fractures
- Management of trauma in the elderly
  —In establishing airway, check for dentures.
  —In assessing breathing, check for rib fracture.
  —In assessing circulation, check blood pressure.
    ~ Consider hypovolemia in older person whose systolic blood pressure is less than 120 mm Hg
    ~ In replacing fluids, slow infusion to prevent congestive heart failure
  —Neurologic assessment should include level of consciousness and status of pupils.
  —Start IV with lactated Ringer's, but use extreme caution in administering IV fluids to prevent overload/congestive heart failure.
  —Monitor cardiac rhythm, check for dysrhythmias.
  —Immobilize the cervical spine before moving the patient.
  —Pad the backboard generously with pillows and/or blankets; best is whole-body vacuum splint.

MEDICAL EMERGENCIES IN OLDER PERSONS

- Acute myocardial infarction
- Symptoms may include the following:
  —Chest pain: declines from 76% (under 70) to 38% (over 85)
  —Dyspnea: 38% (under 70) to 43% (over 85)
  —Syncope: increases from 9% (under 70) to 18% (over 85)
  —Stroke: 2% (under 70) to 7% (over 85)
  —Confusion: 3% (under 70) to 19% (over 85)
  —Weakness: 7% (under 70) to 10% (over 85)
  —Dizziness: 6% to 5%
  —Palpitations: 4% to 1%
  —Vomiting: 18% to 16%
  —Sweating: 36% to 14%
  —Silent: remains about 2% to 3%
- Congestive heart failure
  —Very common among elderly
  —Presentation may be atypical
    ~ Acute confusional state (reduced cerebral oxygen)
  —History of multiple episodes of nocturnal confusion ("sundowning")
  —Blisters on the legs: translucent, multiple, often large
    ~ Result from sleeping in a chair at night, maintaining increased hydrostatic pressure in already edematous legs
  —Crackles often heard at the lung bases in the elderly, without pathology
- Delirium
  —Acute confusional state
    ~ Common presenting sign in the elderly
    ~ Occurs in up to 25% of hospitalized elderly
    ~ Can be associated with almost any physical condition, drug toxicity
    ~ Often begins abruptly, at night
    ~ All mental functions become disordered: memory, thinking, judgment, perceptions.
    ~ Hallucinations are common.
    ~ Usually disoriented as to time and place
    ~ Level of consciousness may be depressed or hyperalert
    ~ Sleep-wake cycles often reversed
- (See Chapter 6 for characteristics of delirium and dementia.)
- Depression and suicide in the elderly
  —Depression is common.
  —About 25% of all suicides occur among people over age 65.
  —Older men, especially unmarried, divorced, widowed, are at highest risk.
  —In assessing depression, ask specifically about thoughts of suicide ("Have you ever thought that you just can't go on any more?").

—If patient answers yes to this question, ask about thoughts of suicide, how he or she might commit suicide, if he or she has a very concrete plan for how suicide would occur; the patient is at very high risk and should be placed on suicide precautions.

- Pharmacologic problems/toxicities in the elderly
  —The elderly consume more than 25% of all prescribed and over-the-counter (OTC) drugs in the United States.
  —More than 80% of elderly take at least one prescribed drug.
  —Those in nursing homes take an average of 5 to 12 different medications daily.
  —Drug reactions account for up to 30% of hospital admissions among elderly.
  —Patients may be taking medications prescribed by more than one physician.
  —The best dosage of a drug is the lowest that will achieve a therapeutic effect.
  —Drugs that most commonly cause toxic reactions in the elderly include the following:
    ~ Digitalis
    ~ Diuretics
    ~ Analgesics, narcotics, aspirin
    ~ Sedative and hypnotic drugs
    ~ Phenothiazines
    ~ Anticoagulants
    ~ Theophylline
    ~ Propranolol
    ~ Quinidine
    ~ Lidocaine
    ~ Steroids
- When transporting an elderly patient to the hospital in an ambulance, it s best not to use the siren unless there is a clear need for it.

BIBLIOGRAPHY

Birren JE, Cunningham WR: Research on the psychology of aging. In Birren JE, Schaie KW, eds: *Handbook of the psychology of aging*, New York, 1983, Van Nostrand Reinhold.

Buhler C: The development structure of goal setting in group and individual studies. In Buhler C, Massack F, eds: *The course of human life*, New York, 1968, Springer.

Caroline NL: *Emergency care in the streets*, ed 5, Boston, 1995, Little, Brown.

Cassel CK, Cohen HJ, Larson EB, et al, eds: *Geriatric medicine*, ed 3, New York, 1997, Springer-Verlag.

Cumming E, Henry W: *Growing old: the process of disengagement*, New York, 1961, Basic Books.

Erikson E: *Childhood and society*, New York, 1950, Norton.

Finucane TE: Geriatric medicine: Special considerations. In Barker LR, Burton JR, Zieve PD, eds: *Principles of ambulatory medicine*, ed 5, Baltimore, 1999, Williams & Wilkins.

Hansen M: *Pathophysiology: foundations of disease and clinical intervention*, Philadelphia, 1999, Saunders, pp 125-130.

Havighurst RJ: *Developmental tasks and education*, ed 7, New York, 1972, David McKay.

Havighurst RJ, Neugarten BL, Tobin SS: Disengagement, personality, and life satisfaction in the later years. In Hansen P, ed: *Age with a future*, Copenhagen, 1963, Munksgaard.

Kart CS, Metress EK, Metress SP: *Human aging and chronic disease*, Boston, 1992, Jones and Bartlett, pp 237-250.

Latchman DS: Transcription-factor mutations and disease, *N Engl J Med* 334(1):28-33, 1996.

Litgow GJ, Kirkwood TBL: Mechanisms and evolution of aging, *Science* 273:80, 1996.

Lueckenotte AG: *Gerontologic nursing*, St. Louis, 1996, Mosby.

Maslow A: *Motivation and personality*, New York, 1954, Harper & Row.

Maslow A: *Toward a psychology of being*, ed 2, Princeton, NJ, 1968, Van Nostrand Reinhold.

McCance KL, Huether SE: *Pathophysiology: the biologic bass for disease in adults and children*, ed 2, St. Louis, 1994, Mosby.

Peek R: Psychological development in the second half of life. In Neugarten B, ed: *Middle age and aging: a reader in social psychology*, Chicago, 1968, University of Chicago Press.

Resnick NM: Geriatric medicine. In Tierney LM, McPhee SJ, Papadakis MA, eds: *Current diagnosis & treatment 2000*, ed 39, New York, 2000, Lange Medical Books/McGraw-Hill, pp 47-70.

Riley MW, Johnson M, Foner A: *Aging and society*, vol 3, *a sociology of age stratification*, New York, 1972, Russell Sage Foundation.

Troncale JA: The aging process: Physiologic changes and pharmacologic implications, *Postgrad Med* 99(5):111-122, 1996.

US Bureau of the Census: Current Population Reports. Special Studies, *65+ in the United States*, Washington, DC, 1996, U.S. Government Printing Office, pp 23-190.

REVIEW QUESTIONS

1. Characteristics of healthy aging include all of the following EXCEPT:
   a. Is a developmental process at the cellular and other subsystem levels
   b. Incorporates age-related structural changes and loss of function
   c. Invariably includes symptoms of dementia
   d. Is a risk factor for specific diseases
2. Presentation of disease in the elderly is usually:
   a. Easy to diagnose because of its defined signs and symptoms
   b. Atypical, with barely recognizable symptoms
   c. Easy to diagnose because most older persons have only one disease
   d. Characterized by severe symptoms and inability to respond to questions

3. Of the following, which symptom is NOT one that most older people present with?
   a. Delirium
   b. Acute confusion
   c. Depression
   d. Weakness

4. Which of the following is NOT a theory of aging?
   a. Genetic mutation theories
   b. Telomere lengthening theories
   c. Oxidative stress theories
   d. Genetic program theories

5. Aging is considered to be/be a process of:
   a. Increasing pathology with advancing years
   b. Genetically determined
   c. Increased cellular atrophy
   d. Progressive, gradual functional decline

6. Many older people today were reared in an era when debilitation and frequent illnesses were considered part of normal aging. As a consequence, they do not seek health care until:
   a. They reach age 75 or more
   b. The disease is at such an early stage as to be undetectable
   c. The disease is at a very advanced stage
   d. The person is brought to the emergency room because of fracture

7. Most older patents:
   a. Cannot provide a reliable medical history because of memory deficits
   b. Often provide too many details for the history to be focused on the presenting problem
   c. Fail to mention extremely pertinent information, considering particular symptoms to be too trivial to be noted
   d. Generally are able to provide quite a reliable history

8. The total percentage of the U.S. population that represents all people over age 65 is:
   a. 7%
   b. 9%
   c. 10%
   d. 13%

9. Aging is considered to be:
   a. A developmental stage
   b. A process
   c. Rapid in onset and progression
   d. A nonlinear process

10. Which of the following is NOT included among biologic theories of aging?
    a. Genetic program theories
    b. Telomerase-mediated theories
    c. Genetic mutation theories
    d. Oxidative-stress theories

11. Which of the following does NOT relate to biologic theories of aging?
    a. Codon expansion
    b. Disposable soma (accumulation of random errors)
    c. Obligate aging
    d. Decreased heat shock response

12. Which of the following is NOT a sociologic theory of aging?
    a. Roles
    b. Behaviors
    c. Values of society
    d. Relationships

13. The sociologic theory that focuses on "behavior" is:
    a. Activity theory
    b. Age stratification theory
    c. Person-environment fit theory
    d. Disengagement theory

14. **True or False.** Psychologic theories of aging are intertwined with both biologic and sociologic theories of aging, and cannot be studied separately.
    a. True
    b. False

15. Maslow's hierarchy of needs shows that motivation to satisfy higher level needs:
    a. Is based on the age of the individual
    b. Is determined by emotional development of the individual
    c. Is stimulated when needs are met at a lower level
    d. Is not sustained throughout the life span of individuals

16. The Swiss psychologist Carl Jung stated that personality comprises three components. Which of the following is NOT included in Jung's personality components?
    a. The ego
    b. The superego
    c. Personal unconsciousness
    d. Collective consciousness

17. Erikson proposed that the life span incorporates stages. The number of stages is:
    a. Three
    b. Five
    c. Seven
    d. Eight

18. Erikson made three divisions of this final stage of life, of which all but one of the following is one of the stages. The one that is NOT a part of the final stage of life is:
    a. Role differentiation versus ego preoccupation
    b. Body transcendence versus body preoccupation
    c. Ego transcendence versus ego preoccupation
    d. Ego differentiation versus work role preoccupation

19. People over 65 years of age have, on the average, this number of disabilities:
    a. 1.5
    b. 2
    c. 2.5
    d. 3.5

20. When performing a history and physical examination on an older person, the nurse practitioner should look for:
    a. Signs and symptoms of aging
    b. Signs and symptoms of specific diseases
    c. Signs and symptoms of hypochondria
    d. Signs and symptoms of cognitive impairments

24

Genetics

The interacting influences of both genetic and environmental factors determine the development of every individual.

TERMS USED IN GENETICS

Acrocentric—term used to describe a chromosome in which the centromere lies close to one end, producing one long and one short arm.

Allele (allelomorph)—alternative form of a gene occupying the same locus on a particular chromosome.

Aneuploid—any chromosomal number that is not the exact multiple of the normal haploid number.

Autosome—any chromosome that is not a sex or mitochondrial chromosome; there are 22 pairs of autosomes in humans.

Bacteriophage—a bacterial virus; these are modified and used as vectors for deoxyribonucleic acid (DNA) cloning.

CDNA—complementary DNA synthesized from a messenger ribonucleic acid (mRNA) template by the enzyme *reverse transcriptase*.

Centromere—the point at which two chromatids of a chromosome are joined, and also where the spindle fibers become attached during mitosis and meiosis.

Character (trait)—an observable phenotypic feature of an individual.

Chromatid—one of two strands, held together by the centromere, that make up the chromosome as seen during cell division.

Chromatin—genomic DNA coiled and supercoiled in association with histone proteins.

Chromosomal aberration—an abnormality in the number or structure of a chromosome.

Chromosome—a thread-like body containing DNA and protein, situated in the nucleus, and carrying genetic information.

Clone—cells having the same genetic constitution and derived from a single cell by repeated mitoses.

Codon—three adjacent nucleotides in a nucleic acid that code for one amino acid.

Concordance—the occurrence of the same trait in both members of a pair of twins.

Deletion—the loss of a part of a chromosome.

Diploid—the number of chromosomes found in somatic cells (i.e., two sets).

DNA ligase—the enzyme that joins two DNA ends together.

DNA polymerase—the enzyme that replicates DNA.

Dominant—term used to describe a trait expressed in individuals who are heterozygous for a particular gene.

Episomal DNA—gene carrying DNA found outside the main genome (i.e., bacterial plasmids, mitochondrial DNA).

Eukaryote—organisms whose genome is bound by a nuclear membrane.

Euchromatin—regions of chromosomes that are not tightly coiled and therefore accessible for gene expression.

Exon—a segment of a gene that is represented in the final spliced mRNA product.

Expressivity—the degree to which the effect of a gene is expressed.

Gene—part of a DNA molecule that directs the synthesis of a specific polypeptide chain.

Gene pool—the total genetic information contained in all the genes in a breeding population at a given time.

Genetic marker—a genetically controlled phenotypic feature used in inheritance studies.

Genetics—the science of heredity and variation.

Genome—the total amount of genetic material in the cell.

Genotype—the genetic constitution of an individual.

Haploid—the number of chromosomes found in germ cells (i.e., one set).

Heterochromatin—condensed chromatin in which supercoiling prevents expression of the encoded genes.

Heterozygote—an individual possessing two different alleles at the corresponding loci on a pair of homologous chromosomes.

Histones—nuclear proteins that hold genomic DNA in coils and supercoils.

Homozygote—an individual possessing identical alleles at the corresponding loci on a pair of homologous chromosomes.

Hybridization—the pairing of complementary DNA or ribonucleic acid (RNA) strands to give DNA-DNA or DNA-RNA strands; for example, it is used to search for particular DNA fragments after Southern blotting.

Intron—a segment of a gene not represented in the final mRNA product because it has been removed through splicing together of exons on each side of it.

Karyotype—the number, size, and shape of the chromosomes in a cell.

Linkage—the co-segregation of two unrelated DNA sequences that are physically close together on the chromosome.

Linkage disequilibrium—the association of particular alleles at two linked loci more frequently than expected by chance.

Locus—the site of a gene on a chromosome.

Metacentric—term used to describe a chromosome in which the centromere lies in the middle.

Monosomy—a state in which one chromosome of a pair is missing.

Mosaics—patients with two different cell lines in their constitution.

Nondisjunction—failure of a chromosome pair to separate during cell division, resulting in both chromosomes passing to the same daughter cell.

Nucleotide—the basic unit of nucleic acids, which is made up of a pyrimidine or purine base, a pentose sugar, and a phosphate group.

Oncogenes—normal genes that, when altered in their structure or expression, contribute to the abnormal growth of cancer cells.

Penetrance—the proportion of individuals with a particular genotype who also have the corresponding phenotype; full penetrance occurs when a dominant trait is always seen in an individual with one such allele, or when a recessive trait is seen in all individuals possessing two such alleles.

Phenotype—the appearance of an individual, resulting from the effects of both environment and genes.

Plasmid—a simple circular DNA molecule derived from bacteria that can be modified and used as a vector for DNA cloning.

Ploidy—term that describes the number of chromosome sets, namely 23 = haploid (1 set), 46 = diploid (2 sets).

Polymerase chain reaction (PCR)—technique for rapid analysis of DNA; oligonucleotide primers corresponding to each end of DNA of interest are synthesized and amplified in genomic DNA, using DNA polymerase.

Positional cloning (or reverse genetics)—methodology used to isolate genes whose protein products are not known but whose existence can be inferred from the disease phenotype.

Prokaryote—organisms whose genome is not bound by a nuclear membrane.

Pulsed-field gel electrophoresis—technique for separation of large fragments of DNA.

Recessive—term used to describe a trait expressed in individuals who are homozygous for a particular gene but not seen in the heterozygote.

Restriction fragment length polymorphism (RFLPs)—when variations in noncoding DNA sequences affect restriction enzyme cleavage sites, DNA fragments of different sizes (RFLPs) will result from enzyme digestion.

RNA polymerase—the enzyme that synthesizes RNA, based on a DNA template.

Sex linkage—genes carried on the sex chromosomes.

"Somy"—term referring to the number of copies of an individual chromosome per cell (e.g., "trisomy"—three copies).

Splicing—removing the introns from an unprocessed RNA molecule.

Synteny—term used to describe genes on the same chromosome.

Transcription—the process by which an RNA molecule is synthesized from a DNA template.

Translation—the process by which genetic information from mRNA is "translated" into protein synthesis.

Translocation—the transfer of a piece of one chromosome to another nonhomologous chromosome.

Trisomy—representation of a chromosome three times rather than twice, giving a total of 47 chromosomes.

Transfer RNA (tRNA)—a molecule that carries a single amino acid (depending on its anticodon) and that brings the amino acid to the ribosome.

Vector—a DNA molecule used to carry DNA regions of interest.

Three types of genetically determined disorders are:

- *Mendelian (single-gene) mutations*—inherited in recognizable patterns.
- *Polygenic (multifactorial) conditions*—in which genetic mutations involve more than one gene, and nongenetic factors interact in ways that are not always clearly recognizable.
- *Chromosomal aberrations (abnormalities)*—including both structural defects and deviations from the normal number.

CONSTRUCTION OF THE PEDIGREE

- The chief method of genetic study shows the distribution of genetic traits among family members.
- Some familial disorders with identical **phenotypes** (observable features) are inherited in different patterns.
- Cleft palate may be caused by
  —Autosomal dominant gene
  —Autosomal recessive gene
  —X-linked recessive gene
  —Multifactorial condition (familial, with no predictable inheritance pattern)
  —In the pedigree chart: each individual is identified with 2 numbers (e.g., II, 3).
  —Generations are identified by Roman numerals (earliest at top, latest at bottom).

—Individuals within generations are numbered from left to right with Arabic numerals.

—A spouse, if included, also has 2 numbers (e.g., III, 5).

—Siblings are arranged by age, the oldest at the left.

—A particular trait or disease is studied beginning with the first affected person, called a **proband, propositus,** or **index case.**

—The siblings of the index case are identified first, then the parents and the parents' brothers and sisters and their children, then the grandparents, and so on.

—The number of relatives included depends on the inheritance pattern of the disease/ condition and the known information about family members.

SINGLE-GENE HUMAN DEFECTS

Single-gene disorders are the easiest to analyze and have been the most thoroughly studied. These may be autosomal or X-linked, dominant or recessive.

Autosomal Dominant Inheritance

- Typical pedigree
- Rules that apply
  —Every affected person has at least one affected parent.
  —Males and females are equally likely to be affected.
  —An affected person marrying a normal individual has an equal number of affected and normal children (on average).
- Normal children of an affected parent have normal children and grandchildren.
  —The trait can appear in every generation.
  —Heterozygotes are affected.
- Variations from above general rules
  —Gene penetrance and expressivity
    ~ Influenced by both environment and by the thousands of other genes that may change the expressivity of the specific gene
    ~ Persons with Waardenburg syndrome can have white forelock, deafness, hypertelorism, and heterochromia of iris; <20% have significant hearing loss. One may have only white forelock, but have children with severe congenital deafness.

~ Rarely, the gene's expressivity is so minimal that no abnormality can be seen clinically; the gene will appear to have skipped a generation. Yet the person with no apparent abnormality can pass the gene to children, who may develop all of the characteristics of a particular inherited disorder. This rare phenomenon is called lack of penetrance. Individuals with minimal expressivity are referred to as having a *forme fruste* of the disorder.

—Pleiotropy ("many forms")

~ A single-gene defect may produce multiple anomalies.

~ With *osteogenesis imperfecta,* which affects connective tissue, there are many variations such as fragile bones because they cannot be normally calcified and hypermobile joints which tend to dislocate easily. Minor abnormalities can go undetected.

—Mutations

~ New mutations are common in autosomal dominant disorders.

~ A germline mutation in one cell, which occurs early in the embryonic life of one parent when only a few germ cell precursors are present, can contribute a large number of affected cells to the developing gonad. In this case, it is impossible to predict the risk for offspring.

~ An example of one outcome from such a mutation is normal parents producing one or more achondroplastic dwarf children.

—Phenocopies

~ Rarely, an individual develops a syndrome exactly like that caused by a fresh mutation, but the individual apparently does not have the mutant gene and does not transmit the disorder to offspring.

~ In this case, the disorder is either not linked to genetic makeup or is caused by a different genotype.

—Sex-limited inheritance

~ Trait that appears in only one sex.

~ Males are usually affected because of X-linked inheritance patterns.

~ Differences between males and females with respect to sex hormones and other physiologic differences can greatly change the expressivity of an allele.

~ Premature baldness is an inherited autosomal dominant trait that is rarely expressed in females, likely because of the effect of female sex hormones.

—Homozygous dominant genotype

~ Occurs in the children of parents who are heterozygous (or homozygous) for the same dominant gene.

~ Parents with the same autosomal dominant abnormality can produce offspring with more severe anomalies than either parent might have.

~ Among these parents are increased numbers of spontaneous abortions and stillborns with multiple anomalies, perhaps showing that two dominant alleles may be potentially lethal.

~ In Huntington's disease, however, there are no phenotypic differences between heterozygotes and homozygotes regarding inheritance; a homozygote would have 100% affected offspring.

Autosomal Recessive Inheritance

• Typical pedigree (Fig. 24-1)
• There is a horizontal pattern in the pedigree, with a single generation affected.
• Consanguinity is an important factor in autosomal recessive disorders because both parents are highly likely to share the same mutant allele.
• Rules that apply
  —If an affected person is born to normal parents, both parents are heterozygotes; on average, $\frac{1}{4}$ of their offspring will be affected, $\frac{1}{2}$ will be heterozygotes, and $\frac{1}{4}$ will be normal.

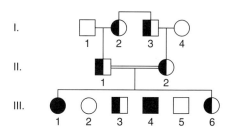

Fig. 24-1 Typical pedigree of autosomal recessive inheritance. (From Beers MH, Berkow R, eds: *The Merck manual of diagnosis and therapy,* ed 17, Whitehouse Station, NJ, 1999, Merck & Co, Inc.)

—If affected siblings derive from a consanguineous marriage, there is strong evidence of recessive inheritance.

—If an affected person marries a genotypically normal person, all offspring will be phenotypically normal heterozygotes.

—If an affected person marries a heterozygote person, on average, $^{1}/_{2}$ of their offspring will be affected, and $^{1}/_{2}$ will be heterozygotes.

—If two affected persons marry, all of their children will be affected.

—Males and females are equally likely to be affected.

—Heterozygotes are phenotypically normal but are carriers of the trait. If a specific protein, such as an enzyme, is identified as the cause of the disorder, the carrier usually has a reduced amount of the protein.

—Most diseases due to homozygosity for autosomal recessive mutant genes are rare, such as inborn errors of metabolism. Affected individuals are homozygous, and each parent is a heterozygote or a carrier.

X-Linked Dominant Inheritance

- Typical pedigree
- Rules that apply
  —Affected males transmit the trait to all of their daughters but none of their sons.
  —Affected heterozygote females transmit the disease to $^{1}/_{2}$ of their children regardless of sex.
  —Affected homozygous females transmit the trait to all of their children.
  —X-linked dominant mutants are very rare; females generally are more mildly affected than males.
  —In nephrogenic diabetes insipidus, females show mild symptoms of polydipsia and polyuria.
  —The X-linked gene for *incontinentia pigmenti* is apparently lethal in males, and causes a peculiar swirled pattern of melanin pigmentation and other anomalies in affected females.
- Because differentiation is difficult between X-linked dominant and autosomal dominant inheritance, large pedigrees are needed, with special focus on offspring of affected males because male-to-male transmission rules out X-linkage.

—New technology is alleviating this problem, as in the case of Alport's syndrome, which is hereditary nephritis with deafness, once considered an autosomal dominant trait. In this condition, affected males are very ill; therefore few males have reproduced. A few years ago, a new X-linked probe showed that the gene is on the X chromosome.

—Similarly, a gene probe can distinguish between the X-linked and the autosomal dominant forms of Charcot-Marie-Tooth disease, which causes peroneal muscular atrophy, making genetic counseling more accurate and helpful.

X-Linked Recessive Inheritance

- Typical pedigree
- Rules that apply
  —Nearly all affected persons are males.
  —The trait is always transmitted through the heterozygous mother, who is phenotypically normal.
  —An affected male never transits the trait to his sons.
  —All daughters of an affected male will be carriers.
  —The carrier female transmits the trait to $^{1}/_{2}$ of her sons.
  —None of her daughters will show the trait, but $^{1}/_{2}$ will be carriers.
- More than 300 traits (most of them diseases) are a result of mutant genes on the X chromosome.
- The male has only one X chromosome; the term hemizygous is used.
- All genes on the X chromosome, recessive or dominant, are expressed.
- An affected female must have the mutant allele in both X chromosomes. This can occur only if her father is affected and her mother is either heterozygous or homozygous for the mutant allele.
- Most X-linked mutants are rare; therefore affected females are very rare.
- One half of maternal uncles of the proband will be affected.
- One half of the maternal aunts will be carriers; therefore some of the proband's maternal first cousins will be affected.
- It can happen that females who are heterozygous for X-linked mutations show varying de-

grees of expression but almost never as severely as the affected hemizygous male.

- A structural chromosomal rearrangement, such as an X-autosome translocation, can occur in an affected female even though she is a heterozygote.

CODOMINANT INHERITANCE

- A trait or disease can be dominant or recessive, not the gene.
- Codominance can be seen only if the phenotypes are qualitatively different, as with blood group antigens (AB, MN), the white blood cell (WBC) antigens, and serum proteins, which differ in electrophoretic mobility (albumin, haptoglobin, and so on).
- Cases such as sickle cell disease cause confusion because heterozygotes are clinically normal and the condition is usually thought to be recessive. If, however, the phenotype is considered to be the sickle cell preparation, which is positive in both heterozygotes and homozygotes, the disorder can be considered dominant. The condition can also be considered codominant in terms of the hemoglobin (Hb) electrophoresis because the ratio of sickle Hb to normal Hb in the heterozygote is about 40:60.

Multifactorial Inheritance

Close relatives usually resemble one another with respect to such characteristics as height, weight, size and shape of nose, other facial features, blood pressure, and "intelligence." Many of these traits occur in a "normal distribution" pattern, which is congruent with determining a trait by a number of genes. Each gene adds to or subtracts from the trait, and each gene acts in an additive way independently of others, with no dominance.

Also, the effects of environmental factors will result in a normal distribution of traits. Variation within populations results from genes and environmental factors acting together to produce a final result. Many relatively common congenital anomalies and diseases are familial, but do not fit the pattern of mendelian inheritance. These affected persons have a predisposition to the condition, but the final result is based on the sum of genetic and environmental influences. First-

degree relatives have a high risk of particular traits because they share 50% of their genes; the risk decreases among more distant relatives, who inherit few of the high-risk genes.

An example is neural tube defects, which include anencephaly, encephalocele, and myelomeningocele, together known as spina bifida. In the North American white population, these conditions occur at the rate of 1.5/1000 live births. Parents, identified at the time of the birth of an affected infant as carrying a relatively large number of high-liability genes, have about a 1/30 chance of producing another affected child. A parent with a neural tube defect has about a 3% to 4% chance of having an affected child. If a couple has two affected children, their risk for having a third affected child rises to 7% or 8%.

Environmental factors unquestionably play a role in spina bifida defects. Research shows that daily oral supplements of folic acid both before conception and during early pregnancy substantially decreases the recurrence of neural tube defects. Other factors may very well be involved. Other examples of multifactorial inheritance include:

- Congenital anomalies of the heart
- Idiopathic epilepsy
- Congenital megacolon (Hirschsprung's disease)
- Cleft lip with or without cleft palate
- Many forms of cancer

Congenital pyloric stenosis has a 5:1 male/female ratio, indicating that the threshold for girls is higher, and that they require more potent liability genes to develop the condition, should have more affected siblings, and have a greater risk of producing affected offspring than a male with pyloric stenosis.

GENETIC HETEROGENEITY

Humans have an enormous capacity to vary, both phenotypically and genotypically. Heterogeneity occurs in almost all inborn errors of metabolism, resulting from different alleles or mutations at different loci (Table 24-1). For example, more than 12 mutations are known to produce the phenotype of Hurler's syndrome, and more than 60 specific causes of congenital deafness are known, both genetic and environmental. Environmental factors, such as smoking, drinking al-

TABLE 24-1
Representative Inborn Errors of Metabolism

Class of Defect	Example	Biochemical Defect	Inheritance
Aminoacidopathy	Phenylketonuria	Phenylalanine hydroxylase	AR
Connective tissue	Osteogenesis imperfecta type II	α1(1) and α2(1) procollagen	AD
Gangliosidosis	Tay-Sachs disease	Hexosaminidase A	AR
Glycogen storage disease	Type I	Glucose-6-phosphatase	AR
Immune function	Chronic granulomatous disease	Cytochrome b, β chain	XL
Lipid metabolism	Familial hypercholesterolemia	LDL receptor	AD
Mucopolysaccharidosis (MPS)	MPS II (Hunter's syndrome)	Iduronate sulfatase	XL
Porphyria	Acute intermittent	Porphobilinogen deaminase	AD
Transport	CF	CF transmembrane conductance regulator	AR

From Pyeritz RE: Medical genetics. In Tierney LM, McPhee SJ, Papadakis MA, eds: *Current medical diagnosis & treatment 1999*, Stamford CT, 1999, Appleton & Lange, p 1537.
AR, Autosomal recessive; *AD,* autosomal dominant; *XL,* X-linked recessive; *LDL,* low-density lipoprotein; *CF,* cystic fibrosis.

cohol, and taking drugs during pregnancy, can have devastating effects.

MITOCHONDRIAL DNA ABNORMALITIES

Mitochondria are intracellular organelles that generate energy via a series of respiratory chain complexes. They contain a unique circular chromosome that codes for 13 proteins, several kinds of RNAs, and a variety of regulating enzymes. More than 90% of the mitochondrial proteins are coded by nuclear genes.

Maternal inheritance is the rule with mitochondrial DNA in that mitochondria are passed on via the ova. Therefore all offspring of an affected female should be affected, and none of the offspring of an affected male.

Variability is common regarding the clinical manifestations and is likely due to mixtures of mutant and normal mitochondrial genomes within cells and tissues.

Conditions associated with mitochondrial DNA abnormalities include the following:
- Chronic progressive external ophthalmoplegia (CPEO)
- A variant of CPEO—Kearns-Sayre syndrome: CPEO, heart block, retinitis pigmentosa, and central nervous system (CNS) degeneration

- Pearson syndrome: sideroblastic anemia, pancreatic insufficiency, progressive liver disease that begins in infancy and is often fatal
- Leber's hereditary optic neuropathy: bilateral visual loss often occurring in adolescence
- Mitochondrial deletion in cells of the basal ganglia occurs in patients with Parkinson's disease, and research shows decreasing respiratory chain efficiency and progressive accumulation of mitochondrial DNA deletions related to aging, indicating that mitochondria have a role in the natural aging process.

GENETICS OF MALIGNANT DISEASE

Information is accumulating about the genetics of types of cancer: molecular genetics techniques confirm the existence of oncogenes (tumor genes), many of which are present in everyone. Normally, they are present and remain inactivated. However, new evidence indicates that the human genome is not as stable as was once thought; when some of these normal genes are relocated, rearranged, or broken as a result of chromosomal translocation or inversion, they may initiate a malignancy.

Although most malignancies occur in genetically predisposed individuals who are exposed to environmental carcinogens, some malignancies clearly show mendelian or multifactorial inheritance patterns.

- Familial polyposis of the colon—autosomal dominant condition
- Retinoblastoma—due in part to autosomal dominant genes
- Neuroblastoma—a malignancy of childhood
- Wilms' tumor—inherited mutation; specific chromosomal deletion (11p13).
- Xeroderma pigmentosum—rare, disfiguring syndrome due to autosomal recessive trait.
- Immunologic deficiency diseases, e.g., agammaglobulinemia—carry a risk of malignancy of the lymphoid system: lymphomas and leukemias.
- Persons with Down syndrome develop leukemia 15 times more often than the general population.
- Carcinoma of the breast occurs significantly more often in daughters whose mothers have had the condition.
- Cancer of the lung—first-degree relatives of persons with lung cancer appear to be significantly more at risk, especially if they smoke cigarettes.

SYNDROMES ASSOCIATED WITH AUTOSOMAL ABERRATIONS

- Down syndrome (trisomy 21, trisomy G, Mongolian)
  —Incidence: 1/2000 live births; 1/40 mothers over age 40
  —Extra chromosome 21 in 95% of cases
- Edwards' syndrome (trisomy 18)
  —Incidence: 1/3000 live births; 3:1 females to males
  —Extra chromosome 18
- Patau's syndrome (trisomy 13)
  —Incidence: 1/5000 births
  —Trisomy of chromosome 13
- Partial trisomy 22 (the cat-eye syndrome)
  —Extra small chromosome 22

DELETION SYNDROMES

- Cat-cry syndrome (cri-du-chat syndrome, 5p-syndrome)
  —Rare
  —Physical and mental development are markedly retarded

- 4p- deletion syndrome
  —Extremely rare
  —Similar to the cat-cry syndrome
  —Survivors are severely handicapped

Syndromes Associated with Sex Chromosome Aberrations

- Gonadal dysgenesis (Turner's syndrome, Bonnevie-Ullrich syndrome)
  —Incidence: 1/3000 live female births
  —Due to the complete or partial absence of one of the two X chromosomes in the female
- Triple X syndrome (47,XXX)
  —Incidence: 1/1000 apparently normal females
  —Affected females have 3 X chromosomes and 2 Barr bodies, or sex chromatin masses
  —Mildly impaired intellect with intelligence quotient (IQ) scores averaging just below 90
  —Difficulty in all subjects compared with siblings
  —Sterility is sometimes present.
  —Several normal XXX females have had offspring who were both chromosomally and phenotypically normal.
- Klinefelter's syndrome (47,XXY)
  —Incidence: 1/700 live male births
  —Formerly thought to be mentally retarded, recent research shows that most of these males are normal in appearance and intellect; however, many have deficits in verbal IQ and reading.
  —Are diagnosed during the course of infertility work-up; all are likely sterile
- The 47,XYY syndrome
  —First described in 1961
  —Formerly thought to be aggressive or violent, but are found in normal populations with the same high frequency as 47,XXY
  —Increased language dysfunction similar to 47,XXY males
- X-linked mental retardation (fragile X syndrome)
  —Among institutionalized persons because of mental retardation, there is a 30% to 50% preponderance of males.
  —Family studies show affected male siblings and maternal uncles, indicating that a group of X-linked mutant genes causes mental retardation without major congenital anomalies.

INDICATIONS FOR CHROMOSOME ANALYSIS

- Congenital malformations
- Mental retardation
- Failure-to-thrive infants
- Small-for-gestational-age infants
- Fetal anomalies detected by ultrasonography
- Ambiguous external genitalia
- Habitual abortion
- Infertility
- Sperm or ova donors
- Cancer cytogenetics

SELECTED GENETIC DISORDERS

Down Syndrome

Etiology
- Trisomy for chromosome 21, due in part to increased predisposition of older oocytes to nondisjunction during meiosis

Incidence
- The risk for Down syndrome increases exponentially with the mother's age at conception, and a marked increase occurs after age 35; by age 45, mothers have 1:40 chance of having an affected child. The risk of other conditions associated with trisomy also increases. Paternal age is not related to trisomy.

Diagnosis
- Diagnosis is usually evident at birth, based on the typical facial features, hypotonia, and single palmar crease. Some serious problems that may be present at birth or develop early in childhood are: duodenal atresia, congenital heart disease, especially atrioventricular canal defects, and leukemia.

Treatment
- The intestinal and cardiac anomalies can be treated surgically, and leukemia responds to conservative management.

Prognosis
- Intelligence varies across a wide spectrum. Many of those with Down syndrome do well in sheltered workshops and group homes, but few achieve full independence in adulthood. An Alzheimer-like dementia often becomes evident in the fourth or fifth decade of life, in those who survive childhood.

Klinefelter's Syndrome

Etiology
- Males with an extra X chromosome

Diagnosis
- These boys appear normal before puberty, but then develop disproportionately long legs and arms, a female cutcheon, gynecomastia, and small testes. Infertility is due to azoospermia; the seminiferous tubules are hyalinized. Mental retardation is somewhat more common than in the general population.

Treatment
- Treating with testosterone after puberty is advisable but will not restore fertility.

Prognosis
- The risk of breast cancer and diabetes mellitus is much higher in men with Klinefelter's syndrome, and most men have learning difficulties.

Marfan's Syndrome

Etiology
- This systemic connective tissue disease is inherited as an autosomal dominant condition. Mutations in the fibrillin gene on chromosome 15 cause the condition.

Diagnosis
- Affected persons are typically tall, with particularly long arms, legs, and digits (arachnodactyly). There is wide variability in clinical presentation. Frequently, joint dislocations and pectus excavatum are seen. Ectopia lentis often leads to severe myopia and retinal detachment. Mitral valve prolapse occurs in about 85% of these persons. Aortic root dilation with aortic regurgitation or dissection with rupture may occur. Diagnosis is based on affected persons having signs in at least two systems (e.g., skeletal, ocular, cardiac).

Treatment
- Children with Marfan's syndrome require regular ophthalmologic evaluation to correct

visual acuity to prevent amblyopia. Annual orthopedic evaluation is scheduled to diagnose scoliosis early, so that bracing may delay progression. Annual echocardiography is required to detect cardiac defects such as aortic diameter and mitral valve function. All patients are given standard endocarditis prophylaxis. Restricted strenuous activity helps to prevent aortic dissection. Replacement of the aortic root with a composite graft when the diameter reaches 50 to 55 mm (normal < 40 mm) prolongs life.

Prognosis

- Those with Marfan's syndrome who do not receive treatment usually die in their forties or fifties, from aortic dissection or congestive heart failure due to aortic regurgitation.

BIBLIOGRAPHY

Beers MH, Berkow R: General principles of medical genetics. In Beers MH, Berkow R, eds: *The Merck manual of diagnosis and therapy*, ed 17, Whitehouse Station, NJ, 1999, Merck Research Laboratories, pp 2470-2480.

Hansen M: Genetic regulation of cellular development, genetic variation and abnormality, Modes of inheritance. *Pathophysiology: foundations of disease and clinical intervention*, Philadelphia, 1998, Saunders, pp 107-118; 135-142.

Iles RK, Kumar PJ: Cell and molecular biology, genetic disorders, and immunology. In Kumar P, Clark M, eds: *Clinical medicine*, ed 4, Edinburgh, 1999, Saunders, pp 125-159.

Jorde LB, Carey JC, Bamshad MJ, et al: *Medical genetics*, ed 2, St. Louis, 1999, Mosby.

Lashley FR: *Clinical genetics in nursing practice*, ed 2, New York, 1998, Springer.

Marx J: Chipping away at the causes of aging, *Science* 287(5462):2390, 2000.

Pyeritz RE: Medical genetics. In Tierney LM, McPhee SJ, Papadakis MA, eds: *Current medical diagnosis & treatment 2000*, New York, 2000, Lange Medical Books/McGraw-Hill, pp 1574-1597.

REVIEW QUESTIONS

1. Tall stature, ectasia, ectopia lentis, and scoliosis are all manifestations of:
   a. Neurofibromatosis
   b. Marfan's syndrome
   c. Myotonic dystrophy
   d. Huntington's disease
   e. Peroneal muscular dystrophy

2. Patients with Down syndrome have increased incidence of all but one of the following problems. Which problem is NOT associated with Down syndrome?
   a. Delayed secondary sexual development
   b. Hypothyroidism
   c. Atlantoaxial instability
   d. Hirschsprung's disease
   e. Cataracts

Questions 3 to 6: Match each of the following chromosomal disorders with its major clinical manifestations:
   a. Trisomy 21 (Down syndrome)
   b. Trisomy 18 (Edwards' syndrome)
   c. Trisomy 13 (Patau syndrome)
   d. XO (Turner's syndrome)
   e. XXY (Klinefelter's syndrome)

3. Short stature, mental deficiency, cardiac defects, hypotonia. _____

4. Short stature, infertility, coarctation of the aorta, nuchal webbing. _____

5. Severe mental deficiency, brain malformations, cleft lip, polydactyly, cardiac defects. _____

6. Tall stature, hypogonadism, long legs, decreased upper/lower ratio of body habitus. _____

Questions 7 to 13: Match each of the following clinical syndromes or conditions with the correct pattern of inheritance:
   a. Autosomal dominant inheritance pattern
   b. Autosomal recessive inheritance pattern
   c. X-linked recessive inheritance pattern
   d. Multifactorial (polygenic) inheritance pattern

7. Hemophilia _____
8. Phenylketonuria _____
9. Cystic fibrosis _____
10. Neurofibromatosis _____
11. Neural tube defects _____
12. Facial cleft anomalies _____
13. Sickle cell anemia _____
14. Which of the following is NOT associated with Mendel's rules of heredity?
   a. Many traits are determined by a pair of hereditary units (genes or alleles).
   b. Gametes (ova or sperm) each receive one of the paired alleles.
   c. There is random sorting of alleles into ova and sperm.

d. Alleles at loci on the same chromosome may segregate together.

e. The pair of alleles is reconstituted by zygote formation.

15. What proportion of families with three children will have all boys?
    a. 1/3
    b. 1/6
    c. 1/8
    d. 1/12
    e. 1/64

16. What is the baseline risk for congenital malformations in the average pregnancy?
    a. 2/10,000
    b. 2/1000
    c. 2/100
    d. 2/10
    e. 2/5

17. The average incidence of common single malformations, such as cleft palate or spina bifida, is:
    a. 1/10,000
    b. 1/5000
    c. 1/1000
    d. 1/500
    e. 1/100

Questions 18 to 22: Match each term with its partial definition.

    a. Heritable change in deoxyribonucleic acid
    b. Alternative form of a gene
    c. Position of gene on chromosome
    d. One gene, multiple effects
    e. Complete set of genes in cell or organism

18. Genome _____
19. Allele _____
20. Mutation _____
21. Locus _____
22. Pleiotropy _____

Questions 23 to 27: Match each description with the correct disorder:

    a. Chromosomal disorders
    b. Single-gene defects
    c. Multifactorial disorders
    d. Somatic cell genetic defects
    e. Mitochondrial disorders

23. Mendelian inheritance _____
24. Human cancers _____
25. Most common type of human genetic disease

    _____

26. Major causes of miscarriages _____
27. Maternal derivation _____

25

Study Skills and Test-Taking Strategies

LEARNING
Definition

Learning is an active process that goes on within the student/learner and it consists of all activities (cognitive, motor, sensory) concerned with acquiring and retaining knowledge, skills, and psychologic characteristics that generate productive thinking, doing, and learning. It is a learned pattern of interrelated physical, cognitive, and emotional attributes that combine to facilitate learning.

MOTIVATION
Definition

The conditions and processes that activate, direct, and sustain behavior.
- Theories on human motivation
  - Human motivation is at its highest when people
    - ~ Are competent
    - ~ Have sufficient autonomy
    - ~ Set worthwhile goals
    - ~ Get feedback
    - ~ Are affirmed by others
  - These are interdependent, and are the minimum components of a self-motivational system of learning.
- Types of motivational behavior (these three elements form the central focus of the study of motivation)
  - Choice
  - Level of involvement
  - Persistence

- Theories about motivation
  - Expectancy-value model
    - ~ Beliefs about one's ability or skill to perform a task
    - ~ Beliefs about the importance and value of a task
    - ~ Feelings about the self or emotional reactions to the task (i.e., affective components)
  - Locus of control model
    - ~ Students who believe that they are in control of their behavior and can influence their environment (internal locus of control) achieve at higher levels.
  - Three aspects of control: internal, external, unknown
    - ~ Students who believe that they control their own outcomes
    - ~ Students who believe that powerful others (teachers, parents) are responsible for their success or failure
    - ~ Students who do not know who or what is responsible for the outcomes
  - Self-efficacy theory
    - ~ Those who believe that the environment is responsive to their actions (that they directly influence outcomes)
      - This belief leads them to higher expectations and to greater persistence in working toward their goals.
    - ~ *Learned helplessness* is seen in persons who are passive, anxious, do not put out effort, and level of achievement decreases.

- Summary of theories
  - All motivation models indicate that a general pattern of perception of internal control results in positive outcomes (i.e., higher achievement, higher self-esteem), whereas sustained perceptions of external or unknown control result in negative outcomes (lower achievement, lack of effort, passivity, anxiety).
  - Some experts say that persistence is the key to success in any endeavor.
    - ~ Persistence is an inner drive or high level of motivation, undeterred by obstacles.
    - ~ Although perception of control is not a personality trait, it is considered to be acquired/learned behavior; persistence ("drive") is considered by some experts to be innate, a genetically derived personality trait.
  - Motivation is a function of classroom contextual factors, and the individual's own construction and interpretation of that context.
  - Individuals have responsibility for their own motivation and learning.
  - Motivation is enhanced by the reciprocal and dynamic interactions among context, faculty, and other students in the class.

CRITICAL THINKING
Definitions

Using logic and reason to make sense of one's world by means of analyzing the thinking/apperception processes that assist us to clarify and understand everything around us. It is the ability to conceptualize, collect, analyze, apply, and evaluate data by means of observation, experience, reflection, reasoning, and communication, leading to beliefs, conclusions, and action. The intended outcomes may include making judgments, choosing among alternative actions, strategic planning, and interpretation of data/evidence to arrive at optimal conclusions/decisions.

- Critical thinking
  - Entails purposeful, goal-directed thinking
  - Is based on the principles of science and the scientific method
  - Is aimed at making judgments based on facts rather than conjecture (guess)
  - Requires techniques that maximize human potential and compensate for errors/problems that occur because of human failure/mistakes
- The critical thinker
  - Is unrelentingly inquisitive
  - Is well-informed in a wide range of areas
  - Trusts his or her own reasoning power
  - Honestly faces personal biases
  - Makes evidence-based judgments
  - Has an open mind toward all issues/topics
  - Logically organizes complex material
  - Evaluates all aspects of a question or problem
  - Carefully selects and adheres to appropriate criteria
  - Is able to focus consistently over time
  - Seeks precise results within circumstantial limits
- Components of critical thinking
  - Identify and challenge assumptions
  - Be aware of the importance of *context* in creating meaning
  - Visualize and explore alternatives
  - Cultivate a reflective skepticism
- Critical thinking skills
  - Interpretation: categorizing, decoding, clarifying
  - Analysis: investigating ideas, developing arguments, analyzing aspects
  - Evaluation: assessing claims, arguments, refutations
  - Inference: query evidence/facts, consider alternatives, derive conclusions
  - Explanation: present arguments, clearly state results, justify procedures
    - ~ Self-regulation: routinely and regularly perform self-examination and self-correction throughout the process
- The process of critical thinking
  - Identify/isolate a problem or question that requires solution.
  - Construct assumptions.
  - Formulate specific, measurable goals and objectives.
  - Develop a detailed time frame.
  - Establish priorities.
  - Develop a method for collecting and organizing information.
  - Determine the significance/value of collected information.
  - Categorize commonalities and differences.
  - Recognize recurring patterns of response.

—Determine stressors and usual adaptation re-
sponses to stressors.
—Discover discrepancies or gaps in informa-
tion.
—Categorize according to relatedness.
—Make inferences based on facts/data.
—Use comparative analysis to assess results.

REASONING

- Judgment
  —Perceptual judgment: making the best choices,
  selections
  —Inferential judgment: right determination of
  significance, value
  —Analytic judgment: categorizing, organizing,
  making relationships
- Inductive reasoning
  —Making generalizations from numbers, evi-
  dence, facts, data, assessments
- Deductive reasoning
  —Developing specific conclusions/actions/de-
  cisions based on general principles of broad
  information

LEARNING STRATEGIES

Learning domains
- Cognitive: thinking, seeing, hearing, touching,
  taking in
- Psychomotor: moving, manipulating, posi-
  tioning
- Affective: feeling, beliefs, values, attitudes
Learning plan
- As far in advance as possible before the actual
  test date, work out a detailed study plan that
  includes all the major topics likely to be on the
  test.
  —Allot specific time frames for each section,
  depending on your level of knowledge about
  each area: allow more time for those areas
  that are least known to you (e.g., neurologic
  disorders)
- Consistently practice positive thinking.
- Overprepare for the examination.
  —Use learning techniques that work for you.
  ~ Reading: reviewing (seeing)
  ~ Reading aloud: review (hearing)
  ~ Writing: review (psychomotor)
    - Use 5 × 8 cards.
    - Use ruled tablet or notebook.

~ Have someone else put questions to you
(interaction).
~ Use CD-ROM or computerized questions
and answers.
~ Respond to questions according to area
(e.g., respiratory).
~ Respond to random questions.
—Study with a person who will also be taking
the examination.
~ Quiz each other.
~ Read aloud to one another.
  - Chapter by chapter
  - Questions/answers with rationale
—Use study aids.
~ Specific review books with questions/an-
swers
~ Record information into audiotape cas-
settes to play at home or while driving.
~ Use algorithms.
~ Use tables, graphs.
~ Use illustrations of biochemical/meta-
bolic processes.
  - Renin-angiotensin system
  - Gas exchange
  - Liver functions
—Practice using different types of questions.
~ Multiple-choice
  - Differentiate types of stems: those with
  complete sentences, those with incom-
  plete sentences, and those with positive
  (do) or negative (don't) polarity.
~ Case study with a set of questions
  - Read carefully.
  - Analyze various parts.
  - Determine what the questions refer to.
  - Requires critical thinking and judgment
~ Structured response questions
  - Matching
  - True-false
~ Restricted response questions
  - Short answer
  - Completion (one word or short an-
  swers)
—Develop your own questions and answers.
~ Focus on areas with which you are *least*
familiar.
~ Construct a Jeopardy-type game (revers-
ing questions/answers is an excellent
tool).
~ Write case studies related to major areas:
respiratory, cardiovascular, and so on.

– Develop questions and answers related to each case study.
—Use all down-time to think about questions and answering them.
~ While waiting for others
~ On bus or subway
~ While driving
~ Before going to sleep
~ While performing "mindless" tasks: washing dishes, folding clothes

TIPS TO USE JUST BEFORE AND DURING TEST

- Attend to own physical/psychologic needs
  —Get a good night's sleep before the examination—you've studied enough!
  —The night before or the morning of the test, avoid drinking too much coffee or tea.
  —Eat a nourishing breakfast: the brain needs glucose to function effectively.
  ~ Drink a large glass of orange juice.
  ~ Eat a bowl of cereal with a sliced banana.
  ~ Eat one or two slices of toast with butter, jam, or jelly.
  —Arrive early at the test center BUT DO NOT RUSH.
  —Select a seat that suits you in terms of
  ~ Lighting
  ~ Placement with respect to others (e.g., not near doorways or common pathways)
  —Wear loose-fitting, comfortable clothes and shoes.
  —Take care of bathroom needs immediately before the examination.
  —Carry in purse or backpack bottled water or other beverage and a small snack.
  —Bring tissues, extra paper, and pen or pencil (or both).
  —Bring a calculator if permitted.
- Considerations during testing
  —Time: calculate the maximum amount of time to spend on each question
  —Mental attitude: maintain positive stance, know that not all questions will count toward final score because some are experimental
  —Similar to a performance by a singer or musician, deep, sustained concentration is required during test taking.
  —Read directions carefully as they appear.

—If an answer escapes you, move on to the next question; succeeding questions may offer clues to a previous unanswered question.
—**Reminder: a computer test does not allow one to go back; the answer must be given the first time.**
—Changing answers on paper-and-pencil tests is usually not a good idea; your first response is usually the correct one.
—On computer tests, changing answers is not possible.
—**Do not read into the question anything that is not there or that you think is intended to be there.**
—Straightforward, concrete answers are the best.
—Use the process of elimination if an answer is not clear.
—On some tests, scores for selecting answers that are totally wrong, or that may in real life prove to be potentially harmful, are calculated separately and count heavily against you.

- Identify the key word in the stem that indicates a priority or focus; match it to the most likely answer.
- Identify the option that is unique or different from other responses.
- Identify potential opposites among options.
- Identify clue(s) in the stem.
- Differentiate equally possible answers.
- Identify key words that indicate positive or negative responses (e.g., do/don't).
- Identify what appear to be "tricky" questions that seem simple; choose the best answer.
- Select answers on the basis of logic.
- Make relationships among questions and answers: there may be a series of questions about one specific area or topic.
- A correct answer may be the "odd" choice, the only one that does not fit in with the others.
- Be cautious about qualifiers such as never, always, usually, frequently, few, and so on.
- Be cautious about totally new words or names; they may be distractors.
- When answers are in rank order (e.g., percentages), the correct one is often between the two extremes.
- Make plans ahead of time to do something special after the examination, as a reward for having done your best in preparing for and in taking the test.

- **Prepare well, have confidence in yourself and your knowledge, answer only what is asked, and GOOD LUCK!**

BIBLIOGRAPHY

Carskadon TG: Student personality factors: psychological Type and the Myers-Briggs Type Indicator. In Prichard KW, Sawyer RM, eds: *Handbook of college teaching: theory and application*, Westport, Conn, 1994, Greenwood, pp 69-82.

Nugent PM, Vitale BA: *Test success: test-taking techniques for beginning nursing students*, ed 2, Philadelphia, 1997, FA Davis.

Prichard PR: Student motivation in the college classroom. In Prichard KW, Sawyer RM, eds: *Handbook of college teaching: theory and application*, Westport, Conn, 1994, Greenwood, pp 23-44.

Walker CJ, Symons C: The meaning of human motivation. In Bess JL, ed: *Teaching well and liking it: motivating faculty to teach effectively*, Baltimore, 1997, Johns Hopkins University Press, pp 3-18.

Review Question Answers and Rationales

1
Health Promotion and Disease Prevention

1. **c.** The primary care setting is the most appropriate for the nurse practitioner to discuss and instruct patients about both specific and more broad-based health care issues and questions. The other settings can be used for health promotion and disease prevention, but are not as amenable to teaching and responding to questions.

2. **a.** We are becoming more aware every year about the effects of genetic factors on individuals' health and disease. Knowing the patient's genetic makeup helps to direct preventive care and to most effectively promote health.

3. **b.** The definition of primary care states this type of care relates to first-contact, comprehensive, and continuing care. While a primary care setting can provide episodic care, the emphasis is on care that encompasses the entire family over time.

4. **d.** The obvious response is that primary care provides information, education, and care for the largest possible group of people.

5. **d.** Health promotion cannot be provided to terminally ill patients. For these patients, primary care health professionals can offer hope, compassion, and pain-free final days.

6. **c.** Primary prevention is used to follow those patients who have specific risk factors for particular disease, e.g., Parkinson's disease or diabetes mellitus, to emphasize health promotion to prevent, for as long as possible, the appearance of signs and symptoms, and then to provide care as early as possible when first symptoms occur, with the goal of prolonging individuals' well-being. Secondary prevention occurs at the time that the patient begins to have signs and symptoms of disease, by treating the condition early to minimize its effects and to teach the patient how best to live with the condition/disease. Tertiary prevention is that stage when comprehensive treatment of the disease is required.

7. **b.** Weight is the only factor in this list that is amenable to change, and thus to promote health. We cannot change the so-called unmodifiable risk factors: age, gender (except by hormone therapy or transsexual therapy and surgery), or genetic makeup (although that may be possible in the future).

8. **d.** In today's age of commercials and advertising in all forms, dissemination of educational materials is possible, on local to global levels. Constraints to patients' receiving health care information include lack of time, resources, and knowledge.

9. **b.** No guarantee of available or effective treatment can be made for any disease, whether identified by screening test or by comprehensive physical evaluation. Screening tests are not one-hundred-percent accurate and may be detrimental to patients only if a test is positive but no therapy is available.

10. **b.** The leading cause of death in the United States is heart disease, which has been at the top of the mortality list for at least 10 years. Much morbidity and mortality related to heart disease is attributable to lifestyles: smoking, alcohol and/or drug use, lack of exercise, and obesity.

11. **c.** Behaviors related to tobacco, alcohol, illicit drug use, and unsafe sexual practices are all preventable causes of significant morbidity and mortality worldwide. Infection from bacteria/microbes is not preventable, but most such conditions are treatable. Chronic diseases may not be readily treated, e.g., rheumatoid arthritis, multiple sclerosis, and other conditions, many of which are inherited problems.

12. **d.** The initial presenting event in patients with coronary artery disease is often sudden death in the form of myocardial infarction (heart attack) or stroke, which is hemorrhage in some part of the brain.

13. **a.** Knowing a patient's family history is a source of potential risk factors that the patient has, but other measures (b, c, and d) are much more beneficial for the patient in maintaining health and preventing serious events from occurring.

14. **a.** The level of low-density lipoprotein considered to be ideal is less than 130 mg/dl. This ideal level has been decreasing over time, based on health statistics regarding heart disease.

15. **c.** Egg whites are high in protein but contain no fat. The other choices have variable levels of fat.

16. **d.** The number of survivors of stroke accounts for the annual cost of care for these patients. The 3.8 million survivors of stroke in the United States indicate that greater knowledge of the characteristics of stroke and its treatment are significant factors in increased survival of victims of stroke.

17. **d.** The cost of care for survivors of stroke is based on the number of survivors and the number of deficits resulting from stroke, e.g., motor, sensory, hemianopsia, dysarthria, dysphasia, and others, each requiring separate rehabilitation methods.

18. **b.** Hypertension is diagnosed in patients whose blood pressure readings are consistently above the accepted upper limits of normal (160/95). Hypertension is the most significant risk factor for stroke, which occurs four times more often in people with blood pressure that is above normal. Fifty percent of persons with a history of transient ischemic attack(s) eventually have a stroke.

19. **d.** The number of people known to be addicted to alcohol or drugs, or both, is 18 million. Statistics show that 75% of Americans drink alcoholic beverages sometimes. Of these, 10% will likely experience problems with alcohol at some point. In 1996, about 2.1 million Americans were users of cocaine, and 600,000 were dependent on heroin.

20. **d.** Persons who are addicted to alcohol are two to four times more likely to die by age 50 than those who do not drink alcohol.

2
Health Care Policy and Professional Issues

1. **b.** Policy is concerned with priorities and goals, allocation of resources, and values, but not with selection of public officials, who are voted into office by citizens.

2. **d.** Public policy is concerned primarily with issues surrounding public safety (e.g., traffic, public transportation, and gun control). Departments of Transportation in cities, counties, and states are responsible for placing warning signs along the highways such as at railroad crossings.

3. **a.** Social policy deals with such issues as age limits for buying tobacco and alcoholic beverages, speed limits, and ensuring that public school lunches are safe and nutritious. Building permits are usually handled by local land use offices.

4. **c.** The federal government determines retirement ages of employees, under the Employee Retirement Income Security Act of 1974.

5. **c.** State nurses associations, like all private, for-profit, or nonprofit organizations, operate under organizational or corporate policy.

6. **c.** Policies are almost invariably developed in response to political activities (politics), based on discussion, public hearings, and debate.

7. **b.** The definition of politics is "influence," in that individuals or groups want to change or influence policies currently in place, or about to be introduced.

8. **c.** The stages of policy making do not include developing strategies. Although specific strategies may be used, these are developed outside the policy-making arena.

9. **c.** Policy analysis requires systematic description and explanation of the causes and results of federal, state, or local action/inaction.

10. **c.** Changes in all areas that affect people are the result of occurrences and conditions of people, e.g., unemployment, economic status, or mortality from various causes that are amenable to change, such as prevention of diseases.

11. **d.** Nurses' influence can be successful because of their numbers; with 2.9 million registered nurses in the United States, they comprise a large group who, if they were to agree on a particular issue, could effectively influence a large segment of the population.

12. **c.** Highly technical nursing care is not a requirement of professional nursing practice. However, in specific areas of treatment, e.g., operating room or intensive care units, knowing technology can effectively improve patient care.

13. **d.** Consumers are becoming increasingly aware of aspects of health care that can be changed to improve level, access, and quality of health care.

14. **d.** Health care in the United States can be delivered only from a geographic perspective in which small, manageable geographic areas are used as a method to effectively and fairly distribute health care to all people.

15. **a.** Quality of care by all health professionals, particularly nurse practitioners, is a serious issue confronting the nursing profession. Many well-designed research studies show that the quality of care delivered by nurse practitioners, who care for those with chronic diseases, is equal to, or better than, care provided by physicians.

16. **b.** The greatest change occurring in the U.S. population is that we are becoming multicultural. The Hispanic population is increasing faster than any other segment of the population, and is now about equal to that of the black population.

17. **b.** In rural areas of the United States, reimbursement to health care providers comes primarily from Medicare, an indication of the rapidly increasing older population residing in these areas.

18. **c.** In rural states, particularly in the western United States, health care is provided largely by telehealth. A major obstacle to providing care across state lines is the need for health care professionals to have concurrent licensure in all states reached by telehealth. Multiple state licensure will ensure greater capability of meeting needs of people in larger geographic areas.

19. **a.** Bills regarding national health care that are introduced in the U.S. Senate and House of Representatives are sponsored primarily by senators and representatives from large, rural areas in the west and south.

20. **d.** All of these actions are necessary for any group of people to make significant changes in today's health care system, e.g., being organized at local, state, and national levels; being active in nursing associations; and being active in nursing's political action committees (PACs).

3
Legal and Ethical Issues

1. **c.** Ethics is best defined in terms of what is good and bad, of moral obligation and duty. Ethical decisions are those made on the basis of what is best for all.

2. **b.** Prioritizing a person's values is known as a personal value system. Value systems develop gradually as one matures, based on personal experiences, family teaching, religious beliefs, and the world around us. These values are what guide our thinking, behavior, and relationships.

3. **c.** A nurse faced with incompetent practice by a colleague usually bases her thinking on the ethical principle of beneficence, which entails obligations to prevent harm, to remove harm, and to do good. Using beneficence, we balance risks, harms, benefits, and effectiveness.

4. **b.** When asked by a patient's wife about a diagnosis of AIDS, the nurse responds based on the ethical principle of justice, which refers to receiving one's due—fairness. Aristotle explicated justice as an egalitarian concept, in which equality is the right of all with respect to benefits in such matters as health care, without considering who can or cannot pay for care.

5. **d.** The precept that it is best to provide the greatest good for the greatest number is known as utilitarianism. This is a theory that is based on the belief that what is useful is good, and determining what is right conduct should be the usefulness of its consequences.

The aim of action is the largest possible degree of pleasure over pain, and the most happiness for the largest number of people.

6. **d.** Ethical dilemmas involving the use of technology that have captured the public's interest involve the two landmark cases (Karen Quinlan [1976], and Nancy Cruzan [1990]), both of which were widely publicized amid much controversy. Both declined into a persistent vegetative state after drug-and-alcohol ingestion in one case, and a car accident in the other. In each case, no Living Will had been executed, and the lower courts, in deciding against removal of ventilators and removal of food and fluid intake by nasogastric tube, favor right-to-life. High-level courts made the decision to terminate life-support means, which resulted in death of both Karen and Nancy. This decision is what both families had requested.

7. **d.** When nurses' personal values are in conflict with professional values, they are required to make decisions that exclude any consideration of their own personal well-being, and focus actions and decisions only on the needs and wishes of patients and families.

8. **c.** Decisions about which patients will receive a donor organ are based on the ethical principle of justice. Justice must result in a fair and just decision about who will receive a donor organ, when donor organs are scarce. The list of organ recipients is maintained carefully and equitably, with each person next in line receiving the next available organ.

9. **c.** The factor that has the most impact about the ethical dilemma "Is health care a right or a privilege" is that of escalating health care costs. Health care access is linked inevitably with health care costs, which have been rising gradually since the 1970s.

10. **b.** The use of advance directives relates to the ethical principle of autonomy, which is that all people have the right to freedom of choice with respect to their own beliefs and wishes about end-of-life decisions.

11. **c.** The statement that best defies malpractice is that which links malpractice and negligence—the omission or commission of an act that results in care that is below the professional standards of due care, as defined in the State Professional Practice Acts.

12. **a.** State boards of nursing are responsible for licensing and registering qualified nurses. Boards also stipulate practice guidelines for all levels of nurses.

13. **a.** The elements required to prove malpractice are duty of care, breach of duty, injury, and proximate cause.

14. **c.** A nurse reports a medication error in which a patient was given a wrong medication, but had ill effects. The necessary element that would prove malpractice, and that is not present in this case, is patient injury. Injury must have occurred, linked to the nurse's action or cause. If no injury occurred, there is no wrongdoing.

15. **d.** In carrying out an order by the registered nurse in charge, the unlicensed assistive person unknowingly contaminates what should have been a sterile area, which causes the patient to develop an infection. The person who delegates tasks to unlicensed assistive persons is responsible for the safety and care of the patient throughout.

16. **c.** Civil law is concerned with negligence and malpractice torts. A tort is a civil wrong, other than breach of contract, in which the law provides a remedy by allowing the injured person to seek damages.

17. **c.** A strategy that nurses can use to prevent being named in a malpractice suit is to establish a trusting relationship with patients and families. Knowing those involved and interacting with them as frequently as possible usually ensures that nurses and other health professionals will not be named in lawsuits.

18. **b.** Criminal law addresses acts by persons or groups that threaten society, e.g., the person or persons who threaten to blow up official buildings.

19. **a.** Licensure is defined as a legal permit that protects the public from unsafe and incompetent health care practitioners. Licensure affirms that the licensed person is qualified to perform designated services.

20. **b.** Informed consent requires that, after the physician has explained the risks and benefits of a particular procedure, the signatures of both the patient and an objective witness

who observes the patient signing the consent form are obtained before the procedure can begin.

4
Respiratory Disorders

1. **b.** Studies about causes of obstructive pulmonary emphysema show that chronic obstructive pulmonary disease is characterized by chronic bronchitis or emphysema, and airflow obstruction that is generally progressive, may be accompanied by airway hyperreactivity, and may be partially reversible.

2. **a.** Treatment of severe or prolonged attacks of asthma that require hospitalization does NOT include the use of sedatives. Antiasthmatic drugs are divided into those used for symptom relief (β-agonists, theophylline, and anticholinergics) and those used for long-term control (corticosteroids, cromolyn/nedocromil, leukotriene modifiers). Sedatives should never be used because they tend to restrict the cough reflex.

3. **c.** The best test to rule out pulmonary emboli is a ventilation/perfusion scan. This is a non-invasive procedure that is used extensively to measure lung function.

4. **b.** The test that measures functional residual capacity shows the volume of air in the lungs at the end of normal expiration when all respiratory muscles are relaxed. Physiologically, it is the most important lung volume because it approximates the normal tidal breathing range.

5. **a.** The most significant symptom experienced by patients with pulmonary edema is dyspnea, which is difficulty breathing and shortness of breath. Acute pulmonary edema is a life-threatening manifestation of acute left ventricular failure secondary to sudden onset of pulmonary venous hypertension. It can occur with either pulmonary or cardiac diseases.

6. **c.** Symptoms/signs of chronic obstructive pulmonary disease associated with emphysema usually include low or normal levels of arterial CO_2. This is due partly to the amount of air that is in the lungs but that is not involved in gas exchange. The asthmatic lungs have this area of "dead space" in which air remains in the lungs. The result is a lower level of carbon dioxide in the blood, due to trapped air in the inflated lungs.

7. **a.** Treatment of chronic airway obstruction lung disease includes primarily bronchodilators such as ipratropium bromide (Atrovent) and β₂-agonists (metaproterenol [Alupent], albuterol [Proventil]).

8. **d.** In the United States, the number of deaths each year from asthma is about 5000. About 12 million persons have asthma. Between 1982 and 1992, the prevalence of asthma increased from 34.7 to 49.4 per 1000 persons. Mortality is 5 times higher in blacks than in whites. The reason for this difference is not known.

9. **a.** The patient with asthma who comes into contact with a triggering agent generally experiences an immediate allergic reaction, or symptoms may develop 4 to 6 hours after exposure to the allergen. These triggers may include house dust mites, cockroaches, cats, and seasonal pollens.

10. **d.** A 25-year-old man came to the emergency room complaining of rust-colored sputum and fever for 2 days accompanied by chills. Physical examination showed dullness and moist wheezes in the left lower chest. The most likely diagnosis is left lower lobe pneumonia. Despite antibiotics, pneumonia continues to be a major health problem, particularly among older persons, with 3 to 4 million cases diagnosed every year.

11. **b.** The statement that best describes squamous cell carcinoma is that it develops in the central bronchi, where bronchoscopy can visualize the growth. Squamous cell carcinoma and adenocarcinoma are the most common types of bronchogenic carcinoma, and each makes up about 30% to 35% of primary tumors.

12. **b.** Both acute and chronic asthma are characterized primarily by airway inflammation. The histopathologic features include denudation of airway epithelium, collage deposition beneath the basement membrane, airway edema, mast cell activation, and inflammatory cell infiltration with neutrophils, eosinophils, and lymphocytes, especially T lymphocytes.

13. **c.** In severe asthma, airflow may be quite limited, and findings on auscultation of the lungs are primarily markedly decreased breath sounds throughout. Severity of asthma ranges from mild-intermittent to severe-persistent. In

mild asthma, the person may have symptoms about twice a week, and experiences few exacerbations. Severe persistent asthma indicates continual symptoms, with quite limited physical activity and frequent exacerbations.

14. **c.** Most viral pneumonias are characterized by fever up to 105° F (40.5° C). Respiratory syncytial virus causes annual outbreaks of pneumonia, bronchiolitis, and tracheobronchitis in the very young. Serious pulmonary respiratory syncytial virus infections have been described in older persons and those who are immunocompromised.

15. **c.** Tuberculosis, an infection caused by *Mycobacterium tuberculosis*, is transmitted among people primarily by airborne droplets from infected persons.

16. **d.** Primary tuberculosis is undetected in about 90% to 95% of cases. In these people, the tuberculin skin test becomes positive, and the infection becomes latent or dormant. The patient with reactivation tuberculosis presents with classic symptoms of fatigue, weight loss, anorexia, low-grade fever, and night sweats.

17. **b.** The initial tuberculosis infection can leave nodular scars in the apices of the lungs. These nodules are called Simon's foci, which are the most common seeds for later active tuberculosis. The frequency of activation seems unaffected by calcified scars of primary infection (Ghon foci) or by residual calcified hilar lymph nodes.

18. **c.** The most high-risk group of people for the development of tuberculosis is persons infected with HIV. HIV infection causes progression to clinical tuberculosis to be more common and rapid. Rather than a 5% to 10% attack rate in 1 to 2 years, the attack rate is 50% within 60 days. If the infection strain is resistant to available drugs, the result is a 50% death rate within a median time of 60 days.

19. **c.** The most common symptom in patients with TB is cough, which may be discounted and ascribed to smoking, a recent cold, or a recent bout of influenza. At first, it is minimally productive of yellow or green mucus, usually on rising in the morning, but becomes more productive as the disease progresses.

20. **a.** Factors that may predict a poor prognosis for those with community-acquired pneumonia include male gender, absence of pleuritic chest pain, involvement of more than one lobe, advanced age, alcoholism, comorbid medical conditions, altered mental status, respiratory rate less than 30/minute, hypotension with systolic less than 90 mm Hg or diastolic less than 60 mm Hg, and blood urea nitrogen of more than 30 mg/dl.

21. **c.** The number of people affected by chronic obstructive pulmonary disease in the United States is estimated to be about 14 million. Grouped together, chronic obstructive pulmonary disease and asthma now represent the fourth leading cause of death, with over 90,000 deaths reported annually. The death rate from chronic obstructive pulmonary disease is increasing rapidly, especially among elderly men who have a long history of smoking.

22. **c.** An FEV_1/FVC ratio of less than 65% indicates chronic obstructive pulmonary disease. FEV_1 = the forced expiratory volume in 1 sec, in liters; FVC = forced vital capacity, which is the volume of air expired with maximal force.

23. **a.** The pathogenesis of asthma includes denudation of airway epithelium.

24. **c.** In patients with asthma, mast cells are important in the acute response to inhaled allergens, but do not play a major role in the pathogenesis of chronic inflammation. Mast cells are constituents of connective tissue and contain large basophilic granules that contain heparin, serotonin, bradykinin, and histamine. These substances are released from the mast cell in response to injury and infection.

25. **d.** Peak expiratory flow meters are used by asthma patients at home, but their usefulness is limited by the lack of normative brand-specific reference values; the fact that peak expiratory flow values vary with gender, age, and height; and the wide variability in peak expiratory flow reference values among individuals.

26. **a.** The differential diagnosis of asthma includes cardiac failure, chronic obstructive pulmonary disease, and aortic aneurysm that impinge on the bronchial airways. These exhibit symptoms similar to asthma.

27. **d.** The prognosis for patients treated for acute bronchitis is excellent. Chronic bronchitis is

characterized by excessive secretion of bronchial mucus and is manifested by productive cough for 3 months or more in at least 2 consecutive years in the absence of any other disease that could cause bronchial secretions.

28. **b.** In March 2000, the U.S. Supreme Court ruled that the Food and Drug Administration could not regulate how cigarettes are sold and marketed. This action therefore makes cigarettes and tobacco products readily available to everyone.

29. **d.** About 87% of all lung cancers are attributable to exposure to tobacco. Studies show that second-hand smoke definitely causes lung cancer.

30. **d.** About 400,000 deaths occur each year in the United States from tobacco-related causes. Many victims began using tobacco products as children.

5
Cardiovascular Disorders

1. **d.** Isolated systolic hypertension, in which systolic pressure is ≥140 mm Hg and the diastolic pressure is ≤90 mm Hg, usually continues to increase until at least age 80. Systolic hypertension is not a discrete entity. It often results from increased cardiac output or stroke volume. In older persons with normal or low cardiac output, it usually reflects inelasticity of the aorta and its major branches (arteriosclerotic hypertension).

2. **b.** The cause of primary hypertension is more than one factor. The actual cause remains unknown. Heredity is a predisposing factor, but no precise mechanism is known. Environmental factors play a role: dietary sodium, obesity, and stress are relevant only in those patients who are genetically susceptible. Pathologic features lead to increased total peripheral vascular resistance by inducing vasoconstriction, to increased cardiac output, or to both (blood pressure = cardiac output [flow] × resistance).

3. **d.** Angiotensin II is a powerful vasoconstrictor. Angiotensin II receptor blocker with a diuretic, although not recommended for initial therapy, may be necessary at some point. Angiotensin II occurs naturally in the body as an octapeptide that is produced by the action of angiotensin-converting enzyme on angiotensin I. Its effects are stimulation of vascular smooth muscle, promotion of aldosterone production, and stimulation of the sympathetic nervous system.

4. **d.** Plasma renin activity is usually normal in patients with primary hypertension, but is suppressed in about 30% of these patients. Renin is an enzyme that converts angiotensinogen to angiotensin I. Suppression of plasma renin activity would tend to increase hypertension.

5. **a.** Secondary hypertension is associated with other conditions, often with renal parenchymal disease such as chronic glomerulonephritis or pyelonephritis, polycystic renal disease, collagen disease of the kidney, or obstructive uropathy. Other associated conditions include Cushing's syndrome, pheochromocytoma, primary aldosteronism, hyperthyroidism, myxedema, coarctation of the aorta, or renovascular disease. Secondary hypertension results from both renin-dependent and volume-dependent mechanisms. In most patients, increased renin activity cannot be detected in peripheral blood. Meticulous attention to fluid balance usually controls blood pressure.

6. **c.** In the early labile phase of primary hypertension, cardiac output is increased. Abnormal sodium transport across the cell membrane wall due to a defect in or inhibition of the Na^+,K^+-ATPase pump, or due to increased permeability to Na^+, has been seen in some cases of primary hypertension. Defects in Na^+ transport have been described in normotensive children of hypertensive parents.

7. **d.** The hallmark of primary hypertension is nephrosclerosis. Nephrosclerosis is defined as fibrosis of the kidney from overgrowth and contraction of the interstitial connective tissue. No early pathologic changes occur, but ultimately generalized arteriolar sclerosis develops and is particularly apparent in the kidneys. Other long-term effects of primary hypertension include left ventricular hypertrophy that becomes left ventricular dilation. Coronary, cerebral, aortic, renal, and peripheral atherosclerosis are more common and more severe in those with hypertension, which accelerates atherogenesis. Hypertension is a more significant risk factor for stroke

than for atherosclerotic heart disease, however. Tiny Charcot-Bouchard aneurysms, often seen in perforating arteries, especially in the basal ganglia, may be the source of intracerebral hemorrhage.

8. **d.** Pheochromocytoma is a tumor of the chromaffin cells that secrete catecholamines: epinephrine, norepinephrine, and L-dopa, which are the major elements in responses to stress. Pheochromocytoma is a functional chromaffinoma, usually benign, derived from adrenal medullary tissue cells; catecholamines secreted lead to hypertension, which may be paroxysmal and associated with attacks of palpitation, headache, nausea, dyspnea, anxiety, pallor, and profuse sweating.

9. **d.** Angina pectoris is caused by coronary artery obstruction. It is usually an excruciating pain in the chest, often radiating up to the neck and down the left arm. The cause is ischemia of the heart muscle.

10. **a.** The clinician, when seeing a patient for the first time who is complaining of chest pain, must differentiate potential causes of chest pain, which include costochondritis; pleuritic pain, which is usually made worse by deep breathing or coughing; dissecting aneurysm, which is difficult to diagnose from the history and physical examination alone; chest wall pain, which may be due to trauma and is exacerbated by coughing; and respiratory causes, which are more difficult to diagnose.

11. **d.** Myocardial infarction is usually (in over 90% of patients) the result of abrupt reduction in coronary blood flow to a segment of the myocardium due to a thrombus from a ruptured plaque, which occludes an artery, resulting in ischemic necrosis in that area of the heart. Spontaneous thrombolysis occurs in about 66% of patients so that, 24 hours later, thrombotic occlusion is seen in only about 30% of patients with myocardial infarction.

12. **c.** The cluster of cells in the heart that forms the primary electrical generator (pacemaker) of the normal heart is the sinoatrial node. The sinoatrial node is made up of hundreds of cells located in the right atrial wall of the heart, near the opening of the superior vena cava. It comprises a knot of modified heart muscle that generates impulses that travel swiftly throughout the muscle fibers of both atria, causing them to contract. Specialized pacemaker cells in the node have an intrinsic rhythm that is independent of any stimulation by nerve impulses from the brain and spinal cord.

13. **c.** Dysrhythmias are usually caused by the following mechanisms, including abnormalities of impulse formation, abnormalities of impulse conduction, and reentry, which is one of the most common dysrhythmogenic mechanisms. Reentry is the reactivation of myocardial tissue for the second or subsequent time by the same impulse. Many experts believe that reentry is the cause of most dysrhythmias.

14. **d.** Bradydysrhythmias arise from abnormalities of intrinsic automatic conduction, primarily in the atrioventricular node and the His-Purkinje network. Purkinje's fibers are a continuation of the bundle branches and extend into the muscle walls of the ventricles; they carry the impulses that contract the ventricles almost simultaneously.

15. **a.** Quinidine is one of the drugs classified as Class Ia. Class I drugs are sodium channel blockers, including older antidysrhythmic drugs such as quinidine. All of this type of drug reduce the maximal rate of depolarization of the action potential and thereby slow conduction. Quinidine prolongs the action potential and refractoriness, as seen on electrocardiogram as QT prolongation. This broad-spectrum drug is effective for the suppression of ventricular ectopic beats and ventricular tachycardia, and for the control of narrow QRS tachycardias, including atrial flutter and fibrillation. It is one of the few drugs that may convert atrial fibrillation to sinus rhythm.

16. **d.** Radiofrequency ablation can be used in over 99% of patients with atrial fibrillation. Radiofrequency is radiant energy of a certain frequency range. For example, radio and television use radiant energy having a frequency between 10^5 and 10^{11} Hz. Diagnostic x-rays have a frequency in the range of 3×10^{18} Hz. Ablation is defined as removal of a body part or destruction of its function by several methods, one of which is radiofrequency.

17. **d.** Reciprocating tachycardias involve accessory pathways. In the most common form,

activation is from atria to ventricles through the normal atrioventricular node, returning via the accessory pathway to the atria (orthodromic), resulting in a narrow QRS tachycardia during which P waves are inscribed *after* the QRS complex (PR > RP). Rarely, conduction is in the opposite direction, resulting in a broad QRS complex, antidromic reciprocating tachycardia. Examples are in Wolff-Parkinson-White syndrome, an accessory pathway that links the atria and ventricles, bypassing the atrioventricular node. A typical electrocardiogram shows a short PR interval and slurred QRS complex (delta wave). Antegrade conduction over the accessory pathway is necessary to create the short PR interval and the delta wave, but retrograde conduction is important for sustaining orthodromic-reciprocating tachycardia. Therefore a concealed accessory pathway (normal PR, no delta wave in sinus rhythm) may support the dysrhythmia. In Lown-Ganong-Levine syndrome, the accessory pathway links the atrium with His bundle tissue, bypassing the atrioventricular node. The PR interval is short, as in Wolff-Parkinson-White syndrome, but the QRS complex is normal. Patients with Lown-Ganong-Levine syndrome have the same type of dysrhythmias as those with Wolff-Parkinson-White syndrome, and treatment is similar.

18. **a.** The end-diastolic volume is influenced by, and can be predicted by, end-diastolic pressure. End-diastolic pressure in the right ventricle is 4 mm Hg on average, with a range of 0 to 8 mm Hg. End-diastolic pressure in the left ventricle is 9 mm Hg on average, with a range between 5 and 12 mm Hg. In the brachial artery, for example, the end-diastolic pressure averages 70 mm Hg, with a range between 60 and 90 mm Hg.

19. **c.** The Frank-Starling principle states that the degree of end-diastolic stretch (preload) within a physiologic range is proportional to the systolic performance of the ensuing ventricular contraction. This principle applies to degree of function based on diastolic muscle length, end-diastolic pressure, and end-diastolic volume in heart failure and other abnormalities, e.g., reduced ventricular contractility due to ventricular hypertrophy or dilatation.

20. **d.** A patient with heart failure, or who has a history of pulmonary edema, should receive fluids at a minimal rate only to restore fluids lost in diaphoresis, urinary output, vomiting, and other losses. Too-rapid infusion of IV fluids in patients with heart failure results in massive congestive heart failure, requiring ventilator support, often for several weeks, and worsening an already weakened heart.

21. **b.** On both short-term and long-term electrocardiogram recordings, sinus rhythm was shown to be remarkably variable. The sinoatrial node, possibly the atrioventricular node, and most of the specialized conducting tissues are capable of automatic (spontaneous) phase 4 diastolic depolarization. The intrinsic pacemaker rate is highest in the sinoatrial node, which dominates the lower, slower latent cardiac pacemakers.

22. **c.** The dysrhythmia that typically shows "sawtooth" electrocardiogram waves is atrial flutter.

23. **b.** Antidysrhythmic drugs continue to be the mainstay of treatment for cardiac dysrhythmias, although many of these drugs have limited effectiveness and often produce side effects. They are divided into four classes according to their electropharmacologic actions: Class I drugs are sodium channel blockers (e.g., quinidine, procainimide, and others). Class II drugs are β-blockers (e.g., propanolol, acebutolol, and others). Class III drugs are potassium channel blockers (e.g., amiodarone, sotalol, and others). Class IV drugs are the slow calcium channel blockers (e.g., verapamil and diltiazem).

24. **c.** The most common chronic dysrhythmia is atrial fibrillation, which can occur spontaneously and is also associated with rheumatic heart disease, atrial septal defect, hypertension, mitral valve prolapse, and cardiomyopathy.

25. **b.** Torsades de pointes is a ventricular tachycardia, defined as three or more consecutive premature beats. The usual mechanism is reentry. The usual rate is 160 to 240 beats/min, which is moderately regular. As with other dysrhythmias, torsades de pointes can occur spontaneously or after quinidine or another drug that prolongs the QT interval. Torsades de pointes has a particularly poor prognosis.

26. **a.** Afterload is determined by all but the degree of relaxation of the chambers of the

heart. The definition of afterload is the resistance (load) against which the left ventricle must eject its volume of blood during contraction. The resistance is produced by the volume of blood already in the vascular system and the condition of the vessel walls.

27. **d.** Risk factors for heart failure include pregnancy, anemia, change in drug therapy for heart failure, coronary artery disease, hypertension, cardiomyopathy, and congenital defects of the heart. Sudden weight gain does not pose a risk for heart failure.

28. **d.** The most frequent cause of right ventricular heart failure is previous left ventricular failure. Volume overload resulting from IV fluids running too fast, which overwhelm the damaged or diseased ventricles, can often cause massive congestive heart failure.

29. **c.** Bed rest is not recommended for patients with deep venous thrombosis because walking activates circulation. Superficial thrombosis requires no specific therapy other than nonsteroidal antiinflammatory drugs to relieve discomfort and warm compresses over involved veins to dilate the veins and improve circulation. For deep vein thrombosis, direct treatment involves prevention of emboli to the lungs or heart and prevention of chronic venous insufficiency. Chronic venous insufficiency results in stasis ulcers in the lower leg, at the ankle, and discoloration of the skin of the lower leg.

30. **a.** Angiotensin-converting enzyme inhibitors improve myocardial performance by lowering venous pressure, reducing levels of circulating catecholamines, and decreasing systemic vascular resistance.

6
Neurologic Disorders

1. **c.** In making a diagnosis, one of the first correlations to make is that between the age of the patient and usual age at onset of neurologic diseases that affect the central areas of the body (trunk and limbs). Differential diagnoses would include those named in the question. However, in reviewing usual age of onset, you find that amyotrophic lateral sclerosis usually begins in those over age 50. Poliomyelitis is seen more often in those younger than 20 years of age, although polio can occur at any age, so it is kept on the list.

Multiple sclerosis can occur in people between 20 and 40 years of age, so this is a definite "perhaps." Usual onset of Parkinson's disease is after age 40. You have narrowed the list of differential diagnoses to two: polio and multiple sclerosis. Next, you look at the usual presenting signs and symptoms for polio and multiple sclerosis. These data definitely point to multiple sclerosis, and that is your working diagnosis, until you have confirmation of a diagnosis from diagnostic tests.

2. **d.** Comparing muscle and sensory reactions on both sides of the body yields essential information, and any asymmetry can provide a working diagnosis such as brain tumor or stroke. The other three areas are not as specific, and all may occur in a number of neurologic conditions.

3. **b.** A positive Babinski is often the only indication of an upper motor neuron disease, and it may indicate a lesion in the pyramidal tract. A positive Babinski can be demonstrated in various ways: (1) absence of an ankle jerk in sciatica; (2) an extensor plantar response with extension of the great toe and adduction of the other toes; (3) a more pronounced concentration of platysma on the unaffected side during blowing or sneezing; (4) pronation that occurs when an arm affected by paralysis is placed in supination; and (5) when a patient in supine position with arms crossed over the chest tries to assume a sitting position, the thigh of the affected side is flexed, and the heel is raised, while the leg on the unaffected side remains flat. These signs all relate to upper motor neuron disease of some type: progressive bulbar palsy, pseudobulbar palsy, progressive spinal muscular atrophy, primary lateral sclerosis, or amyotrophic lateral sclerosis.

4. **a.** Festination is a common characteristic seen in those with Parkinson's disease.

5. **c.** A positive test, in which the patient is asked to stand straight, with feet together and eyes open, then closed, but cannot maintain balance, indicates cerebellar ataxia.

6. **c.** The seventh (facial) nerve is damaged when a lower motor neuron lesion develops, resulting in paralysis of both the lower and upper facial muscles.

7. **d.** Diffuse inflammation results in global disorders of the cerebral cortex. Organic cerebral

dysfunction may be focal (space-occupying lesions, stroke, trauma, scars, maldevelopment) or global (metabolic-chemical disorders, disseminated structural lesions such as diffuse inflammation, vasculopathy, disseminated malignancy).

8. **c.** The frontal lobes influence learned motor activity, and the planning and organizing of expressed behavior. Patients with large basal frontal lesions lose the ability to show emotions, and therefore exhibit apathetic behaviors.

9. **b.** The parietal lobes are dominant in spatial relationships, integration of awareness of the trajectories of moving objects, position of body parts, language recognition, and word memory.

10. **b.** The most characteristic symptom of tension headache is pain that is felt as pressure from a tight band around the head. Typically, these headaches can last from 30 minutes to 7 days, are nonpulsating, mild-to-moderate in severity, bilateral, not aggravated by exertion, and are not accompanied by nausea, vomiting, or sensitivity to light, sound, or smell.

11. **c.** The noncharacteristic sign or symptom of migraine is that the headache is not affected by walking upstairs or performing other routine activities.

12. **a.** The risk factor that is not characteristic of migraine is that of age of onset. Of the 24 million Americans who experience migraine headaches, onset began in most between the ages of 10 and 40.

13. **b.** Giant cell arteritis is not characterized by frontal headaches. Temporal (giant cell) arteritis is a chronic inflammatory disease of large blood vessels, particularly those with a prominent elastica, involving mainly the carotid (cranial) arteries. Symptoms of giant cell arteritis include severe pain in the temporal or occipital areas.

14. **c.** The major cause of seizures in older people is cerebrovascular disease. Another often overlooked cause is withdrawal from alcohol. Beginning 12 to 48 hours after cessation of intake of alcohol, patients may exhibit tremors, weakness, sweating, hyperreflexia, and gastrointestinal symptoms. Some patients have tonic-clonic seizures, usually not more than two in short succession.

15. **a.** A first-line drug used to treat and to prevent seizures is the antiepileptic drug phenytoin (Dilantin). No single drug controls all types of seizures. Patients seldom require more than one drug. About a dozen drugs may be used, some of which are add-on drugs to augment a principal drug. Another commonly used drug is phenobarbital. All have side effects, which is why drug therapy must be tailored to individual patients based on reactions, effectiveness, and side effects.

16. **b.** Parkinson's disease usually begins in people between the ages of 35 and 45. Often, patients will have the disease for several years before it is diagnosed. They account for unsteady gait, occasional falls, and early tremors to aging, hurrying, and other external causes.

17. **b.** Onset of delirium is always sudden, whereas dementia occurs gradually over several months. Causes are variable. Delirium can occur in people with a normal brain, but is more common in those with underlying brain disease such as dementia. It is also more common in the elderly likely due to changes in neurotransmitters, cell loss, and concomitant disease. Symptoms fluctuate rapidly, often within minutes, and may be worse late in the day ("sundowning"). The person is often confused (delirium is also known as an acute confusional state). Some may become quiet and withdrawn, whereas others become agitated or hyperactive.

18. **c.** People tend to think that delirium and dementia are similar. The one characteristic that occurs in delirium that does not occur in dementia is clouded consciousness, which is the most prominent symptom in delirium. The other areas mentioned (**a**, **b**, and **d**) are typical of patients with dementia.

19. **a.** One characteristic that is not found in those with Alzheimer's disease is the *absence* of the epsilon4 allele, which decreases the risk for Alzheimer's disease in the white population. The other statements about Alzheimer patients are true.

20. **c.** Cerebral cortex dysfunction can be grouped into **focal** and **global**. The one factor listed that is not a cause of focal disorders is diffuse inflammation. This condition, however, is a primary cause of global disorders of the cerebral hemispheres.

21. **b.** Apraxia and amnesia may be caused by either focal or diffuse (global) brain dysfunction.

22. **a.** Wernicke's aphasia is a subtype of receptive (sensory) aphasia in which the patient speaks fluently, but includes meaningless phonemes, and does not know the meanings of words or the relationships among words. The typical speech of a person with Wernicke's aphasia is "word salad."

23. **d.** Statistics show that those who experience episodic tension headaches have fewer than 180 episodes each year. This is a high number of such headaches. These patients should probably be evaluated for comorbid condition(s) that may be causing tension headaches.

24. **c.** Older patients with migraine equivalents (ischemic symptoms without headache) should be evaluated for the occurrence of transient ischemic attacks because ischemia is often related to cardiovascular conditions.

25. **b.** Ergotamine is a drug commonly prescribed for patients with migraine headaches because of its vasoconstrictor action, which often decreases vascular pressure that could instigate migraine, or act as a factor in the duration of migraine.

26. **a.** Cluster headache is classified separately from migraine because of its different therapy. These are of short duration, lasting from 15 to 180 minutes, and are always unilateral, invariably the same side of the head. Accompanying symptoms include severe pain often in one eye, with tearing, photophobia, congestion of the nose, and ptosis in the affected eye. The pain of cluster headaches has been described as "bone-crushing," and usually leaves the patient unable to function for the time of greatest pain, in the first 10 to 30 minutes.

27. **b.** Giant cell arteritis is described as a disease of the large arteries, primarily the cranial arteries that branch off the carotid arteries. The diagnosis is confirmed by biopsy of the temporal artery. Treatment is based mainly on prednisone, which the patient takes for about a year.

28. **c.** Polymyalgia rheumatica is defined as severe pain and stiffness in the neck, shoulder, and pelvic girdle. The erythrocyte sedimentation rate is markedly increased in these patients, many of whom also experience nonspecific systemic symptoms. Diagnostic tests show no evidence of muscle weakness or muscle disease on electromyography or biopsy. There may be a relationship between polymyalgia rheumatica and giant cell arteritis.

29. **c.** Bladder cancer can be missed in perimenopausal women who have intermittent urethral bleeding, which can easily be mistaken for vaginal bleeding.

30. **a.** The cause of trigeminal neuralgia (also known as tic douloureux) is thought to be compression of the fifth cranial nerve (trigeminal nerve) root. Trigeminal neuralgia is described as bouts of excruciating, lancinating pain, lasting between seconds and 2 minutes, along the distribution of one or more of the nerve's sensory divisions, usually the maxillary.

7
Gastrointestinal Disorders

1. **b.** Upper endoscopy is the "gold standard" in diagnosing peptic ulcer disease. Essentially, all patients with upper tract bleeding should undergo upper endoscopy, which has three benefits: (1) it identifies the source of the bleeding; (2) it identifies the risk of rebleeding; and (3) it provides for endoscopic therapy such as cautery or injection to stop bleeding.

2. **a.** The pathogenic role of *Helicobacter pylori* in peptic ulcer development is that, if one excludes nonsteroidal antiinflammatory drugs and Zollinger-Ellison syndrome as causes of peptic ulcer disease, 100% of duodenal ulcers are caused by *H. pylori*. When this was first suggested over 10 years ago by a researcher studying gastrointestinal diseases, physicians and others at a national conference absolutely rejected the possibility that an organism could cause peptic ulcer disease. Further research by others proved the validity of the original research studies.

3. **c.** When empirically treating peptic ulcer disease, it is important to remember that a response to treatment does not preclude the possibility of gastric ulcer or carcinoma. These should also be ruled out by meticulous diagnostic testing.

4. **d.** Patient education programs for those with peptic ulcer disease should include advice to stop smoking, reduce alcohol intake, avoid aspirin and nonsteroidal antiinflammatory drugs, and eliminate those foods that cause

distress (e.g., fruit juice, and spicy and fatty foods). Milk, once a mainstay of ulcer therapy, does not help healing of ulcers and actually promotes gastric acid secretion.

5. **d.** The patient's typical posture in acute pancreatitis is sitting up, with the upper body bent forward. This posture is in response to the severe abdominal pain that radiates straight through to the back. Biliary tract disease and alcoholism account for ≥80% of hospital admissions for acute pancreatitis.

6. **a.** An objective physical finding in patients with acute pancreatitis is Cullen's sign, which is the appearance of faint, irregularly formed hemorrhagic patches on the skin around the umbilicus. The discolored skin is usually blue-black and becomes greenish-brown or yellow. Cullen's sign may appear 1 to 2 days after the onset of anorexia and the severe, poorly localized abdominal pains that are characteristic of acute pancreatitis. It is also associated with massive upper gastrointestinal hemorrhage and ruptured ectopic pregnancy.

7. **c.** Proton pump inhibitors are not used in treating acute pancreatitis. Patients with severe acute pancreatitis are treated in the intensive care unit. Fasting is maintained for 2 weeks, and sometimes for up to 4 weeks. Parenteral H₂ blockers are given. Other drugs are given to reduce pancreatic secretion: anticholinergics, glucagon, somatostatin, but which have no effect on the course or outcome of the disease.

8. **c.** Pain is controlled by giving meperidine 50 to 100 mg intramuscularly q3-4h if normal renal function is maintained. Morphine causes the sphincter of Oddi to contract and should not be given.

9. **c.** In diagnosing irritable bowel syndrome, crampy pain and constipation are the most common symptoms.

10. **b.** Older patients with abdominal disorders are usually more difficult to diagnose and treat because they usually present with vague symptoms and often little or no abdominal pain.

11. **c.** If acute diverticulosis is suspected, the best and safest diagnostic approach is to order abdominal and pelvic computed tomography with contrast. Diverticula are small outpouchings in the large bowel, often as a result of fecal impaction, particularly in older persons. Bleeding may ensue due to rupture of diverticula. Invasive procedures, such as lower endoscopy, should not be done.

12. **b.** Treatment for gastroesophageal reflux disease occurs in phases. Phase II therapy consists of drug therapy. This condition indicates incompetence of the lower esophageal sphincter. Patients with moderate symptoms that occur daily or several times a week are treated with either an H₂-receptor antagonist: ranitidine or izatidine 150 mg, famotidine 20 mg, cimetidine 400 to 800 mg. Promotility drugs include cisapride, metoclopramide, and reduce reflux by increasing lower esophageal sphincter pressure, thus enhancing esophageal acid clearance and gastric emptying. Patients should be advised not to lie down within 3 hours after meals and to raise the head of the bed on 6-inch blocks to help reduce reflux.

13. **c.** The direct cause of esophageal varices is portal hypertension. These are seen in 50% of patients with cirrhosis, but only 30% of these patients develop serious bleeding from the varices. Bleeding esophageal varices have a higher morbidity and mortality rate than any other source of upper gastrointestinal bleeding. Over 60% of these patients who bleed are dead within 5 years.

14. **a.** Crohn's disease, one of the two major forms of nonspecific inflammatory bowel disease, affects all parts of the gastrointestinal tract from the mouth to the anus. It most commonly affects the distal ileum and colon. The cause is not known, but evidence suggests that a genetic predisposition leads to an unregulated intestinal immune response to an environmental, dietary, or infectious agent.

15. **a.** When ulcerative colitis is confined to the rectum, constipation is not present. This condition is a chronic, inflammatory, and ulcerative disease that arises in the colonic mucosa, and is characterized most often by bloody diarrhea. The patient is advised to avoid raw fruits and vegetables that decrease mechanical trauma to the inflamed colonic mucosa and may lessen symptoms. In those with mild or moderate disease that does not extend proximally beyond the splenic flexure, remission may be achieved with a hydrocortisone edema rather than oral corticosteroid therapy.

16. **a.** Vegetarians are less likely to develop diverticulosis. Treatment attempts to reduce segmental spasm by means of a high-roughage diet, supplemented with psyllium seed preparations or bran.

17. **c.** The hallmark of painful diverticular disease is left lower abdominal tenderness and mass. Perforation of a colonic diverticulum results in an intraabdominal infection that varies from microperforation (most common) with local inflammation to macroperforation with either abscess or generalized peritonitis.

18. **b.** Histologic changes are irreversible in chronic pancreatitis. Plain films show calcifications due to pancreaticolithiasis in 30% of affected patients. Pseudocysts may develop. These changes are irreversible in many patients, and account for typical signs and symptoms of chronic pancreatitis: anorexia, vomiting, nauseam constipation, flatulence, and weight loss. Abdominal pain is often recurrent or persistent in the left upper quadrant with referral to the upper left lumbar region. Narcotic addiction is often an outcome of the disease.

19. **c.** The pain of cancer of the colon develops gradually, in the later stages of the disease. Adenocarcinoma of the colon and rectum grows slowly, and a long interval elapses before it is large enough to produce symptoms. Early diagnosis and treatment depend on routine examination. Treatment consists of wide surgical resection of the colon cancer and regional lymphatic drainage after the bowel is prepared. When surgery is not curative, limited palliative surgery may be indicated; median survival is 7 months.

20. **c.** The condition that is associated with difficulty in initiating swallowing is myasthenia gravis, a disease characterized by episodic muscle weakness caused by loss or dysfunction of acetylcholine receptors. Dysphagia is a common symptom, resulting in serious problems with swallowing. Eventually patients develop respiratory paresis that requires complete respiratory support.

21. **d.** Those patients with abdominal pain who require detailed evaluation are men and women older than 55. It is people in this age group who begin to develop serious diseases such as cancer and other abdominal diseases.

22. **c.** Visceral pain results from spasm or stretching of the covering or wall of a hollow viscus. Gas pains are commonly felt in the abdomen, when the bowel is distended.

23. **c.** Abdominal pain is associated with enlarging tumors, with inflammation in any part of the abdomen or organs enclosed within the peritoneum, and also with familial Mediterranean fever. Abdominal pain is not associated with hyperlipidemia.

24. **b.** Restlessness and pacing often indicate pain from gallbladder disease. Movement may lessen the colicky pain, which comes and goes at first, then becomes severe and localized in the right upper quadrant, often radiating to the right lower scapula.

25. **b.** Achalasia occurs as a result of inability of a muscle to relax, particularly the cardiac sphincter muscle of the stomach, resulting in slowed peristalsis. It may be caused by a malfunction of the mesenteric plexus of the esophagus that results in denervation of esophageal muscle. It can occur at any age but most commonly occurs between ages 20 and 40. Initially, forceful dilation of the sphincter is successful in about 85% of patients, although repeated dilations may be needed.

26. **d.** The preferred diagnostic test for diffuse esophageal spasm is videoesophagram, which provides detailed visualization of the entire esophagus by rapid- sequence method.

27. **a.** One of the risk factors for gastroesophageal reflux disease is a low basal lower esophageal sphincter pressure (10 to 30 mm Hg). Patients with esophageal strictures or Barrett's esophagus usually have an incompetent lower esophageal sphincter (<10 mm Hg), resulting in free reflux or stress reflux during abdominal straining, lifting, or bending. Barrett's esophagus is a condition in which the squamous epithelium of the esophagus is replaced by metaplastic columnar epithelium containing goblet and columnar cells, perhaps resulting from chronic reflux-induced injury to the esophageal squamous epithelium

28. **d.** The percentage of patients with cirrhosis who have esophageal varices is 50%.

29. **c.** In patients with duodenal ulcer, the pain is not present in the morning on awakening. Epigastric pain (dyspepsia) is the hallmark of peptic ulcer disease and is present in 80% to

90% of patients. However, pain is not sensitive or specific enough to serve as a reliable diagnostic criterion. Less than 25% of patients with dyspepsia have ulcer disease on endoscopy. Classic features of peptic ulcer pain are rhythmicity and periodicity. The pain, described as "dull, gnawing, aching," fluctuates in intensity throughout the day and night. About 50% of patients report pain relief from eating or from antacids.

30. **a.** Hemorrhoids are not varicosities of the rectal venous plexus but are caused by proximal displacement of anal tissues, known as anal pads, which permit the rectum to expand or contract as necessary for comfortable defecation to occur.

8
Kidney and Urologic Disorders

1. **b.** The unique system that the kidneys have involves the free ultrafiltration of water and nonprotein-bound, low-molecular-weight compounds from the plasma, and the selective reabsorption and/or excretion of these as the ultrafiltrate flows along the tubule.

2. **a.** There are about 1 million nephrons in each kidney. About 1300 ml of blood passes through the 2 million glomeruli every *minute*. This is 25% of cardiac output. The kidneys are extremely busy organs. Every day, they process by ultrafiltration between 170 and 180 liters of water and the outgoing small-molecular-weight constituents of blood.

3. **b.** The countercurrent hypothesis states that a small difference in osmotic concentration at any given point between fluid flowing in opposite directions in two parallel tubes that are connected in a hairpin manner is multiplied many times along the length of the tubes. The descending limb of the loop of Henle is permeable to water and impermeable to sodium. The fluid moves in the opposite direction as it flows up the ascending loop of Henle, which is impermeable to water but permeable to sodium. This opposite-direction movement causes a large osmolar concentration difference between the corticomedullary junction and the hairpin loop at the tip of the papillae; the result is a countercurrent multiplication and a much greater concentration of urine at this point.

4. **c.** When the glomerular filtration rate falls, it reduces the kidneys' ability to eliminate waste products, and to regulate the volume and composition of body fluids. This result is reflected in a rise in the blood level of urea or the plasma level of creatinine, and a reduction in measured glomerular filtration rate.

5. **c.** The filtration rate of the kidneys decreases $\geq$50% before evidence for this dramatic change is seen in the blood and plasma studies (urea and creatinine elevations). The body is well protected by this reserve capacity to excrete those constituents that must be excreted to maintain homeostasis.

6. **b.** Once it is elevated (because of decline in glomerular filtration rate), creatinine is a better guide to glomerular filtration rate than is urea. In addition, serum creatinine is a good way to monitor further deterioration in the glomerular filtration rate. However, a normal serum urea or creatinine does NOT indicate a normal glomerular filtration rate.

7. **c.** The glomerular filtration rate must be measured to define the exact level of renal function, particularly when the serum urea or creatinine is within normal range.

8. **d.** The "gold standard" among physiologists to measure glomerular filtration rate is the inulin clearance. This test is neither practical nor necessary in the clinical setting. The most widely used method of determining glomerular filtration rate is creatinine clearance. The usual practice is to collect a 24-hour urine sample and then measure a single serum creatinine value during the 24 hours.

9. **a.** Erythropoietin is a glycoprotein that is produced primarily by the kidneys. It is the major stimulus for erythropoiesis (production of red blood cells). A decrease in erythropoietin therefore results in anemia, which is a normochromic, normocytic anemia. An increase in erythropoietin results in polycythemia, or an overabundance of red blood cells in the blood, as occurs naturally when a person moves from a low-altitude geographic location to a high-altitude location, where oxygen is decreased. The body responds by producing more red blood cells to carry more oxygen.

10. **b.** Nonsteroidal antiinflammatory drugs inhibit prostaglandin synthesis by the kidneys. Prostaglandins are important to maintain

renal blood flow and glomerular filtration rate during decreases in both of these by vasoconstrictors such as angiotensin II, catecholamines, and α-adrenergics. Inhibition of prostaglandin synthesis causes further reduction of glomerular filtration rate, sometimes sufficiently severe to cause renal failure.

11. **b.** Proteinuria is one of the most common signs of renal disease. A dipstick measurement for proteinuria is easy and inexpensive. If a repeated dipstick test is also positive for protein, a 24-hour urine collection should be measured and tested.

12. **b.** Computed tomography is used primarily for detecting renal tumors. If the results are not clear, or are ambiguous, magnetic resonance imaging is done as follow-up to obtain more details on which to base a diagnosis.

13. **d.** Microalbuminuria is an early sign of diabetic glomerular disease. To correct this, tighter glucose control and angiotensin-converting enzyme inhibitor therapy are instituted.

14. **c.** Cholesterol and lipid stones are formed primarily in the gallbladder. The most common calculi seen in the urinary tract are calcium oxalate or phosphate. Struvite stones consist of triple phosphate (magnesium ammonium phosphate).

15. **a.** Patients with a single calcium calculus, uncomplicated by infection or obstruction, require only limited evaluation: plasma calcium concentration on two occasions to look for hyperparathyroidism, and an intravenous urogram to rule out any anatomic abnormality (e.g., medullary sponge kidney). The patient should receive instructions about fluid intake of more than 2 L/day, and when to call the care provider if specific symptoms occur: flank pain, or pain in the costovertebral angle, or pain in the lumbar or lower abdominal areas, which would indicate renal colic.

16. **c.** The normal urinary tract is sterile and thus very resistant to bacterial colonization. The meatus into the urethra is large enough for organisms to enter. The normal pH of blood is between 7.28 and 7.42, which is moderately alkaline. A pH of 6.9 is very acid (high level of H^+ ion concentration). The pH of urine is often at the low end of the scale (between 4.5 and 7.0), and quite acid, which may inhibit growth of pathogens. There seems to be no correlation between infec-

tions of the urinary tract and the manner of wiping the area after voiding or defecation.

17. **d.** Intrinsic renal causes of acute renal failure are associated with prolonged renal ischemia from hemorrhage, surgery, or a nephrotoxin. Prerenal causes of acute renal failure include excessive diuresis, hemorrhage, gastrointestinal losses, ascites, burns, low cardiac output, low systemic vascular resistance, or increased renal vascular resistance. Postrenal causes include ureteral obstruction, both intrinsic and extrinsic, and bladder obstruction. Renal causes include problems within the kidneys themselves: tubular injury, acute glomerulonephritis, tubulointerstitial nephritis, and acute vascular nephropathy from vasculitis, malignant hypertension, microangiopathy, and atheroembolism.

18. **d.** The survival rate for patients with acute renal failure is about 60%, despite aggressive nutritional and dialytic therapy. In many patients, the course of the illness is erratic, changing from day to day, dependent largely on the patient's response to nutritional and pharmacologic factors, as well as fluid intake.

19. **a.** A history of pulmonary emboli is not one of the risk factors for chronic renal failure. The other conditions listed cause direct injury to components of the kidney: the basement membrane, kidney vasculature, and tubules and/or glomeruli.

20. **d.** When the patient's serum creatinine concentration level reaches ≥1.5 to 2 (usually "2" is the magic number), progression to the chronic stage of renal failure seems certain. However, diagnosis becomes more difficult as the patient develops end-stage renal disease.

9
Hepatic and Biliary Disorders

1. **d.** Jaundice is a yellowing of the skin, sclerae, and other tissues caused by excess circulating bilirubin. It is seen best in the sclerae, or white part of the eye. A detailed history and physical examination are crucial because diagnostic errors usually result from inadequate clinical judgment and overreliance on laboratory data.

2. **d.** Healthy people produce about 250 to 350 mg of bilirubin daily, of which 70% to 80% derives from the breakdown of senescent red blood cells. The remaining 20% to 30% (early-labeled bilirubin) comes from other

heme proteins located primarily in the bone marrow and liver.

3. **c.** Splenomegaly is the hallmark of hypersplenism, and spleen size correlates directly with the degree of anemia. Many hematologic abnormalities are associated with liver disease. The primary mechanism is a sieve-like action resulting in red blood cell sequestration. The degree of anemia is compounded by a dilutional component resulting from the plasma volume expansion associated with splenomegaly.

4. **d.** Cholestasis (obstructive jaundice) is a clinical and biochemical syndrome that results when bile flow is impaired. Laboratory tests for cholestasis have limited value. The most typical abnormality is a disproportionately high serum alkaline phosphatase.

5. **c.** The incubation period of viral hepatitis caused by hepatic virus A is 15 to 50 days. Hepatitis A virus invariably disappears after the acute infection and, unlike hepatitis B and C virus infections, has no known chronic carrier state and plays no role in the production of chronic hepatitis or cirrhosis.

6. **a.** A major sign of viral hepatitis is clay-colored stools. However, signs and symptoms of viral hepatitis are extremely variable, ranging from asymptomatic infection without jaundice to a fulminating disease and death in a few days.

7. **c.** The differential diagnosis of hepatitis includes other viral diseases such as infectious mononucleosis, cytomegalovirus infection, and herpes simplex infections; spirochetal diseases, such as leptospirosis and secondary syphilis; brucellosis; rickettsial diseases, such as Q fever; drug-induced liver disease; and shock liver (ischemic hepatitis).

8. **b.** Chronic hepatitis is that which lasts from 3 to 6 months. This type is characterized by elevated aminotransferase levels for more than 6 months, and develops in 1% to 2% of immunocompetent adult patients. Over 80% of patients with hepatitis C develop chronic hepatitis. Cirrhosis may develop in up to 30% of those with chronic hepatitis C, and 40% of those with chronic hepatitis B. These two groups are also at risk (3% to 5%/year) of hepatocellular carcinoma.

9. **a.** The best treatment for chronic hepatitis C is recombinant human interferon alfa-2b, or alfa-

2a. The dose of each is 3 million units three times a week for 24 weeks, along with "consensus" interferon (a synthetic recombinant interferon derived by assigning the most commonly observed amino acid at each position of several alpha interferon subtypes), given in doses of 9 mg three times a week. These drugs induce biochemical, virologic, and histologic improvement, with return of alanine aminotransferase to normal, loss of hepatitis C virus ribonucleic acid from serum, decrease in hepatic inflammation, and sometimes regression of fibrosis, in up to 50% of patients.

10. **d.** Continuing therapy for patients with chronic hepatitis C is recommended for 12 to 18 months.

11. **b.** Alcoholic hepatitis is characterized by acute or chronic inflammation and parenchymal necrosis of the liver. Although alcoholic hepatitis is often a reversible disease, it is the most common precursor of cirrhosis in the United States. Cirrhosis ranks among the most common causes of death of adults in America.

12. **d.** In the United States, the 3-year mortality rate among those who recover from acute alcoholic hepatitis is 10 times greater than for people who are healthy.

13. **a.** Cirrhosis is characterized by a fibrous covering of the lobes. Liver biopsy shows macrovesicular fat, polymorphonuclear neutrophil infiltration with hepatic necrosis, and Mallory bodies (alcoholic hyaline).

14. **b.** After alcohol, the most common causes of cirrhosis are chronic hepatitis B and C.

15. **c.** Esophageal varices are caused by portal hypertension, which causes increased pressure in the portal venous system. The portal vein is formed by the superior mesenteric and splenic veins. It drains blood from the abdominal gastrointestinal tract, spleen, and pancreas into the liver. The portal vein provides about 75% of the liver's blood flow, and about 60% of its oxygen. The most significant complication of portal hypertension is acute variceal bleeding, most often from the distal esophagus.

16. **c.** The maximum dosage of spironolactone for patients with cirrhosis who do not respond to salt restriction is 400 mg/day. This diuretic drug helps to eliminate water, along with sodium, from the body to decrease the amount of ascites.

17. **b.** Liver transplantation is recommended for selected patients with cirrhosis. In many patients, other effects of alcohol in the vascular system, esophagus, and gastrointestinal tract may be severe enough to disallow liver transplantation.

18. **d.** The percentage of patients with severe hepatic dysfunction from cirrhosis (serum albumin <3 g/dl, bilirubin >3 mg/dl, ascites, encephalopathy, cachexia, upper gastrointestinal bleeding) who survive 6 months is 50%.

19. **b.** Primary biliary cirrhosis is a chronic disease of the liver characterized by autoimmune destruction of intrahepatic bile ducts and cholestasis. The onset of symptoms is insidious, and usually occurs in women aged 40 to 60.

20. **c.** The major symptom in primary biliary cirrhosis is pruritus, perhaps due to a buildup of toxins in the skin.

21. **b.** One of the most significant laboratory findings that should lead to a work-up and diagnosis of primary biliary cirrhosis is a greatly increased alkaline phosphatase level. The disease must be differentiated from chronic biliary tract obstruction, carcinoma of the bile ducts, primary sclerosing cholangitis, sarcoidosis, drug toxicity (e.g., chlorpromazine), and chronic hepatitis.

22. **b.** The major physiologic aberration in Wilson's disease is excessive absorption of copper from the small intestine, and excessive deposition of copper in the liver and brain. Wilson's disease is a rare autosomal recessive disorder that usually occurs between ages 10 and 30. It is a potentially reversible disorder if recognized and treated early.

23. **c.** The most common cause (90% of cases) of acute cholecystitis is gallstones (cholelithiasis). It occurs when a stone becomes impacted in the cystic duct and inflammation develops behind the obstruction.

24. **c.** The typical pain in acute cholecystitis occurs in the right hypochondrium with radiation to the infrascapular area, just beneath the shoulder blade. The pain that occurs in an acute attack usually begins after a large or fatty meal. In uncomplicated cases, the pain may gradually subside over 12 to 18 hours.

25. **c.** The most reliable imaging procedure to diagnose acute cholecystitis is plain films of the abdomen, which may show radiopaque gall-stones in 15% of cases. ^{99m}Tc hepatobiliary imaging, using iminodiacetic acid compounds, known as a hepatobiliary imaging imino-diacetic acid scan, shows the obstructed cystic duct. This test is reliable if the bilirubin is under 5 mg/dl, with 98% sensitivity and 81% specificity.

26. **d.** Chronic cholecystitis is far more common than acute cholecystitis. Chronic cholecystitis results from repeated episodes of acute cholecystitis or chronic irritation of the gallbladder wall by stones.

27. **d.** Complications of chronic cholecystitis include "strawberry gallbladder," in which the villi of the gallbladder enlarge due to deposits of cholesterol, and become visible to the naked eye, appearing as though the gallbladder is filled with strawberries; cholangitis with Charcot's triad of symptoms (intention tremor, nystagmus, and scanning speech); and gangrene of the gallbladder.

28. **d.** Gallstones are present, often without symptoms, in about 20% (20 million) of the U.S. population. Symptoms may occur from time to time but usually subside without treatment, although eventually surgery may be necessary.

29. **c.** Gallstones are classified by chemical composition such as cholesterol and calcium bilirubinate.

30. **b.** Cholecystectomy is the treatment of choice for patients with symptomatic cholelithiasis and is relatively easy with the laparoscopic procedure, which allows for complete resolution of symptoms because the gallbladder is removed.

10
Endocrine Disorders

1. **b.** The hypothalamic gland is now known to be the final common pathway that receives input from virtually all other areas of the central nervous system, and directs input to the pituitary.

2. **a.** Hormones are classified according to chemical structure as proteins, glycoproteins, polypeptides, amines, and steroids. The protein hormones (insulin, pituitary, hypothalamic, parathyroid) are water-soluble and generally circulate in free (unbound) forms. Lipid-soluble hormones are transported in blood primarily bound to proteins designated as carrier or binding proteins.

3. **d.** These include corticotropin-releasing hormone, gonadotropin-releasing hormone, growth hormone–releasing hormone, prolactin-releasing-inhibiting hormone, prolactin-releasing hormone, and thyrotropin-releasing hormone. The hypothalamic hormones therefore control at least part of the four broad categories of body function: reproduction, growth and development, maintenance of homeostasis, and energy production, utilization, and storage during metabolic processes.

4. **b.** Biologically active hormones are those that are not bound to proteins, and are therefore "free" hormones. These hormones (e.g., thyroxine) circulate freely in the blood and the amounts of free hormones can be determined by specific laboratory measures.

5. **c.** The ability of a cell to respond to a particular hormone depends on the presence of specific receptors for that hormone on or within the cell. Cell hormone receptors are proteins that bind with the circulating hormone; hormone-receptor binding is the first step in eliciting a response from the cell.

6. **b.** Diabetes mellitus is the most common endocrine disorder, affecting at least 8 million Americans. About the same number is estimated to have undiagnosed diabetes mellitus.

7. **b.** Drugs that can simulate endocrine disorders include licorice (hypertension, hypermineralocorticoidism); amiodarone (hyperthyroidism); and antibiotics (polyarteritis). Diuretics do not simulate endocrine disorders, although diuretics have side effects and can cause particular conditions (e.g., hypercalcemia).

8. **a.** Clinical syndromes that result from autoimmune diseases that affect the endocrine glands include pernicious anemia, Addison's disease, and Graves' disease. Acromegaly is not related to autoimmune diseases.

9. **c.** Hypopituitarism and the resulting decrease or absence of specific hormones include the strong relationship between hypothalamic and pituitary hormones: gonadotropin-releasing hormones, growth hormone–releasing hormone; somatostatin, thyroid-releasing hormone; prolactin-releasing hormone, follicle-stimulating hormone, luteinizing hormone, thyroid-stimulating hormone, adrenocorticotropic hormone.

10. **c.** Diabetes insipidus is caused by a deficiency of vasopressin (antidiuretic hormone), or an inability of the kidneys to respond to antidiuretic hormone. The condition may be acquired, familial, idiopathic, neurogenic, or nephrogenic.

11. **c.** Causes of polyuria, other than diabetes mellitus, include lithium therapy, which inhibits thyroid hormone synthesis and secretion, and can cause goiters in some people; decreased synthesis of antidiuretic hormone; decreased release of antidiuretic hormone; vasopressin (antidiuretic hormone)-resistant polyuria, a congenital nephrogenic diabetes insipidus (usually X-linked recessive); acquired nephrogenic diabetes insipidus due to chronic renal disease; systemic or metabolic disease such as amylasemia, amyloidosis, hypercalcemic or hypokalemic nephropathy, or sickle cell disease; or osmotic diuresis due to glucose levels in diabetes mellitus, or poorly resorbed solutes (mannitol, sorbitol, urea).

12. **a.** Primary hypothyroidism is considered to be an autoimmune disease. Its cause does not include thyroid-stimulating hormone deficiency, increased thyroid hormone, or vitamin D excess.

13. **c.** One of the major physiologic effects of thyroid hormones is that they increase red blood cells. Another significant effect is that they increase protein synthesis in virtually every body tissue. T_3 increases oxygen consumption primarily by increasing the activity of the sodium pump (Na^+,K^+-ATPase), in tissues responsible for basal oxygen consumption: heart, liver, kidneys, and skeletal muscles.

14. **c.** Hyperthyroidism is also known as thyrotoxicosis. This is a condition encompassing several specific diseases, characterized by hypermetabolism and elevated serum levels of free thyroid hormones.

15. **b.** Graves' disease is an autoimmune disease. It is characterized by hyperthyroidism and one or more of the following: goiter, exophthalmos, and pretibial myxedema. The disease has a chronic course with remissions and exacerbations.

16. **a.** The most common form of hypothyroidism is primary. Hypothyroidism is thought to be an autoimmune disease, usually occurring as a result of Hashimoto's thyroiditis and associated with a firm goiter or, later in the

disease process, a shrunken fibrotic thyroid gland with little or no function.

17. **b.** One of the most prominent complications of aggressive thyroid therapy for hypothyroidism is congestive heart failure. The patient may also develop increased susceptibility to infection. Megacolon has been seen in patients with long-standing hypothyroidism.

18. **d.** The adrenal glands' three zones produce the following: **Aldosterone,** a mineralocorticoid, is secreted by the zona glomerulosa, the outer layer of the adrenal cortex. It stimulates the renal tubule to reabsorb sodium and excrete potassium, protecting against hypovolemia and hyperkalemia. **Cortisol** is the major glucocorticoid secreted by the middle zona fasciculata and the inner zona reticularis of the adrenal cortex. Cortisol counters insulin effects, tending to cause hyperglycemia by inhibiting insulin secretion and by increasing hepatic gluconeogenesis, substrate being provided by the increased amino acids made available by cortisol's inhibition of protein synthesis in muscles. **Androgens** are produced in the adrenal cortex, mostly by the inner zona fasciculata. Testosterone and androstenedione are the major functional androgens secreted by the adrenal. Their secretion causes adrenarche, which precedes gonadal androgen secretion and stimulates the first sexual hair of puberty.

19. **b.** After adrenalectomy, cortisol secretion is increased in a complication known as Nelson's syndrome, in which the pituitary gland continues to expand, causing a marked increase in adrenocorticotropic hormone and β-melanocyte-stimulating hormone secretion, resulting in severe hyperpigmentation.

20. **b.** Addison's disease is also known as adrenocortical insufficiency. Steroid replacement therapy must be lifelong. Replacement is usually 15 to 20 mg of cortisol (or equivalent) daily. The simplest and least expensive therapy is 12.5 mg (one half of a 25-mg cortisone tablet) twice daily. An alternative is 10 to 15 mg of cortisol (hydrocortisone) twice daily.

21. **c.** The hallmark of primary hyperparathyroidism is hypercalcemia. The disease is caused by hypersecretion of parathyroid hormone, usually by a parathyroid adenoma.

22. **a.** Cushing's syndrome most often occurs as a primary disease caused by destruction or dysfunction of the adrenal cortices. It is characterized by chronic deficiency of cortisol, aldosterone, and adrenal androgens. Hyperpigmentation is often present, and can be subtle or strikingly dark. The darker color appears first in folds of skin on the hands and other areas.

23. **c.** Repeated normal values of free cortisol in 24-hour urine collections make the diagnosis of Cushing's syndrome suspicious. In about 70% of patients who are diagnosed with Cushing's syndrome, which refers to the manifestations of excessive corticosteroids, usually due to excessive doses of glucocorticoid drugs, the condition is really due to Cushing's disease, caused by adrenocorticotropic hormone hypersecretion by the pituitary gland. The underlying cause is often a small, benign pituitary adenoma.

24. **c.** The classification of diabetes mellitus is different from the old system, which was based on insulin dependence. The newer classification is based on etiology of the disease. Type 1 diabetes mellitus is due to pancreatic islet B-cell destruction, predominantly by an autoimmune process; these patients are prone to ketoacidosis. Type 2 diabetes is the more prevalent form, and results from insulin resistance, mainly caused by visceral obesity, with a defect in compensatory insulin secretion.

25. **d.** The main consumer of glucose in the body is the brain, which is essential for efficient cell function.

26. **c.** Type 2 diabetics comprise more than 90% of all diabetics in the United States. Circulating endogenous insulin is sufficient to prevent ketoacidosis but is inadequate to prevent hyperglycemia in the face of increased needs owing to tissue sensitivity. The cause of this type of diabetes is unknown.

27. **a.** Factors relating to onset of type 2 diabetes include abdominal-visceral obesity and genetic influence as seen in monozygotic twins over 40 years of age, in whom concordance develops in over 70% of cases within a year whenever one twin develops type 2 disease. Environmental factors may be involved regarding food patterns. Many of these patients do take in excessive calories, however. Tissue insensitivity to insulin is noted in most type 2 patients regardless of weight.

28. **a.** Corticosteroid therapy can affect every body system. Prolonged treatment with systemic glucocorticoids causes adverse effects that can be life-threatening. Major side effects include insomnia, personality change, weight gain, muscle weakness, polyuria, kidney stones, diabetes mellitus, sex hormone suppression, occasional amenorrhea, candidiasis and other opportunistic infections, osteoporosis with fractures, or aseptic necrosis of bones, particularly of the hips.

29. **d.** One of the classes of drugs that may cause hypercalcemia is loop diuretics.

30. **c.** The most common cause of hypocalcemia is renal failure. The others listed can also cause hypocalcemia but are not as common as kidney disease.

11
Acid-Base, Fluid, and Electrolyte Disorders

1. **c.** In healthy males, water makes up between 50% and 60% of lean body weight, in all compartments—intracellular, interstitial fluid, and plasma. Total body water in healthy females makes up between 45% and 50% of lean body weight. Small amounts of water are contained in bone, dense connective tissue, and epithelial secretions (e.g., digestive secretions and cerebrospinal fluid).

2. **c.** Water molecules move freely across permeable membranes only when there is NO solute present. The other three answers are not relevant: molecular weight, size of cell membrane, or presence of NaCl (a solute).

3. **b.** Water tends to stay in the solute-containing compartment because there is less free diffusion across the membrane, thus inhibiting the movement of water across the membrane. Most of the magnesium in the cell is bound and osmotically inactive. The specific compartment is not relevant; it's the one with the most solute that will hold onto the water.

4. **c.** There is less bicarbonate in intracellular fluid. Extracellular fluid comprises both plasma and interstitial fluid, because both are outside of cells. The healthy adult contains about 11.2 L of interstitial fluid (16% of body weight), and about 2.8 L of plasma (4% of body weight). Plasma and interstitial fluid have similar chemical compositions and, together with intracellular fluid, help to control the movement of water and electrolytes through the body. Some of the ionized components of extracellular fluid are protein, magnesium, potassium, chlorine, calcium, and certain sulfates.

5. **d.** The sodium-potassium-ATPase (adenosine triphosphatase) pump largely restricts sodium to the extracellular fluid, and potassium to the intracellular fluid. Therefore, movement across the cell membrane is possible, but only in a limited (restricted) way, depending on many factors and the type of disease present.

6. **c.** This type of solution is distributed equally to all compartments, whereas one liter of 0.9% saline remains in the extracellular compartment and is therefore the treatment of choice for extracellular water depletion, since sodium keeps the water in this compartment.

7. **b.** Schrier states that the fullness of the arterial vascular compartment (the effective arterial blood volume is the primary determinant of renal sodium and water excretion. Sufficient circulatory volume must be present to maintain body fluid homeostasis. Without this pressure, water and sodium are not "pushed" out of the kidneys in sufficient quantities to maintain the correct balance (homeostasis). A person who has lost a great deal of blood, for example, cannot excrete sodium and water from the kidneys in sufficient amounts to remain in a normal electrolyte state. When the effective arterial volume is expanded, the kidneys can excrete sodium in amounts greater than 100 mmol/L.

8. **d.** Sodium reabsorption occurs in both the proximal and collecting tubules, not in the distal tubule or the loop of Henle, both of which are flow-dependent to allow for sodium, potassium, and chloride transport, whereas other substances are used for sodium reabsorption in the proximal and collecting tubules (e.g., angiotensin and noradrenaline in the proximal tubule, and aldosterone and atrial natriuretic peptide in the collecting tubules).

9. **a.** Vasodilators, not vasoconstrictors, are involved in body water homeostasis, which is maintained by thirst, and the urine concentrating and diluting functions of the kidney. These functions are controlled by intracellular osmoreceptors, primarily in the hypothalamus, to some extent by some volume receptors in capacitance vessels close to the heart, and by

way of the renin-angiotensin-aldosterone system. The osmoreceptors sense changes in the plasma sodium concentration and osmolality, and then act on both thirst and the release of antidiuretic hormone (vasopressin). Antidiuretic hormone increases the water permeability of the (normally) impermeable cortical and medullary collecting tubules, to promote water reabsorption in the collecting tubules.

10. **c.** Loop diuretics cause urate to be *retained*, which can cause gout. The other components listed are excreted in larger amounts by the action of loop diuretics. Loss of potassium can, of course, lead to hypokalemia. Magnesium is also excreted, which could lead to hypomagnesemia. However, the loop diuretics do cause sodium chloride and water to be excreted, to decrease water overload, and cause increased venous capacitance, which rapidly improves the status of patients with left ventricular failure.

11. **b.** Increased sodium causes water to be retained, and the formation of edema in body tissues; increased amounts of body water result from increased sodium. Decreased lymphatic drainage would help to reduce total body sodium and water, and decreased venous tone would enable the veins to expand slightly, and to thus hold larger amounts of blood, which is to be avoided in patients who are retaining water.

12. **c.** Sodium and water are combined, and both are lost at the same time, which leads to extracellular volume depletion rather than expansion. With water, potassium is lost. When loop diuretics are given, they retain urate, which can cause gout. In some cases, relatively more sodium than water can be lost, resulting in hyponatremia.

13. **d.** Healthy kidneys can excrete up to 25 L of urine a day, all other factors also being normal. Water intake would have to be excessive for the kidneys not to be able to function normally.

14. **b.** Symptoms of hyponatremia occur when the effective plasma osmolality falls to ≤240 mOsm/kg, regardless of the underlying cause. The rate of the decrease may be as important as the magnitude of the decrease; symptoms may occur at somewhat higher plasma osmolality if the change occurs rapidly.

15. **a.** Restricting water to 1 to 2 L/day is one of the first orders for patients with symptomatic

hyponatremia. Diuretics should be used, to hasten excretion of water and NaCl. Hypertonic intravenous solutions should be administered with great caution; no more than 22 ml only if necessary. Emergency dialysis may also be considered if other measures fail. The goal is to treat the underlying problem (e.g., renal insufficiency), and replace sodium and potassium deficits.

16. **c.** Whereas diabetes mellitus is not a risk factor, central diabetes insipidus is. Other risk factors are renal disease, severe burns, excessive sweating, or any condition that creates loss of body water, with high plasma sodium concentration.

17. **d.** Whereas the other symptoms may help to differentiate low potassium, particularly signs of muscle dysfunction such as cramping and fasciculations, the laboratory evidence of a low plasma potassium level is definitive.

18. **c.** Any patient with mild encephalopathy and unexplained dementia, depression, or psychosis should be suspected of having a slowly developing hypocalcemia. In prolonged hypocalcemia, papilledema and cataracts may occur.

19. **c.** Excessive exogenous vitamin D produces increased bone reabsorption and increased intestinal calcium absorption and hypercalciuria. Sarcoidosis is seen in up to 20% of patients with hypercalcemia; other granulomatous diseases include tuberculosis, leprosy, berylliosis, and histoplasmosis. Immobilization (e.g., prolonged bed rest) can cause hypercalcemia due to accelerated bone resorption, which results in osteoporosis.

20. **d.** When metabolic alkalosis is associated with extracellular fluid volume depletion, the urine chloride is almost always low (<10 to 20 mEq/L), but urine Na may exceed 20 mEq/L. Sodium chloride is used with caution in these patients, and particularly in those who tend to develop volume overload, perhaps because of renal insufficiency. In most cases, potassium chloride is the preferred choice for chloride replacement.

21. **b.** Brain cellular water content is elevated in both acute and chronic hyponatremia. In acute hyponatremia, brain cells cannot adjust their tonicity nearly as well, and swelling results. Thus symptoms of central nervous sys-

tem dysfunction are more common, and mortality is substantially greater in acute hyponatremia than in chronic hyponatremia.

22. **c.** A major symptom in patients with hypernatremia is thirst. The absence of thirst in conscious patients with hypernatremia suggests an impaired thirst mechanism. Those unable to talk may be unable to communicate thirst and their need for water. The nurse should make certain that there is water available and that the patient can help him/herself. There are often signs/symptoms of central nervous system dysfunction due to brain cell shrinkage: excitability, confusion, seizures.

23. **a.** Cardiac toxicity is often the first indication of hyperkalemia. Electrocardiogram changes include shortage of the QT interval and tall, symmetric peaked T waves. If the hyperkalemia progresses, the electrocardiogram records nodal and ventricular dysrhythmias, widening of the QRS complex, PR interval prolongation, and disappearance of the P wave. As the patient's condition worsens, the QRS complex degenerates into a sine wave pattern, followed by ventricular asystole or fibrillation.

24. **d.** If no electrocardiogram abnormalities are seen, and if the plasma K is not greatly elevated, sodium polystyrene sulfonate in sorbitol is given—15 to 30 g in 30 to 70 ml of 70% sorbitol PO q4-6h. This medication acts as a cation exchange resin, and removes K through the gastrointestinal mucosa.

25. **c.** Two characteristic signs of tetany are Chvostek's and Trousseau's signs. Chvostek's sign is an abnormal spasm of the facial muscles elicited by light taps on the facial nerve in patients who are hypocalcemic. Trousseau's sign is a carpal spasm induced by inflating a sphygmomanometer cuff on the upper arm to a pressure exceeding the systolic blood pressure for 3 minutes. A positive sign is seen in patients with hypocalcemia and hypomagnesemia.

26. **a.** Symptoms of hypocalcemia result primarily from neuromuscular irritability. Muscle cramps involving the back and legs are common complaints. Slowly developing, insidious hypocalcemia may produce mild, diffuse encephalopathy, indicated by unexplained dementia, depression, or psychosis. Papilledema sometimes occurs and cataracts may develop after prolonged hypocalcemia. Severe hypocalcemia with plasma Ca <7 mg/dl (<1.75 mmol/L) may cause tetany, laryngospasm, or generalized convulsions.

27. **d.** Hypercalcemia may be caused by excessive bone resorption, primary hyperparathyroidism, or other causes: malignancy with bone metastasis, vitamin D toxicity, multiple myeloma, hyperthyroidism.

28. **c.** Phosphorus is one of the most abundant elements in the human body. Most phosphorus is complexed with oxygen as phosphate (PO_4). About 85% of the 500 to 700 g of phosphate is contained in bone, where it is an important constituent of the crystal hydroxyapatite. In soft tissues, phosphate is found mainly in the intracellular compartment and is an integral component of several organic compounds such as nucleic acids and the phospholipids of cell membranes.

29. **a.** The most common cause of clinically significant hypomagnesemia is inadequate intake and impairment of renal or gut absorption. It is seen in association with prolonged parenteral feeding, usually combined with loss of body fluids via gastric suction or diarrhea.

30. **c.** The Henderson-Hasselbach equation is used to determine plasma pH. Plasma bicarbonate and CO_2 concentration and pH are chemically related to one another, as shown by the Henderson-Hasselbach equation.

12
Hematologic Disorders

1. **b.** Among causes of anemia, blood dyscrasias do not result in anemia. This group of disorders is defined as morbid states resulting from the presence of abnormal materials in the blood that usually affect blood cells or platelets.

2. **a.** Classification of anemia by mean corpuscular volume includes all of those listed except normocytic, which describes the shape of red blood cells in a blood smear seen by microscope.

3. **d.** The most common cause of iron deficiency anemia is blood loss, which can be either massive hemorrhage at one time, or minimal loss of blood over weeks or months, e.g., bleeding gums, menstrual bleeding. Marrow reserve is limited and depletion can occur from almost any site of bleeding, large or small.

4. **c.** Total body iron for women is 35 mg/kg. Most (70% to 95%) of the iron is present in hemoglobin in circulating red blood cells. One milliliter of packed red blood cells (not whole blood) contains about 1 mg of iron.

5. **b.** A 70-kg man has about 2100 mg of iron in his circulating blood. In women, the red blood cell volume is about 27 ml/kg. A 50-kg woman has about 1350 mg of iron in red blood cells. About 200 to 400 mg of iron is present in myoglobin and nonheme enzymes. The amount of iron in plasma is negligible. Other than in circulating red blood cells, the major location of iron is the storage pool; iron is deposited either as ferritin or as hemosiderin, found in macrophages. There is a wide range in the average amount of storage iron (0.5 to 2 g), but about 25% of women in the United States have none.

6. **d.** The presence of mild anemia indicates an underlying disorder such as chronic infection or inflammation, cancer, or liver disease. If a person shows typical symptoms of anemia (fatigability, tachycardia, palpitations, tachypnea on exertion), a physical examination is warranted to discover the reason for anemia.

7. **b.** In iron-deficiency anemia, the total iron-binding capacity rises in response to the decreased number of red blood cells. The serum ferritin becomes abnormally low, <30 μg/L, indicating absent iron stores. Serum ferritin is a highly reliable indicator of iron deficiency.

8. **a.** Anemia of chronic disease is seen in rheumatoid arthritis. This type of anemia is characterized by low serum iron, low total iron-binding capacity, and normal or increased serum ferritin (or normal or increased bone marrow iron stores). In cases of significant anemias ($<60\%$ of baseline), coexistent iron deficiency or folic acid deficiency should be suspected.

9. **c.** Patients undergoing hemodialysis usually have both iron and folate deficiency.

10. **d.** The thalassemia anemias are hereditary disorders that occur because of defective hemoglobin synthesis due to reduction in the synthesis of globin chains (α or β), which causes reduced hemoglobin synthesis, eventually producing a hypochromic microcytic anemia.

11. **a.** Diagnosis of thalassemia is by quantitative hemoglobin studies. Thalassemias are considered to be hypoproliferative anemias, hemolytic anemias, and anemias related to abnormal hemoglobin.

12. **d.** Treatment of α- and β-thalassemia minor is not required, because these persons are clinically normal. α-Thalassemia is due primarily to gene deletion, causing reduced α-globin chain synthesis. Because all adult hemoglobins are alpha-containing, α-thalassemia produces no change in the percentage distribution of hemoglobins A_{12}, A_2, and F.

13. **d.** Liver vitamin B_{12} stores are sufficient to supply the body's needs for 3 to 5 years. Because vitamin B_{12} is present in all foods of animal origin, dietary vitamin B_{12} deficiency is extremely rare and seen only in vegans—strict vegetarians who avoid all dairy products, meat, and fish.

14. **c.** The usual dose of vitamin B_{12} therapy is 1000 μg intramuscularly two to four times/week. Therapy is needed for those patients who have had abdominal surgery such as gastrectomy, which eliminates the site of intrinsic factor production necessary for binding with vitamin B_{12} and absorption in the ileum, then is transported through the plasma and is stored in the liver; blind loop syndrome causes competition for vitamin B_{12} by bacterial overgrowth in the lumen of the intestine; surgical resection of the ileum eliminates the site of vitamin B_{12} absorption.

15. **a.** Inadequate amounts of folate ingested during pregnancy result in neural tube defects such as spina bifida.

16. **b.** Sickle cell disease (Hb S) affects 0.15% of the black population in the United States. Sickle cell disease is an autosomal-recessive disorder in which an abnormal hemoglobin leads to chronic hemolytic anemia with a variety of severe clinical consequences.

17. **c.** In a married couple, if both partners have the sickle cell trait, the chance of their offspring having sickle cell disease is 25%. The hemoglobin S gene is carried in 8% of American blacks, and one birth out of 400 in these couples produces a child with sickle cell anemia.

18. **a.** Patients with sickle cell disease who experience a thrombotic crisis are treated with hydration and narcotics. These episodes are repeated from onset of the disease during the first year of life when clusters of sickled cells

occlude the microvasculature of the involved organs. The episodes may last for hours to days, and produce acute pain and low-grade fever.

19. **c.** Disseminated intravascular coagulation is a very serious coagulopathy caused by overstimulation of both clotting and anticlotting processes. Disseminated intravascular coagulation can be caused by many serious illnesses, including sepsis (especially with gram-negative bacteria but possible with any widespread bacterial or fungal infection), severe head injury, obstetric complications (amniotic fluid embolus, septic abortion, retained fetus), cancer (acute promyelocytic leukemia, mucinous adenocarcinoma), and major hemolytic transfusion reactions.

20. **b.** Acute leukemia is a malignancy of hematopoietic progenitor cells. The malignant cell loses its ability to mature and differentiate. These cells proliferate in an uncontrolled fashion and replace normal bone marrow elements. Radiation and some toxins (benzene) are leukemogenic.

21. **c.** Most of the clinical findings in patients with leukemia are due to replacement of normal bone marrow by malignant cells. Most patients, when first seen, have been ill for days or weeks. Bleeding, usually due to thrombocytopenia, occurs in the skin and mucosal surfaces, with gingival bleeding, epistaxis, or menorrhagia.

22. **a.** A blast cell is any immature cell (e.g., erythroblast, lymphoblast).

23. **a.** Most patients with acute leukemia are first treated with combination chemotherapy of daunorubicin and cytarabine to achieve complete remission. Effective therapy produces aplasia of the bone marrow, which takes 2 to 3 weeks to recover. During this period, intensive supportive care, including transfusion and antibiotic therapy, is required. Once remission occurs, several different types of postremission therapy are potentially curative.

24. **b.** Chronic lymphocytic leukemia is a clonal malignancy of B lymphocytes (rarely, T lymphocytes). The disease is usually indolent, with slowly progressive accumulation of long-lived small lymphocytes. These cells are immunocompetent and respond poorly to antigenic stimulation. Clinical manifestations are

immunosuppression, bone marrow failure, and organ infiltration with lymphocytes.

25. **d.** The median survival is 5-6 years, although 25% survive for 10 years or longer. It is important to reassure these patients that they can live a normal life for many years. Those with stage III or IV disease have a median survival of less than 2 years.

26. **d.** Chronic myelogenous leukemia is a myeloproliferative disorder characterized by overproduction of myeloid cells. The myeloid cells retain the capacity for differentiation, and normal bone marrow function is retained during the early phases. The disease usually remains stable for years, and then transforms to a more overtly malignant disease.

27. **b.** The hallmark sign in chronic myelogenous leukemia is a strikingly elevated white blood cell count due to overproduction, which may be greater than 500,000/μl.

28. **b.** The only cure for chronic myelogenous leukemia is allogeneic bone marrow transplantation. Young patients (60%) who have bone marrow transplantation have long-term survival and appear to be cured.

29. **c.** The incidence of Hodgkin's disease is characterized by a bimodal age distribution: those in their twenties and those over 50. This disease is a group of cancers characterized by Reed-Sternberg cells in an appropriate reactive cellular background. The nature of the malignant cell is a subject of controversy. The diagnosis is made by lymph node biopsy.

30. **c.** Non-Hodgkin's lymphoma is characterized by painless lymphadenopathy and malignant monoclonal proliferation of lymphoid cells in sites of the immune system, including lymph nodes, bone marrow, spleen, liver, and gastrointestinal tract.

13
Gynecologic Disorders

1. **c.** Premenstrual syndrome affects women primarily between the ages of 25 and 40. Although not a serious condition, the effects of premenstrual syndrome are felt by a large number of women, resulting in lost time at work and considerable physical and psychological symptoms.

2. **c.** Typical symptoms of premenstrual syndrome include bloating, ankle edema, breast

pain, pelvic pain, headaches, emotional lability, irritability, depression, and anxiety. Weight loss is not a sign of premenstrual syndrome.

3. **a.** The cause of premenstrual syndrome is unknown. It appears to be related to fluctuations in levels of estrogen and progesterone, causing fluid retention that likely accounts for many of the symptoms that these patients have. Recent studies show that women with premenstrual syndrome metabolize progesterone differently, producing less allopregnenolone, a neurosteroid that enhances γ-aminobutyric acid–A ($GABA_A$) receptor function in the brain and that has anxiolytic effects. Production of pregnenolone, which has an opposite effect in the brain, may be increased.

4. **b.** The cause of dysfunctional uterine bleeding is overgrowth of endometrium due to estrogen stimulation without adequate progesterone to stabilize growth; this occurs in anovular cycles. Anovulation associated with high estrogen levels commonly occurs in teenagers, in women aged late thirties to late forties, and in extremely obese women or those with polycystic ovary syndrome.

5. **c.** Tests that are usually done for patients with dysfunctional uterine bleeding include complete blood count, coagulation time, sedimentation rate, thyroid function tests, and cervical smears for cytologic studies and culture. Blood glucose is usually done to rule out diabetes, and a pregnancy test is done to rule out miscarriage with retained placental tissue or ectopic pregnancy.

6. **a.** Other causes of dysfunctional uterine bleeding are excessive drug or alcohol use, myomas, and stress. Ultrasound is used to evaluate endometrial thickness and to diagnose intrauterine or ectopic pregnancy or adnexal masses. Endovaginal ultrasound with saline infusion sonohysterography is used to diagnose endometrial polyps or subserous myomas.

7. **b.** In cases of intractable bleeding, danazol 200 mg qid is sometimes used to create atrophic endometrium. Premenopausal patients with abnormal uterine bleeding include those with submucous myomas, infection, early abortion, or pelvic neoplasms. History, physical examination, and laboratory findings identify those patients who require definitive

therapy. A large group of patients remains, most of whom have dysfunctional uterine bleeding on a hormonal basis. Hormones used to treat these patients include progestins, which limit and stabilize endometrial growth. For younger women who are actively bleeding, any of the combination oral contraceptives are given four times daily for 1 or 2 days, followed by two pills daily through day 5, then one pill daily through day 20; after withdrawal bleeding occurs, pills are taken in the usual dosage for three cycles.

8. **d.** In older women, the test/procedure that is done prior to beginning hormonal therapy is a dilation and curettage.

9. **b.** Postmenopausal vaginal bleeding is any vaginal bleeding that occurs 6 months or more after menses have ceased. Any bleeding of this kind should be thoroughly investigated. The most common causes are endometrial proliferation, hyperplasia, endometrial or cervical cancer, and taking estrogens without added progestin.

10. **d.** Carcinoma of the cervix is considered by many experts to be a sexually transmitted disease. Cancer appears first in the intraepithelial layers (the preinvasive stage, or carcinoma in situ). Preinvasive cancer (CIN III) is a common diagnosis in women 25 to 40 years of age and is etiologically related to infection with the human papillomavirus. An estimated 2 to 10 years are required for carcinoma to penetrate the basement membrane and invade the tissues. After invasion, death usually occurs within 3 to 5 years in untreated or unresponsive patients.

11. **b.** The risk of cervical cancer is inversely related to age at first intercourse. The risk rises with the number of sexual partners and the frequency of intercourse.

12. **b.** Human papillomavirus infection is closely associated with cervical intraepithelial neoplasia. Current data indicate that cervical infection with the human papillomavirus is associated with a high percentage of all cervical dysplasias and cancers. Over 60 human papillomavirus subtypes are recognized, of which types 6 and 31 tend to cause mild dysplasia, while types 16, 18, 31, and others cause higher grade cellular changes.

13. **d.** Staging of cervical carcinoma ranges between 0 and IVB. In Stage I, carcinoma is

strictly confined to the cervix. IA1 and IA2 are used to define diameter and depth of the growth in millimeters (mm). Stage IVB involves the spread of cancer to distant organs.

14. **c.** Emergency treatment for vaginal hemorrhage due to cervical cancer includes wet vaginal packing, emergency irradiation, or ligation of the uterine or hypogastric arteries. Ligation and suturing of the cervix is not done because it does not control hemorrhage from blood vessels.

15. **d.** Overall 5-year survival rate for carcinoma of the cervix is 68% in white women and 55% in black women. The difference may be because black women do not seek medical care as early as white women.

16. **d.** Five-year survival rate in patients with stage IV cervical cancer is less than 20%. The cause of death is the widespread invasion of the cancer into many body organs.

17. **d.** The second most common cancer of the female genital tract is adenocarcinoma of the endometrium. An estimated 33,000 cancers of the endometrium are detected each year. Endometrial cancer accounts for 8% of all cancers in women, and almost 50% of all new gynecologic cancers. Only 13% of cancer deaths result from endometrial carcinoma, about 4000 each year, despite its high prevalence.

18. **d.** Patients' increased risk of endometrial cancer from estrogen replacement therapy lasts for 10 years after stopping estrogen hormone therapy. However, with the now widely used combination of estrogen and progestin, this length of time is decreased. It is too early to know the impact of combination hormone replacement therapy on prevention of osteoporosis in postmenopausal women.

19. **c.** Diagnostic tests done in patients with suspected endometrial cancer include histologic examination of tissue from the endometrium obtained by use of the Pipelle endometrial suction curette, then chest x-ray, transvaginal sonography, and sigmoidoscopy, to detect metastasis of cancer from the uterus to other organs.

20. **c.** Early diagnosis and treatment of endometrial cancer result in a 5-year survival rate of 85%.

21. **b.** Endometriosis is a nonmalignant disorder caused by aberrant growth of endometrium outside the uterus, particularly in the dependent parts of the pelvis and in the ovaries. It is a common cause of abnormal bleeding and secondary dysmenorrhea. Its causes, pathogenesis, and natural course are poorly understood.

22. **a.** In endometriosis, functioning endometrial tissue may be present in the posterior cul-de-sac, in the peritoneal or serosal surfaces of abdominal organs, and in surgical scars. Endometrial tissue is never found in bone.

23. **b.** Among fertile women, about 10% to 15% experience signs and symptoms of endometriosis. The prevalence is three or four times that in infertile women. During the woman's regular menstrual cycles, the endometrial tissue outside the body acts the same as that in the uterus, causing discomfort and pain depending on the amount of tissue involved.

24. **d.** The number of women who eventually develop ovaria cancer is 1 in 70. Most ovarian tumors are benign, but malignant ovarian tumors are the leading cause of death from reproductive tract cancer. In women with no family history of ovarian cancer, the lifetime risk is 1.6%. In those with one first-degree relative with ovarian cancer, the risk is 5%; in those with two first-degree relatives, the risk rises to 7%. Women with *BRCA1* gene mutations have at least a 50% lifetime risk of ovarian cancer.

25. **c.** Polycystic ovary syndrome is an endocrine disorder characterized by chronic anovulation with resulting infertility. These women have a relatively steady state of high estrogen, androgen, and luteinizing hormone levels rather than the fluctuating levels seen in ovulating women. The condition is manifested in hirsutism (70%), obesity (40%), and virilization (20%). About 50% of women have amenorrhea, 30% have abnormal uterine bleeding, and 20% have normal menstruation.

26. **d.** Menopause is considered to be established when menses have not occurred for 12 months. The age of onset of menopause is highly variable, ranging from early forties to about 55. The average age at menopause in Western societies is now 51 years.

27. **d.** The true failure rate of oral contraceptives is 3%.

28. **a.** New evidence from case-controlled studies done in the United Kingdom indicates that

risk of myocardial infarction associated with oral contraceptives is not present.

29. **d.** Failure rates with use of the progestin minipill are reported to be 1% to 4%.

30. **c.** The postcoital contraceptive pill mifepristone (RU 486), developed in France, is now available in the United States.

14
Reproductive Disorders

1. **c.** The endogenous substances that cause transformation of the perineum to include a penis, penile urethra, and scrotum that contains the testes are androgens. Androgen is a generic term for an agent, usually a hormone, such as androsterone and testosterone, that stimulates activity of the accessory male sex organs, encourages development of male sex characteristics, or prevents changes in the latter that follow castration. Natural androgens are steroids, derivatives of androstane. Adrenal androgens are androgenic hormones that originate in the adrenocorticoids: dehydroepiandrosterone and its sulfate, androstenedione, and 11β-hydroxyandrostenedione.

2. **c.** The ducts of the female embryonic genital tract that form the fallopian tubes, uterus, and vagina are the mullerian ducts, so named because they were identified by Johannes Muller, a German anatomist (1801-1858).

3. **d.** The effects of testosterone are to produce male secondary characteristics, to maintain libido, and to produce anabolism, which is the process in the body that builds up complex chemical compounds from smaller, simpler compounds (e.g., proteins from amino acids). Testosterone does not stimulate luteinizing hormone–releasing hormone that is secreted by the hypothalamic/pituitary network.

4. **c.** Precocious puberty is defined as the appearance of secondary sex characteristics before the age of 9.

5. **b.** Café-au-lait areas of pigmentation on the skin are characteristic of Forbes-Albright syndrome, which is a pituitary tumor in a patient without acromegaly that secretes excessive amounts of prolactin, producing persistent lactation.

6. **a.** The causes of male hypogonadism include renal failure, Leydig cell agenesis, and chemotherapy or radiation therapy. Congenital absence of Leydig cells is a cause of male

pseudohermaphroditism associated with ambiguity of the external genitalia.

7. **c.** There is a high probability that all 47,XXY males are sterile. This chromosomal abnormality is termed Klinefelter syndrome, which occurs in one of 800 live male births. The extra X chromosome is maternally derived in 60% of cases., The affected persons tend to be tall, with disproportionately long arms and legs. They often have small, firm testes, and about one third develop gynecomastia. Puberty usually occurs at the normal age, but often facial hair growth is light. Clinical variation is great, and many 47,XXY males are normal in appearance and intellect. Sterility in these men is usually discovered in the course of an infertility workup.

8. **a.** Normal levels of testosterone are present in such conditions as hypergonadism, hypopituitarism, and hypothalamic disorder, but low levels are seen in hypogonadism. Hypogonadism is characterized by inadequate gonadal function, manifested by deficiencies in gametogenesis and/or the secretion of gonadal hormones, resulting in atrophy or deficient development of secondary sexual characteristics and, when occurring in prepubertal males, in altered body habitus such as short trunk and long limbs.

9. **b.** Replacement of testosterone in males is effective in preventing or reducing the risk of osteopenia and vasomotor instability, increasing libido, and preventing impotence. Potential adverse effects include fluid retention, acne, and sometimes transient gynecomastia. Men with hypogonadotropic hypogonadism who want to develop spermatogenesis are treated with menopausal gonadotropins that contain 75 IU each of follicle-stimulating hormone and luteinizing hormone, 1 to 2 vials intramuscularly three times/week, with 2000 IU of human chorionic gonadotropin intramuscularly three times/week, both of which must be continued for at least 3 months to effect spermatogenesis. Alternatively, pulsatile subcutaneous administration of gonadotropin-releasing hormone via a portable infusion pump may be tried if there is sufficient gonadotroph reserve such as in Kallmann syndrome characterized by hypogonadism due to deficiency of hypothalamic gonadotropin-releasing hormone.

10. **d.** In females, the 28-day menstrual cycle is imposed by the higher brain centers, and involves neuroendocrine regulation through pulsatile secretion of luteinizing hormone and follicle-stimulating hormone, which is determined by the pulsatile secretion of gonadotropin-releasing hormone. Ovarian hormones modulate the frequency and amplitude of the luteinizing hormone and follicle-stimulating hormone pulses, which vary throughout the menstrual cycle. Normal reproductive function depends on complex hormonal communication between endocrine and target organs.

11. **a.** The number of follicles selected to become a mature graafian follicle, capable of being fertilized, is one. In the ovulatory phase of the menstrual cycle, luteinizing hormone is massively released from the pituitary gland due to estrogen feedback. As luteinizing hormone levels increase, estradiol levels decrease while progesterone levels continue to rise. The luteinizing hormone surge results in complete maturation of the follicle and the release of the ovum from the mature graafian follicle, which occurs about 16 to 32 hours after the luteinizing hormone surge.

12. **d.** When implantation of the fertilized egg occurs, human chorionic gonadotropin production maintains corpus luteum function until 1 to 12 weeks' gestation, when estrogen and progesterone are produced in sufficient amounts by the placenta to maintain the life of the fetus.

13. **a.** The percentage of women who are infertile have a history of pelvic inflammatory disease, intrauterine device use, ruptured appendix, lower abdominal surgery, or ectopic pregnancy. Any of these, particularly pelvic infections, cause adhesions in the fallopian tubes, which obstruct the transit of the fertilized ovum through the tubes to the implantation site in the endometrium of the uterus.

14. **b.** Other causes of infertility are amenorrhea or anovulation, intercourse that does not occur at the time of ovulation, and treated hypogonadism in the male. In cases of unexplained infertility, the woman is given clomiphene citrate for 3 to 4 cycles to enhance ovulation, together with human chorionic gonadotropin to trigger ovulation and intrauterine insemination on the next 2 days. If no pregnancy occurs, the woman is given gonadotropins intramuscularly or subcutaneously daily beginning on cycle day 3 or 5. When 1 to 4 follicles are ≥17 mm, human chorionic gonadotropin is given to induce ovulation; insemination occurs within the next 2 days. Treatment with the combination of clomiphene and gonadotropins increases probability of conception by 10% to 15% per cycle. If no pregnancy occurs after 3 to 4 cycles, assisted reproductive techniques are recommended (e.g., in vitro fertilization or gamete intrafallopian tube transfer) for women who have normal tubal function.

15. **c.** Women who have antisperm antibodies are instructed to use condoms for 6 months. The immunobead test is the most common test for detecting antisperm antibodies that bind to immunoglobulin G and immunoglobulin A on the sperm head, midpiece, and tail. Another test is the hypoosmotic swelling test, which results in changes in the sperm. If the expected changes do not occur, the sperm are considered to be abnormal.

16. **c.** Anovulation prevents pregnancy; however, ovulation can be induced by clomiphene citrate therapy (see answer 14). Infertility affects about one of five couples in the United States. The financial burden and time commitment required for diagnosis and treatment of infertility can cause marital strife. Despite all efforts, some couples do not achieve pregnancy, and should consider when to stop treatments and when to consider adoption.

17. **a.** The sensitivity of the menstrual cycle to disruptions in, for example, hormone levels is extremely acute. Any change in hormonal level causes response in the cycle.

18. **d.** The Stein-Leventhal syndrome, more commonly known as polycystic ovary syndrome, is a condition that is benign. The syndrome is characterized by amenorrhea or irregular menses, mild obesity, and hirsutism, typically beginning in the pubertal years but worsening with time. The cause may be a neoplasm that can be treated definitively.

19. **b.** Turner's syndrome is caused by a sex chromosome abnormality. Another name for this condition is Bonnevie-Ullrich syndrome. The condition occurs in about 1 in 4000 live female births. The sex chromosomal abnormality causes complete or partial absence of one

of the two sex chromosomes, producing a phenotypic female. Ninety-nine percent of these 45, X conceptions are miscarried, Eighty percent of live newborns with monosomy X have loss of the paternal X. While mental deficiency is rare, many have some domination of certain perceptual abilities and score poorly on performance tests and in mathematics, even though they score average or above in verbal intelligence quotient tests. Ninety percent have gonadal dysgenesis with failure to go through puberty, develop breast tissue, or begin menses. Replacement with female hormones will bring on puberty.

20. **d.** For maturation, spermatogenesis requires 72 days. Spermatogenesis is a continuous process and is most efficient at 34° C (93.2° F); exposure to excessive heat or prolonged fever within 2 to 3 months of evaluation for infertility can adversely affect sperm count, motility, and morphology.

15
Immunologic Disorders

1. **b.** The immune system is a biochemical complex, known because of its biologic and chemical components. Its complexity, organization, and integrated system could have it be, in addition to a biochemical system, also cellular, reactive, and protective complexes.

2. **a.** The local barriers provide chemical and mechanical defenses through the skin, the mucous membranes, and the conjunctivae. The inflammatory reaction draws polymorphonuclear leukocytes and neutrophils to the site of injury/invasion, where phagocytes engulf the bacteria or virus.

3. **b.** The central nervous system is not considered part of the immune system. However, phagocytes, including neutrophils and monocytes in the blood, are widely distributed, and macrophages are strategically placed at the interfaces of tissues with blood or cavitary spaces, e.g., the alveolar macrophages in the lungs, Kupffer cells in the liver sinusoids, synovial cells in the lining of the coronary sinus, and mesangial phagocytes in the kidneys.

4. **b.** The humoral immune response produces antibodies to react with specific antigens, and is particularly effective against bacterial and viral invasions. This system uses B cells to produce appropriate antibodies. The humoral response may begin immediately, or as long as 48 hours after the invasion, depending on several factors, including the status of the host's defenses and the virulence of the invading organisms.

5. **d.** Natural immunity is present at birth, does not require a previous encounter with the offending substance, and does not develop memory. The natural immunity system makes up the fast-reacting, "front-line" defenses, including both physical and chemical barriers, together with the components of the immune system.

6. **c.** The cellular component of the specific (adaptive) immunity is the lymphocyte. Lymphocytes are "programmed" by particular lymphoid organs to carry out specific functions.

7. **b.** All lymphocytes originate from the bone marrow. Lymphocytes and monocytes secrete cytokines, which are nonimmunoglobulin polypeptides that are involved in cell-to-cell communication, coordinate antibody and T-cell immune reactions, and amplify immune reactivity.

8. **a.** All blood cells are derived from a pluripotent stem cell in the bone marrow, the site of hemopoiesis in mature mammals. The primitive cell types have no specific function, divide rapidly, and, under the influence of various cytokine signals, differentiate into myeloid precursors, producing neutrophils, eosinophils, and monocytes (lymphoid cells). Pre-B lymphocytes remain in the bone marrow to mature, but those cells destined to be T lymphocytes travel to the thymus to develop further.

9. **b.** The lymphocytes, generated in bone marrow as a primitive cell type, travel to the thymus to develop into mature T cells.

10. **d.** Tonsils function similarly to lymph nodes. They are located in the nasopharyngeal tract, and are therefore well placed to combat airborne antigens. They are composed primarily of B cells.

11. **b.** In humans, major histocompatibility complex is a cluster of genes located on the short arm of chromosome 6. It encodes a series of molecules known as the *human leukocyte antigens*. These structures are defined as antigens because they can be recognized by cells of the immune system, were first seen to be impor-

tant in transplantation reactions, and determine the acceptance of an organ or tissue graft between individuals.

12. **a.** Cytokines, nonimmunologic polypeptides, are secreted by monocytes and lymphocytes in response to interaction with a specific antigen, a nonspecific antigen, or a nonspecific soluble stimulus such as an endotoxin or other cytokines. Cytokines comprise a large group of low-molecular-weight proteins that are secreted by various cell types, and that are involved in cell-to-cell communication, coordinating antibody and T-cell immune reactions, and amplifying immune reactivity. Cytokines include colony-stimulating factor, interferons, interleukins, and lymphokines.

13. **d.** Neutrophils have receptors for both the *Fc* (a part of an antibody that has been split by a proteolytic enzyme) and the *Fab*; the Fc represents the relatively constant region, rather than the Fab portion that contains the binding sites. The Fc portion is also identified as the crystallizable fragment and complement components, which bind tightly to the coated particle. The opsonization process results in increased force of adhesion between the particle (organism) and phagocyte, further activating the cell and promoting phagocytic ("killing") activity.

14. **c.** Impaired host defenses are a major cause of opportunistic infections, such as patients who have received immunosuppressive drugs, or are debilitated because of infections such as HIV/AIDS. Examples of opportunistic infections include candidiasis and Kaposi's sarcoma.

15. **c.** Although the "whole body" can be affected by immunodeficiencies, these deficiencies are grouped under congenital, acquired, phagocyte, antibody (B-cell defects), and T-cell deficiencies. Immunoglobulin deficiencies may occur also, such immunoglobulin A deficiency or immunoglobulin G subclass deficiency.

16. **b.** The CD4+ T lymphocytes are the cells most affected by HIV. In addition to these cells, a second receptor is required for fusion/viral entry—the CXCR4 in lymphocytes, and CCR5 in cells of the monocyte/macrophage lineage; these are both chemokine receptors.

17. **d.** The progressive and severe depletion of CD4+ "helper" lymphocytes is the most char-

acteristic feature of immunologic abnormalities. In the healthy person, these cells orchestrate the immune response by responding to antigen; they proliferate and release cytokines, particularly interleukin-2, which then results in proliferation of other reactive T-cell clones, including T-cytotoxic cells that eradicate viral infections. Therefore the severe depletion of the CD4+ helper lymphocytes makes the body virtually incapable of mounting an effective response to HIV and other infections.

18. **b.** Autoimmune disease occurs when the immune system fails to recognize the body's own tissues as "self," and mounts an attack on them (immunologic abnormalities). Autoimmune diseases include rheumatoid arthritis, type 1 diabetes, thyroiditis, multiple sclerosis, and many others. Amyotrophic lateral sclerosis (Lou Gehrig disease) is a degenerative disease of the motor neurons, characterized by weakness and atrophy of the muscles of the hands, forearms, and legs, and eventually involving most of the body and face. Recent evidence suggests implication of viral infection in amyotrophic lateral sclerosis, and the possibility that it too may be an autoimmune disease, but this has not been conclusively proven and such a connection must wait for further investigation.

19. **c.** Immunodeficiency diseases comprise a group of diverse conditions caused by one or more immune system defects, and characterized clinically by increased susceptibility to infections resulting in severe, acute, recurrent, or chronic disease. Immunodeficiency is relatively rare in clinical practice, unlike some diseases that are caused by immunologic abnormalities such as rheumatoid arthritis and other autoimmune diseases, and allergies, which are commonly seen in practice. The incidence of *symptomatic* primary immunodeficiency is estimated to be 1:10,000 persons, with about 400 new cases seen each year.

20. **d.** Immunodeficiency has no common cause, but a single gene defect is often implicated, which can lead to a missing enzyme, (e.g., adenosine deaminase), a missing protein (e.g., complement component deficiencies), or developmental arrest at a specific differential stage (e.g., pre-B-cell arrest in X-linked agammaglobulinemia). Chromosome locations of the defective genes have been identified for

many of the primary immunodeficiencies, but the precise biologic abnormality in most of these illnesses is unknown.

16
Oncologic Disorders

1. **d.** At least one third of the populations in developed countries will probably develop cancer at some time in their lives. The precise number is difficult to know for certain, but most authorities indicate that one third or more will have some type of cancer at some time. For example, currently, the people of England and Wales have a very high rate of lung cancer because of the large number who smoke. These figures may diminish slowly over the next several decades as people learn how dangerous tobacco use is.

2. **c.** Cancer cells proliferate uncontrollably, extend rapidly, and can invade all types of tissue in the body: skin, muscle, bone, others. The cancer cells lack differentiation, as normal cells do, microscopically. Extension of a cancer can, if untreated, extend throughout the body in a random fashion because no controls limit its growth or extension.

3. **c.** Mutations in genes are responsible, in part, for the growth and reproduction of malignant cells. These mutations, after the quantity or behavior of the proteins, encode by growth-regulating genes and alter cell division. Two major categories of mutated genes are oncogenes and tumor suppressor genes. The activation of oncogenes is not clearly understood, and many factors may contribute (e.g., chemical carcinogens in tobacco smoke, infectious agents such as viruses).

4. **c.** The ras gene is abnormal in about 25% of cancers. The Ras protein, which is encoded in the ras gene, regulates or signals cell division. In most circumstances, the ras gene is inactive, but in malignant cells, the Ras protein is active and signals cells to divide, even though they should not.

5. **c.** Protein kinase enzymes have not been found in pancreatic cancer but have been found in many other cancers, including those listed. Advances in molecular biology have greatly increased our knowledge about the structure and function of malignant cells.

6. **b.** Chromosomal abnormalities are found in particular human cancers. For example, about 80% of patients with cell-mediated lympholysis have the Philadelphia (Ph) t(9:22) chromosome. Molecular scientists believe that normal cells undergo chromosomal changes (e.g., loss of alleles) that result in cells' becoming malignant. Other changes may also take place, but this is probably the initial change.

7. **c.** Proliferation, although occurring in cancer development, is not included in the steps that occur in chemical carcinogenesis. Initiation is the stage in which a cell experiences a carcinogenic event that may potentially cause the cell to develop into a neoplastic clone. In the promotion phase, which is reversible, the continued existence of the neoplastic clonal multiplication depends on a chemical or agent (cocarcinogen) with little carcinogenic activity. In progression, irreversible growth of altered (neoplastic) cells occurs.

8. **c.** Patients who show a complete remission of a cancer, or a complete response to therapy, have a potential cure. These patients may appear to be completely cured but could still have cancer cells in their body that may, in time, cause recurrence. Complete cure depends on length of time since treatment; if 10 years pass without any sign of recurrence, most specialists say that the cancer has been cured.

9. **b.** Methotrexate is a classic folic acid antagonist, is structurally quite similar to folic acid, and binds preferentially to dihydrofolate reductase, the enzyme responsible for the conversion of folic acid to folinic acid. Methotrexate is widely used to treat solid tumors and hematologic malignancies and to treat nonmalignant conditions such as rheumatoid arthritis.

10. **b.** Cytosine arabinoside is used almost exclusively to treat acute myeloid leukemia and remains the backbone of therapy for this malignancy.

11. **c.** Myeloma is an osteolytic neoplasm that affects only bones in the body. The bones most commonly affected are the flat bones of the skull, the vertebrae, the ribs, and the pelvic bones. This is a complex disease that reflects the interrelationships among bone destruction that causes vertebral collapse; bone marrow infiltration that causes anemia, neutropenia, and thrombocytopenia; and renal

impairment caused by a combination of factors such as deposition of light chains, hypercalcemia, and hyperuricemia.

12. **d.** Most bronchogenic carcinomas are endobronchial, and patients usually present with a cough, with or without hematemesis. In patients with chronic bronchitis, increased intensity and intractability of preexisting cough suggest a neoplasm. Bronchial narrowing may cause air trapping with localized wheezing.

13. **d.** About 2,009,000 new cases of prostate cancer are diagnosed every year. Prognosis depends on such factors as grade, stage, and pretreatment prostate-specific antigen level; for patients with low-grade, organ-confined tumors, survival is almost the same as that for age-matched controls without prostate cancer. If prostate cancer is diagnosed in men over the age of 80, no therapy is recommended because these patients will likely die of causes other than prostate cancer, which progresses quite slowly.

14. **c.** Cigarette smoking accounts for over 50% of bladder cancers in both sexes. In many, the cause is metastasis of a primary cancer from another location such as the prostate or uterus. The prevalence of bladder cancer is increasing, probably because of the increased numbers of smokers throughout the world.

15. **d.** One in eight persons in the United States will develop breast cancer if they live to be 95. Older age does not diminish the risk of breast cancer, as many people believe. Rather, the risk is greater in older people. Women are usually affected, although men can develop breast cancer, too, which may be a metastasis from lung or other cancer sites. However, in older people, breast cancer usually progresses more slowly than in the young and vital.

16. **a.** Only about 5% of women who develop breast cancer carry one of the two genes that cause breast cancer, which does not support the belief that almost all breast cancers are genetic. Other risk factors are increasing age, early menarche, late menopause, or a late first pregnancy. The magnitude of risk is still not known for certain but may be as high as 50% to 85% by age 80.

17. **a.** Cervical cancer is essentially a cancer of young women. It can be considered a sexually transmitted disease because age of first intercourse and the number of sexual partners are directly related to the development of cervical cancer. Cigarette smoking is also implicated in this cancer, as is human papillomavirus types 16, 18, 33, 35, and 39.

18. **d.** Ovarian cancer occurs mainly in perimenopausal or postmenopausal women over the age of 50. However, ovarian cancer at one time was linked to mothers who had taken diethylstilbestrol during pregnancy. Since this drug was taken off the market, the incidence of ovarian cancer in young women (teens to twenties) has decreased markedly. Ovarian cancer is rarely diagnosed in the early stage, and so is usually far advanced by the time a diagnosis is made; 75% of women present with advanced stage disease.

19. **c.** Endometrial cancer is the most prevalent gynecologic malignancy and occurs primarily in women in their fifties and sixties. About 34,000 new cases were diagnosed in 1996. Risk factors include a history of infertility, anovulation, late menopause (<52 years), exogenous estrogen, uterine polyps, and a combination of diabetes, hypertension, and obesity.

20. **a.** The major risk factors are older age; low-fiber, high-protein, high-fat diet; high alcohol consumption; family history; smoking; sedentary lifestyle; and exposure to radiation or asbestos. While this malignancy usually occurs in people over the age of 50, it does occur with distressing frequency in younger people in their thirties and forties. Slightly more women than men are affected and often clusters in families. These cancers are primarily adenocarcinomas that tend to grow slowly; therefore the cancer is usually large by the time it produces symptoms. However, a surgical cure is possible in about 70% of patients.

17
Musculoskeletal Disorders

1. **b.** Erosive osteoarthritis affects the distal interphalangeal joints of the fingers (Heberden's nodes), and the proximal interphalangeal joints (Bouchard's nodules). Bony enlargement occurs in the distal interphalangeal joints, and bony overgrowth in the proximal interphalangeal joints. Cervical and lumbar vertebrae are also affected. The metacarpophalangeal joints of the thumbs,

and the wrists, are not usually affected in osteoarthritis.

2. **a.** Osteoarthritis causes chronic degeneration of the joints of the hip and knee—the weight-bearing joints. Osteoarthritis (type 1, post-menopausal osteoarthritis) usually occurs between the ages of 51 and 75. Reduced estrogen leads to elevated serum levels of interleukin-6 and perhaps other cytokines, which may result in increased bone resorption. The morning stiffness that is associated with osteoarthritis lasts for no longer than an hour; morning stiffness associated with rheumatoid arthritis lasts several hours, typically.

3. **b.** Osteoporosis is mainly a metabolic disease, with components such as calcitonin, estrogen, parathyroid hormone, 25-hydroxyvitamin D, cytokines, calcium, and potassium involved in the condition.

4. **c.** Hypochromic, microcytic anemia may be caused by nonsteroidal antiinflammatory drugs, which are used to treat pain associated with osteoarthritis. Many clinicians recommend taking hormone replacement therapy and calcium supplements to help to preserve bone tissue.

5. **d.** Antinuclear antibodies are seen most often in patients with systemic lupus erythematosus. Some drugs (e.g., hydralazine, procainamide, β-blockers) produce positive antinuclear antibody tests and, occasionally, a lupus-like syndrome associated with antihistone antibodies.

6. **c.** Nurses and other health care professionals must be careful not to attribute signs and symptoms of osteoarthritis in patients who may have diseases such as cancer, multiple myeloma, or osteoporosis.

7. **a.** The major goal of osteoarthritis therapy is to preserve joint function. Flexion of the hands in warm water, a walking program for weight-bearing joints, and eliminating prolonged periods of rest in bed are measures that are helpful in maintaining near-normal flexibility and function in all joints.

8. **c.** Acetaminophen (Tylenol) is the usual first medication suggested to treat pain associated with osteoarthritis. Addition of other analgesics should be delayed as long as possible because most drugs prescribed for patients with osteoarthritis have side effects, or are not helpful in some people.

9. **b.** The disability that occurs in patients with rheumatoid arthritis is much more pronounced and incapacitating than the pain and stiffness experienced by patients with osteoarthritis.

10. **b.** Gout, a type of acute arthritis, affects primarily the peripheral joints, including the great toe. Attacks of gout are associated with feasting and drinking that accompany special holidays or celebrations.

11. **c.** Gout is caused by both acquired and genetic factors. Usually, the family history reveals other members of the family who had gout.

12. **a.** The risk of crystal deposition and acute attacks of gout increases with the degree of hyperuricemia, which can be caused by overproduction or underexcretion of uric acid—often both.

13. **b.** The "gold standard" for diagnosing gout is the appearance of urate crystals in fluid aspirated from a joint.

14. **b.** Colchicine is effective, but side effects have reduced its use. It may be given for 24 hours, beginning at the start of the acute attack. The dose is 0.5 or 0.6 mg by mouth every hour until pain is relieved, or until side effects occur, e.g., nausea, diarrhea.

15. **a.** Nonsteroidal antiinflammatory drugs have become the treatment of choice for acute gout. Indomethacin is often used, but other nonsteroidal antiinflammatory drugs are likely to be as effective. Indomethacin is given in 25 to 50 mg doses by mouth every 8 hours until symptoms subside, usually in 5 to 10 days.

16. **b.** Diuretics should not be prescribed for persons with gout because they may decrease the clearance of uric acid from the kidneys.

17. **c.** Colchicine is used to prevent attacks in older men who may have chronic renal failure and require diuretics, and have a history of multiple attacks of gout. Generally, the higher the uric acid level and the more frequent the attacks, the more likely it is that chronic medical therapy will be beneficial.

18. **a.** Uricosuric drugs are prescribed for those who have underexcretion of uric acid. These include probenecid and sulfinpyrazone. They act by blocking tubular resorption of filtered urate and reducing the metabolic pool of urates.

19. **a.** Xanthine oxidase inhibitors such as allopurinol are used in patients who have hyperuricemia because of overproduction. Dosage depends on the serum uric acid level.

20. **d.** Shoulder function involves the thorax, 3 bones, and about 30 muscles. Injury can cause severe pain and limited movement. Exercises to strengthen the uninjured muscles while allowing the tendons time to heal help to maintain muscle tone, yet provide recovery time for the tendons.

21. **c.** The most common cause of shoulder pain in adults is rotator cuff tendinitis. The rotator cuff holds the humeral head in the glenoid fossa of the scapula. The patient should avoid pushing movements and instead should perform pulling movements, if movement does not cause pain. Surgery may be necessary if the injury was severe, if there is a complete tear of the rotator cuff, or if the tendons do not heal within 6 months.

22. **c.** The primary steps in diagnosing shoulder problems and a comprehensive history and physical examination. Experienced orthopedists can accurately diagnose muscle and joint problems by having the patient perform several movements, some against pressure.

23. **b.** In some patients, carpal tunnel syndrome may be the presenting manifestation of rheumatoid arthritis, which is classified as a diffuse connective tissue disease. Systemic lupus erythematosus is another condition under this classification.

24. **a.** One of the major risk factors for low back pain is deficient or chronic poor-quality sleep. Any back pain must be diagnosed so that appropriate treatment can be given. Causes can include sprain or strain of back muscles, or more chronic and serious problems such as osteoarthritic, fibromuscular, or ankylosing spondylitic processes of the lumbosacral area.

25. **d.** The "tender points" seen in patients with fibromyalgia number nine pairs at different places on the trunk and limbs. The condition occurs mainly in women and may be caused or intensified by physical or mental stress, poor sleep, trauma, or exposure to dampness or cold. Muscles, areas of tendon insertion, and nearby soft tissues are most affected.

26. **b.** Rheumatoid arthritis is now considered to be a serious systemic disorder with 5-year sur-

vival similar to stage IV Hodgkin's disease or triple-vessel coronary artery disease.

27. **c.** The drugs that are now the "gold standard" to treat rheumatoid arthritis are the cytotoxic or immunosuppressive drugs methotrexate, azathioprine, and cyclosporine, which are also used to treat patients with cancer.

28. **a.** The most common cause of Reiter's syndrome is *Chlamydia trachomatis* infection, which is usually sexually transmitted. A dysenteric type of Reiter's syndrome is caused by *Shigella*, *Salmonella*, *Yersinia*, or *Campylobacter* organisms from the gastrointestinal tract.

29. **b.** Psoriatic arthritis is a form of arthritis associated mainly with psoriasis of the nails, hands, and feet, especially the distal interphalangeal joints of the fingers and toes. Remissions are frequent, often complete. In other patients, the disease becomes chronic and may progress to severe crippling.

30. **c.** The most common characteristic of systemic lupus erythematosus is joint involvement. Of patients with systemic lupus erythematosus, 90% are young women. It is described as a chronic inflammatory connective tissue disease that may involve joints, kidneys, serous surfaces, and vessel walls. Antinuclear antibodies are found in the serum of most patients, indicating the likelihood of autoimmune reactions.

18
Dermatologic Disorders

1. **b.** The dermatologist's first step is to identify the skin lesion, then to consider the degree of contagion, if any, and the type of treatment required. Diagnosis may require other tests, e.g., skin biopsy or skin scrapings, to confirm the suspected diagnosis.

2. **a.** The basement membrane is an amorphous extracellular layer closely applied to the basal surface of epithelium and also investing muscle cells and Schwann cells; it is thought to be a selective filter, and to serve both structural and morphogenetic functions. It is composed of 3 layers: lamina lucida, lamina densa, and lamina fibroreticularis a matrix of collagen, of which type IV is unique to this membrane, and several glycoproteins.

3. **b.** If a blister (a raised lesion containing serous fluid) normally measures less than 5 mm it is

called a vesicle. If it is equal to or greater than 5 mm, it is called a bulla (blister).

4. **c.** Cellulitis is inflammation of subcutaneous, loose connective tissue. Erysipelas is a specific, acute, superficial cutaneous cellulitis caused by β-hemolytic streptococci, and characterized by hot, red, edematous, brawny, and sharply defined eruptions. It is usually accompanied by severe constitutional symptoms, e.g., pain on movement.

5. **c.** Impetigo is a contagious, superficial pyoderma caused by *Staphylococcus aureus* and/or group A streptococci, seen most often in children. The skin lesions begin with a superficial flaccid vesicle that ruptures and forms a thick, yellowish (honey-colored) crust.

6. **d.** A furuncle, commonly called a boil, is a localized, pyogenic infection usually caused by *S. aureus,* and originating deep in a hair follicle. The boil gradually comes to a "head" that opens and drains pus. The core of the infection usually must be manually removed by pressure such as used in squeezing a pimple or blackhead.

7. **b.** Contact dermatitis is a T-lymphocyte–mediated dermatitis (type IV hypersensitivity) from skin contact with a specific allergen or irritant. The skin reaction often takes the form of the allergen contact (wrist bracelet, T-strap sandals).

8. **a.** Ringworm of the skin is an infection caused by dermatophytes—fungi that invade only dead tissues of the skin or its appendages (nails, hair, stratum corneum).

9. **c.** Candidiasis (moniliasis), a common infection of the skin, is found primarily in intertriginous and mucocutaneous areas, where heat and maceration produce a fertile environment: axillae, umbilicus, groin, inframammary areas, and gluteal folds.

10. **c.** Scabies is a transmissible ectoparasite infection characterized by superficial burrows, intense pruritus, and secondary infection. Scabies is caused by a mite, *Sarcoptes scabiei.* The impregnated female tunnels into the stratum corneum and deposits her eggs along the burrow. The larvae hatch within a few days.

11. **b.** Warts (verrucae) are common, contagious, epithelial tumors caused by any one or more of at least 60 types of human papillomavirus. They usually disappear over time with no treatment, but there are over-the-counter preparations available that may speed the healing process.

12. **a.** Acne is an inflammatory disease of the pilosebaceous glands characterized by comedones, papules, pustules, inflamed nodules, superficial pus-filled cysts, and (in extreme cases) canaling and deep, inflamed, sometimes purulent, sacs. Interaction among hormones, keratin, sebum, and bacteria determines the course and severity.

13. **d.** Rosacea is a chronic, inflammatory disorder that occurs mainly on the central areas of the face—cheeks, forehead. It develops most often in older (over 40) persons with very light skin. The characteristic red areas, telangiectasia, erythema, papules, and pustules vary, with occasional "flares" that subside. Treatment is topical metronidazole gel or cream, or broad-spectrum oral antibiotics.

14. **d.** Pityriasis rosea occurs most often in young adults. The cause is unknown, but mycoplasma, a picornavirus, and human herpesvirus 7 have been isolated. A herald patch, 2 to 7 cm in diameter, usually appears first, followed in 5 to 10 days by eruption of rose- or salmon-colored round or oval patches that may be slightly scaly with a raised border (collarette). The plaques are generally localized to the trunk and disappear within 4 to 5 weeks without treatment and without recurrence.

15. **c.** Lichen planus is a recurrent, pruritic, inflammatory eruption characterized by small, discrete, polygonal, flat, violaceous papules that may coalesce into rough, scaly patches. Although the cause is unknown, some drugs (e.g., arsenic, bismuth, gold) may cause this or a similar eruption.

16. **a.** Basal cell carcinoma is the most common type of skin cancer. More than 400,000 new cases are reported every year in the United States.

17. **a.** Squamous cell carcinoma is often seen in people who are exposed to direct sunlight for long periods. The incidence in the United States is 80,000 to 100,000 new cases every year. The difference between basal cell and squamous cell cancers is that squamous cell cancer of the tongue or oral mucosa frequently has metastasized before it is diagnosed.

18. **d.** Malignant melanoma may also result from exposure to sun in light-skinned people. About 25,000 new cases occur each year in

the United States, and 6000 deaths. About 40% to 50% of malignant melanomas arise from pigmented moles.

19. **b.** Sebaceous (holocrine) glands in the dermis usually open into hair follicles and secrete an oily semifluid (sebum) into the hair follicle and skin.

20. **c.** Breslow's index is one of two classifications used to evaluate stage I melanomas. The measurement is the thickness of the melanoma from the granular layer of the epidermis to its greatest depth, and indicates how broad and deep the area of excision, for biopsy or removal, should be.

21. **a.** Lentigo maligna melanoma arises from Hutchinson's freckle (a tan patch on the skin that grows slowly and becomes mottled, dark, thick, and nodular).

22. **c.** Survival rates in patients with malignant melanoma are determined by the thickness of the tumor at the time of diagnosis.

23. **b.** Kaposi's sarcoma is caused by herpesvirus type 8.

24. **d.** Since 1981, aggressive Kaposi's sarcoma has occurred in at least 33% of patients with AIDS. Treatment of Kaposi's sarcoma does not prolong life in most patients because infections dominate the clinical course of AIDS.

25. **a.** Warts occur most often on sites that are subject to trauma, e.g., fingers, elbows, knees, face.

26. **c.** *Candidiasis* is usually limited to both skin and mucous membranes.

27. **c.** The most common type of *Candida* infections are those that appear in intertriginous areas.

28. **d.** Stasis dermatitis is associated primarily with venous incompetency such as the lower legs and ankles.

29. **a.** Signs and symptoms of contact dermatitis range from transient redness to severe swelling with bullae.

30. **c.** A significant risk factor for cellulitis is a break in the skin, particularly in the lower legs.

19
Eye Disorders

1. **c.** An ophthalmologic emergency is gonococcal conjunctivitis because corneal involvement may rapidly lead to perforation. It usually is acquired through contact with infected genital secretions. Diagnosis is confirmed by stained smear and culture of the discharge. If the cornea is not involved, a single intramuscular dose of ceftriaxone, 1 g, is effective. When the cornea is involved, a 5-day course of parenteral ceftriaxone, 1 to 2 g daily, is required. These patients should also be tested for other sexually transmitted diseases, e.g., chlamydia, syphilis, and HIV infections.

2. **a.** The cause of inclusion conjunctivitis is a species of *Chlamydia* (*C. trachomatis*, serotypes D-K). This organism is a common cause of genital tract disease in adults. The eye is usually involved after accidental contact with genital secretions. The infection occurs most frequently in sexually active young adults. Treatment should include both eye and genital infections, as appropriate.

3. **a.** The appearance of purulent, creamy yellow discharge from the eyes in a patient with conjunctival hyperemia is a sign of bacterial conjunctivitis. The most common organisms are staphylococci, streptococci (particularly *Streptococcus pneumoniae*), *Haemophilus* species, *Pseudomonas* species, and *Moraxella* species. All of these may produce copious purulent discharge. In severe cases, examination of stained conjunctival scrapings and cultures is recommended. The infection is usually self-limited, and lasts between 10 and 14 days if untreated. A sulfonamide 10% ophthalmic solution or ointment, instilled in the eye, will usually clear the infection in 2 to 3 days.

4. **b.** Conjunctivitis that causes symptoms such as mucopurulent discharge, tearing, local irritation, and eyelids sticking together during sleep is an acute viral conjunctivitis—"red eye." It is commonly seen in children, who may contract the infection from contaminated swimming pools. Local sulfonamide therapy may prevent secondary bacterial infection. Warm compresses reduce discomfort of eyelid swelling. The infection usually lasts at least from 1 to 3 weeks.

5. **d.** The reason that corticosteroid pharmaceutical preparations are NOT recommended for the treatment of eye infections or other eye problems is that these drugs cause corneal ulceration.

6. **c.** Blepharitis is inflammation of the lid margins with redness, thickening, and often formation of scales and crusts or shallow

marginal ulcers. The disease can be caused by bacterial or seborrheic dermatitis, or abnormal meibomian gland secretions, and is often associated with acne rosacea. An antibiotic eye ointment such as bacitracin or gentamicin is given for 7 to 10 days. Seborrheic blepharitis can be improved by eyelid hygiene: scrubbing the eyelid margins with a cotton swab dipped in a solution of water to which has been added 2 to 3 drops of baby shampoo.

7. **b.** Corneal ulcers occur as a result of local necrosis caused by invasion of bacteria, fungi, viruses, or *Acanthamoeba*. Treatment with topical trifluridine 1% eye drops nine times/day, or vidarabine 3% ointment five times/day is effective. For some patients, acyclovir 400 mg five times/day is indicated.

8. **c.** An external hordeolum is a localized infection of a sebaceous gland in the eyelid. Warm compresses will cause the area to open and drain. Healing occurs spontaneously within a few days.

9. **d.** Uveitis is inflammation of any component of the uveal tract: iris, ciliary body, or choroid. Anterior uveitis is usually the most symptomatic. The patient presents with pain, redness, photophobia, and decreased vision. Signs of anterior uveitis include pupillary miosis and injections of the conjunctiva adjacent to the cornea. Complications of uveitis are many, some very serious. Patients with uveitis should be referred immediately to an ophthalmologist.

10. **c.** In 40% of patients with uveitis, an underlying systemic disease such as syphilis may be present. A complete evaluation should be conducted by an ophthalmologist.

11. **d.** A key diagnostic test used by the ophthalmologist when there is a suspicion of corneal trauma is fluorescein staining and slit-lamp examination.

12. **d.** The immediate treatment for chemical burns of the eye is irrigation of both eyes with copious amounts of normal saline or lactated Ringer's solution, if available, or plain tap water.

13. **a.** The most serious emergency situation involving the eye(s) is sudden partial or complete loss of vision. The cause could be detached retina, vitreous hemorrhage, age-related macular degeneration, or central and branch retinal vein or artery occlusions. All patients with loss of vision, particularly that which occurs suddenly, should be taken immediately to an ophthalmologist or hospital.

14. **d.** Among persons over 65 years of age, the percentage who have some degree of opacity of the lens of the eye is 95%. Cataract is often the cause, and can be treated surgically quite easily. Usually, cataracts occur in both eyes, not simultaneously, as a rule.

15. **c.** Glaucoma is characterized by increased intraocular pressure. Patients should be evaluated regularly for glaucoma, particularly older persons. Two types of glaucoma are open-angle glaucoma and acute (angle-closure) glaucoma. Both are more common in older people, and both are treatable.

16. **a.** One of the major risk factors for retinal detachment is hypertension. Cataract extraction and myopia (near-sightedness) are also associated with detached retina. About 80% of uncomplicated cases can be cured with one operation; another 15% will need repeat surgery, and the remaining 5% never reattach.

17. **b.** Treatment for detached retina is the operation called scleral buckling, performed only by a retinal specialist. Laser photocoagulation treatment may be used at the discretion of the surgeon. The goal is to close the retinal tears and create permanent adhesion between the neurosensory retina, the retinal pigment epithelium, and the choroid by the use of cryotherapy to the sclera.

18. **d.** The area of decreased vision in people with macular degeneration is central vision. Peripheral fields and therefore navigational vision are always maintained, though these may become impaired by cataract formation, which can be surgically corrected.

19. **a.** The procedure that most likely will result in permanent cure of patients with primary acute angle-closure glaucoma is laser peripheral iridotomy.

20. **b.** Refractive surgery is being performed on more persons, allowing them to have near-normal vision without glasses or contact lenses.

21. **a.** Risk factors for primary open-angle glaucoma include older age, family history, and black race. A normal intraocular pressure is not a risk factor for glaucoma.

22. **b.** The most useful signs/symptoms to diagnose angular blepharitis are hyperemia, excoriation, and maceration. Scarring is not relevant to diagnosis of the condition.

23. **a.** The risk factors for seborrheic blepharitis include dandruff of the eyebrows and/or scalp, poor hygiene, especially around the eyes, and presence of staphylococcal blepharitis. Age is irrelevant in diagnosing this type of blepharitis.

24. **c.** In meibomian gland dysfunction, inflammation and swelling occur in only one upper lid. There is usually an area of infection with redness, swelling, and discomfort. Warm compresses will help to localize the infection and facilitate rupture and draining, which will achieve healing within a few days.

25. **a.** The most frequent cause of orbital cellulitis is infection of nearby sinuses, usually the ethmoid sinus. Treating sinusitis prevents cellulitis of the orbit.

26. **d.** Internal hordeola involve the Zeis and Moll glands of the eye.

27. **c.** The most predominant symptom of detached retina is sudden partial or complete loss of vision in one eye. In patients who have had one detached retina, the chance of detachment in the other eye is about 25%.

28. **c.** Trachoma must be treated in the early stages to prevent blindness. Trachoma is a chronic conjunctivitis from *Chlamydia trachomatis,* characterized by progressive exacerbations and remissions, with conjunctival follicular hyperplasia, corneal neovascularization, and scarring of the conjunctiva, cornea, and eyelids. The disease is endemic in poverty-stricken parts of North Africa, the Middle East, the Indian subcontinent, and Southwest Asia. Trachoma, if untreated, results in total blindness.

29. **b.** Inclusion conjunctivitis caused by *C. trachomatis* D-K is seen most often in sexually active young adults who are not aware of the danger of contamination of the hands from genital secretions, and then touch or rub their eyes.

30. **c.** The cause of many corneal ulcers is incomplete eyelid closure, as happens with some older people as they sleep, or as a result of ptosis of the lower eyelids. Eye drops should be used often to keep the cornea wet. Wearing eye patches at night would also be beneficial.

20
Ear, Nose, and Throat Disorders

1. **c.** Diagnosis of middle and inner ear disorders is made primarily by the clinical picture (symptoms). These include acute and chronic otitis media, otosclerosis, and trauma—middle ear; and sensory hearing loss, tinnitus, vertigo, and diseases of the central auditory and vestibular systems—inner ear.

2. **b.** The ear canal consists of cartilage covered by skin, and therefore it is highly protected from damage that may result from objects being put or pushed into the ear, usually by toddlers or young children. Cerumen may obstruct the ear canal, but can be removed by flushing gently with water from a small syringe.

3. **c.** The middle ear begins at the tympanic membrane. Patients with middle ear problems may present with a variety of symptoms: feeling of pressure, excruciating pain, otorrhea, diminished hearing, and vertigo. Symptoms may result from infection, trauma, or disturbed pressure relationships secondary to eustachian tube obstruction.

4. **d.** The cone of light that is reflected from the tympanic membrane begins at the umbo. Examination of the ears provides experience in identifying parts of the middle ear. The examiner should look carefully at the external ear and the ear canal, in which may be seen external otitis, furuncle, or swimmer's ear. A bulging tympanic membrane almost invariably indicates middle ear infection.

5. **a.** Hearing is possible because of vibrations of air that cause the tympanic membrane to move slightly, causing the fluid to vibrate and result in movement of the stapes, which activates the acoustic nerve.

6. **d.** The cochlear nerve is a part of the eighth cranial nerve. Hearing tests involve this nerve.

7. **b.** Pain in acute sinusitis is due to relative negative pressure in the sinus (vacuum sinusitis).

8. **d.** The major purpose of the labyrinth of the middle ear is to maintain the person's balance by sensing position and movements of the head. Patients with labyrinthitis suffer from acute onset of continuous, usually severe, vertigo that lasts several days to a week, and is accompanied by hearing loss and tinnitus. During the recovery period, which may

be several weeks, rapid head movements may precipitate transient vertigo.

9. **c.** In the primary care setting, hearing impairment can be adequately determined by means of the patient's history, repeating words of the examiner, and testing with a tuning fork. If any question remains, the patient can be referred to an audiologist for further testing.

10. **a.** Treatment of acute sinusitis includes steam inhalation, saline nasal irrigations, and surgery, if the patient does not respond to other therapy. Long-term use of vasoconstrictors is not recommended because the blood supply is diminished with their use.

11. **a.** Two classifications of hearing loss are used. They are conductive and sensorineural hearing loss. Conductive hearing loss results from dysfunction of the external or middle ear. Four obstacles may cause impairment of the passage of sound vibrations to the inner ear: obstruction, middle ear effusion, otosclerosis, and ossicular disruption. Sensorineural hearing loss results from deterioration of the cochlea, usually due to loss of hair cells from the organ of Corti. Causes of cochlear deterioration include noise trauma, ototoxicity, and aging (presbycusis).

12. **d.** Conductive hearing loss usually results from external or middle ear disease.

13. **b.** The basis for using Weber's test is that a unilateral conductive hearing loss with normal bilateral ear function produces a softer sound in the unaffected ear.

14. **c.** Evaluation of hearing by means of audiometric testing results in determination of the precise level of hearing loss by using sounds that vary in intensity (dB).

15. **a.** A major cause of acute suppurative otitis media is *Streptococcus pneumoniae.*

16. **c.** Antibiotic therapy for acute otitis media must be given for at least 10 days, to ensure that the infection is entirely cured.

17. **a.** In chronic otitis media, there is conductive hearing loss because the tympanic membrane is unable to vibrate.

18. **c.** Meniere's disease is associated with conditions that affect the vestibular apparatus in the inner ear.

19. **c.** Treatment of acute pharyngitis is uncertain because of the difficulty of differentiating between viral and bacterial infection.

20. **a.** Several systemic illnesses are associated with ear, nose, and throat symptoms. Included among these is infectious mononucleosis, which usually begins as an upper respiratory infection, sore throat, and congestion.

21. **b.** The differential diagnosis of cerumen impaction includes external otitis, bony overgrowth in the canal, and foreign body in the canal. Otitis media is not among the differential diagnoses for cerumen impaction.

22. **c.** External otitis is seen frequently in swimmers' ears. The canal is often filled with exudate with some crusts, limiting the examiner's ability to see all of the tympanic membrane.

23. **d.** A sign of gout, either past or present, is tophi, seen on the external ear as small hard lumps under the skin of the auricle.

24. **a.** Sudden severe pain followed by bleeding, partial or complete loss of hearing, tinnitus, and purulent discharge that develop within 24 to 48 hours are signs and symptoms of ruptured tympanic membrane.

25. **b.** Relative negative pressure, retraction of the tympanic membrane, displacement of the light reflex, and immovable tympanic membrane are signs and symptoms of serous otitis media.

26. **c.** Treatment for serous otitis media includes Valsalva's maneuver by the patient, a trial of antibiotic therapy, and myringotomy. Instillation of any type of eardrops is not recommended in these patients.

27. **d.** The condition that produces progressive conductive hearing loss in young adults with normal tympanic membrane is otosclerosis, which is usually a hereditary condition of unknown cause in which irregular ossification occurs in the ossicles of the middle ear, especially the stapes, resulting in hearing loss. It is first noticed when the patient is between age 11 and age 30. Women are affected twice as often as men. Stapedectomy is usually successful in restoring hearing.

28. **c.** Recurrent, severe vertigo, sensory hearing loss, tinnitus, and a sensation of fullness or pressure in the ear are signs and symptoms of Meniere's disease. The cause is distention of the endolymphatic compartment of the inner ear. The primary lesion appears to be in the endolymphatic sac, which is likely responsible for endolymph filtration and excretion.

Although the precise cause of hydrops has not been established, two known causes are syphilis and head trauma. The classic syndrome is episodic vertigo that lasts from 1 to 8 hours; low-frequency sensorineural hearing loss; tinnitus, usually low-tone and "blowing" in quality; and a sensation of aural pressure. Symptoms come and go, depending on the fluctuating endolymphatic pressure. Caloric testing shows loss or impairment by thermally induced nystagmus on the involved side.

29. **b.** Lesions of the eighth cranial nerve (acoustic) and central audiovestibular pathways produce neural hearing loss and vertigo.

30. **a.** Acoustic neuroma arises from Schwann cells. The neuroma is benign, and may be unilateral or bilateral. As it grows in size, symptoms may include tinnitus, progressive hearing loss, headache, facial numbness, papilledema, dizziness, and an unsteady gait.

21
Infectious Diseases

1. **d.** Viruses such as those that cause hepatitis B and herpes infections stay in the body for years, but can reactivate and cause disease long after the initial infection began. A typical example is the chickenpox virus caused by the varicella zoster virus that can cause herpes zoster ("shingles") years after the person had chickenpox.

2. **b.** A biologic vector is usually an arthropod in which the infecting organism completes part of its life cycle. A mechanical vector transmits the infecting organism from one host to another but is not essential to the life cycle of the parasite. A carrier is a person who harbors and spreads an organism that causes disease in others but does not become ill him/herself.

3. **b.** The infections that can be transmitted from animals to man are known as zoonoses. Zooparasites are any kind of parasitic animal organism. The other two (arthrophones and zoopaths) are fiction. Arthropods can transmit malaria and other diseases by mosquito bite; ticks can transmit Rocky Mountain spotted fever or Lyme disease.

4. **d.** The skin covers our entire body and acts as a major defense against invasion of organisms. Most of our body systems have their own defense mechanisms (e.g., respiratory tract filtering system, the acid pH of the stomach, and the acid pH of the vagina. The mucous membranes that are kept moist by secretions that contain antimicrobial properties are also a barrier against infection.

5. **d.** Transformation alone does not affect resistance of the body to antimicrobial drugs. Transformation is the transfer of large fragments of "naked" deoxyribonucleic acid into a bacterium. Successful transformation and transduction, in which transfer of deoxyribonucleic acid occurs via a bacteriophage vector, depend on the integration of the new deoxyribonucleic acid into the recipient of chromosomal deoxyribonucleic acid.

6. **c.** A fever of at least 38.3° C (101° F), present for at least 3 weeks without its cause being discovered, despite intensive investigation for at least 1 week, is termed *fever of unknown origin.*

7. **d.** Malaria typically has fluctuating fever as a major symptom. The old Latin terms of "tertian" and "quartan" were used to describe recurrent fevers. Other infections almost always have fever as a symptom, but in those infections, the fever remains relatively stable, or can increase or decrease, but does not come and go.

8. **b.** A systemic infection caused by bacteria is known as bacteremia, or bacteria that have invaded the bloodstream and are therefore being carried to every organ and tissue in the body. The systemic inflammatory response syndrome was previously know as sepsis syndrome, similar to bacteremia. Infected blood will invade the lymphatic system. Hemodynamic instability occurs in patients with septic shock, and refers to hypotension and other signs of shock typical of sepsis.

9. **c.** Although cellulitis occurs, it is not among the three most common skin infections. These are all caused by bacteria, primarily *Staphylococcus aureus* and *Streptococcus pyogenes* (group A hemolytic streptococcus). Bacteria are present in the skin lesions (vesicles); if any of these break, bacteria spread out to infect other nearby areas.

10. **b.** Before antibiotics, most patients with severe infection were treated in the hospital, with strict isolation precautions. Quarantine occurs when a person has been exposed to a

communicable disease and is kept apart from others so that the disease does not spread to others during the highly contagious stage, which usually precedes onset of symptoms. Although many patients with erysipelas died, many more recovered, but full recovery often took several weeks.

11. **c.** Infected persons who harbor organisms that are spread to others but do not, themselves, develop symptoms are identified as carriers. Streptococcal carrier state is possible. In the early, acute stage of infection, patients are sickest and exhibit the most symptoms. A chronic stage of streptococcal infections does not occur. Delayed symptoms (complications) may occur at least 2 weeks after the acute stage has ended, and the patient at first appears to be recovering. *Streptococcus* is also a cause of toxic shock syndrome.

12. **d.** In cold weather, pneumococci normally inhabit the respiratory tract of apparently healthy people. The organisms are spread by droplets that are coughed or sneezed into the atmosphere. Some of these patients develop tracheobronchitis, bronchopneumonia, or lobar pneumonia. Individuals' immune state and general health are the most important factors in warding off infection.

13. **c.** All gram-negative organisms may be implicated in gastrointestinal infections, including *Salmonella, Shigella, Escherichia, Klebsiella, Enterobacter, Serratia, Proteus, Providencia, Yersinia,* and other, less common, genera. Many experts say that *Proteus mirabilis* causes most human infections, which may be true because the organisms are found in soil and water, and are among the normal flora of feces.

14. **c.** The *Helicobacter pylori* organism is now considered the primary cause of peptic ulcer disease. The organism is found in 10% of healthy people under age 30, in 60% of healthy people over age 60, and in 90% of people with a duodenal ulcer. This discovery, first presented at a scientific meeting in the late 1980s, was discounted then but has since been fully accepted by all scientific areas.

15. **d.** The white-footed mouse is the primary animal reservoir for the spirochetal organism *Borrelia burgdorferi*. In the United States, the preferred hosts for adult ticks who carry the organism from the white-footed mouse are deer. In Europe, the preferred hosts of adult ticks are sheep.

16. **c.** Men who live in highly congested areas and are between the ages of 25 and 44 form the group in whom the incidence of tuberculosis is highest. Many factors influence the incidence of tuberculosis in this group: crowded conditions, close contact with those who have the disease, living conditions, general health status, and other, similar factors.

17. **a.** To live and reproduce, viruses must invade other cells, whether bacterial, plant, or animal, where they are able to replicate their own deoxyribonucleic acid, thus reproducing other viral organisms. The other cells lose their identity.

18. **a.** HIV-1 is a retrovirus that causes HIV infection, which progresses to AIDS—acquired immunodeficiency syndrome. There are over 200 viruses, many of which cause disease in humans. Estimates of the number of Americans infected with AIDS show it as about 700,000. This estimate has been scaled down from prior estimates, based on recent AIDS incidence data.

19. **b.** Molluscum contagiosum is among several new venereal diseases that have developed recently, and is more prevalent than the "historic five": syphilis, gonorrhea, chancroid, lymphogranuloma venereum, and granuloma inguinale. The most prevalent sexually transmitted diseases today are chlamydia, genital and anorectal herpes and warts, and trichomoniasis. In 1995, the worldwide incidence of gonorrhea was estimated to be over 250 million cases, and about 400,000 in the United States. Chlamydia affects about 500,000 people in the United States every year, but only 10% to 20% of cases are reported.

20. **b.** Gallbladder stones do not occur because of chlamydial infection, although the organism can cause infection in the perihepatic peritoneum, which stimulates cholecystitis. Chronic pelvic infection due to chlamydial infection can cause ectopic pregnancy and infertility. Reiter's syndrome, which is characterized by arthritis with skin and eye lesions and noninfectious recurrent urethritis, occurs most often in men as a complication of chlamydial infection.

22
Psychosocial Disorders

1. **c.** Of patients in primary care settings in the United States, the percentage who have a psychosocial disorder is 30%. This is a significant number of people who suffer from psychosocial disorders, caused either by psychological or functional/organic factors. The clinician's task is to determine the actual cause, and to treat the patient appropriately.

2. **d.** Social factors that are frequently associated with psychosocial illness include personal loss, such as death of a loved one, loss of job, loss of home; a major recent change, such as a move to another city or state, or beginning a new job; and stress, often unexpected and acute, such as a weather disaster, serious accident, or other damage to people or property.

3. **b.** Personality is defined as long-established attitudes and patterns of behavior that are based largely on one's genetic makeup, background, religion, level of education, and other factors. It is who we are as individuals.

4. **a.** Coping mechanisms are used by people to adapt to life stresses. They are used to protect ourselves from threats, either real or imagined, or from actual danger to our body or our psyche.

5. **d.** The American Psychiatric Association has developed a particular approach to formulate psychosocial problems, known as the five-axis system. In very broad terms, Axis I refers to clinical disorders; Axis II refers to personality disorders and mental retardation; Axis III refers to general medical conditions; Axis IV refers to psychosocial and environmental problems; and Axis V refers to global assessment of functioning.

6. **c.** Psychotherapy consists of verbal and behavioral processes used to relieve patients' symptoms and resolve patients' intrapersonal and interpersonal conflicts. Psychoanalytic psychotherapy uses many of the tools of psychoanalysis such as free association, dream analysis, and transference. This method involves the development of a close professional relationship between the therapist and the patient that may continue for variable lengths of time—months to years—that it takes to help the patient resolve what may often be deep-seated problems.

A second kind of psychotherapy is the short-term, dynamic therapy that is completed in about ten sessions, the goal of which is to provide resolution of problems effectively, without going through a complete personality overhaul that was usual in classic analytic therapy as developed by Freud.

7. **b.** Transference occurs when patients transfer expectations to the therapist regarding how they consider that the therapist should respond to them as their parents did during their growing-up years.

8. **a.** Countertransference occurs when the physician or therapist develops positive or negative expectations regarding the patient, based on past experiences of the therapist with other people—parents, siblings, friends, or other patients.

9. **c.** Patients with somatoform disorders express their emotional distress in somatic complaints, thinking that they have a serious or an incurable physical disease. These patients exhibit signs and symptoms similar to the physical disease that they believe they have. The practitioner must carefully, but meticulously, ask questions that will elicit as much information as possible about relationships, financial status, home situation, and stresses of any kind, to differentiate what is physical and what is psychologic.

10. **c.** Supportive counseling serves two purposes—to help the patient with medical problems that may be present, and to cope with the stresses of life (family, occupational, other).

11. **b.** Dysmorphic disorders are conditions in which the person places undue emphasis on a particular physical characteristic (e.g., hair, skin, nose).

12. **d.** Anxiety encompasses a wide range of feelings and fears, including physical symptoms such as palpitations, profuse sweating, and restlessness (pacing). Anxiety may begin as a mild sense of impending disaster, but is usually more acute and the patient is in a state of intense anxiousness and near-panic, with accompanying physical signs (those listed), shortness of breath, chest pains, dizziness, and a feeling of being enclosed and unable to get out of a situation.

13. **c.** Obsessive-compulsive disorder is characterized by repetitive, purposeful, but senseless

actions such as washing hands 100 times a day. Patients cannot adequately explain why they perform the actions, only that they must do them.

14. **c.** Most psychosocial disorders must be present for a specific period of time before a definitive diagnosis can be made. The period of time is variable, but is usually 6 months.

15. **d.** Personality evolves from a combination of inborn factors: intelligence, temperament, sociability, emotionality, and relationships with parents and others. We are also finding that genetic makeup plays a major role in personality.

16. **d.** The impact of depressive disorders on public health is extremely severe. By any measurement, depressive conditions are major public health problems. In a medical outcome study of community-dwelling people, the *poor functioning uniquely associated with depressive symptoms* was comparable with or worse than that uniquely associated with nine major chronic medical conditions: arthritis, advanced coronary artery disease, recent myocardial infarction, angina, back problems, severe lung problems, gastrointestinal disorders (ulcers or inflammatory bowel disease), diabetes, and hypertension.

17. **c.** The risk for first-degree relatives to develop a major depressive disorder is 10% to 15%. Bipolar disorder and affective disorder are the two psychologic conditions most commonly seen in family members.

18. **d.** The only drug that has been unequivocally established as effective in preventing relapses in patients with bipolar disorder is lithium. Most patients tolerate the drug well.

19. **c.** Even with modern therapy, the majority of patients with severe major depression may not fully recover for 2 years. During the period of illness, the patient or the patient's family should remain in close touch with the physician, who may be able to change drug regimens or suggest other ways to lessen the severity of depression or shorten its effects.

20. **a.** The cause of schizophrenia is unknown. The American Psychiatric Association lists the major features of the disorder as the presence of certain psychotic features for a significant length of time (i.e., 6 months). It is considered to be a lifelong disorder.

21. **b.** Disorders formerly called "affective" disorders are now termed depressive disorders. These can be differentiated into several categories, depending on the type of depression. Bereavement usually results in an adjustment disorder, perhaps with minor depression, but the period of grieving is not considered to cause major depression. Major depression, if it should occur during the period immediately after a major loss of some kind (e.g., child, spouse, parent, home), is not typical and should be treated specifically as a major depression. Subcategories of major depression include major depression with atypical features (hypersomnia, lethargy). Major depression with a seasonal onset is identified as seasonal affective disorder. Major depression can occur in the postpartum period, usually within 2 weeks to 6 months after the birth of a child.

22. **c.** Persons with depressive symptoms function more poorly than those with any one of nine major chronic medical conditions: arthritis, advanced coronary artery disease, recent myocardial infarction, angina, back problems, severe lung problems, gastrointestinal disorders, diabetes, and hypertension.

23. **a.** Patients who have terminal illnesses and who may fear death are overwhelmed with feelings of helplessness. They feel totally incapable of making any changes in the situation, and often become unable to do anything, becoming more and more withdrawn.

24. **d.** Bereaved persons usually show at least partial recovery from grief by 5 months. At that point, they begin to want to go out and do their usual tasks such as grocery shopping. They still have periods of deep sadness, but these periods become less frequent and less prolonged.

25. **b.** Most patients with depression who seek professional help do not complain of emotional (depressive) symptoms. They are much more likely to complain about sleeplessness or vague aches and pains. The practitioner must work slowly with the patient to elicit symptoms of feeling sad, unable to enjoy things that formerly were quite pleasurable.

26. **a.** St. John's wort was the subject of several articles and discussions not so long ago, and touted as a "natural antidepressant." Studies show that the plant has some antidepressive properties, but its full effects are not known.

Like most alternative therapies, if they make the patient feel better, and cause no harm, then the patient can be encouraged to use them.

27. **c.** Dementia is characterized by cognitive decline. The practitioner must assess the patient as to the likely cause of the dementia, particularly if it is treatable. Three causes of treatable dementia are medication toxicity, depression, and thyroid disease.

28. **c.** Signs and symptoms of schizophrenia include loss of contact with reality, hallucinations, and delusions. These patients do not exhibit emotion, either sadness or exuberance. They tend to withdraw into their own little world. Hallucinations are usually auditory, often of a derogatory nature. Delusions may be grandiose, during which patients believe themselves to be powerful and influential, or persecutory in nature.

29. **b.** In 1973, the American Psychiatric Association stated that homosexuality was no longer considered to be a psychiatric disorder because for most it is not a matter of choice but is physiologically determined.

30. **b.** "Core gender identity" reflects a biologic self-image—the conviction that "I am a male," or "I am a female," which is usually well developed by age 3 or 4. Gender dysphoria refers to the development of a sexual identity that is the opposite of the biologic one.

23
Care of the Aging Adult

1. **c.** Symptoms of dementia are not associated with healthy aging. Most individuals at any age have increased life expectancies. Only 30% of those over age 85 are impaired in any activity required for daily living, and their life expectancy at that point is another 6 years.

2. **b.** Older persons usually exhibit mild signs and symptoms of even quite serious conditions, e.g., pneumonia or fracture. Impaired compensatory mechanisms often result in these patients presenting with very early diseases that have few signs and symptoms at that point.

3. **a.** Delirium is generally not among symptoms that older persons have at the time of the visit to the clinic. Rather, symptoms are more vague, and do not relate to any particular disease; acute confusion, depression, weakness, and syncope are the most common presenting symptoms, making clinical diagnosis difficult. Careful questioning of the patient and family members may yield clues to possible causes of the patient's illness.

4. **b.** Telomere shortening occurs, and is considered one theory of aging, but not telomere lengthening. Telomeres, the ends of chromosomes, appear to shorten with each cell cycle in body cells. Telomere shortening is therefore relatively continuous throughout the life of each cell.

5. **d.** Older people are not prone to increasing pathology as they age, although they are at increased risk for particular diseases, e.g., cancer. Research has not conclusively determined that aging is related to genetic make-up. Some conditions are related to increased cellular proliferation, such as cancer and hyperplasia, but not to increased cellular atrophy. In general, aging is accepted as a progressive decline in ability to function as they did in earlier decades; the body slows down but does not necessarily develop pathology.

6. **c.** Many older people were taught not to complain about vague aches and pains, and that these are a part of normal aging. They frequently neglect their health and ignore signs and symptoms that may be serious. When they do seek care, their disease is advanced and therefore more difficult to treat.

7. **d.** Contrary to what many people believe, most older persons are able to provide accurate information about their health history, although exact dates may be lacking. Their memories for events are usually sound, particularly for events that stand out in people's lives, such as the birth of a child, serious illness, or hospitalizations.

8. **d.** People over age 65 comprise about 13% of the total population. The most rapidly growing segment of the older population is the 85+ group. Those over age 65 account for more than 12% of the population, estimated at 33 million, with a net gain of more than 1000 every day. In the year 2030, when post–World War II baby boomers reach age 80, more than 70 million Americans (>20%) will be age 65 or older. Those over 85 years

of age will make up a greater proportion of the population than they do now.

9. **b.** The process of aging is probably linear, although it may also be intermittent, and is certainly gradual. We are aging from the time of conception, and nothing is known now about how to stop or to slow the process.

10. **b.** Telomerase is involved in biologic theories of aging but is not a separate theory itself.

11. **a.** One biologic theory of aging is programmed loss of genetic material, also called codon restriction, not codon expansion. The multiple theories of biologic aging indicate that we do not know, right now, how the process of aging is carried on.

12. **b.** Although behaviors are intrinsic to roles and relationships, the word is not used in terms of sociologic theories.

13. **d.** Disengagement theory focuses on withdrawal behaviors, stating that as people age, they tend to withdraw from social contacts and become more reclusive. Although this type of behavior may be true for some older people, it is not true of the majority of older persons.

14. **a.** Birren, who has done extensive research on the psychologic aspects of aging, said that psychologic theories are invariably intertwined with both biologic and sociologic theories, and thus cannot be studied in isolation.

15. **c.** Everyone, throughout their lives, has the same needs, and these needs are met in the same way. One cannot progress toward satisfying needs at a higher level until needs associated with the lower level are achieved. Part of the process involves maturation and education.

16. **b.** The superego is not one of Jung's components of personality. The three that Jung focuses on include the ego, the personal consciousness, and the collective consciousness.

17. **d.** Erikson divided the life span into eight stages, beginning with infancy and progressing to "old age," by developing a stage focused on the "old-old"—those over 80.

18. **a.** The first choice listed is not identified as one of the divisions of the stage of old-old persons. The goal of the final stage of life is for the older person to accept the inevitability of death, but not to dwell on the thought of

death in a negative way. Death is part of the life cycle, and many older people welcome it after a lifetime of unceasing work.

19. **d.** The majority of people over age 65 were diagnosed with 3.5 health problems. In examining older people, the clinician needs to remember that most older people will have symptoms of more than one disease.

20. **a.** The only characteristic listed that is true of dementia is that it develops gradually, often over years, whereas delirium occurs suddenly, often in response to infection, fever, other illness, or other events that significantly impact on the person.

24
Genetics

1. **b.** Characteristics of patients with Marfan syndrome include tall stature, ectopia lentis, long limbs, joint laxity, and cardiovascular defects such as aortic aneurysm or mitral valve prolapse. The cause is an autosomal dominant inheritance resulting from mutation in the fibrillin-1 gene on chromosome 15q. Abraham Lincoln had Marfan syndrome.

2. **a.** Patients with Down syndrome have increased incidence of several problems resulting from a chromosomal dysgenesis consisting of a constellation of abnormalities due to triplication or translocation of chromosome 21. Abnormalities may be any combination: mental retardation without delayed sexual development, growth retardation, flat hypoplastic face, small low-set ears, fissured and thickened tongue, pelvic dysplasia, broad hands and feet, stubby fingers, heart disease, and increased evidence of Alzheimer's disease by age 40.

3-6: Matched chromosomal disorders and clinical manifestations.

3. Short stature, mental deficiency, cardiac defects, hypotonia. **a—Down syndrome.**

4. Short stature, infertility, coarctation of the aorta, nuchal webbing. **d—Turner's syndrome.**

5. Severe mental deficiency, brain malformations, cleft lip, polydactyly, cardiac defects. **c—Trisomy.**

6. Tall stature, hypogonadism, long legs, decreased upper/lower ratio of body. **e—Klinefelter's syndrome.**

7-13: Matched pattern of inheritance and clinical syndromes/conditions:

7. **c**—X-linked–recessive inheritance pattern.
8. **b**—autosomal-recessive inheritance pattern.
9. **b**—autosomal-recessive inheritance pattern.
10. **a**—autosomal-dominant inheritance pattern.
11. **d**—multifactorial (polygenic) inheritance pattern.
12. **d**—facial cleft anomalies.
13. **b**—autosomal-recessive inheritance pattern.
14. **d.** Alleles at loci on the *same* chromosome are not associated with Mendel's rules of heredity. Alleles may segregate together
15. **c.** The proportion of families with three children in which all three are boys is 1:8 (1.25%).
16. **c.** The baseline risk for congenital malformations in the average pregnancy is 2:100.
17. **c.** The average incidence of common single malformations such as cleft palate or spina bifida is 1:1000.

18-22: Matched term and partial definitions:

18. Genome **e**—complete set of genes in cell or organism.
19. Allele **b**—alternative form of a gene.
20. Mutation **a**—heritable change in deoxyribonucleic acid.
21. Locus **c**—position of gene on chromosome.
22. Pleiotropy **d**—one gene, multiple effects.

23-27: Matched descriptions with correct disorder:

23. Mendelian inheritance—**b** single gene defects.
24. Human cancers—**d** somatic cell genetic defects.
25. Most common type of human genetic disease—**c** multifactorial disorders.
26. Major causes of miscarriages—**a** chromosomal disorders.
27. Maternal derivation—**e** mitochondrial disorders.

Index

leukemia(s)—cont'd
  acute myelogenous (AML),
      335, 336, 337, 399
  acute promyelocytic, 336, 337
  chronic, 337-341
  chronic lymphocytic (CLL),
      337-339
  chronic myelogenous (CML),
      339-341, 399, 405
  hairy cell, 338
  lymphoma, 339
  monocytic, 336
  prolymphocytic, 338, 339
leukocytosis, 340
leukoplakia, laryngeal, 540-541
levodopa (L-DOPA)
  for Parkinson's disease,
      146-147
  problems with, 147-148
levonorgestrel, 366
Leydig cell aplasia, 378
liability, in tort law, 30
lice infestation, 472-473
licensure, 32
  interstate, 26
lichen planus, 482-483
licorice, 288
lidocaine, 95-96
lipemia, 209
lipodermatosclerosis, 287
listeriosis, 563
lithium, 629-630
lithotripsy, 235
litigation, 31
liver disorder(s), 219-232
  cirrhosis as. *See* Cirrhosis.
  hepatitis as. *See* Hepatitis.
  jaundice as, 219-220
  oral contraceptives and, 362
  pain in, 164t
  secondary diabetes mellitus
      from, 272b
  tumors as, 362
  Wilson's disease as, 231-232
liver function tests, 220t
living wills, 32
low back pain, 438-440. *See also*
    specific causative
    disorders.
  acute
    management of, 440b
    patterns of, 439t
  causes of, 438b
  physical examination in, 439t
low-density lipoprotein levels, 4t

lower limbs
  ankle
    impingement of meniscoid
        body, 441
    sprain, 441-442, 441t
  examination of, 427b
  foot disorders
    Athlete's foot, 470-471
    in fibromyalgia, 443
    prophylactic care, 114
    ulcers of, in sickle cell disease,
        332
lower motor neuron disease,
    127
  gait in, 126
  upper motor neuron lesions
      compared, 121
Lown-Ganong-Levine syndrome,
    101
lumbar puncture, 128
lung cancer, 10, 61-64
  bronchiogenic carcinoma, 407-
      409
  paraneoplastic syndromes in,
      63, 63t
  screening for, 10
lung volumes, 41t
  in COPD, 42-44, 43t
luteal phase deficiency, 375
luteinizing hormone deficiency,
    246
luteinizing hormone-releasing
    hormone, 245
  in male sexual development,
      371
luteinizing hormone-releasing
    hormone analog, 372
Lyme disease, 571-573, 573b
lymphocytes, 391
lymphokines, 401
lymphoma(s), 341-344
  Burkitt's, 342-343, 344
  classification of, 343b
  Hodgkin's disease as, 341-342
  mucosa-associated lymphoid
      tissue, 344
  non-Hodgkin's, 342-344,
      405
  T-cell, 399
Lynch syndrome, 420

M

macule, 463
magnetic resonance angiography,
    128

magnetic resonance imaging
    (MRI)
  in kidney disorders, 201
  in neurologic disorders, 128
  in respiratory disorders, 39
  in shoulder pain, 435
major depressive disorder, 624-
    628. *See also* Depression.
  diagnosis of, 625b
  treatment of, 626-628
    antidepressants in. *See*
        Antidepressants.
major histocompatibility com-
    plex, 389-390
maladaptive personalities,
    614-619
male reproductive system
  disorders of, 376-381
  physiology of, 371-372
malignancies. *See* Oncologic
    disorder(s).
malignant melanoma, 485-487
Mallory-Weiss syndrome,
    172-173
malnutrition, refeeding after, 289
mammography, 413, 414
managed care, ethics and, 36
manic depressive disorder,
    623-630
  manic episodes in, 628-629,
      628b
  drugs and substances associ-
      ated with, 625b
manometry, esophageal, 167
Marfan's syndrome, 667-668
Maslow's hierarchy of human
    needs theory, of aging,
    649-650
mastectomy, 414
mastoiditis, 530-531
measles vaccination, 182-183
measles virus, 182-183
medroxyprogesterone acetate
  for contraception, 363
  for dysfunctional uterine bleed-
      ing, 349
  for endometrial hyperplasia,
      350
  for endometriosis, 355
  for polycystic ovary syndrome,
      359, 384, 385
megestrol, 247
Meibomian gland dysfunction,
    497-498
  chalazion as, 499